THE ENCYCLOPEDIA OF

HIV AND AIDS

Second Edition

Sarah Barbara Watstein, M.L.S., M.P.A.
Stephen E. Stratton, M.S.L.S., M.A.

Foreword by
Evelyn J. Fisher, M.D.

☑®
Facts On File, Inc.

The Encyclopedia of HIV and AIDS, Second Edition

Facts On File, Inc.
132 West 31st Street
New York NY 10001

Library of Congress Cataloging-in-Publication Data

Watstein, Sarah.
The encyclopedia of HIV and AIDS/Sarah Barbara Watstein, Stephen E. Stratton;
foreword by Evelyn J. Fisher.—2nd ed.
p. cm.
Previous ed. has title: The AIDS dictionary.
Includes bibliographical references and index.
ISBN 0-8160-4808-8 (hc.: alk. paper)
1. AIDS (Disease)—Dictionaries. I. Watstein, Sarah. AIDS dictionary.
II. Stratton, Stephen E. III. Title.
RC606.6.W385 2003
616.97'92'003—dc21
2002035220

Facts On File books are available at special discounts when purchased in bulk quantities for businesses, associations, institutions, or sales promotions. Please call our Special Sales Department in New York at (212) 967-8800 or (800) 322-8755.

You can find Facts On File on the World Wide Web at http://www.factsonfile.com

Text and cover design by Cathy Rincon

Printed in the United States of America

VB Hermitage 10 9 8 7 6 5 4 3 2 1

This book is printed on acid-free paper.

For those waiting on the other side of the rainbow.

—Sarah Barbara Watstein

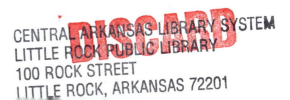

For Rob Harris, my partner, who gave up his on-line shopping
for several months as I worked on this dictionary,
and who has been very supportive throughout the process.

—Steve Stratton

CONTENTS

FOREWORD

In the early 1980s patients began coming to my office for treatment of symptoms and illnesses that were later defined as AIDS. Infections, illnesses, and cancers that were not seen before, particularly combined in the same people, suddenly had familiar names. Patients wanted to understand what was wrong with them. They had never heard of these infections, but now had to live with them. Patients also wanted to learn as much as possible in order to try and stay alive when no one, including doctors, knew a great deal about HIV. In the 20 plus years of the HIV/AIDS epidemic, patients have educated themselves about the virus and the opportunistic infections (OIs) that accompany it. Many patients advocated early in the epidemic for better access to information and a voice in their treatment. With the involvement of the patient in the treatment and drug approval process has come the need for the patient to understand the mechanisms of the virus and the many illnesses and medications available for their treatment.

This encyclopedia provides a way for patients, friends, family, and patient advocates to educate themselves about HIV/AIDS, OIs, and many other areas related to HIV in 2003. I have read through the entries with the authors; they cover a wide variety of cultural, medical, personal, social, and pharmacological issues that are vital to understanding HIV and AIDS. I do not necessarily agree with everything the authors have selected for inclusion in the book but respect that the decisions are theirs and recognize that HIV and AIDS information covers more subject areas than just medicine. The second edition is a necessary update to keep the material correct—and timely.

However much time the authors have spent on this book, readers must realize that it will always be out of date. The changes that occur in medicine happen quickly these days. More is learned about HIV/AIDS each day, and material is outdated daily. I want to remind readers that this book should not be used for self-diagnosis or treatment. The information presented here is general in nature and does not apply to individuals. People need to consult with their personal physician and HIV/AIDS specialists before receiving any type of medical treatment.

Remember, HIV is still a serious virus that causes illness and death. To date there is no medicine to rid the body of the virus and no cure. Educate yourself with this book and other information sources. There are medicines that can help keep a person healthy for much longer than was possible in 1981, but these drugs are not easy to take and have many side effects. Protect your health through safe sex practices. If you are HIV positive, protect your health through adherence to your treatment plan as suggested by your doctor. Use the information in this book to protect and educate yourself and others.

—Evelyn J. Fisher
Associate Professor of Internal Medicine,
Virginia Commonwealth University

ACKNOWLEDGMENTS

No two people write a dictionary of HIV/AIDS by themselves—the field is too vast, complex, and changing. The authors owe so much to so many who contributed ideas, stimulation, challenges, and constructive criticism. We particularly wish to acknowledge the patience and understanding of our friends, colleagues, and family, who were always there with words of support and encouragement, cups of coffee, and an occasional meal to facilitate our all too often nose-to-the-grindstone posture during the development and production of this work. Additionally, we express deep appreciation and admiration to those who have contributed to the knowledge that has found its way into this volume—the many current and past friends and acquaintances who have worked on the front-lines with people who have HIV/AIDS, practitioners, and health care providers, and, of course, the many we have known who are HIV-positive. It is they, who daily confront the challenges, who contribute the most in volume and precision to the lexicon of HIV/AIDS.

—Sarah Barbara Watstein

I want to mention several friends who have helped me over the course of the 20 years of this epidemic, in a variety of ways. Some of these people are not around any longer, but I still think about all of them, living or not, often: Rodney Blair, Richard Towler, Robert Wright, Tommy Lee, Jerry Griffin, Jeffrey Helyer, Larry Wyatt, Joyce Sherman, Rich Healy, and Patrick Yankee. I also thank the people at the various organizations where I have volunteered my time: Wellness Networks—Huron Valley (now the HIV/AIDS Resource Center) (http://comnet. org/local/orgs/harc/); Osborne Association AIDS in Prison Project (http://www.osborneny.org/aids_in_ prison_project.htm); Richmond AIDS Consortium, Community Advisory Board (http://views.vcu.edu/ hiv/research/racsite/); and Terry Beirn Community Programs for Clinical Research on AIDS (http://www.cpcra.org). Of course I want to thank Sarah, too, for giving me the opportunity to help her on this book.

—Steve Stratton

INTRODUCTION

Projections made in an early July 2002 issue of *The Lancet* medical journal by a group of experts from the United Nations AIDS agency, the World Health Organization, the United States Census Bureau, Imperial College in London, and the Futures Group International were staggering—45 million more people worldwide will be infected with the AIDS virus in the next eight years—between 2002 and 2010. Make no mistake—the global prevalence of HIV infection and AIDS is sobering indeed. Today—two plus decades into the pandemic—we know that HIV prevention works. And we know that access to effective prevention is one of the key challenges to effective prevention. "Knowledge is power" is a slogan that has been bandied about in recent years in many circles; indeed, its relevance has far exceeded its initial application. Within the context of HIV/AIDS this much is clear—being informed is one of the key components of effective prevention.

A compilation and clarification of the language of HIV/AIDS, this encyclopedia is a tool and a reference source for all who wish to be more knowledgeable about HIV/AIDS. It is a reference source for those who work with, or are concerned about, HIV/AIDS. A book such as this one serves several purposes. It records the linguistic status of HIV/AIDS at a period in time. It is a record of how concepts and ideas are communicated. It is also a record of the nomenclature of HIV/AIDS at a given time, captured by the authors' study of its literature. Note that this book is not a substitute for prompt assessment and treatment by experts trained in the diagnosis and treatment of HIV/AIDS.

This encyclopedia continues the spirit and intent of *The AIDS Dictionary*, published by Facts On File in 1998. *The Encyclopedia of HIV/AIDS* consists of hundreds of entries addressing a wide range of topics, including the basic biological and medical aspects of the disease, as well as terms that capture many of the financial, legal, and even cultural, political, and social ramifications of the pandemic. Once again, we realize that many of the topics are controversial, and we believe we have presented those topics in a fair and balanced manner. The appendixes have been completely updated, with a current statistical snapshot of the pandemic and an updated bibliography, as well as selected resources available by phone or on the Internet for students, researchers, general adult readers, and persons with HIV/AIDS. Cross-references are used throughout to facilitate access and further understanding.

Its entries are as diverse as the field of HIV/AIDS itself. It addresses the basic science and epidemiology of HIV/AIDS as well as transmission and prevention, pathology, and treatment. For example, readers interested in physical pathological conditions or those interested in mental health will not be disappointed. The encyclopedia also considers terms that are pertinent to government and activism, and policy and law. Readers interested in the complex social and cultural dimensions of the pandemic will also find much of interest here, as will those seeking information about the global epidemic.

The *Encyclopedia of HIV and AIDS* is a sensitive and comprehensive—although not exhaustive—survey of terms. As with the first edition, every effort has been made to ensure that the information in this work is accurate and up to date; again, however, we note that HIV/AIDS is a field that is so vast and rapidly changing that it is not possible to guarantee that there are no errors. As was noted in the earlier edition, readers seeking definitive answers will not find them in this or any other book on this subject. To the best of our knowledge, there is no reference work to date that contains definitions of all the terms and phrases that the HIV/AIDS lexicon comprises.

As we noted in the acknowledgments, no two people write an encyclopedia of HIV/AIDS by themselves—the field is too vast, complex, and changing. Compiling this work, however, was a much different process from compiling its predecessor, in large measure because of the vast amount of HIV/AIDS information available on the World Wide Web today—more than four years after the publication of the first edition. Today the Web provides those interested in HIV/AIDS with enormous resources—bibliographical and statistical resources alongside geospatial data and full text research reports as well as newspaper and scholarly journal articles. Today the challenge to stay current, to stay abreast of developments in the field of HIV/AIDS, is at once more manageable and more unwieldy because of the Web. The authors hope that readers will find this book to be a good jumping-off point in their search for information about HIV/AIDS, a springboard to further inquiry and research in both print and Web-based sources. Note that entries are alphabetized following a word-by-word mode. Alphabetization is interrupted after the first word; hyphens, slashes, and apostrophes are ignored.

We hope that this work increases understanding of HIV/AIDS. Despite its inherent limitations, this encyclopedia is dedicated to assisting both students and general adult readers as they seek an increased measure of knowledge about HIV/AIDS. Please send comments to The Authors, *The Encyclopedia of HIV and AIDS*, c/o Facts On File, 132 West 31st St., New York, New York 10001-2006.

—Sarah Barbara Watstein
—Stephen E. Stratton

abacavir Also known by its trade name Ziagen or 1592U89. A NUCLEOSIDE ANALOG REVERSE TRANSCRIPTASE INHIBITOR (NRTI) approved in late 1998. It is structurally similar to ZIDOVUDINE (AZT). Clinical trials show that in NAIVE patients abacavir has a profound potency, similar to that of a PROTEASE INHIBITOR. However, it is not so effective in treatment-experienced patients. Resistance analysis shows that the likelihood of failing to respond to abacavir increased according to the number of mutations on the REVERSE TRANSCRIPTASE of an individual's HIV regardless of whether those mutations specifically reduced sensitivity to the new drug. HIV with four or more reverse transcriptase mutations had little or no susceptibility to abacavir. The intricacies of abacavir, or NRTI, resistance have yet to be understood fully; abacavir may not work well in people who have failed other NRTI drug regimens. About 3 percent to 5 percent of all people treated with abacavir have an allergic reaction to the drug. Symptoms of allergic reaction to abacavir are fever, difficulty in breathing, rash, and blistering inside the mouth. People suffering this reaction within the first few days of taking abacavir must stop taking the drug and never take it again. Reactions to the drug can be life-threatening and get worse if the drug is restarted or attempted a second time. Other normal side effects are headaches and nausea. Abacavir's well-tolerated dosing regimen (one tablet twice a day with no dietary restrictions) makes it a good drug for new simplified treatment regimens, which are particularly important in improving patient adherence, one of the most significant clinical challenges in HIV treatment today. Abacavir combined with EPIVIR (3TC) and Zidovudine has been approved by the FDA and sold as TRIZIVIR.

abdomen Area of the body between the thorax (chest) and the pelvis. Contains vital organs such as the stomach, lower part of the esophagus, small and large intestines, liver, gallbladder, spleen, pancreas, and bladder and reproductive organs.

Abelcet Abelcet is a new form of amphotericin B, in which the drug molecules are combined with lipid (fat) molecules. This combination seems to reduce the toxicity and side effects of amphotericin B. Its use is approved for patients who cannot tolerate treatment with amphotericin B. It is used to treat invasive fungal infections, such as ASPERGILLOSIS or CRYPTOCOCCOSIS.

ablative surgery Surgery performed on peripheral nerves, the spinal cord, the brain, or the brain stem to reduce or eliminate pain through permanent disruption of nerve pathways. Ablative surgery is used only as a last resort to pain relief because it cannot be undone.

abortion Induced premature termination of pregnancy; almost always done before the fetus reaches the stage of viability (ability to live outside the womb). The legal threshold of viability differs from state to state but is usually 20 to 24 weeks. Some premature NEONATES younger than 24 weeks or weighing less than 500 grams are viable. Symptoms commonly experienced during abortion include uterine contractions, uterine hemorrhage (sometimes including tissue), dilatation of the CERVIX, and ejection of fetal material. Abortion done at the request of the mother is *elective abortion,* in contrast to *therapeutic abortion,* done when the mental or physical health of the mother would be endangered by continued pregnancy or when the fetus is known to have, in standard medical parlance, "a condition incompatible with life." Abortions can be induced by drugs, suction, scraping of the lining of the uterus, injection of a sterile hypertonic solution into the amniotic cavity, or surgery. Premature terminations of pregnancy that occur spontaneously are called miscarriages. Prior to the 1970s abortions were often done in unsanitary offices, in private homes, or in other nonmedical locations. Currently some states require a 24-hour waiting period before an abortion can be performed, particularly for women below the age of 18. The drug mifepristone (also known as Mifeprex or RU-486) was approved in 2000 for usage in the United States but so far has been little used.

abscess Pus-filled cavity in any part of the body that occurs as a result of disintegration or displacement of tissue. A serious complication of PELVIC INFLAMMATORY DISEASE.

abstinence Going without or refraining voluntarily, particularly from indulgence in food, alcoholic beverages, or sexual activity (some people include masturbation in this definition, others do not). Sexual abstinence is an option people have exercised for a variety of reasons ranging from moral or religious conviction to fear of pregnancy or disease. Some people, including some religious orders, practice celibacy, or permanent abstinence from all sexual activity (historically, the term *celibacy* has also been used to mean simply the state of being unmarried). Some couples practice abstinence as a means of contraception: In "natural" family planning, periodic abstinence is practiced during the fertile period of the woman's menstrual cycle.

Sexual abstinence is one means of avoiding AIDS and other SEXUALLY TRANSMITTED DISEASES. Some people opt never to have sex with anyone before or outside of permanent, exclusive sexual relationships, rather than renounce sex entirely; but for society generally, as history and everyday observation show, abstinence has not been found to be a practical or effective means of preventing infection. Today, emphasis is placed on changing sexual behavior and reducing the risk of infection through sexual contact. The positive aspects of SAFE SEX are stressed instead of emphasizing the negative aspects of UNSAFE SEX.

ABT-378 See LOPINAVIR.

ABV A standard cancer chemotherapy treatment. It is made up of the three drugs adriamycin, bleomycin, and vincristine. It is given INTRAVENOUSLY.

accelerated approval The abbreviated regulatory process under which the U.S. FOOD AND DRUG ADMINISTRATION (FDA) grants conditional marketing approval for a new drug on the basis of early clinical testing data. Accelerated approval allows pharmaceutical manufacturers to bring to market as quickly as possible drugs for the treatment of serious or life-threatening diseases such as HIV/AIDS and is based on relatively short-term evidence of laboratory "markers" of effectiveness (see SURROGATE MARKERS). The agency requires that drug makers provide more substantial proof of effectiveness after drugs are on the market, according to the more stringent traditional criteria, including adequate information on definitive endpoints such as disease progression and mortality rates. It could withdraw approval if such evidence is not forthcoming. ACT-UP activists were the main push behind the development of FDA guidelines that allowed accelerated approval beginning in 1992; ddI and ddC were the first drugs brought to market through this process. Some AIDS activists later questioned the wisdom of accelerated drug approvals. They complained that the accelerated approval caused corporate pharmaceutical giants to put on the market products that had safety problems before they could be discovered in clinical settings. Accelerated approval has adapted to change over the years since it began. ENDPOINTS for clinical studies have changed to reflect the control that PROTEASE INHIBITORS have had on AIDS. Studies used to evaluate drugs for accelerated approval must involve at least 400–500 patients over a period of at least six months of taking the drug with no outstanding safety issues.

access to injection equipment See NEEDLE ACCESS.

access to legal services Part of the American ideal is that everyone has the right to legal services when they are necessary. Nonetheless, people with HIV have sometimes been denied this right. There are several reasons for this. First, in terms of its scope, incidence, transmissibility, and the challenges it poses to society as a whole, HIV is unlike other illnesses with which our modern society has dealt. Second, because of its unique characteristics, the degree of ignorance about the disease remains high, and the degree of fear even higher. The legal system, after all, is run by people who are subject to the same ignorance and fear as everyone else. Additionally, persons with HIV disease have special problems that they bring to the legal system. And the system may indeed be really trying to provide such persons with an equal opportunity at fairness by giving them a helping hand in order to equalize their chance at justice with the chance enjoyed by persons not infected with HIV. In general, the courts have been slow in recognizing these special problems, for instance, protecting the privacy of people with AIDS (PWAs), weighed against the need to protect the public from transmission of HIV; balancing risks to the defendant and the public in determining the sentence for a PWA convicted of a crime; dealing with the fears of court personnel about courtroom contact with PWAs; and introducing new aspects of old issues of discrimination in employment, housing, public accommodations, and schools.

The American Bar Association's (ABA) Policy on AIDS was adopted in August 1989. It sets forth four principles. First, the judiciary and the organized bar should encourage attorneys and judges to become knowledgeable about HIV and its related legal issues and should provide appropriate education and training in these areas. Second, the judiciary and the organized bar should support the allocation of additional private and public resources, including the further development of pro bono activities, for the delivery of legal services to individuals affected by HIV. Third, attorneys should not refuse to represent clients or limit or modify their representation of clients because of the clients' known or perceived HIV status. Fourth, judicial or administrative proceedings involving participants known or perceived to be HIV-infected should be conducted in the same fashion as any other such proceedings. Extraordinary safety or security precautions should not be undertaken based solely upon the participants' known or perceived HIV status.

access to medical care The degree of ease with which the consumer can secure health services. Along with AVAILABILITY, access is a key criterion used to measure the adequacy of a health care system. Access, especially early in the course of their illness, is a particularly important issue for those infected with HIV, who require a broad array of services at all times. Early access to drugs and therapies for the treatment of HIV infection includes access to promising treatments before full marketing approval. Historically, within the context of HIV/AIDS, pharmaceutical companies and government agencies alike have been unenthusiastic if not hostile towards early treatment access.

accessory cells See ANTIGEN PRESENTING CELL.

accessory molecules Membrane GLYCOPROTEINS of the Ig superfamily on certain T cell surfaces, additional to the T cell receptors themselves, regulating adhesion between T cell and ANTIGEN-PRESENTING CELLS (APCs).

acemannan A freeze-dried powder form of juice extracted from the aloe vera plant (trade name Carrisyn). Aloe vera has been used for centuries for its healing properties, especially for burns. Also known as Ace-M, it is a complex carbohydrate that has been shown to have a broad spectrum of action against viruses that infect warm-blooded animals and HIV IN VITRO. Two clinical studies involving HIV patients in the early 1990s showed no ill effects from use of the drug. However, they also showed no positive effect on the immune system produced by using the drug.

acetaminophen A synthetic drug with antipyretic (antifever) and ANALGESIC actions similar to aspirin. It does not have the anti-inflammatory or antirheumatic actions of aspirin. It is available without a prescription. As a prescription medicine,

it is used in combination with stronger pain relievers for the treatment of moderate-to-severe pain.
It is also used in a number of cold and flu products
in combination with ANTIHISTAMINES, deconges-
tants, and sleeping medications. Acetaminophen
is available in many forms and doses, under many
trade names.

achlorhydria   The absence of free hydrochloric
acid in the gastric juices, a result of atrophy of the
gastric mucous membrane. Also called gastric
anacidity. May be associated with CARCINOMA, gastric ulcer, pernicious anemia, ADRENAL INSUFFI-
CIENCY, or chronic gastritis.

acid-fast   Resistant to decolorization with acidi-
fied organic solvents after staining with a dye. This
property is used as the basis of a test for identifying
acid-fast bacilli (AFB) such as MYCOBACTERIUM
TUBERCULOSIS and other MYCOBACTERIA.

acid-fast bacillus   See ACID-FAST.

acidophilus   Bacteria that help maintain or
restore a supportive bacterial environment in an
intestinal tract affected by disease and ANTIBIOTICS.
Acidophilus also may be useful in preventing CAN-
DIDIASIS (thrush) in the throat, mouth, and vagina.
Most HIV-positive people have some form of digestive imbalance at some time. Daily acidophilus supplementation is suggested to prevent or mitigate
such problems. Among the benefits of acidophilus
are production of significant amounts of folic acid,
vitamin B_{12} and other B-complex vitamins, reduction of intestinal gas and diarrhea and increased
production of lactase, leading to improved digestion of dairy products. Acidophilus is found in
yogurt and is available in capsule form in health
food stores.

acids   See ACQUIRED COMMUNITY IMMUNE DEFI-
CIENCY SYNDROME.

**acquired community immune deficiency syn-
drome (ACIDS)**   An early name for what is now
called ACQUIRED IMMUNODEFICIENCY SYNDROME
(AIDS).

acquired immune deficiency syndrome   An early
name for what is now called ACQUIRED IMMUNO-
DEFICIENCY SYNDROME (AIDS).

acquired immunodeficiency syndrome (AIDS)
An infectious disease characterized by failure of the
IMMUNE SYSTEM and caused by the HUMAN IMMUN-
ODEFICIENCY VIRUS (HIV), one of a large group of
IMMUNODEFICIENCY viruses (IVs) widespread among
primates and other mammals. The now universal
acronym was first used by the Centers for Disease
Control and Prevention (CDC) of the U.S. Public
Health Service in the fall of 1982. AIDS and HIV
are not the same: AIDS is best understood as the
latest stage of the illness resulting from infection
with HIV, characterized by the appearance of dif-
ficult-to-treat OPPORTUNISTIC INFECTIONS and malignancies, which profoundly decreased immunity is
unable to control. HIV is the virus itself. People can
carry the virus for many years before their
immune system is weak enough to be diagnosed
with the diseases that make up an AIDS definition.
See AIDS CASE DEFINITION; SYNDROME.

ACTG   See AIDS CLINICAL TRIALS GROUPS.

activated lymphocytes   LYMPHOCYTES that have
been stimulated by specific ANTIGEN or nonspecific
MITOGEN.

activated macrophages   Mature MACROPHAGES in
a metabolic state caused by various stimuli, especially PHAGOCYTOSIS or LYMPHOKINE activity.

active immunity   Resistance to a disease resulting
from the production of ANTIBODIES in a person who
has been inoculated with an ANTIGEN. See PASSIVE
IMMUNITY.

activism   The practice of direct action or involvement as a means of achieving political or other
social or civic goals. In recent decades, activism has
emerged as an effective way for those without
great financial resources or political clout to participate in public debate over issues as diverse as institutionalized racism, class bias, reproductive rights,
sexism, heterosexism, or ableism.

AIDS activism is a way to respond collectively and constructively to the epidemic in all of its enormity and complexity, keeping it alive as an urgent public issue. It serves many specific purposes. Perhaps most importantly, AIDS activism empowers persons with HIV/AIDS by helping them organize around, and even figure out what their issues are. For both individuals and groups, it provides a means to fight discrimination and to overcome, or begin to overcome, a history of powerlessness. It provides a constant challenge to government agencies, social service providers, the medical establishment, the media and the public.

On the HIV/AIDS issue, letter writing, postcard campaigns, leafletting, conducting safe-sex "tupperware" parties for adults, setting up information tables outside high schools, creating videotapes, questioning public officials, and, for gays and lesbians, forcing colleagues and families to confront an issue they may have preferred to evade by "coming out," are all forms of activism. ACT-UP (AIDS COALITION TO UNLEASH POWER), formed in 1987 in New York by a group outraged at the government's mismanagement of the AIDS crisis, was one of the earliest and still probably the best known AIDS activist group.

Significantly, although AIDS activism has not decreased, in recent years there have been far fewer of the kind of attention-getting acts that deliberately disrupt some public function or ceremony. The reason is that earlier efforts have succeeded in putting AIDS on the public agenda. AIDS activists are now consulted by the CDC and other agencies on health policy, to the benefit of the public. Although many have taken issue with some of the tactics employed by organized activist groups in their early years, most would agree that they have served a good purpose.

activity   The ability in a drug, to control or inhibit a PATHOGEN. Activity may be determined in the laboratory and differs from EFFICACY, which is the ability of a treatment to alter the course of clinical disease.

ACTU   See AIDS CLINICAL TESTING UNIT.

ACT-UP   See ACTIVISM; AIDS COALITION TO UNLEASH POWER.

acupressure   Based on the principles of ACUPUNCTURE, this ancient Chinese technique involves the use of finger pressure, rather than needles, on specific "chi" points on the body to relieve tension and stress, as well as menstrual pain, cramps, arthritis, headaches, and eyestrain. Acupressure is also said to prevent and combat colds, improve muscle tone, boost energy levels, and be generally useful in preventive health care.

Acupressure, like acupuncture, is intended to relieve muscular tension, increasing the flow of blood—and therefore of oxygen and nutrients—to tissues throughout the body. This helps promote physical calmness and mental alertness, and aids in healing by removing waste products. Many researchers now believe that acupuncture and acupressure trigger the release of ENDORPHINS, neurochemicals that relieve pain. Both techniques have been used with some success to provide relief to people with HIV and AIDS.

acupuncture   A Chinese medical therapy in which needles are used to press "chi," or energy, points on the surface of the body. Traditional Chinese medical theory holds that energy imbalance is the cause of all illness. Acupuncture seeks to diagnose such an imbalance before a detectable physiological impairment occurs. Acupuncturists focus on helping patients balance the chi energy within and between the five major organ systems: the heart, lungs, liver, spleen, and kidneys. To restore health, an acupuncturist uses long, very thin needles as "antennas" to direct chi to organs or functions of the body. The needles can also be used to drain chi where it is excessive, and to decrease or increase moisture and heat. The acupuncturist does this by selecting points along the body's fourteen "meridians" that affect the functioning of specific organs and puncturing and stimulating tissue at these locations. The needles penetrate to just below the epidermis and do not draw blood or cause discomfort. Sometimes heat is used, along with massage or electrical impulses.

The World Health Organization (WHO) currently recognizes more than forty medical problems, ranging from allergies to arthritis and AIDS, that can be helped by acupuncture treatment. Acupuncture has become a respectable therapy in

American hospitals in the last 20 years, and is used to reduce pain in patients with sore throats, sickle-cell anemia, dysmenorrhea, aftereffects of dental surgery, hysterectomies, chronic back disorders, migraine headaches and other ailments. It has been used successfully to induce cessation of smoking and to treat alcoholism and opiate addiction. Acupuncture has also been used to reduce pain in patients undergoing cancer chemotherapy and, of course, HIV/AIDS and related opportunistic infections and diseases.

In most states of the United States, acupuncturists must be medical doctors and have certification from the National Commission of Acupuncturists. However, some states do not regulate the practice at all. It is advisable to check a practitioner's credentials before a visit.

An acupuncturist generally uses a history and physical examination of the patient in making a diagnosis. In addition to asking questions, he focuses his attention on the character of the pulse and the appearance of the tongue. Sophisticated biological testing is not employed. The goal of the history and the physical is to assess the balance of yin and yang in the patient, and to guide the acupuncturist in selecting the correct chi points for a particular condition. Several treatments may be required over a period of weeks or months. The goal of therapy is to correct deficiencies or excesses of chi, thus restoring health. See ACU-PRESSURE.

acute   In medicine, this term describes intense short-term symptoms or illnesses that either resolve or evolve into long-lasting chronic disease manifestation.

acute aseptic meningitis   See MENINGITIS.

acute encephalopathy   See ENCEPHALOPATHY.

acute HIV exanthem   A severe skin eruption or rash that manifests itself as a result of HUMAN IMMUNODEFICIENCY VIRUS.

acute HIV infection   See PRIMARY HIV INFECTION.

acute phase proteins   SERUM PROTEINS whose levels increase during infection or inflammatory reactions. See INFLAMMATION.

acute phase reactions   Increases in certain PLASMA PROTEINS in response to almost any disease process that causes tissue damage. The blood sedimentation rate is influenced by these increases, as is the synthesis of C-reactive protein. The reaction is induced by INTERLEUKIN-1, interleukin-6, and TUMOR NECROSIS FACTOR. This factor is important in prompting the body defenses against MICROORGANISMS.

acute PID   See PELVIC INFLAMMATORY DISEASE (PID).

acute salpingitis   See PELVIC INFLAMMATORY DISEASE; SALPINGITIS.

acyclovir   A NUCLEOSIDE ANALOG like AZT, acyclovir is an ANTIMICROBIAL and ANTIVIRAL drug approved for use against HERPES SIMPLEX I (fever blisters, cold sores), herpes simplex II (genital herpes), HERPES ZOSTER (shingles), CYTOMEGALOVIRUS (CMV), and EPSTEIN-BARR VIRUS. Acyclovir was often used as an adjunct to AZT early in the AIDS EPIDEMIC, although the effectiveness of the combination was never proved in clinical trials. This use of acyclovir has generally stopped. The belief that acyclovir might work together well with AZT grew out of observations in the first major AZT study. In that study, it was noted that patients who also were using acyclovir suffered significantly fewer OPPORTUNISTIC INFECTIONS than those who used AZT alone. This led some researchers to suspect that acyclovir might strengthen the effect of AZT, perhaps allowing AZT to be used at lower doses than were then common. This combined use of the two drugs promised to reduce AZT's side effects. Other researchers suspected that acyclovir was merely helping control the effects of the opportunistic infections for which it was known to work (herpes, CMV, etc.). Side effects include arthralgias, DIARRHEA, headache, nausea, vomiting, and dizziness. Psychosis may be seen at high doses. Topical administration (ointment) may cause burning and stinging; skin may become hypersensitive with subsequent use. Combined use with the drug probenecid increases the half-life of acyclovir by decreasing its excretion from the body. Increased antiviral activity has been seen in combination with ALPHA-INTERFERON in vitro. Combination with NEPHROTOXIC drugs increases the risk of nephrotoxicity. High IV doses in combination with other bone marrow suppressant agents (i.e., high-dose trimethoprim/sulfamethoxazole) may induce blood DYSCRASIAS. Acyclovir is available for oral (considered most effective), intravenous, and topical administration. It is marketed under the trade name Zovirax. It has been supplanted by many doctors in HERPES treatment with VALACICLOVIR, which does not require as many daily doses to do the same amount of work.

ADA See AMERICANS WITH DISABILITIES ACT.

ADAP See AIDS DRUG ASSISTANCE PROGRAM.

adaptation Adjustment of an organism to a change in internal or external conditions or circumstances. In ophthalmology, it refers to an adjustment of the eye to various intensities of light, accomplished by changing the size of the pupil and through chemical changes inside the eye. In psychology, the term means a change in quality, intensity, or distinctness of sensation occurring after continuous stimulation of constant intensity. In dentistry, adaptation is the proper fitting of dentures or orthodontic bands to the teeth, or closeness of a filling to walls of a cavity.

adaptive immunity A series or complex of host defenses characterized by extreme specificity and memory mediated by ANTIBODY or T CELLS. See IMMUNITY.

ADC See AIDS DEMENTIA COMPLEX.

ADCC See ANTIBODY-DEPENDENT CELL-MEDIATED CYTOTOXICITY.

addiction Although there is disagreement among authorities as to how inclusive this designation should be, addiction is generally recognized to be a state of intense dependence upon a substance that chemically alters the functioning of the central nervous system, characterized by uncontrollable use of the substance, tolerance for its pleasure-giving effects, and manifestations of withdrawal symptoms when it is withheld. These features constitute physical dependence—a state of physical incorporation of the substance into the fundamental biochemistry of the brain. Habitual repeated behaviors such as overeating, reading, and television-watching are sometimes loosely referred to as addictions, but the term is properly used to indicate physiological need to experience the effects on the central nervous system of the addictive substance.

In regard to alcohol and drugs, addiction is distinguished from other noncompulsive ways of use such as *experimental* (trying a drink or a drug to see what it does); *social* or *recreational* (using a drink or a drug to enhance an activity or an event); *situational* (using a drink or a drug for a specific temporary pharmacological effect, such as relaxation of tension); and *intensified* (daily use without signs of compulsion).

The life of addicts is one of compulsion. Seven stages of addictive behavior have been noted. First, use of the addictive substance so that the user loses awareness of the amount and frequency of use. Second, the effects of the substance become unpredictable. Third, use becomes indiscriminate, and the user is no longer careful about the circumstances in which he or she uses it. Fourth, the user exhibits fear of abstinence and acts to secure or protect his supply; he feels better simply by having the substance in his possession. Fifth, the user develops a peer support group of fellow users and may reject nonusers. Sixth, where circumstances (such as the illegal status of some addictive substances) encourage them, the user develops self-protective, often pathological behaviors, including lying, stealing, and cheating, and may also engage in trafficking. Finally, the user develops the destructive physical and psychological effects of the prolonged use at toxic levels of the addictive substance—most commonly alcohol, tobacco, or a narcotic drug.

Addison's disease A disease resulting from a disorder of the adrenal glands, resulting in deficiency or lack of secretion of adrenocortical HOR-MONES. It may be a result of TUBERCULOSIS or autoimmune-induced adrenal disease. Its symptoms include occasional discoloration of the skin and mucous membranes, irregular patches of vitiligo (depigmentation of the skin), black freckles over head and neck, fever, tumors, HEMORRHAGIC NECROSIS, weakness, FATIGUE, HYPOTENSION, NAUSEA, vomiting, ANOREXIA, weight loss, and sometimes HYPOGLYCEMIA. If not treated, it is usually fatal. See ADRENAL FUNCTION and ADRENAL INSUFFICIENCY.

adefovir Adefovir dipivoxil is the first available drug in a new class of drugs called NUCLEOTIDE REVERSE TRANSCRIPTASE INHIBITORS or nucleotide analogs. Nucleotide analogs work against a virus's reverse transcriptase enzyme as do the nucleoside analog drugs such as AZT, ddI, ddC, d4T, and 3TC. The difference is that the nucleoside analogs have to go through complicated chemical processing inside cells in the body in order to work against HIV. Adefovir goes through a simpler chemical process because it already contains a phosphate group that most of the NUCLEOSIDE ANALOGS do not have and must acquire once in the body. Adefovir is a close "relative" of the drug TENOFOVIR; both are produced by Gilead Sciences. Studies initially showed that adefovir added some extra benefit to the highly active antiretroviral therapies (HAART) regimen. However, serious side effects of the drug were too likely at the dosage required for effectiveness against HIV, and the FDA rejected Gilead's approval request for the drug in relation to HIV treatment in 1999. Adefovir continues to be prescribed for use against HEPATITIS B (HBV). It has been very effective in treating HBV in clinical trials, at a much lower dose than used against HIV. Studies have shown adefovir can lower HBV viral levels by 99 percent. The main side effects are nausea, diarrhea, and liver problems. Kidney problems have also been seen. This latter problem is the main reason the drug cannot be used against HIV. Drug studies showed adefovir caused FANCONI'S SYNDROME in close to 40 percent of those on the drug at the levels prescribed for HIV. Kidney function should be monitored if you are taking this drug. Adefovir is produced as a pill, taken once a day. Because adefovir reduces the amount of L-carnitine, a natural substance in the body needed for getting energy into muscles, you must take a daily L-carnitine supplement with adefovir. (Also known as Preveon, bis-POM PMEA, and Hepsera.)

adenine Adenine is one of the four bases that make up DNA. Adenine bonds only with THYMINE (A-T or T-A), one of the other bases, to form what is called a purine base. The other two bases, GUANINE and CYTOSINE, also only bond with each other (G-C or C-G), to form what is called a pyrimidine base. The complementarity of these bondings ensures that DNA can be replicated (i.e., that identical copies can be made to transmit genetic information to the next generation). This bonding process is known as BASE PAIRING.

adenine arabinoside See VIDARABINE.

adenopathy Swelling or enlargement of the LYMPH NODES.

adenosine Adenosine is a NUCLEOSIDE of ADENINE. It is one of the constituents of RNA that HIV uses to replicate itself. The drug DIDANOSINE (ddI) is an ANALOG of adenosine that blocks the replication of the virus at the adenosine nucleoside. Scientists are unsure why adenosine plays a role in mediating sleepiness. They now know that the reason caffeine keeps people awake and affects sleep patterns is that it blocks adenosine receptors in the brain. Studies are under way to evaluate possible new sleeping pills made from adenosine.

adenosine triphosphate (ATP) The chemical created by the MITOCHONDRIA of the cell from the sugar, fat, and oxygen in the cell. Cells use this ATP as needed to provide energy for their activities.

adenovirus One of a group of closely related VIRUSES that can cause infections of the upper respiratory tract, such as the common cold and "pink-eye." Other adenoviruses can cause gastrointestinal illness or urinary tract infections. These viruses have also appeared in latent infections in some people. Many types of adenoviruses have been isolated and designated by number. In addition to human adenoviruses there are animal types. Some adenoviruses may induce malignant tumors in experimental animals.

adherence The act or state of adhering; in the context of HIV/AIDS, sticking closely to a prescribed treatment regimen. The importance of maintaining adherence to highly active antiretroviral therapies has received considerable attention since the advent of highly active antiretroviral therapies (HAART). However, if these treatments are not used properly (i.e., doses are repeatedly skipped, taken at lower than prescribed dosages, or not taken at scheduled intervals), drug RESISTANCE will develop more rapidly, and the potential benefits of combination therapy can be lost. Moreover, resistance to one drug may also result in decreased effectiveness of other drugs of the same class (CROSS-RESISTANCE). This is particularly true in regard to protease inhibitors.

Adhering to a treatment regimen is difficult under the best of circumstances. The triple combinations used with HIV disease can require that a person take a dozen or more antiviral pills per day, with specific timing and dietary requirements. Some HAART strategies have reduced the pill burden to one or two pills a day. When a person must also use preventive or maintenance doses of drugs for opportunistic infections, the total daily pill count can soar. Keeping track of one's medication becomes a major activity. Maintaining perfect adherence to today's complex treatment regimens is difficult. Studies have shown that there are many possible explanations for failure to adhere to treatment regimens, including forgetting to take a dose, sleeping through a dose, being away from home, changing one's therapy routine, being busy, sickness, experiencing side effects, or being depressed. The degree to which nonadherence is tolerable and the speed with which it contributes to drug failure is unclear. Additionally, it can vary from patient to patient how best to encourage and maintain adherence over time. Key components of these strategies are planning, support, and commitment.

adhesion The binding, or "sticking" of migratory LEUKOCYTES to endothelial or structural cells by the interaction of complementary adhesion PROTEINS.

adipocyte A fat cell.

adipogenesis The formation of fat or fatty tissues in the body. More specifically it is the process whereby STEM CELLS mature into ADIPOCYTES. Some PROTEASE INHIBITORS interfere in the process somehow, causing redistribution of fat within an HIV patient's body. See LIPODYSTROPHY.

adipose Fat.

adjustment disorder A maladaptive reaction to an identifiable psychological or social stress that occurs within three months of the onset of the stressful situation. The reaction is characterized by impairment of function or symptoms in excess of the norm for that stress. The symptoms may be expected to remit either when the stress ceases, or a new, more functional adaptation is achieved.

adjuvant Assisting. In medicine, a drug added to a therapy to increase the effectiveness of the treatment. In immunology, one of a variety of substances, including inorganic gels such as alum, aluminum hydroxide, and aluminum phosphate, that increase antigenic response (see ANTIGEN). A compound capable of potentiating an immune response.

adjuvant analgesic drug A drug that is not primarily used as an ANALGESIC but that research has shown to have independent or additive ANALGESIC properties. It is often used for additional relief in HIV or cancer treatment. One example of an adjuvant analgesic drug is nortriptyline, a TRICYCLIC ANTIDEPRESSANT, which is also used to treat NEUROPATHY pain.

administration In medicine, the introduction of a drug or chemical into the body.

administration, route of The method—INTRAVENOUS, oral, INTRAOCULAR, or other—of introducing a drug or chemical into the body.

administrative law judge (ALJ) An outside, impartial officer appointed to hear disputes and render decisions regarding the administrative determinations of many state and federal government agencies. An applicant who has been turned down for benefits in a SOCIAL SECURITY ADMINISTRATION (SSA) program, for instance, may request an ALJ hearing.

adolescence The period in which full sexual development occurs, between the onset of puberty and sexual maturity. It is characterized by physical growth, the appearance of secondary sexual characteristics, intense and wildly changeable emotions, and strong sexual urges (sometimes known as "raging hormones").

This development is a gradual process and its timing varies among individuals. It is defined by the National Library of Medicine as ranging from ages 13 to 18, but other institutions and disciplines hold that it ranges as broadly as from ages 11 to 25.

adoption The assumption of complete parental responsibility for children by persons who are not the natural parents. Formal adoption is an exhaustive legal procedure.

adrenal function The action performed by the ADRENAL GLAND.

adrenal gland One of two ENDOCRINE GLANDS located on the top of the kidneys; each consists of an adrenal cortex, which secretes cortisol and aldosterone, and an adrenal medulla, which secretes epinephrine and norepinephrine

adrenal insufficiency Abnormally low or decreased production of adrenal corticoid hormone by the ADRENAL GLAND. ADDISON'S DISEASE is the result.

adriamycin See DOXORUBICIN.

adult day services Day-long social service and care programs for incapacitated adults, on the model of senior citizens' or children's day care programs. Sponsored by the Department of Veterans

Affairs (formerly the Veterans Administration [VA]).

adult respiratory distress syndrome (ARDS) A form of restrictive lung disease caused by increased permeability of the pulmonary capillaries or the alveolar EPITHELIUM, characterized by the presence of an abnormally large amount of fluid in the tissue. The condition often develops after severe infection, trauma, or systemic illness. It has approximately a 50 percent fatality rate.

adult services Social services such as counseling, home chore aid, meals-on-wheels, discharge planning, program placement, drug abuse treatment, and so on, provided to adult welfare recipients as well as to some moderate-income aged and disabled people.

adverse event A side effect or result of treatment for an illness. In CLINICAL TRIALS government agencies rank adverse events on a scale. The NATIONAL CANCER INSTITUTE (NCI) uses a 0–5 scale

0 = No adverse event or within normal limits
1 = Mild adverse event
2 = Moderate adverse event
3 = Severe or undesirable adverse event
4 = Life-threatening or disabling adverse event
5 = Death related to an adverse event

The AIDS CLINICAL TRIALS GROUP (ACTG) Adult Adverse Experience Grading Table uses a I–IV scale.

   I = Mild, usually transient, and requiring no special treatment or interference with the patient's daily activities
  II = Moderate, may interfere with daily activities but can be controlled with simple therapeutic measures
 III = Serious, interrupts daily activities and requires systemic drug therapy or other intervention
 IV = Life-threatening, intolerable, and unacceptable, causing the patient to be in imminent danger of death

adverse reaction See ADVERSE EVENT.

Advil   See IBUPROFEN.

advocacy   In regard to social services and health care, action taken on behalf of individuals by themselves or others to ensure appropriate access to and availability of such services.

adynamia   See ASTHENIA.

aerobic   Requiring the presence of air or free oxygen for life, for example, aerobic bacteria.

aerobics   Shortened form of *aerobic exercises.* Any form of repeated exercises such as jogging, swimming, or cycling that stimulates the heart and lungs, thereby increasing the intake of oxygen in the body. Aerobics are a good way to decrease cholesterol levels and build lean muscle mass, both important for HIV-infected people on a HAART regimen.

aerosol   In medicine, the action by which a drug, such as PENTAMIDINE, is turned into a fine spray or mist by a nebulizer for administration by inhaling. See ADMINISTRATION, ROUTE OF.

aerosol pentamidine   See PENTAMIDINE.

AETC   See AIDS EDUCATION AND TRAINING CENTERS (AETC) PROGRAM.

AFB isolation   A specific type of hospital isolation for persons with acute MYCOBACTERIUM TUBERCULO-SIS. Its purpose is to prevent the spread of infection during the infectious phase of the disease. See ACID-FAST.

AFDC   See AID TO FAMILIES WITH DEPENDENT CHILDREN.

AFDC foster care   FOSTER CARE for children who originated in families receiving benefits under the AID TO FAMILIES WITH DEPENDENT CHILDREN (AFDC) program. It includes MEDICAID coverage of the children.

affected community   Persons living with HIV and AIDS, and any other related individuals, including their families, friends, and advocates, whose lives are directly influenced by HIV and all of its psychological and physical ramifications.

affective   Pertaining to feelings, emotions, or mental states.

affective disorder   Any disorder of affect, that is, of the feelings or emotions, characterized by mood swings and depression. It is not caused by, but may accompany, other physical or mental disorders. Affective disorders are common in HIV/AIDS patients.

Africa   There were estimated to be 40 million cases of HIV/AIDS in the world as of the end of 2001, according to the United Nations (UN). Of that number, 28.5 million, or 71.25 percent, of the world's cases are in sub-Saharan Africa. Seventeen million Africans have died since the HIV plague began in the early 1980s. The disease in Africa has taken the heart of the populations of these countries. Children are left orphaned, and parents must bury their adult children before caring for their sick grandchildren.

Cultural norms in Africa have made it difficult to openly discuss the problem. Sex is generally not discussed openly in Africa, and leaders are afraid to talk about the issue. Early on in the epidemic, some leaders denied that AIDS existed in their country. In Malawi, where 850,000 people are infected with HIV, it was illegal to publicly discuss AIDS until 1994. In Kenya, a former president said it is improper to discuss usage of condoms, and he asked all Kenyans to stop having sex for two years to stem the tide of the disease. In Swaziland, where 33 percent of the adult population is infected, King Mswati III has ordered young women to abstain from sex until at least 19 years of age and not to wear trousers so they do not encourage attention from young men. They are to wear a "don't touch" tassle that alerts boys to their vow of chastity. The king has also imposed on young women a five-year ban from having sex. However, the king violated his own order, choosing a 17-year-old high school student as his eighth wife shortly after issuing his decree.

Instead of discussing how to protect their populations, some African leaders are merely encouraging their populations not to engage in sex. Some do not believe that HIV/AIDS exists. President Thabo Mbeki of South Africa has repeatedly called into question the existence of AIDS. Policies he has initiated have downplayed the epidemic and routed money to fight other tropical illnesses, such as malaria and tuberculosis.

This lack of discussion has caused people with AIDS to be thrown out of their homes, beaten for bringing shame on their families, and fired from their jobs. Family members of people with HIV/AIDS falsely claim that their sick relatives who are ill or dying have TB, malaria, diarrhea, or pneumonia. Religious or cultural beliefs cause people to say the sickness afflicting them or family members is the result of jealousy from neighbors, witchcraft, retribution for some evil committed, or vengeful ancestors come to curse their descendants. Similar beliefs around the world contribute to the avoidance of discussion of the causes of this illness.

This disease has been particularly horrific in southern Africa, where in many cases population growth is in negative numbers and life expectancy has fallen below the age of 30. Botswana is the worst affected. This country has southern Africa's highest per capita income, and it also has the highest percentage of adults that are HIV positive: nearly 39 percent. According to UN studies, the situation in neighboring countries is nearly as critical: In Zimbabwe, 33 percent of adults are infected; in Swaziland, 33 percent; Lesotho, 31 percent; Namibia, 23 percent; Zambia, 21 percent; and South Africa, 20 percent. A study released in early 2003 by the government of Swaziland has increased the UN numbers to an estimated 38 percent HIV rate among adults in this small country of 1 million people. Life expectancy in Botswana has fallen, for the first time since 1950, to 39 years. Without the advent of AIDS the life expectancy in Botswana would be 72 years. Six other countries also have life expectancies under 40. They are Swaziland, 39; Zimbabwe, 39; Rwanda, 39; Angola, 38; Zambia, 37; and Malawi, 37. Five countries—Botswana, Mozambique, Lesotho, Swaziland, and South Africa—will experience negative population growth from AIDS by 2010, according to reports by USAID, a U.S. government aid agency. South Africa also had more HIV/AIDS infected citizens—5 million—than any nation on earth at the end of 2001.

The rest of Africa has fared only slightly better. Ten percent of the adult population of the Ivory Coast is HIV positive. Nigeria, Ethiopia, and Kenya all have more than 2 million residents who are HIV positive. The Central African Republic, Cameroon, Kenya, Malawi, and Rwanda all have 9 percent or more of their populations infected with HIV. In addition rates of HIV infection in western and central African countries have seen large increases in the past two years. Angola has seen the HIV infection rate of women in pregnancy clinics jump from 1.2 percent in 1995 to 8.6 percent in 2001.

The bright spots have been few and far between in Africa. Uganda, where the disease first came to light in Africa, has lowered its adult prevalence rate from 8.3 percent in 1999 to 5 percent in 2001. Uganda has implemented major education campaigns about AIDS and how to prevent it. However, Uganda still has close to 1 million children orphaned from the disease. In Zambia, prevalence rates among urban and rural women have also dropped in the last two years, giving hope that this country may be making some headway in educating its citizens.

Compounding these statistics is the poverty of the region. Drugs that are available in the Western countries are generally not available in Africa. South Africa has just been forced through its court system to provide access to specific generic drugs, against the policies set by the current government. Botswana, with grants from the Bill and Melinda Gates Foundation, has begun offering medicines to its populace. However, Zimbabwe for example, has not been able to provide medications because of their high cost. Western pharmaceutical companies have for the most part not allowed these countries to manufacture generic equivalents of their expensive and patented AIDS medications. The governments in southern Africa do not have the financial resources necessary to encourage manufacture of these items or the means to pay for their citizen's health costs.

To further compound the problem, in the years 2000–2002, the harvests of most of the nations in southern Africa were adversely affected by a severe drought. Except in South Africa, the region is experiencing the worst famine seen in these countries. Angola and Zimbabwe have exacerbated the situation by forcing farmers off their fields, hampering agricultural production. Policies in Angola, to starve rebels, and in Zimbabwe, to eliminate white ownership of farms, have created the combination of hunger and HIV that could easily kill more of their population.

The UN and Western medical organizations have stated that the problem of AIDS has not leveled off as anticipated a few years ago. Indeed, they now admit it has become much worse than they thought possible. Life expectancies are now thought likely to drop below 30 years of age in several countries by 2010. The extent of death and illness has not been seen since the plague entered Europe in the Middle Ages. International public and private monies are currently being sought by the UN for a large Global AIDS Fund that the UN hopes will be able to increase knowledge of the disease and ways to prevent its transmission. However, donations by the United States, the richest nation, have not been forthcoming as anticipated. The United States promised $1 billion in 2001 to the fund but had not delivered as of the end of 2002. In addition, The U.S. ranks only ahead of three of the 14 donor nations to the fund. Luxembourg, New Zealand, and nine other countries rank higher in per capita donations to the fund. Many AIDS ACTIVISTS have begun condemning the United States for lack of action is this arena. See MIDDLE EAST AND NORTH AFRICA.

African swine fever A viral disease caused by an IMMUNODEFICIENCY-distinct agent, first isolated in Africa. It has also been found in Brazil, Cuba, the Dominican Republic, Haiti, and western Europe. Early in the AIDS epidemic it was suspected to be the causative agent of the acquired immunodeficiency syndrome.

agammaglobulinemia Total or near-total absence of gamma globulin, a protein part of the blood rich in antibodies, caused by certain genetic diseases or HIV infection. Immunoglobulin injections can relieve the problem temporarily but must be repeated often throughout someone's life if the disease is inherited or until some restoration of the immune system's functioning has occurred, as through HAART treatment.

age In psychology, the stage of development reached by an individual, as expressed in terms of the chronological age of an average individual at a comparable stage of development or accomplishment.

Agenerase See AMPRENAVIR.

agent Something that causes a biological, chemical, or physical effect. BACTERIA that cause a disease are agents of that disease; medicine administered to treat a DISEASE or illness is a therapeutic agent.

agonist A chemical substance capable of binding with a receptor on a cell's surface to induce a full or partial pharmacological response. All drugs are agonists, either full or partial agonists. The opposite of antagonist.

AHG See FACTOR VIII.

A.I.D. See ARTIFICIAL INSEMINATION.

aid and attendance A term used by the DEPARTMENT OF VETERANS AFFAIRS (VA) to designate the home chore aid a disabled veteran pensioner must purchase because he or she is too incapacitated for daily living activities and for which he or she is therefore eligible for a higher pension income.

Aid to Families with Dependent Children (AFDC)
One of a number of federal welfare programs that used to provide temporary financial assistance to needy families with dependent children. The principal agency designated to carry out welfare, the Department of Health and Human Service's Administration for Children and Families' (ACF) Office of Family Assistance (OFA), saw its mission transformed by the Personal Responsibility and Work Opportunity Reconciliation Act of 1996. This law was designed to "end welfare as we know it," in the words of President Bill Clinton. Beginning July 1, 1997, AFDC ended, and the new TANF program

replaced AFDC, among other programs. See TEMPO-
RARY ASSISTANCE FOR NEEDY FAMILIES (TANF).

**Aid to the Permanently and Totally Disabled
(APTD)** A federal-state welfare program for poor
disabled persons. It was replaced by the federal SUP-
PLEMENTAL SECURITY INCOME (SSI) program in 1974,
but the term is still used in some states to refer to
STATE SUPPLEMENTARY PAYMENT (SSP) programs.

AIDS See ACQUIRED IMMUNODEFICIENCY SYNDROME.

AIDS advocacy organization See COMMUNITY-
BASED ORGANIZATION.

AIDS and cultural analysis See CULTURAL ANALY-
SIS AND AIDS.

AIDS and cultural discourse See CULTURAL
ANALYSIS AND AIDS; AIDS DISCOURSE.

AIDS buyers' club Any of a network of outlets
that provide access to alternative treatments, often
on a cost-plus basis. Typically a nonprofit organization set up by persons with HIV or AIDS, a buyers'
club helps its members buy nutritional and other
products, especially those not readily available
elsewhere, at wholesale prices. Buyers' clubs also
protect their members by making more sophisticated product selection and purchasing decisions
than individuals would be likely to do on their
own and negotiating better prices. They often have
products independently tested, helping members
avoid shoddy products.

Clubs also share information and negotiate as a
unit when necessary, so they provide the power
of a national network, one entirely dedicated to
serving the interests of HIV positive people and
finding the best treatments available. Buyers'
clubs serve an important quality control function
in the marketplace.

Their importance also goes beyond their role in
the market. They often serve as treatment-oriented
support groups. Members share information not
only about products but about physicians, clinics,
and therapies, including all kinds of conventional,
experimental, or alternative treatments. These
grassroots groups fill the gap left by major AIDS

support organizations that have usually refused to
allow their support group to focus on treatment
information.

In practice, buyers' clubs vary widely. Some of
the smaller ones skip the considerable paperwork of
incorporating as a nonprofit, so technically they are
for-profit businesses even if they do not actually
make money. Some clubs will ship products; others
are not set up to do that. Some need to collect
money in advance before placing orders; others
have stock on hand. Clubs are located throughout
the United States, and in foreign countries as well.

AIDS case definition As with any disease, a consistent definition was developed for AIDS so that the
CENTERS FOR DISEASE CONTROL AND PREVENTION (CDC)
could track its spread and implement strategies to
prevent the transmission of infection. In 1982, the
CDC developed a surveillance case definition for this
syndrome focusing on the presence of opportunistic
infections. The AIDS case definition was expanded
in 1985 to include a total of 20 conditions. Four of
these conditions were cancers: KAPOSI'S SARCOMA
and three distinct types of LYMPHOMA. The remaining
conditions were opportunistic infections—those
caused by bacteria, fungi, protozoa, and other infectious agents—that an intact immune system can
usually manage but take advantage of the "opportunity" provided by weakened immunity to proliferate
in the body. By the mid-1980s all states and many
localities were requiring all health care providers to
report AIDS cases to their local health departments.
These cases, and only these cases, were included in
the CDC's surveillance reports of AIDS diagnoses
and fatalities. On the basis of the CDCs experience
(in the early and mid-1980s) with people with HIV,
at the time predominantly gay men, the AIDS case
definition systematically excluded women, injection
drug users, low-income people, and other populations. These people with AIDS were, in turn, unable
to be officially diagnosed as having AIDS. Although
the way in which the CDC defines AIDS may seem
remote from the daily lives of people with HIV, it
does, in fact, have a profound impact on their access
to health care and benefits. For example, many entitlement programs determine an individual's eligibility for benefits according to whether or not she or
he has CDC-defined AIDS. In addition, as a second

example, federal and state funds are often allocated on the basis of the CDC-defined AIDS cases reported. At issue, therefore, are when an HIV infection becomes AIDS and when AIDS becomes disabling. In 1987 the CDC added three more illnesses to their list of defining conditions: extrapulmonary tuberculosis (TB outside the lungs), WASTING SYNDROME, and HIV effects on the CENTRAL NERVOUS SYSTEM (ENCEPHALOPATHY or DEMENTIA). These three additions resulted in a one-quarter increase in reported AIDS cases, primarily among heterosexual African American and Latino individuals. These new cases also included high numbers of injecting drug users. In 1992, bowing to increasing public pressure from patients, health professionals, activists, and others, federal officials proposed an expanded definition of AIDS that included a laboratory test of immune function and added three illnesses (invasive cancer of the cervix, pulmonary tuberculosis, and two or more episodes of bacterial pneumonia) to 23 other complicating ailments listed in the 1987 definition. The proposed definition also included any adult infected with HIV who had 200 or fewer CD4 cells per cubic milliliter of blood, or about one-fifth the normal level. No such measurement was part of the original definition. The expansion of the AIDS definition to include the gynecological symptoms and diseases of women with HIV paved the way for research and treatment for women-specific infections. The new definition went into effect in 1993 and resulted, as was predicted, in a significant increase in the number of cases designated as AIDS cases. The change did not have a significant impact on insurance and other benefits because Social Security Administration officials do not rely on the CDC definition in determining disability. In addition, the CDC considers an additional two illnesses when defining AIDS in children. These are multiple, recurrent bacterial infections and LYMPHOID INTERSTITIAL PNEUMONIA. Definitions of AIDS vary in different countries and generally are made by the government health department.

AIDS classification   The CDC, since 1993, has used a table to classify the seriousness of the clinical case definition for AIDS. This table was part of the revision that declared that anyone who has a CD4 cell count below 200/mm^3 has AIDS. The table is divided into nine sections; by following the column on the left side, it can be seen that a person's CD4 T-cell count is divided into three categories. The row across the top is divided into three sections also. These are divided by the clinical complications a HIV-positive person has experienced. By this classification any person who is labeled A3, B3, C1, C2, or C3 is defined as having AIDS.

CLINICAL CATEGORIES		
A Asymptomatic, Acute HIV or Persistent Generalized Lymphadenopathy	**B** Symptomatic, Not A or C Conditions	**C** AIDS Indicator Conditions

CD4+ T-cell Categories	A	B	C
1) >500/mm^3	A1	B1	C1
2) 200–499/mm^3	A2	B2	C2
3) <200/mm^3	A3	B3	C3

In Category A one or more of the following have occurred:

1. Asymptomatic HIV infection
2. Persistent generalized lymphadenopathy
3. Any accompanying illness or history of acute HIV infection

Category B consists of symptomatic conditions in an HIV-infected adolescent or adult that are not included in Category C.

1. Conditions attributed to HIV infection or indicative of a defect in cell-mediated immunity
2. Conditions that are considered by medical personnel to have a clinical course or require management that is complicated by HIV infection

Conditions that occur in Category B include but are not limited to

Oral candidiasis
Vulvovaginal candidiasis
Cervical dysplasia (moderate or severe)
Constitutional symptoms such as fever or diarrhea lasting more than a month
Oral hairy leukoplakia
Herpes zoster, shingles
Idiopathic thrombocytopenic purpura

Pelvic inflammatory disease
Peripheral neuropathy

Category B conditions take precedence over Category A conditions.

Category C: for classification purposes once a category C complication has occurred, a person remains in category C.

Candidiasis of the bronchi, trachea, or lungs
Candidiasis of the esophagus
Cervical carcinoma, invasive
Coccidioidomycosis, disseminated or pulmonary
Cryptococcoses, extrapulmonary
Cryptosporidiosis, chronic intestinal
Cytomegalovirus
Encephalopathy
Herpes simplex, chronic ulcers of longer than a month's duration
Histoplasmosis, extrapulmonary or disseminated
Isosporiasis, chronic intestinal
Kaposi's sarcoma
Lymphoma, primary brain
Lymphoma, immunoblastic
Mycobacterium avium complex or *Mycobacterium kansasii,* disseminated or extrapulmonary
Mycobacterium tuberculosis, any site
Other *Mycobacterium* species, extrapulmonary or pulmonary
Pneumocystis carinii pneumonia
Progressive multifocal leukoencephalopathy
Pneumonia, recurrent
Salmonella septicemia, recurrent
Toxoplasmosis of the brain
Wasting syndrome due to HIV

In children below the age of 13 the following two illnesses are also used for Category C classification:

Multiple, recurrent bacterial infections
Lymphoid interstitial pneumonia/pulmonary lymphoid hyperplasia

AIDS Clinical Testing Unit   The site at which AIDS drug trials are performed in the AIDS CLINICAL TRIALS GROUP, a division of the NATIONAL INSTITUTE OF ALLERGY AND INFECTIOUS DISEASE (NIAID).

AIDS Clinical Trials Group (ACTG)   Also known as AIDS Clinical Trials Unit (ACTU). A nationwide, multicenter clinical trials network that tests new drugs and treatment strategies for adults and children infected with HIV that is sponsored and administered by the National Institute of Allergy and Infectious Diseases (NIAID). The ACTG was established by NIAID in 1987 and remains the largest network of its kind in the world. The specific goals of the ACTG are three-fold: to evaluate innovative therapeutic strategies and interventions to control HIV infection and its complications; to facilitate rapid translation of basic research into clinical research and practice; and to provide a flexible resource for state-of-the-art, multidisciplinary clinical trials that address the goals and objectives of NIAID's therapeutics research agenda. NIAID contracts with institutions such as hospitals, academic medical centers, and so forth to perform the actual drug trials through a grant process, with a principal investigator controlling the trial.

The ACTG is an outgrowth of NIAID's first major programs for the evaluation of potential treatments for people with AIDS, which began in the summer of 1986. The original 36 AIDS Clinical Trials Units included two sites that enrolled children with AIDS. Additional pediatric sites were added between 1988 and 1989, and again in 1992. After a competitive renewal in 1992, the ACTG grew to include 35 adult and 22 pediatric AIDS Clinical Trial Units. in addition to a statistical and data analysis center and an operations office. More than 35,000 adults and 6,000 children and adolescents have enrolled in ACTG clinical trials ranging from early single-site safety studies to large-scale, multicenter efficacy trials.

In 1993, NIAID conducted a comprehensive evaluation of the ACTG to assess its mission, scientific agenda, and future direction, as well as the group's organizational structure and efficiency. This review was carried out by an external scientific review panel that evaluated the ACTG's scientific plans, and NIAID staff working group that assessed organizational and managerial issues. Both review groups recommended that the leadership of the ACTG be strengthened, giving it increased authority and accountability for development and management of its scientific program. The reviewers also recommended that the ACTG place greater emphasis on pathogenesis-based clinical research.

These recommendations and others, including the separation of the Adult ACTG from the Pediatric ACTG, were incorporated into a Request for Applications for the competitive renewal of Adult ACTG, published in August 1994. Three types of applications were solicited: one for prospective AIDS Clinical Trials Units, one for a Coordinating and Operations Center, and another for a Statistical and Data Management Center. Two separate committees were convened to review the three types of applications. Applications recommended for further consideration went through a second level of external peer review by the National Advisory Allergy and Infectious Diseases Council, before a final decision was made on the sites that would be funded. Among the criteria considered in the review process were the scientific and technical merit of the applications, the qualifications of key personnel, experience in multicenter HIV/AIDS clinical research, adequacy of plans for inclusion of women and minorities, and a demonstrated ability to accrue a certain number of patients each year.

Today, the ACTGs remain the largest network of their kind in the world. A consortium of academically affiliated clinicians responsible for conducting a large portion of clinical research of AIDS in the United States constitutes the backbone of the ACTGs. Medical centers throughout the United States that conduct clinical trials of drugs for treating people with HIV infection are also members of the consortium. Specifically, the drugs are for treating opportunistic infections or tumors as well as HIV itself, and for stimulating the immune system. ACTGs are funded federally through the National Institutes of Heath.

ACTG trials have been the source of most of the information currently available on how best to treat people with HIV infection and related diseases. ACTG research also has defined the standard preventive therapies and treatments for many opportunistic infections. When a drug is given ACTG status it means that a specific protocol and a series of sites were chosen to carry out government-funded clinical trials of the drug in order to study the drug's effect in people living with HIV/AIDS.

AIDS Coalition to Unleash Power (ACT-UP)
An AIDS activist organization founded in 1987 in New York City. Composed mainly of young gays and lesbians with a desire to be politically active, ACT-UP quickly became the strongest and best known organization of its kind. In its heyday, ACT-UP had to move its weekly New York meeting from a small community center in Greenwich Village to a more commodious auditorium at the Cooper Union. There, at what was then the epicenter of AIDS activism, as many as 700 people would show up, pumping each other full of a take-no-prisoners fervor and plotting brash demonstrations that would halt traffic, heckle politicians, and guarantee prominent coverage on the evening news. From interrupting trading at the New York Stock Exchange to disrupting a sermon by Cardinal O'Connor inside St. Patrick's Cathedral, its nervy tactics became a staple of television news. Its leaflets and logos formed a sort of visual iconography in many cities, including New York, where it used to be difficult to use an automated teller machine without seeing a decal bearing a pink triangle and the caveat "silence = death," or to walk a few blocks without seeing a rendering of a bloody handprint. Indeed, in its heyday in New York just about every possible target was zapped, and many of those demonstrations made the newspapers and the television news.

Several big moments in ACT-UP's history merit mention. In March 1987, at ACT-UP's first demonstration, 17 members were arrested on Wall Street as 250 protested drug company profiteering and other issues. In April 1989 four ACT-UP members were arrested after barricading themselves inside a Burroughs Wellcome office in North Carolina to protest the high cost of AZT. In September 1989 seven ACT-UP members interrupted trading on the New York Stock Exchange floor. In December 1989 some 4,500 people converged on St. Patrick's Cathedral in New York City to protest church opposition to safer-sex education and legal abortion. A total of 111 people were arrested, including 43 inside for disrupting a sermon by Cardinal O'Connor. In October 1992, while the AIDS quilt was on display in Washington, ACT-UP mourners broke through police lines and threw ashes of people who had died of AIDS on the White House lawn.

ACT-UP served a variety of purposes, not the least of which was to train a whole generation of activists in a range of social-change work and advocacy. ACT-UP demanded increased financing for medical research and accelerated drug development; today, much of this has come to pass. In March 1987, when ACT-UP held its inaugural demonstration on Wall Street, the annual budget allotted by the National Institutes of Health for AIDS research was about $290 million and AZT was the only antiviral AIDS drug that was approved by the FOOD AND DRUG ADMINISTRATION. As of fiscal 2003, the annual research budget was an estimated $2.7 billion, and there were 20 approved ANTIVIRAL drugs, including seven PROTEASE INHIBITORS, which seem by far to be the most effective medications to date. Moreover, the time from initial development of a drug to its availability to patients has been cut from about seven or eight years to less than three. ACT-UP was a compelling force behind these changes. Above all, ACT-UP irrefutably accomplished its bedrock goal: to make Americans pay some attention to AIDS. It did this with such unmitigated gall and undeniable panache that in New York, San Francisco, Los Angeles, and many other cities, ACT-UP turned into the coolest club to which homosexuals could belong. And it did this while surviving on donations and the sale of T-shirts and artwork.

Today, ACT-UP is a shadow of its former self. This reflects, in part, the deaths of many of its leaders, the infighting that fractured the group, the seemingly inevitable mellowing of any radical movement, and the degree to which the armies that amassed to battle AIDS traveled a spectrum of grief from anger to acceptance. It also is because ACT-UP's energy did not so much dissipate as disperse, with members marching off in different, more specialized directions and with an array of other AIDS-related organizations spun off from or inspired by it. Most interestingly, and perhaps most significantly, it also reflects the extent to which the protesters once clamoring at the dining room door have gained a place at the table. See ACTIVISM.

AIDS dementia complex (ADC) See HIV ENCEPHALOPATHY.

AIDS denialism AIDS denialists believe that HIV is not the cause of AIDS. AIDS denialism has occurred since the late 1980s, when AIDS denialists began spreading the message that it was not the virus making people sick, but other factors, including anti-HIV drugs such as AZT. AIDS denialists were partly right, in that though not the cause of AIDS, the early nucleoside analogs sometimes made people ill. The drugs could also delay disease and improve survival as long as they continued to work against the virus (until resistance had set in). But at the time, it was much harder to determine when the drugs were, or had stopped, working because viral load tests were not available to clinicians for patient management. Instead, people were kept on therapy until clinical progression or major drops in CD4 cell counts, long after the drug's effectiveness had worn off. At that point, the nucleoside analogs were merely toxins that probably did cause more harm than good. The AIDS denialism movement became rather quiescent around the time the protease inhibitors appeared and when triple combination therapy was shown to decrease HIV levels, and the incidence of AIDS-related opportunistic infections and death dramatically. This seemed to prove once and for all that HIV caused AIDS and that keeping the virus suppressed kept the disease at bay. In the late 1990s the AIDS denialist movement gradually began picking up steam, at roughly the same time that the very visible signs of lipodystrophy appeared. The prominent AIDS denialist journalist Celia Farber essentially blames lipodystrophy on protease inhibitors. She also asserts that the protease inhibitors were approved mainly as a result of Dr. David Ho's theory that eradication might be possible if the virus were fully suppressed by potent therapy. She ignores the body of clinical evidence of reduced opportunistic infections and reduced AIDS-related mortality rate that led to marketing approval of ritonavir and the other protease inhibitors. Instead, she notes only reports of drug toxicity. Eventually, she returned to old AIDS denialist rhetoric, denying HIV's causative role in AIDS. Treatment journalists generally agree that sensationalism sells magazines and that AIDS denialism makes their jobs communicating the complex issues surrounding the long-term side effects of HIV treatment more difficult. They note that people should be warned about how debilitating these side effects can be when making their treatment decisions and stress the importance of doing so without panicking patients.

AIDS denialist   Someone who does not believe that the HIV virus is the root cause of the illness AIDS. Over the 20 years that AIDS has been recognized as a disease many different people have proffered various explanations for the cause of the illness.

After the discovery of the virus and how it worked, many still believed that this explanation was incorrect. Today there are individuals and groups that do not hold that the HIV virus causes AIDS or illness. They believe any number of other viruses, drugs, or government germ warfare are responsible these illnesses.

Dr. Peter Duesberg has written many books and articles on his theories that state that illegal drug use leads to AIDS. He has reportedly had himself injected with HIV to prove it does not cause AIDS. San Francisco ACT-UP (not part of the nationwide ACT-UP network) holds that HIV does not cause AIDS and that HIV medications are the culprit in killing people. President Thabo Mbeki of South Africa publicly doubts whether AIDS is caused by HIV and suggests it is the result of whites wanting to kill black Africans. Boyd Graves, a lawyer from California believes he has uncovered proof that HIV is derived from research done in the United States with the Visna virus from sheep. He believes it is part of a continuing eugenics program the United States government funded through the Special Virus Cancer Program, which created the virus and injected it in humans through hepatitis B vaccines tested in gay and African populations. Results of an official government investigation can be found on the Internet, http://www.gao.gov/new.items/d02809r.pdf.

Denialists often stand in the way of new research, proper treatments, and social advancement in the prevention of HIV transmission by propagating beliefs that cause others to ignore health warnings and education campaigns. Denialists also, however, cause researchers to check their facts, create understandable reports to explain their findings, and force everyone in HIV research to be able to prove theories concerning the virus.

AIDS discourse   The complex of formal speech and writing that examines what HIV and AIDS have been made to mean socially and culturally, both in the lives of the people and communities coping with AIDS and HIV infection, and in society as a whole; the totality of informed discussion about AIDS. See CULTURAL ANALYSIS AND AIDS.

AIDS Drug Assistance Program   Program that provides life-sustaining and life-prolonging medications to low-income individuals with HIV who have no other means of paying for these drugs. ADAPs are the most heavily utilized AIDS programs in the nation. More than 80,000 people were served by ADAPs in June 2002 alone, with expenditures of $70 million. Some states have slightly different names for the federally mandated program.

Although an average of 80 percent of ADAP funding comes from the federal government, individual ADAPs are administered by the states and require some additional amount of state funding if they are to offer more than bare bones drug coverage. The list of medications provided by the ADAPs varies considerably from state to state. Traditionally poor states in the Southeast and Rocky Mountain areas often have financial shortfalls and lack of easy access to these services.

Federal ADAP funding was increased by $68 million in 2002, bringing total state and federal spending to $898 million. This amount was believed to be approximately $130 million short of the total required to assure medication assistance for everyone needing it. This meant that most, if not all, ADAPs would run out of money toward the end of 2002. Budgets for 2003 had not been finalized for ADAPs as of this printing. However, word from several states was that funding would be cut in 2003 to help reduce the state budget shortfalls that many states are currently experiencing. Pressure on ADAPs is expected to increase as new drugs such as pegylated INTERFERON, ATAZANAVIR, and ENFUVIRTIDE become available. Additional pressure could come from increasing unemployment, lack of insurance, a steady number of new HIV infections, side effects increasing the number of medications needed, and the tight budgets of state Medicaid programs.

For 2003, President George W. Bush proposed flat funding ADAP (no increases). Advocates for ADAP say a push in Congress for an Emergency Supplemental Request to increase federal funding is needed right away. If no supplemental funding is received in 2003, shortfalls will return funding per capita to levels to those of the mid-1990s, when many people were simply unable to receive the HAART drugs that became available, due to their cost. This would then add the United States to a large list of countries that cannot or do not fund medications for HIV positive people. With the Federal shortfalls, and state cutbacks ADAPS may resort to waiting lists or other restrictions. Debates about increasing contributions to ADAP funding are expected in most states. For more information, see the annual National ADAP Monitoring Report released by the Kaiser Family Foundation in April of each year (http://www.kff.org). For detailed information on each state's individual ADAP, contact the AIDS Treatment Data Network/The Access Project (http://www.aidsinfonyc.org/network/access).

AIDS education and training centers   See AIDS EDUCATION AND TRAINING CENTERS (AETC) PROGRAM.

AIDS Education and Training Centers (AETC) Program   The National AIDS Education and Training Centers Program was established in 1987 to increase the number of health care providers who are effectively educated and motivated to counsel, diagnose, treat, and manage individuals with HIV infection and to assist in the prevention of high-risk behaviors that may lead to infection. The program conducts targeted, multidisciplinary HIV education and training programs for health care providers through a network of 15 regional centers and 75 associated sites. Information dissemination efforts emphasize electronic communication and include cosponsorship of the quarterly national HIV Clinical Conference Call series. The program began with four AETCs that focused on educating providers about the epidemiology of AIDS and methods to identify groups at increased risk of infection. By 1991, in response to the growth of the epidemic, the program had increased the number of regional AETCs, which serve all 50 states,

the Virgin Islands, Puerto Rico, and the six U.S. Pacific Jurisdictions (Guam, Marshall Islands, Palau, Federated States of Micronesia, American Samoa, and the Northern Marianas). Clinical training of primary care providers (physicians, nurses, dentists) became the primary focus, with a secondary emphasis on training providers in mental health and allied fields. Most resources have been concentrated on areas of high HIV incidence. Over 700,000 training interactions have taken place through the AETCs. Allocation of program resources and scheduling of activities are based on a comprehensive local, state, and regional needs assessment. The http://www.aids-ed.org/ National Resource Center website is especially helpful for health care practitioners who may not be familiar with HIV or AIDS or who practice in rural areas.

AIDS enteropathy   Any intestinal disease appearing in a person with AIDS.

AIDS, origin of   See HIV, ORIGIN OF.

AIDS orphan   A child or youth who has lost parents, foster and adoptive parents, grandparents, siblings, friends, neighbors, or other crucial caregivers to the AIDS epidemic. AIDS orphans generally do not have the disease themselves and are not viewed as patients by the medical community. Often unable to share their family secrets and losses, they are often invisible to service communities, schools, churches, and courts. Few professionals seem to be helping to plan for their futures, or even recognize that they exist. CONFIDENTIALITY and disclosure, custody and placement, benefits programs, and bereavement are some of the issues these children and youth face. An additional challenge these children and youth face is that the general public is not well educated about the issue.

Children and youth whose lives are touched by the HIV/AIDS epidemic confront not one epidemic but two: as the disease spreads, so does the epidemic of indifference to the children's and youths' plight. The indifference arises in part from ignorance. Breaking society's silence about these children who must struggle to survive AIDS in their families is one means of arresting the epidemic of indifference. It is noted that there are numerous national organizations that provide useful information to HIV-affected children and youth and their families.

AIDS prodrome   Any sign or symptom indicative of the onset of AIDS.

AIDS quilt   See QUILT.

AIDS service organization (ASO)   A nongovernmental, nonprofit group that provides services such as medical care, counseling, legal and housing assistance, and access to food banks to those infected with HIV. The first was the GAY MEN'S HEALTH CRISIS (GMHC), created in New York City in 1981 by the playwright Larry Kramer and others. Today, ASOs are the principal institutional vehicles of volunteer, community-based AIDS prevention and care efforts. Though they may operate at a local, regional, or national level, most of these organizations are quite small, staffed and supported by a remarkable variety of activists, including gay men and lesbians, social and health care workers, and others affected and infected by HIV. ASOs have for years been central to society's response to AIDS. When initially government response was nonexistent, ASOs served as the only place that PWAs could receive any assistance. The future of ASOs will revolve around funding and the need for constantly replacing volunteers, as they tire, burn out, or die. Since the introduction of HAART several midsize ASOs in the United States have folded as a result of clients' not needing their services. What happens in the age of HAART and government focus on nondisease issues will have considerable influence on ASO functioning in the future of the epidemic.

AIDS Treatment Evaluation Units (ATEU)   Original name of the AIDS CLINICAL TRIALS GROUP, established by the National Institute of Allergy and Infectious Diseases in 1986 to test new AIDS-related drugs.

AIDS virus   In medical literature, HIV, the virus responsible for AIDS, is called by various other names dating from early in the AIDS epidemic. Though it continues to be debated, the basic terminology has been fairly well standardized.

AIDS-associated retrovirus (ARV)   Isolates of the retrovirus that causes AIDS. See HUMAN IMMUNODEFICIENCY VIRUS (HIV).

AIDS-associated virus (AAV)   An early name for HUMAN IMMUNODEFICIENCY VIRUS (HIV).

AIDS-defining diagnosis   See AIDS CASE DEFINITION.

AIDS-defining illness   One of a number of serious illnesses that occurs in HIV-positive individuals and contributes to a diagnosis of AIDS. See ACQUIRED IMMUNODEFICIENCY SYNDROME; AIDS CASE DEFINITION.

AIDSLINE   AIDSLINE is the National Library of Medicine (NLM) database of published literature on AIDS and HIV. It is updated weekly with journal citations, and monthly with citations from AIDS newsletters and public health materials. It began in 1980 when the NLM began tracking articles on HIV and AIDS. In 2002 the NLM merged AIDSLINE with its other databases into one large database divided into citations, meeting summaries, and books (http://gateway.nlm.nih.gov).

AIDSphobia   A term coined to denote an unrealistic fear and dread of the acquired immunodeficiency syndrome and of those afflicted with it.

AIDS-related complex (ARC)   A health condition in which some of the signs and symptoms of HIV infection (stages 1 to 5) have appeared, but none of the opportunistic infections associated with AIDS. At the onset of the epidemic the term designated the condition of HIV-infected individuals not diagnosed with AIDS but with compromised immune systems and decreased T-CELL COUNTS. The term is no longer officially recognized by the CDC.

AIDS-related condition   A serious stage of HIV infection characterized by opportunistic infections other than those clearly associated with AIDS. In effect, a variety of AIDS.

AIDS-related virus (ARV)   A strain of HUMAN IMMUNODEFICIENCY VIRUS (HIV) found in HOMOSEX-

UAL men in 1984 in Atlanta, Georgia. This was one of the names given the virus responsible for AIDS early in the epidemic, before the terminology was standardized.

AIDSspeak   A vernacular created by public health officials, politicians, and AIDS activists to discuss issues related to the pandemic. Among its characteristics is the use of nonjudgmental language.

airborne transmission   Process by which an infectious AGENT passes through the air from a CARRIER to others in the form of tiny inhalant droplets. Typically the process begins with a sneeze or a cough.

AL-721   An immune stimulant believed to inhibit the replication of the HIV virus, AL-721 was, prior to the marketing of AZT, the unofficial, "underground" treatment of choice for people with AIDS. This inexpensive egg-based compound was developed in 1979 at Israel's Weitzmann Institute of Science to remove cholesterol from cell walls. Use of AL-721 was discarded after a single, tiny, loosely-controlled clinical trial at St. Luke's-Roosevelt Hospital in New York. Most research on AL-721 has been done outside of the United States.

alanine aminotransaminase (ALT)   A LIVER ENZYME that plays a role in PROTEIN metabolism. Elevated SERUM levels of ALT are a sign of liver damage from disease or drugs. ALT is also known as SGPT (serum glutamic pyruvic transaminase).

alcoholism   ADDICTION to alcoholic beverages. A primary chronic disease with genetic, psychosocial, and environmental factors influencing its development and manifestations. A progressive disease, alcoholism can cause physical, psychological, and social harm and can be fatal.

alitretinoin   Also known by the trade name Panretin and ALRT-1057. Alitretinoin is used as a topical treatment for cutaneous AIDS-related Kaposi's sarcoma when there is no need for oral or intravenous medication. Patients should not also use the insect repellent DEET when using this drug and should not use this drug if they are allergic to retinoid drugs.

alkaline phosphatase   An ENZYME produced in the liver as well as in bone and other tissues. Elevated SERUM levels of the enzyme are indicative of LIVER disease, bile duct obstruction in particular.

allele   Any alternate form of a GENE located at a particular CHROMOSOME. Each allele is an individual member of a gene pair that is inherited from a parent. Alleles are responsible for hereditary variation.

allergen   A protein or HAPTEN that induces the formation of anaphylactic antibodies and may precipitate an IMMUNE RESPONSE; a substance that causes an ALLERGIC REACTION. Among common allergens are inhalants (dusts, pollens, fungi, smoke, perfumes, odors of plastics); foods (wheat, eggs, milk, chocolate, strawberries); drugs (aspirin, antibiotics, serums); infectious agents (bacteria, viruses, fungi, animal parasites); and contactants (chemicals, animals, plants, metals).

allergic dermatitis   See ATOPIC DERMATITIS.

allergic eczema   See ATOPIC DERMATITIS.

allergic reaction   Physiological response triggered by an ALLERGEN. See ALLERGY.

allergy   A hypersensitivity to an ALLERGEN (an environmental HAPTEN OR ANTIGEN), resulting in tissue inflammation, fever, organ dysfunction, and other physiological manifestations. The most common allergic reactions are on the skin and in the respiratory and GASTROINTESTINAL TRACTS.

allogeneic (allogenic)   Having a different genetic constitution. The term is often used to refer to intraspecific (within a species) genetic variations.

allopathy   The method of treating disease by the use of treatments that produce effects different from the effects produced by the disease. Opposite of HOMEOPATHY. Most doctors in Western countries practice allopathy.

all-trans-retinoic acid   A drug used to treat cancer. It is administered orally. All-trans-retinoic acid is the first successful differentiating agent for the treatment of patients with acute promyelocytic leukemia. The drug is a vitamin A derivative that works by prodding MALIGNANT leukemic cells to differentiate or "mature" into normal blood cells, which subsequently die. There are not many side effects; in some patients retinoic acid syndrome, a potentially serious complication characterized by fever, weight gain, and heart irregularities, develops. The syndrome must be diagnosed early and treated with CORTICOSTEROIDS. Researchers are currently studying the use of the drug against Kaposi's sarcoma and LYMPHOPROLIFERATIVE DISORDERS.

aloe vera   A plant of the genus *Aloe*, a member of the lily family. There are at least 120 known species of aloe, many of which have been used as botanical medicines. The sap and rind portions of the aloe vera leaf contain analgesics, antiinflammatory compounds, minerals, and beneficial fatty acids. Aloe vera is widely known as a skin moisturizer and healing agent, especially in treating cuts, burns, insect stings, bruises, acne, poison ivy, welts, ulcerated skin lesions, eczema, and sunburns. It has also been used to treat stomach disorders, ulcers, and many colon-related disorders, including colitis. Aloe juice may be used to treat food allergies, varicose veins, skin cancer, and arthritis as well. Aloe vera may help stop the spread of some viruses, such as HERPES SIMPLEX I and II, VARICELLA ZOSTER VIRUS, pseudorabies virus, and the influenza virus.

alopecia   Hair loss. In HIV hair loss can result from use of drugs for treatment of the virus in some individuals. Alopecia also occurs in other diseases that use similar strong CHEMOTHERAPY. Other types of alopecia are caused by a variety of skin and hair follicle diseases. They can all occur in men, women, and children.

alpha interferon (IFN-α)   Alpha interferon is a natural protein secreted by immune cells in response to viral infection. A manufactured version of IFN-α is approved to treat Kaposi's sarcoma and genital warts, hepatitis B, and hepatitis C. Alpha interferon has been shown to be effective in preventing replication of the human immunodeficiency virus IN VITRO (in the laboratory). Its TOXICITY significantly limits its use IN VIVO (in the living body). A current study under the auspices of the National Institute of Allergy and Infectious Diseases is investigating whether low-dose oral alpha interferon (LDOAI) therapy is effective in reducing the symptoms of AIDS. The use of LDOAI in the United States has been controversial, in part because the data about its effectiveness are conflicting and in part because LDOAI products are sometimes used to the exclusion of other therapies of proven value. Large multicenter randomized placebo-controlled trials have shown that LDOAI provides no benefit in fighting HIV, the virus that causes AIDS, or in improving the immune system function of those infected. Nonetheless, LDOAI products have been used in the United States, particularly in African American communities, on the basis of reports that these agents have beneficial effects on HIV-related symptoms, weight loss, and severity of opportunistic infections associated with HIV infection. Alpha interferon has many side effects, including severe nausea; diarrhea, flulike symptoms, such as fever, chills, muscle pain, and joint pain; and a reduction in number of blood cells, called anemia or neusion. Rare cases of severe depression leading to suicide have been reported. Side effects can lessen over time, as the body gets used to the treatment. (Trade names include Roferon, Intron-A, and Wellferon.)

alprazolam   A triazolo-benzodiazepine antianxiety agent. (Its trade name is Xanax.)

ALRT-1057   See ALITRETINOIN.

ALT   See ALANINE AMINOTRANSAMINASE.

altered mental state   A changed functional state of mind—as manifested in behavior, appearance, speech, memory, judgment, and responsiveness to stimuli of all kinds—that is markedly different from an individual's norm.

alternative delivery   A term used to denote a method other than the usual method of getting a medication into the body. If a tablet is the usual method of drug delivery then patch or intravenous delivery would be an alternative method.

alternative delivery system (ADS) A term coined to describe a variety of health care forms other than the traditional fee-for-service model, such as health maintenance organizations (HMOs) and preferred provider organizations (PPOs).

alternative health care See ALTERNATIVE TREATMENT.

alternative insemination See ARTIFICIAL INSEMINATION.

alternative medicine Approaches to medical diagnosis and therapy that have been developed outside the established standards, practices, and institutional sites of conventional medical science. Included are a great number of theories and "systems," including therapeutic NUTRITION, CHIROPRACTIC, HOMEOPATHY, structural, energetic therapies and MIND-BODY THERAPIES; traditional non-Western ethnomedicinal system such as CHINESE MEDICINE and AYURVEDA, which combine botanical medicine with other applications; other uses of botanical substances; and various treatments that simply have not been accepted by the medical establishment. This is not to say that, were these methods subjected to scientific study, all of them would be found to be ineffective. Alternative medicine has been variously called "natural," "complementary" (the preferred term in Europe), and numerous other terms referring to elements of a particular modality or tradition. "Alternative medicine" is not equivalent to "HOLISTIC medicine," a more narrow term.

Traditional ethnomedicinal systems are typically holistic, meaning that they aim to treat the whole person rather than a specific disease or symptom and that they therefore address not only the physical patient but also the mind and spirit. It is typically assumed that each individual possesses an innate healing capacity (an "immune system" in the broadest sense), and the goal of such treatment generally is to reinforce this, restoring strength and "balance" to weakened systems with a variety of natural modalities: foods, herbs and other botanicals, "body work," detoxification, and so on, tailored as much as possible for the individual. The

use of alternative therapies for AIDS grew out of this same eclectic mix.

alternative therapy See ALTERNATIVE TREATMENT.

alternative treatment Generally, therapy with procedures or agents that are not approved by the Food and Drug Administration (FDA) or other certifying authority. Alternative medical treatments have been used by a significant proportion of people with HIV, often to complement approved treatments. Some alternative treatments have been investigated in laboratory settings and observational studies, and a few have undergone clinical trials; others are being used without having undergone any studies. Alternative treatments are available for a variety of conditions, including weakened immune system, stress, drug abuse, mental disorders, common health problems, pregnancy, childbirth and infant care, dental care, eye, ear, nose and throat disorders, cancer and heart disorders, and aging. Alternative medicine combines many different Eastern and Western medical specialties: AYURVEDA medicine, CHINESE MEDICINE, ACUPUNCTURE and ACUPRESSURE, NUTRITION, exercise, NATUROPATHIC MEDICINE, HOMEOPATHY, botanical medicine, CHIROPRACTIC, and MASSAGE. Although all these methods have been lumped together in the generic category "alternative health care," they differ substantially from each other in philosophy, modality, cost, and other important ways. Although often touted as nontoxic, some herbs or nutritional supplements can have significant toxicities if used in sufficient quantities. Additionally, just as there is no universal language, so no single medical system or tradition—Eastern or Western, ancient or modern, scientific or unscientific—can provide the magic lantern that reveals all the mysteries of the human body. All alternative treatments share one similarity—very little is known about their activity in the human body and their usefulness in treating AIDS, even those that seem beneficial.

In 1992, for the first time in the then eight-year history of the International Conference on AIDS, alternative and traditional indigenous medicines had a prominent place. Politically, that year marked a change in the course of the conference toward greater attention to alternative or traditional treatments, in addition to mainstream pharmaceutical industry drugs. Many physicians and researchers believe that as time passes and the limitations of Western medicine become more defined, it is increasingly important for there to be cooperation among different medical traditions.

In 1993, partly as a response to the growing popularity of alternative medicine in the United States, President Clinton signed into law on June 14, 1993, the National Institutes of Health Revitalization Act, now known as Public Law 103–43. In the law, Congress permanently established the Office of Alternative Medicine (OAM) within the Office of the Director of National Institutes of Health. The purpose of the OAM is "to facilitate the evaluation of alternative medical modalities, including acupuncture and Oriental medicine, homeopathic medicine and physical manipulation therapies."

Some members of the AIDS community dismiss all alternative treatments, regardless of evidence demonstrating efficacy, and others defend all alternative treatments, regardless of evidence demonstrating lack of efficacy or toxicity. The reality seems to be that some alternative treatments may be effective, some are clearly ineffective, and most are in some degree toxic. The chief difficulty with using alternative treatments is a lack of empirical data. In the absence of the usual university, government, or corporate sponsorship of scientific research into them, there is no infrastructure that systematically addresses the potential benefits and risks of alternative treatments.

Since toxicity studies on most alternative treatments have not been conducted, it must be assumed that they may be toxic. There is no legal or regulatory mandate to disclose negative side effects. It must be kept in mind that profit is as big a motive for the marketers of "alternative" medicines as it is for the conventional pharmaceutical industry.

Access is also an issue with regard to alternative approaches to AIDS treatment. Alternative medicine, with its roots in traditional ethnomedicine, has the reputation of being a "new age" phenomenon, of interest mainly to the affluent middle class. This is due to its fringe status, which means that insurance and entitlement programs do not cover it, rather than to any lack of interest on the part of lower-income people. Increasing the availability of potentially useful treatments is directly related to their gaining wider acceptance among the medical and insurance industries.

Among the most common alternative agents are plants and plant extracts, derived from natural products or medicinal herbs. These are used for their possible antiviral properties and antibacterial and antifungal activity in the treatment of opportunistic infections. They include acemannan, astragalus, bitter melon, blue-green algae, burdock, garlic extract, glycyrrhizin, hypericin, iscador, maitake mushroom, mulberry roots and seeds, pine cone extracts, red marine algae, shiitake mushrooms, Siberian ginseng, traditional medicinal herbs, trichosanthin, and woundwaret.

Nutritional supplements are used in an attempt to restore natural levels of nutrients, to enhance resistance to opportunistic infections, and, when taken in high doses, to treat various HIV/AIDS-related conditions. Vitamins, minerals, and other substances in this category include BETA-CAROTENE, calcium, FOLIC ACID, iron, vitamins B_6 and B_{12}, VITAMIN C, vitamin E, ACIDOPHILUS, colostrum, COENZYME Q10, L-lysine, N-ACETYLCYSTEINE, and SELENIUM.

Dietary management is used to maintain or improve general health. Special regimes, such as those eliminating refined sugar or yeast to prevent or treat fungal infections, can be used as prophylaxis or treatment.

Physical techniques are used to treat certain conditions, relieve physical symptoms, and improve comfort and the quality of life. They can be combined with other therapies without fear of interactions with medication. Treatments include acupuncture, chiropractic manipulation, hydrotherapy, and massage.

Spiritual and psychological approaches seek to provide a holistic balance to complement other treatment strategies for HIV/AIDS. Although benefits are highly individual and subjective, they can contribute to an overall state of health. Treatments include hypnotherapy, meditation, psychotherapy, spiritual healing, stress reduction, and visualization.

Other treatments include ASPIRIN, colonics, dehydro-epiandrosterone (DHEA) DNCB (dinitrichlorobenzene), ozone therapy (super oxygenation), passive immunotherapy, shark cartilage powder, shark liver oil, snake venom, and thymus extracts.

ALVAC-HIV   A trademarked name for a genetically engineered HIV VACCINE. It is made with a live weakened CANARYPOX virus that has had genes of noninfectious parts of HIV inserted into it. When the canarypox virus infects a human cell, the cell begins making HIV proteins. These proteins are not infectious but fool the immune system into mounting an immune response to HIV. Canarypox can infect but not grow in humans; as a result, this type of LIVE VECTOR VACCINE is safe to use. The ALVAC-HIV is currently in PHASE I and II trials across the United States, in Thailand, and other countries.

alveolar proteinosis   See PULMONARY ALVEOLAR PROTEINOSIS.

alveolus (pl. alveoli)   Any small, saclike cavity in the body, such as an air cell of the lung or an erosion or ulcer in the gastric mucous membrane. Also, the socket of a tooth.

Alzheimer's disease   A chronic, organic mental disorder; a form of presenile dementia due to atrophy of the frontal and occipital lobes of the brain. Onset is usually between age 40 and 60. Its effects include progressive irreversible loss of memory, deterioration of intellectual functions, apathy, speech and gait disturbance, and disorientation. Its course may take from a few months to four or five years to progress to complete loss of intellectual function.

Ambien   See ZOLPIDEM.

AmBisome   See AMPHOTERICIN B.

ambulatory care   Care treatment provided to ambulatory (mobile, not hospitalized) patients.

Amcill   See AMPICILLIN.

AMD-3100   AMD-3100 is an experimental ENTRY INHIBITOR developed by AnorMED, Inc., in Canada. It was being investigated as an injectable drug. Tri-

als and development have been suspended as a result of heart arrhythmias at higher doses and poor viral suppression at lower levels.

ameba   See AMOEBA.

amebiasis   A parasitic intestinal infection caused by tiny unicellular microorganisms called AMOEBAS, especially *Entamoeba histolytica*. Many patients remain asymptomatic, but the disease is generally characterized by dysentery with diarrhea, weakness, prostration, nausea, vomiting, and pain. One serious complication is amebic hepatitis.

amebic dysentery   Infection with *Entamoeba histolytica*. Also called hepatic AMEBIASIS.

amebic hepatitis   Amebic abscess of the liver caused by infection with *Entamoeba histolytica*.

amenorrhea   Absence or suppression of menstruation. Amenorrhea is normal before puberty, after menopause, and during pregnancy and lactation. Primary amenorrhea is the failure of the menstruation cycle to begin at puberty; this may result from a congenital defect in the reproductive organs. The term usually refers to a condition caused by reasons other than these. Secondary amenorrhea is the suspension of menstruation after it has been established at puberty, and may result from an illness, a change of environment, or irradiation or removal of the uterus or ovaries. It is also associated with certain metabolic disorders (obesity, malnutrition, diabetes) and certain systemic diseases (SYPHILIS, TUBERCULOSIS, nephritis). Amenorrhea may also result from emotional causes (excitement, anorexia nervosa), pituitary disorders (hormonal imbalance of estrogen, progesterone, or FOLLICLE-STIMULATING HORMONE), or eating disorders (OBESITY, ANOREXIA).

America Responds to AIDS   An AIDS education campaign launched in 1988 by the Centers for Disease Control and Prevention (CDC) to promote public awareness.

American Association of Blood Banks   Association comprising blood banks and individuals that promotes blood banking, operates a clearinghouse for the exchange of blood and credits for blood, conducts educational and training programs, and supports and sponsors research.

Americans with Disabilities Act (ADA)   Signed into law on July 26, 1990, by President George H. W. Bush, this legislation guarantees equal opportunity for, and prohibits discrimination against, persons with disabilities in employment, public accommodation (essentially every type of business and service provider), transportation, state and local government and services, and telecommunications. In the ADA the term *disability* describes a broad range of conditions often inappropriately taken into account by employers and businesses. The ADA definition of disability is not the same as that used to establish eligibility for benefit programs under other legislation. The ADA prohibits discrimination against all people with disabilities, specifically including people with HIV disease, defined to include everything from asymptomatic HIV infection to full AIDS. The ADA prohibits discrimination by all public employers and private employers with 15 or more employees. The ADA also protects against discrimination people who are perceived as having or somehow carrying HIV disease. These could include friends, family members, lovers, caretakers of people with AIDS (PWAs); or volunteers serving the PWA community. Under the ADA, an employer may not refuse to hire someone simply because she or he has HIV disease; nor may it fire someone or refuse to a promote someone simply because he or she has HIV disease. In other words, an employer may not discriminate against an otherwise qualified person with HIV disease. To be qualified, an individual must be able to perform all the essential functions of a job, despite his or her HIV. This includes being well enough to get to work on a regular basis and to perform the job adequately. Under the ADA, an employer must make "reasonable accommodations" for persons with disabilities. This means that the employer has a responsibility to make changes in a job that will help the person perform it adequately. This could include establishing flexible work schedules and allowing a person time off for medical treatment. An employee, however, must request such accommodation. Furthermore, under the ADA, an employer only has to make "reasonable" accommodations that will not impose an "undue hardship" on it. An employer who shows that it would be a significant difficulty or expense to make a certain accommodation does not have to make it. The ADA treats the testing issue as well. An employer may not require that an employee take an HIV ANTIBODY TEST unless the employer proves that the test results are relevant to the employee's performance of the job. The act does allow the HIV antibody test to be included in a general physical examination, if one is required, after a conditional offer of employment is made to a job applicant. But the test may not be selectively administered in a discriminatory manner, and the employer may not withdraw the conditional offer of employment unless the test results indicate that the applicant is no longer qualified for the job. The ADA does not apply to the federal government, but a very similar statute, the REHABILITATION ACT OF 1973, does apply to the executive branch. The ADA also does not mention housing because there is already a federal law, the FAIR HOUSING ACT (as amended by Congress in 1989), that prohibits discrimination against people with disabilities (including HIV disease) in the sale and rental of private housing. Beyond employment issues, the ADA further prohibits discrimination based on disability in "public accommodations." In the ADA, that term *public accommodations* denotes not only its traditional meaning—hotels, restaurants, theaters, convention centers, and such—but virtually every type of business or service provider in the country, including doctors, dentists, pharmacists, and even lawyers. These public accommodations may not discriminate in the delivery of goods or services against a person because that person has HIV disease or because the person is regarded as having HIV disease or associates with persons with HIV disease. The employment portion of the ADA (Title I) is enforced by the Equal Employment Opportunities Commission (EEOC). The public accommodation provision of the ADA (Title III) can be enforced by filing a lawsuit in court or, in some instances, by filing a complaint with the Department of Justice, which is empowered to undertake an investigation and compliance review. The public entity portion of the ADA (Title II) is enforced by the Department of Justice. For the first few years of enforcement, there was some question whether the ADA included people with AIDS or HIV. In 1998 that question was resolved in the case of *Bragdon v. Abbott* (524 U.S. 624). In this case a dentist stopped filling a cavity of a patient when he learned the patient was HIV-positive but displayed no symptoms. The Supreme Court held that the dentist could not discriminate against the patient because HIV is "a physical . . . impairment that substantially limits one or more of [an individual's] major life activities." The court agreed that treating the patient in the dentist's office would not have posed a direct threat to the health and safety of others. This case was considered a major victory by ADA and HIV activists.

amikacin   An ANTIMICROBIAL, AMINOGLYCOSIDE ANTIBIOTIC, amikacin is indicated for *MYCOBACTERIUM AVIUM* COMPLEX (MAC) and multidrug-resistant MYCOBACTERIUM TUBERCULOSIS. Side effects include NEPHROTOXICITY and OTOTOXICITY. Amikacin should not be used with other nephrotoxic drugs such as AMPHOTERICIN B, vancomycin, loop diuretics and other aminoglycosides, or with other ototoxic drugs. Amikacin may potentiate the effects of neuromuscular blockers. (Its trade name is Amikin.)

amino acid   Any of 20 major nitrogen-containing acids that are the building blocks for proteins and are required for human growth. All proteins found in humans are linear chains of these 20 amino acids. Occurring freely within organisms, amino acids contain an amine group and a carboxyl group. There are hundreds of amino acids found in nature.

amino acid therapy   A questionable form of AIDS therapy available outside the United States, especially in Mexico. Results have not been proved in research to be effective or long-term. Amino acid therapy consists of the oral or intravenous administration of one or more of the essential AMINO ACIDS.

aminoglycoside   One of a number of ANTIBIOTICS derived or synthesized from species of *Streptomyces* bacteria.

aminosalicylic acid   An antituberculosis drug believed to delay development of bacterial resistance. Its effectiveness is greatly enhanced when used in combination with STREPTOMYCIN and ISONIAZID (INH).

amitriptyline   A tricyclic antidepressant. Although the FOOD AND DRUG ADMINISTRATION (FDA) has not approved such use, it is sometimes given to HIV-infected people to reduce the pain associated with peripheral neuropathy, a condition characterized by numbness, tingling or pain in the feet, legs, arms, or hands. It is thought to work by increasing the concentrations of neurotransmitters called serotonin and norepinephrine in the brain.

This class of antidepressants is usually taken over a long period of time; amitriptyline should not be taken by people who have HIV ENCEPHALOPATHY because it may cause acute delirium. Additionally, most antidepressants increase the risk of seizures in people susceptible to them. Because seizures are not uncommon in HIV disease, people who are infected with the virus should be cautious about taking all antidepressants, including those in the tricyclic class.

Amitriptyline is available in tablet and injectable form. The most common side effects include sleepiness, blurred vision, disorientation, confusion, hallucinations, muscle spasms, seizures, dry mouth, constipation, difficult urination, worsening glaucoma, and sensitivity to bright light or sunlight.

amniotic fluid   The transparent, almost colorless liquid contained in the inner membrane (amnion) that holds a suspended fetus. It protects the fetus from physical impact, insulates against temperature variations and prevents the fetus from adhering to the amnion and the amnion from adhering to the fetus. Amniotic fluid is continually absorbed and replenished; about one third of the water in the amniotic fluid is replaced each hour.

amoeba (pl. amoebae)   A one-celled, microscopic protozoan organism, found in soil and water, that may infect humans, causing AMEBIASIS. It sends out fingerlike projections of protoplasm (pseudopodia) that enable it to move about and through which it obtains nourishment. The pseudopodia also keep the shape of the amoeba in constant flux. Amoebae reproduce by binary fission, with the nucleus dividing by mitosis.

amoebiasis See AMEBIASIS.

amoebic dysentery See AMEBIC DYSENTERY.

amoebic hepatitis See AMEBIC HEPATITIS.

amoxicillin An antibiotic drug; semisynthetic derivative of ampicillin effective against a broad spectrum of gram-positive and gram-negative bacteria. In people with HIV, amoxicillin is used specifically to treat bacterial inflammation of the sinuses (sinusitis), diarrhea caused by salmonella, and vaginal ulcers (chancroid) caused by *Haemophilus ducreyi*. Amoxicillin works by interfering with a susceptible bacteria's ability to build cell walls. It is converted by the body into AMPICILLIN. The primary difference between the two is that amoxicillin is resistant to acid in the stomach, which means that more of the active drug gets into the intestines where it is absorbed.

Amoxicillin is generally well tolerated. The most common side effects are minor and include rashes, heartburn, nausea, vomiting, or diarrhea. These side effects are likely to occur in people who are allergic to penicillin or have a history of allergy, asthma, or hay fever. Rarely, some people taking amoxicillin experience agitation, anxiety, insomnia, dizziness, confusion, or behavioral changes.

In recent years, bacteria have become more resistant to amoxicillin and other penicillin-type antibiotics. Resistance may occur more frequently in the HIV-positive population because of their widespread use of such drugs. In cases of resistance additional antibiotics that kill bacteria by a different mechanism are often needed. (Trade names include Amoxil, Moxicillin, Wymax, and Augmentin. Augmentin is amoxicillin plus clavulante.)

Amoxil See AMOXICILLIN.

amphetamine One of a group of organic compounds that act as CENTRAL NERVOUS SYSTEM stimulants. Their action resembles that of adrenaline, one of the body's natural hormones. Sometimes referred to as speed, amphetamines if abused may lead to psychological dependence, producing symptoms ranging from restlessness to psychosis in severe cases. Amphetamine and its close chemical analogs METHAMPHETAMINE and dextroamphetamine have been used to treat hyperactivity in children, narcolepsy (uncontrollable sleeping episodes), and obesity. However, these legal uses are currently limited. The preparation most commonly used is the sulfate, marketed in tablet and capsule form. Some PROTEASE INHIBITORS are known to increase the amount of amphetamine in the body, causing many unexpected health problems including possible death from overdose.

amphotericin B An antibiotic, amphotericin B is the standard treatment for many infections caused by fungi, including those that affect people infected with HIV: *CANDIDA*, *CRYPTOCOCCUS*, *HISTOPLASMA*, *COCCIDIOIDOMYCOSIS*, and *ASPERGILLUS* species. People with HIV are routinely given amphotericin B for initial treatment of severe cryptococcosis, histoplasmosis, aspergillosis, blastomycosis, and coccidiosis. Amphotericin B is available in intravenous, topical, and liquid forms. It is one of the most toxic antibiotics known. Amphotericin B is metabolized slowly and can be found in urine up to seven weeks after treatment. The drug works by attacking the cell walls of the fungi. Because human and fungal cell walls contain similar compounds, amphotericin B's side effects may be a result of the drug's attacking human cells as well. The most important side effects are kidney damage, anemia, disturbances in the balance of electrolytes, nausea and vomiting, headache, fever and chills, alteration in blood pressure, changes in appetite, and phlebitis or inflammation of the vein into which the drug is injected. These reactions are usually most severe with the first few doses and usually diminish with subsequent treatment. The serious kidney toxicities caused by amphotericin B are most evident when treatment lasts six to 10 weeks or longer. Many of these side effects can be reduced in severity or eliminated by stopping the drug, by continuing the drug in a lower dose, or by taking other medications at the same time to counteract them. Medications that affect kidney functions, such as AMINOGLYCOSIDE antibiotics, FOSCARNET, and PENTAMIDINE, should be prescribed to patients using amphotericin with extreme caution. Because of amphotericin B's toxicity, other drugs, such as ITRACONAZOLE and FLUCONAZOLE, are preferred in situations in which they are considered likely to be as effective or nearly as effective. One potentially more effective and safer alternative to standard amphotericin may be liposomal amphotericins. In these "high-tech" versions of the drug, amphotericin is encapsulated in tiny fat globules known as liposomes. LIPOSOMAL AMPHOTERICIN must be administered through intravenous infusion as the standard drug is, but it is hypothesized that the LIPOSOMES may be preferentially absorbed at the sites of infection, thereby preventing most of amphotericin's side effects and potentially extending the length of time amphotericin therapy can be tolerated. (Its trade name is Fungizone.)

ampicillin   A semisynthetic penicillin, this broad-spectrum antibiotic is effective against various gram-negative and gram-positive bacteria. Predominantly used in the treatment of urinary system and urinary tract infections, it is also used to treat prolonged bronchial infections. (Trade names are AMCILL, OMNIPEN, POLYCILLIN, and Principen.)

ampicillin sodium   Monosodium salt of ampicillin. (Trade names include omnipen-N, polycillin-N, and Principen-N.)

amplification   Multiplication of a virus either through the body of an individual host or through a population of hosts. Extreme amplification is the multiplication of a virus everywhere in a host, partly transforming the host into a virus. Host here refers to an organism supporting a parasite in or on its body and to its own detriment.

ampligen   A non-nucleoside drug found in the late 1980s to be ineffective against AIDS. Previously it had been thought to have the activity of both an antiviral and an immunomodulator.

amprenavir   FDA-approved PROTEASE INHIBITOR used in treatment with other HIV ANTIRETROVIRAL medications. It was the fifth protease inhibitor approved. Dosage is difficult as it involves administration of eight pills twice a day, with or without food. Amprenavir is a sulfa drug, a type of drug to which many people are allergic. A well-known sulfa drug is Bactrim (see TMP/SMX). A person who has had allergic reactions to Bactrim is likely to have a reaction to amprenavir. In about 25 percent of the people taking amprenavir some allergic reaction to the drug has developed initially. Sometimes it can be overcome by continued exposure to the medication; other times it develops into a bright red rash on the skin, which has caused some people to stop taking this drug. About 1 percent of people taking amprenavir experience a reaction called Stevens-Johnson syndrome (SJS). Stevens-Johnson syndrome is a type of allergic reaction called an erythema, a redness of the skin due to congestion of the capillaries, causing flulike symptoms and severe lesions under the skin. It can be fatal. Major side effects of the drug are nausea, vomiting, diarrhea, headache, stomach pains/gas, skin rash, and numbing sensations on the skin, particularly around the mouth. The numbing sensations are generally temporary. Each tablet contains a large amount of vitamin E. People taking amprenavir should not use vitamin E supplements. Vitamin E causes thinning of the blood, so people who are using blood thinners should discuss use of amprenavir with their doctor before starting the drug. Amprenavir does not seem to cause increased fat levels in the blood thus far. However, the studies have not been under way as long as other drug studies so this effect may not occur as time passes. People taking amprenavir should have their TRIGLYCERIDE and CHOLESTEROL levels checked regularly to monitor this effect. (Its trade name is Agenerase.)

One AIDS drug currently being scrutinized is fosamprenavir, a PI hopeful from GlaxoSmithKline. Fosamprenavir is specially designed to be taken up by the gut and then immediately processed into amprenavir before being sent into the bloodstream. The *fos* indicates the difference between having to take 16 pills a day and only two pills a day. Improved tolerance and fewer side effects have also been noted with fosamprenavir. On its own, fosamprenavir given twice a day can produce viral suppression comparable to nelfinavir without the troublesome rise in triglycerides. Boosting from ritonavir is also possible once a day.

amyl nitrite   A fluorocarbon that, inhaled, dilates the blood vessels, producing a temporary "rush" or "high." Used to treat angina and asthma, it has become popular for enhancing sexual experience. Known as "POPPERS."

amyl nitrite inhalant   See ISOBUTYL NITRITE INHALERS.

amylase   A starch-splitting enzyme secreted by the salivary glands and the pancreas to aid digestion of food. An increase in amylase serum levels may indicate pancreatitis, a possible life-threatening consequence of ddI.

anabolic   A metabolic process that builds new tissue in the body. See CATABOLIC.

anabolic steroids   Anabolic steroids are testosterone derivatives designed to increase strength and muscle mass. Testosterone performs these functions in the body, but its masculinizing effects make it an inappropriate therapy for men who already have normal testosterone levels, or for women. The synthetic anabolic steroids, such as nandrolone, oxandrolone, methandrostenolone, and oxymetholone, were designed to be less masculinizing than testosterone and are often used to treat men with AIDS. These men often have low testicular function or testosterone deficiencies caused by HIV suppression of normal endocrine-gland function or by drugs (like KETOCONAZOLE) used to treat opportunistic infections. These deficiencies are associated with weakness and loss of lean tissue mass.

Weight loss is a common symptom in people with HIV. It can be caused by opportunistic infections that interfere with the ability to absorb nutrients. Oral problems such as thrush or dry mouth may contribute to decreased food intake. Weight loss can also be caused by a poorly understood condition called HIV-related wasting, where lean muscle mass is lost even when a person is eating properly.

Oral and injectable testosterone have long been available to treat testosterone deficiencies. The oral form is metabolized by the liver and can cause serious liver toxicities, so it is infrequently used. Injectable forms of the drugs are used more commonly, but they cause transient high levels of the drug in the blood, which may increase the risk of side effects.

Anabolic steroids have the advantage of being dramatically cheaper than most therapies being studied for HIV-related wasting. The ability of anabolic steroids to increase muscle mass and break down fat in healthy, exercising people is well-documented and doctors can legally prescribe therapeutic doses. Despite the numerous anecdotal reports of steroid use in people with HIV-related wasting, its long-term safety and efficacy has yet to be established in controlled studies. Additionally, for treatment of HIV-related weight loss, anabolic steroids are only effective for men with abnormally low testosterone levels. Consequently, before initiating treatment, physicians usually measure their patients' testosterone levels. For maximum effect against wasting, both adequate nutrition and exercise should be combined with anabolic steroid therapy. The drugs make cells ready to build tissue, but they have little effect without the proper building blocks (especially protein) and exercise. Use of steroids by people with no urgent medical reason for it, however, is considered extremely dangerous. Aside from undesirable potential side effects such as (in women) hirsutism, masculinization and clitoral hypertrophy, such use affects immune system functioning and has been associated with muscular deterioration and brain cancer.

Anadrol   See OXYMETHOLONE.

anal eroticism   Finding sexual enjoyment in the stimulation of one's own or a partner's anus.

anal intercourse   Sexual intercourse involving the insertion of one partner's penis into the other's anus. The person who inserts his penis into the anus of his partner is performing insertive, or active, anal intercourse. The partner is experiencing passive anal intercourse. Anal intercourse without a condom with an infected partner carries a high risk for HIV infection and other sexually transmitted diseases (STDs) because it often causes small tears in the rectal tissue and other internal injuries, through which infected semen can enter the bloodstream. Generally speaking, a condom does not offer quite the same protection in anal intercourse as in vaginal intercourse. Because the anus is usually tighter than the vagina, the condom may slip or break more easily. Lubricants are used to reduce friction and lessen the chance of small, unseen tears in the anus. Lubricants are essential because the anus does not produce enough mucus, unlike the vagina, to allow insertion without tearing of the anus.

anal intraepithelial neoplasia Also called anal neoplasia (AIN). AIN is an abnormal cell growth, a lesion, of the ANUS that may develop into cancer. The term *neoplasia* itself does not mean cancer. It is an abnormality that is benign or malignant. It is known that AIN is more prevalent in people who have been exposed to the HUMAN PAPILLOMAVIRUS (HPV), both men and women. It also occurs more often in women and gay males than in heterosexual men. HPVs includes more than one hundred distinct types of viruses. Not all of the types are thought to have links to particular abnormalities in tissue.

AIN has many similarities to cervical neoplasia in that the progression and location in particular tissue are similar. AIN generally shows up initially as a lesion in the transformation zone of the anal canal, where the anus meets the rectum. Similarly, most occurrences of cervical neoplasia first appear in the transformation zone of the cervix, where the exocervix (outer cervix) joins with the endocervix (inner cervix). These regions have the same type of epithelial cells in areas where the initial lesions are found. The epithelium is the thin layer of cells that cover internal and external body surfaces.

People who are HIV-positive have a higher rate of AIN than people who are not HIV-positive. With the extended lifespans of people with HIV since the advent of HAART, it is thought that more people with HIV infection may have possible problems with AIN in the future. No treatment guidelines for AIN have ever been issued by the U.S. Public Health Service. Therefore, all treatments for AIN are considered experimental. Typically people who have small, low-grade lesions are monitored every six months for any changes to the tissue. People with middle-grade lesions may be treated with laser removal or cryogenic freezing and removal of the lesion. Treatment of major lesions or lesions that have changed into cancers most likely entails chemotherapy.

Treatment with HAART may decrease the occurrence of AIN. It is not known whether AIN acts predominantly as an OPPORTUNISTIC INFECTION (OI) in HIV-positive people or not. Occurrence of most OIs has been reduced among patients who are on HAART therapy. Preliminary studies do show that HIV-positive patients having HAART treatment has reduced progression of lesions when compared to HIV-positive people not on HAART.

People who have been exposed to HPV or have had anal or cervical warts should consider having at least an annual anal cytology test. This test is similar to a cervical screening in women. Swabs are taken of anal tissue and sent to a lab for examination. Although this is currently not an official screening protocol, because of lack of government guidelines, the rates and similarities between cervical cancer in women and anal cancer in gay men dictate such a screening. Rates of cervical cancer have dropped significantly since initiation of regular screenings. Rates of anal cancers may also drop as much if physicians understand the risk and similarities and are not afraid to discuss the issue with patients.

anal sex See ANAL EROTICISM; ANAL INTERCOURSE.

analgesic A compound that reduces or relieves pain without reducing consciousness. Tylenol, ASPIRIN, and the OPIATES are examples of analgesic drugs.

analogue Alternate spelling of *analog*. A molecule that resembles another structurally and that can normally be substituted for the original molecule. NUCLEOSIDE ANALOGS imitate molecules that HIV needs to copy DNA and replicate itself, thereby blocking the process.

anal-oral sex See ANILINGUS.

anamnestic response See SECONDARY IMMUNE RESPONSE.

anaphylactic shock See ANAPHYLAXIS.

anaphylaxis A systemic allergic reaction (also called anaphylactic shock) of immediate hypersensitivity to a drug or other antigen that results in life-threatening respiratory distress usually accompanied by shock and collapse of blood vessels. Symptoms include acute respiratory distress; hypotension; edema; rash; tachycardia; pale, cool skin; convulsions; and cyanosis. If untreated, unconsciousness and death may be the outcome. Edema can be life-threatening if the larynx is involved, since air flow is obstructed with even minimal swelling.

Anaphylaxis occurs in nearly all vertebrates. It results from sensitization of tissue-fixed mast cells by cytotropic antibodies following exposure to an ANTIGEN.

androgen A HORMONE or synthetic substance with masculinizing (androgenic) effects. TESTOSTERONE is an androgenic hormone.

anecdotal evidence Evidence, or potential evidence, that is based on reports of specific individual cases. It is not as reliable or reproducible as clinical evidence that is based on large, controlled clinical studies.

anemia A condition in which the hemoglobin content of the blood (carried in the red blood cells), is less than that required to meet the oxygen demands of the body, producing fatigue and other symptoms. The condition may be caused by too few red blood cells, too little hemoglobin, or both. Because variables such as lifestyle, location, age, and sex can influence red cell and hemoglobin concentrations, it is not possible to state that anemia exists when the hemoglobin is less than a specific value. If the onset of anemia is slow, the body may adjust so well that there will be no functional impairment even though the hemoglobin may be less than 6 gm/100 ml of blood. Symptoms, in addition to fatigue, include pallor of skin, fingernail beds, and mucous membranes; weakness; vertigo; headache; sore tongue; drowsiness; general malaise; dyspnea; tachycardia; palpitation; angina pectoris; gastrointestinal disturbances; amenorrhea; loss of libido; slight fever.

Anemia is not a disease; it may be a symptom of various diseases or of malnutrition. When the reduction of red blood cells, responsible for delivering oxygen to all parts of the body, is severe, the result is fatigue. Anemia can be triggered by HIV infection, an opportunistic infection, or by several of the drugs commonly taken by people with AIDS. Drugs often responsible include trimethoprim-sulfamethoxazole, other sulfa drugs, PENTAMIDINE, AMPHOTERICIN B, and AZT. When anemia is severe, it can be corrected with transfusions. When drugs are responsible, the drugs can be reduced in dose or discontinued.

anergic See ANERGY.

anergy The lack of reaction to ANTIGENS; a state of impaired or absent CELL-MEDIATED IMMUNITY, diagnosable through administration of a common skin test. Used of T-CELLS, the term refers specifically to the lack of response to a normally stimulatory MHC-PEPTIDE complex on an ANTIGEN-PRESENTING CELL.

angiogenesis The formation of new blood vessels. Tumors and KAPOSI'S SARCOMA lesions stimulate angiogenesis to supply themselves with blood.

angular cheilitis See PERLECHE.

angular cheilosis See PERLECHE.

angular stomatis See PERLECHE.

anilinctus See ANILINGUS.

anilingus Sexual activity involving contact between the mouth and the anus; anal-oral sex. Also called anilinctus.

animal models Drug trials done in animals prior to human studies. For example, tests of various substances in standardized genetic strains of mice or the tests of HIV VACCINE in CHIMPANZEES.

anion An ion carrying a negative charge; it is attracted by, and travels to, the anode (positive pole). It is the opposite of cation. Examples include acid radicals and corresponding radicals of their salts.

anion gap A concept used to estimate electrolyte (anion and cation) levels in the serum and conditions that influence them. The anion gap ranges from eight to 18 mEq/L in normal patients. If the anion gap is high, one possibility is that the individual has LACTIC ACIDOSIS of some kind.

anogenital wart Raised skin in the anal or genital region occurring as a response to infection with PAPILLOMA virus.

anomanual intercourse Sexual contact involving placing a hand in a partner's anus. After insertion the hand is made into a fist and a thrusting motion is made.

anonymous testing Persons who decide to get tested for HIV may want to do so anonymously. Centers for such testing have been established in many cities. The standard procedure is to assign a testee an i.d. number before testing, so that the testing agency never knows his or her personal identity. Test results are identified only by the number and cannot be traced. No name or other identification is required, taken, or reported. Anonymous testing differs from confidential testing, in which a testee's doctor and others in his or her office know the test results, which become part of the testee's private medical record.

Locations of anonymous testing centers are available through any AIDS hot line or local public health service. Tests are often free of charge.

anorectal disease A PATHOLOGICAL condition of the anus and rectum, or the area joining the two, which is manifested by a characteristic set of clinical signs and symptoms.

anorexia Lack or loss of appetite for food (sometimes known as inappetence). This is common in the onset of fevers and systemic illnesses, certain psychiatric illnesses, depression, and malaise, and in disorders of the alimentary tracts, especially the stomach. It also is a common result of alcoholic excesses and drug addiction. Many drugs and medical procedures have the undesired side effect of causing malaise with concurrent anorexia.

Because anorexia is a common HIV disease-related complication, a patient's appetite is a key piece of clinical information; causes of inappetence may include undiagnosed or untreated opportunistic infections. Many drugs used against HIV have side effects that include nausea and anorexia. As the number of medications given to an HIV/AIDS patient grows, the impact on his or her overall well-being, including nutritional status, must continually be reassessed. Small, frequent meals and calorically dense foods and beverages are often recommended; shared meals and changes in eating place are encouraged, and NUTRITIONAL SUPPLEMENTS are frequently indicated. In many cases, patients learn to prepare their own high calorie/high nutrient drinks, significantly reducing their cost.

Anorexia is a symptom or side effect of a serious health problem. *Anorexia nervosa,* often referred to simply as anorexia, is a serious (psychological) disorder in itself, the pathological absence or *suppression* of appetite. Unlike the anorexia suffered by so many patients with HIV/AIDS, cancer and other illnesses, anorexia nervosa is not associated with the presence of any physical illness.

anoscope A long narrow tube with lenses at both ends, used to examine the rectal walls closely.

Antabuse See DISULFIRAM.

antagonist A drug or medication that neutralizes or counteracts another substance. See AGONIST.

antenatal Occurring before birth.

antenatal diagnosis A determination of the health and genetic status of a fetus. Methods include amniocentesis, chorionic villus sampling, cell culture, biochemical methods, nonstress testing, oxytocin challenge test, biophysical profile, amnioscopy, amniography, and ultrasound. See PARENTAL TESTING.

antepartum care See PRENATAL CARE.

anthelmintic A medication used to treat infection caused by helminths. Helminths are parasitic worms, such as tapeworm, trichinella, hookworm, or pin worm. The drugs work by stopping reproduction by the worms and encouraging their expulsion through the intestinal tract. Studies indicate that from 4 percent to 15 percent of the population in the southeastern United States is infected with hookworm. Worldwide many hundreds of millions of people are infected with various helminths.

anthrax An acute infectious bacterial disease caused by *Bacillus anthacis.* It generally attacks cattle, goats, horses, or sheep but may be passed on to humans through contact with infected animals, their discharges, or contaminated animal products. Failure to properly treat anthrax may be fatal. Also called CHARBON, MILZBRAND, and SPLENIC FEVER.

anthroposophic medicine Medicine practiced according to anthroposophy, an occult spiritual system developed by the social philosopher and mystic Rudolf Steiner (1861–1925). Anthroposophic medicine attempts to take into account the spiritual as well as the physical components of illness. A treatment regime may include herbal and homeopathic medicines as well as special dietary practices, art therapy, movement therapy, massage, and specially prepared baths.

anti-anxiety drugs An umbrella term for a number of compounds (also called anxiolytic drugs), including the BENZODIAZEPINE drugs and the muscle relaxant MEPROBAMATE, that are used for reducing anxiety. They are sometimes referred to as minor TRANQUILIZERS.

anti–B cell monoclonal antibody A specific MONOCLONAL ANTIBODY that is used to target B cell LYMPHOMAS. By using the monoclonal antibody to transport specific drugs (CHEMOTHERAPY) to the diseased cells, doctors attempt to increase the amount of the drug reaching the infected or diseased areas of the body. It is also used to fight EPSTEIN-BARR VIRUS infections in patients who have had major transplantation surgery.

anti-B4 blocked ricin Anti-B4 blocked ricin is a MONOCLONAL ANTIBODY that is currently under investigation for treatment in HODGKIN'S DISEASE and NON-HODGKINS LYMPHOMA. Anti-B4 is linked to ricin, a potent IMMUNOTOXIN derived from the castor bean. The anti-B4 attaches to most lymphoma cells but not to normal tissue; then the ricin kills the lymphoma cells. Ricin is chemically altered so that it has only a slight effect on normal tissues. Preclinical studies of anti-B4 blocked ricin in monkeys demonstrated that its main toxicity is elevation of liver enzyme levels. It is currently in PHASE I/II trials in humans. The therapy is given as a seven-day, around-the-clock continuous infusion.

antibacterial Destructive of the growth of BACTERIA; any agent that has such an effect.

antibiosis An antagonistic process or relationship between living organisms, specifically MICROORGANISMS. This natural destructiveness, or antibiotic activity, is the basis for the effectiveness of ANTIBIOTIC drugs.

antibiotic Pertaining to ANTIBIOSIS, the natural destructiveness of some microorganisms against others; any of a class of drugs that exploits this phenomenon to fight microbial infections.

Antibiotics are made from natural substances and incorporate specific living microorganisms (in relatively weak solution) that kill or inhibit the growth of those causing infection. Effective antibiotic drugs have been developed for use against most BACTERIA, fungi (see FUNGUS), PARASITES and VIRUSES that cause infection in humans. Some of the antibiotics most frequently given to the HIV-infected include TRIMETHOPRIM-SULFAMETHOXAZOLE (TMP/SMX) and other sulfa drugs, PENTAMIDINE, KETOCONAZOLE, AMPHOTERICIN B, PYRIMETHAMINE, GANCICLOVIR, ACYCLOVIR, PENICILLIN, ERYTHROMYCIN, NYSTATIN, CLOTRIMAZOLE, and AZT.

In recent years it has become clear that antibiotics have been overused. The consequence is that the infectious organisms they once destroyed have evolved strains resistant to them. See DRUG RESISTANCE.

antibiotic resistance See DRUG RESISTANCE.

antibiotic therapy See ANTIBIOTIC.

antibody A chemical substance developed by the immune system to fight an infectious agent found in the body. Specifically, antibodies are members of a class of proteins known as immunoglobulins, which are produced and secreted by B-lymphocytes in response to the presence of specific antigens. For most antigens, the B-lymphocytes take one or two weeks to produce antibodies; for HIV the time required may be months. Immunoglobulins can be found in the blood or secretory fluids. Although antibodies share many properties, each one is highly specific. Once a specific antibody is formed in response to a specific antigen, the cell has a "memory" of this event. This "memory" usually renders the person immune to the specific substance or microorganism in the future.

The presence of antibodies may be linked to vaccination, previous infection, perinatal transfer of bodily fluids between mother and fetus, or unknown exposure. The body also possesses natural antibodies that react without apparent contact with a specific antigen. Antibodies neutralize toxins and interact with other components of the immune system to eliminate infectious microorganisms for the body. In AIDS, these antibodies are usually not effective in neutralizing infection.

At the dawning of the AIDS epidemic, scientists had a very simplistic view of the immune system: antibodies, antibodies, and more antibodies. Now they are finding that the human immune system is much more complicated than they previously imagined. Most people are familiar with antibodies and believe that they provide protection against the opportunistic infections in AIDS. It is now known that production of antibodies enables viral and other microbial pathogens to flourish because it does not destroy the infected cells that are the source of infection, but only temporarily controls cell-free or cell-surface infectious microbes. The other arm of the immune system, cell-mediated immunity, is critical in controlling and clearing the infectious agents that cause opportunistic diseases in AIDS. See CELL-MEDIATED IMMUNITY; CELLULAR IMMUNITY.

antibody envy An accusation sometimes leveled at HIV-negative individuals who seek to express or explore the damage the AIDS epidemic has done to those not infected. The expression of an opinion, or even a simple assertion of fact or statement of an issue, may enrage some who are HIV-positive or have an AIDS-related illness, as if the HIV-negative had no right to speak publicly. When they do they may be accused of "robbing" resources from the "truly needy." Such accusations serve to divide and discourage those who wish to help, and to minimize and discount the severity of the impact of the epidemic in the lives of those who are HIV-negative and in the community as a whole.

antibody therapy The use of antibodies to treat patients with IMMUNODEFICIENCY. This is done by using PARENTERAL IMMUNE GLOBULIN.

antibody-dependent cell-mediated cytotoxicity A form of LYMPHOCYTE-MEDIATED cytotoxicity in which an effector cell kills an antibody-coated target cell, presumably by recognition of the Fc region of the cell-bound antibody through an F C RECEPTOR present on the EFFECTOR lymphocyte.

antibody-dependent cellular cytotoxicity Direct killing of an infected cell by antibody-coated lymphocytes.

antibody-mediated immunity Immunity that results from the activity of antibodies dissolved in BLOOD, LYMPH, and other body fluids that bind the ANTIGEN and trigger a response to it (also called humoral immunity). It involves the activation of B cells (see B LYMPHOCYTE). B cells become activated when they come into contact with a foreign substance, such as bacteria, fungi, or viruses, and transform into plasma cells and begin creating antibodies to the foreign substance (ANTIGEN). They also have the ability to clone themselves, becoming "antibody factories." Plasma cells remain in the body in lymph and other tissues and create antibodies for specific antigens. Within a few hours, a resting B cell is transformed into a plasma cell with the ability to produce more than 2000 antibodies per second. It used to be believed that antibodies were all that acted in immunity. In the past few years, it has become known that the production of antibodies enables viral and other microbial pathogens to flourish because it does not destroy the infected cells that are the source of infection, but only temporarily controls cell-free or cell-surface (extracellular, exogenous) pathogens. Flu, colds, and many common viral and other infections are controlled by antibody-mediated immunity. See CELL-MEDIATED IMMUNITY.

antibody-negative Not having been infected with a particular ANTIGEN, such as HIV, at any time and therefore not having developed antibodies to it; a blood test result showing this to be the case. See ANTIBODY; ANTIBODY-POSITIVE; ANTIBODY TESTING.

antibody-positive Having been infected with a particular ANTIGEN, such as HIV, at some time, and developed antibodies to it; a blood test result showing this condition to exist. See ANTIBODY; ANTIBODY-NEGATIVE; ANTIBODY TESTING.

antibody testing A clinical procedure used to determine the presence of an ANTIBODY in the blood. In the case of HIV, because it takes some time after infection for antibodies to develop, the tests currently in use are not foolproof. Experts disagree about the time it takes, but most people infected with HIV develop antibodies within six months. The chance of testing error is minuscule but not nonexistent. The preliminary test currently in use for HIV antibodies, the ENZYME-LINKED IMMUNOABSORBENT ASSAY (ELISA), is designed to err in the direction of a positive reading. Such a result must be confirmed with a second test, usually the WESTERN BLOT test. See ANTIBODY; ANTIBODY-NEGATIVE; ANTIBODY-POSITIVE.

anticoagulant A substance that delays or counteracts blood clotting (coagulation).

anticonvulsant Preventing or relieving convulsions; a drug that does so.

anti-D Anti-D polyclonal antibody is an IMMUNE GLOBULIN blood product used to achieve a temporary and occasionally long-term elevation of the platelet counts. It is used for treatment only in Rh-positive people (approximately 85 percent of the population). The anti-D coated-red cells succeed in blocking the spleen's destruction of IDIOPATHIC THROMBOCYTOPENIC PURPURA–coated platelets, thus increasing platelet counts. Significant increases in platelet counts occur within one to three days with peak counts observed eight days after infusion. The effects last approximately one month. People who have shown allergies to blood products should not receive infusions of anti-D. Anti-D is also used in hemolytic disease of the newborn, which occurs when the blood type of the mother is Rh-negative and that of the baby is Rh-positive. Rh factor is a specific protein on the outside of the red blood cells. (The trade name for the anti-D product is WinRho SDF.)

antidepressant Any of a wide range of drugs used to treat psychological depression. They are given to elevate mood, counter suicidal thoughts, and increase the effectiveness of psychotherapy. Before the introduction of these drugs in the late 1950s, most patients with major depression had no choice but hospitalization; only 45 percent improved after one year. In contrast, 80 percent to 90 percent of people suffering depression can expect significant relief with one of the medications now prescribed. Antidepressants act on the flow of the neurotransmitters epinephrine, serotonin, and norepinephrine across neural synapses. There are three main groups of antidepressants, the MONOAMINE OXIDASE INHIBITORS (MAO inhibitors), the cyclic antidepressants, and the selective serotonin reuptake inhibitors (SSRIs).

MAO inhibitors include Eutonyl, Eutron, Furoxone, Marplan, Matulane, Nardil, and Parnate. MAO inhibitors cause several adverse reactions that are due to the way they are absorbed in the body. People taking MAO inhibitors should not consume certain fishes and meats, soy products, legumes, some dairy products, or any alcoholic beverage. MAO inhibitors also interact with numerous prescription and over-the-counter medicines. Check with your doctor about any interactions if you are prescribed an MAO inhibitor. Overdose, which can cause cardiovascular problems and death, can occur.

Cyclic antidepressants, including the group known as tricyclic antidepressants, include amitriptyline (Elavil), nortriptyline (Pamelor), imipramine (Tofranil), doxepin (Sinequan), desipramine (Norpramin), and trazodone (Desyrel). A major side effect of these drugs is dry mouth. Other SIDE EFFECTS can include constipation, weight gain, changes in sexual desire and ability, dizziness, and fatigue. A side effect of some drugs in this class has been the relief of nerve pain (neuropathy). These drugs, the ADJUVANT ANALGESIC DRUGS, specifically nortriptyline and amitriptyline, are used specifically for neuropathy. Usually the amount used for this treatment, however, does not produce all these side effects. Overdose can occur and can cause heart arrhythmias, delirium, and death.

SSRIs, including fluoxetine (Prozac), setreline (Zoloft), and paroxetine (Paxil), are a more recent group of antidepressants. They work in blocking the flow of serotonin across neural synapses, the parts of your brain that send instructions to other parts of the brain. There are much fewer side effects of SSRIs, including very few involving cardiovascular problems. Common side effects include nausea and sexual effects. These medications have proved very popular in the past decade, and many people use them because they cause fewer side effects.

There are other antidepressants that do not fit into these three categories. A well-known one is bupropion (Wellbutrin, Zyban), which is also used in smoking cessation treatment.

antidiarrheal   Tending to prevent or suppress diarrhea; a substance used to prevent or treat diarrhea.

antidiuretic hormone   See VASOPRESSIN.

antiemetic   A drug that stops or lessens nausea and vomiting.

antifungal   Acting against FUNGUS; any agent that kills or inhibits the growth or reproduction of fungi or is used to treat fungal infections.

antigen   A foreign substance, usually a protein, that stimulates an immune response. Autoantigens are antigens on the body's own cells. Antigens on all other cells are called foreign antigens. Antigens include proteins, toxins, or other substance or microorganism that the body's immune system

recognizes as foreign and attempts to destroy. Specific substances called antigen receptors are found on the surfaces of both B LYMPHOCYTES and T LYMPHOCYTES. These antigen receptors make possible the reaction of B and T lymphocytes to antigens. Without the antigen receptors, the lymphocytes cannot respond to the presence of antigens and no immune response can take place.

antigen processing   The conversion of an antigen by proteolysis into a form in which it can be recognized by lymphocytes.

antigen processing cell   See ANTIGEN-PRESENTING CELL.

antigen test   A test that looks directly for the presence of a virus in the body rather than for antibodies to that virus. An antigen test for AIDS looks for HIV.

antigen-binding site   The part of an immunoglobulin that binds an antigen.

antigen-presenting cell (APC)   Also called an accessory cell or an antigen processing cell. T LYMPHOCYTES are part of the immune system involved in identifying ANTIGENS. However, in order for an antigen to be recognized by a T lymphocyte, it must first be processed and "presented" in a form the T cell can recognize. This is the function of an APC. APCs include MACROPHAGES, DENDRITIC CELLS, FOLLICULAR DENDRITIC CELLS, ENDOTHELIUM, and LANGERHANS CELLS. First an APC engulfs an antigen. Then the enzymes of the APC break the antigen into smaller pieces called peptides, which bind on the surface of the APC with class I or II MAJOR HISTOCOMPATIBILITY COMPLEX (MHC) molecules. The helper T cells can then recognize the antigen linked with the MHC and bind to it.

antigenic shift   Changes over time in the surface antigens of certain viruses, caused by genetic mutations.

antigenicity   The condition of being able to produce an IMMUNE RESPONSE to an ANTIBODY.

antihemophilic factor   Blood coagulation FACTOR VIII. It is available commercially under the trade names Antihemophilic Globulin, Hemofil, Hemofil F, and Profilate.

antihemophilic factor A   See FACTOR VIII.

antihistamine   Any of various drugs that counteract histamine in the body; often used to relieve the symptoms of allergic reactions and colds.

anti-idiotype antibody   A vaccine strategy that is being used in HIV vaccine research. Antibody molecules can assume almost any shape at all. Scientists therefore can take an antibody to the HIV antigen and make copies of it. Then you have an antibody that resembles the HIV antigen. These antibodies are injected into an animal, and that animal's immune system responds by making antibodies to the antibodies. The way this process works for vaccine research is that these new antibodies (known as the anti-idiotype) in the animal are nearly identical to the original antigen (HIV). Giving these anti-idiotype antibodies to humans should allow their immune system to produce antibodies that fight off what resembles an HIV antigen, but in reality is a harmless antigen. It should induce this immune response so the body is protected against invasion by antigens that resemble HIV. This method works in theory on humans and has worked in animals for a variety of viruses, including HBV, rabies, Newcastle disease virus, and feline leukemia virus.

anti-infective   Acting against infection; a drug designed to do so. Many such drugs, including ANTIVIRALS, ANTIBACTERIALS, ANTIFUNGALS, and ANTIPROTOZOALS, are used widely in AIDS treatment to prevent the onset of opportunistic infections. The use of most of these drugs, even in short-term treatment of acute illness, has been shown to have a negative impact on cell-mediated immune functions by decreasing lymphocyte populations and impairing T-cell function. Long-term use of unlikely combinations of drugs has not, to date, been evaluated for possible synergies that may result in profound immunosuppression. Con-

ceivably, these side effects could prove to be lethal to an already immune-compromised individual.

Weakening of the immune system has also been found to occur in antiviral regimes targeting primary HIV infection itself. The development of resistance to and immunosuppression caused by AZT is now understood to be a consequence of widespread antiviral therapy.

anti-inflammatory   A substance that counteracts or suppresses inflammation. There are two types of anti-inflammatory drugs: STEROIDS, such as cortisone, and NONSTEROIDS, such as aspirin.

antimanic drugs   Agents that prevent or arrest mania, a mental disorder characterized by irrational excitement and hyperactivity, which sometimes appears in people with AIDS.

antimicrobial   An agent that destroys or prevents the growth of microorganisms such as bacteria, fungus, or parasites.

antimoniotungstate   A drug found to be poisonous to the blood when tested for possible use in treating infection with HIV. The drug was developed in the 1970s as a potential treatment for CREUTZFELDT-JAKOB disease. It acts by inhibiting REVERSE TRANSCRIPTASE.

antineoplastic   Preventing the development, growth, or spread of malignant cells; an agent that has such effect.

antioxidant   A substance that may prevent FREE RADICALS (chemicals with free electrons, or oxidants) from causing cell damage. VITAMINS A, C, and E are antioxidants.

antioxidant therapy   Treatment with ANTIOXIDANTS, substances that tend to reduce damage caused by the presence of oxidants in the blood.

"Renegade" oxygen atoms, known as FREE RADICALS or singlet oxygen, have been shown to damage the cellular component of the immune system. Many people living with immune deficiencies therefore attempt to reduce such damage by supplementing their diets with antioxidant nutrients and vitamins. This is a part of an approach to illness known as orthomolecular medicine. Antioxidants have been used to reduce stress, to treat Alzheimer's and cancer, for lens functioning, macular degeneration, and to reduce heart disease.

Oxygen free radicals are produced by several unavoidable factors in our environment. Toxins, highly processed foods, large amounts of saturated fats in our diets, and, significantly, stress, can cause oxygen in the blood to degenerate from its stable and useful form. Antioxidant therapies seek to remedy deficiencies caused by these factors, decrease damage to the immune system and, speculatively, slow down the aging process. Orthomolecular therapeutic agents include BETA-CAROTENE (a nontoxic form of VITAMIN A that can be stored in the body); COENZYME Q10 (a nutrient used in Japan as an anticancer agent); GERMANIUM (a fossilized plant product used widely in Japan as a cancer preventative); GLUTHATHIONE peroxidase (a complement to superoxide); SUPEROXIDE DISMUTASE (one of the basic building blocks of the body's antioxidant response, usually extracted from wheat or barley sprouts); VITAMIN C (probably the most widely used orthomolecular therapeutic agent, and also the most controversial); and vitamin E and SELENIUM (two minerals that must be combined to function optimally, essential to cell and tissue repair). In addition to supplementing their diets with antioxidant nutrients and vitamins, many people chose to add antioxidant foods to their diets; yams, butternut and winter squash, pumpkin, carrots, spinach, broccoli, iceberg lettuce, endive, kale, tomatoes, cantaloupe, apricots, mango, and papaya are good sources of antioxidants.

antiprotozoal Tending to kill or inhibit the multiplication of single-celled microorganisms called PROTOZOA; a drug that has such an effect.

antipsychotic Tending to alleviate the symptoms of psychotic disorders; any drug that has such an effect. Major tranquilizers, including especially phenothiazine derivatives such as chlorpromazine (trade name Largactil) and thioridazine, are used primarily in the treatment of schizophrenia and other disorders involving psychotic symptoms. Lithium compounds are used primarily in the treatment of bipolar (manic-depressive) disorder.

Psychosis is a common manifestation in the late stages of AIDS.

antiretroviral Active against RETROVIRUSes; a drug that has such activity. Antiretroviral drugs reduce the replication rate of retroviruses such as HIV and are widely used in the treatment of HIV-infected persons. The first antiretroviral drug approved by the FOOD AND DRUG ADMINISTRATION was AZIDOTHYMIDINE. The most commonly used are ZIDOVUDINE (AZT), DIDANOSINE (ddI), and ZALCITABINE (ddC).

Antiretroviral therapy can reduce the risk of death in asymptomatic patients with intermediate-stage HIV disease. Moreover, research has shown that ddI alone, ddI in combination with AZT, and ddC in combination with AZT are all superior to AZT alone in preventing serious consequences of HIV infection, including CD4+ T-CELL decline, whether or not there has been previous treatment with AZT.

Today, preferred regimens generally include two or three drugs, based on the patient's condition. Often, the three-drug combination includes a PROTEASE INHIBITOR. MONOTHERAPY, almost invariably with ddI, is a reasonable alternative for patients who refuse a heavier regimen or show intolerance for AZT. To date, there is little data to support rational decisions about whether to employ antiretroviral therapy. Often, a combination of symptoms and SURROGATE MARKERS (CD4 and viral load) is considered. CD4 and VIRAL LOAD values considered to indicate such treatment vary widely among physicians. Some rely on algorithms to determine when to start. Patients' lifestyles, preferences, and ability to comply are also taken into account. In the absence of sufficient information, some physicians are relying on their own and others' clinical experience to guide them in the development of new treatment modalities.

Decisions to stop or switch therapies most often involve toxicity and adverse events. Others are based on combinations of symptoms and surrogate markers, patients' requests, and poor compliance. Many physicians discontinue antiretroviral regimens when the side effects are judged to exceed the potential benefits. This is fairly common in very advanced illness, when the need to treat CMV and MAI and to prevent PCP is more urgent than

antiretroviral therapy. Others stop when no further benefit is demonstrated or there's more benefit from PROPHYLAXIS alone.

The waning effectiveness that has been seen in
antiretroviral therapy over time is generally attributed to the emergence of drug-resistant strains of
HIV (see DRUG RESISTANCE). Many researchers hope
that combination therapy will increase the time
necessary for resistant strains of virus to emerge.
In the meantime, it has been shown that dual-
resistant HIV that can replicate in the presence of
both AZT and 3TC is indeed possible, and that
dual-resistant virus can be detected one year after
the addition of AZT to the regimen of symptomatic
HIV-infected individuals undergoing 3TC monotherapy. This acquisition of dual-resistant virus
may in part account for the return of viral load to
pretreatment levels in those treated at first with
3TC monotherapy and then AZT/3TC combination
therapy, although this does not always mean that
the combination will lose its antiviral effect. And
until a patient develops dual-resistant virus, the
combination of AZT and 3TC generally does continue to have anti-HIV activity.

Guidelines for the use of antiretroviral agents in
HIV-infected adults and adolescents are available
on the website of the HIV/AIDS Treatment Information Service (ATIS) and can be reached at
http://www.hivatis.org.

antiretroviral therapy   See ANTIRETROVIRAL.

antisense   A synthetic segment of DNA or RNA that
will bind to a specific DNA or RNA sequence, interfering with the functioning of that particular gene.
Antisense drugs are designed to block viral genetic
instructions, marking them for destruction by cellular enzymes, in order to prevent the building of a
new virus or the infection of new cells. Antisense
therapy, a type of GENE THERAPY, and the first to enter
clinical studies, attacks the RNA of the HIV virus.

An understanding of the antisense mechanism
requires an understanding of VIRAL INFECTIONS. All
viral infections, including AIDS, can be described
as acquired GENETIC diseases. Viruses are packages
of genetic material that insert themselves into
DNA, the double-stranded chain of genes inside
the nucleus of every cell, and transform the cell
into a factory for producing new copies of the

virus. Each sequence on the DNA provides the
blueprint for the production of a specific protein.
In order to produce proteins, the DNA must transmit its information to a messenger RNA (mRNA)
molecule, also known as the sense strand. The
mRNA uses this information to organize the building and assembly of proteins into the finished
product, usually essential cellular components but,
in the case of infected cells, new copies of HIV. An
antisense drug carries the opposite message to a
specific sense strand. Antisense drugs attach to
mRNA, and thereby block the production of particular proteins at the genetic level.

Traditional drugs that attack proteins in anti-HIV
treatments include reverse transcriptase, protease,
and other familiar drugs. However, proteins are
large, complex structures that are produced in massive quantities by infected cells. In order to be successful, traditional drugs must disable every copy of
the protein. Traditional drugs often attack healthy,
normal proteins as well, in a process known as toxicity. Antisense technology, by attacking a single
mRNA strand that is responsible for producing large
quantities of single protein, may be a more efficient
way of eliminating large quantities of unwanted
proteins at once, and, since an antisense drug binds
only with its exact opposite, it is extremely specific
and should produce minimal toxicities.

While proteins are large and complex, RNA is
composed of various combinations of just four
well-known amino acids—adenosine, cytosine,
thymidine, and guanosine. Since the genes of HIV
have been extensively studied by molecular biolo-
gists, researchers can design antisense compounds
aimed at specific mRNA molecules that produce
proteins essential to HIV's survival. Antisense has
not yet become clinical reality, due partly to tech-
nological and partly to fiscal challenges. Few clinical trials have actually begun, and clinical efficacy
is far from certain. Nonetheless, the pharmaceutical industry has devoted significant resources to
antisense. Its proponents believe it will radically
transform medicine and open new possibilities for
the treatment of AIDS and other viral diseases.

antisense therapy   See ANTISENSE.

anti-TNF monoclonal antibody   A drug that
blocks the action of TNF. TNF occurs naturally in

the body, particularly in people with activated immune systems. TNF is believed to be one of the causes of wasting and inflammation in HIV-positive people. Several studies are under way to test anti-TNF drugs' effect on HIV-positive people. See TUMOR NECROSIS FACTOR.

antiviral Tending to destroy a virus or inhibit its replication; a drug that has such activity. Among the antiviral agents studied or in use against the HIV virus are AL-721, AMPLIGEN, Ansamycin, ACYLOVIR, DESCICLOVIR, GONCICLOVIR, AZIDOTHYMI-DINE (AZT), RETROVIR, Compound S, BWA S900, ZIDOVUDINE (ZDV), ddC, 8-bromoguanasine, FOS-CARNET, HPA-23, ALPHA-INTERFERON (IFN-A), RIB-ARIN, RIBABUTINE, silicotungstate, PEPTIDE T, susamin, and tilorone.

antiviral resistance The developed resistance of a virus to a specific ANTIVIRAL agent.

antiviral therapy See ANTIVIRAL.

Antivirogram A trademarked name for a particular PHENOTYPIC ASSAY. It measures the quantitative ability of a particular drug to inhibit growth of the patient's virus, as compared to a sample of WILD-TYPE virus. It is the only PHENOTYPIC ASSAY that works in all GROUP M subtypes of the virus and provides a full report on all genetic sequences of the virus in the patient. Results are given in FOLD RESISTANCE measures.

anus Terminal opening of the alimentary tube for the elimination of feces. Also the body opening used for ANAL SEX. Slang terms include *asshole, butt hole, bung hole, bussy* (boy pussy), and *manhole.*

anxiety Distress or uneasiness of mind caused by fear of danger or misfortune. Also, a state of apprehension and psychic tension occurring in some forms of mental disorders. Anxiety consists of a somatic, physiological side and a psychological side. Disturbed breathing, increased heart activity, vasomotor changes, musculoskeletal disturbances such as trembling or paralysis, and increased sweating are some of the unpleasurable characteristics of anxiety. The psychological side of anxiety

includes ". . . a specific conscious inner attitude and a peculiar feeling state characterized (1) by a physically as well as mentally painful awareness of being powerless to do anything about a personal matter; (2) by presentiment of an impending and almost inevitable danger; (3) by a tense and physically exhausting alertness as if facing an emergency; (4) by an apprehensive self-absorption which interferes with effective and advantageous solution of reality-problems; and (5) by an irresolvable doubt concerning the nature of the threatening evil, concerning the probability of the actual appearance of the threat, concerning the best objective means of reducing or removing the evil, and concerning one's subjective capacity for making effective use of those means if and when the emergency arises." (Piotrowski, Z. *Perceptoanalysis,* Macmillan, New York, 1957). Anxiety is contrasted with fear, a reaction to a real or threatened danger.

anxiolysis Sedation or hypnosis used to reduce anxiety, agitation, or tension.

anxiolytic Active against anxiety; or agent that has affect. See ANTI-ANXIETY DRUGS.

APC See ANTIGEN-PRESENTING CELL.

aphasia A defect or loss of the ability to speak or write or to understand spoken or written language, which is due to injury or disease of the brain.

aphtha (pl. aphthae) Single or multiple recurrent, well-defined white or cream colored ulcers, in the mouth or on the lips. These can also be called canker sores. This condition can be painful, particularly during eating.

aphthous Pertaining to or characterized by, APHTHA.

aphthous ulcer A single or multiple ulcer of the inside of the mouth that tends to recur. The ulcers are shallow and are often accompanied by soreness and pain. They usually last one to two weeks. Although their cause is unknown, they have been seen often in HIV-positive people. Treatment with a number of medications may be attempted to try to find what is successful for individual patients. THALIDOMIDE is an experimental drug proven helpful in a number of severe cases, although a topical corticosteroid is generally used.

apoplexy   See   CEREBROVASCULAR   ACCIDENT; STROKE.

apoptosis   A metabolic process driven by cellular enzymes, in which a cell's chromosomes and then the cell itself breaks down into fragments—a part of cellular suicide. In the immune system, apoptosis is a process that eliminates unneeded cells. Some researchers believe that accidental apoptosis may be the way that CD4 cells become depleted in HIV disease, rather than through direct killing by HIV.

appeals council   The Social Security Administration's inhouse "supreme court" for further appeals of decisions made by ADMINISTRATIVE LAW JUDGES after hearings. Appeals almost always consist of file reviews rather than new in-person hearings.

appellate court   Any court above the trial court level in either a state or the federal court system; it hears cases on appeal from the trial court.

APTD   See AID TO THE PERMANENTLY AND TOTALLY DISABLED.

AR-623   A lipid encapsulated INTRAVENOUS form of TRETINOIN that is used in the treatment of KAPOSI'S SARCOMA. See TRETINOIN.

ARA-A   See VIDARABINE.

ARA-C   See CYTARABINE.

ARC   See AIDS-RELATED COMPLEX.

ARDS   See ADULT RESPIRATORY DISTRESS SYNDROME.

area under the curve (AUC)   A measure of total exposure or total effect, such as total drug concentration. It is defined by charting on a graph the change in a particular variable over a period of time and calculating the area between the curve and the horizontal axis (which represents elapsed time from the start of the study). Blood levels of drug and viral load during treatment are two numbers frequently quantified by the AUC.

arenavirus   Any of a group of RNA viruses consisting of multishaped virions that have four large and one to three small segments of single-stranded RNA. The presence of ribosomes gives the virions a sandy appearance. The principal virus in this group is the lymphocytic choriomeningitis (LCM) virus. Also included are the American hemorrhagic fever viruses and the Lassa fever virus. The LCM virus rarely infects humans, but when it does, the disease is usually a mild form of meningitis. The Lassa virus causes a highly contagious, severe febrile illness and may be fatal. Rodents typically serve as hosts for these viruses.

arm   One of two or more treatment alternatives in a drug trial.

armamentarium   A collection of drugs or other treatments for a particular disease or condition.

aromatherapy   ALTERNATIVE TREATMENTS using essential oils (the volatile oils distilled from plants) to treat emotional disorders such as stress and anxiety as well as a range of other ailments. Applied by a massage method, the essence is directly inhaled and is said to circulate over the pathways of the nerve centers of the spine. The oils are also absorbed into the body through the skin. This method is thought to work better than ingesting the oils in pill form. Although this process is of unproven medical value, many of the herbs and other plants are known to have medicinal properties have long been used in traditional medicine, and their derivatives in modern drugs. Aromatherapy is often used in conjunction with massage therapy, acupuncture, reflexology, herbology, chiropractic, and other holistic treatments.

artemisia   An herb (*Artemisia annua,* also known as qing hao), that has been used as an antimalaria treatment in China since before A.D. 340. More recently, an extract of the herb, artemisinin, or qinghaosu (QHS), has shown efficacy against malaria. Studies have suggested that artemisinin and its derivatives may also have a place as anti-toxoplasmic agents.

arteriosclerosis A general term for the thickening, hardening, and blockage of the walls of blood vessels. This generally occurs over time as fats, cholesterol, fibrin, platelets, cellular debris, and calcium are deposited in the artery wall. Gradually these substances build up, and eventually they narrow and block the artery, similarly to scales forming on the insides of pipes. The minerals, particularly calcium, cause the hardening of the arteries. If the coronary arteries are involved, this process leads to pain and potential heart attacks. If leg arteries are involved, it leads to pain in walking and potential gangrene from loss of blood flow. Strokes may occur if the blockages occur in the brain. Risk factors such as (1) elevated levels of cholesterol and triglyceride in the blood, (2) high blood pressure, and (3) smoking all accelerate the process of vascular disease. Diseases such as HIV disease, which produce an element of inflammation in tissues, further add to these risks. See META-BOLIC TOXICITY.

arthralgia Pain in a joint.

arthritis A clinical condition characterized by inflammation of the joints. It is associated with a large number of different disease processes.

artificial insemination The introduction by instrumental means of semen containing viable spermatozoa into the vagina or uterus to induce pregnancy. To be safe, sperm banks are requested to test sperm donors for HIV at the time of donation, freeze and quarantine the sperm, and test the donor again six months later. If both HIV tests are negative, the sperm can then be thawed and used. It is generally recommended that all women who want to use artificial insemination to become pregnant should be certain that the donor—whether known to them or not—has been screened for HIV antibodies. Individuals considering artificial insemination should talk to their doctors or call their sperm banks to discuss the procedures they use to protect their clients from HIV infection. Women inseminated with HIV-positive semen are at risk of getting the infection and passing it on to their babies.

ARV See AIDS-ASSOCIATED RETROVIRUS.

ascending disease Certain sexually transmitted diseases (STDs) that start in the CERVIX and move up to the pelvic organs.

asceticism See ABSTINENCE.

ascomycetes The largest class of *Eumycetes,* the true fungi. They are characterized by a sac that encloses the spores. Included in this group are yeasts, mildews, blue molds, and truffles.

ascorbic acid See VITAMIN C.

aseptic meningitis See MENINGITIS, ACUTE ASEPTIC.

Asia In comparison to Africa, Asia has been relatively less hard hit by HIV infection. The virus arrived relatively late in most of Asia compared to other regions of the world. It also has never shown the growth in rates of infection evidenced in some other regions of the world. There were believed to be 6.6 million people in this region with HIV disease at the end of 2001. One million of them were infected in that year according to United Nations (UN) statistics.

The disease has spread predominantly through injection drug use (IDU) and unsafe sexual practices. Some regions of Asia have similar problems to Africa. In India, for instance, large parts of the population in some areas of the country are migrant workers. These people, generally men, are away from their families for months at a time. When they are away, they fill their social time with alcohol, drugs, and sex outside their predominant relationship. Upon returning home for a vacation, these workers often then infect their wives, who become pregnant and pass on the virus to children. India also has a large immigrant population of Eastern European and Russian woman sex workers who have assisted in spreading HIV. In other countries often the only way a family can earn money is to send their young children to work in brothels. In Thailand, Burma, and Cambodia young people serve tourists from around the world who arrive in the region for sex vacations. This has increased the spread among the sex workers and among visiting workers and tourists heading home to other parts of Asia. Sexual mores have also changed in many of these countries. In addition to a burgeoning gay movement in the region, Southeast Asia has always had a role for transsexual boys who serve as sex workers, from Burma and Thailand to India and Malaysia. These are all populations that have seen large increases in HIV in the last few years.

It was considered good that only three countries showed a rate of infection in the adult population above 1 percent, Cambodia, Thailand, and Myanmar. In these nations the outbreak has been spread by individuals who use unsafe sexual practices and injection drug users (IDUs). These countries are on traffic routes for the "Golden Triangle" heroin production area in Asia. IDUs have already caused significant outbreak of HIV in these countries. HIV prevalence rates of IDUs in this area of northern Burma, Thailand, southern China, and far eastern India are above 40 percent. Even in Nepal, IDUs show an infection rate above 50 percent. Many experts agree that the virus is still relatively new to the area, and every where that HIV outbreaks have started, it began in particular populations and then spread quickly to other areas of the population. In Myanmar IDUs and sex workers have HIV prevalence rates of 60 percent and 40 percent, respectively. The national rate of infection overall in Myanmar ranges from an estimate of 1 percent according to the military government to above 5 percent according to the government in exile of Daw Aung San Suu Kyi.

Since the late 1990s growth in the spread of the virus has increased dramatically in other parts of Asia. India and China have both had large numbers of new cases of HIV/AIDS. Both of these countries have large populations, and though a rate of infection at 0.1 percent in China and 0.8 percent in India does not sound high, it represents close to 1 million people in China and 4 million in India. The total is equivalent to that of a metropolitan area with the population of Houston. China is having the first outbreak of HIV disease that is the direct result of blood *donation*. Almost 20 percent of AIDS cases in China are the result of selling of blood by poor rural Chinese. The blood dealers in China reuse needles and after separating plasma pool the blood of the population before sending that blood back into the donor's veins. Many rural Chinese sold their blood to earn

money, and currently many of these same people are suffering from HIV disease–related illnesses.

In China particularly the spread of HIV is believed to be increasing. The country has been very hesitant to acknowledge AIDS at all. Stories in the world media indicate that very few Chinese know what AIDS is or how it is spread. Interviews with sex workers in China indicate that men pay more for sex without condoms so the workers feel they must perform without them. When one doctor in Henan province, where a large number of the donation-derived AIDS cases exist, offered free AIDS test kits to the local clinic, the government refused to allow them to be used. The doctor went back anyway with some tests, according to a report, and found that 80 of 140 people he tested had positive test results. Officially HIV rates in China jumped 67 percent in the first six months of 2001. Prevalence among IDUs in some areas of China is known to exceed 70 percent. Populations of sex workers have tested positive at rates as high as 11 percent. For these reasons, experts expect HIV rates in China to continue to increase.

In India HIV is believed to be spreading into the general population. Rates of infection in postnatal clinics run from 1 percent to 3 percent across the country. Rates of infection at SEXUALLY TRANSMITTED DISEASE (STD) clinics in India exceed 10 percent. India already has more HIV-infected citizens than any other country except South Africa. India has also seen significant numbers of IDUs infected in both the eastern and western parts of the country, as those areas abut the heroin production areas of the Golden Crescent of Afghanistan and Pakistan and the Golden Triangle of Southeast Asia. IDU rates of infection in those areas top 70 percent.

In other countries religion has stopped discussion of AIDS. In Indonesia and Malaysia, policies have often prevented discussion of sexual activities or mores of the population. A government employee in Indonesia was fired in 1998 for saying publicly that the sexual activity of youths had increased dramatically in recent years. Government spokespeople said that the minister had no right to say such things. In Indonesia the rate of infection had remained very low 15 years into the outbreak affecting the rest of the world. But since the mid 1990s that has changed. Sex workers in parts of Indonesia now register rates of infection of 20 percent, up from less than 1 percent in 1995. HIV infection rates at drug treatment centers in Jakarta, the capital, jumped from 15 percent in 2000 to above 40 percent in mid-2001.

Sex work also occurs at significant levels in the Philippines and Bangladesh, where rates had been low up through 2001. However, injection drug usage is fairly high in both countries, and some health care workers in those countries expect the rate to increase soon. The Philippines also is a country with a large number of men who work overseas. Twenty-five percent of the AIDS cases in the Philippines and Bangladesh have been in workers returning from abroad.

Thailand and Cambodia have both shown some ability to contain the virus. Both countries have offered extensive campaigns of education to their populations. New cases of AIDS in Thailand dropped from 143,000 in 1991 to 29,000 in 2001. This is a tremendous decrease in new cases. Despite it, AIDS remains the leading cause of death in Thailand. In Cambodia the national rate of infection dropped from 4 percent in 1999 to 2.7 percent in 2001. Cambodia has adopted a 100 percent condom usage advertising campaign and has also enacted human rights laws to protect HIV-positive people. Japan, Mongolia, and Korea to date have very low rates of infection. All three of these countries have rates of infection below 0.001 percent. With strong education programs, these countries may still be able to avoid the worst of the spread in Asia.

In other nations, UN reports suggest that epidemics are waiting to happen. There are many foreign Laotian workers living in Thailand. There are many Nepalis working in India. Interisland migrations in Indonesia are quite common, and laborers often work on one island and live in another part of the country. All these scenarios could lead to future problems for these nations. Bangladesh, fearing such transmission routes and an epidemic, has launched massive education campaigns to teach people about HIV and to encourage condom usage. Nepal has seen condom usage among long-distance truckers and sex workers increase dramatically since an education program began. Whether these preventive measures work will be seen in the not too distant future.

One response among corporations in India is that drug manufacturers have been making triple drug combination medicines in generic form. This makes the drugs available at a lower price than is paid in the West. These drugs are also exported to Africa in some cases. A triple drug combination in India can run about $500 U.S. a year. Cipla Ltd., a pharmaceutical giant in India, has agreed to sell at cost drugs to India and African governments. It has also agreed to provide free for two years the drug nevirapine, which helps prevent the vertical transmission of HIV from mother to child. Other Indian companies have followed suit: Hetero Drugs Ltd and Aurobindo, Ltd are trying to stay competitive in the Indian and world market. The Indian companies currently have patent laws different from those of the United States that allow them to manufacture the same drug as long as they do not use the production method of an international patent holder. This policy led them to decide that they would provide access to HIV drugs for the less developed world. India's laws change to conform to international standards in 2005, so this may be a short-term policy. It is hoped that it will allow the government to stabilize the death and infection rates, as that of Brazil has through similar actions.

ASK1   Abbreviation of *apoptosis-signal regulating kinase 1*. This is a poorly understood cellular chemical that is believed to trigger a cell to self-destruct. It is found at the site of injuries and trauma in the body. It is also important to the ability of HIV to cause cell death around HIV-infected cells.

ASO   See AIDS SERVICE ORGANIZATION.

aspartate aminotransferase (AST)   A LIVER ENZYME that plays a role in PROTEIN metabolism. Elevated SERUM levels of AST are a sign of liver damage from disease or drugs. AST also is known as serum glutamic oxaloacetic transaminase (SGOT).

aspergillomycosis   See ASPERGILLOSIS.

aspergillosis   An infection caused by the fungus *Aspergillus,* characterized by granulomatous lesions in the tissues or on any mucosal surface. Symptoms include fever, chills, difficulty breathing, and coughing up blood. The infection can spread through the blood to other organs and cause lesions of the skin, ear, nasal sinuses, or lungs, as well as occasionally the bones, meninges, heart, kidneys, or spleen. If the infection reaches the brain, it may cause dementia. Also called *aspergillomycosis.*

Aspergillus A genus of fungi in the family Moniliaceae. After sexual development, it is classed with the asomycetes. This genus includes several species of molds, some of which are opportunistic pathogens. See ASPERGILLOSIS.

aspirin An anti-inflammatory drug (acetylsalicylic acid, a derivative of salicylic acid). It occurs as white crystals or powder. It is one of the most widely used ANALGESICS and antipyretics. Because it is so widely available, it is often misused. Prolonged use will cause gastrointestinal irritation and bleeding in some individuals.

assay The chemical analysis of a substance or mixture to determine its constituents and the relative proportion of each. In biology, the estimation of the strength of a drug or substance by comparing its effects in test animals to a reference standard.

asset level The standard used in needs-based programs to determine eligibility for benefits. Only those with assets below the set amount are eligible.

assets The total value of money and personal and real property owned by a benefits applicant.

AST See ASPARTATE AMINOTRANSAMINASE.

astemizole An antihistamine drug used for the treatment of allergies. Astemizole cannot be taken when taking KETOCONAZOLE, all PROTEASE INHIBITORS, macrolide antibiotics (clarithromycin), selective serotonin reuptake inhibitors (see ANTIDEPRESSANT), and several other drugs. In 1999, the manufacturer of astemizole stopped making the medication for sale in the United States and withdrew all hismanol products from that market as a result of serious side effects the drug caused when taken with numerous medications. It is still available in other countries. (Its trade name is Hismanol.)

asthenia A lack or loss of strength. A debility or any weakness, but especially one originating in muscular or cerebral (brain) disease. It can also be called adynamia.

asthma A condition characterized by recurring sudden attacks of paroxysmal shortness of breath, accompanied by coughing and wheezing. The wheezing is caused by spasmodic contractions of the bronchi (bronchial tubes) or by swelling of the bronchial mucous membrane. Asthma may be an allergic reaction or be caused by other factors, such as physical, mental, or emotional stress; fatigue; and pollutant irritants. Severe attacks may be life-threatening.

astragalus An herb *(Astragalus memranaceious)* used in China, reportedly for the purpose of "boosting" the immune system and preventing chemotherapy-related bone marrow suppression and nausea. In the former Soviet Union and in Japan it is used to treat heart attacks and strokes. The active substances are taken from the root of the plant. Studies have reported that an extract of astragalus, Fraction 3 (F3), has stimulated immune responses in the test tube and in animal studies. Clinical trials of astragalus in people will determine whether such effects can be duplicated in the body. Astragalus is believed to be nontoxic, but there are reports that it can trigger low blood pressure and increase the amount of urine produced, resulting in dizziness and fatigue. Overdosing of astragalus may cause immunosuppression, and plants from different sources may vary in quality and produce different results.

as-treated analysis A type of CLINICAL STUDY analysis that only looks at data from those participants who completed that particular study. See INTENT-TO-TREAT ANALYSIS.

asymptomatic The absence of symptoms of a disease or infection. An asymptomatic person feels healthy, and may be healthy. It is possible, however, to be ill and be asymptomatic; this condition is generally associated with the early stages of an infection. See ASYMPTOMATIC INFECTION.

asymptomatic infection   An early stage of an infection in which the patient has no physical symptoms. Long-term asymptomatic HIV infection has been associated with high levels of antibodies to HIV core proteins and the absence of HEPATITIS B markers. No association with unsafe sex has been found. Additionally, no association between psychological coping skills and slower disease progression has been found.

ataxia   A lack of muscular coordination, causing a stumbling walk, speech problems, tremors, and other neurological impairments. It is caused by a variety of spinal cord SYNDROMES and seen most often in HIV-positive people with MYELOPATHY.

atazanavir   Protease inhibitor also known as Zrivada and BMS 232632. This drug is currently in the final phases of testing. The developer, Bristol-Meyers-Squibb has filed papers for the approval of atazanavir with the U.S. Food and Drug Administration (FDA). It is expected to come before the approval board by June of 2003. As of December 2002, atazanavir is in an expanded access program, allowing people to receive the medication free of charge prior to FDA approval, if they are failing their current regimen of medications.

Known side effects of atazanavir include diarrhea and elevated levels of bilirubin, a liver enzyme. Diarrhea was experienced by about 30 percent of research subjects. Bilirubin is the liver enzyme that causes jaundice. A person with high levels of bilirubin may experience a yellowing of the eyes, nails, and skin. The high bilirubin levels were not associated with any liver damage in patients. Research has shown that patients with HBV or HCV coinfection did not suffer liver problems from the rise in bilirubin levels. In some studies hyperbilirubinemia was experienced by 50 percent of the patients.

Atazanavir will also be available to patients that have experienced high LIPID levels on other protease inhibitors and have not been able to lower them effectively while on HAART. Unlike other PIs, atazanavir has not shown the large increases in triglycerides and cholesterol. It has been shown to increase HDL, the "good" cholesterol, that can help prevent heart disease. Atazanavir has also been effective at lowering VIRAL LOAD and raising CD4 counts in patients. It has a high BIOAVAILABILITY, so it can be taken as one pill, one time a day.

Atazanavir has the ability to boost the levels of several other PIs in the blood in the same way that ritonavir is used to raise levels of some drugs. This has the possibility of reducing the number of other pills taken in combination with atazanavir.

ATEU   See AIDS TREATMENT EVALUATION UNITS.

athlete's foot   A fungal infection of the foot caused by various dermatophytes.

atopic dermatitis   A chronic inflammation of the skin of unknown cause and characterized by severe itching leading to scratching or rubbing, which in turn produces lesions. Individuals affected generally have a hereditary predisposition to irritable skin. Also called ALLERGIC DERMATITIS and ALLERGIC ECZEMA.

atopic diathesis   An allergic condition that makes the body tissues more susceptible to certain diseases.

atopic eczema   See ATOPIC DERMATITIS.

atopy   A genetically determined state of hypersensitivity to common environmental allergens, mediated by IgE antibodies.

atorvastatin   A lipid level–lowering drug used to lower a person's cholesterol and/or triglyceride level, when diet and exercise are not effective. The trade name is Lipitor. See STATINS.

atovaquone   A recently licensed oral drug for treatment of mild-to-moderate cases of PCP as well as for salvage treatment of TOXOPLASMOSIS. Its absorption is highly dependent on ingestion with food, especially fatty food, which increases its absorption four- or fivefold. Atovaquone is known to have many drug interactions, some of which result in synergistic or additive effects against the toxoplasma parasite. It is known to be synergistic with AZITHROMYCIN, CLARITHROMYCIN,

PYRIMETHAMINE, and RIFABUTIN against this parasite. Atovaquone should be used with caution along with FLUCONAZOLE and RIFAMPIN, since they can lower atovaquone blood levels. Atovaquone itself can lower AZT blood levels, though to date the clinical significance of this reduction remains unknown. (The trade name is Mepron.)

ATP   See ADENOSINE TRIPHOSPHATE.

atrophy   A wasting away; a decrease in the size of a cell, tissue, or organ; to undergo or cause atrophy. Atrophy may result from death and resorption of cells, diminished cellular proliferation, pressure, ischemia, malnutrition, decreased activity, or hormonal changes.

attachment inhibitors   A class of drugs that use some type of mechanism to block the binding of HIV to healthy human cells. See PRO-542.

attenuation   Thinning or weakening of strength or virulence of pathogenic microorganism. An attenuated virus is a weakened virus whose ability to infect or produce disease is potentially reduced.

atypical squamous cells of undetermined significance (ASCUS)   Abnormalities in the cells on the surface of the CERVIX, an aberration that turns up on PAP TESTS. Three approaches to managing this mild abnormality include COLPOSCOPY (a procedure in which the clinician examines the cervix through a lighted, binocular-like magnifying instrument and biopsies abnormal areas), "watchful waiting" (repeating the Pap test every six months), and testing the cells in the smear for the strains of HUMAN PAPILLOMA VIRUS (HPV) that are associated with progression to cancer.

In 1997, the National Cancer Institute launched a nationwide study to evaluate these three approaches. Its two principal purposes are to determine whether watchful waiting is a reasonable alternative to colposcopy (if so, many women would be spared the inconvenience and discomfort of the procedure) and to discern whether HPV testing can predict which types of cells will revert to normal and which will progress to high-grade SQUAMOUS INTRAEPITHELIAL LESION.

AUC   See AREA UNDER THE CURVE.

Augmentin   The trade name of a combination (amoxicillin and clavulanate) penicillin-related medicine widely used to treat bacterial infections by killing bacteria or preventing their growth. It is available in tablet, chewable tablet, and liquid formulations. Augmentin is often used to treat PELVIC INFLAMMATORY DISEASE, sinus infections, urinary tract infections, and rashes that occur with HIV. It often causes diarrhea in patients.

Australia   See OCEANIA.

autoantibody   An antibody produced by B CELLS in response to an altered self antigen on one type of the body's own cells, that attacks and destroys these cells; an antibody to self-antigens (autoantigens). Autoantibodies are the basis for autoimmune diseases.

autocatalysis   A phenomenon in which the rate of a chemical reaction is increased through the catalytic action of the products of the reaction itself. Autocatalysis is the process by which PROTEASE is able to cut itself loose from the other components of the larger, inactive viral protein.

autocrine system   The process by which a cell produces a hormone that then influences the cell's own growth.

autoimmune disease   An ailment caused by an IMMUNE RESPONSE against an individual's own tissues or cells. Among many such diseases are rheumatoid arthritis, diabetes mellitus, multiple sclerosis, and lupus.

autoimmune mechanism   The response that produces AUTOIMMUNITY, in which the body recognizes itself as foreign and forms antibodies against its own tissues. See ANTIBODY.

autoimmunity   Immunity to self-ANTIGENS (autoantigens); the loss of normal tolerance by the immune system of self-antigens on the surface of the body's own cells. B CELLS are activated to produce autoantibodies against these autoantigens, causing the destruction of normal tissue. Exactly why LEUKOCYTES do not normally react with self-antigens is not known.

autoinoculation The transfer of microorganisms from one location of the body to another, typically by the hands. The term is used to describe the contagiousness of such organisms as the virus that causes MOLLUSCUM CONTAGIOSUM. It can also refer to injection of some of the body's cells back into the body. Usually autoinoculation is a treatment in which cells are removed from one's body, treated or altered medically, and then reinjected into the body. Using one's own cells helps prevent or reduce antibody formation.

autologous transfusion See TRANSFUSION.

autopsy An examination of the body after death, including organs and tissues, in order to determine the cause of death or pathological changes. Also called NECROPSY or POSTMORTEM EXAMINATION.

autovaccination Vaccination with autogenous vaccine, or autovaccine, made from organisms taken from a patient's own tissues; vaccination resulting from the transfer of a virus or bacteria from a sore of a previous vaccination to a break in the skin elsewhere.

availability In regard to health care, the degree to which services, including facilities and personnel, are in place and readily accessible to all consumers.

average In statistics, the average is reached by adding up all of the numbers in a particular result and dividing that number by the total number of results added. For example, in a study of five people whose ages are 20, 22, 30, 39, and 40 years, the average age of the people in the study is 30.2 years. Also known as the mean. See MEDIAN.

Avlosulfon See DAPSONE.

award letter Letter or form from a government agency informing an applicant of approval for benefits and, if applicable, how much those benefits will be. SOCIAL SECURITY DISABILITY INSURANCE (SSDI), SUPPLEMENTARY SECURITY INCOME (SSI), and DEPARTMENT OF VETERANS AFFAIRS (VA) notifications almost always state that disability is a basis for eligibility. AID TO FAMILIES WITH DEPENDENT CHILDREN (AFDC), GENERAL ASSISTANCE (GA), MEDICAID, and FOOD STAMP PROGRAM award letters may not explicitly state that incapacity or disability is a basis of eligibility.

Ayurveda An Indian spiritual tradition more than 5,000 years old. Ayurvedic tradition holds that illness is a state of imbalance among the body's systems that can be detected through such diagnostic procedures as reading the pulse and observing the tongue. Nutrition counseling, massage, therapy, natural medications, and other modalities are used to address a broad spectrum of ailments, from allergies to AIDS.

azathioprine An immunosuppressive agent created from a cytotoxic chemical substance and used for the prevention of transplant rejection in organ transplantation. It is also under investigation for use in the treatment of autoimmune diseases. (Its trade name is Imuran.)

azidothymidine (AZT) [zidovudine (ZDV)] The first and best-known anti-HIV drug, and still the primary ANTIVIRAL agent used against HIV. Though the nomenclature has changed—the correct name for this drug is now zidovudine (ZDV)—it is still almost universally referred to as AZT, a practice followed in this encyclopedia. See AZT.

azithromycin An ANTIBIOTIC drug that prevents the growth and multiplication of susceptible organisms by interfering with their formation of essential proteins. It is used in the treatment of certain upper respiratory tract infections (streptococcal pharyngitis and tonsilitis), certain lower respiratory tract infections (acute bronchitis and PNEUMONIA), certain skin infections, and nongonococcal URETHRITIS and CERVICITIS due to CHLAMYDIA trachomatis. It may also have activity against MYCOBACTERIUM AVIUM COMPLEX, TOXOPLASMOSIS, and CRYPTOSPORIDIOSIS. Possible side effects include nausea, diarrhea, dizziness, sensitivity to sunlight, and vaginal CANDIDIASIS. (Its trade name is Zithromax.)

AZT (azidothymidine) [zidovudine (ZDV)] A NUCLEOSIDE ANALOG used to slow replication of HIV. AZT was the first and is still the primary ANTIVIRAL drug used to combat the human immunodeficiency virus. AZT is a synthetic THYMIDINE (one of the basic components of DNA), and inhibits the virus's growth and development.

AZT is approved for the initial treatment of HIV infection in adults with CD4 counts of less than 500 and for children over three months old. It is also approved for preventing maternal-fetal HIV TRANSMISSION. Multiple investigations have shown that ASYMPTOMATIC patients with absolute CD4 counts of less than 500 benefit from taking AZT, slowing the decline in their CD4 counts and delaying the development of opportunistic infection, but it has not been demonstrated to prolong long-term survival. AZT is indicated for symptomatic HIV disease and is superior to DIDEOXYINOSINE (ddI) and DIDEOXYCYTIDINE (ddC), as first-line therapy. While there is still some controversy regarding the optimal time to initiate therapy, offering asymptomatic patients the option of initiating AZT when their CD4 counts are under 500 is recommended. Patients with CD4 counts of more than 500 may also benefit from AZT.

It is known that AZT and other nucleosides lose effectiveness over time, especially in advanced HIV disease. The reasons for this are not fully understood, but appear to relate to incomplete suppression of viral replication and consequent development of DRUG RESISTANCE, decreased drug PHOSPHORYLATION, and the development of syncytium-inducting (SI) viral phenotypes.

AZT is especially vulnerable to the emergence of genetic mutations that produce resistance because it belongs to a class of drugs known as REVERSE TRANSCRIPTASE INHIBITORS. These drugs block HIV's reverse transcriptase enzyme, which the virus uses to help insert its genes into the genetic material of healthy, uninfected cells. Reverse transcriptase inhibitors thus impede the spread of HIV into new cells, but they do nothing to stop the production of new virus in cells that already harbor their viral agents. Moreover, it is now clear that there are large numbers of HIV-containing cells at nearly every stage of infection, especially in the LYMPH-NODES, and therefore a steady production of new HIV particles, some of which inevitably contain mutations conferring resistance to AZT.

At first it seemed a good idea to administer as much AZT as possible as early as possible in HIV infection, but this intuitive notion has run up against the complex realities of an interaction among a limited and toxic therapy, a rapidly mutating virus, and a declining immune system. Real-world experience indicates that AZT has an impact on health and survival that lasts for a year or so and then fades, no matter at what stage of immune deficiency the treatment is started. Another intuitive notion that has proven not to be true is that patients with HIV could benefit from AZT for a year or so and change to another drug, with equal results. Experience has shown, however, that such patients do poorly on their second drugs. The reason these replacement drugs perform comparatively poorly is not clear. The continued toll of HIV and opportunistic infections plus AZT's accumulating side effects may leave the immune system less functional than before AZT therapy, regardless of actual CD4 count. Also, AZT-resistant HIV may be more mutable than AZT-sensitive strains of the virus, making resistance to new drugs emerge more quickly.

The primary toxicity of AZT is hematologic. When AZT treatment is first started, patients seem to get a boost to their immune system, but then, inevitably, there's a rapid decline. This is called a rebound effect. AZT is a toxic chemical, and when a TOXIN is introduced into the blood, the supply of red blood cells is killed off. To compensate for that loss, the bone marrow, where the blood cells are made, produces at a higher level. The loss increases, however, as long as treatment with AZT is continued, until the supply is below the level it was at before treatment. So for the short term, if the bone marrow is in reasonably good shape, it can compensate for the initial loss. But as cells are continually killed off, the damage exceeds the ability of the remaining intact cells to produce more. Patients develop ANEMIA, with fewer white and fewer red cells than before AZT treatment. The time it takes for this decline to occur varies among individuals.

Patients tolerant of AZT generally develop a mild macro-CYTOSIS with or without anemia in two months. This is not a reason to discontinue treatment with AZT. Normocytic anemia may develop and is of greater concern because it may precede severe anemia. In cases of severe anemia, AZT is reduced or discontinued, and TRANSFUSIONS given as needed. Severe persistent anemia may respond to ERYTHROPOIETIN. There may also be other causes of anemia, particularly infections. Patients with persistent or severe recurrent anemia are candidates for alternate ANTIRETROVIRAL therapy such as ddI or ddC.

In pregnant women, AZT may reduce transmission to babies by lowering HIV levels, though it is not clear when in pregnancy or labor it should be administered. Most mother-to-child transmission seems to take place at the time of birth, but a significant amount of IN UTERO transmission is also thought to occur. AZT may function as a primary prophylaxis in fetuses and newborn babies, preventing infection of any of their cells. This would argue for administering AZT prior to birth as well as afterward. The long-term dangers AZT poses for birth defects and other health problems for children is unknown.

Major side effects, such as NEUTROPENIA, limit therapy. Recent studies indicate that AZT may be continued safely until the absolute neutrophil count declines to below 750. GROWTH stimulating FACTORS may be considered at this point, but alternative therapy with ddI or ddC may be preferable.

Common side effects of AZT include headache, insomnia, and gastrointestinal symptoms and are often seen soon after beginning therapy. They generally resolve in a few weeks with symptomatic treatment, but will occasionally require discontinuation of AZT (see AZT INELIGIBILITY). Some clinicians initiate therapy at a low dose and increase it gradually until the target dose is reached, a practice that appears to mitigate some of the headaches and gastrointestinal distress. Taking AZT with meals may also minimize such complaints, and these can be affected by other drugs taken simultaneously. Drugs that decrease AZT concentrations may decrease antiretroviral activity. Insufficient viral inhibition and lack of a CD4 response may be a sign of this problem. Drugs that lower AZT levels include RIFABUTIN and CLARITHROMYCIN, the two most common agents used for MAC prevention.

Drugs that increase AZT concentrations in the blood reinforce AZT's suppression of bone marrow, resulting in increased hematologic toxicity, producing anemia and neutropenia. Drugs that increase AZT levels include Bactrim, FLUCONAZOLE, and probenecid.

Drugs with hematologic toxicity similar to AZT's have to be used with caution, since if given simultaneously, the combination may lead to enhanced anemia or neutropenia. Such drugs include Bactrim, DAPSONE, FLUCYTOSINE, GANCICLOVIR, INTERFERON, PENTAMIDINE, PYRIMETHAMINE, and SULFADIAZINE and CHEMOTHERAPIES such as DOXORUBICIN.

AZT failure   The status of a patient who has taken at least 500 mg per day of AZT for more than six months and whose condition is worsening.

AZT ineligibility   The status of an HIV-infected patient who may not be administered AZT owing to a condition such as low WHITE BLOOD CELL count or severe ANEMIA, or the simultaneous administration of an incompatible drug.

AZT ineligible   Prohibited from taking AZT for medical reasons. See AZT INELIGIBILITY.

AZT intolerance   Abnormal SENSITIVITY or ALLERGY to AZT; inability to endure treatment with the drug. AZT intolerant patients may experience the same common side effects of AZT (headaches, nausea, hypertension, and a general sense of feeling ill) as AZT tolerant patients, but these do not disappear after a few weeks of therapy as they generally do in the AZT tolerant. The AZT intolerant may also experience more serious side effects (ANEMIA, GRANULOCYTOPENIA, MYOPATHY). AZT intolerance may occur in people with a known allergy to the drug and in those with kidney or liver disease.

AZT intolerant   Abnormally sensitive to, and unable to endure treatment with, AZT; patients who have such sensitivity. See AZT INTOLERANCE.

AZT monotherapy   The administration of zidovudine (AZT) to an HIV-infected person, unaccompanied by other drugs. The effectiveness of monotherapy is known to decline over time, since the HIV virus gradually becomes resistant to the drug. There is now research evidence that combination drug therapies will so reduce HIV replication that strains resistant to multiple medications may not evolve. See COMBINATION THERAPY; MONOTHERAPY; SEQUENTIAL MONOTHERAPY.

AZT resistance The ability of the body to resist the effects of AZT. Resistance to AZT may predict more rapid disease progression. Studies have shown that the presence of AZT-resistant HIV in the body translates into poorer physical health in general, even in individuals who have switched to another drug. The reasons for this continue to elude researchers. It may be that AZT resistance is a sign that the virus has gained greater mutability, helping it to respond quickly to challenges posed by new drug therapy or immune defenses.

One way to get around the problems posed by resistance to AZT and related drugs, researchers speculate, is to find a therapy that attacks the virus at a different, more vulnerable point in its life cycle. Protease inhibitors block the assembly of HIV particles as they bud out from an infected cell and hold promise as such a therapy. Simultaneous resistance to different protease inhibitors may be more difficult for HIV to achieve. Studies of protease inhibitor compounds have reported that viral resistance may develop at a slower pace than with NUCLEOSIDE ANALOGS such as AZT, ddI, and ddC.

AZT resistant Having developed resistance to the antiviral activity of AZT; those HIV-positive patients in whom the virus has developed such resistance and for whom the drug is no longer working well.

It is believed that the AIDS virus may develop resistance after a year or more, though this point is still under investigation. It is not feasible to do viral cultures for every potential subject to prove that viral resistance to AZT has in fact developed. There may be other reasons that explain the declining effectiveness of AZT in any given case. See AZT RESISTANCE.

AZT tolerance The ability to tolerate treatment with AZT without serious side effects (anemia, granulocytopenia, and myopathy). They may experience the drug's more common side effects (or symptoms due to anxiety about taking it), including headaches, nausea, hypertension, and a general sense of feeling ill, but these generally disappear after a few weeks. Side effects occur more frequently in people taking high doses of AZT or in people with more advanced disease at the time therapy is started. See AZT INTOLERANCE.

AZT tolerant Able to endure treatment with AZT; patients who have this tolerance. See AZT INTOLERANCE; AZT TOLERANCE.

AZT worrisome An informal term for those who are on AZT and not intolerant, but who show signs, short of a major opportunistic infection, that the drug is beginning to fail; those apprehensive about AZT generally and the implications of taking it.

Patients on AZT therapy may continue to experience HIV-related symptoms, OPPORTUNISTIC INFECTIONS, and declining IMMUNE-SYSTEM function, in addition to the side effects of the drug itself. Controversies exist about when to begin AZT therapy, continue it and add or change to other therapies. All these factors—added to the trauma of being infected with HIV in the first place—create understandable unease, anxiety, and apprehension. The AZT worrisome may also include friends and family of patients who are using this drug.

AZT/ddI treatment COMBINATION THERAPY with AZT and ddI. Both drugs appear to prevent the AIDS virus from replicating, and ddI is in fact a chemical relative of AZT. Their relationship may also be synergistic, meaning that the combination may work better than would be indicated merely by adding their separate efficacies. There does not appear to be cross resistance—strains of the virus which have become resistant to AZT are not automatically resistant to ddI, so ddI may be effective in patients for whom AZT no longer works well.

AZT-experienced Having taken AZT or other ANTIVIRAL drugs. See AZT-NAIVE.

AZT-naive Never having taken AZT or any other ANTIRETROVIRAL drug; those who have never taken such drugs. See AZT-EXPERIENCED.

B

b₂-microglobulin   See BETA-2 MICROGLOBULIN.

B & D   Also written as B/D and BD. Short for bondage and discipline, a sexual practice that involves sadomasochistic (S & M or SM) activities such as whipping or flogging. Even though partners usually signal when an activity exceeds pleasurable limits, such practices expose participants to considerable risk. Emotional and physical safety and disease prevention are increasingly common subjects of discussion in S & M literature, and such practices are increasingly common among those who participate in such activities. Bleeding, abrasion, infection, and bruises can sometimes result from activities in B & D. Any time the skin is broken, there is the risk of disease transmission and infection. Any equipment used in these activities needs to be thoroughly cleaned before and after each use so any viruses or bacteria are not passed from person to person, regardless of how slight the likelihood may seem. If beating or whipping is involved, avoid the kidney and abdomen areas. If restraint is used, check to make sure blood flow is not cut off. Never exceed the limits that have been set before initiating the activity or that are restated during the activity.

B cell   See B LYMPHOCYTE.

B lymphocyte   A type of white blood cell (also called a B cell) responsible for producing antibodies to attack certain diseases. B lymphocytes are distinct from T lymphocytes (including CD4 cells, also called T4 cells), which are also part of the immune system, but work against a different group of microbes using different mechanisms. B lymphocytes are formed from pluripotent stem cells in the BONE MARROW that migrate to the spleen, lymph nodes, and other peripheral tissue where they come into contact with foreign antigens and become mature functioning cells. Mature B cells independently identify foreign antigens and differentiate into antibody-producing plasma cells or memory cells. Plasma cells are the only source of immunoglobulins (antibodies).

baboon bone marrow   See BONE MARROW TRANSPLANTATION.

bacillary angiomatosis   A bacterial illness commonly called cat scratch fever. It is caused by two varieties of *Bartonella* bacteria. *Bartonella henselae* is the known cause of cat scratch fever. *Bartonella quintana* is the known cause of trench fever, which was first diagnosed in soldiers in Europe during World War I. *B. henselae* is a bacterium that causes a minor infection in cats, passed usually through flea bites. It is generally seen in patients that live with cats. *B. quintana* has typically been seen in homeless people in the United States, it is passed by body lice. Most people that contract bacillary angiomatosis report being scratched or bitten by cats, but it is the flea bites that pass the bacteria. The bacteria causes a self-limiting, mild infection in healthy people.

In people with compromised immune systems, especially people who are HIV positive, it is characterized by the eruption of lesions both on and below the skin. As the number of lesions increases, patients may develop fever, sweats, chills, poor appetite, vomiting, and weight loss. If untreated, patients die from complications of the disease. It can be diagnosed from blood tests developed in the 1990s. It is sometimes mistaken for Kaposi's sarcoma because it, too, is a disease of the blood vessels. The lesions, papules, or nodules are usually purplish to bright red. They do not turn white when pushed on, and they do not generally occur on the palms, soles, or in the mouth. Continued infection can cause the blood vessels to grow out of control and form tumorlike masses in skin, bone, liver, and other organs. It can be successfully treated with antibiotics for a period of three to four weeks. Patients with cats in their homes should treat the animals for fleas, so the illness is not repeated.

bacille Calmette-Guérin (BCG) vaccine A vaccine containing a bovine-derived live attenuated strain of mycobacterium that has been used in countries other than the United States as immunization against human tuberculous.

baclofen A drug used to control muscle spasms. The most common side effect is drowsiness and, in large doses, severe sedation, lack of coordination, and lowered functioning of the heart and lungs. (The trade name is Lioresal.)

bacteremia The presence of bacteria in the blood. Medical workers define three types of bacteremia: transient, intermittent, and continuous. Transient bacteremia occurs after actions such as brushing teeth or cleaning a wound on the skin. Intermittent bacteremia is usually associated with an undrained abscess. Continuous bacteremia, also called SEPSIS, can be caused by a number of bodily infections or through venous or arterial CATHETERS. It is produced by flora from the skin that migrates into the body through the catheter.

bacteria A class of single-celled MICROORGANISMS characterized by a lack of distinct cellular components. They may be aerobic or anaerobic, motile or nonmotile, and may exist independently, in decaying matter, or as parasites. Those that can cause disease in humans are called pathogenic bacteria.

bacterial culture See CULTURE.

bacterial infection The state or condition in which the body or part of it is invaded by bacteria that have multiplied and caused injurious effects.

bacterial pneumonia An inflammation of the lungs caused by bacteria. Although PNEUMOCYSTIS CARINII PNEUMONIA (PCP) is more widely associated with AIDS, bacterial pneumonia also occurs frequently among HIV-infected persons. Community-acquired bacterial infections of all sorts often affect persons with HIV, both women and men. Bacterial pneumonia is also common in pregnancy and may be more common in HIV-positive pregnant women. Symptoms of bacterial pneumonia include fever, wet cough, and chest pain. Some infections are easily treated with standard oral or intravenous antibiotics, while some lead to life-threatening complications. Pneumococcal vaccination (along with annual influenza vaccination) has been recommended for people with HIV disease with more than 200 T4 cells, although its effectiveness in HIV disease is unknown. Other strategies for dealing with persons at risk include cessation of smoking, the use of trimethoprim-sulfamethoxazole, immunoglobulin therapy, and antimicrobial prophylaxis. See PNEUMONIA.

bacterial vaginosis One of three major causes of vaginal discharge. (The others are *Candida* and *Trichomonas* species.) Bacterial vaginosis produces a change in the normal bacterial flora of the vagina. The direct cause of the change is not known, and it is unclear whether it is contagious. The condition is called vaginosis instead of vaginitis because there is no apparent inflammation. Bacterial vaginosis causes a discharge that is often malodorous but does not typically cause itching. This problem has led to slang terms that refer to women as "fish" or statements about "fishy" odors of the vagina. Treatment typically employs metronidazole.

bacteriophage A virus that infects bacteria. Bacteriophages are found throughout nature and have been isolated in excrement, polluted water, and sewage. They are regarded as "bacterial viruses." The phage particle consists of a head composed of either RNA or DNA and a tail by which it attaches to a host cell.

bacterium See BACTERIA.

Bactrim See TRIMETHOPRIM-SULFAMETHOXAZOLE (TMP-SMX).

baculovirus   An insect, arachnid (spiders), and crustacean (shellfish) virus used in the production of some HIV vaccines that are being designed. It does not infect higher life forms such as monkeys or humans. See VACCINE; VACCINE DEVELOPMENT.

bad debt   In the medical industry, unpaid hospital bills, which may include in-house charity care, Hill-Burton cases, and balances in which a hospital charges more than MEDICARE, MEDICAID, or insurance contracts allow.

bad sex   Cultural analysis fueled by the AIDS epidemic often pits "good sex" against "bad sex." These terms refer not to the subjective quality of a sexual experience but, in this context, to "safe" and unsafe practice.

People do not "catch" AIDS. They may be infected with HIV, which over a period of time may or may not cause AIDS, but they will do so only through very intimate physical contact, when bodily fluids are passed from one body to another. People do not "catch" HIV through causal social contact. With the proper precautions, nobody has to "catch" HIV. Current AIDS prevention activities, rather than emphasizing the negative aspects of bad or unsafe sex, emphasizes the positive aspects of good or safe sex. The positive approach stresses that even if sexual behavior patterns have to be changed to prevent infection, they can still lead to satisfaction and complete erotic fulfillment, and may even lead to greater intimacy and mutual understanding between partners. While bad or unsafe sex can also lead to satisfaction and erotic fulfillment, it increases the risk of contracting HIV (as well as other sexually transmitted diseases) during sexual contact. Bad sex includes such behaviors as impromptu, unprotected sexual encounters or engaging in frequent, non-relational unprotected sex. In this context, bad sex is also approaching sex with fear and anxiety, avoiding the facts, and making negative choices about how one lives one's life.

BAL   See BRONCHOALVEOLAR LAVAGE.

band   An immature NEUTROPHIL is called a band or band cell.

barbiturates   Drugs derived from barbituric acid and commonly used to treat insomnia, anxiety, and seizures. All barbiturates affect the central nervous system. Low doses cause mild sedation, and high doses can lead to deep coma. When barbiturates are used for sedation, they remain effective for only about two weeks, unless doses are escalated. This is because tolerance to these drugs develops quickly. As a result, alternative drugs are generally preferred to treat insomnia. Barbiturates' most important roles are prevention of delirium tremens (the DTs) that results from alcohol withdrawal and in the induction of anesthesia. The major side effects are symptoms of central nervous system depression, including drowsiness, depression, lethargy, and hangovers, as well as stomach pain, allergic reactions, and fever. Prolonged use of high doses of the drug can cause physical dependence, psychological dependence, and tolerance. Discontinuing use of barbiturates can cause withdrawal symptoms similar to those experienced by an alcoholic who has abruptly stopped drinking. Examples of barbiturates include amobarbital (trade name Amytal), pentobarbital (trade name Nembutal), phenobarbital, and secobarbital.

bareback sex   UNPROTECTED anal SEX among HIV-positive gay men, many of whom appear to believe that we are in the twilight of the AIDS epidemic and that they will not be infected with HIV—or that if they are infected, they will not die. Bareback sex was a phenomenon of the late 1990s (which became a popular topic of discussion on the Internet). The late 1990s witnessed better HIV treatment and alarming rates of new HIV infection among gay men. There is generally believed to be a connection, even if it is impossible to say that it is one of direct cause and effect. There is little doubt that attitudes toward AIDS have been changing, and that some gay men are engaging in unsafe sex at higher rates than before the advent of PROTEASE INHIBITORS. This is particularly true among young gay males who may not have experienced the crisis of the disease in the early to mid-1980s. Unprotected sex can have serious consequences. Even if both partners are infected, one partner may not have had opportunistic infections, and he may contract one. Another major concern is that someone with a strain of HIV that responds well to drugs could have the virus change to a drug-resistant one introduced by a sexual partner. AIDS educators fear that unsafe behavior may have an effect on HIV-negative men as well, by eroding their negative views about being HIV-positive. For men who prefer to return to condomless intimacy, this trend only accentuates that attitude. Some argue, however, that some unsafe sex has been occurring all along and that the availability of protease inhibitors and combination therapies may simply be focusing attention on it. Although barrier-free sex may be occurring more often these days, participants must be educated to recognize the inherent dangers of these activities.

Baridol See BARIUM SULFATE.

barium A soft metallic element of the alkaline earth group. Barium sulfate is used as a contrast medium in X-ray examinations of the gastrointestinal tract. The barium outlines the anatomical forms, allowing irregularities to be spotted.

barium sulfate A compound used during X rays and (CT) scans to assist medical personnel to detect masses, tumors, or other abnormalities of the esophagus, stomach, small bowel, and colon. Barium sulfate is radiopaque, which means it is visible under x-ray technology. It is given either as a milky drink or as an enema. Sometimes it can cause severe constipation or impaction, so eliminating the barium after a procedure is very important. Laxatives may be used to encourage elimination of all the barium sulfate.

barrier See CONTRACEPTIVE; SAFE SEX.

Bartholin's duct A duct that drains one of the two BARTHOLIN'S GLANDS, located at each side of the vaginal opening; also called the ductus sublingualis major. CYSTS or abscesses may form in Bartholin's duct as a result of an acute infection such as GONORRHEA or CHLAMYDIA and may become a recurrent or chronic ABSCESS, secondary to obstruction in the duct. The cystic mass may be small or large, sterile or infected, asymptomatic or very tender. Treatment is with local heat or sitzbaths, along with a broad-spectrum antibiotic where purulence is noted.

Bartholin's gland One of a pair of glands located at each side of the vaginal opening; drained by BARTHOLIN'S DUCT. Also called the glandula vestibularis major. They secrete lubricating mucosal fluid for the vagina and the vulva.

basal cell A type of cell found in the innermost layers of the skin.

basal-cell carcinoma The most common, and least lethal, form of skin cancer. It usually develops on areas of the skin exposed to sunlight. It commonly appears as a small nodular bump that is raised from the surrounding skin and has a pearly quality. Small basal-cell carcinomas can resemble MOLLUSCUM CONTAGIOSUM, which is occasionally found in HIV disease. It can also appear as a firm scarlike patch. Basal-cell skin cancer is very slow-growing and seldom fatal. Diagnosis requires the removal of some tissue for a biopsy (a microscopic examination for cancer cells). Frequently, if the cancer is small, the biopsy also removes the cancer. However, if the area is sizable, more tissue may have to be removed until there are "clean margins." Treatment depends on the size of the tumor, the type of tumor, and the general health of the patient. Treatment is generally surgery to remove the cancer. The main cause of basal-cell carcinoma of the skin is ultraviolet radiation from the Sun.

base pairing The process, during genetic replication, in which nucleic acid bases pair with their opposites. Every base pair contains one purine and one pyrmidine. Adenine and thymidine are always paired, as are guanine and cytosine. The result of this pairing is that two different nucleic acid molecules with complementary sequences wrap around each other to form a double helix. The double helix is the basic shape of DNA.

baseline The beginning point of a CLINICAL TRIAL, just before a volunteer starts to receive the experimental treatment undergoing testing; the point at which BASELINE VALUES are determined.

baseline CD4 count The BASELINE VALUE of CD4 at the start of a clinical trial or the beginning of a course of treatment. The CD4 COUNT was once believed to be a complete SURROGATE MARKER, but current diagnostic and prognostic technology suggest otherwise.

baseline value   The initial measurement of a crucial SURROGATE MARKER or indicator, made at the start of a clinical trial or a course of treatment as a reference point for later measurements, allowing for assessment of results.

basic research   Basic or pure research in the sciences; not product oriented.

basket   Slang term for the protuberance of the male sex organs.

basophil   A blood cell that has high-affinity RECEPTORS for IgE and generates inflammatory mediators in ALLERGY; a granular leukocyte characterized by the possession of coarse, bluish black granules of varying size that stain intensely with basic dyes. It represents less than 1 percent of all leukocytes.

bathhouse   The gay liberation movement of the 1970s spawned a sex industry, with bathhouses and sex clubs, back-room bars, bookstores, porno theaters, and other businesses, all of which advertised in local gay papers. Of these, bathhouses and sex clubs remained major centers of gay sexual activity through the mid-1980s and were vital to the social cohesiveness and economic viability of gay communities in large cities like Los Angeles, New York, Paris, and San Francisco.

Bathhouses were sex emporiums, sprawling sex palaces characterized by a complete focus on the physical aspect of sex. Labyrinthine hallways, private rooms with doors, private cubicles, dark back rooms, dim lights that encouraged orgies, and dormitories where group sex was conducted were commonplace. Sex was oriented toward eroticism and the exchange of semen. Frequent, nonrelational, anonymous sexual behavior was de rigueur. Bathhouses were also havens for anal intercourse. The only limit to promiscuity was stamina.

Bathhouses were designed to make many partners available to all—ensuring that everyone had a high chance of being infected. By the early 1980s, virtually every study on sexually transmitted diseases had shown for years that gay men who went to bathhouses were far more likely than others to be infected with whatever venereal disease was going around. While AIDS would have crept through the United States without bathhouses, bathhouses guaranteed the rapid spread of AIDS among gay men. By the early to mid-1980s, common sense dictated that they be closed down. The inevitable impassioned bathhouse controversy is one of the gay political landmarks of the early to mid-1980s. The controversy pitted bathhouse owners against public health officials, businesspersons against politicians, spokespeople of the gay rights movement against "concerned individuals," community leaders against physicians, government against media. The challenge of balancing public health and private rights was at the heart of the controversy. The issue ultimately became one, however, not of civil liberties, but of money. In his book *And the Band Played On,* Randy Shilts writes, "The bathhouses weren't open because the owners didn't understand they were spreading death. They understood that. The bathhouses were open because they were still making money."

In the early 1980s many bathhouse owners agreed to put out brochures and post notices about AIDS. Others rallied against steps to impede bathhouse sex. In the face of increasing pressures (to support AIDS education, to impose regulations to ban high-risk sexual activity, to shut down), many owners joined forces and formed organizations such as the Northern California Bathhouse Owners Association, protesting that gay businesses should not be singled out for harassment during the AIDS crisis. Inspections of bathhouses increased, as did publicity, and attempts to close them down. By the mid-1980s, support for the facilities had steadily dropped within the gay community. Gay America's changing response to the AIDS epidemic, and the subsequent business decline, ultimately proved lethal for many bathhouses and private sex clubs.

BCG   See BACILLUS CALMETTE-GUÉRIN.

BCX-34   A purine nucleoside phosphorylase inhibitor, similar to hydroxyurea. It did not prove helpful against HIV in trials and was discontinued by the maker, BioCryst Pharmaceuticals.

bDNA assay   See BRANCHED DNA ASSAY.

bedsore   A sore most often due to pressure from confinement in bed or from a cast or splint. There are four stages of manifestation. First is skin redness, warmth, or tenderness usually near a bone. The second stage is a blister or break in the skin that is red. The third stage involves an ulcer or sore that extends down to the muscle or fat of a person, beyond the layers of skin. A fourth stage bedsore extends all the way to the bone; the area is white or black and may involve fluid draining.

Emaciated or weak HIV/AIDS patients and those who must remain immobile because of orthopedic or similar problems are especially likely to have bedsores. These are generally located in areas over bony prominences only thinly covered with flesh, such as the end of the spine, hips, heels, elbows, and shoulder blades. The number one cause of bedsores is infrequent change of position of someone who is bedridden or bound to a wheelchair. Persons with HIV/AIDS are more likely to experience bedsores if they have any of the other predisposing causes: injury or illness that weakens circulation of the blood and interferes with mobility, prolonged fever, paralysis, cardiac diseases, nephritis; diabetes, or anemia, poor nutrition, poorly made beds, beds containing irritating bits of debris and lack of cleanliness are other causes.

Patients should be turned or moved on a regular schedule, several times a day. Generally treatment entails keeping the bed dry and clean, relieving pressure as soon as the first signs of redness appear, and using prescribed medication strictly as directed. Maintenance of proper nutrition, chemical or surgical débridement of ulcers, use of sheepskin or a substitute under a vulnerable area, and use of a special air bed are also generally recommended.

behavioral techniques   One of several types of activities that constitute effective HIV prevention. Others include HIV treatment interventions and other medical interventions, such as timely treatment of STDs, substance abuse treatment, and psychiatric and mental health treatment for persons with psychological disorders or severe mental illness. Behavioral techniques include the promotion of voluntary HIV counseling and testing, prevention case management of HIV-infected persons and those at risk for infection, health education and risk reduction counseling of adolescents, injection drug users, people with STDs, men who have sex with men, and women at risk for infection; street and community outreach for those at risk; school- and prison-based health education and risk reduction counseling; and implementation of syringe exchange programs.

behavior, risky   See RISK BEHAVIORS.

beneficiary   The person(s), institution(s), trustee(s), or estates named to receive death benefits, if any, from insurance or annuity contracts.

benefit   SOCIAL SECURITY, welfare, MEDICAID, MEDICARE, food stamps, housing, and drugs are among the financial, health care, nutrition, and other public welfare benefits that are available to persons with HIV/AIDS. These benefits are also available to the indigent, disabled, or elderly who are eligible for them. Unlike the traditional poor, disabled, and elderly who have long had institutional support to help them access benefits, persons with HIV/AIDS and their advocates often have virtually no personal knowledge of public benefit programs or their eligibility rules. Today, most persons with HIV/AIDS and their advocates are aware that the programs available to them are often complicated and obscure and vary widely from jurisdiction to jurisdiction. Working within the current American social benefits system is often difficult, frustrating, and enormously intimidating.

Major federal benefits programs include AID TO FAMILIES WITH DEPENDENT CHILDREN (AFDC); AZT DRUG ASSISTANCE; EMERGENCY ASSISTANCE (EA); the FOOD STAMP (FS) PROGRAM; GENERAL ASSISTANCE (GA); GENERAL MEDICAL ASSISTANCE; the HILL-BURTON PROGRAM; LOW INCOME HOME ENERGY ASSISTANCE (LIHEA); Medicaid; Medicare; the SOCIAL SERVICES BLOCK GRANT program; SOCIAL SECURITY DISABILITY INSURANCE (SSDI); SUPPLEMENTAL SECURITY INCOME (SSI); STATE SUPPLEMENTARY PAYMENTS (SSPs); and the TEMPORARY EMERGENCY FOOD ASSISTANCE (TEFA) PROGRAM. Benefits may also be obtained from the DEPARTMENT OF VETERANS AFFAIRS (VA).

benign In medicine, noncancerous (of a growth).

benwa balls A sex aid consisting of small metal or plastic balls that are placed in the vagina.

benzodiazepine Any of a class of drugs commonly used to treat anxiety, insomnia, seizures, and painful muscles. In general, all benzodiazepines act in similar ways and seem to be equally effective. Most physicians prefer benzodiazepines to BARBITURATES and MEPROBAMATE for treating anxiety and tension. When given at effective doses, they are less addictive and produce less sedation. Major side effects are drowsiness, loss of coordination, confusion, dizziness, and fainting. People taking benzodiazepines should be aware that the drug may impair their ability to perform activities that require mental alertness and physical coordination. Benzodiazepines can also cause physical dependence and symptoms of severe withdrawal if stopped suddenly after regular use over a substantial time. These drugs include alprazolam (trade name Xanax), diazepam (trade name Valium), flurazepam hydrochloride (trade name Dalmane), lorazepam (trade name Centrax), temazepam (trade name Restoril), and triazolam (trade name Halcion).

benzoyl peroxide A class of skin cleaners that are used in the treatment of skin infection and acne due to their ANTIBACTERIAL and ANTIFUNGAL properties.

bequest Personal property left to another by will.

bestiality Sexual interest in/or contact with animals. Also called *zoophilia*.

beta cell One of the cells making up the islets of Langerhans, in the PANCREAS. Beta cells secrete the HORMONE insulin. BASOPHILIC cells in the anterior lobe of the pituitary are also called beta cells.

beta-carotene Beta-carotene is a member of a larger family of nutrients termed carotenoids. There are more than 500 of these substances. Examples are lutein and zeaxanthin, found in spinach, kale, and broccoli; and lycopenes, found in tomatoes and pink grapefruit. It is believed that the interaction of various carotenoids and other nutrients—phytochemicals—helps prevent disease. The specific reactions are not all known but are currently being studied. Beta-carotene is a carotenoid that is converted into VITAMIN A in the body. It is a red-orange substance found in leafy dark green vegetables such as spinach, beet greens, and kale and yellow or deep orange vegetables and fruits, such as butternut squash and cantaloupe. People who take VITAMIN A supplements often substitute beta-carotene because unlike vitamin A, beta-carotene is water-soluble, so it does not build up in the body and cause problems. Initial research derived from dietary histories—mostly involving beta-carotene from foods—suggested that it could lower the risk of cancer and possibly other diseases. There was no evidence of adverse effects other than potential to turn skin slightly yellow or orange, an effect that is harmless and disappears when doses are lowered. In 1996 in the United States, a study (the CARET Study) examined the effect of beta-carotene on people at higher risk for lung cancer: people who were smokers, former smokers, and asbestos industry workers. The study was halted after it became clear that the people taking the beta-carotene supplements in the study actually had significantly higher (28 percent higher) rates of lung cancer than those *not* taking the beta-carotene. A similar study in Finland showed similar results. The bottom line is that persons should not use beta-carotene supplements if they are a smoker or an ex-smoker. The mix of chemicals in the smoke and the beta-carotene have since been shown to disable the beta-carotene and cause it to build up in the body, where it is typically broken down by vitamin C. However, vitamin C levels in smokers are very low and do not take care of the job, causing dangerous levels of beta-carotene. Beta-carotene can still be received in a safe natural form by eating plenty of leafy green vegetables. Small amounts in multivitamins are also considered harmless.

While small increases in dietary vitamin A may stabilize blood cells so their immune abilities may be enhanced, an excess of vitamin A may harm immune response. For this reason, vitamin A should be replaced with beta-carotene, which as an antioxidant, has its own potential to fight disease. The body excretes any excess amounts not absorbed, eliminating the risk of toxicity experienced with vitamin A. In laboratory tests, beta-carotene can stimulate immune cells so that they are better able to fight off such infections as CANDIDA ALBICANS, the sort that multiply in AIDS patients. Adding beta-carotene to suspensions of immune cells called NEUTROPHILS more than doubled the kill rate of *Candida*.

beta-2 microglobulin (β2M) A LYMPHOCYTE membrane protein that is tightly bound to the surface of all cells with a nucleus. β2M is released into the blood when a cell dies. Elevated β2M levels occur in a variety of diseases and cancers. They are associated with immune activity. Although β2M activity is nonspecific for HIV infection, there is a weak correlation between elevated β2M levels and progression of HIV disease.

beta-2 microglobulin test A test that doctors use to monitor the immune status of someone who has the HIV virus.

bezafibrate An antihyperlipidemic drug that can control high triglyceride levels in people when diet and exercise have not worked. It is in the class of drugs known as FIBRATES. There are potential side effects of all of these drugs, which include elevated liver enzyme levels and a myostitislike illness that impairs renal function. These drugs also typically do not lower the cholesterol levels in patients and can be given with a STATIN in cases of high cholesterol levels. (Trade name is Bezalip.)

BHT See BUTYLATED HYDROXYTUOLENE.

bi See BISEXUAL.

BIA See BIOELECTRICAL IMPEDANCE ANALYSIS.

Biaxin See CLARITHROMYCIN.

bicyclam A member of a group of chemical compounds that affect HIV's ability to bind with healthy cells. See FUSION INHIBITOR.

B.I.D. (*bis in die*) Latin phrase that translates as "twice daily." The letters *B.I.D.* often appear in a pharmacist's or doctor's prescription instructions.

bidirectional transmission See TRANSMISSION.

bile-acid resins A class of drugs that have been shown to reduce LDL "bad" cholesterol by 10 percent to 30 percent in HIV-negative people; examples include cholestyramine (Questran) and colestipol (Colestid). These drugs bind with cholesterol in the intestines and prevent it from being absorbed into the bloodstream. The cholesterol is then removed from the body with each bowel movement. Bile-acid resins are often used in combination with other lipid-lowering drugs. This is because bile-acid resins can actually cause triglyceride levels to increase. Side effects of these drugs include stomachaches, bloating, flatulence (farting), heartburn, and constipation. Another problem with bile-acid resins is that they should be taken two hours before other medications, including antiretrovirals. This can be challenging for HIV-positive people who are already overwhelmed by a two- or three-times-daily medication schedule. Bile-acid resins have not yet been studied in HIV-positive patients with increased lipid levels associated with lipodystrophy.

bilirubin The orange-colored or yellowish pigment in bile. It is carried to the liver by the blood. It is produced from hemoglobin of red blood cells by RETICULOENDOTHELIAL CELLS in bone marrow. It is changed chemically in the liver and excreted in the bile via the duodenum. As it passes through the intestines, it is converted into urobilinogen by bacterial enzymes, and most of it is excreted through the feces. If urobilinogen passes into the circulation, it is excreted through the urine or reexcreted in the bile. The accumulation of bilirubin leads to jaundice in many cases. An elevated level in blood serum is an indication of liver disease or drug-induced liver impairment. The normal value for bilirubin is 0.1 to 1.5 milligrams per liter of blood.

binding antibody In HIV studies it is an ANTIBODY that attaches itself to some part of the HIV. The binding antibody may or may not cause the death of the virus.

binding site The spot where two things join together. HIV requires two binding sites before it can fuse with the cell's membrane and begin replication. The virus locates the protein CD4 and locks on to the immune cell. Then, depending on whether the cell is a macrophage or a lymphocyte, the virus uses CHEMOKINE RECEPTORS to attach itself fully into the host cell. Once that has happened, replication of the virus can begin. HIV uses a protein called GP120 to bind to the body's immune cells.

bioavailability   The extent to which an oral medication or food supplement is absorbed in the digestive tract and is available for the body's use. Some medications are more bioavailable than others. Some have bioavailability affected by other food or body processes. This is why some medications are prescribed for use on an empty stomach or why particular foods must not be eaten when the medicine is prescribed. These measures ensure the drug's bioavailability in the body. If a drug has low bioavailability, then much of it is destroyed by stomach acid, or is not absorbed in the small intestine, or is removed by first-pass metabolism in the liver. The amount of drug taken in a pill is calculated to correct for this so that the amount actually needed enters the blood. Once drugs are past the liver, the bloodstream carries them throughout the rest of the body in about one minute. In order to work, they have to move from the bloodstream into the infected cells. Some generic drugs have different bioavailability from that of their patented counterparts because of minor manufacturing differences. Switching to generic drugs should be monitored to determine whether changes in bioavailability occur.

bioelectrical impedance analysis (BIA)   A simple painless procedure that enables a doctor or health care provider to analyze the amounts of fat, muscle, and water in the body. For persons with HIV disease, the loss of weight, specifically of lean body mass (LBM), which is also known as fat-free mass (FFM), can be very serious. FFM is muscle as well as the metabolically active tissue in the organs. The loss of LBM may be an indication of wasting. Without the proper amount of LBM, the body does not function properly, and with the loss of one-third or more, death can result. If the loss of lean body mass is significant, measures to reverse the loss may be necessary. Using anabolic agents such as steroid hormones and human growth hormone in conjunction with resistance exercise and good nutrition can be beneficial. In addition to indicating how much LBM an individual has, BIA can give information about hydration status. Hydration, or the amount of water in the body, is very important for overall health.

BIA can be given in a doctor's office and takes only a few minutes. The test is performed with the individual lying down. Electrodes are placed on the wrist and the ankle on one side of the body. Then a small electrical current is passed through the body and measurements are made. The electrical current is so small that it cannot be felt at all. After the information is collected, it is entered into a computer, which calculates the percentages of fat, muscle, and water in the body according to height, weight, sex, and age. A single BIA measurement is not as important as tracking of BIA over time, to show trends in a person's body composition.

bioenergetics   A kind of psychotherapy based on the idea that repressed emotions and desires create chronic muscular tension, diminish vitality and energy, and thereby wound the psyche. Through physical exercises, breathing techniques, or other forms of emotional-release work, combined with "talk therapy," therapists attempt to loosen "character armor" and restore natural well-being.

biofeedback   A technique of monitoring minute, normally imperceptible metabolic changes in one's own body, such as temperature changes, heart rate, and muscle tension, with the aid of sensitive machines, for the purposes of exerting control over them consciously. By visualizing, relaxing, or imagining, while observing light, sound, or metered feedback, one is said to be able to learn to make subtle adjustments to achieve a more balanced internal state. For some people this can be an effective way of controlling pain. The technique is also used for stress-related conditions, such as asthma, migraines, insomnia, and high blood pressure.

biological cofactor   Any physico-chemical variable, such as the effect of a toxin or vitamin deficiency on the rate of HIV progression, that influences the pace, and perhaps the direction, of HIV's course.

biological response modifier (BRM)   Any agent that boosts the body's immune system by stimulating it, modifying it, or restoring it. There are many types of BRMs, some produced naturally in the body, others made synthetically. The major biological response modifiers are antibodies, MONOCLONAL ANTIBODIES, VACCINES, COLONY-STIMULATING FACTORS, and CYTOKINES, which include the INTERFERONS and INTERLEUKINS.

biological warfare   An alternative theory of the origin of AIDS that holds that AIDS is the result of the deliberate manipulation of human genes to defeat the body's immune response, as part of a program of biological warfare. The culprit is typically said to be the Pentagon or the now defunct Soviet Union. In some parts of Africa and among some people in the United States it is alleged to be an attempt to kill all people of African descent. Today, the theory that AIDS was created for or used as biowarfare, a descendant of any of a number of germ warfare programs, has been banished beyond the periphery of respectability. Numerous articles describing medical research and reports by the medical establishment and the press, including many "alternative" publications that cover AIDS extensively, have shown this legend not to be accurate or true.

biomaterial dumping   The sale in bulk and at a price below the domestic market price of a natural or synthetic substance that is compatible with living tissue and is suitable for surgical implantation, especially in a foreign market.

biomedical discourse   See BIOMEDICINE; CULTURAL ANALYSIS AND AIDS.

biomedicine   The practice of medicine based on the application of the natural sciences, especially biology and physiology.

biopsy   A procedure in which a small sample of some tissue or organ is removed for laboratory examination under a microscope. The microscopic changes in tissue often indicate a diagnosis, and stains and CULTURES for MICROBES will often reveal the infecting organism. Many biopsies are performed with long needles with special tips that are pushed into an area or organ. A biopsy may be performed on an outpatient basis when the area to be biopsied is near the surface or in the lungs or gastrointestinal tract and can be reached with an ENDOSCOPE, an instrument passed through the mouth or anus. The biopsy of organs deep within the body may require a surgical procedure. Means of obtaining tissue for biopsy include aspiration (by use of a needle attached to a syringe); needle (by use of a needle with a hollow point); punch (by use of a hollow punch); brush (by use of a brush); and endoscopic.

birth control pill   A drug taken by women to achieve contraception. It works by preventing ovulation.

birth defect   A congenital anomaly.

birth rate   The number of live births in one year for each 1,000 persons in the population.

bisexual   Although most people are exclusively heterosexual or homosexual in orientation during their entire adult lives, there is also a vast number of people who are both—those whose sexual desires are aroused, often or occasionally, in fantasy or in fact, by both men and women. People in this group are known as bisexuals. Slang terms include bi, versatile, and AC/DC.

bis-POM PMEA   See ADEFOVIR.

biting   In October 1995, the *New York Times* reported that a 91-year-old man in Florida, had become infected with HIV after a prostitute bit his hand. Prior to that incident, there was apparently only one previous case on record of HIV being transmitted through a bite. Health officials do not believe that the 1995 case will significantly change the way scientists think the disease is spread. Apparently, both cases involved the spreading of blood between the persons involved. The CENTERS FOR DISEASE CONTROL AND PREVENTION claims that no cases of HIV TRANSMISSION are clearly attributable only to saliva, and states that there has been a number of reports of bites from people infected with HIV that did not spread the infection. Officials at the CDC do not keep statistics on such bites, as they do on cases in which people are stuck by needles that have been used by someone infected or presumed to be infected with HIV. If bites and saliva were important in the transmission of HIV, however, many more cases attributable to such facilities would have been identified among the cases reported to date.

Bites by children rarely draw blood or break the skin. Federal health recommendations say the type of educational and health care setting in which children with HIV are placed should be determined by their behavior, neurological development, and physical condition, and by the way they could be expected to interact with other children in a given setting. The recommendations call for the decision to be made on a case-by-case basis by a team including the child's doctor, parents or guardians, public health workers, and school officials.

bitter melon *Momordica charantia* is a member of the Cucurbitaceae (gourd) family and a relative of squash, watermelon, muskmelon, and cucumber. It is also known by other names in various parts of the world: bitter gourd, balsam pear (United States), *fu kwa* (China), *kerala* (India), *nigai uri* (Japan), and *ampalaya* (Philippines). In the Amazon region and parts of Asia this plant's leaves and fruit are used as herbal medicines for a variety of purposes, including inducing abortions, treating fevers, infections, and colic; and acting as an antidiabetic. Scientists have extracted several active proteins from bitter melon, including MAP-30 and alpha- and beta-momorcharin. Tests have not been conducted on humans with any of these proteins, so claims about usefulness in HIV treatment are questionable. Bitter melon is often sold as an herb or pill at health food stores. People should be particularly careful about using bitter melon if they are hypoglycemic as it is used for diabetes treatment in China.

blackout A sudden loss of consciousness; condition characterized by a temporary loss of con-

sciousness and failure of vision due to reduced blood circulation to the brain; a period of total memory loss induced by prolonged ingestion of alcohol and drugs.

bladder A membranous sac or receptacle for a secretion, as the GALLBLADDER. Used alone, the term commonly refers to the urinary bladder.

blanc fixe See BARIUM SULFATE.

bleach Ordinary chlorine bleach is highly effective in killing HIV within minutes. It is recommended for killing any virus or other microbe that may be present in such body fluids as blood, saliva, and stool. Mixed in water at a strength of 1:10 (one part bleach in ten parts of water), it can be applied to surfaces or on clothes.

bleomycin A chemotherapeutic drug used in the experimental treatment of AIDS-associated KAPOSI'S SARCOMA (KS). Specifically, any of a group of antibiotics produced by a strain of *Streptomyces verticillus*. Commonly used in conjunction with other chemotherapies for treatment of HODGKIN'S DISEASE and NON-HODGKIN'S LYMPHOMAS, squamous cell carcinomas of the head and neck, testicular carcinoma, and uterine cervix carcinoma. Fever, nausea, and vomiting are common side effects. Other side effects include occasionally fatal dose-related pneumonia, pulmonary fibrosis, and severe skin reactions.

blind test A trial of a drug or form of therapy in which one group of patients will receive the drug or therapy being tested and another group will be given a placebo or ineffective therapy; neither group knows which is which. In a "double blind" test those conducting the test are also "blinded." Blind tests are designed to prevent patients' or testers' judgment from being influenced by their expectations.

blinding See BLIND TEST.

blindness The leading causes in the United States are cataract, glaucoma, and age-related macular degeneration. In AIDS, blindness can be caused by

CYTOMEGALOVIRUS (CMV) retinitis or CRYPTOCOCCAL MENINGITIS.

blood The fluid that circulates through the heart, arteries, veins, and capillaries, carrying nourishment, ELECTROLYTES, HORMONES, vitamins, ANTIBODIES, heat, and oxygen to the tissues, and taking away waste matter and carbon dioxide. Human blood is composed of fluid (plasma) in which are suspended red blood cells (erythrocytes), which carry oxygen; white blood cells (leukocytes), which help make up the immune system; platelets (thrombocytes), required for coagulation; fat globules; and a great variety of chemical substances, including carbohydrates, proteins, hormones, and gases such as oxygen, carbon dioxide, and nitrogen. Blood consists of approximately 22 percent solids and 78 percent water. See BLOOD PLASMA.

blood bank A facility for the collection, processing and storage of whole blood and certain derived components for transfusion.

Blood is mixed with adenine-supplemented citrate phosphate dextrose and is stored at 4°C (39°F). Heparin may be used as a preservative. Banked blood should be used as soon as possible because the longer it is stored, the fewer red blood cells survive in usable form. Ninety percent of the red cells survive up to 14 days of storage, but only 70 percent remain after 24 days.

blood cell differential Can also be called blood differential; a blood test that measures relative numbers of white blood cells and the amount of various types of the white blood cells. It can also be used to measure changes in the size and shape of red blood cells (ERYTHROCYTES), which can be of greater importance than changes in the total white and red blood cell counts. Ascertaining changes in the proportions of the different kinds of white blood cells helps to diagnose different diseases and disease processes. Proportions that are considered normal are neutrophils, 40 percent to 60 percent; lymphocytes, 20 percent to 40 percent; monocytes, 2 percent to 8 percent; eosinophils, 1 percent to 4 percent; basophils, 0.5 percent to 1 percent; band, 0 percent to 3 percent.

blood clot A coagulated mass of blood. See COAGULATION.

blood count The number of red and white blood cells and platelets in a unit of blood. It is determined by a relatively simple, inexpensive standard test, in which the red blood cells are stained as well as counted, to reveal their size, shape, and hemoglobin content. Blood for testing is usually taken from a vein, but a drop from the heel, fingertip, or earlobe may also be drawn. The blood is examined through a microscope and counted manually or electronically. Normal red cell counts may vary from 4 to 6 million per unit (one cubic millimeter [cu mm]) for men; for women, slightly lower; and for newborn babies, higher. A low red cell count is called ANEMIA; a low white cell count is called LEUKOPENIA; a low platelet count is called THROMBOCYTOPENIA. People infected with HIV commonly have low red counts, low white counts, and low platelet counts. A normal white cell count is 5,000 to 10,000 per unit for adults; children may have higher values.

Although blood counting is believed to be 90 percent accurate, there is recent evidence that electronic counting may yield false undercounts.

blood donation Giving of blood to be used for transfusion. Today, the Centers for Disease Control and Prevention, the Food and Drug Administration, and blood-banking organizations do not accept blood or plasma donations from persons in the following groups: those with clinical or laboratory evidence of HIV infection; men who have had sex with another man at least once since 1977; persons who have been prostitutes since 1977; users of intravenous drugs for nonmedical purposes; hemophiliacs who have received clotting factor concentrates; residents of sub-Saharan Africa or the islands off the coast of Africa (unless known to be HIV-1- and HIV-2-negative); those with sexual contact with any member of the specified groups. In addition, several other groups are also denied the opportunity to donate blood for various reasons, for example, citizens who have lived for more than six months in Great Britain (for fear of variant–CREUTZFELDT-JAKOB disease) and people with various forms of HEPATITIS (because of contagiousness). The following additional groups are asked to refrain from blood donation because there is a small, but real, risk that they may be infected with HIV: recipients of a blood transfusion or a blood component; those with tattoos, ear piercing, or acupuncture performed with a non-sterile needle; persons stuck with a needle in a health care setting; persons who have had sexual contact with a prostitute. All blood is tested in most Western countries before being used in medical settings, so the probability of contracting any illness from blood or blood products in North America or Western Europe these days is almost zero.

A frequently asked question in the first decade of the AIDS epidemic was, Can I get AIDS from donating blood? The answer in Western countries is no: you cannot. There is a big difference between donating blood and receiving a blood transfusion. Donating blood involves having blood taken out of one's own body. The needle used is sterile and is never reused. The only blood a donor has contact with is his or her own. It is not possible to contract anything that one does not already have, including HIV/AIDS, by donating blood. However, in developing nations, needles are reused in blood donation, and this practice has caused the spread of HIV in some countries. In particular, stories emerged from China in 2000 about many thousands of people with AIDS who had received the virus through infected needles reused in blood donation drives in rural parts of the country.

blood giving   Donating blood. In recent years, discrimination and "the greater good" have collided over blood giving. Gay men, in all practical senses, are prohibited from donating blood in the United States because of a U.S. Food and Drug Administration (FDA) policy first formulated in the mid-1980s, when the HIV epidemic was new, the nation gripped in panic, and HIV testing still in development. In recent years, this policy has come into sharper focus because individual gay men, but not, notably, major gay or HIV organizations, have raised objections to local blood drives as discriminatory. The debate has become so heated at many universities that several now prohibit the Red Cross or other blood banks from organizing blood drives on their campuses. Since the nation faces a severe shortage of blood, questions continue to be raised about the policy that otherwise healthy gay men are prohibited from blood donation. Under-

standing the issues requires taking a look back at the early years of the epidemic, understanding current patterns of HIV transmission, estimating the numbers of gay men in the United States, and examining how the nation's blood supply is collected and regulated. Today, although blood safety is assured by what is in essence a three-stage safety system, what rankles gay men is that any homosexual activity since 1977 results in what is essentially a lifetime ban on blood donation. One of the challenges facing the Blood Products Advisory Committee of the FDA is to formulate a policy based on science that recognizes epidemiological reality but also is perceived as less discriminatory and stigmatizing by healthy gay men. Revisions of the gay blood donation policy may be delayed as a result of the discovery of human herpesvirus 8 (HHV-8), a recently discovered virus thought to be the cause of Kaposi's sarcoma (KS). The widespread prevalence of HHV-8 among gay men, helps explain the baffling concentration of KS among gay AIDS patients but not heterosexual AIDS patients. Data emerging on HHV-8 show that it has a similar epidemiological profile to that of HIV. HHV-8 is most likely transmitted orally, but no blood test is routinely available to detect those who have it. In Africa, where HHV-8 is epidemic, the virus seems to be acquired in childhood. HHV-8 has also been transmitted through kidney transplant and dialysis procedures. To date it is not known whether HHV-8 can be transmitted through a blood transfusion. Until more is known about HHV-8 transmission, change in the gay blood donation policy is unlikely.

blood lipid level   Levels of lipids (fats) measured in routine blood chemical tests. Cholesterol and triglycerides are the main types of lipids measured in these tests. Special lipid panels are available to measure the occurrence of the two main forms of protein-bound cholesterol—LDL and HDL cholesterol—which are sometimes referred to as "bad" and "good" cholesterol, respectively. These terms arise from the fact that high LDL levels increase the risk of heart attacks and stroke, whereas high HDL levels are associated with a decreased risk of these conditions. Very high triglyceride levels can be a concern in the short term because of the risk of pancreatitis, and there may be a longer-term increased risk of heart attack and stroke associated with high triglyceride levels. Many persons on combination therapy have abnormally high blood lipid levels, particularly of triglycerides. High LDL and low HDL cholesterol levels also seem to be relatively common in patients on protease inhibitors and may increase the risk of heart attack and stroke. It is not known whether and how protease inhibitors cause lipid level elevations. Some researchers have suggested that the drugs act to inhibit the function of human protease enzymes and thereby affect the function of other proteins involved in lipid metabolism. Protease inhibitors are also known to affect the function of the cytochrome P450 system, a set of liver enzymes that metabolize drugs and other substances. These effects of cytochrome P450 are the reason many drugs interact with protease inhibitors. Researchers have also theorized that the effects of protease inhibitors on cytochrome P450 may affect the body's metabolism of lipids, leading to level elevations. Further research is ongoing in an attempt to sort this out. Many physicians are now testing blood lipid levels on a regular basis in their patients who are using protease inhibitors. These blood tests are optimally done in the fasting state, since food elevates lipid levels, especially triglyceride levels. Dietary management of elevated lipid levels may be tried, but many persons ultimately need medication to lower lipid levels. Doctors prescribing cholesterol level–lowering drugs must be aware of all of the other medications that the patient is taking because of the potential for drug interactions with protease inhibitors.

blood plasma The liquid part of the blood, containing minerals and proteins. See BLOOD SUPPLY; PLASMA.

blood pressure The pressure exerted by the flow of blood on the wall of the arteries. The flow is determined by a number of factors: the force of each heartbeat; the elasticity or resilience of the walls of the arteries; the amount of blood flowing through the arteries at any time; the viscosity (thickness) of the blood; the amount of various substances in the blood (such as protein, sodium, and certain hormones and enzymes, including adrenalin and renin); the functioning of the autonomic or sympathetic nervous system in response to changes in posture, emotional stress, and other stimuli; as well as age and general state of health. The blood pressure is altered during every heartbeat, reaching its highest point when the heart muscle is most contracted and its lowest point when the heart muscle relaxes after each heartbeat. In medicine, the heart muscle contraction is the *systole,* and the highest point of one's blood pressure is the *systolic* point. The momentary resting phase of the heart is *diastole,* and the low point of one's blood pressure is the *diastolic* point. The difference between these two pressures is called the blood pressure.

blood product Any natural or artificial substance taken or derived from the blood, to be used in medical procedures. There are two major types of blood products. The first type is obtained from whole blood itself and includes both blood cells (red cells, platelets, and buffy coat elements) and PLASMA. The second type is derived from separating the plasma (a process called fractionation) into components, such as albumin, immune serum globulin, and factor VIII (antihemophilia factor).

Today, decreasing the transmission of HIV through blood and blood products remains an issue of prevention. Four key methods have been identified: donor selection, laboratory testing, appropriate usage, and viral inactivation. When relying on the general population for blood donations, no screening method will ever be totally failsafe. However, appropriate education, counseling, and well-designed questionnaires are all emphasized. In addition, voluntary blood donation has proved to be much safer than paid or otherwise remunerated donations. All donors should be tested for HIV. In practice, however, this approach is thwarted by lack of structures, services, funding, and coordination. When HIV prevalence is especially low in the general donor population, other approaches—such as pooling samples of blood for testing—may be considered.

Guidelines should be strictly followed to ensure that blood and blood products are not used unless absolutely necessary. In many countries, for example, transfusions are prescribed in situations in which blood substitutes such as volume expanders could be used instead, but these alternatives are not always available or affordable. As a final measure, heat processing can ensure viral inactivation of certain blood products, including plasma. All of the foregoing models—donor selection, laboratory testing, appropriate usage, and viral inactivation—are interdependent: one cannot be ignored without reducing the efficacy of the others, hence the need for comprehensive, coordinated blood transfusion services. See BLOOD; BLOOD BANK; BLOOD DONATION; BLOOD SUPPLY.

blood screening   Each year 12 million units of blood are donated in the United States. Every single unit is tested to make certain that it is not infected with HIV and other diseases. If infected blood is found, it is destroyed.

blood splash   An accidental scattering of blood that comes into contact with an individual.

blood sugar   Glucose dissolved in the blood. Normal level is from 60 to 100 mg per 100 ml; it may rise after a meal to as much as 150 mg/100 ml.

blood supply   The amount of blood stored in blood banks and hospitals and available for use. Blood and blood products are exchanged and sold through an international network. The major commercial interest is in PLASMA, and the industry is well developed, particularly in the United States. The American plasma industry has been strongly criticized in the past, particularly for its practice of obtaining plasma in developing countries.

The practice of obtaining plasma from donors in poor countries for the benefit of those in rich countries is considered morally abhorrent by many and has been less free, and in some places eliminated altogether, in recent years. The lack of a universal labeling or an enforced marketing code for blood also works to increase potential for abuses.

blood supply safety   The advent of HIV has raised new concerns about the safety of the BLOOD SUPPLY in the United States. Although safety has been a concern since the practice of TRANSFUSION began,

AIDS places a serious stress on the supply system. Early in the epidemic, suspicions arose that AIDS could be transmitted by transfusion. In the spring of 1983, cases of AIDS diagnosed among HEMOPHILIACS were thought to be related to CLOTTING FACTOR concentrates made from contaminated blood. Although the etiologic or causative agent of AIDS had not been identified in the early 1980s and no specific diagnostic tests were available, these cases prompted BLOOD BANKS and collection organizations to institute a variety of precautions. These included efforts to exclude donors who were members of groups at high risk for AIDS, tests that measured factors considered to be surrogate markers for AIDS (such as ANTIBODY to HEPATITIS B core ANTIGEN and T-LYMPHOCYTE ratios), increased use of AUTOLOGOUS transfusion, and the reduction of unnecessary transfusions. After HIV, the etiologic agent of AIDS, was identified and blood tests became available in 1985, HIV ANTIBODY TESTS became standard as well.

Despite the high sensitivity of these tests, they do not detect all infected blood. A variable length of time elapses between infection with HIV and development of a detectable antibody response. Generally, this is no more than a few months, but studies have found that it may be as long as three years. Blood collected from an infected donor during this so-called "window" period may test negative and thus go undetected. For this reason, although HIV antibody tests have vastly improved the safety of the blood supply, they cannot eliminate all possibility of transfusion-associated HIV infection.

Additional methods to detect infected blood continue to be explored to increase the sensitivity of serologic testing. These include methods based on recombinant-DNA technology, synthetic peptides, and gene-amplification techniques. Other safeguards involving improved donor screening and recruitment are also being evaluated and implemented.

The major organizations active in efforts to improve global blood supply are the Red Cross, the World Health Organization, and the International Society of Blood Transfusion.

blood test   A diagnostic laboratory analysis of a sample of blood taken from a vein, usually in the arm, to determine the chemical, physical, or serological characteristics of the blood or some portion of it. Blood tests can help in the diagnosis and treatment of a host of conditions and to monitor a patient's progress once in treatment.

Specific blood tests are performed to ascertain blood cell differential, blood pressure, clotting factors, blood grouping, blood type, and blood matching, volume, and as a measure of electrolytes, fats, gases, blood urea nitrogen, and viscosity.

blood transfusion The process of replacing blood in the body with whole blood or blood products, taken from others. See TRANSFUSION.

blood work Phrase used to refer to the numerous tests that require that blood be drawn from a patient and the results of those tests be evaluated.

blood-brain barrier The barrier between circulating blood and brain tissue, formed by astrocytes (fibrous cells) and brain capillaries, which prevents harmful substances in the blood from damaging brain neurons. The phrase also refers to the relative resistance to diffusion of molecules across the unfenestrated capillaries of the brain, whose cells have tight junctions, and the fatty astroglial cell sheath surrounding the capillaries. The latter obstructs polar solutes more than it does such lipid solutes as psychoactive drugs. This presents a problem in treating HIV infection in the brain because treatments must cross it to be effective. Research is being done to find ways to disrupt the barrier temporarily so that drugs and other treatments can penetrate it.

blood-retina barrier The barrier that prevents the passage of most substances from the blood to the retina, making it difficult to treat eye disease with systematically administered medicines (e.g., pills and intravenous infusions). Fibrous cells and many capillaries screen out the large molecules that are often present in complex antiviral drugs.

blotting A technique for analyzing a tiny portion of the primary structure of genomic material (DNA or RNA) by applying electric current to the blood plasma, to separate the different components in blood. Northern blot techniques are used to analyze small portions of RNA. Southern blot analysis techniques are used in molecular genetics to analyze small portions of DNA. The WESTERN BLOT TEST is a method for analyzing PROTEIN ANTIGENS and antibodies that is often used to confirm a diagnosis of AIDS. In testing for HIV it is the antibodies to the various components of HIV that the Western blot detects. See AIDS-DEFINING DIAGNOSIS; GENE; GENETIC RESEARCH.

blue balls A painful condition of the testicles resulting from prolonged sexual stimulation without ejaculation.

blue-green algae A generic name for the algae (Cyanobacteria) found in most wet places. Spirulina is an edible variety commonly available as a food supplement at health food stores. Scientists have reported that extracts from *L. lagerheimmi* and *R. tenue*, two specific types of blue-green algae found only off the islands of Hawaii and Palau, contain sulfolipids that they believe have a cytotoxic (cell-killing) effect on HIV. However, no research has been conducted with humans. It is unknown whether spirulina contains such sulfolipids. It has not been shown to have any direct benefit against HIV, though it is rich in amino acids and minerals.

BLV See BOVINE LEUKEMIA VIRUS.

BMS 232632 See ATAZANAVIR.

board-and-care home A publicly or privately operated residence that provides personal assistance, lodging, and meals to two or more adults unrelated to the operator. Also called custodial, domiciliary, personal-care, adult foster-care, congregate, old age, community, and rest homes. Rents are paid from residents' private incomes, and—for the needy—with SSI and SSPs.

body cell mass (BCM) The functional mass of the body where metabolic activity takes place. It consists of muscle tissue, organs, as well as red cells and other tissue cells. It is the part of the body responsible for oxygen consumption and production of carbon dioxide. A minimal amount of body cell mass must be maintained by the body to support its day-to-day activities plus fight infection. Loss of body cell mass is called WASTING.

body composition The components that make up the body. The skeleton, water, blood, muscle, fat, and LEAN BODY MASS all constitute the body's composition. Some people on ANTIRETROVIRAL medications have had abnormal changes in their body composition, such as shifting of body weight, accumulation of fat in particular spots of the body, bone density changes, and other noticeable changes. See METABOLIC TOXICITY.

body fat Changes in body habitus—accumulation of fatty tissue in areas such as the trunk, the neck, the breasts, and the upper back, accompanied by atrophy of adipose tissue in the face (Bichat's fat pad), the limbs, and the pelvis/butt—remain a mystery. Their probable cause, pathogenesis, and prevalence are the focus of ongoing research; treatments for the underlying cause and/or preventive strategies are still unavailable.

body fat redistribution syndrome A set of symptoms related to the abnormal loss of body fat from some areas of the body, most often the face, extremities, and butt, and accumulation of body fat in other areas, generally the back of the neck, shoulders, breasts, and stomach. See METABOLIC TOXICITY.

body fluids The total amount of water in the human body varies from 50 percent of body weight in obese individuals to 70 percent in the non-obese. The principal compartments for body fluids are intracellular and extracellular. A much smaller segment, the transcellular, includes fluid in the tracheobronchilial tree, the gastrointestinal tract, the bladder, cerebrospinal fluid, and the aqueous humor of the eye. Of the various liquids found in the human body, such as blood, breast milk, cervical secretions, saliva, semen, sputum, sweat, tears, urine, and vaginal secretions, only blood, breast milk, semen, and vaginal secretions

have been found to contain concentrations of HIV high enough to infect another person. Saliva, sweat, tears, and urine have not been shown to transmit HIV.

body mass index (BMI) An index used to judge the relation between a person's height and weight. The BMI is a person's weight in kilograms divided by height in meters squared. The resulting number correlates strongly with total body fat in adults. The National Heart, Lung and Blood Institute has a quick BMI calculator at http://www.nhlbisupport.com/bmi/bmicalc.htm

boil An abscess or furuncle, which is an acute circumscribed inflammation of the subcutaneous layers of the skin glands or hair follicles. Boils can be painful as a result of the pressure from the buildup of fluid in the abscess. Boils are most commonly due to localized infections with staphylococci.

bone marrow The inner, spongy substance in the center of the bones that produces all of the red blood cells (ERYTHROCYTES), most of the white blood cells (LEUKOCYTES), and all of the platelets (THROMBOCYTES). It is now believed that all blood cells derive from primitive stem cells in the bone marrow. Damage to the bone marrow makes an individual far more susceptible to infections. Bone marrow is located throughout the skeletal system.

Bone marrow plays a significant role in the development, diagnosis, and treatment of cancer. Bone marrow can be withdrawn (by placing a needle in the hip bone) and analyzed to detect abnormalities in the production of red blood cells, white blood cells, or platelets.

bone marrow depression See BONE MARROW SUPPRESSION.

bone marrow suppression Bone marrow suppression (or depression) is a condition characterized by the decreased ability or inability of the bone marrow to make white blood cells, red blood cells, and platelets. Such reductions result in anemia, bacterial infections, and spontaneous or excess bleeding. Bone marrow suppression is a side effect of many anticancer and antiviral drugs and a major factor in determining the frequency of treatment and the amount of such drugs given to patients. It also occurs through the course of HIV disease itself. Bone marrow suppression is usually reversible, if derived from a particular drug, but not from a disease. Because persons who have below-normal blood levels are at greater risk for infections, anemia, and bleeding, they are generally advised to take the following preventive measures: wash hands frequently, always before eating and after using the bathroom; use an electric shaver rather than a razor, to prevent cuts; do not squeeze or scratch pimples; clean any cuts or scrapes immediately with warm water and soap; clean the rectal area gently but thoroughly after bowel movements.

bone marrow transplantation A supportive treatment in which healthy bone marrow is removed from a donor and transfused into a recipient. Bone marrow transplantation is an effective treatment for some cancers, among them LEUKEMIA and LYMPHOMA. The main purpose of the treatment is to enable the patient to be given very large, and potentially more effective, doses of chemotherapy or radiation. Such doses cause severe damage to the bone marrow; by replacing the damaged marrow, the patient regains the ability to fight off infections. There are three types of bone marrow transplantation: autologous (the patient's own marrow is harvested before chemotherapy, cryopreserved, and reinfused); allogeneic (the marrow is from a sibling, parent, or compatible unrelated donor); and syngeneic (the marrow is from an identical twin). In treatment for HIV/AIDS all of these types of bone marrow transplantation have been tried. In addition, in a highly publicized case, transplantation from a baboon to a human has also been conducted. All of the various transplantations have failed because the new bone marrow cells become infected shortly after entering the new body. In relation to the baboon cells, they seemingly died shortly after transplantation and had no effect on the patient.

Side effects, usually short term, of the high doses of anticancer drugs and/or radiation therapy can include nausea, vomiting, irritation of the lining of the mouth and gastrointestinal tract, lowered blood count, damage to vital organs, hair loss, and loss of appetite. Long-term side effects, which are usually results of anticancer drug and radiation treatment, can include infertility, early menopause, cataracts, and secondary cancers. A patient may experience any of several complications as a result of this treatment, including infections and bleeding, most often from the nose or mouth, under the skin, or in the intestinal tract. Liver disease may also develop in the weeks and months that follow the treatment. In addition, graft-versus-host disease (GVHD) is a frequent complication of allogeneic bone marrow transplantation. In GVHD, the donor's bone marrow attacks the patient's organs and tissues, increasing the likelihood of infection and impairing the ability of the body to function. Around half of allogeneic bone marrow transplantation patients suffer some type of GVHD. Most of the cases are short term and mild. Some cases turn out to be chronic and more severe. GVHD does not result from autologous transplantation.

boost To restimulate a primed immune system; giving a vaccine to a person who already has received at least one dose of a similar vaccine.

booster A second or later dosage of a vaccine given to increase the immune response to the antigen. The booster vaccine may or may not be the same strength as the initial vaccine.

booting The procedure practiced by intravenous drug users in which the syringe is emptied into the vein and then blood is drawn into the empty syringe to wash away any remaining drug then reinjected into the vein. It assures the drug user that all of the drug is injected. Booting increases the risk for transmission of the HUMAN IMMUNODEFICIENCY VIRUS by providing increased contact between the blood and the syringe.

bootleg drugs Drugs which are produced, carried, or sold illegally.

bottom In SEXUAL INTERCOURSE, a slang term for the partner whose body is penetrated by the other.

In regard to sexually transmitted diseases, *bottom mentality* means wanting not to have to deal with negotiation over safety; it's the job of the top to be responsible for that. See TOP.

bottom mentality   See BOTTOM.

bovine leukemia virus (BLV)   A virus found in cattle that is similar in structure to the HUMAN T-CELL LEUKEMIA virus.

brachioproctic intercourse   Penetration of the rectum with the hand and forearm to induce sexual stimulation. Also called FISTING or FIST-FUCKING.

brain cancer   Any primary cancerous tumor in the brain. Brain cancer is relatively rare. There are many different types of brain tumors, only some of which are cancerous. A malignant tumor can spread to other parts of the brain; although a benign brain tumor does not spread, it can be equally devastating because the skull cannot expand to accommodate the mass growing inside. Some benign tumors become malignant. Two types of brain cancer affect HIV-infected people: primary CENTRAL NERVOUS SYSTEM (CNS) LYMPHOMA and metastatic systemic lymphoma in the brain. Other brain cancers are extremely rare in HIV patients. The symptoms of a brain tumor can vary, depending on the part of the brain affected. The most frequent signs of a brain tumor are subtle changes in personality, memory, and intellectual performance that may not be noticed. A common symptom is a headache, not necessarily persistent or severe. Nausea and vomiting unrelated to food consumption occur in about a quarter of people with a brain tumor. Procedures used in the diagnosis of brain cancer are X RAYS, CT SCAN, SPINAL TAP, EEG, cerebral angiography, pneumoencephalography, and MRI. Brain cancers are classified according to the types of cell in the tumors and their histologic grade (how different the tumor cell is from the cells that are near it). Treatment depends on cell type, location of the tumor, general state of health of the patient, and other factors. The three types of treatment currently being used are surgery, radiation therapy, and chemotherapy; biological therapy is being studied in clinical trials. A 2002 study in Michigan has shown that brain cancers have

reduced in occurrence after the beginning of HAART.

brain imaging   The use of X-RAY or nuclear techniques to produce an image representative of the brain.

brain lesion   Any abnormality in the brain tissue.

brain scan   A form of brain imaging using CT SCAN or MRI. These tests may be run with or without staining dyes. Radioisotopes are no longer used in brain scans as they were in the past.

brain tumor   A growth of tissue in the brain. See BRAIN CANCER.

branched chain DNA (bDNA) assay   See BRANCHED DNA ASSAY.

branched DNA assay (bDNA test)   A blood test developed by the Chiron Corporation that measures the amount of HIV, or other viruses, in blood PLASMA. The result is called the VIRAL LOAD. The test uses a signal amplification technique. This means the test creates a glowing signal that shows brightness depending on the amount of viral RNA present. The test results are stated as virus particles per milliliter of plasma (number/ml). The result of the bDNA test is generally about half the number indicated by the POLYMERASE CHAIN REACTION (PCR) TEST, which uses a different technique to measure viral load.

breakthrough infection   An infection that is caused by an infectious agent although the person has been trying to avoid infection through a vaccine. The infection may be caused by exposure to the infectious agent during or shortly after the vaccination (as in VARICELLA ZOSTER) or before the completion of all doses of a vaccine (as in HEPATITIS B).

breakthrough pain   Flare-ups of pain during an illness that are not controlled by a patient's pain medication. This term generally is used when a patient is on a long-acting or narcotic medication such as OxyContin. In these cases, shorter-acting doses of the same medication are used to control the breakthrough pain, or a stronger medication such as morphine may be used.

breast   Area of the chest surrounding the nipple. In women this area may be enlarged and is the source of milk production.

breast cancer   Malignant growth (neoplasm) of the breast. In the United States, breast cancer is the leading cause of death in women between the ages of 30 and 50 and is second only to heart disease as a cause of death in women over 50. Approximately one woman in 10 will develop breast cancer in her lifetime. About 1,000 men develop breast cancer each year. See BREAST TUMOR.

breast mass   See BREAST CANCER; BREAST TUMOR.

breast milk   See BREAST-FEEDING.

breast tumor   A growth of tissue, or neoplasm, in the breast. Most such breast masses are found either by a woman on self-examination or inadvertently by her sexual partner. Routine breast exams will also uncover breast tumors. The majority are benign. It is currently unknown if breast cancer rates, which have been increasing, are altered by HIV infection.

Axillary lymphadenopathy may be associated with breast pathology. Many HIV-positive women have PERSISTENT GENERALIZED LYMPHADENOPATHY (PGL), a condition common in cases of HIV, in which multiple lymph glands are swollen for a long period. Bilateral axillary nodes may be a part of PGL. However, a new node, singular node, or change in the size of a previously noted node may be significant and require node biopsy. It may represent pathology or infection in the breast, elsewhere in the chest, or systemically. The stage of HIV infection must be considered to generate an appropriate differential for evaluation of any singular lymph nodes. Breast exams are the key to management. At the time a breast exam is to be performed, inquiry should be made regarding breast pain, nipple discharge, axillary nodes, lumps, and changes in the skin of the breasts. A

mammogram may be a useful adjunct to the diagnosis of a mass. Ultrasound is often used in differentiating a tumor from a cystic mass.

HIV-positive women should be offered routine mammography on the same schedule as other women. The most widely accepted schedule is baseline mammogram at age 35–40; annual or biannual mammograms for women in their 40s and annual mammogram for all women over 50. See MAMMOGRAPHY.

breast-feeding   Nursing at the breast. A baby can get HIV from its mother: during pregnancy (before birth), during delivery (the most common way babies are infected), and through breast-feeding.

Exclusive breast-feeding is giving the baby breast milk only. Breast milk is very nutritious and helps protect a baby from diseases. It can also help a mother and baby bond. It may help a baby who is born infected stay healthy and avoid germs from formula feeding. A women is less likely to become pregnant while exclusively breast-feeding, which therefore helps her to space her children. Breast-feeding can increase the risk of HIV transmission. A baby is at greater risk of getting HIV through breast-feeding if the mother breast-feeds her baby for a long time; becomes infected with HIV while breast-feeding; gets cracked or bleeding nipples; gets mastitis; is very sick, or has a high viral load or a low CD4+ count, or has a lot of virus in her breast milk.

Replacement or formula feeding is giving the baby formula only. There is no HIV in formula. A baby born HIV-negative can stay HIV-negative. Others can help feed the baby if the mother needs a rest, gets sick, or has to go away for work or other reasons. Various common problems are related to formula feeding: infections from germs in water used to mix formula or from spoiled formula, which can be extremely dangerous; formula-fed babies miss the health benefits of colostrum and many of the nutrients in breast milk; people may wonder why a woman is not breast-feeding and ask whether it is because she has HIV; mixing too little formula or too much formula can make a baby sick; it requires work to boil water and keep all utensils clean every time a baby is fed; formula is expensive; and a woman who does not breast-feed resumes menstruation and becomes fertile sooner. According to the World Health Organization (WHO), babies in developing countries who are fed on formula are up to six times more likely to die of conditions such as diarrhea and respiratory infections than breast-fed babies are.

Mixed breast-feeding is giving the baby breast milk and other drinks, such as formula, glucose water, or traditional medicines. In many places, mixed feeding is the social norm. Note, too, that mixed feeding (breast milk plus formula) is the most dangerous method, because formula feeding can irritate the lining of the baby's stomach, making it easier for the HIV in breast milk to enter and cause an infection.

In the United States and other developed nations, HIV-positive women are advised not to breast-feed and to use formula instead. This is because most women in these regions have easy access to formula, clean water for mixing and washing, and refrigeration. Women in developed regions can usually get health care if the baby becomes sick to prevent a case of diarrhea from becoming fatal. Although formula feeding may be the obvious choice for preventing HIV transmission, it is not easy to use. During the first years of the epidemic, in developing countries, where many people do not have access to clean water, HIV-positive women were often advised to breast-feed their babies to protect them from the health problems related to formula feeding. Today, some people still consider that the best advice; others feel that women should have more information, more choices, and better access to affordable formula.

Whichever method a woman chooses, there are ways she can make it safer. Breast-feeding exclusively for six months or less is less risky—the risk of a baby's getting HIV from breast-feeding increases the longer the baby is exposed to HIV in the breast milk. When breast-feeding is stopped at six months, the risk of transmission is reduced—some say to as little as 5 percent (compared to 14 percent with longer periods of breast-feeding). Second, HIV drugs can reduce the risk of a baby's being infected by breast milk by reducing the viral load in the mother and her milk and by improving the mother's health. However, HIV transmission can still occur through breast-feeding, and, in the United States, HIV-positive women on therapy are

encouraged to formula feed. Most women in developing countries do not have access to HIV drugs. Some studies are considering giving HIV drugs to the mother (or the baby) throughout the breast-feeding period to reduce the chance of HIV transmission to infants. Broader campaigns are working to make HIV drugs available to all HIV-positive people worldwide. Other options and strategies include modification of full fat cow's milk; heat treatment (pasteurization) of breast milk; and reliance on alternative breast milk sources, (e.g., another woman breast-feeds the baby or breast milk is obtained from another woman or from a milk bank). However, this assumes that the woman has tested HIV-negative, is still HIV-negative, and will not become infected with HIV for as long as she is providing milk.

breathwork   "Breathwork" is a general term for a variety of quasi-therapeutic techniques that use patterned breathing to promote physical, mental, and/or spiritual well-being. Some techniques use the breath in a calm, peaceful way to induce relaxation or manage pain, whereas others use stronger breathing to stimulate emotions and emotional release.

breeder   Pejorative gay slang term for a HETERO-SEXUAL.

broad-spectrum   In pharmacology, effective against a variety of MICROORGANISMS.

broad-spectrum antibiotic   A substance that kills or inhibits the growth of a range of different organisms and can be used to combat diseases and infection. See ANTIBIOTIC.

bronchi   See BRONCHUS.

bronchitis   An inflammation of the bronchial tubes, or bronchi, the air passages that extend from the windpipe to the lungs. A virus, heavy smoking, or the inhaling of dust or airborne chemicals can cause the inflammation. When the bronchial tissue is irritated to the point of illness, the tiny hair lining the bronchi, which typically trap these irritants, stop working. Consequently, the air passages become clogged by debris and irritation increases. In response, a heavy secretion of mucus develops; the mucus causes the characteristic heavy, wet cough of bronchitis.

bronchoalveolar lavage (BAL) The introduction, by use of a fiberoptic bronchoscope, of a sterile saline fluid into the lung in order to remove secretions, cells, and protein from the lower respiratory tract. In HIV it is used to diagnose PNEUMO-CYSTIS CARINII PNEUMONIA (PCP). BAL is also used to treat cystic fibrosis, pulmonary alveolar proteinosis, and severe asthma with bronchial obstruction due to mucus plugging.

bronchoscopy Examination of the bronchi through a bronchoscope, an endoscope designed to pass through the trachea to allow visual inspection of the tracheobronchial tree. Bronchoscopy is often used to detect PNEUMOCYSTIS CARINII PNEUMONIA (PCP). The flexible fiberoptic tube is also designed to permit the passage of an instrument that can be used to obtain tissue for biopsy or to remove a foreign body from the tracheobronchial tree.

bronchus (pl. bronchi) One of the two main branches leading from the trachea to the lungs, providing the passage-way for air movement.

brush biopsy Removal of tissue from the body by use of a brush. See BIOPSY.

Bucast Also known as MDL 28574A and Celgosivir. It is an ANTIRETROVIRAL derived from an Australian tree, *Castanospermum australe*. It has been tested in phase I and II trials in humans. The drug appears to inhibit the action of a viral enzyme called glycosidase, which is used by the virus to build the protein envelope that surrounds and protects it.

budding A method of asexual reproduction common in lower animals and plants, including many of the fungi that invade the human body, in which a budlike appendage grows from the side or end of the parent and develops into a new organism. The bud may remain attached, or it may separate and live independently of the parent.

buddy Generally, a volunteer caregiver who works with a person with HIV or AIDS, providing or arranging for an array of services, such as home care, daily living needs (personal hygiene, clothing, bed linens, etc.), transportation, and personal or social support. A buddy provides comfort and assistance and helps a person afflicted with HIV/AIDS maintain as much personal dignity as is possible with this disease. Many AIDS service organizations support some form of buddy system. Buddies often begin working with persons with HIV or AIDS that they do not know. Often, more than one buddy will be assigned to a patient. A patient's needs, capabilities, and limitations from one day to the next generally determine the care and support that are provided. Buddy training and ongoing buddy education are often required of all persons who volunteer as caregivers. Most AIDS service organizations offer buddy support meetings to help buddies deal with stress and burnout, as well as their own grief.

buddying Being a buddy to someone; in the context of HIV/AIDS being a friend or working with someone with HIV/AIDS. Generally, it is the pairing of a healthy individual with someone who is ill under the auspices of an AIDS service organization or social service program. The healthy buddy is on call in the event of emergency, assists with the activities of daily living, and provides companionship. People decide to become buddies for different reasons; most agree that, regardless of motivation, being a buddy yields great joy and love.

buffalo hump The term used to describe the abnormal accumulation of body fat at the back of the neck and top of the shoulders. It is thought to be caused by the use of ANTIRETROVIRAL medications over an extended period. See METABOLIC TOXICITY.

buffered Coated or encased in a special substance that allows easier absorption of a medication by neutralizing the acidic environment of the stomach.

bug-chaser The slang term for someone who eroticizes catching HIV or AIDS from a sexual partner. This person often goes out to bars, or other locations, looking for a sexual partner who will have unprotected sex with him or her. In discordant relationships, an HIV-negative partner might be referred to as a bug-chaser if he or she regularly seeks unprotected sex with the partner or lover.

bulletin board   See BULLETIN BOARD SYSTEM.

bulletin board system (BBS)   An online "space" where computer users can exchange information. Once connected to a BBS, users can post messages, read messages left by others and reply to them, and find and copy files. Other BBS services may include online games, chatting, and database searching. There are thousands of bulletin boards around the world, each with its own area of interest. Many offer access free of charge; for others there is a nominal fee. Online bulletin boards have been a major factor in the maintenance of an international AIDS community.

The growth of a network of AIDS-related computer bulletin boards in the early 1990s both constituted and fostered the emergence of a new kind of activism. They allow specialists to share information with other clinicians, patients, and the "lay learned"—individuals who, dissatisfied with the lack of progress in AIDS research, have taken it upon themselves to learn the basic science and engage credibly in the ongoing dialogue on AIDS therapies. The online bulletin boards also allow discussion between scientists and activists, as well as individuals attempting to develop alternative treatment options. The evolution of this dialogue has had a strong impact on the AIDS treatment development agenda. This global exchange disseminates instantaneously the latest research in immunology and other disciplines relevant to the design of AIDS treatments.

Many online bulletin board systems make available the texts of primary AIDS publications, abstracts of medical journal references on AIDS, government reports, and the daily summaries of the Centers for Disease Control and Prevention. Rather than having to wait for the lengthy process of medical journal publication, professionals and others in this way have available instantaneous

peer review of their theories and proposed treatment regimens by tens of thousands of researchers and practitioners, as well as by knowledgeable PWAS. Many bulletin board systems also sponsor online AIDS-related conferences.

bupropion   A drug made by Glaxo-Welcome that is used both as an antidepressant and as a smoking cessation treatment. It must be taken at a lower dose than typical if you are taking RITONAVIR, as this drug increases the amount of bupropion in the body. There are two side effects of bupropion that are important in HIV patients. One is weight loss. Twenty-eight percent of the people who take this drug lose weight. HIV patients must be carefully monitored on this drug so they do not lose excessive weight. Second, this drug can disrupt sleep. Doses should not be taken after 3 P.M. to decrease this side effect. (Trade names are Welbutrin and Zyban.)

Burkitt's lymphoma   A small noncleaved (undivided) cell LYMPHOMA, also referred to as Burkitt's or Burkitt's-like lymphoma. It normally occurs in children and is rapidly progressive. In the United States, Burkitt's lymphoma makes up a significant portion of undifferentiated B-cell lymphomas in children. The most common sites of occurrence in Americans are the neck and the digestive system. It is often associated with the Epstein-Barr virus (a herpes virus) and chromosomal abnormality. Burkitt's is also seen as a form of aggressive lymphoma in AIDS patients, particularly in Africa, where Burkitt's is a more common disease. Children who have Burkitt's lymphoma most often display abnormal protrusion of the eyeballs and facial swelling. See NON-HODGKIN'S LYMPHOMA.

burnout   A condition resulting from chronic stress, characterized by physical and emotional exhaustion and sometimes physical illness. As the number of people affected by AIDS continues to grow, the emotional, psychological, and physical toll on professional and volunteer AIDS caregivers also increases. Many are confronting burnout. Depression, anger, and despair are some of the emotional effects of AIDS-related burnout.

AIDS caregivers, both professionals and others, face unique demands and stresses. All must cope daily with the risk of accidental exposure, continuing social stigmata associated with the disease, inadequate resources, and the lack of effective treatments or cure, as well as complex ethical and legal issues and the devastating impact of watching young patients die. It is not surprising that emotional responses to these stresses—sometimes referred to as "bereavement overload" or "chronic mourning"—should affect them. Some may also be dealing with AIDS in their own lives, through the illness and death of friends, colleagues, and partners, or because they themselves are infected or ill.

The effects of burnout are both personal and institutional. Burned out caregivers may experience difficulty functioning, psychological distress, and poor health. Where the rate of staff burnout is high, institutions suffer low morale, communication breakdown, internal conflict, decreased productivity, absenteeism, and high turnover. Furthermore, when staff attempt to distance themselves emotionally, become cynical, or limit contact, AIDS patients and their families also suffer.

Strategies to address burnout include creating formal and informal support groups, developing coping and stress management skills, and providing professional development opportunities. All help individuals bolster or renew their inner resources. Institutional responses can also support both patients and staff, without requiring the costly overhaul of established systems. Such institutional responses include restructuring workloads, benefits and time schedules, improving communication at all levels, and acknowledging the difficulties facing staff.

Busse-Buschke disease   See CRYPTOCOCCOSIS.

butch   Slang term, formerly gay but now in common use, to describe someone or something as stereotypically masculine.

butyl nitrite inhalant   A liquid compound that dilates blood vessels and reduces blood pressure when inhaled. It is used recreationally to produce a brief high. Unlike AMYL NITRITE, butyl nitrite does not require a prescription. Also called RUSH and POPPERS. See ISOBUTYL NITRITE INHALERS.

butylated hydroxytuolene (BHT)   A food preservative widely used to prevent rancidity in fat-containing foods. It is believed to strip LIPID-coated viruses of their protective envelope, leaving them susceptible to recognition and destruction by the immune system. It is also thought to remove the binding proteins that viruses use to penetrate cell membranes. Medical researchers have found that BHT greatly reduces the progression of NECROSIS in doxorubicin-induced skin ulcers.

buyers' club   A nonprofit group that makes available "underground" drugs (drugs not approved by the Food and Drug Administration and thus not available in the United States). Many of these drugs are used abroad for purposes not related to AIDS or HIV infection and their effectiveness as treatment for these conditions is only speculative. Many underground groups, some of which are approved in other countries and some not, carry nutritional supplements and vitamins, as well as minerals, enzymes, and herbal or Chinese therapies. Persons considering joining a buyers' group should ask questions and explore thoroughly the standards and procedures of any group offering unapproved therapies before buying a drug from them. Buyers' clubs offer those infected with HIV the opportunity to take drugs that might not otherwise become available for years, but the drugs are untested and could be useless or toxic.

The Food and Drug Administration has had long-standing concerns about buyers' clubs' activities. The lack of physician involvement in the medical care of their clients; the sale of injectable products of unknown purity, sterility, and strength; the sale of products with unknown sources of manufacture; and the promotion, distribution, and commercialization of unproved and potentially dangerous products are among the agency's interests.

In 1993, it wrote to a number of AIDS buyers' clubs expressing official concern about "certain" activities. This was the first time the agency made a stab at formally defining its relationship with the clubs. The agency noted that it had, in the past, articulated a policy regarding importation of drugs for personal use, under which it may exercise what it refers to as "enforcement discretion." It noted further that many buyers' clubs have taken the position that their activities fall under the policy. And it announced several courses of action designed to "explore the feasibility of allowing continuation of the beneficial aspects of the personal use importation policy while at the same time, preventing serious abuses of this policy . . ." The agency claimed it would intensify communications with interested parties in an effort to catalog those products, not yet legally available in the United States, that may have the greatest potential for benefit to people with HIV. It also promised to explore alternatives.

Buyers' clubs were designed as guerrilla activity, intended to spark systemic reform. Issues of access and regulation of bootleg drugs acquired through the underground and increased access to genuine drugs through an expanded testing program have dominated this arena since the AIDS crisis began. Many argue that insofar as it is the government's responsibility to protect people with HIV (and others too) from being harmed or taken advantage of, regulation in this arena is appropriate and even welcome.

buyers' group   See BUYERS' CLUB.

buy-in   The procedure, effectively mandatory since 1969, whereby state MEDICAID programs pay Part B MEDICARE premiums for those eligible for both programs; by extension, sometimes used to denote the pre-1989 practice whereby states paid Medicare deductibles and coinsurance, as well as premiums, for those on both programs. See QUALITY MEDICARE BUY-IN for the newly expanded mandatory buy-in provision.

bystander lysis   COMPLEMENT- or CYTOKINE-mediated LYSIS of cells in the immediate vicinity of an immune response, which are not themselves responsible for the activation. Also known as *bystander effect*.

cachectin A factor present in serum; causes wasting and is identical to TUMOR NECROSIS FACTOR alpha.

cachexia A state of ill health, malnutrition, and wasting that may occur in many chronic diseases, certain malignancies, and advanced pulmonary tuberculosis.

CAF See CELL ACTIVATED FACTOR.

calanolide A Compound derived from a latex tree that works as a nonnucleoside reverse transcriptase inhibitor (NNRTI) and shows some anti-HIV activity. Manufactured by Sarawak MediChem Pharmaceuticals, it is currently in phase II Clinical Trials.

calcitonin A hormone from the thyroid gland important in bone and calcium metabolism.

calcium Calcium is the most abundant mineral in the body and the fifth most abundant substance. In the body, about 99 percent is deposited in the bones and teeth. The remaining 1 percent is involved in the soft tissues, intracellular fluids, and blood. Calcium is used in the development and maintenance of bone structure and rigidity. It functions among other ways, in the clotting process, nerve transmission and muscle stimulation, parathyroid hormone function, and metabolism of vitamin D. To function properly, calcium must be accompanied by magnesium, phosphorus, and vitamins A, C, D, and very possibly E. Bone stability requires vitamin A, magnesium, and fluoride. Calcium is found with magnesium, sodium, phosphorous, strontium, carbonate, and citrate.

The major function of calcium is to act in cooperation with phosphorous to build and maintain bones and teeth. Another important function is the storage of the mineral in the bones for use by the body. The calcium state of the bones is constantly fluctuating according to the diet and to the body's needs. The 1 percent of ionized calcium that circulates in the fluids of the body is small but vital to life. It is essential for healthy blood and eases insomnia, and its delicate messenger ions help regulate the heartbeat. Along with calcium, magnesium is needed to properly maintain the cardiovascular system.

In addition, calcium assists in the process of blood clotting and helps prevent the accumulation of too much acid or too much alkali in the blood. It also plays a part in the secretion of hormones. It affects neurotransmitters (serotonin, acetylcholine, and norepinephrine), nerve transmission, muscle growth, and muscle contraction. The mineral acts as a messenger from the cell surface to the inside of the cell and helps regulate the passage of nutrients in and out of the cell walls. Calcium aids in the body's utilization of iron and helps activate several digestive enzymes (catalysts important for metabolism).

When concentration is too high, hormones and vitamin D make sure that calcium is deposited in its storage place in the bones. When it is too low, the imbalance is corrected in several ways: the kidneys, which slow excretion; in the bones, which control the release of needed amounts; and in the intestine, which encourages absorption. Calcium stored in the bones supplies the bloodstream, which is unaffected by dietary intake. However, a calcium dietary deficiency will diminish the stores of the bones after a number of years.

The best sources are natural. Milk and dairy products are dependable sources with the exception of cottage cheese. Additional sources include canned sardines and salmon with their bones; tofu; oysters; broccoli; mustard greens; kale; parsley; watercress; almonds; asparagus; brewer's yeast; blackstrap molasses; cabbage; carob; figs; filberts; prunes; sesame seeds; yogurt; whey; collards; goat's milk; kelp; oats; and whole-wheat bread. However, to get the needed amounts without consuming large amounts of food, supplements must be taken.

To date, calcium has not been identified as one of the nutrients that may be directly beneficial in the treatment of HIV/AIDS; however, it may be beneficial in treating a variety of ailments, and, therefore, have an indirect benefit to persons with HIV/AIDS. For example, it is a natural tranquilizer and tends to calm the nerves. The production of energy and the maintenance of the immune system benefit from calcium. Supplements along with vitamin D have a strong preventative effect on colorectal cancer. Calcium participates in the structuring of DNA and RNA and activates the digestive system. By lowering cholesterol, the mineral is thought to be beneficial in the treatment of cardiovascular disorders. It is a recognized aid for muscle cramps in the feet and legs. Arthritis, structural rigidity often caused by depletion of bone calcium, may be helped with regular supplements of calcium, although this has not been proved scientifically. Along with estrogen, it has been successfully used in the treatment of osteoporosis. High intakes of calcium may relieve the symptoms commonly associated with aging—bone pain, backaches, brittle teeth with cavities, tremors of the fingers, etc.

calcium antacid A compound used to neutralize stomach acid and relieve heartburn, acid indigestion, esophageal reflux disease, and other conditions related to stomach upset. Aluminum hydroxide is the ingredient most commonly used in antacids. Because it may cause constipation, aluminum hydroxide is often combined with magnesium, which has a balancing laxative effect. Calcium-containing antacids have become more popular recently, in part because their manufacturers have marketed them as calcium supplements to prevent osteoporosis in women. Some antacids also contain a chemical called simethicone, which is used to reduce the gas that may be caused by the reaction of the aluminum or magnesium salts with the stomach acid. In HIV disease, antacids should be used carefully because they reduce the absorption of a number of drugs that combat HIV or opportunistic infections and require acidity in the stomach.

calcium channel antagonist See CALCIUM ENTRY BLOCKER.

calcium channel blocker See CALCIUM ENTRY BLOCKER.

calcium entry blocker Any of group of drugs that act by slowing the influx of calcium ions into muscle cells, resulting in decreased arterial resistance and myocardial oxygen demand. These drugs are used in treating angina hypertension and supraventricular tachycardia, but may cause hypotension. They have been shown to provide protection against coronary artery disease. Included in this group are nicardipine, nifedipine, verapamil, and diltiazem.

call girl See PROSTITUTE.

camptothecins Potent anticancer compounds that also have incidental antiviral activity, including against HIV.

canarypox A virus that infects birds and is used as a live vector for HIV vaccines. It can carry a large quantity of foreign genes. Small studies with a canarypox-based vaccine combination have been conducted by a variety of governmental agencies, including the National Institutes of Health (NIH). Disappointing results impacted the government's plans to launch a large international 11,000-person, $80-million trial of an HIV vaccine in 2003. Another large trial was slated to start in Thailand in 2002; responsibility for this trial would be shared by the NIH and the Royal Thai Army. This trial is designed to see whether the canarypox combination can cut HIV infection rates in half. Although proving that it would be terrific, researchers caution that the problems start if some smaller, ambiguous degree of protection is reported. In theory, even a modestly protective vaccine could have a significant impact on the pace of the epidemic over many years and large populations. However, they question what that news would do to ongoing or planned trials for more sophisticated vaccine candidates, and they note that an ethical quandary over the "best proven treatment" would change the landscape for testing vaccines. John McNeil, an architect of the canarypox study, estimated that the planned 16,000-person Thai trial could balloon to require 100,000 people if there were a standard vaccine in the picture. The U.S.-Thai collaboration on HIV vaccine research dates back a decade and is part of a longstanding partnership that has also tackled malaria and dengue virus. An effective vaccine for tuberculosis, malaria, or pneumococcal infections would have dramatic health benefits for millions of people—with and without HIV.

canarypox virus A virus that does not cause disease in humans and that is used in vaccine research, including HIV vaccine research. Canarypox virus cannot grow in human cells, an important safety feature.

cancer The uncontrolled, or malignant, growth of the cells of the tissues of any organ in the body. Cancers can destroy the tissues surrounding them by depriving normal cells of nourishment and space. Cancer cells can form a mass, or tumor, that can invade and destroy normal tissues, and can spread to different parts of the body through the bloodstream or lymphatic system. Cancers that arise in EPITHELIAL tissues are called CARCINOMAS. Cancers that arise from mesenchymal tissues are classed as SARCOMAS. Leukemias are also classed as malignant growths. Depending on the site, diagnosis is made by various means, including BIOPSY; roentgenography, including COMPUTERIZED AXIAL TOMOGRAPHY (CT scanning); MAMMOGRAPHY; ultrasound; cytology, such as the Papanicolaou test; and palpation for lumps. Some of these techniques and devices can detect an increase in the size or change in the shape of an organ, but cannot tell if such alteration is due to benign or malignant growth. There are various systems of classifying and staging cancers according to the extent and prognosis of tumors. There is no cure for cancer, but there are some effective methods of treatment, including surgery, chemotherapy, radium, and radiotherapy.

Candida A group of yeastlike fungi that develop pseudomycelia (rootlike structures) and reproduce by budding. Part of the normal flora of the mouth, skin, intestinal tract, and vagina, *Candida* species can become clinically infectious in immunocompromised people. Oral or recurrent vaginal candida infection is an early sign of immune system deterioration, diabetes, or steroid use. HIV-infected women have vaginal CANDIDIASIS more often than non-HIV-infected women; HIV infection should be considered a possibility in recurrent or severe cases.

Candida albicans The most commonly found species of CANDIDA, and the most frequent cause of CANDIDIASIS.

candidemia The presence of cells from a CANDIDA fungus in the blood, a result of a *Candida* infection, or CANDIDIASIS, in the MUCOUS MEMBRANE of the mouth, throat, intestines, or vagina.

candidiasis A condition produced by infection with a fungus of the genus CANDIDA, most often *Candida albicans,* that can affect the skin (dermatocandidiasis) and nails, MUCOUS MEMBRANES of the mouth (thrush or oral candidiasis), respiratory tract and lungs (bronchocandidiasis), esophagus (esophagitis or esophageal candidiasis), gastrointestinal tract and vagina (vaginitis or vaginal candidiasis), and other tissues. It is most often found in the mouth and esophagus and is usually nonlife-threatening and treatable. Candidiasis is commonly seen in people with suppressed immune systems, whether or not they are HIV-infected. Candidiasis of the esophagus, trachea, bronchi, or lungs is frequently the first opportunistic infection associated with AIDS. In people who do have HIV infection, candidiasis is especially common, sometimes severe, and likely to recur. In such cases patients may experience only temporary symptomatic improvement with the use of antifungal agents and require almost constant therapy for at least one year after presentation. Many women with HIV infection experience severe, recurrent vaginal *Candida* infections before any other signs of IMMUNE DYSFUNCTION. Among women with HIV infection, unexplained oral and vaginal candidiasis appear to indicate advanced disease and a severely compromised immune system. ULCERATIONS from these disorders may increase the risk of TRANSMISSION in the woman who is HIV negative.

The location of *Candida* infection indicates the state of the immune system. Vaginal candidiasis may precede oral candidiasis (thrush) and may be the first sign of immune dysfunction. As immune suppression becomes worse, the primary site of the *Candida* infection may change from the vagina to the mouth and pharynx and later to the esophagus and gastrointestinal tract in severely immunocompromised women. Vaginal candidiasis may be accompanied by generalized lymphadenopathy, localized HERPES SIMPLEX, depletion of T-HELPER CELLS, and ANERGY.

Despite the presence of oral LESIONS, patients are often asymptomatic during early stages of a candidal infection. Some complain of oral discomfort, a burning sensation when eating or an altered sense of taste. Oral candidiasis is commonly seen as whitish furry or cheesy exudates on the buccal mucosa, gingiva, tongue, or palate. There may be an erythematous (reddish) base noted after scraping the lesion. Occasionally, the typical white exudate is absent and the only finding is inflamed or atrophic oral mucosa. Diagnosis is made by scraping the lesion and examining the collected material under a microscope. Mycelia will be evident. Several therapies are available for oral candidiasis: CLOTRIMAZOLE and NYSTATIN are commonly recommended topical therapies. Systemic therapy with KETOCONAZOLE, FLUCONAZOLE, or ITRACONAZOLE is also available. Many clinicians are quick to institute therapy with fluconazole hoping that there may be some additional prophylactic effect against other fungal infections.

Esophageal candidiasis typically presents as ODYNOPHAGIA or DYSPHAGIA. Many patients complain of anterior chest pain exacerbated by swallowing. Oral thrush may or may not be present. Esophageal candidiasis may occur in patients taking topical therapy for oral candidiasis. A presumptive diagnosis may be made in patients with odynophagia that responds to empiric treatment. Barium swallow may reveal esophageal ulcerations suggestive of candida, but it is not diagnostic. Definitive diagnosis is made by ENDOSCOPY with BIOPSY and pathologic or cytologic evidence of *Candida*. For most patients with odynophagia or dys-

phagia, fluconazole or ketoconazole are the treatments of choice. Patients who have had esophageal candida may relapse after treatment and may require continuous systemic low-dose prophylaxis.

Vaginal yeast infections can usually be treated topically, with a cream or suppository that is inserted into the vagina before bed nightly for three to seven nights. Several are available over the counter (without prescription) such as Monistat-7 or Gyne-Lotrimin. If such treatments fail to relieve the symptoms and eradicate signs of infection, women should be checked for the possibility of a different infection. If no other infection exists, and yeast infection is confirmed, the oral azole agents (such as ketoconazole or fluconazole) may be required. Frequent use of the azole agents for treatment in women with very low T-cell counts, however, is problematic. Research has shown that these women are at risk for development of infection with a resistant strain of *Candida* species. These so-called resistant infections will fail to respond to treatment with azole drugs and may require treatment with topical or intravenous AMPHOTERICIN B, a drug with multiple and sometimes severe side effects. For this reason, it is felt that it is best to use topical treatment for vaginal candidiasis first and to limit the use of azole drugs as much as possible to prevent development of resistant strains. For vaginal candidiasis, exams every six months are warranted. Studies indicate that the ACIDOPHILUS bacteria found in yogurt may reduce candidal infection in the vagina.

Candida species resistant to ketoconazole and fluconaxole have been reported. Amphotericin is required for treatment of resistant strains.

cannabinoids Components of cannabis, including tetrahydrocannabinol (THC). See CANNABIS.

cannabis A plant that contains tetrahydrocannabinol (THC), the active ingredient in marijuana. Medical uses of cannabis, or THC, include stimulation of appetite and reduction of nausea.

capitation A method used by managed care plans to reimburse providers. Unlike the traditional fee-for-service system, which pays providers per service, the capitation system pays a fixed amount per capita, regardless of the type and amount of services provided. This means that doctors get the same amount of money for a person they never see as for someone to whom they provide many services. Capitation provides an incentive to avoid expensive procedures, in theory through early detection and preventive care. Managed care plans often lack adequate outreach and culturally appropriate health education and HIV prevention services.

capravirine (AG 1549, S-1153) An experimental nonnucleoside reverse transcriptase inhibitor from Agouron Pharmaceuticals, a division of Pfizer.

capreomycin Antibiotic used to treat MAC and TB. Side effects include anorexia, thirst, excess urination, red blood cells in urine, anemia, and hearing loss.

capsid A part of some viruses that surrounds the genomes and protects them from the environment.

carbohydrate An organic molecule made up solely of carbon, hydrogen, and oxygen. Carbohydrates may be made up of only one or two components (mono- or disaccharides, also called "sugars") or complex chains of repeating units (polysaccharides or "starches," also the "cellulose" in plant cell walls).

carcinogen A substance or agent that can cause the growth of cancer.

carcinoma A NEOPLASM or malignant TUMOR that arises in the epithelial tissues. Carcinomas tend to infiltrate tissue and METASTASIZE. These abnormal growths may affect almost any organ or part of the body and spread by direct extension, through lymphatics or through the bloodstream. Generally differentiated by location of occurrence in the body, etiology, appearance, or composition, there are many different types of carcinomas. See CANCER.

cardiac abnormalities Abnormalities of the heart.

cardiomyopathy Any disease of the MYOCARDIUM, the cardiac muscle that forms the walls of the chambers of the heart.

cardiopulmonary resuscitation (CPR) The restoration of breathing and heartbeat in a person in which these have stopped. CPR is a form of first aid whose goal is to provide oxygen quickly to the brain, heart, and other vital organs until appropriate, definitive medical treatment can restore normal heart and pulmonary function.

There is a prescribed sequence of steps for CPR. To be certain CPR is required, a patient's state of consciousness and cardiac and pulmonary function must be assessed. A patient may be questioned to test responsiveness. Once it is determined that CPR is necessary (and medical help is called for) the patient is positioned for access to face and anterior chest. Rescue breathing is begun using mouth-to-mouth techniques. In order to prevent transmission of disease from the patient to one administering CPR, a bag, valve, mask, or other device should be used rather than direct mouth-to-mouth contact. The Heimlich maneuver is often used to clear the airway of a foreign body. External chest compression is done if there is no pulse and there is cardiac arrest.

care The provision of accommodation, comfort, medical treatment, protection, and custodial concern, as needed. In medicine, the five basic types of care are ambulatory, emergency, primary, secondary, and tertiary.

care plan A formal written plan for nursing, auxiliary services, and other services and activities for a patient to be conducted by hospital, home health agency, residential treatment center, or other health facility. It is used as a guide for treatment and rehabilitation and to evaluate the patient's needs and progress.

caregiver Professional health care providers (physicians, nurses, social workers, therapists) or personal care providers (family, friends, spouses, significant others, volunteers) who work with persons who are ill or incapacitated.

Compassion, courage, and caring are attributes associated with those who care for people with

AIDS. Training for volunteer caregivers often covers the medical aspects of HIV/AIDS, coping (including stress and burnout), counseling, and practical matters, such as home care, paperwork, or dealing with institutions. Care of caregivers themselves is also a concern of nurses, social workers, and others who manage chronic patients. Generally, caregivers are in need of emotional support and comfort because of the extreme stress of their lives.

Caribbean   Outside sub-Saharan Africa the Caribbean region has a higher percentage of its population HIV-positive than any place in the world. HIV disease was first seen in the Caribbean in HAITI in the very early 1980s. Since then the rate of infection has reached 2 percent across the region. More than 300,000 people have died in Haiti alone since the start of the epidemic. Approximately 500,000 people in the Caribbean region are now believed to be HIV-positive. More than 87 percent of these people reside in two countries, Haiti and the Dominican Republic.

As in developing regions around the world, population migration is considered a large factor in the Caribbean region spread of HIV. Many of the region's residents must seek employment outside their country in a Western economy and consequently are away from their home and families. This is believed to have been the factor that introduced the virus to Haiti, travel by the men to work in the United States, where access to drugs and prostitution was easier, followed by travel home to spread the virus among their family. Statistics reveal that approximately 12 percent of urban Haitians and 5 percent of rural Haitians are infected. Already the epidemic has left more than 200,000 orphans in Haiti, according to UNAIDS. The numbers have been nearly as bad in the Bahamas, where close to 4 percent of the population is infected. It is the leading cause of death in both Haiti and the Bahamas. Tourism is another factor in the spread of the virus. The Caribbean is region that has an excess of relatively wealthy tourists who are marketed on the "sexiness" of the region. This has led to trade in sex that has increased over the same years that the epidemic has arrived. Many island residents see the sex business as a way to earn a good deal of money much more quickly than by working in a field or factory.

This idea has led to rates of infection for teenage women five times higher than those of similarly aged men. This would indicate that these women are earning money sleeping with older men.

The Caribbean region is made up of 30 island nations and territories and four mainland countries and territories that share a common cultural heritage with the islands. The four mainland countries are Guyana, French Guyana, and Suriname in South America and Belize in Central America. The region has a mosaic of different problems that have spread the virus. In Puerto Rico, for instance, the virus was almost completely an IDU illness up through the end of 2001. In Barbados, where the rate of infection has reached nearly 2 percent, the illness is spread solely through sex and no IDU cases have been reported. Heterosexual sex represented four of every five cases of the virus. Trinidad and Tobago also report a predominant spread through heterosexuality. The rate of infection in Trinidad and Tobago is above 1 percent. Other countries that have rates of infection above 1 percent are Suriname, Guyana, Jamaica, Dominican Republic, and Belize.

In some of these countries the numbers continue to rise. In clinics for pregnant women in Guyana, the rate of infection has reached 7 percent. Elsewhere in Guyana, 50 percent of sex workers, 22 percent of people seeking medical care for other STDs, and 3 percent of blood donors were HIV-positive. Reasons vary from country to country. Many people in the Caribbean who have been polled believe that AIDS is a gay disease. Often heterosexuals do not see themselves as targets for the virus. However, other surveys show that men having sex with men account for up to 20 percent of the cases in the Caribbean; in Trinidad and Tobago those statistics are accurate. As in many Latin countries the focus is placed on being macho or the active partner, so these people do not often see themselves as gay and do not discuss having sex with men. Women from the Caribbean say that the macho attitudes of the men lead them to have many affairs, with women and men. Women are culturally not able to use condoms because of restrictions placed on them by the men. Another way that talk is discouraged are regulations such as those in Jamaica, where strict laws require anyone who is HIV-positive to list all of his or her sex partners so the government can notify them. People report not being tested so that they do not have to discuss the number of people with whom they are currently having sex.

There are few bright spots in the Caribbean. One is the Dominican Republic, where HIV-positive rates have remained steady since big increases in the early 1990s. In the Bahamas, the last few years have shown a somewhat positive story as the rate of infection has dropped in the main populace. Then there is Cuba's story. Cuba is a relatively isolated country. It is believed that although Cuba had cases early, they were among soldiers who were returning form Africa, rather than sex workers or IDUs. Cuba began screening all blood supplies before other countries in the region did (1986). Cuba also made it a policy to segregate and quarantine everyone who tested positive. Cuba also began treating everyone with AIDS with strong medical care. The result is that just 0.02 percent of Cuba's population is HIV-positive today. Cuba has since relaxed the requirement of quarantine. Many HIV-positive people live at home but travel to the health clinics for their medications. However, many HIV-positive individuals choose to move to the clinics. They are given all their food and medicines, and Cuba has begun to provide some of the HAART medications free of charge. These are all reasons that induce HIV-positive people to segregate themselves in Cuba and keep the virus levels low in that country.

Caribbean governments, except the Cuban government, were initially slow to respond to the HIV spread. In 2001, the Caribbean Community (CARICOM), the economic development and trade group for the region, initiated agreements between the governments to work toward slowing the progress of HIV through the region. The World Bank has begun funding programs of education and prevention on some islands. The Dominican Republic has started a program, as has Grenada. The World Bank has several other programs awaiting approval from various governments. In mid-2002 several large private pharmaceutical companies agreed to lower drug prices for antiretrovirals for the region. GlaxoSmithKline, Hoffman-LaRoche, Boehringer Ingelheim, Bristol-Meyers Squibb, Merck, and Abbott stated that prices of some medications would now be up to 90 percent lower. The prices were based on the ability to pay in Jamaica.

This policy has upset some leaders, as countries where the epidemic is worst, such as Haiti and Guyana, have much lower income levels than exist in Jamaica.

carotenoids A class of carotenes, such as beta-carotene.

carrier 1. A person who shows no signs or symptoms of disease but who is infected with a contagious disease. This person is capable of spreading the infectious organism to others. 2. Anything that passively carries infectious organisms. 3. A substance that, when combined with another (transport) substance is capable of passing through cell membranes.

Infectious organisms may be carried by people, by animals, air, food, insects, soil, and water. Carriers may be active, convalescent, genetic, healthy, incubatory, intermittent, or passive.

Carrisyn See ACEMANNAN.

case An instance of disease. A shorthand, somewhat depersonalized way to refer to a patient or client and the medical, psychological, or social problem he or she presents to a health care provider.

case advocacy Argument on behalf of or attempts to find a solution for a person or persons with a unique set of problems or service needs. It is distinguished from class advocacy, which is arguing on behalf of or attempting to find a solution to the problems or service needs of an entire population.

case control In epidemiology, a study in which index cases are matched to comparison cases in an attempt to discover risk factors or exposure.

case definition (of AIDS) See AIDS CASE DEFINITION.

case history The complete medical, family, social, and psychiatric history of a patient up to the beginning of treatment for his or her present illness. Case histories are used in the practice of medicine, psychiatry, and psychology to help rule out and pursue probable cause of illness and disease.

case management A system under which a patient's health care and social services are coordinated by one or more individuals familiar with both the patient's needs and community resources. Components of the system include patient or client assessment, treatment planning, referral, and follow-up. The goals of case management are the provision of comprehensive and continuous service and the coordination of payment and reimbursement for care in a manner designed to reduce inpatient costs by providing access to outpatient services and consideration by the insurer or other third-party payer of benefit reimbursement for services and supplies not typically covered. See CASE MANAGER.

case manager One who directs or coordinates CASE MANAGEMENT. Insurers or other third-party payers may have counterparts, also called case managers, who review treatment plans and authorize exceptional benefits in high-cost cases.

case summary A summary of the essentials of a patient's illness, treatment, and prognosis. The interpretations of the health professional preparing the summary may be included.

case-control study A retrospective study that starts with the identification of people who have a disease or condition (the cases) and those who do not (the controls). Researchers then look for information about the exposure that the cases and controls had to some factor or factors under investigation.

casual contact Contact with other people in the course of normal, nonintimate everyday activities and behaviors such as going to school, talking, working, eating, playing, studying, hugging, or shaking or holding hands. Casual contact is distinct from intimate, specifically sexual contact, which involves exposure to or sharing of body fluids.

Casual contact implies contact closer than chance passing on a street or sharing a seat on a bus. Being or dwelling in the same physical environment as an HIV-infected person, wearing that person's clothing, using that person's furniture, or touching or hugging or otherwise exposing the surface of the skin to that person's are all instances of casual contact. Casual contact can also include sitting on a toilet seat, touching a doorknob, or using a public telephone after someone who is HIV-positive or has AIDS. Casual contact is considered without risk of infection with HIV.

casual sex Sexual intercourse with a person whose sexual history is not known and with whom one has not established a permanent, closed sexual relationship.

CAT scan See COMPUTERIZED AXIAL TOMOGRAPHY.

catabolic Refers to metabolic processes that break down tissue in the body.

catalase A naturally occurring antioxidant.

categorically needy In MEDICAID parlance, those who receive Medicaid because they receive, are eligible for, or are deemed eligible for AFDC, SSI, or SSPS.

category A A drug for which adequate and well-controlled studies of pregnant women fail to demonstrate a risk to the fetus during pregnancy.

category B A drug for which animal reproduction studies fail to demonstrate a risk to the fetus, but adequate and well-controlled studies have not been conducted.

category C A drug for which safety in human pregnancy has not been determined and animal studies either have had positive findings for fetal risk or have not been conducted. Pregnant women should not use category C drugs unless the potential benefits outweigh the potential risk to the fetus.

category D A drug for which there is positive evidence of human fetal risk based on adverse reaction data from investigational or marketing experiences. In certain cases, the potential benefits from the use of this drug in pregnant women may be acceptable despite its potential risks.

category X A drug for which studies in animals or reports of adverse reactions in humans have indicated that the risk associated with its use clearly outweighs any possible benefit for pregnant women.

cathartic   An active purgative, producing bowel movements.

catheter   A tube made of a flexible material, such as silicon rubber, which is used when it is medically necessary to introduce fluids to or drain fluids from the body. Many people with HIV illness need a catheter for intravenous infusions of medication or nutrition. A catheter is inserted directly into a sac, cavity, or vein and can be used to administer drugs (it is this function that concerns us here). A peripherally inserted central catheter (PICC) line is usually inserted into a vein in an arm and is used for periods of up to three months. This type of catheter does not need to be surgically implanted and can be inserted at home by a trained nurse. For longer periods, catheters are surgically implanted directly into a central vein in the chest. These are called central venous catheters and can be used for months or years.

When infusions are begun, the first few administrations are usually given through a regular INTRAVENOUS (IV) line, not a catheter. An intravenous line is a small tube that extends about one inch into a vein and about half an inch outside the skin. It ends in a heplock, a small chamber that contains heparin, a substance that keeps blood from clotting, allowing the catheter to remain open. The heplock can be reused for two to three days. After that, a midline, long-line or peripherally-inserted central catheter is likely to be inserted. A midline catheter is inserted into a vein in the arm like an IV line, but the tubing extends about 6 inches. Midline catheters can be used for up to six weeks and cannot be used for long-term total parenteral nutrition, chemotherapy, or to draw blood. A long-line catheter consists of a tube inserted into the arm and then threaded up the arm into a big vein near the heart. Long-line catheters can be used for up to three months.

The most common complication of midlines and PICC lines is phlebitis (inflammation of the vein), in which the skin overlaying the vein becomes warm, red, and painful. The catheter will then usually be removed and replaced in another vein. The irritation may be caused by the catheter itself or by the medication. Over time, people may run out of good peripheral veins, and an indwelling central line (also known as a right atrial catheter or venous access device) becomes necessary. Another complication of both midlines and PICCs is that they can "migrate out," that is, the end of the catheter within the big vein near the heart can be dislocated to a smaller vein. When this occurs, the line usually has to be replaced.

The major complications of central venous catheters are bacterial infections. The catheter exit site and impurities in infusion liquids are potential ports of entry for bacteria. Local infections at the exit site, without tenderness along the tunnel, usually can be treated locally. Tunnel infections may require catheter removal and replacement on the other side of the chest.

The Hickman catheter is the most common of the indwelling central venous catheters. The Hickman catheter is a modification of an earlier catheter developed by a Dr. Broviac in 1973 for the purpose of infusing total parenteral nutrition. The Hickman has a wider tube and thicker tube wall than the Broviac catheter and is more widely used today. The Hickman consists of a long internal tube that extends from a vein above the heart through a "tunnel" in the chest to what is called an exit site. About one inch before the exit site there is a small Dacron cuff that serves as an anchor and barrier to infection.

Catheters may have one or more separate external tubes or "lumens" branching from the catheter outside the body. Each lumen is four or five inches long and ends in a rubber cap. When the catheter is used a needle is inserted in this cap. The lumens are looped and taped to the chest when not in use. Many catheters used today by people with HIV illness have two lumens so that two procedures can be done simultaneously. The Groshong catheter is a newer version of the Hickman, in which the internal catheter tip is closed. Instead of an open tube, there is a valve or slip on the side of the tube. The valve remains closed when not in use. During an infusion, the pressure of the incoming fluid opens the valve, letting the fluid enter the bloodstream. When suction is applied, this negative pressure causes the valve to open inward, letting blood flow through the catheter into the syringe. A Groshong catheter does not need heparin flushes, slightly simplifying routine maintenance procedures. The valve is intended to minimize blood backflow problems. The Groshong's tube is not as wide as the Hickman's. As a result, more time is needed for procedures such as infusions.

The internal tubing of the port is the same as that extending outside the body; a "port" made of metal or a synthetic material is placed mid-chest under the skin. The skin is punctured with special needles every time the port is used. There are no external components to the port. Initially, the skin over the port may be bruised and sore from the operation, but often becomes numb after a couple of weeks. Ports are most suitable for medication administered once or twice a month, but are now being used for daily procedures by people with HIV illness.

Ports are attached to four of five inches of silicone tubing with a clamp and rubber cap at one end and a needle at the other. The needle is inserted through the skin into the port, creating a temporary lumen. Medication is inserted by a needle into the tube's rubber cap, not the port itself. Ports are available with either one or two chambers, however the double size is somewhat large. When two "channels" are considered appropriate, surgeons often prefer to use an indwelling catheter instead of a port. A recent development is a port that can be placed in the forearm under the skin, instead of in the chest.

Institutional contracts with suppliers may determine whether Hickmans or Groshongs are used. Some hospitals do not consider PICC lines cost-effective, and patients go directly from intravenous lines to indwelling central venous catheters. Not all systems are available at every hospital.

There are some clear-cut advantages to one system or the other (catheters vs. ports), and also some relative advantages depending on medical indications. A significant disadvantage of the port is that it must be surgically removed. Also, an infected Hickman catheter can be removed on the spot in an emergency room, while a port requires transfer to an operating room for surgical removal. This can cause a delay in removing the source of the infection.

Some people don't like to stick themselves with needles, and so prefer catheters where the needle goes into the lumen through a rubber cap, not

their skin. When made of stainless steel or titanium, ports interfere with diagnostic imaging (MRI and CT scans) and radiation. People with significant visual impairment cannot handle ports. When two lumens are indicated rather than one, surgeons often prefer Hickmans or Groshongs to ports, although double ports are available. At advanced stages of illness, people might not be able to insert the special needles used with ports and will need assistance. In addition, when people lose a lot of weight, the port becomes quite prominent, particularly if it has two reservoirs.

There are no absolute disadvantages to Hickman-type catheters. However, there are relative disadvantages. The lumens are visible to the patient and to others. More equipment is entailed. This involves keeping track of supplies (dressings, swabs, injection caps) and their delivery. These are also needed with ports, but in smaller amounts. Swimming with a Hickman is not possible. Nursing visits may be needed more often to check on procedures and the condition of the exit site. These are primarily practical and aesthetic disadvantages, and while far from trivial, they are not in the same league as potential port-related major medical problems. All of these disadvantages also apply to ports if the needle and attached tubing are left in place for several days at a time.

CBC   See COMPLETE BLOOD COUNT.

CCNU (Lomustine)   CCNU is one of the older chemotherapy drugs; it has been in use for years. CCNU is a capsule taken orally. It is most commonly used in the treatment of lung cancer, multiple myeloma, and brain tumors. The type and extent of a cancer determine the method and schedule of administration of the drug. This decision is made by the medical oncologist. CCNU is normally administered every six to eight weeks. The degree and severity of the side effects depend on the amount and schedule of the administration of CCNU. Low white blood counts, low platelet counts, anemia, hair loss, lung damage, and diarrhea are some of the most common and significant ill effects.

CCR5   A seven-looped protein structure that normally occurs on the surface of certain immune system cells and acts as a chemokine receptor site. CCR5 is the second receptor necessary for macrophage-tropic HIV to bind to and enter a cell. The other receptor is CD4. People who lack CCR5 receptors seem to be very resistant to HIV infection and, if infected, have a slow progression to AIDS.

CD See CLUSTER OF DIFFERENTIATION.

CD2 cell See ACCESSORY MOLECULES.

CD4 A protein whose presence on the surface of a human cell allows HIV to attach to and enter, and thus infect, a cell. CD4 RECEPTORS are present on CD4 CELLS (HELPER T CELLS), MACROPHAGES, and DENDRITIC CELLS, among others. Normally, CD4 acts as an ACCESSORY MOLECULE, forming part of a larger structure through which T CELLS and other cells signal each other.

It has been hypothesized that CD4 alone is not able to allow HIV or HIV-infected cells to fuse with target cells and infect them. Several lines of evidence have suggested that one or more cofactors, presumably also molecules on the surface of target cells, are necessary for HIV fusion and entry. Recent data indicate that a second molecule, fusin, also is required for fusion and entry of certain strains of HIV into cells. See ANTIGEN; RECEPTOR.

CD4 cell A white blood cell (LYMPHOCYTE) with CD4 molecules on its surface; a CD4-positive (CD4+) cell.

Each type of white blood cell plays a specific role in the immune system. The CD4 cell modulates the immune response to an infection through a complex series of interactions with ANTIGEN presenting cells (MACROPHAGES, DENDRITIC CELLS, and B CELLS) and other types of lymphocytes (B cells and CD8 CELLS). The CD4 cell is also known as the T-helper cell or HELPER T CELL.

CD4 cell count The number of CD4 CELLS per cubic millimeter of blood. This measurement is the most commonly used SURROGATE MARKER for assessing the state of an HIV-infected patient's immune system. The CD4 cell count frequently indicates the stage of HIV infection. As the count

declines, the risk of developing OPPORTUNISTIC INFECTIONS increases. The trend of several consecutive CD4 cell counts is more important than any one measurement.

Recent findings indicate that the immune system's army of CD4+ T cells not only declines in overall size during the course of HIV disease but also becomes progressively less diverse as specific CD4+ T cells programmed to fight different invaders are lost. Furthermore, these depleted cell types may not be immediately restored by therapies such as anti-retroviral drugs or interleukin-2 (IL-2) that can increase an HIV-infected person's overall CD4+ T cell count. Rather, such therapy, at least in the short term, appears to boost only the cells that were present when therapy began. These findings argue for treatment early in the disease, before elements of the immune system are significantly depleted. The data also suggest that drugs to prevent opportunistic infections may remain important even for patients with CD4+ T cell counts that are rapidly increasing in response to therapy, because these individuals may be missing part of their CD4+ T cell repertoires.

The normal range for CD4 cell counts is 500 to 1500 and patients should be tested every six to twelve months if counts are higher than 500. If the counts are lower, testing every three months is advised. The CD4 count is a relatively expensive test, but it is an important way of monitoring the state of the immune system. Counts vary considerably, however; the same laboratory performing multiple tests on the same specimen can find counts that vary by as much as 20 percent. The count is also influenced by a variety of other medical conditions apart from HIV infection. As a result, although the CD4+ count is frequently used to assess progressive disease, changes in the count are sometimes difficult to interpret.

A few years ago, there seemed to be a sound scientific rationale for using CD4 cell counts to predict treatment response. They provided most of the evidence justifying the approval of ddI, d4T, and ddC in combination therapy. Little, however, can be said definitively about the clinical benefit of these drugs, and it has become increasingly apparent that CD4 is a poor "surrogate" for predicting results. A 1994 study retrospectively analyzing the outcomes of a number of randomized trials found that CD4 cell counts actually obscured the clinical results, highlighting the importance of empirical validation in assessing the information derived from such tests.

CD4 lymphocyte   A white blood cell with CD4 molecules present on its surface. See CD4 CELL.

CD4+ percent   The percentage of total lymphocytes made up by CD4 cells. A common measure of immune status that is about 40 percent in healthy individuals and that can be below 20 percent in persons with AIDS.

CD4, synthetic   Soluble genetically engineered CD4 designed to be injected into the blood to inactivate the HIV virus by covering all its "plugs" before they can find real "sockets." CD4 molecule is very expensive to make, and breaks down so fast that it has to be taken—by injection, every four hours.

The efforts to develop synthetic CD4 are the first attempts to develop a potential AIDS therapy by employing recombinant DNA technology (gene-splicing) to focus on a part of HIV's life cycle. Scientists have taken the CD4 protein's gene-encoding program and inserted it into cells that then manufacture more. The idea is that flooding the body with synthetic CD4 might decoy the virus, sparing healthy T-CELLS from infection and destruction. So far, at least, CD4 doesn't seem to be producing auto-antibodies (nor has it been found to be toxic).

CD4-IgG2   A recombinant human fusion protein being studied as a treatment for HIV. See FUSION PROTEINS.

CD4-positive (CD4+)   A designation indicating the presence of CD4.

CD4-positive (CD4+) cell   A cell on whose surface molecules of CD4 are present; a CD4 CELL.

CD4-positive (CD4+) cell count   See CD4 CELL COUNT.

CD4-positive (CD4+) lymphocyte   See CD4 CELL.

CD4-positive (CD4+) percentage   The proportion of CD4+ CELLS in relation to the total number of LYMPHOCYTES in a quantity of blood (standard specimen unit is one cubic millimeter). As HIV infection progresses, the percentage decreases. A significant drop in the CD4 CELL COUNT reflects significant damage to the immune system.

CD4-to-CD8 ratio   The ratio of CD4 to CD8 cells. A common measure of immune system status that is approximately 1.5 to two CD4 cells to one CD8 cell in healthy individuals and falls as CD4 cell counts fall in persons with HIV infection.

CD8   A protein present on the surface of some white blood cells, or LYMPHOCYTES. CD8 seems to be necessary to the CYTOTOXIC function of these cells, which are crucial to the working of the IMMUNE SYSTEM. See CD8 CELL; T-LYMPHOCYTES.

CD8 cell   A white blood cell (LYMPHOCYTE) with CD8 molecules on its surface; a CD8-positive (CD8+) T CELL. Most CD8 cells are thought to consist of SUPPRESSOR/CYTOTOXIC lymphocytes, which play a crucial role in determining IMMUNE RESPONSE. Some recognize and kill cancerous cells and those infected by intracellular pathogens (some bacteria, viruses, and mycoplasma).

In addition to killing HIV-infected cells directly by a process called CYTOLYSIS, these cells also secrete soluble factors that suppress HIV replication in blood and lymph nodes taken from HIV-infected people. It is hypothesized that part of the CD8 suppressor phenomenon is due to the secretion by CD8+ T cells of signaling molecules called beta-CHEMOKINES, which normally recruit inflammatory cells to the site of an infection. Three of these molecules, known as RANTES, MIP-1a and MIP-1B, apparently block HIV replication by occupying receptors necessary for the entry of MACROPHAGE-tropic strains of HIV into their target cells.

Halting of AIDS progression is thought to be associated with stable CD8 CELL COUNTs over time; despite declines, in some cases to zero, in CD4 CELL COUNTS. It is speculated that stable CD8 cell counts may be a common denominator in cases of long-term survival. As a result, therapies have been developed based on techniques of increasing CD8 cell counts in symptomatic individuals. Approaches have included a KAPOSI'S SARCOMA treatment called CD8 cell expansion, in which CD8 cells are removed from the blood and cultivated in culture by adding the protein INTERLEUKIN-2. The cultivated cells are then reinjected into the patients' bloodstream. Another method is modification of the body's biological response. DINITROCHLOROBEN-ZENE (DNCB) is a powerful stimulator of an immune response called DELAYED-TYPE HYPERSENSITIVITY, which is known to control intracellular infections; topical application of it has been shown to raise the levels of CD8 cells and natural killer cells consistently and nontoxically among compliant patients.

CD8 cell count   The number of CD8 CELLS per cubic millimeter of blood; an important measurement of IMMUNE SYSTEM status.

CD8 cell expansion   A treatment that involves growing an HIV-infected patient's CD8 CELLS outside the body, in order to increase his CD8 CELL COUNT.

CD8 lymphocyte   A white blood cell with CD8 molecules on its surface. See CD8 CELL.

CD8-positive (CD8+)   A designation indicating the presence of CD8.

CD8-positive (CD8+) cell   A cell on whose surface molecules of CD8 are present; a CD8 CELL.

CD8-positive (CD8+) cell count   See CD8 CELL COUNT.

CD8-positive (CD8+) cell expansion   See CD8 CELL EXPANSION; CD8 CELL.

CD8-positive (CD8+) lymphocyte   See CD8 CELL.

CDC definition   See AIDS CASE DEFINITION.

ceftriaxone   A broad-spectrum antibiotic. Ceftriaxone is used for bacterial infections of the lower respiratory tract, skin, urinary tract, bones and

joints, abdomen, and blood. It is also used for PELVIC INFLAMMATORY DISEASE and MENINGITIS. It is generally not the first-choice therapy for most bacterial infections because it cannot be taken orally. It is particularly useful against infection in the brain or other part of the central nervous system, when the bacteria is resistant to penicillin or the oral cephalosporins. Ceftriaxone weakens the cell walls of newly formed bacteria. Common side effects include pain, tenderness, or hardness at the injection site. Rash, itching, fever or chills, blood-clotting disorders, and deficiencies in red or white blood cells occur less frequently. (The trade name is Rocephin.)

cefuroxime   An antibiotic used to treat bacterial infections of the ear, respiratory tract, skin, sinuses, bones and joints, and urinary tract. Cefuroxime belongs to the cephalosporin class of antibiotics. The most common side effects include diarrhea, nausea, vomiting, and abdominal pain; these occur more frequently at higher doses. This drug works by preventing susceptible bacteria from building strong cell walls.

Cefuroxime is available in tablet, oral suspension, and injectable solution form. These are taken up differently by the body and require different doses. The oral suspension is intended primarily for children. Tablets are used for mild-to-moderate infections and injection for more serious infections. (Trade names are Ceftin, Kefurox, and Zinacef.)

celibacy   Abstention from sexual intercourse. Also, in a somewhat old-fashioned usage, the state of being unmarried.

cell   A microscopic unit of protoplasm containing a nucleus and bounded by a membrane. The cell is the smallest independent unit of life that is capable of performing all living functions, and the smallest unit making up larger living organisms.

cell cycle   The phases that a cell goes through in dividing, and specifically the period during which events involved in nucleation and reproduction are completed. In proliferative cells this includes all the events taking place between the completion of one round of mitosis and CYTOKINESIS and the next.

Cells that have begun to differentiate have generally left the cell cycle for good.

The molecular details of the cell cycle have been the subject of intense research in recent decades, not least because of their implications for our understanding of the origins of many cancers. In both normal and cancer cells a cell growth cycle can be divided into discrete phases. The two key phases of the cell cycle are the S phase, during which DNA is synthesized, and the M phase, the period of actual division, or mitosis. Both of these points can be measured or marked on an individual cell. Active cells are dynamic, and cancer may be thought of as a disorder of cells that are constantly dividing. Chemotherapy is thought to be effective only when cells are dividing, and certain drugs target this phase of the cell cycle in a specific way. On a basic cellular level, this is how anticancer drugs work.

cell line   A collection of cells that divide continuously in culture. They may be either monoclonal or polyclonal and may have been transformed naturally or be an artificial hybridization.

cell surface receptor   A molecule on the cell's surface that binds with various substances, causing changes in the activity of the cell. See RECEPTOR.

cell-activated factor (CAF)   A so-far-unidentified substance that is secreted by activated CD8 cells and that inhibits HIV replication within cells. CAF activity seems to be high in long-term nonprogressors but low in patients who have rapid disease progression.

cell-mediated immunity (CMI)   The process of the IMMUNE SYSTEM through which the destruction of foreign material (ANTIGEN) is performed by specific defense cells (NEUTROPHILS, MACROPHAGES, NATURAL KILLER CELLS, EOSINOPHILS, and other WHITE BLOOD CELLS) rather than by ANTIBODIES. It is sometimes referred to as cellular immunity. CMI is controlled by T CELLS, as opposed to B CELLS. T cells are produced in the bone marrow, as are B cells, but mature in the THYMUS. From the thymus T cells are produced and move out in the body to attack the specific antigen for which they are produced. Once the T cell attaches itself to the antigen, a wide vari-

ety of defense mechanisms take place. Often these mechanisms involve the various white blood cells mentioned earlier. CYTOKINES are released at the site of T-cell activation; these in turn enhance further T-cell production and activation. These T cells are often called EFFECTOR cells; they include CD4 and CD8 cells. CD4 cells attract MONOCYTES, MACROPHAGES, and GRANULOCYTES, which cause CYTOTOXICITY to the antigen. CD8 cells are directly toxic to the invader themselves. In HIV, the virus invades certain T cells, causing problems in the cell-mediated immunity response. In the early days of immunology research, CMI was considered to be primarily, if not entirely, a DELAYED-TYPE HYPERSENSITIVITY (DTH) reaction against microbial antigens during certain experimental and clinical infections. Research in recent years has shown that CMI is a highly complex immunologic event, expressed not only in DTH but also in a number of infections by a variety of foreign material. CMI has yet to be understood fully despite recent intensive research. See ANTIBODY-MEDIATED IMMUNITY.

cellular immunity   The mechanism of immunity that does not involve antibody production, but rather the destruction of foreign antigens by the activities of T CELLS and MACROPHAGES. The human immune system, which protects the body from infections and tumors, consists of two "arms," HUMORAL IMMUNITY (effected by soluble antibodies secreted by B CELLS into the body fluids) and cellular, or cell-mediated immunity (effected by cells, especially T cells, and their secretions). The primary effector cells are activated macrophages, NATURAL KILLER CELLS, and CYTOTOXIC T CELL lymphocytes. It is the natural function of these cells to destroy all infected and abnormal cells, including HIV-infected CD4 cells. These effector cells are activated by DELAYED-TYPE HYPERSENSITIVITY (DTH). Cellular, or cell-mediated, immunity is critical in controlling and clearing the agents that cause OPPORTUNISTIC INFECTION AND DISEASE in AIDS; these and the neoplasms seen in AIDS, as well as HIV itself, are cellular infections and can be controlled only by cellular immunity.

Defective cellular immunity was the first recognized hallmark of AIDS in 1981 and is a prerequisite to disease progression. Researchers have concluded that the opportunistic infections and neoplasms seen in AIDS, including HIV, flourish when cellular immunity is suppressed and humoral immunity is dominant. They also believe that an imbalance between the two, with humoral immunity dominant, may actually predispose individuals to HIV infection. Successful treatments for AIDS must therefore be able to stimulate cellular immunity and suppress humoral immunity. Stimulation of cellular immunity will probably be the only means by which HIV infection may be made a chronic, rather than fatal, disease. Most of the current approved treatments and prophylaxis for HIV and opportunistic infections are IMMUNOSUPPRESSIVE—they impair cellular immunity.

censoring A term used in survival or time-to-event analyses to denote an individual who has not experienced the event of interest as of a specific point in follow-up, such as time of interim analysis. The process by which patient outcome data cannot be obtained beyond a specific point in time.

Center for Infectious Diseases (CID) A constituent part of the CENTERS FOR DISEASE CONTROL AND PREVENTION (CDC).

Centers for Disease Control and Prevention (CDC) The federal public health agency serving as the center for preventing, tracking, controlling, and investigating the epidemiology of AIDS and other diseases. The agency performs epidemiological study and surveillance of disease, mortality, and morbidity, and develops and conducts programs for disease prevention. The CDC CASE DEFINITION of AIDS can be understood as the legal definition of AIDS; it is the standard for reporting AIDS cases in the United States and for determination of eligibility for welfare and health benefits.

central nervous system (CNS) The part of the nervous system that controls intelligence and emotion. In human beings and other vertebrates it consists of the brain and the spinal cord and the protective membranes (meninges) surrounding them. See PERIPHERAL NERVOUS SYSTEM.

Central Asia See EASTERN EUROPE AND CENTRAL ASIA.

central nervous system damage The central nervous system is composed of the brain, spinal cord, and meninges. Although HIV can infect monocytes and macrophages, they appear to be relatively resistant to killing. However, these cells travel throughout the body and carry HIV to various organs, especially the lungs and the brain. Persons living with HIV often experience abnormalities in the central nervous system. Investigators have hypothesized that an accumulation of HIV in the brain and nerve cells or the inappropriate release of cytokines or toxic by-products of these cells may be the cause of the neurological manifestations of HIV disease.

central nervous system lymphoma See PRIMARY CENTRAL NERVOUS SYSTEM LYMPHOMA.

cerebrospinal fluid (CSF) The fluid found within the cavities of the brain and surrounding both the brain and the spinal cord. A sample of this fluid is often removed from the body for diagnosis purposes by a lumbar puncture (SPINAL TAP). The fluid is analyzed for cancer cells or evidence of other disorders.

cerebrovascular accident (CVA) A STROKE. A general term most commonly applied to cerebrovascular conditions that accompany either ischemic or hemorrhagic lesions. These conditions are usually secondary to atherosclerotic disease, hypertension, or a combination of both. Also called APOPLEXY or simply a "shock."

cervical atypia Abnormalities or irregularities in cervical cells.

cervical cancer Malignant neoplasm (growth) in the CERVIX, or neck of the uterus. Cervical cancer may occur at any age from puberty on. The mortality rate increases with age. Risk factors include early age at first intercourse, multiple sexual partners, more than five pregnancies, and a history of SYPHILIS or GONORRHEA. Women whose mothers took DES while pregnant are also at risk. It is suspected that an oncogenic factor, most probably a virus, is transmitted sexually, and the HUMAN PAPILLOMA VIRUS is thought to be an important factor.

COLPOSCOPY and regular PAP (Papanicolaou) tests after a woman becomes sexually active are two means of diagnosis.

Cervical cancer may be present for up to ten years before symptoms appear. The most common symptom, when the cancer is at a more advanced, invasive stage, is abnormal bleeding (which can be a symptom of other diseases as well).

Cervical cancer develops progressively in several stages through which it spreads throughout the cervix, the pelvic areas and other parts of the body. Treatment depends on the stage of the cancer, general state of health of the patient, and other factors. As with other cancers, radiation, surgery, and cytotoxic agents are used.

The best way to screen HIV-positive women for cervical cancer has long been a matter of debate. Medical reports through the years have documented that women with HIV have a greater risk of cervical cancer than noninfected women, and that it progresses more rapidly and tends to recur after treatment. The accuracy of the Pap smear, the standard method for detecting abnormalities that might develop into cervical cancer, has recently been called into question, particularly in the case of women with HIV. These women frequently have lower genital tract infections that may obscure test results. In colposcopy, a low-power microscope (colposcope) is used to examine the cervix, and if suspect tissue is observed, a biopsy is performed for further evaluation. Colposcopy has traditionally served only as a corroborative test in women with abnormal Pap smears, but in recent years some medical authorities have urged that cervical colposcopy be part of the routine management of HIV-positive women regardless of the findings of previous Pap smears.

Cervical cancer is now regarded as a totally preventable disease. AIDS activists and many health care providers believe that cervical cancer represents not an individual or a medical failure, but a system failure. They believe that all women should receive gynecological care as part of their routine primary care.

cervical cap   A contraceptive device for women that works like a small diaphragm over the CERVIX. It is held in place by suction.

cervical disease   Any disease of the cervix, particularly HUMAN PAPILLOMA VIRUS (HPV), a sexually transmitted virus certain strains of which are known to cause precancerous growths in the cervix (CERVICAL INTRAEPITHELIAL NEOPLASIA, or CIN). See CERVICAL CANCER.

cervical dysplasia   An abnormality in the size, shape, or organization of the cells on the cervix (the head and neck of the uterus). On a Pap smear report, dysplasia is referred to as cervical intraepithelial neoplasia (CIN) or squamous intraepithelial lesion (SIL). Cervical dysplasia is usually first discovered by Pap smear, in which cells are swabbed from in and around the cervical os (opening of the cervix). Dysplastic changes in the Pap smear result are rated as low-grade or high-grade. High-grade lesions are considered precursors to cervical cancer; the significance of low-grade dysplasia has not been established. If undetected, cervical dysplasia may progress to a more severe lesion; thus any abnormal finding should prompt further examination.

Cervical dysplasia and cervical cancer are strongly associated with, and believed to be caused by, specific subtypes of the sexually transmitted virus called human papillomavirus (HPV). Other subtypes of HPV cause genital and anal warts in men and women. HIV-positive women have a high rate of persistent HPV infections, and a higher rate than HIV-negative women of types of HPV that are associated with the development of high-grade dysplasia and cervical cancer. Numerous studies have also documented that HIV-positive women are more likely than HIV-negative women to have cervical dysplasia. The strong association between HPV infection and cervical dysplasia, the finding that HIV-positive women are more likely to have persistent HPV infection of the specific subtypes associated with dysplasia, and the much higher incidence of dysplasia of HIV-positive women all suggest that HIV-related immunosuppression either increases the risk of persistent HPV infection or changes the natural history of HPV-related disease. The documentation of increased rates of cervical dysplasia prompted the CDC to add invasive cervical cancer to the AIDS surveillance case definition in 1993. However, much remains unknown about the incidence and natural history of the disease in HIV-positive women.

Cervical cancer is largely a preventable disease. Screening by Pap smear for all sexually active women can identify those with dysplastic precursor lesions so that they can be treated and monitored before more serious disease develops. With the high rates of HPV infection and dysplasia known to exist in the HIV-infected population, screening, early diagnosis, treatment, and careful monitoring are crucial. With no medical intervention available to prevent HPV infection and disease, regular Pap smears, lower genital tract inspection, and appropriate colposcopic follow-up and treatment of abnormalities are the best hope for preventing serious disease in women with cervical dysplasia. Colposcopy is performed to evaluate atypical and dysplastic smears. At this point, there is not a consensus of opinion regarding optimal frequency of Pap smears or the management of abnormal findings in HIV-positive women. Note that there are a number of methods for destroying or removing dysplasia from the cervix. These include cryotherapy (tissue destruction by freezing), laser therapy (tissue destruction by laser), loop excision (tissue removal by a "loop" of wire adjusted to be slightly larger than the size and shape of the affected zone of the cervix and the visible lesion), cone biopsy (removal of a cone of tissue from in and around the cervical os, either by traditional surgery or by laser), use of isotretinoin (experimental, an oral drug), and use of 5-fluorouracil (experimental, a topical cream). However, dysplasia can recur after treatment, especially in HIV-positive women.

Studies indicate an increase in prevalence of cervical dysplasia among women living with HIV. Additional studies have documented that a higher prevalence is associated with greater immune suppression. HIV infection may also adversely affect the clinical course and treatment of cervical dysplasia and cancer. See CERVICAL CANCER; CERVICAL INTRAEPITHELIAL NEOPLASIA.

cervical intraepithelial lesion Localized damage or abnormality, resulting from disease or trauma, in the tissue of the CERVIX. Such LESIONS can be benign (noncancerous) or malignant (cancerous).

cervical intraepithelial neoplasia (CIN1, CIN2, CIN3) Dysplasia of the cervical epithelium, often premalignant (i.e., precancerous), characterized by various degrees of hyperplasia, abnormal keratinization (forming of horny epidermal tissue), and condylomata. It may progress to involve deeper layers of the epithelium. It is classified by severity: grades 1, 2, and 3 represent progressive stages of a pathological condition. Grade 3 (CIN 3) represents CARCINOMA in situ (i.e., stage 0 of cancer of the cervix). PAP SMEAR or COLPOSCOPY generally reveals CIN. Considerable evidence implicates human papillomavirus (HPV) in the development of CIN. Immunosuppression may also play an important role in facilitating infection or persistence of HPV in the genital tract and progression of HPV-induced neoplasia. See CONDYLOMA; NEOPLASM.

cervical secretion HIV was first detected in the cervical secretions of HIV-infected women in 1986. Scientists reported that the virus might be cultured from secretions throughout the menstrual cycle, an indication that the presence of virus was not solely the result of contamination with menstrual blood. The probable source of HIV in cervical secretions is infected cervical tissue. The cells most often infected were MONOCYTE/MACROPHAGES and ENDOTHELIAL cells. In male-to-female TRANSMISSION of HIV, contact with infected semen could lead to local infection of susceptible cervical cells. Replication of the virus in those cells might precede systemic infection with HIV. Female-to-male transmission probably results from the sloughing of infected cervical cells into cervical and vaginal fluids. HIV infection of the uterine CERVIX might also explain some cases of viral transmission from mother to newborn.

cervical squamous cell abnormalities See SQUAMOUS CELL CARCINOMA.

cervicitis Inflammation of the CERVIX. Cervicitis may be asymptomatic and is generally diagnosed by inspection. Symptoms, when present, include vaginal discharge that increases just after menstruation, intermenstrual bleeding, postcoital bleeding, a burning sensation during urination, and low back pain. The cervix appears red and friable on examination. It often bleeds when touched with a cotton applicator or cervical spatula. A purulent exudate is often observed. CERVICAL CANCER can also give this appearance. Most infectious cervicitis is due to sexually transmitted infection, often CHLAMYDIA, GONORRHEA, or TRICHOMONAS. In HIV-positive women, viral infections may be isolated from cervical secretions and may cause local infections including CYTOMEGALOVIRUS, HERPES SIMPLEX virus, and even HIV itself. All vaginal infections should be treated and followed up.

cervicovaginal lavage (CVL) A technique in which a saline solution is sprayed into the vaginal vault and recovered for testing. CVL can be used to determine HIV viral load in genital tract secretions.

cervix The lower end of the uterus which protrudes into the vagina. Various contraceptive devices, such as the cervical cap and the diaphragm, do their job by blocking off this cervical opening and thus preventing the egg-hunting sperm from entering the uterus. Also called *cervix uteri.*

cesarean section The removal of a fetus by means of an incision into the uterus, usually by way of the abdominal wall. It may be performed by an extraperitoneal or intraperitoneal abdominal route. Indications for cesarean section include an abnormally large fetus (too large to be delivered through the pelvic outlet), an abnormally small pelvis, or a combination of these factors. A breech presentation of the fetus may also be an indication that a cesarean section is needed.

challenge In vaccine experiments, the exposure of an immunized animal to the infectious agent. Challenge experiments are never done in human HIV vaccine research.

chancre A primary sore or lesion at the site of entry of the bacteria that causes SYPHILIS.

chancroid An ulcerative lesion caused by *Haemophilus ducreyi.* Chancroids usually begin with a sensitive and inflamed pustule or ulcer with multiple, abrupt edges, a rough floor, and yellow

exudate, purulent secretion. The incubation period is approximately three to five days. Chancroids may affect the penis, urethra, vulva, or anus. Multiple lesions may develop by autoinoculation. Types include transient, phagedenic, giant, and serpiginous. Chancroids usually present as painful ulcers accompanied by tenderness and inguinal lymphadenopathy. Women with cervical chancroid tend to have multiple ulcers, with an average of four. Diagnosis based only on history and physical exam is often inaccurate. Culture for *H. ducreyi* is warranted for both diagnosis and reporting purposes. SYPHILIS, HERPES SIMPLEX, and HIV coinfection should also be considered in the differential diagnosis.

Chancroid lesions have been identified as a major risk factor for heterosexual spread of HIV through ulceration. Genital ulcers are thought to act as portals of entry for the virus from male genital secretions. Women may be unaware of the presence of ulcers.

ERYTHROMYCIN or CEFTRIAXONE usually satisfactorily treat chancroid. Treatment failure is more common in HIV-infected patients, especially single-dose treatment. As the susceptibility of *H. ducreyi* varies by geography, response should be monitored clinically and by susceptibility patterns.

charbon Infection with *Bacillus anthracis.* See ANTHRAX.

charity care coordinator A financial counselor.

chart review A retrospective way of collecting data that involves looking over patients' medical records.

chastity The state or quality of being chaste, or abstention from sexual intercourse or sexual relations. In a more general sense, chastity also refers to moral purity.

chemokine Glycoproteins that activate and direct the migration of white blood cells to sites of inflammation. They have been implicated in various viral illnesses, including HIV. There are two main subfamilies of chemokines, the CXC and the

CC chemokines, and two smaller families. CELL-SURFACE RECEPTORS for chemokines are used by HIV, along with the CD4 molecule, to enter the cells it infects. The CXCR5 receptor and the CCR4 receptor are the two chemokine receptors that HIV can use to infect T cells. Each chemokine binds to a specific chemokine receptor on white blood cells (monocytes, lymphocytes, basophils, and eosinophils). Several drug companies are working on producing drugs that may be able to block the chemokine from attaching to the receptor. It has been learned that some people of European descent do not have the CXCR5 chemokine receptor in their T cells. This seems to protect them from getting HIV despite repeated infection by the virus. The virus does not have the required binding site to reproduce itself. The number of people in the general population that lack this chemokine receptor is 1 percent or less.

chemotaxis   The movement of additional white blood cells to an area of inflammation in response to the release of chemical mediators by NEUTROPHILS, MONOCYTES, and injured tissue. For instance, the movement of LEUKOCYTES toward the chemicals produced by an immune reaction.

chemotherapy   The use of chemical agents in the treatment or control of disease, generally malignancies. Used colloquially most often to refer to the treatment of cancer with anticancer drugs, highly toxic medications that destroy cancer cells by interfering with their growth or preventing their reproduction. Generally, the smaller the tumor the more effective the chemotherapy is. The larger the tumor, the greater the number of cancer cells and the greater the possibility that some of the cells will become resistant. Chemotherapy may also be used to prolong life when a cure is improbable and to provide palliation (relieve symptoms).

There are a number of types of chemotherapy drugs, including alkylating agents, antimetabolites, anticancer antibiotics, plant alkaloids, hormones, and others. To be as effective as possible, different types of chemotherapy drugs are frequently used together (COMBINATION CHEMOTHERAPY). In that way, as many cell phases as possible will be vulnerable at the same time. In addition, chemotherapy

can be used alone or along with other treatments such as radiation therapy, surgery, and/or biological therapy. When chemotherapy is used along with other treatments, it may be given before surgery to reduce the size of the tumor so that the surgery can be more effective. Chemotherapy may also be given after the primary treatment, as adjuvant therapy, to destroy any remaining cancer cells. The type of chemotherapy given a patient, and the dose, is determined by a number of factors, including the kind of cancer, the stage it has reached, the objective of the treatment, and the medical condition of the patient. Chemotherapy has many side effects, ranging from unpleasant to life-threatening, depending upon, among other things, the degree of toxicity of the particular drug. Nausea, vomiting, diarrhea, and constipation are common.

Chemotherapy can treat cancer throughout the body systemically. Administration may be oral, by IV, by injection (into a vein, the membrane lining the abdomen, a muscle, an artery, a body cavity, or the spinal fluid), or by topical application. Chemotherapy may be given on any schedule that has proved to be effective.

child and family services   Social services provided to children and their parents, such as counseling, home chore aid, child rearing, housekeeping training, and abuse treatment. Child and family services may be provided to welfare recipients and may also be provided to other modest-income families, by government agencies or private charitable or social service organizations.

childbearing age   The period of a woman's life between puberty and menopause during which she is capable of bearing a child.

children   Human beings between infancy and puberty. AIDS was first described in children in 1982, a year after the syndrome was first identified in adults. By 1992, HIV disease was the seventh leading cause of death in children one to four years old in the United States. Today, early diagnosis and antiretroviral treatment and use of prophylactic drugs for protection against opportunistic infections have enabled some HIV-infected children to live into their teens.

To some extent, HIV disease in children resembles HIV disease in adults; however, in many ways, pediatric HIV disease is very different, as noted:

- The course of the disease is more uncertain in children. Some children born with HIV progress to advanced disease in three years; others live into their teens with few signs of illness.

- The immune system is still developing and maturing in infants and children. In addition, infants possess a higher number of CD4 lymphocytes than adults, and the number of their lymphocytes changes at rates different from those of adults during disease progression. All this adds to the complexity of determining the timing and course of antiretroviral therapy.

- The amount of virus in the blood of infants during acute HIV infection is higher than it is in adults. In addition, the levels of free virus in the blood of HIV-infected infants decline more slowly than do those of adults, often taking three to four years to reach a baseline level.

- Advances in antiretroviral therapy for children lag those made for adults. This happens in part because new treatments for pediatric HIV disease must be tested through clinical trials conducted in children to show that treatments are safe and that the dose is correct for children in various age groups. Because the number of HIV-infected children is much smaller than the number of infected adults, enrolling the number of children needed to complete a pediatric trial takes longer. For this reason, it is important that as many HIV-infected children as possible receive treatment through clinical trials. In addition, pharmaceutical companies appear less interested in pediatric clinical trials because children represent a much smaller commercial market for new drugs.

- In many children lymphatic infiltrating pneumonitis, a chronic lung disease uncommon in adults, develops.

- HIV-related cancers, which occur frequently in adults, are much less common in children. Kaposi's sarcoma, a common cancer in adults, is extremely rare in children.

- HIV infection in children is complicated by a number of unique social and psychological factors. More than 98 percent of HIV infections in children result from mother-to-child—perinatal, or vertical—transmission. In all perinatal infections, the mother is infected. Often, the HIV-infected child's caregiver is a single mother who struggles to care for her HIV-infected child while infected herself. HIV-infected children often are members of homes already troubled in many ways.

Discussion of the diagnosis of infection in infants and children must include mention of the source of HIV infection in children and consideration of the screening of infants and the role of CD4 lymphocyte counts in HIV-infected children. The source of HIV infection in children has changed considerably since the beginning of the HIV epidemic in 1981. In the first years of the epidemic, some children contracted HIV through transfusions of then-untested blood; others, born with hemophilia, contracted it through contaminated clotting factors. The testing of blood for antibodies to HIV, which began in the United States in 1985, and the use of heat-treated or genetically engineered clotting factors have virtually eliminated these sources of infection. Today, nearly every new case of HIV infection among children in the United States and worldwide occurs through perinatal transmission, that is, during pregnancy, delivery, or breast-feeding. Today, the rate of mother-to-infant transmission is being dramatically reduced in the United States with the use of AZT in pregnant HIV-infected women before and during delivery, and in their infants for six weeks after birth. Clinical trials are now under way to determine whether the use of a combination of antiretroviral drugs in HIV-infected pregnant women will reduce perinatal transmission even further.

All children born to HIV-infected mothers test HIV-positive at birth by the standard HIV antibody test. But about three-fourths of these children are not infected with HIV. Non-HIV-infected newborns can nevertheless test positive because certain antibodies produced by the mother pass into the fetus's blood during pregnancy. Traces of these maternal antibodies remain in the child's blood for up to 18 months. Only after the child reaches the age of 18 months does the HIV antibody test reliably reveal whether a child is HIV-infected or not, that is, whether he or she produces his or her own antibody in response to HIV infection. Unless the truly HIV-infected infants can be identified within the first few weeks of life, all infants born to infected mothers will be given PNEUMOCYSTIS CARINII PNEUMONIA (PCP) prophylaxis to prevent this life-threatening infection in the 25 percent of them who are truly HIV-infected. To reduce this problem the Centers for Disease Control and Prevention recommends first identifying pregnant women who are HIV-infected and then screening their newborns by using new tests that identify the presence of the virus itself, rather than antibodies to it, in blood. These new tests can accurately identify 90 percent of truly HIV-infected infants within the first month or two of life.

Note that HIV-infected children are subject to most of the opportunistic infections that can occur in adults. Some that are particularly notable in HIV-infected children are bacterial infections, candidiasis and other fungal infections (oral candidiasis, esophageal candidiasis, other fungal infections such as ringworm and athlete's foot), herpesvirus infections, measles virus, *Mycobacterium avium* complex, *Pneumocystis carinii* pneumonia, and tuberculosis. Diarrhea, lymphoid interstitial pneumonitis, and HIV encephalopathy are other important conditions in children with HIV disease.

Since the beginning of the AIDS pandemic, the treatment of infants and children with HIV infection has presented unique problems. Even before the introduction of antiretroviral drug therapy when the standard of care for patients was palliative, the management of HIV infection in infants and children was especially difficult. Many of the drug treatments and therapies used to delay or treat opportunistic infections in adults were not readily applicable to the care of pediatric patients. Moreover, whereas the appropriate dosages for most drug treatments are well established for adults, the dosages that are safe and effective for children and infants are not always known. These difficulties continued when antiretroviral agents were introduced in the late 1980s. It was not until the late 1990s that most of the antiretroviral agents used to treat adults became available in pediatric formulations. Thus, the first formal clinical trials of HAART in children were begun in 1997, years after the same trials were carried out in adults. The preliminary results show that infants and children with HIV infection can benefit from HAART as adults

do. These trials have also raised the question of timing: when should HAART be started in these patients? In adults this same question has long been a source of controversy among HIV clinicians. Some argue that drug therapy should be started as soon as the condition is diagnosed, under the mantra, "HIT EARLY, HIT HARD." The rationale is that the sooner HAART is started, the less the immune system will be damaged and the better off the patient will be in the long run. Others strongly disagree. They note that there is no evidence that starting HAART sooner or later has any effect on survival rates. Starting HAART later, when the first symptoms of AIDS appear, might spare patients both the agony of taking pills for years and the toxic effects of drugs, while possibly providing the same benefits of extending survival relatively free of symptoms. These differences in medical opinions apply only to those patients receiving care during the chronic stage of HIV infection. There is far less disagreement among physicians regarding when to initiate HAART among newly infected individuals in the acute stage of the disease—immediately. It has now been theorized that those patients who start a regimen of antiretroviral drugs may be able to reduce critical damage to their immune systems. Moreover, it has also been theorized that in at least a few patients who have been started on HAART at the acute phase immune responses that can suppress HIV without the assistance of drug therapy can later develop. Note that viral suppression without drug therapy is largely unrealistic. The acute stage of HIV infection mimics other, more innocuous infections or gives rise to no symptoms at all. Thus, very few adult patients are diagnosed with acute infection and reach the attention of HIV specialists. Over time, few adults are likely to benefit from this strategy.

In pediatric HIV infection, diagnosis during the acute stage is the norm, not the exception. The great majority of infants are infected in utero near term or during the birth process. Thus, most of those infected with the virus have recently acquired it. See BREAST-FEEDING; PEDIATRIC HIV; PREGNANCY; TRANSMISSION.

chimpanzee Because of their genetic similarity to humans, chimpanzees have often been used in HIV and other medical research (chimps are the only other primates that can be infected with HIV-1, although it does not make them ill). However, because of habitat destruction in their native Africa, theirs is an endangered species. Decreased numbers and high cost have limited their use in recent years.

China See ASIA.

Chinese herbs Herbs used routinely in therapy, including treatment of HIV, by practitioners of traditional CHINESE MEDICINE. Some commonly used natural herbal products—ASTRAGALUS *mongholicus, Acanthopanax senticosus* and *Eleutheroccocus senticosus, Panax notoginseng,* aconitum, *Artemisiae annua, Tripterigium wilfordii,* and *Echinacea purpurea*—are clearly active immunologically, and can modulate, potentiate, or suppress immune response. It is important to note that the immunological effects may not be due to the purified versions or extracts of the herbs, but to their entire compositions, possibly including unknown and unrecognized substances. Many researchers and clinicians observe that Chinese medicine can hope to function in full partnership with Western medicine only if it heeds the most recent discoveries in immunology. To date, critical analyses of the use of Chinese herbs for HIV are lacking, and the jury is still out on the use of Chinese therapeutics for HIV.

Chinese medicine The practice of the Chinese system of medicine dates back more than two thousand years, making it the oldest medical tradition in the world. Chinese medicine combines empirical experience with a philosophical theory. Unlike Western medicine, which is derived solely from scientific methods of observation and investigation of physical disease, Chinese practice is founded on a holistic view of the mind-body's innate ability to maintain health and to heal itself should illness occur. This view sees the universe as a living organism, and the human body as a microcosm of that larger organism. In contrast, Western medicine tends to view the human body mechanistically and has evolved its practice based on the assumption that the body is a machine with essentially separate but linked components. Rather than dealing only with discrete components of the human organism, the Chinese approach is one of "aligning" the functions of the organs and internal systems as a whole, promoting the dynamic balance of energy polarities crucial to good health and well-being. Much Western research on certain aspects of Chinese medicine, particularly on the properties of traditional herbs, has been conducted in recent years, but so far it has not led to the development of any useful therapies for HIV/AIDS.

chiropractic The chiropractic system of physical therapy is based on the premise that the spine, literally the backbone of the body, is also the "backbone" of health: subluxation (misalignment) of the vertebrae caused by poor posture or trauma or pressure on the spinal nerve roots, which may lead to diminished function and illness. The chiropractor seeks to analyze and correct these misalignments through spinal manipulation or adjustment.

Though chiropractic has its roots in nineteenth-century pseudoscientific theories, it has proved of some use for those with ailments specifically related to muscle tension, pinched nerves, and so forth.

Chlamydia A sexually transmitted bacterial infection that is caused by *Chlamydia trachomatis*. It produces infection in the cervix and often spreads to the pelvic organs. Asymptomatic infection is common; other clinical symptoms include abnormal discharge and symptoms of urethritis; if untreated, 10 percent–40 percent of cases develop into PELVIC INFLAMMATORY DISEASE. It can cause great damage to pelvic structures, resulting in PELVIC INFLAMMATORY DISEASE, tubo-ovarian abscesses, and tubal infertility. Diagnosis is made by culture (cell-based), antigen detection, DNA probe, and PCR/LCR. It can be transmitted perinatally and is a frequent cause of conjunctivitis and pneumonia in newborns. In terms of prevalence, clinical presentation, diagnosis, and treatment in HIV-positive women, there is no difference when they are compared with HIV-negative women. Recommendations for the management of sex partners are the same as for gonorrhea—sex partners should be treated for both gonorrhea and chlamydia if their last sexual contact occurred within 60 days before the diagnosis or onset of symptoms. Note too that if a patient's most recent sexual contact occurred more than 60 days before the onset of symptoms, her most recent sexual partner should be treated. Intercourse should be avoided until treatment is completed and symptoms have been resolved. It is generally recommended that the initial medical evaluation of HIV-positive women include screening for chlamydia as well as for vaginitis, urinary tract infection, syphilis, and gonorrhea—along with a complete menstrual, sexual, obstetrical, and gynecological history and breast and pelvic exams. Some evidence suggests that sexually transmitted infections, including gonorrhea and chlamydia, are more common in HIV-positive women, but it is not clear yet whether this is a result of HIV infection or of high-risk behavior that is also responsible for acquisition of HIV infection itself.

chlamydial infection   See CHLAMYDIA.

chloral hydrate   Chloral hydrate is a sedative used to treat insomnia. It is usually taken fifteen to thirty minutes before bedtime. Using chloral hydrate regularly for more than two weeks often reduces its effectiveness. Major side effects include stomach irritation, residual sedation, and hangover. Chloral hydrate should be used with great caution by people who are depressed, who are suicidal, or who have a history of drug abuse.

chloramphenicol   A broad-spectrum antibiotic used to treat a number of bacterial infections, including salmonella, meningitis caused by *Haemophilus* influenza, rickets, and cholera. Chloramphenicol prevents multiplication of susceptible bacteria by preventing them from making strong cell walls and essential proteins. There are significant toxicities with chloramphenicol, so it should only be used when necessary, for serious infections caused by organisms that are resistant to other antibiotics or when other antibiotics are not tolerated.

In HIV-infected people, chloramphenicol is most frequently used to treat salmonella infections that cause severe diarrhea. Salmonella is more common in people with AIDS than in the general population. In people with healthy immune systems the infection is rarely treated, but symptoms tend to be

much more severe in immunocompromised people and require intervention. Chloramphenicol is available in tablet, ointment and injectable form. Although rare, the most serious side effect of chloramphenicol is BONE MARROW SUPPRESSION. (Trade names Chloromycetin and Elase-Chloromycetin.)

Chloromycetin   See CHLORAMPHENICOL.

chlorpheniramine   An antihistamine used to treat allergic reactions such as hay fever, hives, and inflammation of the eye, among others. It is also taken to prevent or treat allergic reactions to blood transfusions or compounds taken to enhance X-ray images. Occasionally it is used as a supplementary therapy to EPINEPHRINE for the treatment of ANAPHYLACTIC SHOCK. In people with HIV, the drug is used to reduce certain drug-induced allergic side effects, including skin rashes, redness, swelling, hives, and breathing difficulties. The drug is available in a wide variety of formulations, including capsules, tablets, syrup, and oral suspension. Drowsiness is the most common side effect. (Trade names include Alermine, Aller-Chlor, Chlor-Trimeton, Comtrex, Histex, and Teldrin.)

CHO (Chinese hamster ovary) cell   A cell used as a "factory" in genetic engineering to make certain subunit vaccines. CHO cells are derived from mammals and are advantageous because they add carbohydrates (a sugar coat) to the protein, much as naturally infected human cells do.

cholangiopathy, HIV   See GALLBLADDER DISEASE.

cholera   A severe contagious infection of the small intestine characterized by profuse watery diarrhea and dehydration, caused by *Vibrio cholerae* bacteria, and commonly transmitted through contaminated drinking water.

cholestasis   Obstruction of bile within the bile duct.

cholesterol   A steroid found in the tissues and blood plasma. Cholesterol circulates in the blood along with a protein (lipoprotein). Low-density lipoproteins (LDLs) take cholesterol from the liver to body tissues, whereas high-density lipoproteins (HDLs) take cholesterol from the blood to be excreted. High levels of LDLs and/or low levels of HDLs are associated with heart disease and arteriosclerosis.

CHOP (Cy, doxorubicin, vincristine, and prednisone) CHOP is one of the most common combination chemotherapy regimens for treating non-Hodgkin's lymphoma. The drugs used in the regimen are cyclophosphamide (brand names Cytoxan, Neosar), adriamycin (doxorubicin/hydroxydoxorubicin), vincristine (Oncovin), and prednisone (sometimes called Deltasone or Orasone). CHOP is administered in cycles of four weeks. A common treatment regimen entails at least six cycles. The exact number of cycles given is dependent on the treatment prescribed by the medical team. These drugs can cause nausea, vomiting, and loss of appetite. There are medications that may lessen chemotherapy-induced nausea. Fatigue is also common during chemotherapy treatment; proper rest and pacing of oneself may be helpful. Treatments can be delayed if the patient has a low white blood cell count (neutropenia). Blood counts can be raised by drugs such as GRANULOCYTE COLONY STIMULATING FACTOR (G-CSF, brand name Neupogen)—a drug used to stimulate the production of granulocytes in the bone marrow. Late effects of non-Hodgkin's lymphoma have been observed. Pelvic irradiation and large cumulative doses of cyclophosphamide have been associated with a high risk of permanent sterility. For up to two decades after diagnosis, patients are at significantly elevated risk of second primary cancers, especially lung, brain, kidney, and bladder cancers and melanoma, Hodgkin's disease, and acute nonlymphocytic leukemia. Left ventricular dysfunction has also been observed as a late effect. Peripheral neuropathy has been observed as a long-term effect.

chromosome One of a set of threadlike structures, composed of DNA and a protein, that form in the nucleus when the cell begins to divide and that carry the genes that determine an individual's hereditary traits. Apart from sex cells (eggs and sperm) and mature blood cells, every cell in the human body contains 23 pairs of chromosomes. One of each pair is inherited from the mother, the other from the father. Each chromosome is a packet of compressed and twisted DNA. Genes are sections of DNA containing the blueprint for the whole body, including such specific details as the kind of receptors cells will have, for example, CD4, CD8, X4, R5, and so on. DNA is made up of a double-stranded helix held together by hydrogen bonds between specific pairs of bases. The four bases, adenine, thymine, guanine, and cytosine (A, R, G, and C), bond to each other in fixed and complementary patterns that give humans and other species their individuality. If a gene is thought of as a sentence, and the nucleotides in DNA as letters, a change or mutation of only one letter can affect the entire sentence of information that DNA gives the cell.

Much has been written about the biological characteristics of the AIDS virus. Today we know, for example, that retroviruses are grouped into three families: oncoviruses, lentiviruses, and foamy viruses. Today we know that HIV is a lentivirus. We know that it contains nine genes, and 9,749 nucleotides, its genetic code. We also know that six HIV genes regulate HIV reproduction and at least one gene directly influences infection. And we know that HIV RNA produces HIV DNA, which integrates into the host cell to become a proviral DNA. We know too that HIV undergoes rapid genetic changes within infected people, that the reverse transcriptase enzyme is very error-prone, that HIV causes immunological suppression by destroying T4 helper cells, and that HIV is classified into major, outlier, and type genetic subtypes. Understanding the basic genetic structure of retroviral genomes is therefore critical to understanding the virus.

chronic A term denoting symptoms and disease that last for an extended period of time without noticeable change. Distinguished from acute.

chronic fatigue syndrome A viral disease of the immune system, usually characterized by debilitating fatigue and flulike symptoms.

chronic idiopathic demyelinating polyneuropathy (CIPD) Chronic, spontaneous loss or destruction of myelin. Myelin is soft, white, somewhat fatty material that forms a thick sheath around the core of myelinated nerve fiber. Patients show progressive, usually symmetric weakness in the upper and lower extremities. Patients with clinical progression of the syndrome after four to six weeks by definition have CIPD. Treatment in most centers consists of giving IV immune globulin for four to five days or using plasmapheresis (five to six exchanges over two weeks).

chronically infected cells   HIV cells that carry the blueprints of the virus in them and therefore continually make new HIV.

CID   See CENTER FOR INFECTIOUS DISEASES.

cidofovir   A nucleotide analog. Cidofovir is approved as a systemic treatment for new or relapsing cytomegalovirus (CMV) retinitis. Cidofovir is not approved to treat other types of CMV infection or CMV in non-HIV-infected people. Cidofovir interferes with the multiplication of CMV, thereby slowing the destruction of the retina (the light-sensitive tissue at the back of the eye) and loss of vision. Note too that it slows, but does not permanently stop, the progression to CMV retinitis. People taking the drug may continue to lose their vision and should have regular eye examinations at least every six weeks to determine whether a change in treatment is required. It may also act against CMV disease in other parts of the body, but there is less clinical evidence to support its use in these cases. Its primary advantage over ganciclovir and foscarnet is that cidofovir is administered intravenously on a weekly or a biweekly basis instead of daily, eliminating the need for an in-dwelling catheter. The chief side effect of intravenous administration is kidney damage, which can be very severe. To protect the kidneys, cidofovir must be administered with probenecid and intravenous hydration. Cidofovir should not be used at the same time as other drugs that are toxic to the kidneys (such as amphotericin B, aminoglycosides [amikacin, gentamicin, streptomycin, erythromycin], foscarnet, and intravenous pentamidine) or by patients with impaired kidney function. Other side effects include neutropenia, fever, nausea and vomiting, headache, and diarrhea. Cidofovir is being tested for activity against Kaposi's sarcoma and pro-

gressive mutifocal leukoencephalopathy (PML). (Trade name is Vistide.)

cimetidine   A drug that blocks the action of HISTAMINE (H-2), a substance secreted by MAST CELLS, and thus inhibits the ability of the stomach to make acid. Once acid production is decreased, the body is able to heal itself. Benefits include control of hypersecretory stomach disorders and effective treatment of peptic ulcer disease, reflux esophagitis, and heartburn. The drug has been shown to have some stimulating effects on the immune system and has been proposed as a treatment for the immune suppression associated with HIV. (The trade name is Tagamet.)

cipro   See CIPROFLOXACIN.

ciprofibrate   An antihyperlipidemic drug that can control high triglyceride levels in people when diet and exercise have not worked. It is the class of drugs known as FIBRATES. There are potential side effects of all of these drugs that include elevated liver enzyme levels and a myositislike illness that impairs renal function. These drugs typically do not lower the cholesterol levels in patients and can be given with a STATIN in cases of high cholesterol levels. (Trade name is Modalin.)

ciprofloxacin (Cipro)   An oral antibiotic approved for the treatment of many common bacterial infections. It is sometimes administered to treat MAC in combination with other drugs. Possible side effects include gastrointestinal upset, seizures, and rash. Concomitant administration of antacids like Mylanta or Amphogel that contain aluminum or magnesium hydroxide can lead to the formation of insoluble chelates (heterocyclic chemical compounds) that prevent the drug's absorption, reducing its level in the blood. Sucralfate, a stomach ulcer remedy, has a similar effect and should not be taken with ciprofloxacin. Ciprofloxacin, in contrast, can increase the absorption and blood levels of theophylline, an asthma remedy.

circulating immune complexes   Circulating immune complexes are formed in the blood when antigens are present in excess amounts. The host produces antibodies against these, forming antigen-antibody complexes. These can mask the surface of a tumor cell and, for example, prevent LYMPHOCYTES from reacting. Immune complexes can cause diseases, such as nephritis and kidney failure.

circumcision   The surgical removal of the end of the prepuce, of foreskin, of the penis. Circumcision is a social or religious custom, usually performed on newborn babies at the request of the parents. The issue of circumcision as it relates to HIV transmission is hardly trivial. It has been suggested that there is a relationship between absence of circumcision and HIV. Studies seem to support such an association but must be interpreted cautiously because evidence may be unavoidably confounded with other factors. Since the late 1800s, it has repeatedly been found that men with SEXUALLY TRANSMITTED DISEASES (STDs) are more likely to be uncircumcised than are men without STDs. Modern investigators have reported that uncircumcised men were more likely than circumcised men to be infected with gonorrhea or syphilis, less likely to have genital warts, and equally likely to have herpesvirus infection. Recently several investigators have reported that uncircumcised men may be more susceptible to HIV infection than are circumcised men.

There have been a number of reports illustrating that the foreskin provides a vulnerable portal of entry to HIV and other pathogens. Additionally, the highly vascularized prepuce contains a higher density of Langerhans cells—the primary target cells for sexual transmission of HIV—than does cervical, vaginal, or rectal mucosa. It has also been shown that the foreskin is more susceptible to traumatic epithelial disruptions during intercourse, which allow additional vulnerability to ulcerative STDs and HIV. Some researchers believe the evidence may be strong enough to warrant considering circumcision for HIV prevention. Published articles and abstracts are few, however, and conclusions are not certain.

circumoral paresthesia   An abnormal touch sensation, such as burning or prickling around the mouth, often in the absence of an external stimulus.

cirrhosis   A chronic disease of the liver characterized by formation of dense perilobular connective tissue, degenerative changes in parenchymal cells, alteration in structure of the cords of liver lobules, fatty and cellular infiltration, and sometimes development of areas of regeneration. In addition to the clinical signs and symptoms inherent in the cause of cirrhosis, those due to cirrhosis are the result of loss of functioning liver cells and increased resistance to flow of blood through the liver. When severe enough, this leads to ammonia toxicity. Cirrhosis may be due to various factors such as nutritional deficiency, poisons, or previous inflammation caused by a virus or bacterium. Therapy depends on the cause and severity of the disease.

In recent years, there has been an increase in awareness of the impact of viral hepatitis on HIV-positive individuals. At the same time, there is increased recognition of the importance of liver disease in HIV-positive patients. Today it is well established that hepatitis and HIV coinfection demands special treatment considerations and consequences. Both hepatitis B and hepatitis C infections can progress to cirrhosis.

The ability of hepatitis B to produce chronic infection has been documented. Note, however, that the body can create long-lasting immunity to hepatitis B in 90 percent to 95 percent of cases, and in only 5 percent to 10 percent of persons does a chronic infection, which can lead to cirrhosis of the liver, develop. Persons with chronic hepatitis B infection along with HIV must be aware of the interaction of the two viruses. Coinfected patients with hepatitis B and HIV should be placed on a HAART regimen that includes lamivudine (Epivir). The best defense against hepatitis B is immunization before acquisition of the disease.

Acute hepatitis C may have symptoms, but many times people do not know they have been exposed to the hepatitis C virus. When a person becomes infected with hepatitis C virus, the virus is able to evade the immune system in 85 percent of cases to sustain a chronic infection. Hepatitis C is able to change its form slightly, and the immune system has a difficult time reacting to the changes. That means that only 15 percent of the acute infections are effectively defended by the immune system. Over a period of 20 years, hepatitis C virus infection progresses to cirrhosis in 20 percent of patients. In some persons with chronic HCV infection liver cancer develops. The effect of HIV on HCV is a two to three times more rapid progression to cirrhosis than in HIV-negative individuals. More HIV-positive persons also have cirrhosis and higher mortality rates than their HIV-negative counterparts. The ability to lower HIV viral load to undetectable levels has no effect on HCV, and protease inhibitors are not active against HCV. Treatment for HCV may have potential impact on the coinfected state. To date there is no vaccination for HCV. The "gold standard" treatment at the present time for HCV is combination therapy. See HEPATITIS.

9-cis   A hormonal treatment for KAPOSI'S SARCOMA developed by Ligand Pharmaceuticals. 9-cis is available as a topical gel. Ligand has also investigated 9-*cis* retonoic acid, which it calls Panretin, in a variety of other malignancies and noncancerous conditions, but its exact mechanism of action is unknown. 9-*cis* retonoic acid is a natural hormone that activates a series of six cellular receptors, three of which trigger cell growth and development while the others cause death by apoptosis in superfluous or apparently malfunctioning cells. 9-*cis* retonoic acid needs direct contact with KS cells in order to work. Tumors resolve layer by layer from the outside when Panretin is applied.

cisplatin (Platinol)   Chemotherapy treatment for tumors. Kidney damage is the most serious side effect.

civil liberties   Fundamental rights of citizens, such as freedom of speech, often guaranteed by law. Also the freedom of individuals to exercise such rights without state interference.

Some of the responses to the AIDS epidemic have included proposals for drastic legal curtailments of individual rights and liberties, purportedly to stop the spread of the disease. Even without such legal action, people with AIDS or HIV have been discriminated against in employment, housing, public accommodations, government services, and other areas. Despite these deplorable actions, which have largely been based on ignorance and fear, there are serious questions about appropriate public response to AIDS, with implications for civil liberties. Why shouldn't employers be allowed to fire people who have AIDS or who test positive for the AIDS virus? If people who carry the virus can infect others through sexual contact, why shouldn't the government require citizens to be tested? Why shouldn't the government have the name of everyone who carries the AIDS virus? Blood tests to detect sexually transmitted diseases have been required as a prerequisite for a marriage license; why is testing for AIDS different? What should be done about a person known to be infected who refuses to refrain from activities that could transmit the virus? Isn't education about AIDS offensive and, for many, obscene?

Civil Rights Act of 1964   The most comprehensive civil rights legislation in the history of the United States. The Civil Rights Act of 1964 mandates equality for all persons in access to public accommodations and facilities, education, and employment, as well as federally assisted public programs of all kinds. Title VII of the act is regarded as the most all-inclusive source of employment rights. All employers who have at least fifteen employees, including state and local governments and labor unions, are subject to its provisions, but it does not apply to the federal government, Indian tribes, certain agencies in the District of Columbia, private clubs, and religious organizations. Its principles have been extended to federal employment, however, by executive order.

Civil Rights Act of 1968   This act proscribes discrimination in the sale, rental, and financing arrangements of most housing. It applies to agents and brokers as well as to owners of properties.

Civil Rights Act of 1991   This law amends the CIVIL RIGHTS ACT OF 1964 to provide greater protection against employment discrimination. The act repudiates recent U.S. Supreme Court decisions limiting civil rights; grants women and disabled persons the right to recover money damages under Title VII of the Civil Rights Act of 1964; and grants congressional employees the protection of Title VII. The 1991 act was a direct outgrowth of the failed Civil Rights bill of 1990, which President George H.

W. Bush had vetoed. The section of the act that raised the greatest concern dealt with money damages for victims of intentional discrimination or harassment based on sex, religion, national origin, or disability. Unlike claims of racial discrimination, claims of these types of Title VII discrimination could result in awards of back pay and reinstatement on a job.

CL-1012 Anti-HIV ZINC FINGER INHIBITOR currently in studies. ZINC FINGERS are a part of HIV that help assemble new viruses as they are leaving an infected cell. When the zinc fingers are blocked, HIV makes copies of itself that are not functional and cannot infect new cells.

clade One of the major largely geographically isolated, HIV subtypes. Classification is based on differences in envelope protein. There are currently three groups of HIV-1 isolates: M, N, and O. Isolate M (major strains) consists of at least 10 clades, A through J. Group O (outer strains) may consist of a similar number of clades. French researchers reported the discovery of a new HIV-1 isolate that cannot be categorized in either group M or O. The new isolate was found in a Cameroonian woman with AIDS. They suggested that this new isolate be classified as group N (for new or for "non-M–non-O"). Clade B makes up the overwhelming majority of HIV in North America and Europe.

clap See GONORRHEA.

clarithromycin An anti-infective macrolide used in the treatment of certain upper respiratory tract infections, some lower respiratory tract infections, certain skin and skin structure infections, and MYCOBACTERIUM AVIUM COMPLEX (MAC) infections, and in the prevention of disseminated *Mycobacterium avium* complex in advanced HIV. Other generally accepted uses include combination antibiotic treatment of duodenal ulcer disease caused by *H. pylori*. Clarithromycin can also have a role in combination therapy of some TOXOPLASMOSIS infections. It works by preventing the growth and multiplication of susceptible organisms by interfering with their formation of essential proteins. Possible risks include mild gastrointestinal symptoms,

drug-induced colitis (rare), and superinfections (rare). (The brand name is Biaxin.)

clearance The elimination of a substance from the blood plasma by the kidneys.

client An individual who has retained or consented to treatment or receipt of services from a professional. In general, the term *"client"* is used by those educated in social services, where *patient* is used by professionals educated in the medical sciences.

Cleocin See CLINDAMYCIN.

client advocacy See CASE ADVOCACY.

client oriented Directed toward the client's or patient's needs and interests; used of medical and social services.

client-centered therapy A method of psychotherapy or counseling pioneered by the American psychologist Carl Rogers in which the therapist refrains from advising, suggesting, or persuading but tries instead to establish empathy with the client by clarifying and reflecting back the client's expressed feelings. The therapist tries to convey an attitude of "unconditional positive regard" in the context of a permissive, nonthreatening relationship. This method of psychotherapy is also called NONDIRECTIVE COUNSELING or therapy.

climax See ORGASM.

clindamycin An antibiotic effective against anaerobic pathogens, microbes that can grow without the presence of free oxygen. In HIV therapy, clindamycin is used primarily in combination with the antimalarial drug primaquine to treat mild-to-moderate PCP in people who have failed with or cannot tolerate TRIMETHOPRIM-SULFAMETHOXAZOLE (TMP-SMX). People with mild cases of PCP often take the oral from of clindamycin immediately. People with moderate cases of the disease sometimes initially receive clindamycin intravenously and then switch to the oral drug. Clindamycin has also proved effective in treating ENCEPHALITIS caused by the protozoal pathogen *Toxoplasma gondii*. Clindamycin has also been used effectively in combination with SULFADI-AZINE and PYRIMETHAMINE to treat TOXOPLASMOSIS. For PELVIC INFLAMMATORY DISEASE, intravenous clindamycin can be combined with intravenous or intramuscular injections of GENTAMICIN to treat acute infection, followed by gentamicin as maintenance therapy to prevent recurrence.

The most common side effect of clindamycin is diarrhea, caused by the growth of a bacterium called CLOSTRIDIUM DIFFICILE. *Clostridium* infection can lead to a condition called pseudomembranous colitis, characterized by abdominal pain, blood diarrhea, fever, and dehydration. *Clostridium* requires direct treatment with oral vancomycin or Flagyl. Use of any agent that just slows intestinal motility may prolong or worsen pseudomembranous colitis by delaying elimination of the toxin made by the bacteria. Furthermore, use of antidiarrheal agents that contain kaolin or attapulgite (Kaopectate) may decrease the absorption of clindamycin, leading to subtherapeutic effects. ERYTHROMYCIN also interacts with clindamycin, by interfering with its mechanism of action against bacteria.

The most significant side effect associated with the use of clindamycin is severe COLITIS, which is a potentially fatal superinfection caused by *Clostridia*. Severe and persistent diarrhea (occasionally bloody) and severe abdominal cramps are the first signs of colitis. (Trade name is Cleocin T.)

clinic   A facility or part of a facility used for the diagnosis and treatment of medical outpatients. Depending on context, "clinic" may include physicians' offices, facilities that serve poor or public patients, or facilities in which graduate or undergraduate medical education is provided. More broadly, clinics may also include complete inpatient and outpatient facilities and resources. Here, the term describes a group practice of specialty and general health care practitioners who have banded together to share resources and increase the marketability of their services.

clinical   Directly observable; diagnosable by observation.

Clinical Alert   The National Institutes of Health in conjunction with the editors of several biomedical journals publish bulletins on urgent cases in which timely and broad dissemination of results of clinical trials could prevent morbidity (sickness) and mortality (death). The Clinical Alert does not become a barrier to subsequent publication of the full research paper. Clinical Alerts are widely distributed electronically through the National Library of Medicine and through standard mailings.

clinical coordinator   The study nurse or other staff person who is primary administrator and contact person for a research effort.

clinical endpoint   The measure of clinical improvement in a DRUG TRIAL.

This subject has been at the center of an ongoing debate about testing and approving new drugs for deadly diseases, particularly AIDS. At issue are the speed with which drugs are evaluated and approved for use, and the criteria for drug efficacy and effectiveness. Traditionally, the Food and Drug Administration (FDA) has evaluated experimental drugs, not by improvements in the patients who receive them, but by the occurrence of OPPORTUNISTIC INFECTIONS (OIs) or death in those who do not. Because the FDA will not approve a drug based solely on SURROGATE MARKERS, such as reduction in P24 antigen or a rise in T-cell count, because it wants statistical proof that a drug is helping people, and because the FDA has traditionally insisted on the slowest measure of clinical improvement—clinical endpoints—trials often take a long time. Activists and researchers as well as scientists have long questioned whether the best way to prove a drug is to wait for deaths and OIs in those who do not receive it. They do not see why a potentially useful drug should be withheld for months or years pending conclusive proof of benefit, after it is already clear that it does show substantial clinical benefit. And many fear that a return to survival as the sole endpoint in studies would also require a return to the routine use of placebo controls, a guarantee of death for the untreated.

clinical latency   The state or period of an infectious agent, such as a virus or bacterium, living or developing in a host without producing clinical symptoms. In respect to HIV infection, infected individuals usually exhibit a period of clinical latency with little evidence of disease, but viral load studies show that the virus is never truly latent (dormant). Even early in the disease, HIV is active within lymphoid organs, where large amounts of virus became trapped in the follicular dendritic cell (FDC) network. Surrounding tissues are areas rich in CD4+ T cells. These cells increasingly become infected, and viral particles accumulate both in infected cells and as free virus.

clinical practice guidelines   Standards for physicians to adhere to in prescribing care for a given condition or illness.

clinical trial   A carefully planned scientific study done to test an experimental medicine in human beings to see if it is safe and effective. Some trials seek to evaluate safety (phase 1), others test effectiveness and short-term safety (phase 2), and others test safety, effectiveness, and dosage level (phase 3). Phase 1, 2, and 3 clinical trials differ in terms of number of patients, length, and method.

At hospitals across the country, the National Institute of Allergy and Infectious Diseases (NIAID), the research arm of the United States PUBLIC HEALTH SERVICE, has set up a group of research centers called AIDS CLINICAL TRIALS UNITS (ACTUs), where these tests take place. The ACTUs together make up the AIDS CLINICAL TRIALS GROUP (ACTG). In addition, doctors who are part of NIAID's COMMUNITY PROGRAMS FOR CLINICAL RESEARCH ON AIDS conduct studies of AIDS drugs at hospitals and clinics in the communities where the impact of the AIDS epidemic is severe. Clinical trials are also sponsored by drug companies, other government agencies, and private research organizations.

clitoris   A small, complex organ located where the inside lips of the vagina meet. It becomes erect, or blood-filled, during sexual excitement. Slang terms include clit, little man in the boat, and jewel in the lotus.

clofazimine   An antileprosy agent sometimes administered in combination with other drugs to treat MAC. It can decrease the rate of RIFAMPIN absorption and thus reduce its effects. In addition, it lowers dilantin levels, which has led to breakthrough seizures. Possible side effects include gastrointestinal upset, skin discoloration, and rashes. (Trade name is Lamprene.)

clonal anergy   The downregulation of the immune response by lack of proliferation of effector and memory LYMPHOCYTES.

clonal deletion   Physical deletion of immune cells such as LYMPHOCYTES from the peripheral repertoire. Also known as *programmed cell death* or APOPTOSIS.

clonal selection   The fundamental basis of LYMPHOCYTE activation, in which an antigen selectively stimulates only those cells to divide and differentiate which express receptors for it.

clonazepam   An antiseizure drug that is used alone or in combination therapy to prevent and treat epileptic seizures. Clonazepam belongs to a class of psychoactive drugs known as benzodiazepines. In general, these drugs are used to treat anxiety and insomnia, but clonazepam is used almost exclusively as an anticonvulsant in people who have not responded to standard therapy. Many develop a tolerance for clonazepam, and the drug often loses it effectiveness after a few months of therapy. To counter the effect, the drug's dosage may be increased or therapy switched to a different anticonvulsant. Seizures may be caused by any of the CENTRAL NERVOUS SYSTEM disorders or infections associated with HIV infection. Toxoplasmosis is the most common cause of seizures in people with AIDS. Clonazepam treats the symptoms of the neurological disorders, not the underlying causes. When seizures are being caused by an opportunistic infection of the central nervous system, therapy should also include appropriate antibiotic, antifungal, or antiparasitic treatment. Clonazepam is available in tablet form for oral administration. The most common side effects are drowsiness, dizziness, unsteadiness, increased salivation, and altered behavior. (Trade name is Trionopin.)

clone   A cell, cell product, or organism that is genetically identical to the unit or individual from which it was asexually derived. Colloquially, by extension, a person or thing that duplicates, imitates, or closely resembles another in appearance.

cloning   The process of producing a clone.

clostridium difficile   A microbe that is a relatively common, and particularly severe, cause of diarrhea in people who take antibiotics. Almost any antibiotic can cause this complication, but the ones that do so most frequently are AMPICILLIN, AMOXICILLIN, CLINDAMYCIN, and a group of drugs called cephalosporins that includes cefixime, cefuroxime, cephalexin, and cefaclor. People who develop diarrhea while taking these or any other antibiotics should stop taking them and call their physicians. A test of stool will determine if Clostridium difficile is the cause. If it is, it can be treated with METRONIDAZOLE or vancomycin hydrochloride.

clot   See BLOOD CLOT; COAGULATION.

clotrimazole   An antifungal drug used primarily during HIV infection as a topical agent for oral and vaginal CANDIDIASIS. (Trade names Gyne-Lotrimin Lotrimin and Mycelex.)

clotting   See BLOOD CLOT; COAGULATION.

clotting factor   A substance in the blood consisting of proteins essential to COAGULATION. Absence of these proteins may lead to prolonged, uncontrollable bleeding, as in HEMOPHILIA.

clotting factor products   See COAGULATION FACTORS.

cluster of differentiation (CD)   One or more cell surface molecules, detectable by MONOCLONAL antibodies, that define a particular cell line or state of cellular differentiation.

Cmax   The maximum concentration of a drug in the body after dosing. Cmax is often associated with side effects. See PEAK LEVEL.

CMI   See CELLULAR IMMUNITY.

Cmin   The lowest concentration of a drug after dosing. See TROUGH LEVEL.

CMV   See CYTOMEGALOVIRUS.

CMV colitis   See CYTOMEGALOVIRUS COLITIS.

CMV esophagitis   See CYTOMEGALOVIRUS ESOPHAGITIS.

CMV gastritis   See CYTOMEGALOVIRUS GASTRITIS.

CMV neurological disease   See CYTOMEGALOVIRUS NEUROLOGICAL DISEASE.

CMV pneumonia   See CYTOMEGALOVIRUS PNEUMONIA.

CMV polyradiculopathy   See CYTOMEGALOVIRUS POLYRADICULOPATHY.

CMV retinis   See CYTOMEGALOVIRUS RETINIS.

CMV viral load   The total amount of cytomegalovirus (CMV) in a person's blood. Data suggest that CMV viral load can be a useful tool in tailoring CMV treatment options to fit each individual, just as HIV viral load is. Studies show that HIV viral load has some predictive value of risk of CMV disease progression and death; predictive value of CMV viral load is much stronger.

CMV viremia   The presence of cytomegalovirus (CMV) in the blood. Data indicate that CMV viremia indicates risk of disease. Some researchers caution that not everyone with a positive qualitative test result progresses to active CMV and argue that it is important to learn how to understand and use CMV viral load to make treatment decisions. Other researchers suspect that CMV viremia is only part of the equation and that CD4 count and HIV viral load may need to be considered as well in determining who is at highest risk for development of active disease. Note that still other researchers go one step further, asserting that CMV viremia is predictive of disease progression and survival.

Methods to detect the presence of CMV include viral cultures, serological testing, pp65 antigenemia, and POLYMERASE CHAIN REACTION (PCR) assay—a method to detect and amplify very small amounts of DNA in a sample. Of the latter, two types of PCR tests exist to date: the viremia or qualitative assays that determine whether a person is CMV-positive or -negative and the quantitative assays that measure viral load.

CNS See CENTRAL NERVOUS SYSTEM.

CNS lymphoma See PRIMARY CENTRAL NERVOUS SYSTEM LYMPHOMA.

Coactinon See EMVIRINE.

coagulation The process by which a liquid becomes a viscous or solid mass; clotting. Normal blood contains chemical compounds, called COAGULATION FACTORS, whose sequential interactions comprise the process of blood clotting. Those with HEMOPHILIA lack these factors. The blood's ability to clot may be impaired by infection.

coagulation factor Any of the chemical compounds in the blood which interact to create the coagulation process, or blood clotting. Factors are designated by Roman numerals and names. They include Factor I, fibrinogen; Factor II, prothrombin; Factor III, tissue factor; Factor IV, calcium ions; Factor V, proaccelerin, an unstable protein substance; Factor VII, proconvertin or serum prothrombin conversion accelerator; Factor VIII, antihemophilic factor; Factor IX, Christmas factor; Factor X, Stuart-Prower factor; Factor XI, plasma thromboplastin antecedent; Factor XII, Hageman or glass factor; Factor XIII, fibrin stabilizing factor. Other factors include prekallikrein, also called Fletcher factor; high molecular weight kininogen, also called Fitzgerald, Falujenc, or William factor, or contact activation cofactor.

When HEMORRHAGE occurs in patients with HEMOPHILIA A, coagulation factor IX is given. Factor VIII is given when hemorrhage occurs in patients with hemophilia B. These factors are available from various sources and special care has been taken to be as sure as possible that they are free of HIV and hepatitis viruses. Many hemophiliacs learn to self-administer these factors to control bleeding episodes.

coalition building See ACTIVISM.

coalition politics See ACTIVISM.

cocaine A bitter white crystalline alkaloid obtained from coca leaves, used medically as a local anesthetic. It is also widely used illicitly for its stimulant and euphoric properties.

Coccidioides A genus of fungus found in semiarid and desert regions of the U.S. Southwest, Mexico, and Central and South America. When airborne it can be inhaled and cause the illness COCCIDIOIDOMYCOSIS.

coccidioidomycosis A respiratory illness caused by inhaling airborne spores of the *Coccidioides* fungus. It is found in semiarid or desert areas. It is also called valley fever, desert fever, and San Joaquin Valley fever. Outbreaks typically follow dust storms, earthquakes, and excavation of desert sites. It is widespread throughout the southwestern United States, Mexico, and Central and South America. It can spread to other parts of the body besides the lungs. It is not spread from person to person.

The illness is seen in three different forms: acute, chronic, and disseminated. The acute infection is often not noticed by most people. Symptoms can be fever, headache, dry cough, malaise, weight loss, and muscle aches. Acute pulmonary coccidioidomycosis is almost always mild, producing few or no symptoms, and resolves without treatment. The incubation period is seven to 21 days. Chronic disease can occur up to 20 years after an initial infection that has not been recognized or treated. Disseminated infection can affect the spleen, lymph system, bones, and heart area. Meningitis is common in disseminated cases. Diagnostic tests and biopsies can be done to check for disease. HIV-positive people often test negative for the disease serologically.

HIV-positive people who have had coccidioidomycosis are typically placed on prophylaxis for life as the fungi can return and cause great problems in disseminated form. Treatment and prophylaxis employ FLUCONAZOLE or ITRACONAZOLE. Approximately 3 percent of a given population in the affected area may contract the disease. It is more common in the immunocompromised in pregnant women, and in people of African descent.

coccidioses A collection of illnesses found in humans and animals caused by the family of protozoa of the coccidian family. Some can be spread between species. Typically they can cause disease in goats, cats, and birds. CRYPTOSPORIDIOSIS, TOXOPLASMOSIS, and ISOSPORIASIS are all illnesses caused by members of the coccidian family. They are often present in humans but do not typically cause major illnesses unless a person is immunocompromised, as in HIV disease.

cock ring A device placed around the base of the PENIS and TESTICLES that aids men in getting and maintaining an ERECTION, thus prolonging sex.

code In a hospital or medical setting, a coded message used to transmit information, usually about a medical emergency, especially when broadcast over a public address system. "Code blue," for instance, alerts an emergency care team to a particular type of emergency, generally cardiac arrest.

codon A three-nucleotide genetic subunit that determines which amino acid is placed at one point in a protein chain. Mutations at specific HIV codons are associated with changes in the amino acid sequence of HIV's proteins and enzymes. Such mutations help HIV evade the effects of antiviral drugs or specific immune responses.

coenzyme Q10 First isolated in cow heart cells, coenzyme Q10 (Co-Q10) is a substance that assists in the oxidation of nutrients within cells to create energy. It is also highly efficient at protecting internal and external cell membranes against oxidation and is sometimes proposed as a complementary therapy to combat AIDS-related conditions. Co-Q10 is found in mammalian tissue, with the highest concentrations in the heart, liver, kidney, and muscle. Co-Q10 levels are abnormally low in people with congestive heart failure and in populations with HIV, muscular dystrophy, periodontal disease, immune dysfunction, and immunosuppression caused by the cancer chemotherapy DOXORUBICIN. To date, no toxicities have been reported from Co-Q10 use.

cofactor A factor other than the basic causative agent of a disease that activates or furthers the action of a disease-causing agent, thereby increasing the likelihood of developing that disease. Cofactors may also increase the progression of a particular disease. Cofactors may include the presence of other microbes, proteins, hormones, genes, genetic predispositions, psychosocial factors such as stress, or environmental issues. With HIV infection, cofactors are only suspected but may include other viruses (like CYTOMEGALOVIRUS), age, genetic resistance, or predisposition and certain hormone-like substances called CYTOKINES, released by LYMPHOCYTES.

cognitive function See HIV ENCEPHALOPATHY; ENCEPHALITIS.

cognitive reappraisal A coping strategy in which patients are taught to monitor and evaluate negative thoughts and replace them with more positive thoughts and images.

cohort In medical research, a group of individuals sharing a demographic or clinical characteristic that is the subject of a study of the EPIDEMIOLOGY or natural course of a disease.

cohort studies Studies that follow groups of similar individuals over time, noting who develops a disease and who does not, and comparing the groups at the end of the study to determine COFACTORS and other elements that may influence outcome. Cohort studies of gay men in San Francisco have determined that behavior modification can influence incidence of HIV infection and reduce the number of new cases.

coil An INTRAUTERINE DEVICE (IUD), a type of contraceptive device considered an effective form of birth control.

coinfection The condition of an organism or individual cell infected by two pathological microorganisms simultaneously. It has not yet been determined whether an additional "super infection" (or "reinfection") with a second strain of HIV occurs at a period of time after initial infection.

coinsurance Under MEDICARE and most health insurance plans, the percentage of allowable charges for a given class of medical care that the patient must pay.

coitus SEXUAL INTERCOURSE. The term is often used with a modifier to distinguish type (e.g., anal coitus, interfemoral [between the thighs] coitus). Slang terms include ball, FUCK, or hump.

coke See COCAINE.

colitis Inflammation of the COLON, the lower part of the large intestine. It is a chronic condition that causes abdominal pain, diarrhea, and other symptoms. Colitis caused by CYTOMEGALOVIRUS is a common development in HIV-infected patients. Cytomegalovirus infects the colon in slightly more patients than it does the esophagus. While there is no typical pattern of CMV-caused gastrointestinal disease, it is often associated with intermittent or persistent diarrhea with cramping, lower abdominal pain, involuntary rectal spasms, and weight loss. The stool may be watery, semi-formed or formed, and may be accompanied by bleeding. In some patients, diarrhea can be quite severe, with up to twenty bowel movements each day, resulting in severe loss of fluid and electrolytes from the body; other patients may have no discernible diarrhea at all. Fevers are common in patients with CMV colitis.

The diagnostic procedure of choice for colitis is COLONOSCOPY, in which an ENDOSCOPE is inserted into the colon through the rectum for a visual examination. A colonoscopy is performed only after the stool has been examined several times for evidence of other pathogens that may be responsible for the symptoms. The colons of patients with colitis appear diffusely inflamed and bleed easily on contact with the endoscope. A BIOPSY is necessary to rule out possible causes.

colon The part of the large intestine between the cecum and the rectum. The colon and the small intestine are commonly the sites of infections that cause diarrhea. To diagnose problems in the colon, common procedures are COLONOSCOPY and SIGMOIDOSCOPY. These procedures permit observation and BIOPSY of the colon by passing a tube through the rectum.

colonization The presence of a microorganism in or on a host without associated disease.

colony-stimulating factor (CSF-1) A protein present in human serum that promotes MONOCYTE differentiation. G-CSF and GM-CSF have similar efficacy, but G-CSF is significantly better tolerated, according to a study that compared the two colony-stimulating factors as acute salvage therapy in advanced HIV-infected individuals with NEUTROPENIA.

coloproctitis Inflammation of the COLON and RECTUM.

colostrum Breast fluid that may be secreted from the second trimester of pregnancy onward, but is most evident in the first two or three days after birth and before the onset of true lactation. This thin yellowish fluid is rich in proteins, calories, antibodies, and lymphocytes, and is low in fat and sugar.

colposcope A magnifying instrument in the form of a flexible fiberoptic tube, used in COLPOSCOPY.

colposcopy Examination of the VULVA, VAGINA, and CERVIX by means of a COLPOSCOPE.

A more accurate alternative to the PAP TEST, colposcopy is a procedure in which the surface of the uterine cervix is examined for cancerous growths through a colposcope, a flexible fiberoptic tube. Colposcopy requires specialized training, as practitioners must be able to recognize diseased tissue visually through the colposcope lens. There have never been enough expert colposcopists to examine regularly every woman with HIV.

When the CENTERS FOR DISEASE CONTROL AND PREVENTION (CDC) began drafting gynecological guidelines for HIV-positive women in 1993, the CDC's advisory group had to choose between a schedule of regular Pap smears and/or colposcopy. The agency settled on recommending repeat Pap smears as a way of countering false-negative individual Paps. AIDS activists feared that HIV-positive women who had to wait six months or more for testing of abnormal Paps would risk contracting cervical cancer and insisted on colposcopy examinations for all HIV-positive women. Health care providers and activists generally agree, however, that, as a practical matter, it may be a more effective use of resources to create the best conditions for successful use of the low-tech Pap test than to put them into the more sophisticated colposcopy technique.

combination antiretroviral therapy   See COMBINATION THERAPY.

combination therapy   The use of two or more therapies administered alternately or simultaneously, in order to achieve maximum results. Different drugs have different ways of working and different side effects; by combining drugs, it is often possible to come up with a more effective treatment with reduced side effects and less risk of developing drug-resistance. Combination therapy is distinguished from MONOTHERAPY (one drug used alone) and SEQUENTIAL MONOTHERAPY (two or more drugs used sequentially, one at a time, with the change either after a fixed amount of time or after a drug has become ineffective). Research has shown that existing therapies such as the NUCLEOSIDE ANALOGS AZT, ddI, ddC, and D4T progressively lose their effectiveness when used alone. There is evidence that combining therapies reduces HIV replication, preventing the evolution of strains resistant to multiple medications.

According to comprehensive *Guidelines for the Use of Antiretroviral Agents in HIV-Infected Adults and Adolescents,* made available by the Department of Health and Human Services in 2001, all people with CDC-defined AIDS should receive combination ANTIRETROVIRAL therapy, preferably with three drugs, including a PROTEASE INHIBITOR. The *Guidelines* recommend starting treatment with three drugs and changing at least two when there are indications that treatment is failing. Treatment with only two drugs is, in general, considered less than optimal. Treatment with only one drug is not recommended. However, zidovudine (AZT) monotherapy is recommended as prophylaxis to prevent HIV TRANSMISSION to newborn babies. It should not be given during pregnancy to healthy HIV-infected women who do not require antiretroviral drugs for their own treatment.

Two drugs have also been shown to be better than one for treating children with symptomatic HIV. Initial therapy using AZT combined with either LAMIVUDINE (3TC) or DIDANOSINE (ddI) has been shown to be far more effective at staving off disease progression or death in children with symptomatic HIV disease than treatment with ddI alone. See CONVERGENT COMBINATION THERAPY.

Combivir   A combination of the NUCLEOSIDE ANALOG drugs ZIDOVUDINE (AZT) and LAMIVUDINE (3TC). Research has shown Combivir works as well as individual doses of the two drugs. Side effects are the same as if the two drugs were taken individually. Dosage is one pill two times a day. It has greatly reduced the number of pills people are required to take in many HAART regimens. It cannot be taken by children or people of low body weight as the dosage is preset for adult weight figures.

communicable   Capable of transmission from person to person (said of a disease or disease-causing organism).

Community Acquired Immune Deficiency Syndrome (CAIDS)   One of the names proposed in 1981–82 for AIDS.

community norms   As a disease associated with activities regarded by many as violations of public morality, AIDS is a controversial subject. Discussion of AIDS is often disturbing, and rational discussion difficult, for this reason. It challenges, or seems to challenge, the boundaries of community norms of behavior and discourse. Any attempt at AIDS prevention through programs of public education has to deal with this problem.

Broadly speaking, there are two positions on disseminating information about AIDS and AIDS prevention. The first may be called the public health viewpoint and advocates providing complete information as widely as possible. The second, more moralistic view is that since the activities that lead to getting AIDS are morally unacceptable, information about them should not be widely publicized. Among people holding this view, advocating abstinence or saying no to drug use are strongly, even exclusively, favored as AIDS prevention techniques. For those holding the first view, vocabulary is important because it may determine the success of any attempt to overcome public discomfort or hostility to honest and open discussion. The language of AIDS has therefore been evolving toward a more neutral or medical-sounding usage. Examples include: prostitutes (now referred to as commercial sex workers); AIDS patients/victims (PEOPLE WITH AIDS); drug addicts (INJECTION DRUG USERS); promiscuity (multiple sex partners).

Community Programs for Clinical Research on AIDS (CPCRA) The Community Programs for Clinical Research on AIDS is sponsored by the National Institute of Allergy and Infectious Diseases of the National Institutes of Health. It was established in 1989 to involve community physicians and their patients in studies of treatments for HIV and comprises 16 research units, consisting of consortiums of primary care physicians and nurses located at 160 sites in the U.S. and additional foreign sites. These research units represent a significant geographic, racial, and RISK-GROUP diversity. Through this diversity, the CPCRA extends greater opportunity for participation in clinical research to those persons underrepresented in traditional, university-based HIV studies.

community residence home care The term for BOARD-AND-CARE HOME services used by the US DEPARTMENT OF VETERANS AFFAIRS

community-based organization Community-based organizations are those organized at a local level, within a community, as close as possible to the individuals they serve. Those concerned with AIDS issues are also called AIDS ADVOCACY ORGANIZATIONS and AIDS SERVICE ORGANIZATIONS (ASOs). They provide services to people with HIV infection, as well as education and prevention programs for the whole community. The leaders of community-based organizations are lay people, not doctors or government officials, although many have physicians as advisers and have a paid professional staff as well as volunteers. Funding usually comes from state governments, private donations, and local fund-raising events.

comorbidity The coexistence of two or more diseases.

comparison trial A trial in which experimental drugs are tested against each other or against an approved drug.

compassionate use A FOOD AND DRUG ADMINISTRATION classification that allows use of an experimental drug by very sick patients who have no treatment options, even though there is insufficient data about the drug's effectiveness to allow licensing. Drugs are provided free under this program, which is also called Open Study Protocol. Often, specific approval of individual cases must be obtained from the FDA for compassionate use of a drug.

compensation In biology, the improvement of any defect by the excessive development or action of another part of the same structure.

competence In psychological evaluation, having the ability to manage one's affairs and to perform in a manner adequate to the demands of a situation; to interact effectively with the environment.

In cell biology, the capacity of embryonic cells to differentiate into a variety of cell types. Also, a cell able to take up DNA and be transformed is described as "competent."

complacency Despite increasingly grim projections concerning the AIDS pandemic and its demographic, economic, and social impact, many people involved in the international AIDS effort believe that the sense of urgency that marked the late 1980s has abated noticeably, at least in industrialized countries. This apparent complacency was identified by the Global Commission on AIDS as one of the critical issues for the 1990s.

There appears to be a number of factors contributing to this phenomenon: unrealistic expectations that the problem will soon be solved by vaccines and drugs; a public view that the epidemic has leveled off or peaked and is declining in industrialized countries; the belief that spread of AIDS among heterosexuals is not a serious problem in industrialized countries; and fatigue about AIDS on the part of the media, politicians, and the public.

In some seriously affected countries, this apparent complacency may actually be a form of denial, as the true dimensions of the disaster become apparent. In other countries, complacency may be the result of the mistaken belief that certain societies are virtually immune to HIV/AIDS because of cultural factors, including religious beliefs and practices. Whatever its roots, complacency is extremely dangerous. It leads to the failure not only of individuals to protect themselves, but also of governments to sustain a high level of commitment and action, especially in regard to public education and other preventive efforts, such as condom distribution. There is particular danger that public complacency in wealthy countries, combined with economic recession, will result in failure to increase the bilateral transfer of funds to poor countries or to sustain or increase contributions to international efforts against AIDS, at the very time when needs are increasing dramatically, especially for the care of the sick and orphaned. In less affluent countries, complacency may lead officials to ignore the need to shift priorities in national spending, perhaps from military and police to health and social services.

Because the mass media clearly have been the major source of public information about AIDS, they obviously have a critical role in combating complacency. Yet the media's primary role is to report information not to persuade the public. Governments and nongovernmental organizations need to persevere in developing and promoting both general and targeted AIDS information to increase public knowledge and maintain public concern.

Finally, organized advocacy must continue to be one of the cornerstones of the AIDS effort if the danger of complacency is to be overcome and AIDS is to remain high on the national and international agendas.

complement See COMPLEMENT SYSTEM.

complement cascade A precise sequence of events, usually triggered by an antigen-antibody complex, in which each component of the complement system is activated in turn, inactivating and occasionally destroying pathogens.

complement fixation test A diagnostic test that distinguishes between forms of serum antibody proteins (called complement) in the blood to identify specific diseases.

Antibodies are formed when the body is exposed to infections. If the antigens (specific causes) of a disease are mixed with a patient's serum, along with specially prepared sheep red blood cells, the antibodies and antigens will combine, and the blood cells will remain whole. If the patient's serum does not contain complement antibodies to a disease, the sheep red blood cells will dissolve (a process called HEMOLYSIS).

complement system Collectively, the 20 plasma proteins involved in specific and nonspecific IMMUNE RESPONSES. The three main functions of the complement system are CHEMOTAXIS (release of chemicals that attract phagocytic cells to an invasion site), opsonization (the coating of an invading cell for easy recognition by phagocytic cells) and the formation of membrane adherence complex (making the invading cell vulnerable to LYSIS).

Complement activation occurs when antibodies bind to an antigen, causing an amplifying cascade of reactions as each complement protein is activated sequentially.

complementary medicine Nonmainstream health care provided in addition to, or instead of, standard medical practice. See ALTERNATIVE MEDICINE.

complementary therapy   A range of services designed to complement traditional medical practice as part of a practitioner's primary care plan for an individual.

complete blood count (CBC)   A screening of the most important cellular components of the blood. A CBC includes the total white blood (leukocyte) count, counts of specific types of white blood cells, red blood cell count, hemoglobin level, and platelet count.

compliance   See ADHERENCE.

compound Q   A substance (also called GLQ223) whose active ingredient is a protein called tricosanthin, extracted from the root tuber of a Chinese cucumber, *Trichosanthes kirilowii*. It is used in China to induce abortions and to treat ectopic pregnancy, hydatidiform moles, and a type of cancer, choriocarcinoma. In China there are three different grades of trichosanthin prepared for injection: crude extract, purified extract, and crystallized, the highest purity. Only the crystallized form can be used safely; the others cause severe side effects.

In late 1988 and early 1989 compound Q generated enormous public and scientific interest, and was touted as an important treatment to watch. In April 1989 there was widespread publicity about a severe adverse reaction to an injected bogus "compound Q," apparently homemade from roots obtained from a health food store. It was also reported that some health food stores were exploiting the situation by promoting a dried root or extract that, they suggested, contained compound Q. The public was warned that the root also contains lectins, which are poisonous when injected (they cause blood cells to clump together, potentially causing heart attacks or strokes). Moreover, compound Q is almost certainly destroyed by drying, so the dried root available in health food stores does not contain the active ingredient anyway.

A potential benefit of compound Q is that trichosanthin, unlike other treatments, kills HIV-infected cells; thus it has the potential to reduce the total amount of infection and not just slow its spread. Physicians and researchers continue to be concerned about toxicity, however. Two kinds have been found. One appears to be dose-related and the other seems to depend on the condition of the patient. Clearly not enough is known to determine the most beneficial use of this substance, or to predict its value as a treatment.

Comprehensive AIDS Resource Emergency Act of 1990   See RYAN WHITE COMPREHENSIVE AIDS RESOURCES EMERGENCY (CARE) ACT OF 1990.

comprehensive care   Care that includes the full spectrum of health, educational, social, and related services.

compromised   Weakened, as in compromised immunity, a decreased ability to resist infection.

computer bulletin board   See BULLETIN BOARD SYSTEM.

computerized axial tomography (CT)   A noninvasive method of examining the brain or other organ by means of scanning it with an X-ray beam repeatedly from different angles, enabling a computer to build up a visual image. This procedure is known as a CT (formerly CAT) scan. CT scans are more detailed than conventional X-ray images. CT scans of the entire body or of parts of it can be done. A person undergoing a CT scan first receives an injection of a CONTRAST AGENT material that shows up well in X-ray images. (Some people have allergic reactions to contrast agents.) He or she is next put into a cylindrical chamber around which a scanner moves, producing three-dimensional images in parallel sections of an inch or less. CT scans, first developed in the 1970s, are an excellent method for detecting tumors, infections, or other changes in the anatomical features of the brain, chest, or abdomen.

Concorde   The Concorde study was a landmark clinical trial that examined the long-term effect of AZT on the survival of HIV-infected but asymptomatic patients. Concorde began in October 1988 and was organized by the British Medical Research Council and the French National AIDS Research Agency, and was conducted in Britain, France, and

Ireland. The trial was the largest randomized, double-blind placebo-controlled AZT study ever conducted. Neither the clinicians nor the participants knew who was given AZT and who was given placebo. Preliminary results were released in a letter to the *Lancet,* the leading British medical journal, on April 3, 1993.

Concorde addresses a fundamental question: does early AZT therapy truly prolong the lives of asymptomatic people?

The study followed nearly 1,800 subjects for an average of three years. At the start, all were HIV-positive and asymptomatic, with a broad range of CD4 counts. Eight hundred and seventy-seven individuals were randomized to receive 1,000 mg per day of AZT from the start, regardless of their CD4 levels ("immediate treatment") and eight hundred and seventy-two were given placebo ("deferred treatment") until they developed symptomatic disease (AIDS or ARC). The two groups were similar in age, sex (15 percent were women), and immunological markers. The trial was designed to show whether it is beneficial to begin AZT treatment of HIV-positive people before symptoms appear. The trial was not designed to provide information on the usefulness of taking AZT for symptomatic HIV disease.

In 1989, an American study was halted after one year when it found that AZT seemed to delay progression of disease in people with a CD4 count of below 500. (This study was too small and too short to examine the effect of AZT on ultimate survival.) The Concorde study was then modified on ethical grounds to allow all participants with a lower-than-500 CD4 count to begin taking AZT. Those who chose to begin AZT once their CD4 count fell below 500, along with those who began AZT because they developed symptomatic disease, were included in the preliminary analysis.

After an average of three years, survival rates did not differ significantly, nor was there a significant difference in disease progression. However, there was a statistically significant difference in CD4 levels between the two arms of the study, which was sustained up to three years. No new or unexpected toxicities were seen.

The authors of the study concluded that "Concorde has not shown any significant benefit from the immediate use of zidovudine (AZT) compared with deferred therapy in symptom-free individuals in terms of survival or disease progression, irrespective of their initial CD4 counts."

Criticisms of Concorde were numerous. Some noted, for example, that the protocol change in 1989, which allowed open label use of AZT for those with less than 500 CD4 cells, may have skewed the results by causing a significant number of those in the deferred treatment arm to receive the same therapy as those in the immediate treatment arm. It was therefore not surprising that there was no significant difference between the two arms. Others noted that since Concorde did not use what is believed to be the optimum dose of AZT, the results did not provide an accurate indication of the potential benefits of AZT. It was also noted that Concorde was a study of AZT MONOTHERAPY, rather than COMBINATION THERAPY, which is widely believed to provide the most beneficial results in anti-retroviral therapy.

Concorde results challenged the belief that the NUCLEOSIDE ANALOGS (the class of compounds that includes AZT, ddI, and ddC) would transform AIDS into a so-called chronic manageable condition. Some of the basic assumptions underlying AIDS drug development evidently needed to be reexamined. Consensus on the central questions in AIDS research was lost.

Concorde also raised questions about the applicability of the current expedited drug approval criteria to treatments for asymptomatics as well those with AIDS disease symptoms. The question was becoming urgent as more and more companies were taking advantage of regulations to develop new therapeutic vaccines, new antiretrovirals, and immunomodulators for asymptomatics as well as those with AIDS disease symptoms. On a broader level, Concorde raised disturbing questions regarding the American AIDS research effort as a whole. Had the point of diminishing returns been reached with the nucleosides? Would it be wiser to use limited AIDS research dollars to develop and test new, more promising classes of compounds? Was there an overall strategy and program for developing anti-HIV therapies? Was the federal government ensuring that the country's AIDS research effort was as effective as it could be? Some activists felt there was evidence of a conspiracy by the manufacturer of AZT to manipulate scientific evidence.

conditional eligibility   The status of those applicants granted temporary SSI benefits even though they have slightly too much in assets, while they attempt to sell some assets. They are required to repay program benefits out of the proceeds. By extension, this term is sometimes applied to situations in which an applicant is granted eligibility, in the SSI or MEDICAID program, despite excess assets, if the assets are essentially unsalable (for instance rural property for which there is no market).

condom   A flexible shield made of latex, polyurethane, or lambskin that is placed over the penis or sex toy during penetration to prevent conception and sexually transmitted diseases. HIV will not go through latex. If a condom does not leak, break, or fall off, it will block the virus. Correct use of a latex condom during every act of intercourse greatly reduces, but does not eliminate, the risk of infection with HIV. Lambskin or "natural" condoms do not offer protection because they are too porous. A condom is also called a bag, boot, french letter, jimmy hat, latex sheath, prophylactic, rubber, and raincoat.

Latex condoms have been proved to be the most effective contraceptive as well as the best protection against sexually transmitted diseases, including HIV. Some are lubricated with a spermicide, NONOXYNOL-9, which decreases the risk of pregnancy if some semen spills outside the condom. However, the extent of decreased risk has not been established. Nonoxynol-9 has also shown to be a skin irritant so some people may find it uncomfortable to use the condoms with it on the surface.

Condoms seldom break when used correctly, but pulling out before ejaculating will add further protection. (Condoms can fail: no condom or contraceptive works 100 percent of the time. The only absolutely sure way to prevent pregnancy and sexually transmitted diseases is not to have sex.) Polyurethane condoms have a slightly higher breakage rate than latex condoms but have proved more comfortable in consumer testing. They are both equally effective at preventing STDs when used properly. Condoms should be used for vaginal, anal, or oral sex, and a new condom should be used for each sex act. Both men and women should learn how to use a condom properly. All latex condoms sold in the United States must meet minimal standards for strength and quality.

Here are the basic instructions for using a condom: Open the package carefully so that the condom is not torn or a hole made with a fingernail. Testing the elasticity will only weaken it. Do not unroll the rubber until putting it on. A drop of water-based lubricant inside the tip of the rubber makes the penis feel better during sex. The shaft of the penis should be free of lubricant to decrease the chance that the condom will fall off. Hold the tip of the condom to squeeze out the air; excess air can cause the condom to break. This leaves room for the semen after ejaculation. When the penis is hard (before sexual contact), place the condom on the tip and roll down all the way. If the man is uncircumcised, the foreskin should be pulled back first.

In vaginal or anal intercourse, use plenty of water-based lubricant, such as K-Y jelly or Wet. Baby oil, cocoa butter, cold cream, Crisco, hand creams or lotions, massage oil, mineral oil, or petroleum-based products such as Vaseline can break down the latex condoms within minutes. This will increase the risk of breaking the condom or injuring internal and external body tissue, which could leave an opening for infection. Lubricants that contain alcohol can also damage latex. Read the label to make sure there is no oil or alcohol in the jelly or lubricant.

However, polyurethane condoms may be used with oil-based lubricants. A lot of lubricant should be used on the outside of the rubber. This will make it slide easier so it will not break. Lubricant can also be put on the vagina or anus. Water-based lubricants may become dry during sex. If this happens, put a little water on the rubber and it will be slippery again. More lubricant can also be used. If during intercourse you or your partner sense burning or itching, discontinue use of the condom and try another type. After ejaculation but before loss of the erection, pull the penis out gently. Hold the condom at the base of the penis while pulling out so that it does not leak or fall off. Take it off carefully so the semen does not spill. Roll it off, starting at the base of the penis. Throw the condom away. Never wear the same condom twice.

Finally, because no one knows for sure how long a virus lives outside the body, it is good to wash after having sex. Avoid further sexual contact with your partner until both of you wash your sex organs and any other areas that have contact with body fluids. If a condom is sticky or brittle or looks damaged, do not use it. Store condoms in a cool, dry place. Do not keep condoms in a wallet, pocketbook, or glove compartment of a car for a long time. Keep condoms out of direct sunlight; heat can make them weak. Condom packages have a date on the outside, the inner wrapping, or the condom itself. This is the date of manufacture, not an expiration date. If condoms are kept in a cool, dry place, they will last about four years, but unless you know exactly how and where a condom has been stored, do not use it more than two years after the date stamped on it.

condyloma   A wartlike growth of the skin, usually seen on the external genitalia or near the anus.

condyloma acuminatum   A projecting warty growth on the external genitals or the ANUS caused by infection with the HUMAN PAPILLOMAVIRUS (HPV). It is usually benign or noncancerous. Condyloma acuminatum is also referred to as GENITAL WART or verruca acuminata.

condyloma lata   The genital lesion that occurs during the secondary stage of SYPHILIS.

confidence interval   The range of possible results within which there is a specific probability that the "real" answer lies. In science papers, confidence intervals give readers a better grasp of trial results than just the P value (the probability that the findings in the study could have occurred as a matter of chance, instead of reflecting a real change from the expected average) alone. The "95 percent confidence interval" or "95 percent CI" is a range of possible results within which you can be 95 percent sure that the "real" answer lies.

confidential information   Confidential HIV-related information is information that a person has been the subject of an HIV-related test, or has HIV, HIV-related illness or AIDS, or any information which identifies or reasonably could identify an individual as having one or more of these con-ditions, including information pertaining to the individual's contacts. In general, confidentiality laws require written authorization for information to be released. This requirement serves to extend the law's coverage beyond the realm of health and social services, because anyone who obtains information pursuant to a written release is fully bound by the law. See CONFIDENTIAL TESTING; PRIVACY.

confidential testing   In regard to HIV testing, confidential testing means that the results of a test are formally restricted to the person being tested and the person or facility performing the test. Confidential test results however, are permanently recorded in a patient's medical charts, and there is always the risk that they may be disclosed without his or her permission. ANONYMOUS TESTING precludes that risk.

confidentiality   See PRIVACY.

conflict of interest (COI)   A conflict of interest occurs in a situation in which professional judgment regarding a primary interest, such as research, education, or patient care, may be unduly influenced by a secondary interest, such as financial gain or personal prestige. Conflicts of interest exist in every walk of life, including medicine and science. There is nothing inherently unethical in finding oneself in a conflict of interest. Rather, the key questions are whether one recognizes the conflict and how one deals with it. Strategies include disclosing the conflict, establishing a system of review and authorization, and prohibiting the activities that lead to the conflict. Note that federal law now covers conflict of interest in science it funds. Two key questions are, Does the government enforce its own regulations? And, What about COI involving people other than scientists?

In the medical world, business-community partnerships have been described as "deadly" and COI has been said to pose a direct threat to many people's health and to create an enormous opportunity for undue financial gain and political power. In this arena, COI has also been described as "omnipresent," as evidenced, for example, by corporate sponsorships of nongovernmental organizations, service organizations, health websites, research teams, and AIDS conferences. In the context of HIV/AIDS, nonprofit organizations are especially vulnerable to COI. As nonprofit organizations rely on the trust of donors, volunteers, and the public, even the appearance of conflict of interest within the organization or on its board can damage the organization's reputation. Even when the conflict does not constitute a legal impropriety, this damage can limit an organization's ability to carry out its mission.

confounding factor   A variable that differs in the treatment and control groups in a study and that has an effect on the results.

congenital syphilis   A syphilis infection that is present at birth.

congregate living   Any one of a number of housing, shelter, or confinement arrangements in which a number of individuals live together.

conjugate   A combination of two molecules, such as hapten and a protein, that can initiate an immune response.

conjugated protein   A protein to which a non-protein portion is attached.

conjugation   A union of bacterial cells in which two individual bacteria or filaments fuse together to exchange or donate genetic material.

conjunctivitis   An inflammation of the conjunctiva, the thin protective membrane on the inner surface of the eyelids and the outer surface of the eye. There are many different types of conjunctivitis, and treatment varies depending on the specific type of infection.

conscious sedation   "Light sedation" during which the patient retains airway reflexes and responses to verbal stimuli.

conservator   See SURROGATE.

conservatorship   See SURROGACY.

constitutional symptoms   Symptoms caused by the impact of an illness on the entire body or constitution are frequently referred to as constitutional symptoms. These include loss of weight, fatigue, fever, diarrhea, night sweats, and malaise over a period of months. Constitutional symptoms are present in many types of infectious diseases, tumors, and other medical conditions, ranging from the serious to the trivial. For people with HIV infection, constitutional symptoms may be a result of HIV infection itself or the result of such opportunistic illnesses as PNEUMOCYSTIS CARINII PNEUMONIA, TUBERCULOSIS, or widespread CMV infection.

consumer   An individual who uses a product or service. In the health care setting, a more general term for *client* or *patient*.

contact infection   An infection resulting from direct or indirect contact with a person who is infected. A contact infection may be transmitted through physical contact with those afflicted with COMMUNICABLE diseases or with utensils handled by them.

contact sensitivity   A type of delayed hypersensitivity reaction in which sensitivity to simple chemical compounds is manifested by skin reactivity.

contact tracing   A technique used in the treatment of AIDS and other sexually transmitted diseases, involving finding and notifying an HIV-positive person's recent and current sexual contacts, either with or without identifying the infected individual.

contagion, fear of   Fear of contracting a disease, by either direct or indirect contact with infected individuals, carriers, or objects they may have touched or passed near. During the early years of the AIDS epidemic, the fear experienced by the uninfected was compounded by the seriousness of the disease, the degree to which it was associated with unpopular or marginal social groups, and misinformation coupled with inadequate efforts to educate the public about the disease and methods of prevention.

contagious The term is used of diseases, referring to the capacity of being spread from one person to another through casual contact. All contagious diseases are also infectious; but some diseases, like TOXIC SHOCK SYNDROME, are infectious but not contagious. HIV is both infectious and contagious, but it is contagious only with specific types of contact.

contain In medicine, to prevent or limit the advance, spread, or influence of a disease.

contamination In medicine, the introduction of disease germs or infectious material into sterile environments or onto sterile objects.

continuity of care Uninterrupted health care provided from initial contact with a physician or clinic through all phases of a patient's medical care needs. The term is frequently applied more narrowly to mean the provision of care from initial contact through recovery from a given illness.

continuous care In health care services, care that is maintained without interruption despite changes in site, caregiver, or method of payment.

continuous infusion Uninterrupted introduction of fluid other than blood into a vein.

contraceptive Against conception; a drug (ORAL CONTRACEPTIVE, INTRAMUSCULAR PROGESTERONE), BARRIER (creams, gels, suppositories, foams, sponges), physical alteration (surgical sterilization), or device (INTRAUTERINE DEVICE, DIAPHRAGM, CONDOM) that tends or serves to prevent conception or impregnation. For HIV-positive women, there are pros and cons of the various choices that need to be taken into consideration. Oral contraceptives have known and unknown interactions with other medications and possibly reduce immune function in immune-compromised women. Diaphragms with spermicide or cervical cap do not prevent, although they may limit, transmission of STDs. Other barriers, such as creams, gels, suppositories, foams, and sponges may be inadequate for contraception or STD prevention unless used with condoms. Intrauterine devices are not a good choice for immune-compromised women because the risk of PID is high. Decisions for permanent sterilization should not be made in the early months, and perhaps the first year, after diagnosis with HIV infection, and in any case bilateral tubal ligation does not prevent the transmission of STDs. Progesterone implants have uncertain hormonal interaction in HIV illness, a slight risk of infection at the site of insertion which may be increased in conditions of compromised immunity, and uncertain interaction with medications commonly used in treatment of HIV infection and they do not prevent the transmission of STDs.

contraindication A condition or circumstance that prevents prescription of a certain treatment to an individual patient.

contrast agent A contrast agent blocks X rays and thereby silhouettes the body parts of interest, allowing their visual imaging. Different contrast agents are used for different procedures; the methodologies for administering contrast agents also vary. Some contrast agents may be administered by way of an INTRAVENOUS (IV) drip; others can be taken orally. In general, contrast agents and not the X rays cause the complications arising from gastrointestinal exams. Allergic reaction is a major consideration when using any contrast agent.

control arm The group of participants in a clinical trial who receive standard treatment or a PLACEBO, against which those receiving the experimental treatment are compared.

control group In experimental design, a comparison group of subjects who, when the independent variable is manipulated, are not exposed to the treatment that subjects in the experimental group are exposed to, but who in other respects are treated identically. This group provides a baseline against which to evaluate the effects of treatment.

controlled study A study in which doctors give a new drug being tested to one group of people, the treatment group, and give another drug or no drug to a second group of people with the same type of illness, the CONTROL GROUP. Then they compare the results of the two groups. Simply put, if people taking the new drug get better and people taking the other drug or no drug do not, the new drug works. If the treatment group does not improve more than the control group, the new drug does not work, or not better than the treatment the control group was taking. If many people in the treatment group get sicker and people in the control group do not, the new drug is not safe.

controlled trial   See CONTROLLED STUDY.

convergent combination therapy   An experimental form of COMBINATION THERAPY based on the 1992–93 research of Yang-kung Chow, a medical student in Boston. Chow's research suggested that a combination of three drugs—AZT, ddI, and either NEVIRAPINE or the pyridinone L679,661—could stop HIV replication completely. The significance of the finding was limited, however, since successful test tube experiments with new drugs often fail in the nonideal condition of the human body. Nevertheless it was a promising line of investigation.

The idea behind convergent combination therapy is to turn one of the virus's greatest strengths—its ability to mutate quickly and become resistant to anti-HIV drugs—against itself. By 1993, it was well documented that HIV can become resistant to single-drug therapy with AZT or ddI, perhaps even simultaneously. However, Chow's research suggested that there may be a limit to HIV's ability to mutate. The combination of three drugs forces the virus either to mutate to resist all three drugs, resulting in a genetically defective virus, or to remain susceptible to at least one of the drugs' antiretroviral action. In either case, HIV replication will be inhibited.

Chow's findings were later contradicted when the virus proved capable of producing viable strains resistant to all three drugs at once. Ambiguous results from a federally funded clinical trial also demonstrated that the virus can sidestep convergent therapy. However, convergent therapy attracted attention back to a class of compounds known as NONNUCLEOSIDE REVERSE TRANSCRIPTASE INHIBITORS (NNRTI), which include a number of different types of drug, including the pyridinones, the

BHAP drugs, and the thiobenzimidazolone (TIBO) derivatives. In 1991 these drugs were found to induce resistance rapidly in HIV, leading to serious doubts about their usefulness. Convergent combination therapy raised hopes that the NNRTIs may ultimately prove beneficial in combination.

cookers   Equipment used in the preparation of some injectable illicit drugs. See WORKS; DRUG ADDICTION; DRUG PARAPHERNALIA LAWS; NEEDLE SHARING; TRANSMISSION.

Cooley's anemia   ANEMIA resulting from inheritance of a recessive trait responsible for interference with the rate of hemoglobulin synthesis.

Coomb's test   A test for antiglobulins in the red cells used in diagnosing various hemolytic anemias.

cooperative clinical trial   Term frequently used to denote a multicenter trial.

coordinating center   A center in the structure of a study that is responsible for receiving, editing, processing, analyzing, and storing data generated in a study and that, in addition, has responsibility for coordination of activities required for execution of the study.

copayment   The amount an insured patient pays for a health service, beyond the amount paid by the insurance or health plan. By extension, a synonym for COINSURANCE.

coping   Dealing effectively with the stress of daily life and the unusual challenges posed by chronic disease, disability, and pain.

copper-7   One of several CONTRACEPTIVE devices known as INTRAUTERINE DEVICES (IUDs).

coprolalia   Talking dirty, usually in an attempt to be sexually arousing.

coprophilia   A sexual interest in feces.

core   The protein capsule surrounding a virus's DNA or RNA. In HIV, p55, the precursor molecule to the core, is broken down into the smaller molecules p24, p17, p7, and p6. HIV's core is primarily composed of p24.

core proteins   The proteins inside a pathogen; in HIV, refers to p17 and p24.

coreceptor   A second cell surface receptor required for entry by a pathogen into a host cell or for initiation of a biological process. HIV requires both the CD4 receptor and a coreceptor (e.g., CCR-5 or CXCR-4) to enter a cell.

correlates of immunity/correlates of protection
The immune responses that protect an individual from a certain disease. The precise identities of the correlates of immunity in HIV are unknown.

corticosteroid   A steroid synthesized in the adrenal cortex from cholesterol. Some are potent hormones. Corticosteroids are immunosuppressive; synthetic corticosteroids are used as short-term treatments for a host of AIDS-related conditions, such as NEUROPATHY, esophageal ulcers, skin rashes, and THROMBOCYTOPENIA. They are combined with other drugs to treat AIDS-related KAPOSI'S SARCOMA (KS), acute *PNEUMOCYSTIC CARINII* PNEUMONIA, and TUBERCULOSIS and to reduce intracranial pressure caused by TOXOPLASMOSIS or CNS LYMPHOMA. Corticosteroids include prednisone, corticosterone, cortisone, and aldosterone and are available in preparations for use intravenously, orally, or by direct application to the skin. The effects of corticosteroids on primary HIV infection have been given little formal study.

Long-term use of corticosteroids has been associated with reactivation of herpes viruses, *Pneumocystis carinii*, tuberculosis, and various fungal infections. Corticosteroid use has also been associated with the development of AIDS-KS, although rarely with the development of KS in other diseases, and it remains unclear if their use increases the risk of developing KS for people with HIV.

Using high doses of corticosteroids for a long time can be dangerous. They reduce the immune system's defenses against certain infections and are sometimes considered especially dangerous for people whose immune defenses are already weakened.

Nevertheless, many of the complications of HIV infection appear to result from an abundant but misdirected immune response; these complications respond well to corticosteroids. In any case it is considered best that these drugs be taken at the lowest possible dose for the shortest possible period.

cortisol   A glucocorticoid hormone secreted by the adrenal gland to moderate stress. Among other things, glucocorticoids promote the breakdown of protein stores in the body to produce sugar (glucose) and can decrease immune system activity. Cortisol levels are high in people with HIV infections, and the hormone has been implicated in WASTING SYNDROME. Recent studies have found that blocking cells' glucocorticoid receptors reduces the proliferation of KAPOSI'S SARCOMA tissue, and that blocking these receptors also might inhibit HIV itself.

cortisone   A CORTICOSTEROID often used to reduce inflammation in the body caused by various illnesses.

Corynebacterium   A genus of the family Corynebacteriaceae. The bacteria are rod shaped, gram-positive and non-motile. Though many species of this genus are pathogens in domestic animals, birds, reptiles, and plants, the most important is the species *C. diptheriae*, the causative agent of diphtheria in humans.

Cotrimoxale   See TRIMETHOPRIM-SULFAMETHOXAZOLE.

cotton wool spots   Areas of yellowish white coloration in the retina, generally seen by doctors and not the patients themselves. When the blood supply to the eye is cut off or slowed, swelling can occur in the retina. The blood supply can be disrupted as a result of various diseases such as diabetes and HIV retinopathy. The swelling causes the outer layer of the retina, made up of nerve cells, to become injured, thus giving rise to these spots. The cotton wool spots do not cause visual problems themselves and often go away on their own if the underlying condition is treated successfully to return the blood flow and reduce the swelling and pressure.

counseling The providing of advice and guidance to a patient by a health professional.

countable income The amount of a potential enrollee's income needs-based programs use to determine eligibility, after exemption of specified amounts or percentages of gross income.

counterstimulation Application of moderate to intense sensory stimulation, such as cold, heat, rubbing, pressure, or electrical current, so as to decrease perception of pain at the same or a distant site.

Coviracil See EMTRICITABINE.

CPCRA An acronym for the Terry Beirn Community Programs for Clinical Research on AIDS. CPCRA is a community-based clinical trials network whose main goal is to obtain evidence to inform health care providers and people living with HIV of the most appropriate use of available therapies in diverse populations across the United States. CPCRA is unique in that their studies are conducted in community settings such as veteran's hospitals, doctors' offices, community health settings, and HMO offices.

CPCRA is funded by the United States National Institutes of Allergy and Infectious Diseases, Division of AIDS (DAIDS), as part of a network of several research groups studying the treatment and prevention of HIV disease (see http://www.niaid.nih.gov/daids/fundedresearch.htm).

crab louse A species of louse (*Phthiru pubis*) that infests the pubic area of the human body. Often called simply *crab*.

crack A crystallized derivative form of cocaine that is ingested by being smoked. Crack is cheap and extremely addictive. Its use became epidemic in the late 1980s and early 1990s and receded in the late 1990s.

crack house A indoor place where individuals gather to smoke crack.

Cranston-Gonzalez National Affordable Housing Act of 1990 A federal housing law that includes a block grant program designed to encourage state and local governments to provide housing for people with HIV. This provision was intended as a measure against discrimination in housing against people with HIV.

C-reactive protein (CRP) A protein released by the body in response to injury, infection, or other inflammatory stimuli. A new assay for CRP has enabled researchers to use this protein as a marker of systemic inflammation. Studies have shown a high correlation between presence of this protein and atherosclerosis. It is one of many predictors for heart disease that doctors use today. An HIV-positive person may see tests for this protein on lab reports. It is a SURROGATE MARKER of LIPIDS in the blood that cause inflammation. It also is useful if a person is already on STATIN drugs, because those drugs lower inflammation, so a person with high CRP numbers after taking statins may be at high risk for further heart disease.

cream, spermicidal Like spermicidal jelly, foams, and vaginal suppositories, spermicidal creams are a form of birth control that are really designed for use with a BARRIER such as a diaphragm, cervical cap, or INTRAUTERINE DEVICE (IUD). Like jellies and vaginal suppositories, creams can be used for extra protection with a condom. Creams come in a tube with a plastic applicator. While jellies are clear, creams are white. Like condoms and jellies, creams are available without prescription at most drugstores. Deposited just outside the entrance to the cervix at the top of the vagina, cream keeps sperm from entering the cervix and kills them as well. Like jellies, creams increase protection against gonorrhea and chlamydia.

creatinine A substance produced by the breakdown of creatine, an important molecule involved in energy transfer within muscle cells. The level of creatinine in the blood and urine provides a measure of kidney function.

creatinine kinase (creatine phosphokinase) An enzyme found in the muscles. High levels in the blood indicate breakdown of muscle tissue. In AIDS, its presence may be diagnostic of myopathy.

crisis intervention Problem-solving activity intended to correct or prevent the continuation of a crisis. Often this is provided by telephone by professional or paraprofessional medical or social workers.

Crix belly The accumulation of fat in the lower abdomen. So called because it was first noted in association with Crixivan (INDINAVIR), although other antiretrovirals or HIV disease itself could also be involved. See LIPODYSTROPHY.

Crixivan See INDINAVIR.

cross-sectional study A study that examines and analyzes predefined variables at a fixed time or over a short period, as opposed to a longitudinal study, which observes patients over time.

crossed treatments Two or more study treatments that are used in sequence, for example, as in a crossover design, or in combination, for instance, as in a factorial treatment structure.

crossover A patient who does not comply with assigned treatment and begins to adhere to one of the other treatments. The patient may be considered to drop in or to drop out of a treatment, depending on the direction of the crossover.

crossover design A treatment design. Patients are given treatments in sequence, and crossover is determined by time, not clinical outcome.

cross-reaction A reaction between an antibody and an antigen other than the one that precipitated its development. The antigen in such cases is closely related to the original antigen.

cross-resistance A phenomenon in which a microbe that acquires resistance to one drug through direct exposure also becomes resistant to one or more other drugs to which it has not been exposed. Cross-resistance occurs because the mechanism of resistance to each drug is the same and arises through identical genetic mutations.

cryoprecipitate A substance obtained from blood, rich in the clotting factors absent in a common form of HEMOPHILIA.

cryosurgery A method involving freezing for removing GENITAL WARTS and treating cervical problems. See CRYOTHERAPY.

cryotherapy The use of liquid nitrogen to freeze and destroy a lesion or growth, sometimes used to induce scar formation and healing to prevent further spread of a condition.

Cryptaz Brand name for NTZ, a drug for treating cryptosporidiosis, an AIDS-defining condition caused by the relatively common, highly infectious protozoan parasite *Cryptosporidium parvum*. NTZ was the first drug used for treating CRYPTOSPORIDIOSIS submitted to the Food and Drug Administration (FDA). Application to the FDA was made in December 1997 by Unimed Pharmaceuticals. Unimed requested that the FDA approve NTZ as an agent to reduce cryptosporidiosis-associated diarrhea. The FDA's Antiviral Drugs Advisory Committee advised against approving NTZ after a May 6, 1998, meeting to review Unimed's application. Weak data were cited as the primary cause of this decision. Drug rejection raised a ruckus among community organizations.

cryptococcal infection A fungal infection in the central nervous system. Acute cryptococcal infection can be treated with intravenous AMPHOTERICIN B followed by oral FLUCONAZOLE. Lifelong maintenance therapy, usually with fluconazole, is necessary to inhibit resurgence of the *Cryptococcus* fungus. Oral FLUCYTOSINE (100 to 150 mg per kilogram of body weight per day) may be used in conjunction with amphotericin, but both drugs have side effects that can limit their use. Liposomal amphotericin has been tried as a safer alternative. Fluconazole and ITRACONAZOLE are other possible options.

cryptococcal meningitis The most common fungal infection attacking the central nervous system in HIV-infected persons. It is the most common cause of acute meningitis in HIV disease. Symptoms include severe headache, confusion, sensitivity to light, blurred vision, fever, and speech difficulties. Left untreated, the disease can lead to coma and death. Diagnosis is established by cerebral spinal fluid tests or blood tests. A major problem is the frequent occurrence of elevated intracranial pressure, which can be relieved by various drainage techniques. Standard treatments are amphotericin B (as induction therapy) and fluconazole (as maintenance therapy). See CRYPTOCOCCAL INFECTION.

cryptococcosis   Cryptococcosis is an infection caused by the fungus CRYPTOCOCCUS NEOFORMANS. In people with HIV it is especially severe, frequently causing MENINGITIS. Common symptoms include headache, fevers, vision problems, and seizures. The diagnosis is usually made by analyzing CEREBROSPINAL FLUID obtained with a SPINAL TAP. The disease is treated with intravenous AMPHOTERICIN B or oral FLUCONAZOLE. When treatment is stopped, the disease tends to recur so that long-term treatment is generally necessary.

Cryptococcus   A genus of usually harmless fungus that causes MENINGITIS in persons with AIDS. Cryptococcal infections are difficult to cure because they keep recurring and the drug treatment is very toxic.

Cryptococcus neoformans   A ubiquitous fungus that is found in soil. When inhaled by those in normal health, the fungus is contained in the lungs. In immunosuppressed people, it can cause disseminated infection. *Cryptococcus* can cause pulmonary, central nervous system, or disseminated infection. In people with AIDS, the most common presentation is MENINGITIS. Cryptococcal infections may be fatal if untreated.

Onset is insidious with fever, nonspecific fatigue, nausea, and vomiting. Headache may be diffuse, frontal, or temporal. ENCEPHALITIS may occur with altered mental status, subtle behavioral changes, memory loss, and confusion. Photophobia, cranial nerve palsies, PNEUMONIA, and painless skin LESIONS may occur. Prostatic abscesses may serve as a reservoir for recurrent infections. Diagnosis is by serum cryptococcal antigen or lumbar puncture. Treatment is generally with AMPHOTERICIN B followed with FLUCONAZOLE. It is believed that there are some patients who, once disease is diagnosed, may be treated initially with oral fluconazole rather than intravenous amphotericin. These patients generally have earlier disease and milder symptoms. Patients with increased intracranial pressure tend to have poorer outcomes. Elevated pressure readings may be managed with frequent lumbar punctures, mannitol, or CORTICOSTEROIDS. Both liposomal amphotericin and itraconazole for treatment of cryptococcosis are currently in clinical trials.

cryptosporidiosis   A highly contagious infection caused by an opportunistic protozoan, the CRYPTOSPORIDIUM, which is found in human and animal feces and which may contaminate public water supplies by way of untreated sewage. Cryptosporidiosis is must commonly seen in cattle and cattle handlers. It usually causes a diarrhea whose severity varies; in persons with normal immune systems the diarrhea is self-limiting, lasting a week or two, but in persons with AIDS, it is severe and results in enterocolitis that can lead to dehydration and malnutrition. Other symptoms of cryptosporidial infection in AIDS can include weight loss, nausea, vomiting, cramping, abdominal pain, and fever. Infection by the parasite usually occurs in the small intestine, but infection of the colon and other areas of the gastrointestinal tract have been observed. In cryptosporidial infection of the bile duct, nausea and vomiting may be more severe. Cases of respiratory cryptosporidiosis have been documented in immunocompromised individuals. In the lungs, cryptosporidiosis resembles PCP.

A diagnosis of cryptosporidiosis is usually established by simply examining the stool under a microscope to detect the parasite. Since it was first identified in people with AIDS in 1982, more than 70 therapeutic agents have been tested, without success. Cryptosporidiosis was originally classified as a veterinary pathogen, or an organism that affects and causes diseases in animals only. Relatively recently recognized as a common cause of diarrhea in humans, *Cryptosporidiosis parvum* is poorly understood. Without a clear understanding of the biology of the parasite, attempts to design rational therapy for the disease have been nearly impossible. Using animals as models for human cryptosporidiosis has, to date, largely been unsuccessful. *Cryptosporidia* do not grow well in the test tube, making it difficult to determine a drug's potential for animal and human testing. The presence of multiple disease-causing organisms in the gastrointestinal tracts of PWAS also confounds efforts to assess the efficacy of anti-cryptosporidiosis drugs. Severe immune dysfunction may also contribute to the stubborn nature of cryptosporidiosis infections to people with AIDS.

There are no standard treatments, but proposed drug therapies include PAROMOMYCIN SULFATE (Humatin), AZITHROMYCIN (zithromax), letrazuril, and various forms of concentrated cow and chicken antibodies. Controlling and minimizing diarrhea while maintaining fluid and electrolyte balance and nutritional status are key components of treatment. Intravenous nutrition is commonly required to provide sufficient calories and hydration. Prophylaxis is debatable, since there is no clear indication of effectiveness. However, some have recommended prophylaxis of 250 mg of Humatin twice a day for people with AIDS and fewer than 50 T4 CELLS, especially those who have diarrhea, weight loss, or previously diagnosed cryptosporidiosis.

Cryptosporidiosis is highly contagious and can be spread from person to person, as well as through contaminated water and food. Transmission can occur through any contact with fecal matter, so good hygiene is crucial. A latex barrier should be used for all forms of anal sex.

Cryptosporidium   A genus of protozoan parasite (plural *Cryptosporidia*) that causes severe, protracted diarrhea. In persons with normal immune systems, the diarrhea is self-limiting and lasts one to two weeks. In AIDS patients, the diarrhea often becomes chronic and may lead to severe malnutrition. Commonly used medications for *Cryptosporidium* include paromomycin or antidiarrheal medications such as loperamide.

crystallography   The study of crystal structure. Used in the study of crystallized viruses.

CSF   See CEREBROSPINAL FLUID.

CT   See COMPUTERIZED AXIAL TOMOGRAPHY.

CT scan   See COMPUTERIZED AXIAL TOMOGRAPHY.

cultural activism   See ACTIVISM.

cultural analysis and AIDS   AIDS is not just an illness. Like every other social or cultural phenomenon, it is represented and understood in language, images, and ways of thinking that are characteristic of a particular culture, or way of life, and within that culture, ways of considering different aspects life (social, sexual, moral) or defining and approaching formal disciplines of study (medical, literary), each with its own set of terms, theoretical concepts and basic viewpoints. (These are sometimes called discourses.) It might be said that AIDS is not only an epidemic of a transmissible lethal disease, but simultaneously an "epidemic" of cultural signification. Cultural analysis seeks to engage AIDS and its meanings in a broad cultural context, beyond the unreflective "news and public affairs" level of discussion, beyond what has been called the tyranny of images circulating endlessly in every medium, to understand what the epidemic and our responses to it tell us about ourselves and our deepest beliefs. Highly visible public information about AIDS (AIDS education in schools, public service announcements on TV, posters in buses or subways, etc.) is a frequent subject of cultural analysis, as is the representation of the epidemic and people with AIDS, in the movies and on TV and in other mass media. Cultural analysis examines the "meaning" of AIDS in the variety of formal and informal discourses in which it has its cultural (as distinct from physical) existence. The discourses of medicine, science and sexual morality are often explored as sites where meaning is constructed. Key words and phrases often under scrutiny include virus, carrier, condone, family, community, general population, gay/homosexual, heterosexual, lesbian, prostitute, PWA (person with AIDS), risk group, risk practice, spread, and victim. On a practical level, such analysis can help us to challenge automatic assumptions, and may help us to modify social responses and avoid the kinds of difficulties that have so far confronted all practical attempts to control the epidemic.

culture   In medical terms, a medium in which MICROBES can grow. HIV is grown in cultures containing LYMPHOCYTES. If a sample of a person's blood is put into such a culture, and HIV grows, the person is infected with HIV.

cunnilinctus   See CUNNILINGUS.

cunnilingus   The use of the tongue or mouth to stimulate the VULVA.

curcumin   An ingredient of the spice turmeric. Laboratory studies have suggested that curcumin inhibits HIV replication by blocking the long terminal repeat region on HIV's genes, but a 1996 clinical trial found no antiviral effect.

cure   A means of healing or restoring to health; remedy. Although the gloom that has pervaded AIDS research for more than a decade has begun to lift a bit, and progress is occurring on several fronts, no one talks of an imminent cure. Scientists in the lab and doctors treating the disease believe they have reached a secondary goal, making the disease manageable.

curette   A spoon-shaped scraping instrument for removing foreign matter from a cavity in the body (curetting).

curse   See MENSTRUATION.

cutaneous   Relating to the skin.

CXCR4 (Fusin)   A seven-looped protein structure on the surface of certain immune system cells that acts as a chemokine receptor site. CXCR-4, which naturally binds to the alpha chemokine stromal cell-derived factor, is the second receptor necessary for T-tropic, syncytia-inducing (see SYNCYTIUM) HIV to enter and infect a cell. The other receptor site for HIV binding and entry is CD4.

cyclobut G   See LOBUCAVIR.

cyclophosphamide (CY)   An IMMUNOSUPPRESSIVE DRUG that at high doses has been used in cancer chemotherapy regimens. In low doses, the drug has well-documented immunomodulatory properties and has been used to treat several immune disorders, including lupus and Wegener's granulomatosis. In people with HIV, cyclosphosphamide is most commonly used in combination therapy for AIDS-related lymphoma. CY has a greater suppressive effect on B CELLS than on T CELLS, and CD8 CELLS are more sensitive to the drug than other T cell subsets.

CY is an alkylating agent, which means that it works by attaching to biologically important molecules such as DNA and RNA, interfering with cell growth and division. Alkylating agents are toxic to rapidly dividing cells, like those in a tumor or in the bone marrow (where blood cells are continually being replaced). CY is one of the most widely used chemotherapy drugs, in part because its toxicity is more specific to malignant cells and less likely to cause severe bone-marrow toxicity than many other alkylating agents. Although CY can be used alone in chemotherapy, it is used more frequently in combination with other drugs. For the treatment of AIDS-related lymphoma CY is routinely used in a combination of drugs called CHOP (CY, doxorubicin, vincristine, and prednisone). It is also used in a combination called m-BACOD (methotrexate, bleomycin, doxorubicin, CY, vincristine, dexamethasone, and leucovorin). People with less progressive disease, no prior AIDS-defining illness, and no bone marrow or central nervous system involvement are more likely to respond. The CD4+ count at the time the lymphoma is diagnosed is the most important predictor of success: people with CD4+ counts above 200 have the best chance of a positive reaction. CY is available in the form of tablets for oral administration and solution for injection.

Side effects are numerous, ranging from sterility, possibly irreversible (in both sexes), to toxicity to the lungs or kidneys. Menstrual irregularity commonly occurs in women who use the drug; this usually reverses after treatment stops. Damage to the bladder is also a common side effect of CY and appears to be related to the size of dose and duration of therapy. Heart damage has been reported, primarily in those receiving high doses—

120 to 270 mg per kg of body weight, administered over a few days. In a few instances, severe and fatal congestive heart failure has occurred. Nausea, vomiting, and temporary hair loss occur frequently. Bone-marrow toxicity that causes reductions in white blood cell count are common. Reductions in the number of platelets and red blood cells develop occasionally but are reversible after therapy stops. Finally, severe toxicity to the lungs or kidneys also occurs occasionally. Rarely, allergic reactions, and death have been reported.

cycloserine   A broad-spectrum antibiotic that has been used in combination with other drugs in treating TUBERCULOSIS. It is contraindicated in patients with epilepsy and in those with depression or anxiety. (Trade name is Seromycin.)

cyclosporine   An IMMUNOSUPPRESSIVE DRUG used to prevent graft rejection in organ transplants. The drug acts specifically against T CELLS in the early stages of activation. Reports on the use of this drug in people with HIV are contradictory. Also called cyclosporine A, CsA for short.

CYP   See CYTOCHROME P450.

cyst   A closed sac or pouch, with a definite wall, that contains fluid, semifluid, or solid material. It is usually an abnormal structure resulting from developmental abnormalities, obstruction of ducts, or from a parasitic infection. See BARTHOLIN'S DUCT.

cysteamine   Used for treatment of a rare genetic kidney disease in children. May work with AZT in preventing HIV from reproducing.

cysteine   An amino acid, one of three components of GLUTATHIONE (GSH). See N-ACETYLCYSTEINE.

cystitis   An infection of the urinary bladder, usually occurring secondary to ascending urinary tract infections. Associated organs (kidney, prostate, urethra) may be involved. May be acute (with frequent and painful urination) or chronic (secondary to another lesion) possibly with pyuria as the only symptom. Antibiotics are useful in treating the infection, but more definitive therapy will be required if the basic cause is a renal calculus (kidney stone) or other obstruction in the urinary tract.

cytarabine   A drug compound (cytosine arabinoside) originally developed as an antileukemic agent and now being used in treating HERPES virus hominis infections that cause either keratitis or ENCEPHALITIS. The first well-controlled clinical trial found that treatment offers no benefit to patients with PROGRESSIVE MULTIFOCAL LEUKOENCEPHALOPATHY (PML). These results came as no surprise, since there were reports that patients treated with cytarabine die faster than those who received no treatment. There has been at least one published case of cytarabine *causing* PML in a person with cancer by suppressing the immune system. Also called ARA-C.

cytidine   A nucleoside of cytosine. Lamivudine (3TC) and dideoxycytidien (ddC) are analogs of cytidine.

cytochrome P450   One of the many different known cytochrome enzymes living in organisms, cytochrome P450 enzymes are a family of enzymes in the liver that metabolize drugs and other fat-soluble substances. The cytochrome P450 enzymes are found in virtually all animals and vary widely in number. They are most active in tissues that have most frequent contact with external materials—the liver, lung, skin, gut, and kidneys—but are found throughout the human body. It is not known how the cytochrome P450 enzymes recognize the chemicals, including drugs, steroids, and other compounds, on which they act. It is known that these chemicals are sparingly soluble in water and that they tend to accumulate in the membranes and water-free structures within cells and tissues. The cytochrome P450 enzymes metabolize these substances in these locations, rendering them more soluble in water and less toxic. Solubilized and detoxified, these compounds can then be dissolved in the blood and transported to the kidneys for elimination. Certain medications, such as RITONAVIR, inhibit some of the P450 enzymes, in particular P450 3A4 (also called CYP3A4), affecting the liver's ability to break down other drugs. This process increases blood levels of any medication taken concomitantly with CYP inhibitor, and dose adjustments are necessary in order to prevent side effects and overdosing. Note that this blockage of cytochromes is the rationale for the use of the PROTEASE INHIBITORS ritonavir and SAQUINAVIR in combination.

cytokine Any of a large number of proteins produced by cells that influence the activity and behavior of themselves or other cells. Some cytokines increase the intensity of an immune response; others suppress it. Some cytokines create an inflammatory response; others quiet such a response. Still other cytokines regulate the development of immune cells in the bone marrow. Cytokines include LYMPHOKINES produced by LYMPHOCYTES and MONOKINES produced by MONOCYTES and MACROPHAGES. INTERLEUKINS, TUMOR NECROSIS FACTOR, and INTERFERONS are also examples of cytokines.

Cytolin An experimental HIV treatment. It is a patented monoclonal antibody that prevents the CD8+ cells in the body from attacking the CD4+ cells, as occurs in HIV disease. The product is used to keep the immune system functioning while antivirals attack the virus. The product is being developed and produced through the funding of several HIV-positive professionals who started a company called CytoDyn. This is unusual, as most HIV-fighting products are produced by major international pharmaceutical companies. It is currently in phase I/II trials in the United States. It is given as an intravenous drip once every month. No final dosing or frequency has been determined yet in the trials. Because Cytolin is a protein, its use may lessen drug interactions and need for numerous drugs in the system.

cytological screening Testing for cell pathology for diagnostic purposes. Cytological tests can detect and identify both normal and abnormal cells, especially cancer cells, in areas that cannot be easily and directly examined. Specimens to be examined may be obtained from body excretions, secretions, and tissue scrapings. Tests make possible a very early diagnosis and treatment of cancer. They can

also indicate hormone activity in the body as well as specific infections and the effect of radiation.

cytology The study of cells. See CYTOLOGICAL SCREENING.

cytomegalovirus (CMV) A virus belonging to the herpes family, and a major PATHOGEN in people with AIDS. Before the appearance of AIDS, it was most commonly associated with severe congenital infection in infants and with life-threatening infections in patients who had undergone bone marrow transplants and other procedures requiring suppression of the immune system. CMV's most common target is the retina—the light-sensitive-tissue at the back of the eyes. If left untreated, CMV RETINITIS causes blindness in the affected eye 90 percent of the time. CMV also infects the gastrointestinal tract, and may involve the entire tract, from mouth to anus, including the liver and pancreas. Most cases of CMV gastrointestinal disease involve the esophagus or colon. CMV can also cause PNEUMONIA or CERVICITIS in women. There have also been reports of CNS and adrenal disease, although the frequency and significance of these conditions are unclear. As a result of these infections, CMV produces considerable illness and greatly affects the survival of patients with AIDS.

Approximately half of the American population over 50 has evidence of past CMV infection, but prevalence appears to be even higher among homosexual men. Most patients who have CMV disease are infected with it long before they become HIV-infected. CMV is typically contracted in infancy and childhood, but patients may also become infected through sexual contact or after receiving infected blood products. In individuals with intact immune systems, infection either goes unnoticed or may provoke a self-limited one-time illness. After infecting a patient, the virus becomes "latent," hiding in the host's cells. Under conditions of immunosuppression, such as with AIDS, the virus may "reactivate" and cause symptomatic disease. This does not usually occur until a patient's CD4 cell count falls below 100, and more typically below 50. CMV infection of the gastrointestinal tract commonly results in inflammation, erosions, and ulceration of the mucosal linings. This may be quite destructive, and occasionally leads to damage throughout the entire wall of the gut; it may cause perforation of the gastrointestinal tract.

Symptoms and physical findings of cytomegalovirus vary from disease to disease. Symptoms of chorioRETINITIS include unilateral visual field loss, blurring of vision, or scotomata. Examination generally reveals whitish areas with perivascular exudates and hemorrhages. A careful search of the entire fundus (base) of the eye is required. Generally, in gastrointestinal disease, COLITIS is associated with abdominal pain and diarrhea. Fever may also be present. ESOPHAGITIS and GASTRITIS most commonly present with pain from the involved structures. Endoscopy reveals ERYTHEMA, submucosal hemorrhage, and diffuse mucosal ulceration. While CMV may be isolated from pulmonary secretions, it is generally believed that it rarely has a true pathologic role in HIV-infected patients. Diagnosis must be confirmed by lung BIOPSY demonstrating histologic evidence consistent with invasive disease. Finally, ENCEPHALITIS, cranial nerve dysfunction, and neuropathies may occur. CMV polyradiculopathy is rare, but characterized by lower extremity weakness, numbness, and bladder dysfunction.

Rapid diagnosis of CMV disease may lead to improved survival. A variety of diagnostic methods have been attempted, but the most useful is microscopic examination of biopsy samples. CMV infection of human cells results in characteristic changes found in these biopsies. CMV-infected cells become enlarged with a so-called owl's-eye appearance; they are typically found in areas with considerable inflammation. Special tests, which involve such staining techniques as IMMUNOFLUORESCENCE and DNA in situ hybridization may be used by experienced pathologists to confirm the presence of CMV cells. Newer procedures, such as POLYMERASE CHAIN REACTION (PCR), which identifies minute quantities of CMV DNA in body fluids and tissue samples, may be helpful. Culture of CMV from bodily fluids probably adds little diagnostic information. Use of radiographic techniques such as barium exams and CT SCANS may reveal defects in the esophagus, stomach, or intestines, but without biopsy of those lesions, diagnosis is uncertain, and treatment premature.

In the absence of therapy, CMV disease is progressive and is associated with a high mortality rate. Early treatment is essential and may alter the course of the disease, including its spread to other locations in the body. Treatment may also prevent severe consequences of CMV disease such as perforation and hemorrhage, which may result in death. The two most commonly used drug treatments for CMV infection are GANCICLOVIR and FOSCARNET. Both are approved by the United States FOOD AND DRUG ADMINISTRATION. Both result in the suppression of CMV, but not elimination. Ganciclovir has been shown to be effective in the treatment of both CMV esophagitis and colitis in patients infected with HIV, resulting in increased time until relapse and increased survival. Ganciclovir causes adverse side effects that lead to discontinuation of therapy in about one third of patients. The most common adverse effects are on the bone marrow, resulting in a decrease in the number of NEUTROPHILS. Ganciclovir may also cause lowering of the platelet count, which can increase the risk of bleeding because of decreased clotting ability of the blood. The risk of toxicity is worsened when ganciclovir is given with AZT. Adverse reactions are decreased when either DDI or DDC are used instead of AZT. Other side effects include headaches, confusion, nausea, vomiting, diarrhea, and possibly testicular damage.

Foscarnet has also been found to be effective in treating CMV disease and appears to inhibit HIV as well. It is as effective as ganciclovir in the treatment of CMV gastrointestinal disease and can be used both in newly infected patients and in patients who have relapsed after therapy with ganciclovir. Foscarnet has a different side effect profile than ganciclovir. While foscarnet does not affect the bone marrow tissues, and therefore can be used concurrently with AZT, it does have a toxic effect on the kidneys that results in passage of excess electrolytes into the urine. Other adverse effects associated with foscarnet include nausea, vomiting, diarrhea, oral and penile ulceration, and seizures.

Standard treatment of CMV disease usually begins with several weeks of ganciclovir. If there is no elimination of the virus from biopsies taken during repeat ENDOSCOPY, or the patient continues to experience severe symptoms, he or she is switched to foscarnet. If there is only a partial response to ganciclovir, the patient can be reinduced with ganciclovir for several more weeks. It may also become necessary to switch between medications when serious toxicity begins.

Maintenance therapy appears to be necessary for the long-term control of symptoms as well as prevention of CMV dissemination to other sites. Maintenance therapy is controversial for CMV gastrointestinal disease, though, in contrast to CMV retinitis. Progression during maintenance therapy requires reinduction. If both medications fail to result in improvement of gastrointestinal CMV disease, then combined treatment is often recommended.

Treatment of CMV disease with oral agents is being considered. This will permit home therapy and decrease the dangers of infection due to permanent indwelling catheters. The benefit of oral therapy on quality of life could be enormous. Both agents appear to have problems with absorption via the oral route. Newer agents, such as a precursor of the anti-herpes drug ACYCLOVIR, called VALACYCLOVIR, are also being studied for treatment and prophylaxis. Valacyclovir is better absorbed than ganciclovir and is completely metabolized to acyclovir, resulting in serum concentrations similar to that achieved by intravenous administration of acyclovir. Another drug called HPMPC is also being studied but appears to be too toxic for routine use. It is associated with severe damage to the kidney, although concurrent use of probenicid may help prevent this.

cytomegalovirus (CMV) disease　Disease caused by infection with CYTOMEGALOVIRUS. See COLITIS; ESOPHAGITIS; GASTRITIS; NEUROLOGICAL DISEASE; PNEUMONIA; POLYRADICULOPATHY; RETINITIS.

cytomegalovirus encephalitis　ENCEPHALITIS caused by CYTOMEGALOVIRUS. Studies have shown that CMV encephalopathy is underdiagnosed. It frequently occurs unnoticed in persons with CMV retinitis. Symptoms include dementia, headache, confusion, and fever. The infection progresses rapidly, leading to death within weeks or months.

cytomegalovirus colitis　COLITIS caused by CYTOMEGALOVIRUS (CMV).

cytomegalovirus esophagitis　ESOPHAGITIS caused by CYTOMEGALOVIRUS (CMV).

cytomegalovirus gastritis　GASTRITIS caused by CYTOMEGALOVIRUS (CMV).

cytomegalovirus neurological disease　NEUROLOGICAL DISEASE caused by CYTOMEGALOVIRUS (CMV).

cytomegalovirus pneumonia　PNEUMONIA caused by CYTOMEGALOVIRUS (CMV).

cytomegalovirus radiculopathy　CYTOMEGALOVIRUS infection of the peripheral nerves and the spinal roots, leading to generalized weakness and paralysis.

cytomegalovirus retinitis　RETINITIS caused by CYTOMEGALOVIRUS (CMV).

cytopenia　A reduction in the number of cells found in a clinical specimen.

cytophilic　Having a propensity to bind to cells.

cytoplasm　The protoplasm of a cell outside the nucleus.

cytopreservation　A technique for preserving cells by freezing (especially CD8 cells) taken from the blood of an AIDS patient for the use by the same patient at a later stage of the disease, when the cells in the patient will have been destroyed or damaged.

cytosine　One of the four bases that make up RNA (which include adenine, guanine, and uracil) and DNA (which include adenine, guanine, and thymine). See CYTIDINE.

cytosine arabinoside　See CYTARABINE.

cytostatic　Having the ability to stop cell growth.

cytotoxic　Having the ability to kill cells; poisonous to cells.

cytotoxic T lymphocyte A type of CD8 or, less often, CD4 LYMPHOCYTE that kills diseased cells infected by a specific virus or other intracellular microbe. CTLs interact with MAJOR HISTOCOMPATI-BILITY COMPLEX (MHC) class I receptors on infected cells and have the prime role in CELL-MEDIATED IMMUNITY.

cytotoxin An antibody or toxin that attacks the cells of particular organs.

Cytovene See GANCICLOVIR.

d4T See STAVUDINE.

dantrolene   Dantrolene is a muscle relaxant. Its most common side effect is muscle weakness that usually disappears after taking the drug for several days. Other side effects include diarrhea, gastric intolerance, depression, insomnia, and frequent urination. Also sold as Dantrium.

DAPD (diaminopurine dioxolone)   It is an experimental guanosine nucleoside analog being developed by Triangle Pharmaceuticals. It has not yet been evaluated by the U.S. Food and Drug Administration (FDA). DAPD is currently in phase I/II trials in the United States. From these preliminary studies in humans, researchers found that DAPD can be effective against viruses with AZT or AZT/3TC resistance. Researchers have also speculated that DAPD may be effective against MULTIDRUG-RESISTANT VIRUS. DAPD is being studied in twice-daily dosing at a variety of dosage levels; 500-mg doses have been very effective in people with resistant virus. Studies combining DAPD with mycophenalic acid, which has been shown to increase the potency of DAPD in laboratory work, are also beginning. (Also known as Amdoxovir.)

dapsone   An antibacterial sulfone administered orally that inhibits or retards bacterial growth in a variety of GRAM-NEGATIVE and GRAM-POSITIVE organisms. It is used in the treatment of dermatitis herpetiformis and leprosy and in the prophylaxis of falciparum malaria. Dapsone is also commonly used for the treatment and prevention of PNEUMOCYSTIS CARINII PNEUMONIA (PCP) in sulfa-intolerant persons and occasionally for the treatment of mycobacterial or other protozoal infections in people living with HIV. Although dapsone is a sulfone and in the same family as sulfa drugs, it does not cause the same reactions as sulfa drugs most of the time it is used. Possible side effects include skin rash, fever, and gastrointestinal upset. In persons who have the hereditary condition GLUCOSE-6 PHOSPHATE DEHYDROGENASE (G6PD) DEFICIENCY, dapsone can cause destruction of red blood cells (hemolysis), resulting in severe anemia. Dapsone also causes reduced absorption of the drug DIDANOSINE. Because it prevents certain bacteria from multiplying but does not kill them, dapsone is usually considered backup therapy for the treatment of mild to moderate PCP in those who cannot tolerate the preferred drugs such as TRIMETHOPRIM-SULFAMETHOXAZOLE (TMP/SMX or Bactrim) or INTRAVENOUS PENTAMIDINE. Similarly, dapsone is considered second-line therapy for the prevention of PCP. Most physicians recommend PCP prophylaxis for HIV-infected individuals with CD4+ counts less than 200. There is no clear consensus on the best dose of dapsone to use to prevent PCP. Dapsone is known to interact with various drugs, including probenecid, RIFAMPIN, and TRIMETHOPRIM. Dapsone used with AZT or GANCICLOVIR may increase the risk of bone marrow toxicity. Dapsone may decrease the effectiveness of CLOFAZIMINE and increase the risk of PERIPHERAL NEUROPATHY when used with ZALCITABINE, didanosine, or STAVUDINE. The most serious side effect of dapsone is anemia. These side effects are dose-related and occur to some extent in almost all people taking the drug but uncommonly are severe enough to stop therapy. PERIPHERAL NEUROPATHY is an unusual side effect of dapsone. Other side effects may include muscle weakness, nausea, abdominal pain, inflammation of the pancreas, vertigo, and blurred vision.

dapsone/trimethoprim A drug therapy combining dapsone and trimethoprim. This combination is common outpatient regimen for the treatment of PNEUMOCYSTIS CARINII PNEUMONIA.

Daraprim See PYRIMETHAMINE.

Data Safety and Monitoring Board An independent committee of researchers, doctors, statisticians, community members, and others who collect and analyze data during the course of a clinical trial. They monitor for any adverse effects, such as any sign that one treatment is significantly better than another, particularly when one arm of the trial involves a placebo. The DSMB also checks for any sign that would warrant modifying or ending the trial or notifying subjects of new information that could affect their willingness to continue in the trial.

databases The federal government provides unlimited free access to its AIDS-related electronic databases. These are maintained by the National Library of Medicine (NLM), a unit of the National Institutes of Health in Bethesda, Maryland, and the largest health sciences library in the world. The library's four AIDS-related databases are Aidsline, which lists references to journal articles, books, audiovisuals, and conference abstracts; Aidstrials, which contains up-to-date information about clinical trials of drugs and vaccines that have been or are being tested; Aidsdrugs, a dictionary of licensed anti-HIV drugs and experimental chemical and biological agents that are being evaluated in clinical trials; and Dirline, which lists organizations and services that provide information to the public about HIV and AIDS. Free access to this information is the result of recommendations made at the National Institutes of Health HIV/AIDS Information Services Conference in June 1993, to increase AIDS outreach, and to reduce barriers to AIDS information. Increases in the National Library of Medicine's AIDS funding enabled the Library to offer this service. Additionally, the National Library of Medicine plans to create a new electronic database to cover publications on research concerning health services.

date of onset The date on which an SSDI, SSI, or MEDICAID applicant first becomes disabled within the meaning of the SOCIAL SECURITY ACT; almost always before the application, first treatment, or even work-cessation date.

daunorubicin hydrochloride An antineoplastic drug, that is, a drug that controls or inhibits the growth of malignant cells. Daunorubicin is a modified form of an antibiotic isolated from a species of funguslike bacterium called *Streptomyces coeruleorubidus*. A potent bone marrow suppressant, the drug inhibits the synthesis of nucleic acids, preventing cancer cells from dividing. Risk of opportunistic infection or bleeding generally increases. When it is used in people taking AZT or GANCICLOVIR, COLONY STIMULATING FACTORS are often used as well to limit bone marrow suppression. With standard INTRAVENOUS administration, fatal congestive heart failure may occur either during therapy or months to years after the drug is used. The risk increases proportionately to the total cumulative dose. Severe MYELOSUPPRESSION occurs when daunorubicin is used in either its standard intravenous form or when encapsulated by liposomes. Reversible hair loss occurs in most people treated with standard daunorubicin. Acute nausea and vomiting occur but are usually mild. Diarrhea has occasionally been reported. Rarely, allergic reactions, including fever, chills, and skin rash, occur. Daunorubicin may make the urine temporarily red. It is typically used for treatment of LYMPHOMA and KAPOSI'S SARCOMA in HIV patients. (Its trade name is Cerubidine.)

DaunoXome Liposomal DAUNORUBICIN, DaunoXome, is currently being tested in clinical trials for KAPOSI'S SARCOMA. In a mechanism that is not completely understood, encapsulating daunorubicin in liposomes increases the concentration of the drug at the tumor site significantly without increasing the concentration of the drug in the blood or other healthy tissues. In theory, it should target more drug against the cancer while limiting the drug's side effects. As yet, large clinical trials have not produced conclusive evidence of the effectiveness of this formulation. DaunoXome's main side effect is NEUTROPENIA, which can be managed with G-CSF (Neupogen).

DCQA/DCTA   An INTEGRASE INHIBITOR that is being studied for activity against HIV. It is known to have in vitro activity against the virus at a dosage level far lower than that for many drugs currently available. DCQA stands for *dicaffeoylquinic acid*. DCTA stands for *dicaffeoyltartaric acid*.

D-D4FC   A nucleoside reverse transcriptase inhibitor (NRTI) under development by Emory University. Although it is related to lamivudine, their resistance codons differ.

DD214   The military discharge certificate (Department of Defense form 214) that all veterans must present when applying for VA services.

ddC   See ZALCITABINE.

ddI   See DIDANOSINE.

DDS   See DAPSONE.

de novo lipogenesis   Formation of fatty acids from excessive levels of dietary carbohydrates in the body as a result of food intake. See LIPODYSTROPHY.

death   Permanent cessation of all vital functions; total irreversible cessation of cerebral function, spontaneous function of the respiratory system, and spontaneous function of the circulatory system; final and irreversible cessation of perceptible heartbeat and respiration. Indicators of death include the cessation of the heart's action; absence of reflexes; cessation of electrical activity in the brain as determined by EEG; manifestation of rigor mortis.

death benefit   The amount payable to a beneficiary at the annuitant's, or insured's death. Also called the survivor benefit.

death rate   The number of deaths per 1,000 of the population occurring in a given area within a specified time.

death with dignity   A natural death allowed to occur humanely with no attempt made to prolong life by artificial means. The concept arose in reaction to the ability of modern medical technology to maintain vital functions in, without improving the condition of, persons who are at the point of death.

decubitus ulcer   See BEDSORE.

deductible   The medical costs a patient must incur before MEDICARE or health insurance coverage begins, usually on an annual basis.

deeming income and assets   The procedure of lumping together the income of separate nuclear family members who live together in common households (even if they claim not to be sharing income), in determining the eligibility of one of them for a needs-based program. For example, the incomes of spouses, or parent and child, living together are mandatorily combined and measured against a two-person eligibility level, rather than against two separate one-person levels.

defendant   The person or entity against whom or which a lawsuit or criminal indictment, is brought.

defense mechanism   A term originating in psychoanalysis, widely used in psychology and psychiatry, for a pattern of feeling, thought, or behavior that arises in response to perceptions of psychic danger, thus enabling a person to avoid conscious awareness of conflicts or anxiety-arousing stressors. Among the most common defense mechanisms are denial, displacement, intellectualization, projection, rationalization, reaction formation, regression, and repression.

definitive diagnosis   A diagnosis established with certainty, without question, as distinct from a presumptive diagnosis, one based on reasonable grounds established by previous experience.

dehydroepiandrosterone (DHEA)   Produced by the adrenal glands, DHEA is the most abundant steroid hormone in the body. The body converts this hormone to whatever particular hormone is needed at any specific time, including testosterone and estrogen. Blood level of DHEA decreases in the body after the age of 20, and by the age of 80, the level of this substance is 5 percent of that of a 20-year-old. It is unclear whether aging causes this decrease or the decrease causes aging. People argue on both sides of this fence, and there has been no medical research done to show what purpose DHEA has, or what role it plays in any disease or aging process. It is sold by prescription and is heralded as a wonder drug by many, who claim that it has many effects, from increasing sexual potency to decreasing the risk of strokes and slowing the process of HIV. DHEA seems to be nontoxic and is available in synthetic form by prescription.

delavirdine   A nonnucleoside reverse transcriptase inhibitor that, like other NNRTIs, chemically combines with HIV's reverse transcriptase enzyme to block the virus's infection of new cells. Delavirdine was approved in 1997 for use in the United States. It was rejected for approval in Europe because it is believed to have no unique benefits when compared to other NNRTIs on the market. Delavirdine works best when used with INDINAVIR. Like other NNRTIs it is not intended to be used as a monotherapy, and in research tests the virus developed resistance in just eight weeks when treated solely with delavirdine. Delavirdine increases blood levels of PROTEASE INHIBITORS (e.g., with indinavir, 400 percent). Delavirdine cannot be taken simultaneously with ddI, as that combination lowers the concentration of both drugs in the body. Delavirdine is generally used to boost a patient's level of protease inhibitors. Delavirdine does cause a rash in perhaps 25 percent of the people taking the drug. The rash generally develops a week to three weeks after initial use of the drug. If the rash does not recede, a doctor should be contacted because the rash may indicate STEVENS-JOHNSON SYNDROME, a severe reaction. Delavirdine cannot be taken with Halcion, Seldane, and several other prescription medications. Check these with a physician. (Trade name is Rescriptor.)

delayed-type hypersensitivity (DTH)   A CELL-MEDIATED immune response producing a cellular infiltrate and edema that are maximal between 24 and 48 hours after antigen challenge. This response includes the delayed skin reactions associated with type IV hypersensitivity. DTH, which is the process involved in the reaction to poison ivy and poison oak, is often used in tests of immune system function. DTH is also used in TB skin tests when a small needle prick is used to test sensitivity to the virus.

deletion   Removal of a gene, from the chromosome, either in nature or in a laboratory. For example, most people have in their chromosomes the CCR5 CHEMOKINE RECEPTOR gene. However, in some one copy of this gene has been deleted. AIDS has been shown to develop more slowly in these people than in those whose receptor genes are intact. People who have both copies of the receptor deleted when they inherit them from their parents are unlikely to contract HIV. Unfortunately, this HIV-protective deletion is found in only a very small number of people of European descent and even fewer people of African or Asian descent. Research continues into ways to use this knowledge in the treatment of HIV/AIDS.

delirium   A condition that involves severe confusion and rapid, often alternating patterns of mental status. Patients can be slow and lethargic one minute and excitable and overactive the next. Patients may not know where they are or how they arrived at their current location. Speech may be incoherent or grossly inaccurate. Emotional states that are greatly different from an individual's normal emotions are also common in delirium. Delirium is generally caused by an ACUTE illness or condition. This means that some disease process or reaction process is affecting the central nervous system. It can be caused by a number of factors: extremely high fever, imbalance in the body's ELECTROLYTES, lack of oxygen to the brain, associated problems of drug use or drug dependence, drug reactions, and poisons. It is treated by first identifying the cause and then eliminating it. If it is a drug reaction, removal of the drugs should bring about relief. If the electrolytes show imbalance, they can be brought into balance. If it is an infection or disease that is causing the problem, then treatment for that illness can affect the problem. Delirium is usually a temporary condition. If treatment is successful in eliminating the root cause, then it will most likely disappear over time and the patient will recover prior activity and functioning level. If delirium is not recognized as the issue and the root cause is not discovered, then 20 percent of people who have such symptoms typically die of the stress on the central nervous system. Delirium is often mistaken for psychosis or other mental disturbances, and other illnesses or acute conditions must be treated and eliminated before possible mental health issues can be addressed.

delta-9-tetrahydrocannabinol (THC)   The psychoactive ingredient in MARIJUANA. A synthetic version is sold as a drug under the name DRONABINOL as an appetite stimulant for HIV/AIDS patients and to relieve the side effects of cancer chemotherapy.

Delta-32 alleles mutation   An allele is a specific variation of a gene. Every gene has two alleles, or types, one allele each inherited from each parent. The alleles for the CHEMOKINE RECEPTOR CCR5 have been shown to be an inherited trait. People that possess that delta 32 (a name for a location along the gene) allele mutation have been shown to have *some* conferred immunity to HIV infection. People that carry the same two alleles for a particular trait are referred to as homozygous. Those that carry two different alleles are termed heterozygous. The CCR5 receptor is a receptor located on the CD 8 T Helper Cells. It is required for many types of HIV in order for the virus to be merged with the human cells. People homozygous for the delta-32 allele are not 100 percent protected because there are varieties of HIV that use other cell receptors, but the CCR5 receptor is the predominate receptor. It has also been shown that those people that are heterozygous for the particular mutation have some immunity from the virus that may slow the progression of the virus. The number of people that are homozygous for this mutation are small. Ranging from less than one percent in Asian, African, and American Indian populations to more than 20 percent of Ashkenazim, Jewish people originally from eastern Europe and the southern Mediterranean.

deltacortisone   See PREDNISONE.

dementia   See HIV ENCEPHALOPATHY.

demography   The statistical and quantitative science dealing with the age, density, distribution, growth, size, and vital statistics of human populations. Demographic study has shown that rates of disease progression and survival among HIV-infected individuals are determined by access to good medical care, rather than by factors such as race, gender, drug use, income, level of education, or insurance status.

demyelinate   To remove or destroy the myelin sheath surrounding a nerve or nerves, interrupting the transmission of nerve impulses.

dendrite   One of many cytoplasmic processes branching from the cell body of a nerve cell and synapsing with other neurons. Several hundred boutons may form synaptic connections with a single cell and its dendrites.

dendritic cells   A set of antigen-presenting cells present in EPITHELIAL structures and LYMPH NODES, SPLEEN, and (at low levels) BLOOD. Dendritic cells are particularly active in presenting antigen and stimulating T CELLS. Four types of dendritic cells are recognized: follicular dendritic cells in the lymph nodes, lymphoid dendritic cells, interdigitating cells, and Langerhans cells of the skin.

denial   The conscious refusal to admit something; an unconscious defense mechanism in which the existence of anxiety-producing realities are kept out of conscious awareness.

Elisabeth Kübler-Ross, the prominent student of death and dying, believes there are five stages people go through after they learn they are dying. These are denial and isolation; anger; bargaining; depression; and acceptance. Kübler-Ross notes that denial, at least partial denial, occurs in almost all patients, not only during the early stages of illness or immediately following an explicit diagnosis but also later on from time to time. She notes that denial functions as a buffer after unexpected shocking news, allows the patient to collect him- or herself, and, with time, mobilize other less radical defenses. Denial is temporary and is replaced by partial acceptance. Kübler-Ross adds that denial maintained until the end does not necessarily bring increased distress, but that most patients do not maintain it too long.

dental dam   A 150 mm (6-inch)-square piece of thin latex, available in dental and medical supply stores made for use in oral surgery. Dental dams are widely used as a barrier for oral, vaginal, or anal sex, by men and women. After being rinsed to remove any talc or other substance, and then dried, the dam is stretched across the entire VULVA (including the CLITORIS, VAGINA, and LABIA) for CUNNILINGUS or the ANUS for ANILINGUS and held in place with the fingers. A water-based lubricant smeared on the side of the shield against the vulva increases sensation and helps to keep the dam in place. Oil-based lubricants weaken latex and can cause dams or condoms to break. Generous lubrication of the vagina or anus also helps to increase pleasure. Dental dams prevent blood, vaginal secretions, or fecal matter from being transferred between partners. Turning the dam inside out during sex will totally defeat the purpose. Similarly, moving the barrier back and forth between the vagina and anus can transfer infections.

Safer sex guidelines targeted toward women who know that their HIV status is positive and who have sex with men stress the use of dental dams and more private barrier methods, such as a sponge, diaphragm, or spermicidal creams or foams, to help decrease infection. Safer sex guidelines for women who know that their HIV status is positive and who have sex with women advise the use of dental dams to cover the vagina or anus for oral sex. Plastic wrap is often recommended as a substitute for a dental dam, if the latter cannot be found. Women who are sensitive or allergic to latex will need to use alternatives.

Some guidelines suggest a dental dam should be used only once, then discarded. Most sources, however, describe ways of cleaning it safely for reuse. Washing it in a 10 percent bleach solution is often recommended, but can cause skin irritation, so washing in a warm solution of mild detergent followed by a cold rinse may be preferred. Dry flat on a clean towel or tissue. Check for holes by holding up against the light. Color codes for each partner can help identify which one is whose. Marking one side avoids confusion over which side should be in contact with the mouth.

deoxynojirimycin   A plant alkaloid that, in the laboratory, inhibits cell-to-cell spread and formation of nucleated protoplasmic mass induced by the HUMAN IMMUNODEFICIENCY VIRUS.

deoxyribonucleic acid (DNA)   A self-replicating molecule, the major constituent of chromosomes, containing the hereditary information transmitted from parents to offspring in all living organisms apart from some viruses (including the AIDS virus). DNA consists of two strands coiled into a double helix linked by hydrogen bonds between the complementary chemical bases that encode the genetic information—between adenine and thymine and between cytosine and guanine. Recombinant DNA is a hybrid DNA formed by joining pieces of DNA from different organisms.

Department of Health and Human Services (HHS)   The cabinet-level federal agency responsible for almost all health and welfare programs; includes the Health Care Financing Administration, PUBLIC HEALTH SERVICE, and SOCIAL SECURITY ADMINISTRATION.

Department of Housing and Urban Development (HUD)   The cabinet-level federal agency that operates the public housing, rent supplement, low-income housing assistance, and FEDERAL HOUSING ACT and HUD mortgage insurance programs.

Department of Veterans Affairs (VA)   A cabinet-level federal agency that operates a variety of income and medical care programs for certain disabled veterans, some other veterans, and in some cases, their dependents.

dependent variable   See VARIABLE.

Depo-Provera   MEDROXYPROGESTERONE acetate.

depression   A decrease or lowering of a functional activity or vital function; a mental state denoted by an altered mood and characterized by feelings of despair, discouragement, guilt, hopelessness, helplessness, inability to cope, low self-esteem, and sadness. Depression often results in withdrawal from activities usually found to be pleasurable. It may also cause sleep disturbances and changes in eating patterns and energy levels; it may range in intensity from a general feeling of "the blues" to major clinical depression. The term *depression* is used to describe various conditions, including transient moods, mild but persistent sadness, and clinical illness. Clinical depression is defined as a cluster of symptoms that occur together daily over a certain period. The main forms of depressive disorder are major depression, which is often episodic, and DYSTHYMIA, which is a milder chronic condition. The diagnosis of major depression, as defined in current psychiatric standards, requires the presence of at least five of nine specific symptoms during one two-week period. These must include either the first or the second of the following: depressed mood, markedly diminished interest or pleasure in almost all activities, significant unintentional weight gain or loss, insomnia or oversleeping, fidgetiness or slowed movement or speech, fatigue or loss of energy, feelings of worthlessness or excessive or inappropriate guilt, diminished ability to think or concentrate, and recurrent suicidal thoughts. The task of diagnosis in an HIV-positive person is complicated, since many of these symptoms can be caused by HIV, HIV-related conditions, or even HIV medications. Furthermore, the diagnosis cannot be made if the disturbance is a "normal reaction" to the death of a loved one. Use of psychomotor tests can usually distinguish depression from any of several other HIV-related conditions. It has been suggested but not demonstrated that HIV itself causes mood changes and that HIV ENCEPHALOPATHY induces depression. Another important question is whether HIV drugs such as AZT induce mood changes. In practice, it is extremely difficult to distinguish between the symbolic effects of starting antiviral treatment and the direct chemical effects. In later stages of HIV illness it becomes even more difficult to identify effects on mood of any one medication, since as a rule many are taken simultaneously. Patients may experience mood changes associated with medication, but no specific impact on mood has been documented. Clinical depression is the most commonly observed psychiatric disorder among people with HIV illness. The available research literature indicates that HIV-positive depressed patients can tolerate standard doses of antidepressant medications such as Prozac. Psychostimulants, such as methylphenidate (Ritalin) or dexedrine, have also been prescribed. Therapy and group therapy can also be of benefit to patients with depression.

dermatitis   Inflammation of the skin.

dermatitis medicamentosa   See DRUG ERUPTION.

desensitization   The process of reducing a patient's allergic responsiveness to an antigen through a protocol of repeated injections of that allergen, or modified allergen. Desensitization procedures have become common when administering BACTRIM for the first time. Also known as *hyposensitization.*

desmopressin acetate   A VASOPRESSIN analog with antidiuretic (water retention) properties used in the treatment of DIABETES INSIPIDUS. Also used before surgery to increase FACTOR VIII (the factor contributing to the intrinsic value of blood coagulation) in hemophiliacs or patients with Von Willebrand's disease. Desmopressin acetate has greater antidiuretic activity than vasopressin but less pressor activity. (Trade names are DDAVP and Stimate Injection.)

detoxification   Reduction of the toxic properties of a poisonous substance; the process of reducing the physiological effects of a drug or other toxic substance in an addicted individual.

detumescence   The process of losing an erection; deflation of the penis.

developmentally oriented care   Care based on an individual's functional level and chronological age. Functional level includes physical, cognitive, psychosocial, and communicative development.

dexa scan (dual energy X-ray absorptiometry scan)   A medical test that uses minimal radiation to scan the density of bones or amount of body fat and muscle mass a person has. A chest X ray uses

10 times more radiation than a dexa scan. A dexa scan is often used to determine changes in a person's BODY COMPOSITION, which is determined before and after a person has taken particular HAART medications that have been shown to cause LIPODYSTROPHY. Dexa scans are generally covered by Medicaid if a doctor prescribes them.

dexamethasone   A synthetic steroid hormone, similar to those produced by the adrenal glands. Like other CORTICOSTEROIDS, dexamethasone has a wide range of biological actions. It is used most frequently for its anti-inflammatory effects, but it is also a potent inhibitor of certain immune responses. Dexamethasone is used to treat a variety of conditions, including arthritis and other rheumatic diseases, connective-tissue disease, respiratory disease, skin disorders, allergic reactions, inflammation of the eyes, certain blood disorders, inflammation of the brain, and, as a palliative, in certain cancers. In people with HIV it is commonly used alone to counteract allergic drug reactions and as part of a combination chemotherapy for the treatment of AIDS-related lymphoma. Dexamethasone is available in a number of formulations, including tablets or liquid, topical creams or lotions, ointments for administration to the eyes, inhalants, and as a solution for injection. Stomach upset, indigestion, and weight gain are common side effects of dexamethasone. More serious side effects usually occur only with high doses taken for prolonged periods. (Trade names are Decadron and SK-Dexamethasone.)

dextran sulfate   A complex sugar compound used in Japan to treat atherosclerosis, and which showed promise in the test tube as a potential synergizer of the effects of AZT. Such an effect would allow for the use of lower, presumably less toxic doses of that drug. In a trial, however, the drug demonstrated no antiviral or clinical immunological efficacy. In addition, physicians in clinical practice have observed severe side effects such as gastrointestinal bleeding, since dextran sulfate breaks down in the body into sulfuric acid.

dextroamphetamine sulfate   Dextroamphetamine sulfate is an amphetamine, which, as with

METHYLPHENIDATE hydrochloride (RITALIN hydrochloride), stimulates the brain. It is usually given to people with AIDS encephalopathy to counter the symptoms of apathy and social withdrawal. The most common side effects are nervousness and insomnia. Both can usually be controlled by decreasing the dose and by not taking the drug late in the day.

DFA   See DIRECT FLUORESCENT ANTIBODY STAINING.

DHEA   See DEHYDROPIANDROSTERONE (DHEA)/ DEHYDROISOANDROSTERONE.

DHPG   See GANCICLOVIR.

DHT   See DELAYED-TYPE HYPERSENSITIVITY (DTH).

diabetes mellitus   A group of diseases characterized by elevated levels of blood glucose (sugar). In the spring of 1997, reports began to surface about a possible association between PROTEASE INHIBITOR use and the development of diabetes mellitus, or worsening of glucose control in persons already diagnosed with diabetes. How protease inhibitors may cause diabetes or worsening of blood sugar control in diabetics is not known definitively. Some researchers have reported elevated levels of insulin in persons on protease inhibitors. Insulin is a hormone made by the pancreas that acts to lower blood glucose levels. Diabetes may result from inadequate secretion of insulin from the pancreas or from defects that make the cells in the body less sensitive to the effects of insulin (insulin resistance). Elevated insulin levels suggest that insulin resistance is present. The body tries to compensate for this resistance by producing more insulin, and if it fails to compensate sufficiently, high glucose levels (hyperglycemia) or actual diabetes may result. Further research is ongoing to determine the frequency of diabetes, risk factors for its development, and reasons why it occurs. There are no definitive guidelines as to whether all persons on protease inhibitors should be monitored for diabetes, but in general, blood glucose levels should be checked periodically. Glucose levels are usually included in routine blood chemical tests. Persons on protease inhibitors should be aware of the usual symptoms of diabetes, which include increased thirst or appetite, increased frequency of urination, unexplained weight loss, and blurry vision.

diacetylmorphine   The chemical designation for HEROIN.

diagnosis   The determination of the nature of a medical condition; the recognition of the presence of a specific disease or infection, usually accomplished by evaluating clinical symptoms and laboratory tests. For AIDS, the presence of antibodies to HIV in the blood is a sign of HIV INFECTION. These antibodies do not destroy the virus, they simply serve as markers of infection. AIDS is diagnosed when opportunistic infections in sites other than the skin and mucous membranes are present.

In 1993, the original classification for HIV infection was revised and the SURVEILLANCE CASE DEFINITION for AIDS among adolescents and adults was expanded. These changes are important to people who do, indeed, have AIDS but under the original criteria were denied certain medical and economic assistance. The revised criteria include persons who have 200 or fewer CD4 cells or T CELLS per cubic mm of blood. The normal level is about 1,000 per cubic mm.

There are issues specific to HIV-infected women—gynecologic concerns, gynecologic infections, menstrual disorders, cervical dysplasia, and neoplasia, etc., as well as issues specific to pregnant HIV-infected women—prenatal care, intrapartum considerations, postpartum considerations, etc. However, the revised classification for HIV infection and expanded surveillance case definition for AIDS among adolescents and adults does not include a different definition for women. There are in the revised classification, conditions that women present and men do not, such as, for example, cervical cancer. See AIDS-DEFINING ILLNESS.

diagnostic   A means by which to measure or evaluate a patient's medical condition.

dialysis   The process of separating out materials in solution by forcing the solution through a semipermeable membrane. Separation is accomplished because different substances have differ-ent rates of diffusion. See HEMODIALYSIS and PERITONEAL DIALYSIS.

diaminodiphenylsulfone   See DAPSONE.

diapedesis   Passage of blood cells, especially leukocytes, by ameboid movements through the unruptured wall of a capillary vessel.

diaphragm   A contraceptive device in the form of a round or dome-shaped latex object resembling a cap or a cup, which is inserted in the vagina to cover the cervix. It is most effective when used with spermicide. It can also be used as part of an STD risk-reduction strategy. For example, safer sex guidelines for HIV-positive women who have sex with men often suggest that if a man won't use condoms that a diaphragm or other barrier method be used, with spermicidal creams or foams, to prevent pregnancy and to help decrease the risk of infection.

diarrhea   A disturbance in bowel movements characterized by abnormally frequent, loose, or watery stools. Diarrhea is often related to a disturbance in the gastrointestinal system.

diarrhea-wasting syndrome   A term sometimes used to refer to the severe diarrhea characteristically associated with HIV INFECTION. The syndrome (diarrhea persisting for at least a month, accompanied by otherwise unexplained weight loss of 10 percent) in conjunction with HIV infection composes an AIDS-defining illness.

didanosine   More commonly known as ddI, it is an anti-HIV treatment in the same class of drugs as ZIDOVUDINE, ZALCITABINE, LAMIVUDINE, STAVUDINE, and ABACAVIR. These drugs are called NUCLEOSIDE ANALOGS. The body breaks down these drugs into chemicals that prevent HIV from infecting uninfected cells in the body. Many studies have shown that using ddI with two other drugs can prevent the virus from developing resistance. Public Health Service guidelines recommend taking didanosine with at least one other NRTI and one PROTEASE INHIBITOR. The most common side effects of ddI include stomach pain and diarrhea. Long-term use of ddI increases risk of PANCREATITIS as well as PERIPHERAL NEUROPATHY. These latter two conditions are also more likely to occur if ddI is combined in treatment with d4T. A once-daily formulation of ddI has been approved by the FDA; studies show similar results to twice a day dosing with the tablets. ddI should not be combined with ddC and should be taken at different times when used in combination with delavirdine, tenofovir, or indinavir. ddI has a tablet form that can be chewed or dissolved in water; the once-daily formulation is a capsule. It is important to take ddI on an empty stomach at least one hour before eating or at least two hours after the last meal. Didanosine has several drug interactions that can cause levels of the drug to fluctuate in the body. Inform physicians of any medication you are taking if they prescribe this medication. It is also approved for children above six months of age with HIV infection. That formula is available in a flavored liquid that must be mixed with an antacid such as Maalox or Mylanta. (Trade name is Videx.)

dideoxycytidine (ddC)   See ZALCITABINE.

dideoxyinosine (ddI)   See DIDANOSINE.

Didox   A RIBONUCLEOTIDE REDUCTASE INHIBITOR, in the same drug class as HYDROXYUREA, under investigation for anti-HIV activity by Molecules for Health, Inc. It has shown promise in animal models of retrovirus illnesses when used alone or in combination with DIDANOSINE (ddI). Didox has been shown in studies to be much less toxic than hydroxyurea. It is also in trials for cancer treatment in Great Britain and is awaiting investigative new drug (IND) status with the NIH in the United States.

diet supplements   There are many different causes for nutrient deficiencies in people living with HIV: the high demand for antioxidants, the increased metabolism that begins in the earliest disease stages, malabsorption because of damage to the intestines, decreased intake of food because of mouth or throat problems, loss of appetite, loss of taste, fever, nausea, and vomiting. The resulting deficiencies are often of important nutrients critical for supporting immune function. The use of antibi-

otics and other medications that destroy the body's "friendly" gastrointestinal bacteria also cause nutrient deficiencies. Gastrointestinal bacteria are necessary for the breakdown and absorption of certain food substances. Without them, foods cannot be digested properly and become useless to the body as a source of nutrients. Moreover, maldigested food may cause other problems, including diarrhea. Gastrointestinal bacteria also produce several different vitamins, including thiamin, riboflavin, niacin, pantothenic acid, vitamin B_6, VITAMIN B_{12}, folic acid, choline, biotin, and vitamin K.

People with HIV are usually advised to take a multiple vitamin–mineral supplement that supplies the basic level of nutrients most important to body function. Many nutritionists believe that additional supplements are necessary. Symptoms that may be related to nutrient deficiencies and may be reversible with appropriate supplementation include serious fatigue, memory loss or other cognitive dysfunction, skin problems, NEUROPATHY, weight loss, loss of the senses of smell or taste, appetite loss, muscle pain or cramps, digestive problems, night blindness, canker sores, constipation, DEPRESSION anxiety, menstrual cramps, and menopausal problems. Many other symptoms in people living with HIV may be related to nutrient deficiencies.

differential diagnosis   Diagnosis based on comparison of symptoms of two or more similar diseases to determine the cause of illness.

Diflucan   See FLUCONAZOLE.

digital-anal sex   Erotic stimulation of the anus with a finger or fingers.

dihydroxpropoxymethyl (DHPG)   See GANCYCLOVIR.

diiodohydroxyquin   See IODIOQUINOL.

Diodoquin   See IODOQUINOL.

dildo   An artificial erect penis used as a sexual aid.

Dinacrin   See ISONIAZID.

dinitrochlorobenzene (DNCB)   A chemical used in color photography processing. DNCB is "contact-sensitizer," which means that it causes an itchy red rash similar to that of poison oak or poison ivy. Some doctors have used DNCB to measure the strength of the immune system: the greater the skin reaction to DNCB, and the faster it appears, the stronger the immune response. Some researchers and HIV activists believe that when DNCB is applied to the skin once a week, it stimulates the immune system to control HIV replication and delay OPPORTUNISTIC INFECTIONS. As with any natural or nonmedical substance there is very little research on DNCB for use in medicine. The studies that have been done have included very few subjects, and often research subjects drop out of studies. The limited research has shown both positive and negative results. Some research shows that DNCB leads to increases in CD8+ cells. These cells are an important part of the immune system. Some studies suggest that DNCB *decreases* the number of CD4+ cells.

DNCB is available as a liquid solution in a variety of strengths. The solution is applied to a two-inch-square area on the skin once a week. Then the area is bandaged and is kept dry for 10 hours. After the first skin response (a red, itchy rash), the strength of the DNCB solution is lowered. Instructions for using DNCB originally provided by community activists indicated that most other therapies can prevent it from working. They discourage the use of all antiretrovirals, acupuncture, and even multivitamins. These unusual instructions have made it difficult for most people to try DNCB, particularly when there is so little evidence to support its use. Little funding is expected for research on DNCB, which is an inexpensive, nonpatentable substance that drug corporations are unlikely to produce. DNCB seems to restore immune responses in the skin that are lost as AIDS develops. However, it is not known whether skin response is a good indicator of overall immune health.

dipstick test   A test to determine the presence of protein, glucose, or other substances in urine by dipping a chemically impregnated strip of paper into a urine sample.

dipyridamole   A blood-thinning drug long used in heart disease, which has also been shown to potentiate the activity of NUCLEOSIDE ANALOG by reducing the entry of competing natural nucleosides into the cell. Further studies are needed to establish the long-term safety and effectiveness of dipyridamole in combination with AZT, although researchers have been unable to secure financial support from the manufacturer, possibly because the drug's patent has expired.

direct fluorescent antibody staining   A type of medical test that is performed on a sample of tissue or fluid from a part of the body. It is used to test for legionella virus infection as well as CHLAMYDIA and SYPHILIS infections. A swab of tissue from the patient is stained for fluorescence to see whether it matches the known fluorescence of the particular virus.

directly observed therapy (DOT)   A process by which a patient takes a medication while under direct observation by another individual. Usually used in antituberculosis treatment.

disability   Qualification for disability benefits under Social Security is based on an individual's medical condition. An individual is considered disabled if, because of such condition, he or she is unable to earn a "substantial" income in work for which he or she is suited. Usually, monthly earnings of $500 or more are considered substantial. Inability to work must be expected to last at least a year, or the condition must be so severe that the victim is not expected to live. The Social Security Administration also decides how a condition affects children's ability to function—to do the things and behave in the ways that other children of the same age normally would.

Social Security works with an agency in each state, usually called a Disability Determination Service (DDS), to evaluate disability claims. At the DDS, a disability evaluation specialist and a doctor follow a step-by-step process that applies to all disability claims, thus assuring a consistent national approach.

First, the DDS specialists decide whether an individual's impairment is severe. This simply means the evidence must show that the disability interferes with the individual's ability to work. The next step is deciding whether the impairment is included in an approved list. This list describes, for each of the major body systems, impairments that are considered severe enough to prevent an adult from doing any substantial work, or in the case of children under the age of 18, impairments that are severe enough to prevent a child from functioning in a manner similar to other children of the same age.

Because HIV research is a dynamic process and medical knowledge concerning the disease and its symptoms is constantly growing, Social Security continually updates its evaluation criteria for HIV infection. If an individual has symptoms of HIV infection that are not specifically included in (or equivalent to) Social Security's current guidelines, then DDS disability specialists will evaluate all medical evidence to determine ability to work. They will be looking for documentation of signs, symptoms, and laboratory findings that can result from HIV infection. They will also look for evidence of restrictions in daily activities caused by HIV infection. If a disability decision cannot be made on medical factors alone, the DDS specialists evaluate a variety of physical and/or mental limitations that may prevent an individual from working.

Recent developments in Social Security's evaluation process include guidelines that recognize that HIV can show up differently in women than in men, and differently in children than in adults, and differently in younger than in older children (13 or above). When assessing the degree to which the disease affects a woman's ability to function, DDS disability evaluators consider gynecological problems such as vulvovaginal candidiasis, GENITAL HERPES, PELVIC INFLAMMATORY DISEASE, and CERVICAL CANCER.

disability discrimination law In the early 1980s, there was no existing body of legal precedent regarding discrimination based on a contagious medical condition. As the epidemic progressed and such discrimination increased against people with HIV/AIDS, the courts and legislatures responded by adapting disability discrimination law to this new problem. The process culminated in 1990 with the enactment of the federal AMERICANS WITH DISABILITIES ACT (ADA), which has become the basic law governing HIV-related discrimination in employment, public services, and public accommodations as its various provisions have gone into effect during the 1990s. The act applies broadly to businesses and individuals providing goods and services to the public, employers of fifteen or more employees, and most federal and state agencies.

Under the REHABILITATION ACT OF 1973, an "individual with handicaps" is "any person who (i) has a physical or mental impairment which substantially limits one or more of such person's major life activities, (ii) has a record of such an impairment, or (iii) is regarded as having such an impairment." The ADA defines a "disability" as "(A) A physical or mental impairment that substantially limits one or more . . . major life activities . . .; (B) a record of such an impairment; or (C) being regarded as having such an impairment." HIV infection and AIDS have come to be considered handicaps or disabilities by most administrative agencies and courts considering discrimination claims.

disability insurance Insurance that replaces income for individuals unable to work because of accident or sickness.

disability-related inquiries Historically, many employers have felt free to request information concerning a job applicant's physical or mental condition. However, with the passage of the Americans with Disabilities Act (ADA), these questions may not legally be asked at an initial interview. Employers may not ask about the existence, nature, or severity of a disability or require a medical examination until after a conditional offer of employment has been made. They may not ask any of the following types of questions: What prescription drugs are you currently taking? Have you ever been treated for mental health problems? How many days were you sick last year? Do you have a disability that may affect your performance on the job? Do you have AIDS? At the preoffer stage, the employer is entitled to ask only about an applicant's ability to perform the essential functions of the job. Congress intended the ADA restriction on preemployment inquiries to prevent discrimination against individuals with "hidden" disabilities, such as cancer, epilepsy, and HIV/AIDS. The ADA prohibition of preemployment questioning and examinations ensures that the applicant's hidden disability not be considered before the assessment of his or her nonmedical qualifications. After a conditional offer is made, employers may require medical examinations and may make disability-related inquiries, if they do so for all entering employees in that job category.

discharge   To release from care by a physician, other medical care worker, or a medical care facility.

The secretion or excretion from the body of pus, feces, urine, etc.; the material thus ejected.

disclosure   The revelation of a diagnosis of HIV or AIDS. Disclosure of such a diagnosis to someone other than a person with the illness involves issues of public health, social convention, and civil liberties. See PRIVACY.

disclosure counseling   The news that one has been infected with HIV isn't easy to receive. Individuals who have tested positive will have many questions about their condition and its impact on their lives. Post-disclosure counseling is intended to help them come to terms with their diagnosis and to prepare them to deal with their illness in a practical way.

Typical questions include: Why me? Am I contagious to others? Is my partner positive? Is he or she immune? What do symptomatic and asymptomatic mean? Whom should I tell? What should I tell my sexual or needle-sharing partners? What should I tell my doctor and dentist, my family, my employer, my insurer? Will information in my medical records be confidential? Advice is offered concerning medical follow-up, staying healthy, and stopping the spread of the disease. The complexities of disclosure may also be addressed. See PRIVACY.

discordant   See SERODISCORDANT RELATIONSHIPS.

discourse   See CULTURAL ANALYSIS AND AIDS.

discrimination   Disadvantageous treatment, either overt or insidious, of individuals or groups that results in the unequal treatment of or the denial of opportunities to these people. The stigma associated with AIDS has prompted, and continues to prompt, a wide range of individual and social reactions to persons with AIDS and HIV infection. HIV-infected people have the same civil and social rights as the noninfected. Examples of these rights include access to justice; public benefits (programs such as Social Security Disability Income and Supplemental Security Income); confidentiality (as regards testing, donor disclosure, and access to donor medical records, etc.); education (the rights of both HIV-infected students to be able to attend public schools and of HIV-infected teachers to be able to remain the heads of their classes, etc.); employment (the rights of persons with HIV/AIDS to work as long as they are able, etc.); free speech (the right to publish and disseminate AIDS education materials, etc.); housing; immigration; insurance (the right to coverage for health care costs, the right to life insurance coverage, etc.); public accommodations; and professional regulation.

Laws related to AIDS, such as statutes enacted and cases reported, are the most visible evidence of how U.S. society is dealing with AIDS- and HIV-related discrimination. Discrimination laws provide a legal foundation for the rights of people with HIV infection and AIDS. Whether or not this foundation is really adequate to ensure that people with HIV infection and AIDS receive the humane treatment to which everyone is entitled as a basic human right is another issue entirely. The statutes provide limited remedies, and their administration frequently takes more time than people with HIV infection or AIDS can afford to wait. Examples of federal protections include the Americans with Disabilities Act, which passed the United States Senate on September 7, 1989, and the Fair Housing Rehabilitation Act of 1973, Public Law 93-12, Section 504. In addition to federal protections, there are a myriad of state and local protections; for example, all 50 states and the District of Columbia have statutes that parallel the federal Rehabilitation Act prohibiting discrimination against handicapped persons.

In 2003, stories began to circulate in mainstream and scientific publications that members of Congress and the George W. Bush administration were more thoroughly reading grant and research applications for what were termed *key phrases* in HIV-related applications. Stories appeared in *Science* and the *New York Times* indicating that phrases such as "men having sex with men," "commercial sex workers," "prostitutes," "transgender," and "needle exchange" were being looked for in e-mails and reports to the CDC and NIH. Staff and program workers report having been warned of using such "sensitive language" by superiors. It is evidence of discrimination that employees are being told to disguise their reports and work to avoid falling under a congressional review. Staff from congressional offices have stopped by some researchers' offices looking to find proof of federal dollars being spent on what the investigators termed *inappropriate, unfavorable,* and *unsafe* lifestyles with tax dollars. Future research may reflect the clampdown on such studies if current social policies are encouraged or not objected to by other congressional staff or the public.

disease   A pathological condition of the body that presents a group of clinical signs and symptoms and laboratory findings peculiar to it and that sets the condition apart as an abnormal entity differing from other normal or pathological body states. Disease is usually tangible and may even be measured. Illness is highly individual and personal.

disease classification   Disease classification is one of many public health measures that are considered technical, yet have direct consequences for human rights. Classification of a disease as contagious, communicable, transmissible, infectious, or sexually transmitted is only the beginning of a process entailing the application of previously existing laws that may mandate compulsory medical examination or hospitalization, restrictions on travel or immigration, or isolation. Classification can also lead to social stigma, as evidenced by the frequent so-called analogies between AIDS and leprosy.

Even though the scientific literature has pleaded for consistency and precision in disease classification, there is still no uniformity regarding AIDS and HIV infection. Some countries classify HIV/AIDS as a communicable disease, others as infectious disease, still others as a viral disease. Many countries have classified AIDS as a sexually transmitted disease. The World Health Organization (WHO) seems to have passively endorsed this latter approach,

arguing that most HIV infections are acquired and transmitted sexually. From the human rights viewpoint, this classification gives public health authorities wide-ranging powers under already existing STD legislation. Coercive and compulsory measures are envisaged in STD; laws are broad, and the stigma associated with sexually transmitted disease means that these laws are rarely challenged.

The main feature of legislation on STDs is their effort to prevent the spread of infection by denying rights to infected individuals. The traditional measures for controlling STDs include compulsory examination, contact tracing, restrictive measures against carriers to prevent further transmission, compulsory treatment and/or hospitalization, and extensive case finding through premarital and prenatal screening. Additionally, immigration regulations enacted for STDs have been applied to AIDS in order to exclude persons who are HIV infected, thus reviving "certificates of freedom from venereal disease."

disease progression   The process of growth, spread and development of symptoms and affects. The median time from HIV infection to development of AIDS in adults is 10 years. Individuals of similar age have highly variable rates of disease progression, a phenomenon that has remained unexplained. A study, reported in *Nature* in April 1996, has found multiple genes or gene combinations in human DNA that appear to influence how long a person with HIV infection remains disease free. The genes encode HUMAN LEUKOCYTE ANTIGEN (HLA), molecules that help regulate the immune response to HIV-1. The study focused on products of the MAJOR HISTOCOMPATIBILITY COMPLEX (MHC), a cluster of genes that includes the HLA region. The MHC is important for immune recognition and for immune responsiveness to foreign antigens such as might derive from HIV-1. HLA (or MHC) class 1 markers, found on the surfaces of all nucleated cells and blood platelets, determine the immunologic acceptability of transplanted tissue. HLA (or MHC) class II markers, expressed on B CELLS, MACROPHAGE, and other immune system cells, are required to initiate an immune response to foreign antigens such as HIV-1. Pieces of these foreign antigens are transported across the cell's interior by products of TAP genes (also in the MHC). This study provides further support to the belief that the immune response to HIV is an important factor in determining the rate of HIV-mediated disease progression.

disinfection The act of freeing of PATHOGENIC organisms, or rendering such organisms inactive, by physical or chemical means. The term is generally applied to inanimate objects. Methods of disinfection include moist heat, radiation, filtration, physical cleaning, and application of chemical substances, including quarternary ammonia compounds (both tincture and aqueous), mercurials, formaldehyde, glutaraldehyde, germicidal soaps, and formaldehyde gas. Three levels of disinfection are covered in the *Centers for Disease Control's Guidelines for Prevention of Transmission of Human Immunodeficiency Virus (HIV) and Hepatitis B Virus (HBV) to Health-Care and Public Safety Workers* (http://www.cdc.gov/mmwr/preview/mmwrhtml/00001450.htm). High-level disinfection destroys all forms of microbial life except high numbers of bacterial spores; intermediate-level disinfection kills MYCOBACTERIUM TUBERCULOSIS (*M. tuberculosis*) vegetative bacteria, most viruses, and most fungi, but not bacterial spores; and low-level disinfection kills most bacteria, some viruses, and some fungi but not *M. tuberculosis* or bacterial spores. The guidelines also spell out methods for cleaning, disinfecting, and sterilizing equipment and surfaces at each level.

disorientation The loss of normal relationship to one's surroundings; confusion about time, place, and identity.

disregards (of assets or income) Amounts, values, or percentages of an applicant's assets or income that needs-based programs do not count in determining eligibility for benefits.

disseminated tuberculosis A contagious bacterial infection caused by the bacteria MYCOBACTERIUM TUBERCULOSIS that has spread to other organs from the primary focus of infection, the lungs, through the blood or LYMPHATIC SYSTEM.

distal Remote, away from the point of origin.

distal symmetric polyneuropathy (DSPN) A disease of the nerves that manifests as subacute onset of numbness or tingling in the fingers or toes. Early clinical signs are bilaterally depressed ankle reflex and impaired sensation in the toes.

distraction The cognitive strategy of focusing the attention on other body or local stimuli to distract the mind from pain and negative emotions that accompany pain.

disulfiram An orally administered drug used in the treatment of alcoholism. Ingestion of alcohol after taking this drug causes severe reactions, including nausea and vomiting, and may endanger the life of the patient. (Trade name is Antabuse.)

diuretic A drug or other agent that promotes excretion of urine, resulting in the loss of water from the body.

Division of Acquired Immunodeficiency Syndrome (DAIDS) DAIDS (http://www.niaid.nih.gov/daids) was formed in 1986 to address the national research needs created by the HIV/AIDS epidemic. It sponsors research into the basic knowledge of the pathogenesis, natural history, and transmission of HIV disease and supports research to promote HIV detection, treatment, and prevention.

DNA See DEOXYRIBONUCLEIC ACID.

DNA polymerase All living organisms have DNA polymerase. It is an ENZYME that plays the main part in the creation of life. It is the part of a living organism that duplicates its genetic information. When a cell divides, DNA polymerase has duplicated all of the genetic material and passed it on to the new cell. In this way, genetic information is passed from generation to generation. One cell has several different polymerases. DNA polymerase alpha does most of the DNA replication when the cell divides. It is the DNA found in all of our chromosomes. DNA polymerase beta is responsible for the daily repair of DNA chains.

DNA polymerase is very efficient in its job and generally makes a mistake in reproduction only once in every billion bases that it creates. The bases that make up DNA are GUANINE, CYTOSINE, THYMINE, and ADENINE. DNA polymerase also checks each base for mistakes and destroys the base if it is wrong.

DNA polymerase gamma is the enzyme that regulates the replication of mitochondrial DNA. In HIV medicine NRTI drugs have been able to inhibit the synthesis of nuclear DNA, thus also inhibiting the replication of HIV. The nucleus of the cell has been shown to repair the damage to the DNA that NRTIs cause. However, mitochondrial DNA is reproduced differently and does not have the ability to repair the damage HAART drugs cause. This inability can lead to self-replicating mistakes in the DNA polymerase gamma that reproduces the mitochondrial DNA.

DNA vaccine A type of VACCINE that uses pieces of the DNA of a virus, instead of the whole virus, to stimulate an immune response against that particular virus. Several DNA vaccines are currently under investigation for AIDS as well as malaria and several other illnesses. There is currently no DNA vaccine in production for human use. See VACCINE; VACCINE DEVELOPMENT.

DNAR See DO NOT ATTEMPT RESUSCITATION.

DNCB See DINITROCHLOROBENZENE.

DNR See DO NOT RESUSCITATE.

do not attempt resuscitation (DNAR) An order somewhat more precise than DO NOT RESUSCITATE (DNR). DNAR indicates resuscitation efforts should not be attempted regardless of expected outcomes of those efforts.

do not resuscitate (DNR) An instruction given by a patient or family member not to administer cardiopulmonary resuscitation to the patient on the apparent cessation of life. Such an order can be made effective both within and outside a hospital setting. DNR implies that if a resuscitation attempt is made, the patient could be revived.

dogfish shark Any of several small sharks that are destructive to food fishes. A compound isolated from dogfish shark has been found to dramatically inhibit HIV replication in the test tube without disrupting CD4+ T cell proliferation and other normal cellular activities. The compound works by blocking a process central to cellular activation—the exchange of ions across the cell membrane. The compound is known as MSI-1436.

domain A region of a gene or gene product.

donor insemination See ARTIFICIAL INSEMINATION.

dormancy The period when an infectious organism is in the body but not yet producing ill effects. See LATENCY.

Dornan Amendment Attached to the 1996 defense authorization bill, a regulation put forth by Rep. Robert K. Dornan (R-Calif.) that would have discharged military service members with HIV and denied them medical benefits. President Bill Clinton reluctantly signed the defense bill into law, but said the Dornan measure was unconstitutional and ordered governmental lawyers not to oppose legal challenges to it. In April 1996, the leadership of both the Senate and House turned against the measure and killed it after it became clear that the U.S.'s military's entire command structure opposed it. Service members with HIV have been banned from combat and overseas duty since the mid-1980s.

dosage The size, frequency, and number of doses of a drug.

dose The amount of a drug that is given at one time.

dose escalation A preliminary clinical trial technique in which the amount of a drug is either periodically increased or increased with each new trial arm that is added. The test is done to determine how a drug is tolerated.

dose ranging A drug trial technique in which two or more different doses of a drug are tested against each other to determine which works best and is the least harmful.

dose-response relationship   The relationship between the dose of a drug, or the extent of exposure, and a response in the body. When there is a dose-response effect, as the dose increases, so does the response.

dosing   Administration or ingestion of a quantity of medicine prescribed to be taken at one time. Once-a-day dosing (once-daily) and twice-a-day dosing (twice-daily) are examples of treatment regimens. It is generally thought that simpler dosing (e.g., once-daily tablets) is easier to remember and makes life easier for the person taking them. Two open questions about once-daily dosing are noted: first, what is the impact of a skipped dose on blood levels? Second, is there a greater risk of development of drug resistance when doses of these less burdensome regimens are missed? With twice-a-day regimens, the catch-up dose enters the blood 12 hours late; with daily dosing a full day passes before drug levels are changed to recommended concentrations.

(–) dOTC   Also known as SPD 754 and formerly BCH-10618, it is an experimental NUCLEOSIDE REVERSE TRANSCRIPTASE INHIBITOR manufactured by Shire Pharmaceuticals. The drug is similar to LAMIVUDINE (3TC) but acts on different parts of the virus. It seems to have good action on HIV in the CENTRAL NERVOUS SYSTEM. It has a synergistic effect when used with AZT and 3TC. It also seems to work after the virus has developed resistance to AZT, 3TC, and some PROTEASE INHIBITORS. It is currently in preclinical trials. Phase II trials of the original formulation of –dOTC were stopped after significant toxicity was shown in some people.

double blind   See DOUBLE-BLIND STUDY.

double standard   See SEXUAL DOUBLE STANDARD.

double-blind study   A kind of clinical study in which neither the experimenter nor the subjects know until after the data have been collected which treatment has been applied to which subjects. This type of study employing an experimental drug and a placebo is used in drug trials to prevent contami-

nation of the results from the biases and preconceptions of experimenters or subjects. Double-blind studies are believed to promote faster and more objective results, since they control for the possibility of bias. Independent review boards (see DATA SAFETY AND MONITORING BOARD) review the study for any concerns or surprises in the results every six to 12 months. These studies typically have a specified duration and do not continue indefinitely. If the review board finds reason, the study may be stopped for negative or positive reasons.

douche   A liquid that is put into a woman's vagina and then expelled in order to cleanse the internal area of the vagina. A douche may be used to rinse out a person's rectum, in which case it is called an ENEMA. In addition to cleansing, it removes healthy vaginal flora and disrupts the pH balance, thus, it may cause later problems created by imbalance in natural flora. There is no evidence that a douche is effective as a postcoital contraceptive. Overuse of douches has been linked to PELVIC INFLAMMATORY DISEASE (PID). A vagina has the ability to cleanse itself, so there is very little reason to use a douche.

douching   Application of a DOUCHE.

down low (dl)   Slang term used to refer to a man who is engaged in MSM relationships in a clandestine or quiet way. Used particularly in urban communities to refer to men who are married, are also having sex with other men, but do not acknowledge the activity or its potential consequences, to family and friends.

Doxil   See DOX-SL.

doxorubicin   A wide-spectrum antineoplastic antibiotic agent. A long-lasting version of doxorubicin, DOX-SL, may prove beneficial to people whose KAPOSI'S SARCOMA does not respond to other approved treatments. Encapsulated in protective LIPOSOMES (fat globules), this drug tends to concentrate in KS lesions, where it is gradually released.

DOX-SL (Doxil)   An antibiotic agent used in chemotherapy for KAPOSI'S SARCOMA, consisting of a preparation of doxorubicin encapsulated in LIPO-SOMES which deliver significantly greater quantities of doxorubicin to the KS lesions than the standard treatment while reducing the drug's side effects. DOX-SL incorporates so-called stealth liposomes, whose polyethylene glycol (PEG) coating gives them greater stability in the bloodstream. Side effects include nausea, vomiting, stomatitis, diarrhea, and hair loss. DOX-SL causes a significant amount of neutropenia, which can be managed with G-CSF (Neupogen).

doxycycline   A broad-spectrum antibiotic of the TETRACYCLINE group. (Trade name is Vibramycin.)

DPC-083   Also known as Al-183. It is an anti-HIV medication. DPC-083 is in a category of HIV medicines called nonnucleoside reverse transcriptase inhibitors (NNRTIs). DPC-083 prevents HIV from entering the nucleus of healthy T cells. This effect prevents the cells from producing new virus and decreases the amount of virus in the body. It is produced by Bristol-Meyers Squibb and is a derivative of their drug EFAVIRENZ. It has been shown to be retained in the bloodstream for long periods and could be used in a once-a-day dosing regimen. Phase II trials are under way in the United States.

DPC 681 and 684   Two PROTEASE INHIBITORS under PHASE I studies. They are believed to be active against resistant virus. Human trials in which dosing and toleration will be learned are just beginning.

DPC 817   An experimental NRTI from DuPont Pharmaceuticals. It is believed to have strong antiretroviral properties. It is in PHASE I trials in humans for dosing studies. It is thought to work against virus that has become resistant to other NRTIs.

DPT vaccine   A vaccine used for diphtheria, pertussis, and tetanus.

drip   See GONORRHEA.

dronabinol   An appetite stimulant composed of synthetic DELTA-9-TETRAHYDROCANNABINOL (THC),

the psychoactive component of MARIJUANA. It is used to treat weight loss caused by loss of appetite in people with AIDS. It is also used to treat nausea and vomiting caused by cancer chemotherapy in people who have not responded to other treatment. Dronabinol affects the central nervous system, altering appetite, mood, thinking, memory, and perception. The effects of dronabinol are the same as those of natural THC, though many people who use this drug say the effect is less than that achieved by smoking marijuana. Both are dose-related, and the response varies from person to person. Consequently, the dose must be individually adjusted. The drug is a central nervous system depressant and may impair a person's ability to drive an automobile or operate dangerous machinery. It should not be used with alcohol or other depressants. It should be used cautiously by people with a history of cardiac disease, since it may cause low blood pressure, rapid heartbeat, or fainting. Because dronabinol affects the nervous system, it may worsen MANIA, DEPRESSION, or SCHIZOPHRENIA. Mood shifts and, less frequently, hallucinations may occur. These effects are reversible and disappear when the drug is stopped. The most common side effects of dronabinol are on the central nervous system, including elation, easy laughing, dizziness, confusion, and drowsiness. Again, these effects are generally dose-related and reversible when the drug is stopped. (Trade name is Marinol.) In Canada and some other countries, a slightly different formulation of the drug is called Cesamet (Nabilone).

drug abuse   The (generally self-administered) use or overuse of a drug in a manner other than that for which it is intended or prescribed. A drug of abuse may be legal or illicit, addictive or not. (In common usage, the terms *drug abuse* and *drug use* are synonymous. The term *drug use* is rarely applied to legitimate medical use of drugs.) Serious drug abusers are those in bad relationships with drugs, those who have great difficulty with them. A large proportion of drug abusers are compulsive, addicted, or chaotic drug users. There are six key relationships between drug use and HIV/AIDS. The first, and most obvious, is that HIV is efficiently transmitted by sharing drug injection paraphernalia.

The second relationship between drug use and HIV/AIDS involves the sex–drug link. The use of COCAINE, for example, in any form has effects on the libido. In early cocaine use, the libido is stimulated, resulting in more sexual activity; with frequent high-dose use of cocaine, the neurochemical dopamine becomes depleted, resulting in a loss of sexual desire. Additionally, many high-dose users of cocaine, for example, crack-cocaine users, begin to sell sex for crack or for money to buy crack. They are often teenagers of both genders and various sexual orientations who enter into unprotected sexual encounters that result in SEXUALLY TRANSMITTED DISEASES, including HIV INFECTION. There is a strong link between sexually transmitted diseases, particularly those that involve genital lesions, and HIV because these infections and lesions seem to facilitate HIV transmission.

A third link between drug use and HIV is that the use of any mood-altering substance often results in unsafe sexual activity. The effects of drugs can reduce inhibition, cloud judgment, result in memory lapses (called "blackouts"), and lead to false feelings of safety and lack of concern about HIV. This is an important link even for those who are experimenters with or only occasional users of drugs of abuse.

A fourth link between drug use and HIV involves the IMMUNOSUPPRESSIVE qualities of some drugs. Alcohol, cocaine, amphetamines, and inhalant nitrates are believed to damage the immune system, leaving frequent users immune suppressed and possibly more likely to have HIV exposure that results in HIV infection. in addition, if drug users do become HIV-infected, HIV spectrum disease may progress faster than in those who do not have a history of immune-suppressive drug use. This effect has not been studied in medical research, and anecdotally doctors have not found any correlation between drug abuse and length of time to an AIDS diagnosis.

The fifth link between drug use and HIV/AIDS is the pediatric connection. The vast majority of pediatric AIDS cases in the United States have resulted from prenatal transmission in which one or both parents are or were needle drug users.

Finally, the role of injection routes and adulterated drugs should not be ignored. The needle route of drug administration results in a hole in the skin.

Since drug users often reuse disposable syringes and needles without proper sterilization, microorganisms can enter the body, where the immune system must deal with them, adding stress to this system. In addition, because of the criminalization of drug use, illicit drugs are generally not pure; they are adulterated, or "cut" with other substances, thus increasing the dealer's profit but with the potential to harm the immune system of the user.

drug addict   A person who is physically dependent on drugs and unable to control his or her craving. See DRUG ABUSE; DRUG ADDICTION.

drug addiction   A dependency on a habit-forming drug, acquired through excessive or continued use. Symptoms of drug addiction are behavioral and physical and include change in personality, loss of appetite, dulled appetite, disturbance in normal sleep rhythm, and weight loss.

Drug addiction is a psychic and physical state encompassing a compulsion to take a given drug on a continuous or periodic basis in order to experience its pleasurable effects or avoid the discomfort of its absence. Tolerance may or may not be present, and a person may be dependent on more than one drug. Drug addicts run a number of serious risks; aside from organ damage and other long-term destructive effects, users may have serious reactions to unknown substances present in illicit drugs, and hepatitis and AIDS can be transmitted through the use of dirty needles and syringes.

drug administration   A regimen, generally ordered by a physician, for taking drugs or other medications. Most medications are taken orally as tablets, capsules, or liquids; some are administered by injection, through intravenous devices, or via inhalant; some may be applied as liquid or ointment directly to an affected area of the body.

drug approval process   The U.S. system of new drug approvals is perhaps the most rigorous in the world. The steps in development and approval of new medicine are basic research and preclinical development, preclinical testing, investigational new drug (IND) application, clinical trials (phase I, phase II, phase III), new drug application (NDA), and approval. Drugs are researched and developed, for the most part, by privately owned pharmaceutical manufacturers. The entire process is regulated and overseen by the Food and Drug Administration (FDA), part of the United States Department of Health and Human Services.

In preclinical testing of a new compound, laboratory and animal studies are done to show biological activity against a targeted disease, and the compound is evaluated for safety. These tests take approximately three and a half years. After completing the preclinical testing, the developer files IND application. The IND shows results of previous experiments, along with information detailing how, where, and by whom the new studies will be conducted; the chemical structure of the compound; the way it is thought to work in the body; any toxic effects found in the animal studies; and the method by which compound is manufactured. In addition, the IND must be reviewed and approved by the FDA's Institutional Review Board, where separate studies will be conducted. Upon approval of the IND, which is effective in 30 days unless the FDA has an objection, the manufacturer may begin to test the new drug on humans. Progress reports on clinical trials must be submitted at least annually to the FDA. Phase I clinical trials take about a year and involve 20 to 80 normal, healthy volunteers. These tests study a drug's safety profile, including the safe dosage range. The studies also determine the way a drug is absorbed, distributed, metabolized, and excreted, as well as the duration of its action. In Phase II clinical trials, controlled studies of approximately 100 to 300 volunteer patients (people with the targeted disease) assess the drug's effectiveness. Phase II trials are designed to demonstrate whether or not the drug is active, to identify the benefits of using it, and to determine whether there is an optimal dose. This phase takes about two years. In phase III clinical trials, hundreds or thousands of patients in clinics and hospitals are administered the new drug and closely monitored by physicians to determine efficacy and to identify adverse reactions. This phase lasts about three years. Under a plan implemented by the FDA in early 1989, phases II and III may be combined to shave two or three years from the process for medicines that show sufficient promise

in early testing and are targeted against serious life-threatening diseases. Additionally, competition has intensified the need to contain costs, resulting in shorter trial times and an increasing number of trials conducted outside the United States. There is also a trend to contract the work of conducting clinical trials to third-party firms that specialize in human research. For new HIV drugs in particular, offshore trials also provide access to larger numbers of previously untreated people than can be found in the United States. Note that the investment required to develop a drug continues to ramp up as each new phase is initiated. Every milestone in the process calls for a business decision about whether to continue to invest money or not. On the basis of a drug's progress and prospects, new capital must be committed to continue development; otherwise the drug is sidelined. For startup biotech companies, new capital may be raised through private or public stock offerings, loans, or sales of commercial rights and licenses. Failures—or "dry holes," as they are known in the industry—have been frequent in recent HIV drug development history. In the rush for market share during the midnineties, some drugs were apparently launched into clinical trials without a full understanding of their limitations, toxicities, and doses. Yet in the pharmaceutical business model, the cost of bad decisions, bad drugs, and bad luck must be recovered by income derived from future products that successfully make it to market.

After the completion of all three phases of clinical trials, if the results successfully demonstrate safety and effectiveness, the developer files an NDA with the FDA. The application must contain all the scientific information that has been gathered. NDAs typically run 100,000 or more pages. By law, the FDA is allowed six months to review a new drug application. In almost all cases, the period between the first submission of an NDA and the final approval exceeds that limit. The average NDA review time for new synthetic molecular entities reviewed in 1991 was 30.3 months.

In recent years, the high cost of drug development has been of increasing concern to a variety of consumer groups. These groups have compared the pretax cost of bringing a new drug to market during the previous decade with the after-tax outlay on research and development (R&D) (which must also cover expenses for unsuccessful candidates) for each successful drug. The wide gap between these estimates has been challenged by numerous groups, for example, the pharmaceutical industry's trade group, Pharmaceutical Research and Manufacturers of America (PhRMA). PhRMA's mission is to defend the drug industry's image and profits. Consumers, fighting unchecked profiteering to reduce the burden of high drug prices on the poor and elderly, challenge the industry's profits and ethics with press releases and lobbying. To counter PhRMA's justification of high profits, consumer organizations routinely underplay the amount and significance of R&D performed by the pharmaceutical industry. Note that in general estimating drug development costs is not easy as a result of a variety of factors, including the fact that corporations have traditionally jealously guarded research expenses, trade secrets, and technology to mask their activity from competitors. In the past, two basic approaches have been used to gauge the outlay needed to bring a drug from laboratory to pharmacy. An estimate can be derived by analyzing several companies' drug development projects individually. A drawback to this method is the reliance on company-supplied figures for research that may not reflect actual expenses. The price of research may also be estimated by using industrywide aggregate figures for R&D, then apportioning costs among the number of drugs actually approved during the study period.

In recent years, soaring drug prices have also been of concern to numerous states (e.g., Massachusetts and Michigan) as well as a variety of consumer organizations. These entities and organizations contend that patient care is being squeezed by high drug prices and runaway health care costs. Unable to sustain ballooning Medicaid drug budgets, some states have told pharmaceutical makers either to lower prices or to face banishment of their products to a list of medications that will require third-party approval before they can be prescribed. Prior approval is a steep hurdle that effectively means that another company's drug gets Medicaid's lucrative business; prior approval can create hurdles for patients as well. Particularly vulnerable are the elderly, the disabled, and people with complicated treatment needs, including those with HIV.

The magnitude of the drug price spiral crisis is illustrated best by tracking recent data on spending on prescription drugs and on Medicaid expenditures on drugs. Shrinking state and federal budgets that have put Medicaid programs under tremendous pressure to hold down costs also contribute to the magnitude of the crisis. Many states have passed laws designed to contain state or consumer drug expenditures, and a number of experiments in tighter administration of public drug spending are under way. These responses are important to watch because trends in Medicaid often soon spread to other public health plans such as ADAP, the states' AIDS Drug Assistance Programs. Reining in mounting drug expenditures is likely to remain a significant challenge for large health care payers in the coming years. Efforts to cut prices and/or cut utilization are bound to increase, as will consumer resistance to perceived or real efforts to deny medication and, undoubtedly, industry's efforts to fight back.

drug dependence   See DRUG ADDICTION.

drug development   See DRUG APPROVAL PROCESS.

drug dosage   See DOSAGE; DOSE.

drug efficacy   See EFFICACY.

drug eruption   See ERUPTION.

drug fever   The elevation of body temperature that occurs as an unwanted manifestation of drug action. Drugs can induce fever by several mechanisms; these include allergic reactions, drug-induced tissue damage, acceleration of tissue metabolism, constriction of blood vessels in the skin with resulting decrease in loss of body heat, and direct action on the temperature-regulating center in the brain. The most common form of drug fever is associated with allergic reactions. It may be the only allergic manifestation apparent, or it may be part of a complex of allergic symptoms that can include skin rash, hives, joint swelling and pain, enlarged lymph glands, hemolytic anemia, or hepatitis. The fever usually appears about seven to 10 days after starting the drug and may vary from low-grade to alarmingly high levels. It may be sustained or intermittent, but it usually persists for as long as the drug is taken. In previously sensitized individuals, drug fever may occur within one or two hours after taking the first dose of medication. If it is the only symptom, doctors often recommend treating through the fever and the body generally adjusts to the medication without much difficulty. Two drugs often used in HIV treatment that may cause this reaction are Bactrim and amphotericin B.

drug holiday   See STRUCTURED TREATMENT INTERRUPTION.

drug interaction   The mutual pharmacological influence of two or more drugs taken concurrently. The influence may be antagonistic or synergistic and may be lethal in some cases. The chance of development of an undesired drug interaction increases as the number of drugs taken increases. People with HIV commonly take several medications at the same time to fight HIV and its related conditions. These drugs can interact, leading to more toxic side effects and reduced effectiveness. (Not all drugs interact in this way, as some may be combined without ill effect.) Vitamin or mineral supplements can also interact with drugs, causing elevations or decreases in drug availability.

Some interactions affect the way drugs are absorbed by the gastrointestinal system. Degree of absorption is highly dependent on stomach acidity and the rate of absorption; drugs that are not absorbed well do not achieve sufficient levels in the blood to exert their effects. Malabsorption can be caused by diarrhea, which is a side effect of some drugs; it can also occur if a coincident therapy increases or decreases the excretion or metabolism of a drug. Drugs with similar toxic effects usually produce combined toxicity, which may contraindicate taking both drugs together. For HIV-infected persons, the most common drug interactions are among antiretroviral drugs and drugs for PNEUMOCYSTIS CARINII PNEUMONIA and fungal infections. Interactions among TOXOPLASMOSIS, TUBERCULOSIS, *MYCOBACTERIUM AVIVM* COMPLEX, and CYTOMEGALOVIRUS medications are also common. There are thousands of potentially significant interactions for patients with HIV infections.

Effects of gender on drug interaction have not been studied extensively. Women in general react differently to some HIV drugs and women also suffer more drug reactions than men. This area continues to be unexplored by research.

A few drugs slow the functioning of the kidneys. This effect increases the blood levels of substances that are normally removed by the kidneys. The most common drug interactions involve the liver. Several drugs can slow or speed the action of liver enzymes. This effect can cause great changes in the blood levels of other drugs that are broken down by the same enzyme.

PROTEASE INHIBITORS and NNRTIs are processed by the liver and can cause many drug interactions. People taking anti-HIV drugs need to be very careful about drug interactions. Other drugs that can cause interactions are antibiotics, specifically those whose names end in the suffix -*mycin;* antifungals, specifically those that end in -*azole;* antacids; and some anticonvulsives. One food in particular that interacts with protease inhibitors is grapefruit juice. A supplement that is known to interact with protease inhibitors is St. John's wort. For people taking protease inhibitors, an often used illegal substance, MDMA, can also cause severe interaction problems that have led to death.

drug patents and pricing   The issue of the pricing of HIV drugs has been important since the creation of the first antiretroviral medicine, zidovudine (AZT). At the beginning of the epidemic, when there were no medications available, the issue of pricing was not important. However, when medications became available, it became clear that the cost was something that would need to be faced. The only people initially able to receive medications were those who were privately insured. The cost of these medications has ranged anywhere from $10,000 to $15,000 (in U.S. dollars) a year since the advent of treatment. After a few years the U.S. government began programs to cover the cost of HIV medications. These programs are called AIDS DRUG ASSISTANCE PROGRAMS (ADAPs).

Prices have been somewhat lower in Europe because of the ability of governments that run health plans to buy in bulk, whereas U.S. insurance companies and private pharmacies must pay full cost. The cost has been high because the companies hold patents that prevent other companies is the U.S. from manufacturing the drugs for 17 years. The patents for these drugs are held by large pharmaceutical companies that seem to seek to earn large amounts of money for their product while not concerning themselves with countries that cannot afford the medications. The companies have shown little interest until lately in lowering costs to allow greater access.

The ability of the multinational pharmaceutical companies to continue to charge these prices while millions of people suffer around the world has drawn fire from a number of sources. Although various solutions have been put forward by governments and individuals, few steps have been taken to get medication that works to people who need it. In 1997, after it became clear that HAART worked to decrease death rates of HIV-positive people, Nelson Mandela began a process to produce affordable generic medications in South Africa. This caused a lawsuit in South Africa by the 39 pharmaceutical companies that make up the International Federation of Pharmaceutical Manufacturers Association. After three years and the loss of millions of lives the multinational corporations dropped the lawsuit. They had in that time been under growing pressure from across the world for not allowing poor countries to provide access to the medication for their people. Through the media attention directed by the South African nonprofit Treatment Action Campaign (http://www.tac.org.za/), people around the world pressured the pharmaceutical companies to drop their case. Large demonstrations at the Durban International AIDS Conference highlighted the problem for many in the world through the media attending the conference.

In addition, about that time Brazil and Thailand began production of their own generic drugs to treat HAART. The costs of providing HAART dropped to less than $4,000 U.S. per person, including the cost of creating the companies to make the drugs. Thailand began exporting their generic drugs, drawing fire from many pharmaceutical companies. In 2001, the Indian pharmaceutical company CIPLA agreed to begin providing HAART treatments to African governments at the price of $600 U.S. per person per year. If nonprofit companies distribute the medications free, the cost is even lower at $350 U.S. per person per year. Groups in Kenya have begun to purchase drugs for distribution after the pharmaceutical giants did not

drop their prices to compete with Indian companies or the inexpensive donations provided by Brazilian corporations.

Finally, in 2002, pharmaceutical companies in the developed countries have begun to lower prices and provide stepped pricing in an attempt to maintain some sense of responsibility. Several pharmaceutical companies at the Barcelona International AIDS Conference agreed to a program through which the cost of HAART per year would be based on the resources of people in the median range of income in the Caribbean region. This would place the costs within the reach of many in Jamaica and the Dominican Republic but may still place them out of the reach of people in Guyana or Haiti. The cost reduction is said to be almost 90 percent of the cost of treatment in the United States.

How long these price reductions last and how long the generic manufacturers can continue producing drugs remain to be seen. Currently international intellectual property rights that are specified in the World Trade Organization (WTO) treaties state that in 2006, patents in one country must be adhered to in all countries that are members of the WTO. Currently India does not accept these regulations; nor does South Africa. Brazil is a member of the WTO but has ignored the requirements along with Thailand. A country that is not part of WTO, Cuba, signed a treaty in 2001 with South Africa to develop and produce jointly generic versions of several HIV medications. Whether an agreement before that agreement goes into production will continue to allow access or whether the costs will return to desired corporate levels remains to be seen.

A faculty member of Yale University and the Brookings Institution, Jean O. Lanjouw, has suggested a proposal to overcome the problems in patents and pricing. Whether this proposal will ever be accepted is yet to be seen. It is difficult to see that multinational corporations would accept a proposal that would limit their profits in any manner. The proposal is to use a procedural change in the patent offices of rich countries: to make pharmaceutical companies choose whether to protect their new drug patents in rich countries or in poor countries—but not in both. For diseases such as cancer, that affect people in both rich and poor countries, companies would choose to protect their patents in rich countries—allowing low-cost generic copies to be sold in poor countries, which are a negligible market in comparison. But for diseases such as malaria, which almost exclusively affect poor countries, companies would choose patent protection in poor countries. In theory prices would not be prohibitive, as the medications would have to be priced for poor countries in order to sell at all.

Treatment activists like Zackie Achmat of South Africa, however, continue to call for generic production of medications. He says that the drug companies' current lowered costs and gifts of medications are neither guaranteed nor sustainable in the long term and will cost more lives in the long run. Treatment has been shown to work, and Achmat believes that treatment needs to be recognized as an essential public good as outlined in World Health Organization economics reports. He has spent several years heading up TAC's program of trying to gain access to medications by the poor of Africa, sometimes from jail.

drug overdose   Literally, any excess dose of a drug, but in ordinary usage, the self-administration, accidental or not, of a potentially lethal amount of a drug of abuse.

drug paraphernalia laws   In effect in virtually every state in the nation, drug paraphernalia laws make it a crime to deliver or possess with intent to deliver, virtually any item that could be used in connection with illegal drug use, with the knowledge that it will be so used. There must be criminal intent to supply or use such items for unlawful purposes in order for there to be a crime. Selling or distributing hypodermic needles and syringes without knowledge that they will be used to inject illicit drugs are not offenses under these statutes.

Drug paraphernalia laws erect formidable obstacles for illicit IV drug users, especially those attempting to comply with public health advice to use sterile injection equipment. (The definition of drug paraphernalia in these laws is so broad that it could conceivably be read to include bleach distributed with the intent that it be used to clean hypodermic needles.) Even if a user can buy sterile equipment over the counter, she or he may be prosecuted under these statutes if it is found in her

or his possession. In order to escape prosecution a user must demonstrate that she or he has a valid medical purpose for it. Drug paraphernalia laws not only significantly limit the supply of sterile equipment on the street but also provide a marked disincentive for users to have sterile equipment. Drug paraphernalia laws therefore constitute a significant barrier to effective public health practices. See NEEDLE PRESCRIPTION LAWS.

drug reaction   Adverse and undesired reaction to a substance taken for its pharmacological effects.

drug receptor   See RECEPTOR.

drug regulation reform   The Kefauver Amendments passed by Congress in 1962 first vested the FOOD AND DRUG ADMINISTRATION, already responsible for the safety of drugs, with the responsibility to ensure their efficacy as well. This mandate is the cornerstone of drug regulation today. Well publicized debates between AIDS activists and the agency concerning the approval of AIDS drugs have attracted media attention since the beginning of the epidemic. Legislative proposals to significantly reshape the mandate of the FDA began to receive serious attention in Washington in 1995. Although the FDA has always claimed a mandate to advance the public health, the responsibility to keep harmful products off the market has always taken precedence over ensuring that helpful products reach the market. Now the balance is starting to shift the other way. Many of the current suggestions for reforming the FDA would significantly alter its authority. Among the items under discussion are measures that would shift more efficacy studies to a "post-market" setting; utilize local INSTITUTIONAL REVIEW BOARDS to review proposals for early human testing (phase I clinical trials) of drugs; privatize certain drug safety reviews by relegating them to independent testing or accrediting institutions; permit the promotion of FDA-approved drugs for "OFF-LABEL" (not prescribed) uses; impose statutory time limits on FDA reviews; harmonize American with international standards; and remove export barriers for non FDA-approved drugs. Although AIDS activists sparked much of the discussion in the first place, their intention has never been to debilitate the agency; like many more traditional consumer groups, they are now worried that many so-called reform proposals would do just that—and what is worse, might actually diminish the number of effective drugs developed in the future. AIDS activists will both continue to play a major role in the FDA reform debate and be key players in the evaluation of FDA reform proposals from the standpoint of people with life-threatening disease.

drug resistance   The ability of disease-causing microorganisms to evade the drugs designed to eradicate them. Microbial resistance has emerged as one of the major problems in treating infectious diseases. Along with other factors (the emergence of new disease agents, HIV infection, and the use of therapeutic drugs that depress the immune system), microbial resistance has helped to raise the rate of illness and death from infectious diseases in the last 15 years. As germs have developed defenses to penicillin and other widely used antibiotics, diseases like pneumonia and tuberculosis, which were once simply and easily vanquished, have become more difficult to eradicate.

It is commonly believed that it is genetic agility that enables bacteria to become resistant. As single-celled organisms, bacteria divide many times a day, and every division provides an opportunity for a DNA mutation. Some mutations create new genes that are harmful to the bacteria. Others result in changes that are beneficial. Bacteria also occasionally pick up a few new genes from their fellows. They can do so through conjugation—a primitive form of sexual activity in which two cells join together and, in the process, may exchange plasmids—gene-carrying structures outside the chromosomes. Genes can also be transferred by viruses that infect bacteria.

Occasionally, genes acquired through mutation, plasmids, or viral infection confer bacterial resistance. Some genes enable the bacteria to make proteins like penicillinase, which deactivate antibiotics. Other proteins serve as pumps to clear antibiotics out of the bacterium before the drugs have a chance to do any damage. Genetic changes may also alter structural proteins that once served as entry or attachment sites for antibiotics, effectively locking the cellular doorway to these drugs. The end result is the same: drugs are ineffective against the bacte-

ria. With antibiotics, most of the bacteria are wiped out, but the fraction that remain, because they carry the resistance gene, survive to reproduce. This scenario repeats to some degree each time an antibiotic is used. If the resistant bacteria become numerous enough to make themselves known, the original antibiotic is likely to be prescribed again. This time, however, it won't work as well; many of the bacteria are impervious to its effects. In this way, many drugs that were once considered fail-safe have been rendered ineffective. In some cases, bacteria that are resistant to one drug can be eliminated with another one. Eventually, though, strains that are resistant to the second antibiotic will spring up.

The proliferation of resistant microbes is a consequence of the overuse of antibiotics. Much of the problem has industrial and commercial origins. These drugs are routinely added to cattle and poultry feed to produce bigger and healthier livestock. However, the practice also turns the animals into a breeding ground for resistant bacteria. We ultimately consume these pathogens as we eat the meat on our tables.

Antibiotics are also more loosely regulated in some parts of the world. They are available over the counter in many countries, and the resultant overuse has produced resistant strains that have been disseminated via international travel.

Microbial resistance can be corrected. When antibiotics are not used for a time, the slower-growing resistant strains lose their advantage and gradually are eliminated. While we as individuals have little influence over the agriculture industry or foreign drug sales, there are a few things we can do to stem the time of bacterial resistance: (1) don't demand antibiotics for colds (most colds are the result of viral infections, which are unfazed by antibiotics); (2) don't take antibiotics to prevent infection (i.e., to ward off traveler's diarrhea or to prevent urinary-tract infections); (3) consider vaccination (immunization with a vaccine called Pneumovax can prevent not only pneumonia and meningitis, but ear and blood infections as well); (4) use antibiotics only as directed; (5) follow a healthy lifestyle; and (6) keep your hands clean.

drug tolerance   A condition in which the body develops the ability to withstand or overcome the effects of a drug and therefore greater and greater amounts are needed to be effective. This can develop, for example, in patients being treated with painkillers or undergoing chemotherapy.

drug trial Also known as a CLINICAL TRIAL; the clinical experiment through which researchers determine the effectiveness of different forms of treatment.

drug use The issue of drug use, particularly in the face of HIV/AIDS. In ordinary usage, synonymous with DRUG ABUSE.

drug user See DRUG ABUSE.

drug-drug interaction See DRUG INTERACTION.

drug-fast See DRUG-RESISTANT.

drug-resistant Resistant to the action of a drug or drugs; drug fast. Said of infectious agents or diseases. Drug-resistant disease, such as multiple-drug resistant tuberculosis and AZT-resistant strains of HIV, are well understood by modern medicine. A resistant bacterial strain can transfer its resistance to other bacterial strains through resistance transfer factors and transposons (transposable genetic elements). It is a public health imperative to prevent endemic levels of drug-resistant diseases through prudent prescription of antibiotics. A basic tenet of medical ethics requires that antibiotics never be prescribed before performing a "culture and sensitivity" test, a set of diagnostic techniques to determine the most effective antibiotic to be used in a given case and the briefest duration of treatment needed to control or cure the illness. Today, the dangers of physicians' presumptive diagnoses and excessive use of antibiotics, antifungals, antiprotozoals, and antivirals are evident in the increasing drug resistances of formerly treatable diseases. Two types of resistance are recognized—immunity and inherent resistance. Immunity is resistance associated with the presence of antibodies having a specific action on infectious microorganisms. Inherent resistance is the ability to resist disease independently of antibodies.

Many of the antimicrobial drugs used indiscriminately today as prophylaxis for HIV/AIDS OPPOR-TUNISTIC INFECTIONS were originally intended to be used only for brief periods, for the treatment of specific disorders proved susceptible to given drugs through culture and sensitivity testing. A closer look at these drugs, many of which are frequently used for lifetime duration in people with AIDS, may be needed. Concern has been expressed, for example, about the immunosuppression inherent in many of these drugs (especially antibiotics and antivirals) and the fact that they are commonly used in combinations of three or more in an already immune-compromised subject.

dry kiss Also called a social kiss; a kiss with no exchange of saliva.

dry sex Sex that doesn't involve mucous membrane or secretion contact.

DSMB See DATA SAFETY AND MONITORING BOARD.

DSPN See DISTAL SYMMETRIC POLYNEUROPATHY.

DTC See DIETHYLDITHIOCARBAMATE; IMUTHIOL.

DTH See DELAYED-TYPE HYPERSENSITIVITY.

dual-energy X-ray absorptiometry See DEXA SCAN.

durable power of attorney See POWER OF ATTORNEY.

duty to warn Within the context of AIDS, there exists both the patient's duty to warn and the practitioner's duty to warn. The standard says that it is the responsibility of a person who is HIV positive or has AIDS to notify one's sexual partner, or partners, that she is infected with a sexually transmitted disease; this notification must occur before engaging in activities by which a disease might be transmitted. Similarly, this standard requires warnings prior to sharing needles. Some argue that this duty is increased if a pregnancy could result from the unprotected sexual encounter because of the risk of transmission of HIV to the fetus. An individual's duty to warn is probably paramount to the therapist's duty to protect, except in those cases where the patient is mentally incompetent to understand the duty to warn or is actually unable to warn his or her partner. It is generally advised that practitioners should educate clients about the duty to warn their prospective partners and to engage only in safe behavior. Practitioners should also encourage and monitor their client's progress in the fulfillment of these duties. If a patient appears uneasy about informing sexual or needle-sharing partners, then the therapist should offer his or her services to counsel the partners of the patient.

Today, there is probably no issue that causes as much consternation among mental health practitioners as does the "duty to warn" or *Tarasoff* duty. At issue in the *Tarasoff I* case is the basic balance between safeguarding the confidentiality of a patient and protecting others from a patient's violent tendencies. Justice Tobriner of the California Supreme Court said in the *Tarasoff I* case, "Protective privilege ends where public peril begins." The case of *Tarasoff v. Regents of the University of California (UC)* (1976) involved a voluntary psychiatric outpatient evaluated and treated at the UC Berkeley Student Health Service. The patient, Prosenjit Poddar, revealed during therapy with a staff psychologist that as a part of his obsession with a Berkeley student, Tatiana Tarasoff, he had fantasies about harming and perhaps even killing her. In addition, a friend of Poddar's revealed to the psychologist that Poddar planned to purchase a gun. During this period, a staff psychiatrist who had originally evaluated Poddar appropriately prescribed a neuroleptic drug. Despite this intervention, both the psychologist and the psychiatrist became concerned about Poddar's violent tendencies. When Poddar discontinued therapy, the two professionals became particularly concerned and determined that Poddar should be evaluated for hospitalization. Upon their request, the campus police went to see Poddar and questioned him about his intentions toward Tarasoff. When Poddar denied any desire to harm her, the police left. Two months later, Poddar stabbed and killed Tarasoff. Tarasoff's parents sued the practitioners and the UC police for the wrongful death of their daughter, arguing that the university had the duty to protect their daughter from the harm threatened by Poddar during his therapy sessions, despite the privacy privilege Poddar could have asserted. The Supreme Court ruled that the Student Health

Service could be found negligent in its duty to protect Tarasoff because it failed to take the necessary steps to insulate her from the harm fantasized by Poddar in therapy sessions. The Court established the basic standard that "When a therapist determines . . . that his patient presents a serious danger of violence to another, he incurs a serious obligation to use reasonable care to protect the intended victim from such danger."

The standard of *Tarasoff*, as later codified in a California statute, allows warning the third party of the patient's threatened violence only when there is a genuine psychotherapist-patient relationship, when the patient has communicated to the therapist a serious and imminent threat of physical violence against another, and when the threat is against a reasonable identifiable victim or victims. In the absence of these elements, the duty to warn or to protect the third party does not arise, and the therapist should be free from liability. If there is a duty to warn or protect under these limited circumstances, the duty shall be discharged through the therapist's reasonable efforts to communicate the threat to the intended victim or victims and to an appropriate law enforcement agency.

Rulings in other duty to warn cases also help to understand how the *Tarasoff* standard applies in the AIDS crisis. A discussion of duty to warn and a decision tree is available in "Assessing dangerousness and responding appropriately: Hedlund expands the clinician's liability established in Tarasoff" by B. H. Gross, M. J. Southard, H. R. Lamb, and L. E. Weinberger (*Journal of Clinical Psychiatry* 48: 1, 1987). Rulings on this question indicate that the *Tarasoff* duty to protect is a fairly limited one, subject to considerations of the clarity of the patient's threat, the actuality of danger to another, the identification of the potential victim(s), the imminence of danger, and the suitability of the patient to other psychosocial intervention to prevent the threatened harm.

Applying these standards to the issues raised by AIDS requires additional analysis. The risk of HIV infection—the "imminent danger"—is still medically unclear. As concerns "unsafe sex" and "unsafe intravenous needle use," what behavior threatens others with "imminent or impending danger"? In addition, although there are clinical reports of people who were infected after one exposure to the virus, there is still a debate about how many sexual or needle exposures are necessary to cause infection. In this context, it is extremely difficult to say what constitutes "imminent danger." Similarly, "imminent danger" cannot include past exposures to HIV. The standard only refers to those future dangers that the practitioner can prevent. A therapist cannot be held liable for failing to prevent infection in those cases in which a patient has exposed a partner to HIV prior to the therapist's knowledge of the possible danger to the partner. Even if a couple becomes aware of the situation, the therapist will probably not be held liable for the HIV infection of the partner, since the partner cannot prove that HIV transmission occurred after the therapist became aware of the couple's sexual practices. The window period after HIV transmission during which antibodies have not formed but HIV is present and may be transmitted complicates the definitive establishment of infection. If testing occurs during the window period, an infected person may test antibody negative.

The standard of "imminent danger" is also obscured by judicial decisions in other states. These courts have interpreted *Tarasoff* more broadly to require psychotherapists and physicians to warn others of the danger their patients may pose if the risk of disease transmission is merely foreseeable. It appears that, at least for now, before a therapist can be held liable for failing to warn the other party of the "imminent danger," he or she would have to know the following facts: the patient is HIV infected; the parties engage in unsafe behavior on a regular basis; such behavior is actually unsafe; the patient intends to continue such behavior even after being counseled to desist by the therapist; HIV transmission will likely occur in the future. Exposure to HIV in any other context would not be an "imminent danger" invoking the practitioner's duty to warn.

A final complicating factor involves the identification of parties. If a patient names only one or a few sexual or needle-sharing partners, a practitioner can easily identify those people who may be warned about a possible exposure to HIV. But when a patient engages in frequent anonymous contacts with large numbers of people, the practitioner probably cannot be held liable for failure to warn these unknown persons. Nonetheless, thera-

pists do have a duty to treat obsessive or compulsive behavior that may endanger the world at large, and, if this therapy fails, they have a duty to take whatever steps toward legal intervention are available in their communities.

Other issues relevant to the duty to warn include liability for improper warning, the disclosure of HIV-related information by medical doctors, standards of knowledge for different types of practitioners, and PARTNER NOTIFICATION or CONTACT TRACING.

dying The condition in which death is imminent.

dying trajectory A graphic representation of the dying process. Time is recorded along the horizontal axis and nearness to death along the vertical axis. The condition of a dying individual is plotted across time, with the resulting curve being the dying trajectory.

dyke A sometimes pejorative term, depending on context, for LESBIAN.

dysesthesia (dysaesthesia) An impairment or a distortion in the senses, especially that of touch. Dysesthesia may be any unusual or unpleasant feeling associated with any area of the body that is generated by touch. In HIV it is most often in relation to PERIPHERAL NEUROPATHY. Affected individuals often report burning feelings or sharp stabs of pain from simple walking or touching of objects with their feet or hands. Some medications may also cause symptoms that can be labeled as dysesthesia. Herpes simplex often causes local dysesthesia for a day or two before the outbreak of a rash occurs.

dysfunction In medicine, abnormal, disturbed, impaired, or inadequate function of an organ or system or failure to function. The term is often used to denote sexual problems and is also applied to social structures, such as the family.

dyspareunia Occurrence of pain in the labial, vaginal, or pelvic areas during or after sexual intercourse. Dyspareunia is caused by infections in the reproductive tract; inadequate vaginal lubrication; uterine myomata; endometriosis; atrophy of vaginal mucosa; psychosomatic causes; and vaginal foreign bodies. Treatment includes specific therapy for the primary disease and counseling with respect to appropriate vaginal and vulval lubrication.

dyspepsia Digestive upset, which may include flatulence, heartburn, nausea, or vomiting.

dysphagia Difficulty in swallowing. The most common cause of dysphagia is an infection by CANDIDA ALBICANS, a fungus that can be easily treated. Less frequent causes are HERPES or CMV infections. In some cases dysphagia has no readily apparent cause. The usual method of finding the cause of dysphagia is ENDOSCOPY, a procedure in which a tube is placed in the esophagus to view and biopsy the lesions. X-ray examinations are also employed. In many cases, neither of these tests is considered necessary; a patient is presumed to have a candida infection if he or she has thrush and if swallowing is painful.

dysplasia Abnormal growth in cells and tissues.

dyspnea Difficult or labored breathing; shortness of breath. Dyspnea is sometimes accompanied by pain.

dysthymia A term used by the American Psychiatric Association to refer to a mild but generally chronic form of depression. It is not the same as major depression. Both conditions do occur in the same people. Major depression is episodic, meaning it is usually a time-specific episode. Dysthymia affects people over a long period, when they never feel good about their lives. Dysthymia tends to run in families. It has been shown to respond well to treatment with antidepressants, but marked improvement may take longer. *Dysthymia* may be the term used to describe someone who is suffering from an ongoing bereavement reaction, as occurred during the years when AIDS deaths were far more numerous in the United States.

dysuria A burning feeling during urination.

EA See EMERGENCY ASSISTANCE.

ear piercing Since the needle used to pierce ears does come into contact with blood, it is possible to become infected with HIV if the needle was previously used on an HIV-infected person and not properly cleaned and sterilized. Most places that pierce ears, however, clean their equipment with alcohol before each use, so the risk of contracting the virus this way is very small.

early access Early access to drugs and therapies for the treatment of HIV infection. This also includes access to promising new drugs and therapies. See EARLY INTERVENTION.

early cases See EARLY HIV INFECTION.

early HIV infection The stage of HIV infection during which no major physical health symptoms are yet present, though emotional or psychological difficulties are likely to develop. Today, considerable attention is paid to early HIV infection for several reasons. First, it is widely recognized that the evaluation and management of early HIV infection is of critical importance. Second, recognition of early infection is becoming more common, due in large part to more widespread HIV testing and earlier diagnosis. Third, the prevalence of early HIV infection is increasing in proportion to later stages of infection. Fourth, early medical and psychosocial intervention is most effective in delaying the onset of life-threatening symptoms and diseases and in maintaining good health. Finally, early patient education often facilitates increased patient involvement in treatment and better access to services and helps prevent further spread of the disease.

Essential components of early HIV care include assessment of immune function; initiation of antiretroviral treatment and prophylaxis for *PNEUMOCYSTIS CARINII* PNEUMONIA; evaluation and management of infection with mycobacterium tuberculosis and syphilis; oral, eye, and gynecologic assessment; and reproductive counseling. Evaluation usually begins with a medical, sexual, and substance-use history, followed by a physical examination with attention to HIV-related complications. Providers caring for adolescents or children need to consider a range of age-specific issues, including assessment of physical maturity, psychosocial aspects of adolescence, and impediments to assessing care. Providers caring for women, including pregnant women, need to be cognizant of a range of gender-specific issues. Finally, providers caring for infants need to be aware of the fact that HIV infection frequently progresses more rapidly in infants and children than in adults, and the disease characteristics are different. Early diagnosis and evaluation of the immune system are vital, and the disease must be managed aggressively.

early intervention Action taken to protect the health of an HIV-infected person before his or her immune system becomes seriously weakened and OPPORTUNISTIC INFECTIONS develop. Because early HIV infection presents itself differently in adults, adolescents, children, and infants, treatment recommendations vary from group to group. Guidelines for primary care providers as well as adults with early HIV infection generally pertain to monitoring CD4 lymphocytes, initiating antiretroviral therapy and *PNEUMOCYSTIS CARINII* PNEUMONIA prophylaxis, testing and preventative therapy for tuberculosis, and testing, and treatment for syphilis. Special considerations for treating early HIV infection in women include Pap smears, pregnancy counseling, and access of women with HIV infection to clinical trials and investigational treatments. Because HIV-infected individuals experience a range of unique oral conditions in addition to dental problems common to all individuals, both specialized and routine oral care is required by individuals with HIV infection. Similarly, because of the wide range of ocular complications associated with HIV disease, specialized and routine eye examinations are required by individuals with HIV infection.

early stopping   A condition or provision incorporated into the design of a clinical trial that enables investigators to terminate patient recruitment or treatment if data accumulated during the trial strongly indicate an adverse or beneficial treatment effect. The term is also used to characterize an action involving termination of a study treatment in a trial because of adverse or beneficial treatment effects.

early treatment   See EARLY INTERVENTION.

Eastern Europe and Central Asia   These two regions are grouped together because they make up what used to be the Soviet Union. They still have many common characteristics despite the wide range of cultures, languages, and religions. Between 1999 and the end of 2001 the number of HIV-positive individuals jumped from 400,000 to well over 1,000,000, nearly tripling in two years. According to UNAIDS, this region is now the area with the fastest-growing AIDS epidemic in the world. In Russia, the number of cases has doubled each of the last four years. The Ukraine has reached a level of 1 percent of their population who are HIV-positive. The Ukraine now has the dubious honor of having more HIV-positive persons than any country in Eastern or Western Europe at close to 300,000. In 1999 Estonia only registered 12 cases of HIV; in 2001 they numbered nearly 1,500. A similar story is also being told in Latvia and Kazakhstan, where numbers that were minimal jumped tremendously in two years. Countries that had no HIV cases two years ago now report many cases. HIV is still new in the areas of Georgia, Kyrgyzstan, Armenia, and Uzbekistan, yet

they are reporting great numbers of IDU spread cases. The countries of the former Soviet bloc now have the highest rate of new infections in the world: a rate higher than Southern Africa's.

According to several sources the region is experiencing this explosion in HIV for several reasons. There is a great deal of unemployment because these countries are all trying to switch to a market economy after many years in a centralized, government-controlled economic system. There are also many people who have gone abroad for work, including large numbers of women who are sex workers in other countries. These people return to their home countries and then spread the virus. In addition, there is a fairly high incidence of intravenous drug use in the countries of the former Soviet Union. It remains the main vector in the Baltic countries and Russia. Although this is the way the virus began in the Ukraine, recently the majority of cases have been spread through heterosexual sex. IDU HIV-positive rates in some Russian cities have exceeded 25 percent. A strong overlap between groups is known to exist in these countries, also. In Serbia 20 percent of sex workers are known to use injection drugs, and nearly 20 percent of men who have sex with men (MSM) are known to be IDUs. In northern reaches of Russia, the city of Murmansk is having an outbreak of HIV, traced to unsafe sex and IDUs. Concern has been expressed about this city in particular because of its location near the border of Finland and Norway, where HIV rates have been very low. The rate of infection at the end of 2001 in Murmansk had increased seven times from the rate in 2000.

Another factor that concerns public health workers is the lack of health facilities or access to health care in these countries. Many of these areas have seen a decline in standard of living since their entrance to market economies. There have been outbreaks of STDs, which would indicate the occurrence of a great deal of unprotected sex. There have also been large outbreaks in this region of several illnesses: tuberculosis, malaria, influenza, typhoid, and others. These outbreaks indicate that health care in these areas has declined considerably. In addition, some of the Central Asian countries have lower rates of literacy and in surveys very few of the sexually active population have known what AIDS is or how to prevent it. Some reports out of Central Asia indicate that workers are often paid in drugs instead of money because drugs are more readily available.

In Romania, a country affected early in the epidemic, struggles continue. Many children were infected early in Romania as a resulted of infected blood that the government had not removed from the market or reused syringes that the medical facilities were forced to use. Many children were left in government care after their parents' death. It has come to light recently that many people in Romania can no longer afford treatment that was available to them. Romania today still has the largest number of pediatric AIDS cases in all of Europe and Central Asia. Although pediatric AIDS cases transmitted by infected of blood or syringes have declined since the early 1990s, adult cases of HIV infection have tripled in the last four years.

In one of the stranger stories of the HIV epidemic, several Bulgarian physicians who had been working in Libya were charged in 1999 with purposely infecting nearly 400 Libyan children as part of a Western spy plot to undermine the Libyan government. The seven doctors and nurses have been held in Libya since that date and the trial has not yet begun.

In Poland, though, officials instituted a strong education program with IDUs and the rate of infection has dropped considerably. Other former communist countries such as Slovenia, the Czech Republic, and Hungary have retained a low rate of infection by instituting strong, broad education programs on HIV. Recent budget increases in AIDS education funding in the Ukraine and Russia might offer some hope to these areas also.

However, experts do not believe that most of the region will be able to slow the epidemic with current levels of funding. In Russia predictions have been made by the director of the Russian Federal Anti-AIDS Center that between 2 percent and 7 percent of the Russian population will be HIV-positive by 2005. The World Bank predicts that by 2005 $10 billion a year will be needed to fund the public education programs necessary to prevent the infection rate from climbing in these poor countries.

eat See ORAL SEX.

Ebola virus disease A disease caused by a virus classed as a member of the family Filoviridae. It is an acute condition characterized by sudden onset of a high fever, prostration, vomiting, and diarrhea, followed by uremia, rash, hemorrhaging, and central nervous system damage. It is usually fatal. The disease can be transmitted by handling tissues and cells from African green monkeys, but in some cases the source of infection is unknown. Its first known victim come from a village near the Ebola River in Zaire (Congo) in 1976.

Clinically, this disease is almost identical to that caused by the MARBURG VIRUS, but the two viruses are not antigenically related. The virus has three subtypes: Ebola Reston, Ebola Sudan, and Ebola Zaire. There is no specific therapy to date.

EBV See EPSTEIN-BARR VIRUS.

Echinacea The leaves and root of the herb *Echinacea* (*E. angustifolia* or *E. prupurea*) have been used by Native Americans for a broad range of pains and illnesses. Echinaecein is the substance that knits skin and prevents germs from penetrating tissues. Possibly the most important aspect of *Echinacea* is its immunostimulant capability for infectious diseases and other conditions like tonsilitis, bladder infections, colds, flu, and boils. The roots of this herb are used as a tonic and blood purifier, as well as for a variety of other conditions, and other pains and wounds. Advocates of the therapeutic value of *Echinacea* have cited test tube and animal studies to support these claims. Injections of purified *Echinacea* are believed to be relatively nontoxic even at high doses, although there have been reports of skin rashes and insomnia. Few clinical trials have been performed using either injected polysaccharides or oral over-the-counter *Echinacea* supplements, the most common form of this remedy, and its effects and ideal dosing are, to date, unknown.

Immunostimulating herbs such as *Echinacea* have become controversial in HIV therapy. A stimulus to CD4+ cells might help the body or might lead to increased replication. Boosting some of the immune system's chemical messengers (CYTOKINES) may help the body, while boosting others may lead to disease progression. Further research in people with HIV is needed.

echocardiography A noninvasive diagnostic technique for examining the heart by directing beams of ultrasonic waves through the chest wall to produce a graphic record of internal cardiac structures. All cardiac valves can be visualized, and the dimensions of each ventricle and the left atrium can be measured. Also called ULTRASONIC CARDIOGRAPHY.

ecstasy   See MDMA.

ecthyma   An ulcerative inflammation of the skin caused by infection and marked by lesions with crusts or scabs. Variable scarring and pigmentation may result.

ectopic pregnancy   Ectopic pregnancy occurs when a fertilized egg attaches itself to tissue outside the uterus. There is usually a poorly developed decidual reaction in the uterus. Symptoms may include amenorrhea; tenderness, soreness, pain on affected side; pallor, weak pulse, signs of shock or hemorrhage; reflected shoulder pain; bluish discoloration of the umbilicus. Ectopic pregnancy may occur in the free abdominal cavity, in the interstitial portion of the tube, in the ovary, or in the fallopian tube (in the interstitial, ampullar, or isthmic portion). Ectopic pregnancy may be unruptured or ruptured. Irregular hemorrhage, vague pains in the abdomen (usually on one side), and amenorrhea may or may not be present in unruptured ectopic pregnancies. Diagnosis at this stage can be made by the usual biological tests for pregnancy. For ruptured ectopic pregnancies without a severe hemorrhage there is severe pain in the lower abdomen with repeated fainting spells. Diagnosis is made by a transvaginal needle puncture into the peritoneal cavity. This will reveal free blood. If bleeding is severe and surgical therapy is not instituted without delay, death may result.

ectropion   A condition in which the outer CERVIX is covered by cells that would normally be found in the inner cervix.

edema   A local or generalized swelling characterized by excessively large amounts of fluid in the body tissues. It may result from increased permeability of the capillary walls; increased capillary pressure due to venous obstruction or heart fail-ure; lymphatic obstruction; disturbances in renal functioning; reduction of plasma proteins; inflammatory conditions; fluid and electrolyte disturbances; malnutrition; starvation; and chemical substances. It may also occur by diffusion.

Education for All Handicapped Children Act   Congress passed the Education for All Handicapped Children Act in 1975 to meet the special educational needs of children who are mentally retarded, hard of hearing, deaf, speech impaired, visually handicapped, seriously emotionally disturbed, or orthopedically impaired, or other health impaired children, including children with AIDS, or children with specific learning disabilities.

EEG   See ELECTROENCEPHALOGRAM.

efavirenz   DuPont Pharmaceutical's once-a-day nonnucleoside reverse transcriptase inhibitor (NNRTI) for combination use with other antiretroviral agents for adults and children with HIV infection. Ways to add efavirenz that are supported by clinical data include combination with only a PROTEASE INHIBITOR, with a protease inhibitor plus one or more NUCLEOSIDE ANALOGS, or with two nucleoside analogs alone. The simplest regimen is to spare the nucleoside analogs and use efavirenz plus a protease inhibitor only. Efavirenz when added to protease inhibitor plus nucleoside analogs provides extra insurance as first-line therapy and succeeds in many instances as SALVAGE THERAPY for people for whom protease inhibitors fail whether because of viral rebound or of side effects. Individuals who do not obtain adequate HIV suppression with protease inhibitors may have no choice but to move to a protease-sparing regimen.

Efavirenz stays in the body for a long time and therefore is taken only once a day. Before replacing a protease inhibitor with efavirenz, one should remember that efavirenz can have toxicities. Efavirenz is associated with a rise in cholesterol and triglycerides, unlike other NNRTIs. First, it is not yet clear whether the lipid abnormalities observed with protease inhibitors are due to these compounds' effect on the liver or are a less obvious side effect or lingering consequence of long-term HIV infection. Besides profoundly inhibiting HIV, efavirenz does affect liver metabolism, in this case by stimulating the CYP3A enzyme pathway that metabolizes many drugs. Aside from various drug interactions, the other side effects are mainly neurological, in particular, dizziness, vivid dreams, and euphoria. These symptoms usually, but do not always, recede after the first month. They can be ameliorated by taking efavirenz at bedtime. One odd neurological side effect is indicated by reports that those on efavirenz can test positive for marijuana use. This can pose serious problems for individuals in certain jobs. Other major efavirenz side effects involve skin rashes, which are almost always mild to moderate and transient. There have been concerns about fetal outcomes of pregnant women exposed to efavirenz. Because of findings in studies with animals, DuPont has issued warnings that women on efavirenz use two methods of birth control (one a barrier method) to prevent pregnancy. Finally, note that a major fear about efavirenz use is its tendency to cause birth defects, which has been observed during trials with animals. (Trade names are Sustiva and DMP 266.)

effector   An organ or part of an immune system that becomes active in response to stimulation.

effector cells   The active cells of the immune system responsible for destroying or controlling foreign antibodies. Also cell or organ by which an animal responds to internal or external stimuli, often via the nervous system.

effervescent tablet   A tablet that fizzes to dissolve when placed in water.

efficacy   Effectiveness; the power or ability to produce intended effects or results, for example the ability of a drug to control or cure an illness. Efficacy should be distinguished from activity, which refers to a drug's immediate effects on a microbe triggering a disease.

eflornithine   An antineoplastic and antiprotozoal drug. It has been used to treat African sleeping sickness. (Trade name is Ornidyl.)

EIA   See ENZYME IMMUNOASSAY.

ejaculate   To release seminal fluid through the penis; the fluid emitted during ejaculation.

ejaculation   The release of semen from an erect penis, during orgasm.

electroencephalogram (EEG)   A record of the electrical activity of the brain obtained by placing electrodes at various locations on the scalp in order to measure the electrical potential. The recording device is called an *electroencephalograph.*

electroencephalography   Amplification, recording, and analysis of the electrical activity of the brain. This technique has proved useful as a diagnostic tool in studying convulsive disorders such as epilepsy and in locating cerebral lesions. The record obtained is called an ELECTROENCEPHALO-GRAM (EEG).

electrolyte   A solution that is a conductor of electricity; a substance that yields ions in solution so that its solutions conduct an electric current. Also ionized salt in blood, tissue fluids, and cells, including chloride, sodium, and potassium.

electrolyte abnormality   A deviation from the normal condition in electrolytes.

electron microscope   A large and very powerful microscope that uses a beam of electrons to enlarge the image of a very small object, such as a virus, and replicate it on a screen.

eligibility criteria   The conditions that determine a person's suitability for a clinical trial or research study. Examples include age, symptoms (of HIV or other illness) exhibited, results of certain lab tests, overall health, and past treatment received. To be suited for a study, a person's health picture has to match all the study's needs. He or she must meet not only the research plan's inclusion criteria (conditions that must be present), but its exclusion criteria (conditions that must be absent). Both the "must have" and the "cannot have" checklists help doctors get clear research results.

Eligibility criteria are generally divided into two sections: inclusion and exclusion criteria. Inclusion criteria specify who can participate; the second criteria specify who cannot. Sometimes it is not clear which category a particular criterion is in. As a general rule, though inclusion criteria define the population the trial intends to represent, and exclusion criteria define the exceptions.

ELISA   See ENZYME-LINKED IMMUNOSORBENT ASSAY.

emaciation   State of being extremely lean. An emaciated person is excessively thin or lacking in normal amount of tissue.

embryopathy   Any pathological condition in an embryo.

Emergency Assistance (EA)   A federal-state welfare program that makes onetime crisis payments to or on behalf of low-income families with children and, in many states, the poor aged and disabled.

emivirine   An experimental NNRTI that is no longer in development. Studies revealed that emivirine caused a more rapid breakdown of other drugs metabolized by the CYTOCHROME P450 enzyme. (Trade names are Coactinon and MKC-442.)

empiric therapy   Treatment based on a clinician's judgment of the patient's symptoms and signs, offered before a diagnosis has been confirmed.

employee benefits   Benefits, given to an employee, apart from salary, as part of his or her employment. Healthcare and financial benefits are the most common employee benefits. These are distinct from public benefits such as Social Security, Medicaid, Medicare, food stamps, and housing. Persons with HIV/AIDS should be aware what benefits are offered by their employers, who is eligible for them, where and how to apply for them, and how to appeal decisions to deny them.

employment discrimination   In the first decade of the epidemic, as AIDS and AIDS hysteria spread, reports of cases involving loss of jobs due to AIDS, or to perceived AIDS, were frequent. Hostility and fear were particularly marked in the workplace and in prisons, where transmission of the disease was particularly feared. Today, employment discrimination, particularly as a way to sever the lifeline of health care benefits, continues to be a primary problem for people living with AIDS. In decisions under the AMERICANS WITH DISABILITIES ACT emerging from the courts in greater numbers in recent years, there has been a perceptible trend toward a rigid, literal definition of the ADA's terms, shrinking the pool of those who can sue. Additionally, large employers have sought to limit the ability of ex-employees on COBRA or disability to sue over job-related discrimination, as have organizations representing employers' interests, such as the Equal Employment Advisory Council. Some argue that fired employees with asymptomatic HIV infection are not "disabled" enough to invoke the ADA. Others have flipped the argument, insisting that those with AIDS and presumptive eligibility for SSI benefits are too disabled to be "qualified employees" under the ADA.

empowerment   For persons who have concerns about staying well in the age of AIDS, empowerment means their taking control, or taking charge, of their own mental, spiritual, and physical health. Most programs of support and guidance for persons with HIV/AIDS, those at risk of infection or those who care for people with HIV or AIDS stress the importance of empowerment.

Taking control or taking charge can, of course, mean different things for different individuals. Research has shown that emotional and mental patterns affect outcome in chronic and life-threatening diseases. Current data strongly suggest that people who succeed in preventing illness or surviving illness longer have certain characteristics in common and employ similar approaches. Rejecting notions of victimhood, making a commitment to life and to wellness, accepting one's true circumstances, and releasing negative emotions are among the strategies most usefully employed by such people.

emtricitabine   An experimental NUCLEOSIDE ANALOG from Triangle Pharmaceuticals. It is in phase III testing as of the date of publication of this book. It has been shown to have antiviral activity against both hepatitis B virus and HIV. It has performed well in studies. One trial was ended early in August 2002 when treatment with emitricitabine had proved superior to d4T treatment when both were used in combination with EFAVIRENZ and ddI. The drug has shown to have a particularly long HALF-LIFE, so it is believed that once-a-day dosing will be possible. Reports at the time of publication stated that Triangle would be seeking approval from the FDA for the drug. The drug is structurally similar to LAMIVUDINE but has been shown to be more potent during studies. Side effects are similar to those of most known HAART medications: headaches, diarrhea, nausea, and stuffy nose. (It is also known as FTC and Coviracil.)

enabling Any action by a person or an institution that intentionally or unintentionally has the effect of supporting or reinforcing an individual's self-destructive behavior.

emulsion A suspension of droplets of one liquid in another liquid (such as oil and water). The two liquids do not actually combine but are instead suspended within one another.

encephalitis An infection of the brain of viral or other microbial origin. Encephalitis commonly causes headaches, fever, seizures, and neurological problems. The diagnosis is frequently made on the basis of symptoms exhibited combined with the results of an examination of the brain by such methods as COMPUTERIZED TOMOGRAPHY SCAN (CT SCAN), MAGNETIC RESONANCE IMAGING (MRI) or ELECTROENCEPHALOGRAM (EEG). Diagnosis can also be made by analyzing the CEREBROSPINAL FLUID obtained by a spinal tap. In people with HIV infection, the usual causes of encephalitis are infection with HIV itself or such opportunistic illnesses as TOXOPLASMOSIS. Encephalitis is distinct from MENINGITIS, which is an infection of the meninges, the membrane surrounding the brain and spinal cord.

encephalopathy Any progressive, degenerative disease of the brain.

encephalopathy, acute Any degenerative disease of the brain, or reversible deterioration of mental status or cognitive function, with a short or relatively severe course.

end-stage disease Final period or phase in the course of a disease leading to a person's death.

endemic Widespread or very common only in a particular place or population. The term may be used of an organism such as a plant, that is native to a region, as well as of disease. Of disease it is used in contrast to EPIDEMIC, which indicates widespread generally.

endocarditis A microbial infection causing inflammation of the heart valves that, if left untreated, may lead to heart failure and death. The most common cause is a bacteria called *Staphylococcus aureus.* It typically starts as a bloodstream infection that then settles into one of the heart valves. Endocarditis has long been associated with intravenous drug use and is a serious problem for HIV-positive men and women who are IV drug users. The most common symptom is fever; other symptoms include heart murmurs, irregular heartbeat, chills, headache, back and chest pain, stomachache, nausea, and vomiting. Endocarditis can lead to many complications in the circulatory system, central nervous system, lungs, kidneys, and brain. Treatment is with a long course of antibiotics. Prophylaxis is usually indicated only in persons who have had endocarditis in the past and who need to have a surgical or dental procedure during which bacteria may enter the blood.

endocervix The lining of the canal of the CERVIX.

endocrine A hormone; pertaining to an internal secretion, or to a gland that secretes directly into the bloodstream.

endocrine abnormality Any deviation in hormonal secretions.

endocrine gland Any ductless gland, such as the adrenal gland or the pituitary gland, that secretes hormones directly into the bloodstream. The endocrine system functions as an elaborate signaling system within the body, alongside the nervous system.

endocytosis The process whereby material external to a cell is internalized within a particular cell. The cell wall invaginates to form a space for the material and then closes to trap the material inside the cell.

endogenous Originating within an organism.

endometrial biopsy A test in which a small sample of tissue is removed from the uterus, often to see if infection is present.

endometriosis The presence of ectopic endometrium, in various sites throughout the pelvis or in the abdominal wall. Pelvic pain, adnexal mass, and infertility are common symptoms.

endometrium The mucous membrane lining the inner surface of the uterus.

endorphins Proteins called polypeptides, produced in the brain, that act as opiates and produce analgesia by binding to opiate receptor sites involved in pain perception.

endoscope An instrument consisting of a tube and optical system for visually examining the inside of a hollow organ or cavity. See BIOPSY; ENDOSCOPY.

endoscopic Performed by means of an ENDOSCOPE; pertaining to ENDOSCOPY.

endoscopy A diagnostic procedure in which an instrument called an ENDOSCOPE, consisting of a flexible tube and optical system, is passed through the mouth, the rectum, or a small incision to examine an internal organ or to obtain a BIOPSY. In people with HIV infection, the most common types of endoscopy are done to examine the lungs (bronchoscopy) and the digestive system. Upper endoscopy of the digestive system involves passing an endoscope through the mouth to examine the esophagus, stomach, or upper small intestine. Lower endoscopy involves passing an endoscope through the rectum to examine the large intestine or colon. Endoscopy requires the expertise of a specialist and can be done on an outpatient basis. See BIOPSY.

endothelium A form of SQUAMOUS epithelium consisting of flat cells that line the blood and lymphatic vessels, the heart, and various other body cavities.

endotoxin A bacterial toxin confined within the body of a BACTERIUM, freed only when the bacterium is broken down.

endpoints The key data items a clinical trial is focused on, or, to put it differently, the data necessary to prove or disprove the trial's central hypothesis. Essentially measurements that must be recorded, they can be events in a person's life that serve as meaningful milestones for deciding whether a treatment is effective. When a hypothesis, or the main question that drives a trial, is proposed, the endpoints are defined as the information necessary to answer that question. If, at the end of a randomized trial, there is a difference between the tallies of endpoints in a treated group and the tallies of an untreated group, it is attributed to the treatment. Usually when an endpoint reaches a certain set magnitude of change from BASELINE, a trial participant is removed from the trial and given an open-label therapy (either a standard treatment or the experimental one being tested).

Endpoints are divided into primary (or main) and secondary endpoints. Generally, but not always, a trial has one primary endpoint. It is the single most important piece of information to be obtained, and trial design decisions should be made to guarantee to the greatest extent possible getting accurate information on the primary endpoint.

In clinical trials of HIV drugs, the term is often misunderstood as meaning the end of the trial or the end of a participant's enrollment in the trial. This can be the case but is not necessarily. Endpoints in HIV treatment trials may include viral load thresholds, CD4 count, serious toxicity, quality of life, opportunistic infections, and death. As we learn more about the long-term effects of HIV and the drugs used to treat it, follow-up after the main endpoints have been reached appears increasingly important to ascertain the overall risk/benefit ratios of various treatments over time.

The single most common endpoint is "progression of disease or death." This does not mean that the trial is trying to kill someone. It refers to the time when a person will end his or her participation in the trial. If a person progresses in his or her disease, the treatment is not working and it is required of medical personnel to help a person receive helpful treatment. So the endpoint for that patient is progression of disease. If a person dies suddenly they will leave the trial. The endpoint of the trial for that person would be their death. The goals of a trial are often different than endpoints. The goal of a trial is often to differentiate between two types of treatment. If more people in one group show progression to disease, then it shows researchers that the treatment is not working. It does not mean people are dying from the trial, but that they left the trial to receive treatment when they progressed.

enema   The injection of a solution into the rectum or colon for the purpose of stimulating bowel activity, for therapeutic or nutritive purposes or to aid in roentgenography; also, a solution so introduced.

energy level   The position of electrons within an atom. Specifically, one of a quantized series of states in which matter may exist, each having constant energy and separated from others in the series by finite quantities of energy. Energy levels in individuals who are HIV-positive or have AIDS vary depending on the stage of HIV infection, medical, psychological, and social interventions, the special conditions of each patient, and other variables.

enfuvirtide   Trimeris Pharmaceuticals' experimental fusion inhibitor. The first in this new class of HIV drugs, enfuvirtide is a synthetic 36-amino-acid linear peptide that inhibits the fusion of HIV to the host cell. After the virus binds to the CD4 cell receptor, a change in the shape of the envelope protein allows HIV GP41 protein to extend into the cell membrane. The gp41 then folds in two, drawing the virus particle and cell together. This action allows HIV to penetrate the cell membrane. Enfuvirtide interferes by binding to gp41 and preventing it from folding. There is no oral formulation of enfuvirtide, and its half-life in the blood is two to three hours. The preferred method of delivery is twice-daily subcutaneous injection. Enfuvirtide slowly diffuses through the subcutaneous fat layer into the bloodstream. Common side effects include irritation at the injection site, fever, and headache.

Manufacturing enfuvirtide is an extremely lengthy and difficult process involving many steps. It is not believed that there will be adequate supplies of the drug available for everyone who might want to use it initially, so the manufacturer has set up a waiting list for people who have received doctor permission to use the drug. Another drawback is that the companies manufacturing the drug, Roche and Trimeris, plan to charge approximately $20,000 a year for the standard dosage for an individual. Many ADAPs, and even private insurers, have already indicated they will be unable to cover the drug in their programs as priced. (The drug is also known as Fuzeon and T-20.)

enhancing antibody   A type of binding antibody detected in the test tube and formed in response to HIV infection that may enhance the ability of HIV to produce disease. Theoretically, enhancing antibodies could attach to HIV virions and enable macrophages to engulf the viruses. However, instead of being destroyed, the engulfed virus may remain alive within the macrophage, which then can carry the virus to other parts of the body. It is currently unknown whether enhancing antibodies have any effect on the course of HIV infection. Enhancing antibodies can be thought of as the opposite of neutralizing antibodies.

enteric   Pertaining to the intestines.

enteric coating   A type of drug formulation in which tablets or capsules are coated with a special compound that will not dissolve until the pill is exposed to the fluids in the small intestine.

enteric disease   Any pathological condition involving the small intestine.

enteric pathogen   Any microorganism or substance capable of producing a disease in the small intestine.

enteritis   An inflammation of the small intestine. In people with HIV infection, the microbes that usually cause enteritis are CRYPTOSPORIDIA, MICROSPORIDIA, *Mycobacterium avium* or Intracellulare, and CMV. These can be detected by examining stools under a microscope or performing a BIOPSY of the small intestine. The most common symptom is diarrhea.

enterotoxin   A toxin produced by or originating in the intestinal contents; an exotoxin specific for the cells of the mucosa, produced by certain species of bacteria that cause various diseases, including food poisoning and TOXIC SHOCK SYNDROME.

enteral   Within or through the intestines.

ENV gene   A gene of HIV that encodes information, allowing the production of the GP160 polyprotein, which later becomes the GP120 and GP41 proteins. See POLYPROTEIN.

envelope   The outer covering of a virus, sometimes called the coat.

envelope gene   The gene that encodes the major virion surface envelope glycoprotein (for the human immunodeficiency virus, this glycoprotein is GP160) and is then processed to form a transmembrane segment (GP41) and a glycosylated external segment (GP120).

envelope glycoprotein   The glycosylated external segment (GP120) of the human immunodeficiency virus. The envelope glycoprotein is the major target for the HIV-neutralizing antibody.

enzyme   A cellular protein whose shape allows it to hold together several molecules in close proximity to each other. In this way, enzymes are able to mediate and promote chemical reactions in other substances with little expenditure of energy and without themselves being altered or destroyed.

enzyme immunoassay (EIA)   Any of several rapid enzyme testing methods for detecting the presence of an antibody or an antigen in tissue by using an enzyme covalently linked to an antigen or antibody as a label. The resulting complex will retain both immunological and enzymatic activity. The pressure of the antigen or antibody indicates infection by a virus or other microbe. The two most common methods are ENZYME-LINKED IMMUNO-SORBENT ASSAY (ELISA) and enzyme-multiplied immunoassay technique (EMIT).

Solid-phase immunoassay involves fixing antibody to the antigen on a polyvinylchloride sheet, putting on a drop of serum (or urine) and washing off after the antigen-antibody complex has had time to form, and then adding a second labeled or fluorescent antibody, this time specific to a different epitope of the antigen. The amount of the second antibody that binds is proportional to the amount of antigen present.

ELISA is similar, but an enzyme instead of the label is attached to a second antibody. This can convert a colorless substance to a colored product, or nonfluorescent to fluorescent, when added. Sensitivities of both methods can be extremely high.

These assays are quite sensitive and specific as compared with the radioimmune assay tests and have the advantage of not requiring radioisotopes and the expensive counting apparatus.

enzyme-linked immunosorbent assay (ELISA) The most common blood test used to detect antibodies against HIV. When the body is exposed to a microbe, the immune system mounts an attack against it and makes antibodies (the molecules that help fight it off) for the specific agent. The presence of these antibodies are indicative of ongoing infection. The ELISA test determines whether antibodies to the AIDS virus are present in the blood, which they usually are within several months of infection.

The ELISA is the first of two standard tests done together to detect antibodies to HIV. It is extremely sensitive and very specific. Sensitivity means that the test specifically detects a particular infection and no other. With ELISA, people who have HIV infection will rarely test falsely negative, whereas people who do not have HIV infection will occasionally test falsely positive. As a result, the ELISA is used as a screening test; blood samples that test positive are tested again with the western blot test. This combination is more than 99 percent accurate in both sensitivity and specificity.

These tests are generally offered free of charge by most health departments. Tests may be anonymous, meaning that the person being tested is not identified, or confidential, meaning that privacy is honored but a record is kept identifying by name the test result.

The ELISA is easily performed, but the western blot is more complicated and often done only by reference laboratories or on certain days of the week. For this reason, the combined results may not be available for several days or even weeks. Test results are usually either positive or negative, but occasionally western blot tests yield results that cannot be clearly interpreted and are considered indeterminate. The usual recommendation for people with indeterminate results is to have the test repeated in two or three months. People at low risk for HIV and with indeterminate results almost never turn out to have HIV infection. The cause of the indeterminate results is not known.

eosinophil Bone marrow-derived GRANULOCYTES (nondividing granular cells) with a limited life span in the blood. They have both secretory and phagocytic functions and may play a specific role in allergies and defense against parasites. Eosinophils are readily stained with eosin, a synthetic red dye used to stain tissues for microscopic examination.

eosinophilic Pertaining to eosinophils; readily stainable with eosin.

eosinophilic folliculitis Late in HIV infection some people experience a red, extremely itchy acnelike skin eruption that appears similar to staphylococcal folliculitis but is not caused by bacteria or fungi. The exact cause of eosinophilic folliculitis is in fact still unknown. The eosinophils are known to be involved in allergic reactions, and they are clustered in the areas of these bumps, but what they are reacting to is not understood. It is most often seen in persons with a CD4 cell count below 200. Treatment is with antibiotics first; if that does not work, Elmite, a treatment for scabies, is tried. It is thought that perhaps the reaction is to the skin mites that live in human hair follicles, and that is the reason why a scabies treatment sometimes seems to work. Occasionally ultraviolet B (UVB) light treatments are also used successfully.

epidemic Occurring in many more people than would be statistically expected during a given time. (Generally used of a disease the term may also be applied to injuries or other events that endanger public health.) Also, a disease that so occurs. We say there is an AIDS epidemic because the disease is spreading very quickly to many segments of the population. Distinct from ENDEMIC, which indicates restriction to a particular place or population. See PANDEMIC.

epidemiology A branch of medical science encompassing the study of the relationship of various factors in the incidence and distribution of a disease or of diseases in a human environment.

epididymitis Inflammation of the epididymis, a tube that lies against the back wall of a testicle and serves as a storage facility for sperm.

epidural Situated within the spinal canal, on or outside the dura mater (tough membrane surrounding the spinal cord); synonyms are *extradural* and *peridural.*

epinephrine A hormone secreted by the adrenal medulla in response to stimulation of the sympathetic nervous system. It causes some of the physiological expressions of fear and anxiety and has been found to be in excess in some anxiety disorders. Epinephrine, which has been synthesized, is also produced by tissues other than the adrenal. Used as a vasoconstrictor to treat cardiac dysrhythmias and to relax bronchioles. It is also used to check local hemorrhaging, to relieve asthmatic attacks, and to prolong the action of local anesthetics. (Trade names are Adrenalin, Bronkaid Mist, Primatene Mist, and SusPhrine.)

epistasis In genetics, the suppression by a gene of the effect of another gene that is not its allele (one of two or more alternative forms of a gene occupying the same position on matching chromosomes; an individual usually has two alleles for each trait, one from either parent).

epistaxis Hemorrhage in the nose.

epithelial cell   An irregularly-shaped cell that has a single nucleus. Frequently two or three are joined together.

epithelium   The layer of cells forming the epidermis of the skin and the surface layer or mucous and serous membranes. The cells rest on a basement membrane and lie closely approximated to each other with little intercellular material between them. The epithelium may be simple, consisting of a single layer, or stratified, consisting of several layers. Cells making up the epithelium may be flat (squamous), cube-shaped (cuboidal), or cylindrical (columnar). Epithelium serves the general purpose of protection, absorption, and secretion, and specialized functions such as movement of substances through ducts, production of germ cells, and reception of stimuli. Its ability to regenerate is excellent, and it may replace itself as frequently as every 24 hours.

epitope   The simplest form of an antigenic determinant present on a complex antigenic molecule, which combines with antibody or T-CELL RECEPTOR.

Epivir   See LAMIVUDINE.

Epogen   See ERYTHROPOIETIN.

Epstein-Barr virus (EBV)   A herpeslike virus that lies dormant in the lymph glands and causes one of the two kinds of mononucleosis (the other is caused by CMV). EBV is also thought to be responsible for CHRONIC FATIGUE SYNDROME. It has been implicated as a causal factor in the development of BURKITT'S LYMPHOMA in Africa. It has also been linked with nasopharyngeal cancer, a common cancer in China. EBV is a common virus which can be a serious opportunistic infection when associated with AIDS. The virus manifests itself in LYMPHADENOPATHY, LYMPHOMA, KAPOSI'S SARCOMA, and other illnesses. EBV has been hypothesized as a CO-FACTOR for AIDS.

equal allocation   See EQUAL TREATMENT ALLOCATION.

equal treatment allocation   A scheme in which the assigned probability in the randomization process for any one treatment is the same as for every other treatment in the trial. A process that ensures that approximately equal numbers of patients receive each treatment.

equianalgesic   Having equal pain-killing effect; morphine sulfate, 10 mg intramuscularly, is generally used in opioid analgesic comparisons.

erection   The engorgement of the PENIS with blood and consequent enlargement and stiffening. Erection can be a sign of sexual excitement.

erogenous zone   Any area of the body that when stimulated increases sexual excitement.

erogeny   Sexuality and sensuality.

erotic   Sexually stimulating; relating to sexual activity or feeling.

erotophobia   The irrational hatred or fear of anything sexual, or guilt over erotic desire. The development of erotophobia has been the response of both the infected and the uninfected to the AIDS crisis.

eruption   An inflammation of the skin characterized by itching, redness, and skin lesions; may be caused by medication as well as by illness. A drug eruption is also called *dermatitis medicamentosa*.

Erythrocin   See ERYTHROMYCIN.

erythrocyte   A circulating red blood cell; a mature red blood cell or corpuscle shaped in the form of a nonnucleated, yellowish, biconcave disk. It consists of a respiratory pigment (hemoglobin) enclosed in a membrane of proteins and lipoid substances. By the nature of its composition, the erythrocyte is adapted to transport oxygen throughout the body.

erythrocyte sedimentation rate (ESR)   The rate at which ERYTHROCYTES (the circulating red blood cells) settle in a well-mixed specimen of blood. The ESR is an indicator of inflammatory disease and other conditions in which the rate is usually elevated.

erythromycin   An antibiotic administered orally, it is effective against many GRAM-POSITIVE and certain

GRAM-NEGATIVE bacteria. It may also be applied topically in the treatment of certain infections. Administered intravenously it is used in the treatment of Legionaries' disease. It is used to treat patients who are allergic to penicillin and in the treatment of penicillin-resistant infections. (Trade name is Erythrocin.)

erythrophagocytosis See ERYTHROCYTOPHAGY.

erythroplakia A reddened velvety patch that may appear in the mouth. It is a precancerous condition. See ORAL CANCER.

erythropoietin (EPO) A protein, made primarily by the kidney, that stimulates red blood cell production. A genetically engineered version has been approved as a treatment for HIV-related anemia. Anemia, which is frequently seen in people with HIV, can be caused by HIV infection itself or as a side effect of treatment. EPO will not be effective if anemia is caused by iron deficiency, infection, cancer, blood loss, and vitamin deficiency. It is not an appropriate therapy for severe anemia and cannot replace the need for blood transfusions. Early treatment of mild anemia with EPO may prevent the onset of severe anemia and the need for blood transfusions. The recombinant version of EPO is available as a solution for IV injection under the trade names Epogen and Procrit.

Escherichia coli (E. coli) A bacterium in the feces that causes most urinary tract infections.

esophageal candidiasis Serious fungal infection in the conduit between the mouth and the stomach (the ESOPHAGUS). Esophageal candidiasis is caused by the same yeast infection that can also infect both the mouth and the vagina. It may start with an infection in the mouth (oral thrush) and spread to the esophagus, causing pain when swallowing, weight loss, and vomiting.

esophagitis Disease of the esophagus is very common in patients with AIDS. Its most common physical symptoms are painful swallowing or the sense of food sticking in the throat. Patients sometimes complain of chest pain or hiccups. These symptoms may result in decreased food intake in patients with normal appetites, dehydration, weight loss, and malnourishment. The diagnostic procedure of choice for esophagitis is upper ENDOSCOPY, in which a lighted scope is passed through the mouth into the esophagus. Esophagitis is primarily cause by CANDIDIASIS. Other possible causes include herpes simplex, CMV, and aphthous ulcers. In esophagitis related to candidiasis a biopsy is the general diagnostic tool used.

esophagoscope A flexible or rigid instrument, equipped with an optical system, inserted into the esophagus for diagnostic and therapeutic purposes (obtaining or removing foreign substances).

esophagoscopy An ENDOSCOPIC examination of the ESOPHAGUS using an ESOPHAGOSCOPE.

esophagus A muscular canal extending from the pharynx to the stomach. The esophagus carries swallowed food and liquids from the mouth to the stomach.

ESR See ERYTHROCYTE SEDIMENTATION RATE.

estrogen Any natural or artificial substance that induces estrogenic activity; more specifically, the estrogenic hormones estradiol and estrone, produced by the ovary; the female sex hormones.

etharnbutol hydrochloride A drug used in treating TUBERCULOSIS and *MICOBACTERIUM AVIUM* COMPLEX (MAC). It is used in combination with other TB and MAC medications. (Trade name is Myambutol.)

ethics A system or set of moral principles. Also, the rules of conduct recognized in respect to a particular class of human actions or governing a particular group, culture, or profession, such as medical ethics. AIDS research and policy development have from the very beginning involved serious ethical issues. Some of the earliest had to do with blood screening policies, the conduct of epidemiological research and surveillance, risk to health care providers, and the duty to warn people with HIV, patient confidentiality, and the conduct of drug trials. Many of these issues are still with us, although in different forms and some with lesser importance. For example, there are no longer debates about screening donated blood, but the questions around clinical trials have broadened, particularly concerning the inclusion of women and minorities. Additionally, because ethicists, at least in the United States, were involved very early on in policy discussions, the response of public health agencies reflected concerns about individual patient rights and standard infectious disease control measures.

Future ethical challenges include managed care, home care, and physician-assisted suicide. Issues raised by managed care, for example, include coverage for new therapies, coverage for alternative treatments, coverage for mental health treatment, and coverage for preexisting conditions. The challenge of optimizing the quality of life raises a range of ethical issues for health care professionals and AIDS service providers, in addition to family and friends of persons with HIV/AIDS. Attention to psychosocial issues and issues of death and dying are as important as both medical management of HIV infection and careful attention to financial matters. The practicalities of self-deliverance and assisted suicide for the dying aside, there are a number of ethical issues raised by physician-assisted suicide.

ethnic groups   See RACE/ETHNICITY.

ethnicity   See RACE/ETHNICITY.

etiology   The cause(s) or origin(s) of diseases; the study of the factors that cause disease.

etoposide   An antineoplastic drug; a semisynthetic derivative of podophyllotoxin, administered intravenously and used to prevent the development, growth, or proliferation of malignant cells.

etretinate   An antipsoriasis drug used in the treatment of severe recalcitrant psoriasis. (Trade name is Tegison.)

Europe   See EASTERN EUROPE AND CENTRAL ASIA; WESTERN EUROPE.

eustachian dysfunction   Abnormal or impaired functioning of the auditory tube (eustachian tube) that extends from the middle ear to the pharynx. When the passage is blocked, OTITIS media may develop.

exclusion criteria   The medical or social standards by which researchers decide not to include certain potential persons in a clinical or research trial. For example, some trials may not include persons who have chronic liver disease or may exclude persons who have certain drug allergies; others may exclude men or women or only include persons with a lowered T-cell count. Exclusion criteria are generally health factors whose presence in a test subject would be undesirable or inappropriate. Often these are established for reasons of safety. For instance, doctors may know or fear that a new drug may worsen the condition of people with a certain illness. It would thus be wrong to allow them to participate in the clinical trial or study and take that risk. See INCLUSION CRITERIA.

exempt assets   Assets that are not considered or counted in determining eligibility under benefit programs such as the SSI and VA pension programs.

exercise   Bodily or mental exertion, especially for the sake of maintaining fitness, training, or improvement. Exercise is a time-proved method for coping with problems of all kinds. Today, virtually all cultures recognize the importance of regularly moving all parts of the body. In India, yogic exercise has played an important role in Ayurvedic medicine for more than 6,000 years. Similarly, in China, exercise has been practiced for 2,500 years using martial arts such as tai chi. Many studies have shown that people who exercise have fewer illnesses than sedentary persons. Vigorous exercise benefits the body both directly and indirectly by stimulating the immune system and enabling people to cope with a variety of stressors and toxins. The psychological benefits are equally as important, and exercise has been successfully used to treat disorders such as depression. Regular exercise is usually part of any holistic medical program because, next to diet, it most effectively produces total body health. Additionally, the healing process works at its best when the body is relaxed and energy is concentrated inward. A part of being able to relax and allow that to happen is exercise and meditation, which not only enhance general well-being but also aid in the overall health of the immune system.

The amount, type, and frequency of exercise to take in order to develop and maintain a state of fitness is an individual matter.

exhibitionism   Sexual interest in exposing one's genitals. Slang term is flash.

exocervix   The outer CERVIX.

exogenous   Developed or originating outside an organism.

exon   The coding segment of a DNA strand.

exotoxins   Toxin released by a microorganism into surrounding growth medium or tissue during growth phase of infection. Generally inactivated by heat and easily neutralized by a specific antibody. It is produced mainly by GRAM-POSITIVE bacteria, such as the agents of botulism, diphtheria, Shigella dysentery, tetanus, and staph food poisoning.

expanded access   Refers to any of the United States FOOD AND DRUG ADMINISTRATION procedures allowing patients who are failing on current treatments for their condition, who are unable to participate in ongoing clinical trials, and who meet certain criteria to take an experimental drug not yet approved for general use. In the program, doctors monitor patient's responses and report the data to the pharmaceutical company sponsoring the drug. Specific types of expanded access mechanisms include parallel track, compassionate use, and treatment IND. Also called *open-label study.*

expedited process   Under a plan implemented by the Food and Drug Administration (FDA) early in 1989, Phases I and II of the U.S. DRUG APPROVAL PROCESS may be combined to shave two or three years from the development process for medicines that show sufficient promise in early testing and are targeted against serious and life-threatening diseases. Phase I clinical trials consist of tests that take about 1 year and involve about 20 to 80 normal, healthy volunteers. The tests study a drug's safety profile, including the safe dosage range. The studies also determine how a drug is absorbed, distributed, metabolized, and excreted and the duration of its action. In Phase II clinical trials, controlled studies of approximately 100 to 300 volunteer patients assess the drug's effectiveness. Phase II clinical trials generally take about two years.

experimental drug   A drug that has not been approved for use as a treatment for a particular condition.

experimental group   In experimental design, a group of subjects exposed to an independent variable in order to examine the causal effect of that variable on a dependent variable.

experimenter bias   See EXPERIMENTER EFFECTS.

experimenter effects   Biasing effects on the results of an experiment caused by expectations or preconceptions on the part of the experimenter.

exposed   According to the provisions of the Public Health Service's HIV Health Care Services Program, the term *exposed* with respect to HIV disease or any other infectious disease means to be in circumstances in which there is a significant risk of becoming infected with the etiologic agent for the disease involved.

exposed, uninfecteds (EUs)   People or animals that have resisted infection after contact with HIV.

expression system   In genetic engineering, the cells into which a gene has been inserted to manufacture desired proteins. Chinese hamster ovary (CHO) cells and baculovirus/insect cells are two expression systems that are used to make recombinant HIV vaccines. In HIV vaccine production, the system is composed of cells into which an HIV gene has been inserted to produce desired HIV.

extracerebral toxoplasmosis   TOXOPLASMOSIS that occurs outside the brain in a disseminated form, with parasites found in the eyes, lungs, blood, bone marrow, muscles, bladder, and heart.

extrahepatic disease   A pathological condition occurring outside of or unrelated to the liver.

eyewear, protective   Safety glasses. See PROTECTIVE EQUIPMENT.

fab (fragment antigen binding) A part of the antibody molecule that contains the antigen-binding site. It is obtained by enzymatic hydrolysis of the antibody.

facilitated DNA inoculation A means of delivering (non-infectious) HIV genes into a patient's blood by direct injection into a muscle, along with an agent that promotes uptake of the genes into the host cells. The rationale behind this strategy is to induce production of HIV proteins by the patient's own cells, which in turn may prompt his or her immune system to produce antibodies and killer T CELLS to fight HIV. The vaccine includes a segment of HIV DNA comprising the ENV and REV GENES, which code for a viral envelope protein and an essential regulatory protein, respectively. This is incorporated into a plasmid construct, which provides the regulatory elements required to express the HIV genes.

factor Any substance or activity required to produce a result; a contributing cause in any action; a gene (hereditary factor).

factor VIII A naturally occurring protein in plasma necessary for normal blood coagulation. A congenital deficiency in factor VIII results in the bleeding disorder known as HEMOPHILIA A. Factor VIII is also called antihemophilic globulin (AHG) and antihemophilic factor A.

factor IX A naturally occurring protein in plasma necessary for normal blood coagulation. A congenital deficiency in factor IX results in the bleeding disorder known as HEMOPHILIA B.

fag Male homosexual, especially one considered effeminate. Fag may also be an abbreviation for faggot. In the 1973 Gay Activists Alliance and National Gay Task Force guidelines on homosexuality, *fag* and *faggot* were listed as terms of abuse. Other terms included *queer, homo, fairy, mary, pansy,* and *sissy.*

faggot A derogatory term for a male homosexual. Usually meant to be insulting, demeaning, and provocative. Gay men, however, have used it of themselves in an ironic fashion. The word *faggot,* which means a bundle of kindling (sticks), became an epithet for a gay man because gay men were used as human torches to burn "witches" in the Middle Ages.

failure to thrive Condition in which infants and children not only fail to gain weight but may also lose it. The organic causes may include almost any severe chronic condition. Non-organic causes include starvation, emotional deprivation, and social disruption.

fair hearing A semi-judicial proceeding before a state welfare officer at which an applicant for or recipient of almost any state-administered benefit can present claims of error, unfairness, misapplication of rules, or other grievances in an attempt to reverse or modify an unfavorable decision.

Fair Housing Act The Fair Housing Act, adopted by Congress in 1968, prohibits discrimination in the sale or rental of housing and in advertising, financing, and brokerage services. Congress amended the law in 1988 to prohibit discrimination because of "handicap." The Fair Housing Act defines "handicap" as a "physical or mental impairment which substantially limits . . . major life activities." People are also protected if they are *perceived* as having a handicap, even if they do not. This definition was taken from Section 504 of the Rehabilitation Act of 1973, which courts have unanimously interpreted to include HIV. The DEPARTMENT OF HOUSING AND URBAN DEVELOPMENT (HUD), which drafted the regulations for administering the act, has concluded that Congress chose the Section 504 definition with the intention of including people with HIV as handicapped people protected by the Fair Housing Act. People subjected to discrimination in violation of the Fair Housing Act may file a complaint with HUD and may bring a lawsuit in a federal court. The attorney general may also bring actions in court to prohibit "a pattern or practice" that violates the Fair Housing Act. See FAIR HOUSING AMENDMENTS ACT.

Fair Housing Amendments Act   This act, adopted in 1988, is an outgrowth of the Fair Housing Act of 1968, which was amended numerous times in the 1970s and 1980s. The Fair Housing Amendments Act was designed to ban housing discrimination based on disability (including any stage of HIV illness) and covers most real estate transactions (financing, rental, sale). The act provides limited exemptions for religious organizations and private clubs, owners of fewer than three units who do not use real estate agents, and owner-occupied buildings with fewer than four units. Under the act, no landlord may evict, refuse to rent to, refuse to renew the lease of, or legally harm in any way anyone with an HIV illness. If it does, an individual has the same right to file a discrimination complaint with a state or city agency as he or she has in a case of employment discrimination, or to sue in federal court.

During the 1970s and early 1980s, most states passed laws prohibiting disability discrimination in employment, housing, and public accommodations. These laws differ widely, however, in their interpretation and application.

fairy   Male homosexual, especially an effeminate one. This 20th-century derogatory term is not as pejorative as fag.

fallopian tubes   Delicate tubes that extend from the ovaries to the upper uterus, through which an egg passes to be fertilized.

false-negative   A test or procedure that indicates that the abnormality or disease being investigated is not present when in fact it is.

false-positive   A test or procedure that indicates that the abnormality or disease being investigated is present when in fact it is not.

famciclovir   A synthetic chemical that mimics one of the building blocks of DNA. Inside the body, famciclovir is converted to the antiviral agent penciclovir. In cells infected with the VARICELLA ZOSTER VIRUS, the drug slows the replication of viral DNA. It has especially high bioavailability and is an approved therapy for shingles. As with other antiviral drugs, it does not rid the body of a virus but acts to reduce the severity and slow the growth of infection. It is available in tablet form under the trade name Famvir.

family-centered care   Health and social-service care that recognizes and respects the crucial role of families in the lives of their members. It supports families in their natural caregiving roles, promotes normal patterns of living, and ensures family collaboration and choice in the provision of services to family members who are sick.

family law   Family law is the name now more commonly used for what was previously called domestic relations law. It encompasses prenuptial agreements, marriages, annulments, divorces, child custody and visitation rights, and other family issues. The American Bar Association's Policy on AIDS makes clear that the organization feels HIV status should not generally be deemed admissible evidence in a family law proceeding, and that when it is it should be considered only in the same manner as other medical conditions. The ABA believes that HIV status should not be deemed admissible evidence for the purpose of determining a party's sexual orientation.

family planning   At one time synonymous with "birth control," family planning is a concept whose purpose is to allow parents to determine the size of families through the spacing or prevention of pregnancies. Numerous social service agencies and voluntary organizations have programs of counseling and assistance in all aspects of family planning. Generally clinicians or counselors offer a supportive discussion of sexuality, safe sex, contraception, and the desire for children. They offer assistance and support for their clients' contraceptive and family planning needs, preferences, and choices, whether the client is HIV-positive or -negative.

When pregnancy is diagnosed and a woman or a couple seeks such assistance, an agency offers nondirective counseling and usually referrals as requested for abortion or prenatal care and information regarding disease transmission and risk to the mother and fetus. For a woman or a couple contemplating pregnancy, it is often important to initiate a discussion regarding feelings and ability to care for an ill child, and the willingness and ability of family members to provide support and assistance in the event of the illness of a parent. In a couple in which one partner is HIV-positive and the other is HIV-negative, further discussion is useful. Is the couple willing to consider options such as artificial insemination or adoption? Is the couple able to limit exposure to HIV during sex by learning fertility awareness techniques and having only limited unprotected sex?

Contraceptive choices for HIV-positive women include oral contraceptives, condoms with spermicides, diaphragms with spermicides or cervical caps, other barriers (creams, gels, suppositories, foams, sponges), intrauterine devices, surgical sterilization, progesterone implants, or intramuscular progesterone. The pros and cons of each choice should be evaluated before selection. See CONTRACEPTIVES.

Fanconi's syndrome   Named for a Swiss pediatrician, Guido Fanconi, Fanconi's syndrome is a renal tubular dysfunction that can be inherited or acquired through kidney damage. The syndrome includes a collection of illnesses that may include rickets, growth failure, aminoaciduria, and excessive urine output. Typically the kidney functions as an organ that filters the blood and keeps the various substances in the blood in balance. The kidney then passes on unneeded substance into the urine for the body to excrete. In Fanconi's syndrome some of the chemicals the body needs to function properly are also passed into the urine. Substances that are lost include vitamin D, glucose, amino acids, small proteins, water, calcium, potassium, magnesium, bicarbonate, and phosphate. When they are lost, the body becomes overly acidic. In acquired cases Fanconi's syndrome is caused by exposure to heavy metals (cadmium, mercury, uranium, and lead), certain prescription drugs, and some other chemical products (Lysol, toluene, and paraquat). In HIV patients, the drug Adefovir has been shown to cause Fanconi's syndrome in some people. The syndrome is generally reversible if detected. Treatment would involve stopping the medication causing the problem or avoiding the substance that caused the symptoms. To encourage this recovery sometimes patients are given sodium chloride (table salt) and antacids to counter the high acidity of the body. The drug AMPHOTERICIN B also causes a condition similar to Fanconi's syndrome.

fatigue   Fatigue, generally measured by patients' responses to questions concerning reductions in daily activity, is one of the most prevalent and most undertreated problems experienced by persons with HIV infection and AIDS. Despite the fact that HIV/AIDS-related fatigue significantly impacts the psychological well-being and quality of life of patients with HIV/AIDS, many physicians tend to ignore it and do not consider it a symptom requiring clinical intervention. The bottom line, however, is that fatigue can be as debilitating as other symptoms.

HIV-related fatigue has a variety of interactive causes, of which psychological distress and depression are just one aspect. Physical symptoms, drug side effects, sleep disturbances, malnutrition and wasting, HIV encephalopathy, hormonal insufficiency (due to low adrenal gland output, for example), and muscular weakness (HIV- or AZT-related myopathy) all contribute to fatigue. Researchers have also noted a small but statistically significant association between fatigue and anemia (low oxygen transport by the blood).

PNEUMOCYSTIS CARINII PNEUMONIA (PCP) and CYTOMEGALOVIRUS and other active opportunistic conditions directly trigger fatigue. Part of this fatigue results from the increase in inflammatory cytokines as the immune system responds to the opportunistic infections, but in addition PCP lowers oxygen levels in the blood by interfering with lung absorption, and CMV can reduce hormonal levels by infecting the adrenal glands.

Addressing the medical causes of fatigue, which may be as simple as switching patients to alternative drugs, can have a rapid, positive effect. A better diet and special nutritional supplementation to combat malabsorption or the special needs of those with chronic infection can be useful in combating fatigue. Raising hemoglobin levels by administering blood transfusions, recombinant erythropoietin, or nutritional therapy also gives people improved energy levels and greater functional capacity. Red blood cell transfusions are a "quick fix" for treatment-associated anemia, but they carry a small risk of immune reactions and transmission of blood-borne infections. Recombinant erythropoietin has the advantage of being free of significant side effects. It requires three weeks to elevate hemoglobin levels, though, and occasional blood transfusions may still be required. Researchers are currently studying the ability of two commercially available psychostimulants (Ritalin and Cylert) to reduce fatigue in ambulatory HIV-positive individuals. Stimulants are considered an umbrella kind of therapy that helps individuals deal with fatigue of any cause; however, they also can interfere with sleep and cause loss of appetite; both effects can further fatigue in the long run.

Physicians suggest that individuals be encouraged to develop their own methods of coping with fatigue, including pacing their daily lives, altering activity–rest patterns, taking frequent rest breaks, and delegating activities to others. Working out at the gym or jogging is a form of natural psychological and physical stimulation, but more moderate exercise such as walking can be helpful, too. People have found such meditative exercise forms as yoga, tai chi, or chi gong very restorative even when their physical capacity is limited by disease. Massage, therapeutic touch, acupuncture, and other alternative therapies that claim to restore the body's "energy balance" also may have a role to play, if only for their meditative aspects, which may relieve mental tension and depression. Finally, psychosocial counseling and support groups can be important for helping the individual to cope with emotional stress or anxiety. Occupational therapy can also be a valuable strategy for distracting an individual from focusing on his or her disease, symptoms, and emotions. Antidepressant medication can be used in cases of recalcitrant depression.

fat redistribution   See LIPODYSTROPHY.

Fc fragment   Small pieces of immunoglobulins (antibodies) used by macrophages in their processing and presenting of foreign antigens to T lymphocytes.

Fc receptor   A receptor present on monocytes and macrophages that bind FC FRAGMENTS of immunoglobulins G and E.

FDA   See FOOD AND DRUG ADMINISTRATION.

FDC   See FOLLICULAR DENDRITIC CELLS.

F-ddA   See LODENOSINE.

fear of AIDS   The exploitation of irrational fears has often resulted in attacks on, or stigmatization of, gays and other heavily affected groups. Media scares have served and continue to serve to fuel both rational and irrational fear of AIDS. The very considerable medical evidence that transmission cannot occur through casual contact seems not to have been registered by large numbers of people. The high level of fear in so many in spite of the small number of cases and deaths so far, relative to the total population, supports the observation that there is no simple correlation between risk and fear.

fecal matter   See FECES.

feces   Solid body waste consisting of food residue, bacteria, exfoliated cells, and mucus, discharged from the intestines by way of the anus. Also called stool, excreta, dejecta, and excrement. The color, form, consistency, and odor of feces vary with disease and diet, and may be indicative of various disorders.

Federal Rehabilitation Act   See REHABILITATION ACT OF 1973.

feline leukemia virus (FeLV) A virus that causes leukemia in cats. FeLV is in the same family of viruses (retroviruses) as HIV. FeLV is in the oncovirus branch of retroviruses, which is different from the lentiviruses, which cause HIV, SIV, and other illnesses. FeLV is not transmissible to humans from cats.

fellatio The sexual act of stimulating a penis orally. Colloquially called a blow job, but the action is more sucking than blowing. See ORAL SEX.

female condom A protective polyurethane sheath that fits into the vagina and provides a contraceptive and disease-prevention barrier for women that is a safe and effective birth control method. The female condom prevents bodily fluids, such as semen, from entering the vagina. The female condom was designed in the mid-1980s by a Danish gynecologist and his wife and developed by an international group of researchers and physicians. Combining features of a male condom and a diaphragm, it consists of soft polyurethane rings. The smaller ring lies inside the closed end of the sheath. It is inserted into the vagina and anchors the condom behind the pubic bone. The larger, outer ring lines the open end of the sheath and, after insertion, hangs outside the vagina.

A woman can insert the female condom as she would a diaphragm. Unlike the diaphragm, however, the inner ring of the condom is made in only one size and need not fit snugly over the CERVIX. The sheath lines the vaginal canal. During intercourse, the external outer end and ring cover the LABIA, preventing skin-to-skin contact with the base of the penis. The inner lining of the sheath is coated with a silicon-based lubricant. Women may add oil- or water-based lubricants on the outside of the sheath to facilitate insertion and on the inside to promote a natural feel during intercourse. Because it is made with polyurethane, the female condom does not deteriorate when used with an oil-based lubricant. Care in placing the female condom over the cervix ensures the condom does not move during sex and slip out of the vagina. An unexpected side effect is that during sex air occasionally becomes trapped between the side of the condom and the wall of the vagina. This can lead to "farting" sounds as the gas is pushed out of the vagina. This should not detract from condom use or efficiency.

The benefits and advantages of a female condom are similar to those associated with a male condom. It provides adequate but not complete protection against pregnancy and STDs. The female condom, like the male condom, is a safe and practical alternative to other forms of birth control, and it need be used only during sex. There are no health risks to either partner. It is safe to use, with no vaginal side effects except infrequent labial itching and irritation. No prescription or medical exam is needed for purchase. It can be obtained in clinics and pharmacies without a prescription or fitting by a health care professional. And, best of all, it gives women control over their own protection. This in itself may be a problem in the developing world, where women have little or no control over sexual protection, birth control, or the financial ability to purchase a female condom.

Problems and disadvantages include the fact that unlike male condoms, which can be bought in many places (drugstores, clinics, adult bookstores, vending machines in public rest rooms, large supermarkets) and are given away in others (health clinics, doctor's offices, retail stores featuring sexual materials, gay bars), female condoms are as yet less easy to obtain and, therefore, to have handy. Female condoms, like male condoms, can also be used incorrectly and thus ineffectively. On rare occasions, the woman or man might be allergic to the polyurethane. Finally, as for its male counterpart and other female barrier methods, it does not appeal to everyone. Cost is a major problem for many potential users. Initially, the plastic female condom sold for about three times the local price of male condoms. Even at half the retail price, the female condom is too expensive for women in developing countries without substantial government and other agency subsidies. Faced with limited budgets, agencies may have to choose between expanding supplies of male condoms and providing female condoms. And availability does not ensure use. As a relatively new product, the female condom may not be accepted easily by women or by health care providers who need information to promote the new method and to advise women accurately. Women need culturally specific instructions and information to understand its benefits, allay concerns about potential side effects, and ensure correct use. They also need advice on convincing men to accept the product. Given the design, the cost, and the objections of men, many women are likely to use the female condom primarily to prevent STDs and only then as a back-up method to the male condom.

The polyurethane condom is the first vaginal barrier method designed specifically to prevent HIV transmission. Modifications are needed to make it more practical and more acceptable to all women, especially to those at highest risk of HIV infection. To reach potential users, the female condom will have to be promoted and widely distributed through the same channels as the male condom. Ensuring availability to women at high risk of sexually transmitted disease is particularly important. Many of the social marketing programs for condoms aimed specifically at AIDS prevention are setting up commercial outlets in places where high-risk behavior is likely to occur, such as hotels, truck stops, and bars. Such outlets ought to sell the female condom as well.

female homosexual   See LESBIAN.

female-to-female transmission   See TRANSMISSION.

female-to-male transmission   See TRANSMISSION.

feminine hygiene products   Vaginal douches, deodorants, and sprays that may encourage or increase risk of infection by destroying the normal flora and secretions of the vagina. They do not prevent pregnancy or STDs.

fenofibrate   An antihyperlipidemic used to control the triglyceride and blood fat levels of patients whose blood fats are not controlled by diet. It has proved particularly good for patients at risk for pancreatitis as a result of high levels of fats in their blood. Fenofibrate interacts with several drugs, including anticoagulants, so people taking this drug must warn their physicians about any medications they are already taking. Fenofibrate used by people who have liver, kidney, or gallbladder disease with attention to blood levels of enzymes related to these organs. It is unclear whether fenofibrate has any impact on the development of heart disease. (Trade name is Tricor.)

fertility   The quality of being productive or fertile; capable of conceiving a baby.

fetish   Object capable of pathologically arousing sexual excitement. This term is an extension of the belief among tribal communities that a specific object carries magical powers.

fetus   The unborn offspring of a human or an animal while in the uterus or within an egg during the latter stages of development. In humans, this period is considered to be from two or three months after conception until birth. Prior to this period, the fertilized egg is called an embryo.

fetus, transmission to   See TRANSMISSION.

fever   Elevation of body temperature above normal. The normal temperature taken orally is 98.6 degrees F (37 degrees C). From one degree above or two degrees below this value is considered within the range of normal. Rectal temperature is 0.5–1 degree higher than oral temperature.

fibrates   A class of drugs that are antihyperlipidimics. Fibrates are fibric acid derivatives. These drugs work by speeding up the chemical breakdown of triglyceride-rich lipoproteins that circulate in the body. They are used in particular to lower levels of triglycerides, which they control better than the STATIN group of drugs. They are not very effective at reducing LDL cholesterol level or raising HDL cholesterol level. The most common side effects are stomach pain, bloating, and nausea. Liver enzyme levels can also become elevated, and a myositislike syndrome, especially in patients with impaired renal function, can occur. Decreased libido and impotence have occasionally been reported. Fibrates can increase the effect of medications that thin the blood, so their use should be monitored closely by the physician. See BEZAFIBRATE; CIPROFIBRATE; FENOFIBRATE; GEMFIBROZIL.

fibric acid derivatives   Fibric acid derivatives (fibrates) include fenofibrate (Tricor) and gemfibrozil (Lopid). These drugs work by speeding the chemical breakdown of triglyceride-rich lipoproteins that circulate in the body. Fibrates are best known for their ability to lower triglyceride levels—by 30 percent to 55 percent in HIV-negative clinical trial participants—but do not offer much in the way of cholesterol level–lowering effects. In turn, fibrates are usually taken with other lipid level–lowering agents, typically a STATIN. Some experts believe that a fibrate-statin combination may increase the risk of rhabdomyolysis, a rare condition in which damage to muscles results in the release of muscle cell contents into the bloodstream, with potential to cause serious damage to the kidneys and other organs. Gemfibrozil is the most commonly used fibrate in the United States; however, experts suggest that HIV-positive people use fenofibrate, because it is not metabolized by the same enzyme system used by many of the PROTEASE INHIBITORS and NONNUCLEOSIDE REVERSE TRANSCRIPTASE INHIBITORS (NNRTIs). In other words, fenofibrate is less likely to have a negative interaction with anti-HIV drugs—at least in theory.

fimbria   The flared end of the fallopian tube, where it meets the ovary. It draws out and delivers the egg from the ovary into the FALLOPIAN TUBES.

financial counselor   A hospital employee who assists indigents in applying for MEDICAID, HILL-BURTON, GMS, or inhouse charity care.

financial planning   Because AIDS is a progressive, debilitating disease, and the longer a person has it, the more likely he or she will become incapable of dealing with routine business, dealing with financial matters is an important part of the practical preparations for future illness and possible death. Responsible financial planning ensures that an individual will not have to deal with financial problems in a crisis. Financial planning involves consideration of disability payments and other benefits to which one may be entitled, such as food stamps, welfare, and MEDICAID, as well as medical insurance. It may involve exploring sources of financial help other than public programs.

finger cot   Generally made of latex and sometimes of plastic or metal, often found in first-aid kits, finger cots are worn to protect fingers from trauma while healing from injuries. For safe sex, they are used to encase a digit for FINGER FUCKING. They can be bought at most medical suppliers and pharmacies.

finger fucking   Moving a finger in and out of the vagina, anus, or mouth in a manner similar to that of a penis during intercourse. See DIGITAL-ANAL SEX.

first-line treatment   The first choice or standard approach in treating a particular virus or infection. The first line of treatment varies with the virus concerned.

fist-fucking   This term is generally used to describe hand-anus contact but can be used to describe hand-vagina contact. See ANOMANUAL INTERCOURSE; BRACHIOPROCTIC EROTICISM; VAGINAL-MANUAL INTERCOURSE.

fisting   The insertion of an entire hand into someone's vagina or anus.

Fitz-Hugh-Curtis syndrome   A complication of gonorrhea and chlamydia in women that attacks the liver.

5-fluorouracil (5-FU) collagen matrix   A cancer chemotherapy drug. Collagen is a structural component of the skin and connective tissue. The collagen matrix was developed to keep the chemotherapy agent in the lesion longer. The drug was tested for use in HIV-negative people with anal or genital warts. It has been reported to be irritating for unknown reasons in HIV-positive people. However, it is occasionally given to men and women after surgery for human papillomavirus (HPV). In these instances, it has been shown to reduce recurrence of neoplasias.

5-FU collagen matrix   See 5-FLUOROURACIL COLLAGEN MATRIX.

flaccid   Soft, nonerect. Used when referring to a man's penis when it is not erect.

flagellation   The striking of oneself or someone else with an object or one's bare hand(s). Flagellation can also include being struck by someone else. Objects include both short implements, such as paddles, riding crops, or doubled-up belts, and more flexible implements, such as cat-of-nine tails, canes, or blacksnakes. Flagellants may be sexually aroused and gratified by either being threatened with pain or having pain administered, or by threatening or inflicting pain. Within the context of HIV/AIDS it is noted that anytime the skin is broken there is risk of disease transmission and infection. This can be minimized by cleaning the area and one's hands and by using sterile objects. A bloodied object should never be reused on another person unless it is sterilized.

flash   See EXHIBITIONISM.

floater   A drifting dark spot within the field of vision. Floaters can be caused by CMV RETINITIS, but may also appear as a normal part of the aging process. An HIV-knowledgeable eye doctor can make a correct diagnosis.

FLT   Also known as 3'-deoxy-3' fluorothimidine. A nucleoside analog drug that was tested in the early 1990s but rejected as a possible treatment because of its fairly high liver toxicity indicated in studies. However, because of viral resistance that has developed against several drugs, FLT is being looked at again for possible testing. The FDA has received initial preinvestigational new drug requests to restart studies of the drug.

fluax   See INFLUENZA VACCINE.

fluconazole   An antifungal drug that is approved for fungal infections, primarily those caused by CANDIDA ALBICANS (thrush or candidal esophagitis) and CRYPTOCOCCUS NEOFORMANS (cryptococcal meningitis), a severe complication of HIV infection. Another fungal infection, COCCIDIOIDOMYCOSIS, can also be treated with fluconazole. Fluconazole can be taken by mouth or vein. Side effects are unusual. Occasional problems are abdominal discomfort, nausea, rash, or signs of liver damage. Fluconazole has many drug-drug interactions with a wide variety of agents, including those frequently taken concurrently by people with HIV: For exam-

ple, RIFAMPIN has been shown to decrease the half-life of fluconazole. Fluconazole may also increase the blood levels of Dilantin, resulting in greater toxic effects for this drug. Levels of drugs used to control blood sugar level are increased when fluconazole is given. Using fluconazole in conjunction with such drugs as chlorpropamide, cisapride, glyburide, and tolbutamide can result in hypoglycemia (low blood sugar level). Additionally, the metabolism of the common anticoagulant coumadin is decreased by fluconazole so that taking both drugs together may prolong coumadin's effect. Finally, blood levels of various drugs (AZT, cyclosporine, Dilantin, and rifabutin) may increase when taken along with fluconazole. This may exacerbate their side effects. Although it is still under study for VAGINAL CANDIDIASIS and other fungal infections, recent trials have shown that weekly doses of fluconazole safely prevented certain common yeast infections, including mucosal candidiasis, the most common fungal infection affecting women with HIV, and was not associated with adverse events or drug resistance. Some doctors are starting people with low T4 cell counts on fluconazole or a related drug, ITRACONAZOLE, as preventive treatment for fungal infections. (Its trade name is Diflucan.)

flucytosine   Known as 5-FC and 5-fluorocytosine, an antifungal, antiyeast drug, administered orally to treat yeast and fungal infections predominantly caused by CANDIDA and CRYPTOCOCCUS species. Flucytosine works by changing the protein production of the fungus and affecting its genetic coding. The unbalanced growth causes the death of the fungus.

Flucytosine is not used much anymore. It requires a large number of pills, too many times a day. It was initially used together with AMPHOTERICIN B to treat cryptoccocal illness. However, the side effects of flucytosine are very difficult to manage in combination with use of amphotericin B. These include bone marrow toxicity, which leads to low platelet, white, and red blood cell counts; nausea; vomiting; anorexia; bloating; diarrhea; and elevated liver enzyme levels. Renal functions can also be tough to manage on this medication. It is easier to manage in combination with fluconazole. The combination of flucytosine and fluconazole is effective in treating cryptococcal meningitis to bring it under control. Flucytosine and fluconazole are both available as tablets, which do not require intravenous use, as amphotericin B does. (Trade name is Ancobon.)

fluid retention   Failure to eliminate fluid from the body because of renal, cardiac, or metabolic disorders, or a combination of these. A low-sodium diet is indicated in cases of fluid retention, since it is caused by excess salt in the body, which causes retention of water to maintain the proper chemical and physical properties of body fluids.

Fluogen   See INFLUENZA VACCINE.

fluorescent treponemal antibody absorption test (FTA-ABS)   A test of the treponemal variety (looking for *Treponema pallidum* the corkscrew-shaped organisms that cause syphilis). False-positive reactions may occur when the patient's serum contains antinuclear factors, rheumatoid factor, or increased globulins. Blood from a vein is tested.

fluorouracil   An antimetabolite used in treating certain forms of cancer. (Trade names are Efudex and Fluoroplex.)

fluoxetine hydrochloride   An antidepressant that is approved for treatment of major forms of depression. It is also used to treat obsessive–compulsive disorder, bulimia nervosa, and premenstrual dysphoric disorder (commonly referred to as PMS). Fluoxetine works by slowly restoring normal levels of a nerve transmitter (serotonin). Possible side effects are decreased appetite and weight loss. Some patients have reported conversion of depression to mania in manic-depressive (bipolar) disorders, but this effect is rare. Although press reports suggested fluoxetine caused major depression and suicidal ideation in many people who used it, a review of literature on this subject reveals that development or intensification of suicidal thoughts during treatment (regardless of the severity of depression) has been documented for many antidepressant drugs in use. Fluoxetine is a SELECTIVE SEROTONIN REUPTAKE INHIBITOR (SSRI), referring to its family of drugs. (Trade name is Prozac.)

flush   A sudden redness of the skin that may be associated with any febrile disease.

fluvastatin   Fluvastatin sodium, is a cholesterol level–lowering drug. It is a member of the STATIN group of cholesterol level–lowering drugs. It reduces elevated total cholesterol level and decreases fat levels of patients with primary hypercholesterolemia and mixed dyslipidemia whose response to dietary restriction of fats and cholesterol, and other nonpharmacological measures, has not been adequate. It may also slow the progression of coronary atherosclerosis of patients with coronary heart disease. It usually is taken once a day at bedtime. People who use this drug should have liver enzyme levels monitored to detect abnormal liver conditions sometimes associated with drugs of the STATIN group. As with all drugs of this nature it should not be used by pregnant or nursing women, as babies need a good concentration of fat and cholesterol from their mother in order to develop properly. Because some drugs interact negatively with fluvastatin, patients using it should inform their physicians of all other medications they are using concurrently. (Trade name is Lescol XL.)

foam barrier   A form of chemical contraceptive; a spermicide-containing foam that is placed in the vagina prior to intercourse. It may be used alone but is most effective in combination with another contraceptive method or device.

fold resistance   Phenotypic testing for HIV is reported in terms of the measure of fold resistance. When lab results state phenotype test results as 20-fold resistance, it means that a sample of HIV grew at a rate 20 times more than the rate of a sample of a specific WILD-TYPE VIRUS. Doctors generally like to see results below 4-fold as this generally means the HAART regimen is effective. Results of 10-fold or greater generally indicate that a regimen is not currently working. The correlation for all HIV antivirals is still unclear. See PHENOTYPE TEST.

folic acid   A member of the VITAMIN B complex necessary for various metabolic reactions. Folic acid is a required supplement to the diet of pregnant women. It is known to prevent congenital birth defects of the neural tube. A standard amount to supplement a pregnant woman's diet is 0.5 to 1 mg folic acid. Inadequate amounts of folic acid lead to anemia. Folic acid is found naturally in green plant tissue, liver, and yeast. Also called folate, vitamin B_9, and vitamin M.

folinic acid   A derivative of FOLIC ACID used to counteract the effects of folic acid antagonists such as pyrimethamine and to treat anemia caused by a deficiency of folic acid. It is also called citrovorum factor, leucovorin, and calcium folinate.

follicle   A small sac or cavity for secretion; a sweat gland in the skin that produces skin oil to keep the skin lubricated. It is also a part of a lymph node. Lymph nodes are made up of multiple follicles.

follicle-stimulating hormone (FSH)   A hormone produced by the anterior pituitary. It stimulates growth of the follicle in the ovary and spermatogenesis in the testes.

follicular dendritic cell (FDC)   A dendritic cell found in the spleen and lymph node follicles. It has long tentaclelike arms that retain antigens on their surface for a significantly long period. The cells' major function is to obtain antigen in tissues, migrate to lymphoid organs, and activate T cells and B lymphocytes. B cells, with T-cell help and FDC costimulation, become B memory cells and antibody-producing plasma cells. These cell interactions are responsible for immunity to disease. It is considered part of the macrophage group of cells. In HIV infection the virus becomes trapped along with the antibodies on the FDC and is transported to the lymph areas of the body. This is one reason why lymphoid tissues are among the major areas of HIV infection. Therefore, although these cells themselves are not believed to be infected generally, they assist the virus in its ability to move through the body.

folliculitis   A common problem in HIV. It is a bacterial infection that is localized in a hair follicle. It can appear around beards, the back of legs, any-where that there is hair. It is commonly due to *Staphylococcus aureus*, generally called "staph." BOILS are a deep hair follicle infection by this organism. Recommended treatment includes soap and water, antiseptics, antibiotic ointment, and oral antibiotics, in ascending order. A type of folliculitis that results from unclean warm or hot water, called spa pool folliculitis, is due to infection with *Pseudomonas aeruginosa*.

Late in HIV infection some people experience a red, itchy, acnelike skin eruption that appears similar to staph folliculitis but is not caused by bacteria or fungi. The exact cause of eosinophilic folliculitis is in fact still unknown. The eosinophils are known to be involved in allergic reactions, and they are clustered in the areas of these bumps, but what they are reacting to is not understood. The condition is most often seen in persons with a CD4 cell count below 200. Treatment first employs antibiotics; then, if they are not effective, treatments for scabies are tried. It is thought that perhaps the reaction is to the skin mites that live in human hair follicles; for that reason scabies treatment sometimes is effective. Occasionally ultraviolet B (UVB) light treatments are also used.

fomites   An inanimate object that can harbor pathogenic microorganisms, therefore serving as an agent of transmission of an infection. Coins, computer keyboards, and kitchen sinks can all be considered as fomites.

fomivirsen   Also known as fomivirsen sulfate. Manufactured by Novartis. Fomivirsen is used for the treatment of CYTOMEGALOVIRUS (CMV). It is an ANTISENSE phosphorothioate oligonucleotide, a new class of drugs that use a unique antisense mechanism to block the replication of mRNA. mRNA is also referred to as a sense structure; hence the term *antisense*. Fomivirsen binds to the mRNA and stops the protein synthesis of the virus, thereby preventing replication. In treatment of CMV, it is given in INTRAOCULAR injections. This process does not cause pain as the eyeball is numbed before the injection. (Trade name is Vitravene.)

Food and Drug Act of 1906   The original legislation giving the federal government regulatory control over food and drugs. It is the basis for federal regulation of testing AIDS drugs. The act prohibited interstate commerce in misbranded and adulterated foods, drinks, and drugs. The power to administer the law was placed in the Agriculture Department's Bureau of Chemistry. Today, the FOOD AND DRUG ADMINISTRATION (FDA) administers a broad range of legislation, including the Public Health Service Act (1944), the Federal Hazardous Substances Act (1960), the Fair Packaging and Labeling Act (1966), the Radiation Control for Health and Safety Act (1968), the Drug Listing Act of 1972, the Infant Formula Act of 1980, the Orphan Drug Act of 1983 and its amendments of 1985 and 1988, the Federal Anti-Tampering Act (1983), the Drug Price Competition and Patent Term Restoration Act (1984), the Prescription Drug Marketing Act of 1987, the Health Omnibus Programs Extension of 1988, the Nutrition Labeling and Education Act (1990), the FDA Revitalization Act (1990), the Safe Medical Devices Act of 1990, the Generic Drug Enforcement Act of 1992, the Mammography Quality Standards Act of 1992, the Prescription Drug User Free Act of 1992, the Dietary Supplement Act of 1992, and the Dietary Supplement Health and Education Act of 1994. See FOOD, DRUG AND COSMETIC ACT (FDC) OF 1938.

Food and Drug Administration   An agency of the United States DEPARTMENT OF HEALTH AND HUMAN SERVICES that regulates the testing, sale, and promotion of pharmaceutical drugs and food products. The agency also approves new medical procedures for marketing based on evidence of safety and efficacy. Early in the AIDS crisis, when the epidemic's disastrous scope could not yet be imagined, AIDS activists pressed the FDA for a faster and more humane response to this public health emergency. In response, the FDA established accelerated approval and expanded access programs. For example, SAQUINAVIR, the first of the new generation of PROTEASE INHIBITOR drugs, was approved in a record three months, the fastest AIDS drug approval ever.

After the Republican victory in the 1994 congressional elections, the new Congress immediately took up the cause of FDA reform as one of its highest priorities. Instead of focusing on manage-

ment problems at the FDA, the Republican Congress set its sights on the Food, Drug and Cosmetic Act (FDC) itself. The FDC gives the federal government the duty to ensure that drugs, biological products, and medical devices are safe and effective for the treatment of specific health conditions and that evidence of that safety and efficacy is accurately presented to the American people. The act fosters an environment in which medical innovation grows out of solid clinical research. People with AIDS, as well as those with other life-threatening diseases, need this research more than anyone to point the way to effective treatments. By seeking to amend fundamental government authority over drug regulation, Congress has focused not on problems at the FDA but on reducing the role of the federal government in medical, pharmaceutical, and clinical research. FDA-regulated industries, which would benefit financially from such reform, initiated a major lobbying and public relations campaign within a month of the 1994 election. In the summer of 1995, patient advocacy groups also joined together in the Patients' Coalition, which includes over 80 leading national organizations. Perhaps as a result, FDA reform legislation has taken longer to move through Congress than many had predicted. Despite numerous hearings held on FDA reform issues in both the House and the Senate during the 104th Congress, legislation has been very slow to emerge. In fact, there is no consensus on FDA reform.

Food, Drug and Cosmetic Act of 1938   A major overhaul of the basic food and drug legislation occurred in 1938 with the passage of the Food, Drug and Cosmetic (FDC) Act of 1938. Signed by President Franklin D. Roosevelt on June 25, 1938, this act broadened the original legislation by extending the regulatory power of the Food and Drug Administration (FDA) to cover cosmetics and medical devices; requiring predistribution approval of new drugs; requiring that tolerance levels be set for unavoidable poisonous substances; authorizing standards of identity, quality, and fill levels for containers for foods; authorizing inspections of factories where regulated products are manufactured; and adding court injunctions to FDA enforcement powers. The FDC has been amended several times since its passage. Examples include the Humphrey Amendment signed in 1951, the Food Additives Amendment signed in 1958, the Color Additive Amendments of 1960, the Drug Amendments of 1962, the Drug Abuse Control Amendments of 1965, the Vitamins and Minerals Amendments of 1976, the Medical Device Amendments of 1976.

food stamp program A federally financed, state-run welfare program that gives low-income persons vouchers (food stamps) with which to purchase food.

foreplay Activities a couple enjoys before sexual intercourse. For many couples these erotic activities are extremely exciting, stimulating, and fulfilling in themselves and are not simply a prelude to intercourse.

fornication Voluntary sexual intercourse between two persons not married to each other.

Fortovase See SAQUINAVIR.

fosamprenavir See AMPRENAVIR.

foscarnet A broad-spectrum antiviral (trisodium phosphonoformate). It is used in treatment of CYTOMEGALOVIRUS that has proved resistant to ganciclovir and against HERPES SIMPLEX virus that is resistant to acyclovir. Possible adverse side effects include kidney toxicity. There are always changes in kidney functions, which therefore must be monitored. Electrolyte imbalance must also be watched for, and it is not unusual for patients to receive supplements of calcium, phosphorus, magnesium, and potassium while on foscarnet. Electrolyte imbalance can lead to seizures. Other side effects include anemia and nausea. Foscarnet concentrates in the urine; people taking this drug are strongly advised to wipe and wash themselves thoroughly after urination to prevent skin ulcers, which can be caused by high concentrations of the drug. Uncircumcised men and women especially need to follow these guidelines. Drinking plenty of water can help alleviate the concentration in the urine somewhat. There does not seem to be any cross-resistance to foscarnet. (Trade name is Foscavir.)

foster care Care of an orphaned, abandoned, abused, or neglected child by adults or facilities acting in place of the children's parents, supervised by welfare caseworkers.

free HIV See CELL-FREE VIRUS.

free radicals A highly reactive molecular fragment that bears one or more unpaired electrons. For some time, it has been known that foods contain more substances than just vitamins and minerals and energy-giving nutrients. There are known nutrient antioxidants like vitamins E and C and selenium, and there are the new nonnutrient antioxidants like the carotenoids, the phytochemicals, and the polyphenols. These substances aid in removing molecules that attack healthy cells in the body and leave it vulnerable to cancer.

The oxygen we breathe and cannot live without can become one of our worst enemies. Excess oxidation is damaging and destructive to the body. Four destructive forms of oxygen have been identified: hydroxyl radical and superoxide radical (the two real free radicals) and the "nonradical reactive species" oxygen singlet and hydrogen peroxide. Destructive oxygen reactions have been linked to at least 50 diseases, including AIDS.

Oxygen reactions take place when an oxidant or free radical is created that has lost one electron and is no longer stable. In its search for stability, the radical grabs electrons from other healthy cells causing the creation of more radicals. When radicals attack fatty molecules, rancidity results, and the stage is set for deterioration and eventual disease. When these free radicals attack DNA molecules and begin to mutate them, conditions become positive for cancer and also for other degenerative conditions including aging. In order for the body to defend itself against free radicals, it produces free-radical scavengers, or endogenous ANTIOXIDANTS. These agents are made by the body and catch and destroy extra free radicals and keep them from creating greater damage. Exercise contributes oxygen to the system and can increase free radicals in the body. A selenium supplement (50 to 100 micrograms) is also thought to be beneficial, as it strengthens GSH (an antioxidant that counters hydrogen peroxide). Studies continue on the benefit of the coenzyme Q10 for those who exercise extensively. A physician should be consulted before any vitamin therapy is begun since side effects occur at large doses.

freebase   A form of cocaine used by addicts in which the hydrochloride salt is alkalinized, extracted with an organic solvent (e.g., ether), and then heated to 90 degrees C. After inhalation, the drug is absorbed rapidly through the lungs.

freebasing   The inhalation of a form of cocaine known as freebase.

freedom of speech   The right of people to express their opinions openly has come under attack, particularly in the area of AIDS education. Numerous attempts have been made at the local, state, and federal levels to control the content of specific AIDS educational materials. There have also been challenges to teachers' resources, such as curriculum guides and textbooks. In some states police have gone so far as to infiltrate AIDS activist organizations to keep them from demonstrating at public events.

French kiss   A kiss that includes tongue contact and exchange of saliva. Also called a *wet kiss*.

fruit   A derogatory 20th-century term for a male homosexual. Often used for humor or irony by gays.

FS   See FOOD STAMP PROGRAM.

FTA   See FLUORESCENT TREPONEMAL ANTIBODY ABSORPTION TEST.

fuck   To have sexual intercourse. *Fuck* is by far the most widely used term for this activity in the English language. In its adjectival form it is also used almost universally as an intensifier, with no particular sexual connection although this usage is considered quite vulgar. See COITUS.

fulminant   A term given to an illness or condition that is severe or aggressive.

functional antibody   An ANTIBODY that binds to an antigen and has an effect. Functional antibodies

cover a viral antigen and kill it. Most viral vaccines stimulate functional antibodies to work.

fundus   The back wall of the eye or the retina.

funduscopy   Visual examination of the retina with an ophthalmoscope.

funerals   Funerals have often been turned into occasions of political protest during the AIDS epidemic, and many political protests have taken the form of mock funerals (for example, plans to scatter human ashes on the White House lawn as a protest of the Reagan Administration's management of AIDS education and treatment research). The obvious reason for this is to demonstrate the nature of the AIDS epidemic and to instill a sense of urgency by showing the consequences of delay, mismanagement, neglect, or callousness by those making and executing public health policy. This tactic has been controversial and has been attacked as tasteless or worse, but those activists who support it say that the direness of the crisis justifies it.

fungal encephalitis   Inflammation of the brain resulting from invasion by a PATHOGENIC FUNGUS.

fungal infection   The state or condition in which the body, or a part of it, is invaded by a PATHOGENIC FUNGUS. Terbinafine, an allylamine antifungal agent, has been shown to be effective in treating HIV-positive patients who have minor skin and nail fungal problems such as tinea pedis (athlete's foot), tinea cruris (jock itch), and tinea circinata (ringworm, not a worm). Other fungal infections that are considered OPPORTUNISTIC INFECTIONS in HIV-positive people include CANDIDIASIS (*Candida* species), CRYPTOCOCCOSIS, coccidioidomycosis (valley fever), and ASPERGILLUS and HISTOPLASMOSIS infections.

Fungicidin   See NYSTATIN.

fungus   One of a group of plants, lacking chlorophyll, that includes yeast, molds, mildew, and mushrooms. Fungi exist parasitically on organic matter and are generally simple in structure and form. Some fungi are single-celled but differ from bacteria in that they have a distinct nucleus and other cellular structures. AIDS patients are especially vulnerable to infection by fungi because of their compromised immune systems. Recently, powerful antifungal agents have been developed for treatment.

furuncle   See BOIL.

furunculosis   The persistent simultaneous occurrence of FURUNCLES.

furunculus   See BOIL.

fusin   See CXCR-4.

fusion   Process by which an enveloped virus joins or merges with the cell membrane; at that instant, the viral genes and proteins that were outside the cell, within a separate virus particle, are inside. The cell is infected and viral replication begins. The molecular events that bring about this fusion were first determined through analysis of the three-dimensional structure of hemagglutinin, the surface protein of the influenza A virus that binds to cells. Recent studies of the three-dimensional structure of parts of the HIV envelope protein suggest strongly that HIV fuses with cells in nearly an identical way. As is hemagglutinin, the HIV envelope spike is a trimeric structure made up of two subunits: the outer gp120 portion, which binds to the cell, and the underlying gp41 subunit, anchored within the HIV envelope. With HIV, and as contrasted with hemagglutinin, the fusion does not take place within endosomes, but at the cell surface. As with hemagglutinin, the outer gp120 portion must undergo a change in configuration or detach to allow the gp41 subunit to pierce or harpoon the cell membrane. But unlike with hemagglutinin, this uncapping of gp41 is not brought about by a change in pH but by the binding of gp120 to CD4 and a chemokine coreceptor. See FUSION INHIBITOR.

fusion inhibitor   A relatively new class of antiretroviral drug used in the fight against HIV and AIDS. So called because it works by preventing the HIV from binding to and entering the human cell. Fusion inhibitors bind to the CD4 receptor, CCR-5 or CXCR4 coreceptor, or cell membrane. When the virus cannot penetrate the host cell membrane and infect the cell, HIV replication within that host cell is prevented. These drugs are also called entry inhibitors and receptor inhibitors. Fusion inhibitors under development currently are administered by subcutaneous injections. Fusion inhibitors seemingly have very few side effects and have been highly effective in reducing viral loads and neutralizing HIV. In vitro studies have shown fusion inhibitors to block both cell-cell and cell-virus fusion. See ENFUVIRTIDE.

future Medicare eligibility date   Two years after the first date of eligibility for SSDI benefits.

Fuzeon   See ENFUVIRTIDE.

G

GAA See GEOGRAPHIC AREAS OF AFFINITY.

GAG gene A gene of HIV that codes for the core protein p55. p55 is the precursor of HIV proteins p17, p24, p7, and p6. GAG is the gene for group-specific antigens (proteins) that make up the viral NUCLEOCAPSID, the inner protein shell surrounding HIV's strand of RNA. A virus commandeers a cell's reproductive apparatus to make more of itself. New-minted particles migrate to the cell wall and push through it, pinching off to freedom in a process called budding. In retroviruses, including HIV, control over budding falls to the *gag* gene. It may also refer to the proteins produced by the gene. Researchers are using the GAG gene in development of an HIV VACCINE. See ENV GENE; POL GENE; POLYPROTEIN.

gallbladder disease Also known as HIV cholangiopathy or acalculous cholecystitis. The gallbladder is a pear-shaped organ on the interior surface of the liver. It acts as a reservoir for bile. Gallbladder disease without stones is commonly associated with late-stage HIV infection, when there are fewer than 100 T cells. It can cause narrowing of the bile ducts and scattered narrowing of the bile ducts inside the liver, thus blocking the flow of bile between the liver and the intestine and resulting in jaundice and pain. It can also cause sclerosing cholangitis. It is not known definitively why HIV-related gallbladder disease occurs, but the condition is frequently associated with such OPPORTUNISTIC INFECTIONS as CMV, CRYPTOSPORIDIOSIS, and microsporidiosis.

Symptoms of HIV-related gallbladder and bile duct disease include severe right-side abdominal pain with fever, vomiting, progressive weight loss, intermittent fevers, swollen glands, jaundice, and diarrhea. The vagueness of these symptoms makes it easy to misdiagnose this disease. The possibility of gallbladder disease without stones must be considered when patients have abdominal pain, especially in the presence of elevated serum alkaline phosphatase level and the absence of jaundice. MRIs are effective for evaluating the presence of bile duct disease. Because of the nature of these infections, actual tissue specimens may be necessary in order to make the diagnosis. ERCP (an endoscopic procedure in which dye is injected into the biliary ducts), removal of the infected gallbladder, and liver biopsy may all be required to identify the infectious agent positively and begin appropriate treatment. If specific organisms can be identified, antibiotic therapy may be necessary. Further treatment, such as surgical removal of the gallbladder or opening of the obstructed bile duct entrance, may be required to eliminate the infectious agent. Removal of the bile duct can help remove reservoirs of infection.

GALT (gut-associated lymphoid tissue) The accumulations of lymphoid tissue associated with the GASTROINTESTINAL tract.

gamma globulin A type of protein found in the blood. It is made up of antibodies. When gamma globulins are extracted from the blood of many people and combined, they can be used to prevent or treat infections. They are used in what are sometimes called vaccines for hepatitis A and chicken pox. Gamma globulins are synthesized by lymphocytes and plasma cells in response to an antigenic challenge. The ability to resist infection is related to concentration of such proteins.

gamma interferon A protein formed by human cells that limits the production of some viruses.

ganciclovir A synthetic antiviral drug used to treat infections caused by CYTOMEGALOVIRUS RETINITIS in immunocompromised patients and occasionally infections caused by HERPES SIMPLEX and other viruses. Licensed by the FOOD AND DRUG ADMINISTRATION in 1989, it is generally used as an INTRAVENOUS drug. The oral form of the drug is not often used now as it is not absorbed well. Ganciclovir is used to delay the progression of existing CMV disease. There is also a fairly expensive INTRAOCULAR implant that works better than both the tablet and intravenous formulation and does not require a catheter. (Patients receiving intravenous ganciclovir must have a central venous line, usually a Hickman catheter, inserted and receive infusions every day for the rest of their lives, an extremely burdensome, time-consuming, and expensive procedure.)

The most important side effects are renal toxicity, low blood counts, and especially NEUTROPENIA, which predisposes to bacterial infections. If neutropenia is severe enough, the dose should be reduced or the drug temporarily stopped. Drugs with similar effects on the bone marrow should not in general be prescribed at the same time unless the benefits are believed to outweigh the risks. If this occurs people, often have G-CSF (Neupogen) added to the regimen to help increase white blood cell production. (Trade name is Cytovene.)

ganglion A mass of nervous tissue located outside the brain or spinal cord; also, a benign cystic tumor developing on a tendon or aponeurosis, sometimes occurring in the back of the wrist or dorsum of the foot; a knotlike mass.

Gantrisin See SULFISOXAZOLE.

gardnerella A bacterium that was at one time thought to cause BACTERIAL VAGINOSIS. It is known to increase in number during that condition but is no longer thought to cause it.

garlic A member of the lily family that has been given the distinction of being called a "wonder drug." It is the world's second oldest medicine; ephedra was the first. It is made up of sulfur compounds; amino acids; minerals such as germanium, selenium, and zinc; and vitamins A, B, and C. Allicin, a sulfur-containing compound, is believed to be primarily responsible for most of garlic's suggested health benefits along with its unique color. Garlic has been used for many medicinal purposes in folk and holistic treatment. Raw garlic is said to be effective against bacteria, parasites, and viruses. It has been claimed to be effective against heart disease and stroke as well as colds and diarrhea. It also contains compounds, including antioxidants, that are thought to be cancer preventatives. It is believed to help lower cholesterol level and blood pressure. It is effective raw and cooked. Today, clinical and basic studies suggest a broad spectrum of potential uses. Some have postulated that garlic works as an ANTIOXIDANT against FREE RADICALS because of its germanium and selenium content. Claims of garlic's effectiveness against AIDS-related OPPORTUNISTIC INFECTIONS are based on in vitro studies that have shown garlic to be an antibacterial and antifungal agent. However, many chemicals have worked against the virus in the test tube and later had no effect on the virus. Eating too much raw garlic, or taking too many garlic pills, can have toxic effects. The high sulfur content can cause dermatitis and can also cause colitis by an overkill of the normal flora of the intestines. In high doses, garlic may inhibit blood clotting and interfere with proper thyroid function. A 2002 study shows that garlic supplements decrease SAQUINAVIR (Fortovase) levels by an average of 51 percent and are therefore likely to reduce saquinavir's anti-HIV activity greatly. This reduction can lead to the rapid development of resistance to saquinavir.

gastric anacidity See ACHLORHYDRIA.

gastritis The stomach is susceptible to the same disease processes as the esophagus, including infection with cytomegalovirus (CMV). Gastritis, or inflammation of the stomach, may be asymptomatic but often results in severe continuous upper abdominal pain, fever, hemorrhage, or obstruction. CMV infection of the small intestine may result in similar symptoms as well as weight loss and diarrhea. Although CMV may infect any part of the small intestine, it rarely does so without involvement of other gastrointestinal organs.

Another cause of stomach pain in HIV-positive people is *Helicobacter pylori,* the bacterium that has been shown to be the cause of stomach ulcers. When HIV disease reaches a later stage, *Helicobacter pylori* that has until then been under control or unnoticed often flares up. Endoscopy reveals whether it is the bacterium causing the discomfort.

gastroenteritis   Inflammation of the stomach and intestinal tract, which can cause abdominal pain and diarrhea.

gastrointestinal   Pertaining to organs of the digestive system, also called the GASTROINTESTINAL TRACT.

gastrointestinal dysfunction   Abnormal, impaired, or inadequate functioning of the stomach and intestines.

gastrointestinal exams   X-ray examinations of the gastrointestinal (GI) tract are used in the diagnosis of a number of complications associated with HIV and AIDS. There are three basic GI tract exams: the upper GI exam focuses on the esophagus and stomach; the lower GI exam, on the small intestine; and the barium enema exam, on the large intestine and bowel. All GI exams require the use of a contrast agent that blocks X rays and thereby silhouettes the body parts of interest, allowing visual interpretation. Contrast agents used for the GI tract are usually composed of a barium sulfate liquid suspension, but iodine- and non-iodine-based contrast agents are also used. The barium mixture has a thick milky consistency and is either swallowed or introduced into the rectum by an enema while the X rays are taken. The contrast agent and not the X rays generally causes any complications arising from the exam. Constipation, rectal bleeding, faintness, weakness, abdominal pain, inability to pass gas, polyuria (excessive urination), nocturia (excessive urination at night), and abdominal distention (extension of the abdomen with pressure) are examples of complications that may arise. Allergic reaction is also a consideration when using any contrast agent.

gastrointestinal (GI) tract   The organs that absorb and digest food, including the mouth, esophagus, stomach, small and large intestines, colon, and rectum.

gay   A term denoting sexual attraction to people of the same sex. As a noun, a woman or man who is sexually attracted to others of the same sex and defines herself or himself, or is defined by others, in terms of sexual orientation. Generally refers to male homosexuals, but may also include homosexual women. See LESBIAN.

gay bowel syndrome   A historic term that was used in the 1970s with the dramatic increase in enteric diseases within the gay community, such as AMEBIASIS and GIARDIASIS. It was used to denote a constellation of intestinal diseases among gay men including proctitis, proctocolitis, and enteritis.

gay lymph-node syndrome   A now obsolete term applied to generalized LYMPHADENOPATHY (with benign reactive changes shown in biopsy) prior to 1981, when the CENTERS FOR DISEASE CONTROL AND PREVENTION published the first description of persistent generalized lymphadenopathy.

Gay Men's Health Crisis (GMHC)   An AIDS service organization (ASO), one of the first, in New York City. In the United States, as in other countries, privately organized prevention programs started before official government programs. In New York City, the threat of HIV was recognized by a small group of men, who, in September 1981, gathered in the apartment of the writer Larry Kramer in order to do something about the new epidemic in their midst. That day they created the Gay Men's Health Crisis (GMHC). In the following two years, after its example, similar organizations were formed in other major United States cities. Today, the GMHC is recognized not only as one of the premier ASOs, but also as a major nongovernmental HIV/AIDS prevention and care organization.

GMHC, like its counterparts elsewhere, has helped and continues to help thousands of homosexual men overcome the isolation and fear associated with a diagnosis of AIDS. Due in large measure to GMHC's work, large-scale behavior changes among gay men occurred in New York City and San Francisco (the San Francisco AIDS Foundation) in the early 1980s. GMHC has succeeded in responding with equal compassion to the needs of other groups besides gay men with a high incidence of HIV infection—persons of color, injection drug users, and women. GMHC's program is evolving in parallel to the evolving AIDS pandemic.

gay plague   In the early years of the epidemic, this term was often used to denote the acquired immunodeficiency syndrome, since gay men were the first infected and for some time constituted the greatest number of reported cases in the United States. It was often used in a derogatory sense.

gay pneumonia   A term used in the early years of the epidemic to denote PNEUMOCYSTIS CARINII PNEU-MONIA. See GAY PLAGUE.

gay-related immune deficiency (GRID)   An obsolete term used in the very early years of the HIV epidemic. One of a group of names used initially to denote the acquired immunodeficiency syndrome. See ACQUIRED IMMUNODEFICIENCY SYN-DROME; COMMUNITY-ACQUIRED IMMUNE DEFICIENCY SYNDROME; GAY-RELATED IMMUNODEFICIENCY DISEASE.

gay-related immunodeficiency disease   See GAY-RELATED IMMUNE DEFICIENCY.

G-CSF   See GRANULOCYTE COLONY STIMULATING FACTOR.

gel   A colloid or jellylike substance. Barrier contraceptives are available in gel form and work like foams and vaginal suppositories. Gels, as other contraceptives, are most effective in combination with condoms.

gemfibrozil   A fenofibrate drug that is used to reduce triglyceride levels in patients. As can all fenofibrates, it can cause a rise in liver enzyme levels and possible myositislike syndrome, especially in patients with impaired renal function. In some people LDL level may rise when they are being treated with this drug. (Trade name is Lopid.)

gender differences   Early in the AIDS epidemic, the number of men with HIV in developing coun-tries vastly exceeded the number of women with HIV. Their relative lack of numbers limited women's participation in early clinical research. This unintended underrepresentation of women in clinical studies has contributed to a less complete understanding of HIV infection in women than in men. Nonetheless, today we do know that women have some manifestations of HIV infection that are different from those of men. These include, among others, VAGINAL CANDIDIASIS, GENITAL PAPILLO-MAVIRUS INFECTIONS, and PELVIC INFLAMMATORY DIS-EASE, a painful condition of the genital tract that may be caused by a number of different microorganisms. The incidence of some malignancies differs in women and men. KAPOSI'S SARCOMA, a cancer affecting skin and lymph nodes, is relatively infrequent in HIV-infected women; abnormalities of the cervical tissue, including a greatly increased incidence of precancerous lesions, are fairly common in HIV-infected women. To date, there is little information concerning differences between women and men in the effects of various therapies directed at HIV infection.

Women also face a number of issues specific to them as women: rape and AIDS, pregnancy, artificial insemination, prostitution, and the incidence of HIV/AIDS in African women. Talking to children about HIV/AIDS is not a gender-specific issue, strictly speaking but it is a burden that falls on women disproportionately. See WOMEN AND PREGNANCY.

gender-specific issues   See GENDER DIFFERENCES.

gene   The basic unit in which is encoded the form and function of a cell or an organism. Chains of genes in ordered sequences make up the DNA of a cell. Genes function either to specify the formation of a protein or part of a protein or regulate or repress the operation of other genes. The complete human genome contains between 50,000 and 100,000 genes.

gene therapy   A distinct emerging form of treatment in which new manufactured genes are inserted into patients to fight disease or correct disorders of genetic origin by compensating for other deficient proteins, inhibiting abnormal cellular functioning, or regulating the expression of other genes. HIV, can be described as an acquired genetic disease. HIV integrates itself into DNA to transform cells so they create copies of itself. HIV-infected cells mostly CD4s and macrophages produce viral proteins and then assemble them into new viruses. Ultimately, viral infection and replication destroy the cell. Research has identified several of the proteins that play a part in the replication of HIV. This includes enzymes such as REVERSE TRANSCRIPTASE, PROTEASE, and TAT. Anti-HIV drugs work by attacking these proteins. For example, drugs such as AZT, ddi, and ddc are aimed at the reverse transcriptase enzyme; the PROTEASE INHIBITOR is aimed at the protease enzyme. The disadvantage of this approach is that it does not halt the production of these proteins at their source. A drug must be given in high doses to disable every copy of the protein and must be given for the lifetime of the patient. Gene therapy, works against the origin of the disease, the HIV genome. Many strategies are being considered to fight HIV at the genetic level. Some scientists are trying to engineer genes that protect a cell from infection; other researchers are creating genes that regulate HIV into harmlessness. Initial in-vitro models are encouraging, but none of these approaches has yet been tested in humans. Theoretically, gene therapy has at least one great advantage over current therapies: the implanted mechanism for fighting disease within our genetic code lasts as long as the host cell. There is great hope for the future that if researchers can manage to implant therapeutic genes into stem cells (the progenitor cells of all blood cells), every blood cell will be immunized against HIV infection. Gene therapy has had some setbacks as deaths of patients have created a strong political reaction. However, research continues into various illnesses and some studies do include human subjects.

gene transfer therapy   A form of GENE THERAPY that has been shown to prolong the survival of critical immune system cells, such as CD4+ T CELLS, that are typically depleted during the course of HIV disease.

General Assistance (GA)   A generic term used for state-local welfare programs for poor persons who are not coverable by the federal SSI and AFDC programs.

General Medical Assistance (GMA)   State and local programs to provide health care to poor persons who are not coverable by the federal MEDICAID program.

general paresis   A progressive form of mental illness caused by neurosyphilis and characterized by gross confusion.

general population surveys   Large-scale, population-based national HIV seroprevalence surveys have been conducted in only a few countries, including Uganda, Rwanda, Côte d'Ivoire, and the former Soviet Union. These surveys are distinct from the population-based sample surveys undertaken in a number of nonnational geographic settings. Data from a national survey provides, to some extent, a more complete picture of the epidemic in a country. However, it has become increasingly recognized that such surveys leave many important questions unanswered.

generalizability   The degree to which a trial's findings can be applied to a wider population outside the trial participants. For any particular study, the answers received refer only to the people who were in that particular trial at that time. Even if the trial were redone with all of the same people at another time, the answer(s) could be very different. As a rule, a study is only useful to the "real world" in proportion to its generalizability.

genetic engineering   The synthesis, alteration replacement, or repair of an organism's basic genetic material by synthetic means.

genetic material   Material found in the cells of living things that is used in reproduction. In regard to AIDS, this is the material in a cell that determines what kind of cell will be created through transcription.

genetic mutation   A change in the character of a gene that is perpetuated in subsequent divisions of the cell in which it occurs. See GENETIC ENGINEERING.

genetic predisposition   Higher-than-normal susceptibility to a condition or disease by virtue of genetic endowment (i.e., heredity).

genetic research   The study and examination of reproduction and heredity and its variance.

genetic variability   The variability in genetic sequences of a life form. In human beings and other forms of higher life there is no more than 5 percent variation in genetic sequences from person to person, cow to cow, or even *Escherichia coli* to *Escherichia coli*. However, viruses have much more variability. Viruses have up to 35 percent difference between individual viruses. Retroviruses in particular have nearly 35 percent mutability. This mutability makes creating drugs or vaccines that can work against all of the possible variations of a particular virus such as HIV difficult. The efficacy of vaccines depends on their capacity to cover an increasingly broad spectrum of variants, as HIV changes from person to person, continent to continent.

The genetic structures of HIV-1 and HIV-2 are similar, However, in HIV-2, the VPU gene is absent and another gene, called VPX, is present. Precise comparative analysis of each genetic element of HIV-1 and HIV-2 has revealed important differences between these two HIV viruses, especially in the ENV GENE. Genetic diversity is a characteristic of viruses, and even more so of retroviruses. Thus, differences in genetic sequence can be observed between variants of the same type of HIV-1 (or HIV-2) found in a given patient.

Recent data have shown that these strain variations occur in a patient during the course of HIV infection, as early as five days after infections and several months after exposures. HIV mutates as it is submitted to selection by the host's immune system. This mutation may be the way the virus avoids destruction by the host's immune defenses. Persistent infections observed in patients may be a consequence of this viral escape mechanism. This variability is not a property of the entire genome. GAG, POL, VIF, and VPR GENES are usually genetically stable. TAT and REV GENES vary, but to a lesser degree than do nef and env genes.

genetically modified organism (GMO)   A relatively new class of plants that, in many ways, rep-resents the growing fusion of science and trade that is happening globally, assembling life sciences, from medicine to food science, under one roof. Biotech plant drugs are one example of GMOs. Today, plant genes are being radically modified to produce a wide range of substances, from insulin to hemoglobin. New lines of pharmafoods are the result of these experiments. Although many individuals still debate uses of conventional AIDS drugs, frontiers of investment and experimentation have already moved light-years ahead. Small-molecule drugs are being passed over for protein drugs, which facilitate broader, longer-lasting, more lucrative patents.

Biopharming represents another point on the continuum. In general, biopharming appears to be a creature of giant corporations, not family farms. Boosters of biopharming insist that their products will be cheaper than current drugs. Examples include edible vaccines against disorders such as hepatitis B and diarrhea, in the form of genetically modified (GM) bananas, corn, tomato juice, lettuce, and potatoes. These foods must be eaten raw (cooking would destroy the vaccines). The use of edible vaccines to treat autoimmune diseases is currently being studied. Enthusiasts insist that edible vaccines could be valuable in developing countries that lack facilities to refrigerate and deliver standard vaccines. Critics point out that it will be hard to provide consistent doses. In discussions of drugbearing plants, concerns over safety and environmental damage have been and continue to be expressed.

In the coming years, people with HIV/AIDS will, undoubtedly, increasingly see the shadow of bioagriculture falling across their lives. For further information, see *The New York Times* on biopharming, http://www.purefood.org/ge/biopharming.cfm, or the British Royal Academy http://www.shef.ac.uk/uni/projects/sfl/textonly/policy/gmfoods.html, or the World News roundup on GM plants: http://www.connectotel.com/gmfood/.

genital herpes   See HERPES GENITALIS.

genital intercourse   Sexual intercourse involving penis-vagina contact.

genital secretions   Body fluids produced by the genitals, including cervical and vaginal secretions.

Examples of other fluids of the body include bile, chyle, chyme, gastric juice, intestinal juice, lymph, menstrual fluids, pancreatic juice, perspiration, saliva, and urine. These secretions can be external (if the material flows out through a duct) or internal (if it is returned to the blood or lymph). The particles of HIV circulate freely in the blood but mainly live in lymphocytes, which are present in most body fluids, such as semen, blood, cervical and vaginal secretions in women, prostatic secretions in men, saliva, even urine, and tears. Any activity or behavior that results in the sharing of bodily fluids in which the virus is found can transmit HIV. How likely one is to contract the disease depends on the particular fluid and other factors. A sufficient quantity of the virus must be present and the virus must penetrate through the skin and into the body. Blood, semen, prostatic secretions, and vaginal and cervical secretions carry the highest concentrations of the virus; saliva, tears, and urine carry minuscule amounts or no HIV. The virus can also be present in male pre-ejaculate, the clear liquid found on the penis before ejaculation.

genital ulcer An ulcerative lesion on the genitals, usually caused by a sexually transmitted disease such as HERPES, SYPHILIS, or CHANCROID. The presence of genital ulcers may increase the risk of transmitting HIV.

genital wart The name given to warts on the VULVA, the vaginal wall, or the CERVIX in women and on the penis of men and on, around, and in the anus of all sexes. Genital warts result from a sexually transmitted disease caused by the HUMAN PAPILLOMAVIRUS (HPV). In men and women, the warts may be single, occur in clumps, or become florid (a large mass). In HIV-positive people they may respond inadequately to treatment. Warts have been linked to more serious diseases, such as CERVICAL CANCER in women and ANAL NEOPLASIA in men and women. In all cases of genital warts in women, a PAP SMEAR and follow-up treatment for HPV infection of the cervix must be conducted. It is now being suggested that men and women also receive anal smears regularly to detect any anal cancers that may develop from lesions caused by HPV. Both cervical and anal cancers are found at

higher rates in HIV-positive people. They are also called condylomata acuminata.

genitalia The reproductive organs. Female genitalia consist of the vagina, clitoris, vulva, uterus, ovaries, fallopian tubes, and related structures. Male genitalia include the penis, testes and related structures, prostate, seminal vesicles, and bulbourethral glands.

genitourinary tract The system involved in reproduction and elimination of urine. In women this consists of the kidneys, ureters, bladder, urethra, uterus, fallopian tubes, ovaries, and vagina. In men it is the kidneys, ureters, bladder, urethra, testicles, prostate gland, vas deferens, and seminal vesicles. The genital and the urinary systems are distinct, but they are so closely related developmentally and functionally that they are often studied and treated together.

genome The total genetic material within a cell or individual, depending upon context. Specifically, the haploid chromosome complement (the complete set of chromosomes) and thus the total genetic information present in a cell.

Retroviral genomes are composed of at least three genes, designated GAG, POL, and ENV. These genes provide genetic coding for the HIV NUCLEOSIDE antigens, REVERSE TRANSCRIPTASE, and surface proteins, respectively. A similar DNA sequence of varying length can be found at each end of the proviral DNA. This sequence contains elements that can promote proviral gene integration in the host cell's genome and expression of these genes. See GENETIC VARIABILITY.

genotype The genetic material inherited from parents; not all of it is necessarily expressed in the individual.

genotypic assay A blood test that determines the genetic sequences of a virus or other organism. Usually it is performed in HIV-positive persons to establish whether certain mutations conferring drug resistance are present. A genotypic test generally costs about $500, and results are usually available within a few days. Most medical health insurance companies cover this test for HIV patients. Generally, genotypic tests require a blood sample from an individual who has a viral load of at least 1,000 copies. A genotypic assay examines the nucleotide base sequence in the genes that produce PROTEASE and REVERSE TRANSCRIPTASE. When the order of nucleotide bases in a patient's virus differs from the order in WILD-TYPE HIV, a mutation exists. See PHENOTYPIC ASSAY; RESISTANCE.

gentamicin   A broad-spectrum antibiotic of the aminoglycoside class that is derived from the fungi of the genus *Micromonospora*. Gentamicin is used to treat bacterial infections of the blood, central nervous system (meningitis), urinary tract, respiratory tract, digestive system, skin, bone, and soft tissue. In women living with HIV, gentamicin is used to treat PELVIC INFLAMMATORY DISEASE, a condition that develops when sexually transmitted infections such as CHLAMYDIA or GONORRHEA are untreated. Gentamicin is available in a variety of forms, including topical cream, eye drops, ointment, and injectable solution. Gentamicin works by interfering with production of proteins in bacteria and ultimately kills them. It is relatively toxic compared to other antibiotics used for similar conditions and is used primarily when less toxic antibiotics are not effective or cannot be tolerated. Gentamicin works best when combined with drugs from other antibiotic classes. Standard gentamicin may be injected intravenously or into a large muscle; intravenous injection is used for severe infections of the blood and for individuals who are in shock. The most serious side effects are kidney toxicity and damage to the eighth cranial nerve, which controls hearing. The risk of these side effects is low in people with normal kidney function using recommended doses; they occur more frequently in people who take high doses for extended periods and those who have a preexisting kidney impairment. (Trade name is Garamycin.)

genus   In biology, the taxonomic division between the species and the family.

geographic areas of affinity (GAA)   A framework to facilitate tracking of the HIV/AIDS pandemic, analyze its impact, and monitor the response to it. The world has been divided into 10 Geographic Areas of Affinity (GAAs). The diversity of these areas is large enough to accommodate variability in modes of transmission of HIV, yet small enough to facilitate analysis. These GAAs are based on two major factors: evolving HIV epidemiology and the operational and programmatic characteristics of the response to the HIV epidemic. The degree of societal vulnerability to the further spread of HIV is an important underlying element. The 10 GAAs include North America, Western Europe, Oceania, Latin America, sub-Saharan Africa, the Caribbean, Eastern Europe, south-eastern Mediterranean, Northeast Africa, and Southeast Asia.

Despite its utility, it is important to note that the GAA system is still based on generalizations and assumptions. The present delineation of the 10 GAAs is therefore only intended as an interim classification. The Global AIDS Policy Coalition (a coalition and committed to tracking the evolving HIV/AIDS pandemic, critically analyzing the global response and encouraging policy analysis and advocacy activities) is commissioning work to develop a more sophisticated classification system which will seek to take into account an even broader range of relevant factors. Their goal is to understand the local, national, and regional features of the pandemic, information critical for generating a more robust and focused global response.

geographic distribution   HIV/AIDS has reached every part of the world. Its extensive spread started in the mid- to late 1970s, and in less than two decades—during the first of which it was unknown and unsuspected—HIV became the first modern pandemic.

geographic variation   Variation in levels of HIV infection, both between and within countries. Seroprevalence surveys have tended to highlight the trends in particular groups and focus on the differentials among populations at different levels of risk. Today we know that HIV is geographically highly clustered. We know, too, that even with adjustments for underreporting and delays in reporting, striking disparities exist in, for example, AIDS mortality among different geographic areas of affinity. To date, the geographical distribution of AIDS has reflected the progression of the pandemic to the developing world. Projections of AIDS continue this trend—geographic variations are important. The range of proportional increases varies significantly by geographic area of affinity.

germanium Discovered in 1886, the mineral germanium, which has an atomic weight of 32 on the periodic table of elements, is not known to be essential to human health. It is a rare element that is never found free in nature. Yet in the early 1990s considerable research into its therapeutic effects on the immune system was carried out in several countries, including the United States and Japan. It must be stressed that organic germanium is not to be confused with inorganic germanium, which is used as a semiconductor and is highly toxic in minute concentrations. Germanium is currently being used as a drug in the treatment of pernicious anemia. There are several papers demonstrating that organic germanium compounds (germanium-32 in particular) have immunity-enhancing properties. It has been reported that two new organic germanium compounds inhibited the growth of certain mouse cancers. The compounds specifically enhance MACROPHAGE activity. A macrophage is a type of immune cell that kills cancer cells. In addition, researchers have been studying the effect of organic germanium compounds in the treatment of HIV. Some patients are claiming that the compound has been helpful; specific research has not been done to confirm these benefits. Claims made by patients and vitamin sales companies range from assertions that germanium increases the numbers and activity of natural killer cells to claims that it keeps white blood counts within normal ranges after surgery or during illness. Some medicinal plants such as *Aloe vera*, garlic, ginseng, comfrey, shiitake mushrooms, and chlorella contain high natural concentrations of germanium. More research is needed to determine the potential of both elemental germanium and the compound germanium-32.

germinal centers A collection of metabolically active lymphoblasts, macrophages, and plasma cells appearing within the primary follicle of lymphoid tissues following antigenic stimulation. Germinal centers are the sites of antibody production and are populated mostly by B CELLS but include a few T CELLS and MACROPHAGES. As HIV infection progresses, the germinal centers gradually decay.

giant cells Large multinucleated cells sometimes seen in granulomatous reactions and thought to result from the fusion of macrophages. They are found in both kinds of marrow, especially red marrow, and spleen; also in tissues that are healing, around foreign bodies, and in the inflammatory reaction to tuberculosis.

Giardia Species of protozoan found in humans. *Giardia lamblia* causes GIARDIASIS. Organisms are transmitted by ingestion of cysts in fecally contaminated matter (water or food) and are found worldwide. *Giardia* species can be passed through oral-genital and sexual contact and during food preparation. The organism is endemic in many day care centers in the United States. The most frequently observed symptoms of infection with *G. lamblia* are diarrhea, fever, cramps, anorexia, nausea, weakness, weight loss, abdominal distension, flatulence, greasy stools, belching, and vomiting. Onset of symptoms begins about two weeks after exposure, and the disease may persist for up to two or three months. There is no known chemoprophylaxis for GIARDIASIS; treatment with metronidazole or albendazole is highly effective.

giardiasis An infection by the flagellate protozoan *Giardia lamblia*. Infection is spread through contaminated food or water. Many cases are asymptomatic. When present, symptoms include anorexia, cramps, diarrhea, fever, nausea, weakness, weight loss, and vomiting. Giardiasis can be passed through oral-genital sexual contact and through food preparation.

gift-giver In the culture of BAREBACKING, this is the person who eroticizes infecting or exposing another person to HIV by sharing his SEMEN.

ginseng Ginseng root is an herb that has been used extensively throughout Southeast Asia and

China for treatment of various disorders. There are three different families of ginseng: the Oriental and American ginsengs *(Panax schinseng)*, the Siberian ginseng *(Eleutherococcus senticosus)* and the desert ginseng *(Rumex hymenosepalus)*. For thousands of years, ginseng has been the most prized of herbal remedies, with a host of alleged benefits, including relief of fatigue, relief of stress, and other systemic benefits.

It has been suggested that *Panax* ginseng may increase natural killer cell activity. *Panax* and *Eleutherococcus* can produce insomnia, diarrhea, nervousness, depression, and skin rash. Ginseng can amplify the effect of certain antidepressant medications and, due to the small amount of estrogens in the plant, can affect menstruation in women.

gland   A group of cells that removes materials from the blood, alters them to produce a specialized substance (such as a hormone), and then releases that substance back into the bloodstream to act in the body.

glans   The head of the penis, the area covered by the foreskin in uncircumcised men.

glial cells   Nonconducting nerve cells, which perform supportive and protective roles for neurones, including astrocytes, oligodendrocytes, Schwann cells, microglia, and ependyma cells. Glial cells are believed to become infected with HIV and may be one cause of HIV ENCEPHALOPATHY.

glitazones   Being studied for the treatment of LIPODYSTROPHY, glitazones belong to a class of drugs called the thiazolidinediones and are best known for their ability to make cells more sensitive to insulin. Glitazones have also been shown to help correct the function of adipocytes (fat cells).

globulins   Simple proteins found in the blood serum that contain various molecules central to immune system function. Immune globulins (IGs) make up preparations used for passive immunization vaccines for the prevention of several illnesses, including chicken pox (VARICELLA ZOSTER), HEPATITIS A, HEPATITIS B, rabies, tetanus, and measles. HIV

and other viruses cannot be transmitted through immune globulin vaccines, as the process of extracting IG from the blood inactivates the virus.

glory hole   A hole in a wall or partition through which a man sticks his penis. The person on the other side then anonymously fellates, masturbates, or otherwise stimulates the penis. This activity can take place in rest rooms, at gay sex clubs, or in other places where partitions exist.

glove   In medical care gloves are used to prevent the contamination of an operative site with organisms from the person wearing the glove and to prevent pathogens from the patient from contaminating the health care worker. These factors are particularly important when the patient has a disease such as HEPATITIS B or AIDS. Medical gloves are generally made of latex. For those allergic to latex, gloves made of polyurethane are also manufactured for these purposes.

GLQ-223   See TRICHOSANTHIN.

glucose   Also sometimes called blood sugar. A form of sugar that is the body's primary fuel. Glucose broken down from food can be converted into energy or stored. Abnormally low (hypoglycemia) or high (hyperglycemia) levels of glucose in the blood often indicate metabolic problems such as DIABETES MELLITUS. Diabetes mellitus occurs when the body cannot use glucose for fuel either because the PANCREAS is not able to make enough INSULIN or because the insulin that is available is not effective. As a result, glucose accumulates in the blood instead of entering body cells.

glucose-6-phosphate dehydrogenase (G-6-PD) deficiency   An inherited enzyme deficiency that can lead to HEMOLYSIS of red blood cells when an affected individual is exposed to drugs with oxidant properties. The drugs most commonly used by HIV patients that can lead to hemolysis in G-6-PD-deficient patients are dapsone, primaquine, and sulfonamides. There are a number of variants of G-6-PD deficiency; approximately 10 percent of men of sub-Saharan African descent and 2 percent of women of sub-Saharan African descent have one variety, and another variety is predominantly found in people of Asian Indian, Mediterranean, and Southeast Asian descent. This second variety can in some people be life-threatening and precludes the use of oxidant drugs, whereas the first variety discussed may not preclude the use of these drugs. There are degrees of deficiency, and not all people from the same areas of the world are affected in the same way. An estimated 200 to 400 million people are affected by glucose-6-phosphate dehydrogenase deficiency worldwide. One unusual aspect of the deficiency is that G-6-PD-deficient individuals are more resistant to the malaria-causing parasite. Screening for G-6-PD deficiency should be done for people who have the appropriate genetic background.

glucosidase An enzyme that catalyzes the hydrolysis of a glucoside.

glutamine Glutamine is classified as a conditionally essential amino acid. This means it generally is found in the body in abundance because the body can make its own supply. However, when the body is unhealthy, particularly as a result of cancer or HIV, levels of glutamine can drop 50 percent or more. Glutamine is particularly important in the function of the intestine. The intestine serves as a place for the body to absorb nutrients but also as a site where the body prevents organisms such as bacteria from entering. The microbes that fill the human intestine use glutamine as their fuel. Supplemental glutamine has been shown to decrease DIARRHEA in HIV and cancer patients, even in diarrhea caused by PROTEASE INHIBITORS. Glutamine has also been theorized to increase absorption of nutrients, thus preventing AIDS WASTING SYNDROME. No side effects have been linked to glutamine supplements.

glutathione A key antioxidant compound required for the smooth functioning of all cells. It is composed of three amino acids: cysteine, glutamine, and glycine. Besides acting as an antioxidant, glutathione is involved in protein synthesis, amino acid transport, and in the recycling of other antioxidants, such as vitamin C. Glutathione, like other antioxidants, may or may not, play a role in slowing HIV disease progression. Study results are often conflicting; the findings that follow illustrate some of the claims made for this antioxidant. A deficiency of glutathione has been linked with shortened survival in HIV-infected individuals who have CD4 counts below 200. In fact, researchers have found that glutathione levels in CD4 cells closely correlate with CD4 count. Researchers have also postulated the use of glutathione replacement therapy in the treatment of HIV infection to enhance the immune system. Other research has shown that NAC, or N-acetylcysteine, is essential for the synthesis of glutathione, and studies have indicated that oral administration of NAC can replenish glutathione stores in people with HIV. Some researchers have inferred that NAC itself may be useful in prolonging survival.

glycine A nonessential amino acid, meaning the body produces enough through its own processes. Glycine helps trigger the release of oxygen to the energy-requiring cell-making process and is important in the manufacturing of hormones responsible for a strong immune system.

glycoprotein Any of a class of compounds in which a carbohydrate group is combined with a protein; any of a class of compounds (including the mucins, the mucoids, and the chondronproteins) consisting of a carbohydrate and a protein. Generally it is a protein molecule that is glycosylated, or covered with a carbohydrate or sugar. The outer-coat proteins of HIV are glycoproteins. The number that follows the abbreviation *gp* in the name is the molecular weight of that glycoprotein.

glycyrrhiza The dried root of *Glycyrrhiza glabra*, known commercially as Spanish licorice. Used as an ingredient of glycyrrhiza fluid extract and glycyrrhiza syrup, both of which are used as flavoring agents in compounding medicine. This substance has a weak cortisone-like action.

glycyrrhizin (licorice root) Glycyrrhizin is a substance isolated from the root of the licorice plant *(Glycyrrhiza glabra or Glycyrrhiza uralensis)*. It is widely used in Japan and is reported to have benefits in the treatment of chronic HEPATITIS B and HEPATITIS C. Some studies suggest that glycyrrhizin produces decreases in fatigue and light-headedness and small improvements in CD4 counts. It may mitigate injury to the liver in patients who are receiving HAART. Studies of glycyrrhizin show that it can cause an increase in blood pressure, potassium deficiency, water retention, and possibly heart complications when taken in high doses.

GM-CSF   See GRANULOCYTE-MACROPHAGE COLONY STIMULATING FACTOR.

GMHC   See GAY MEN'S HEALTH CRISIS.

go both ways   See BISEXUAL.

golden shower   Urination on a sex partner, or being urinated on, for sexual pleasure. See UROPHILIA.

gonad   A gland or organ that produces reproductive cells in animals; a general term for a gamete-producing gland, including both the female ovary and male testis.

gonorrhea   A sexually transmitted, or venereal, disease (STD or VD) caused by the bacterium *Neisseria gonorrhea*. It is transmitted when a mucous membrane or warm, moist part of a carrier's body comes into contact with similar tissue on another's. Symptoms include a puslike discharge from the penis in men or the cervix in women, and lower abdominal pain and fever in women. Other parts of the body (heart, throat, joints, rectum, and skin) may also be affected. If not treated, gonorrhea can cause severe infection and sterility. Penicillin, orally or by injection, is standard treatment for gonorrhea. Tetracyclines and cephalosporins are also used. Slang terms include the *clap,* a *dose,* and the *drip.*

gossypol   A toxic chemical that is yellowish in appearance and found in cottonseed. Gossypol is detoxified by heating. Gossypol is used by men as a contraceptive agent in China. It has had some anti-HIV activity in test tubes, as many chemicals have, and has been investigated as a potential viricide (like NONOXYNOL-9) that may reduce the risk of HIV transmission during sexual intercourse. Research into development of synthetic molecules modeled on gossypol that might inactivate the HIV in a patient's blood continues.

gp   See GLYCOPROTEIN.

gp41   A GLYCOPROTEIN on HIV's outside envelope that anchors GP120. It plays an important role in HIV infection of CD4+ T cells by easing the fusion of the virus membrane and cell membrane. The HIV ELISA test detects antibodies to gp41.

gp120   A GLYCOPROTEIN on HIV's envelope that binds to the CD4+ molecules and CHEMOKINE receptors on cells' outside membrane. Free gp120 in the body may be toxic to cells, by causing CD4 cell depletion in the immune system through APOPTOSIS and neurological damage leading to HIV ENCEPHALOPATHY. It is one of the areas of focus in vaccine development because it is the outer part of the virus that encounters antibodies.

gp160   A GLYCOPROTEIN made from HIV RNA. A precursor to the HIV envelope proteins GP120 and GP41, it is divided by viral enzymes into the two envelope proteins at a late stage of viral assembly.

grade I, II, III, or IV adverse event   See ADVERSE EVENT.

graft-versus-host (GVH) reaction   The clinical and pathologic sequelae of the reactions of immunocompetent cells in a graft against the cells of the histoincompatible and immunodeficient recipient.

gram-negative   See GRAM'S STAIN.

gram-negative bacteria   See GRAM'S STAIN.

gram-positive   See GRAM'S STAIN.

gram-positive bacteria   See GRAM'S STAIN.

Gram's stain   A differential method of staining bacteria for classification purposes. It is one of the first tests run on samples that a doctor takes to see what illness may be affecting a patient. It is a reasonably easy test to run and can be done in many doctors' offices. It gives an initial idea of what a particular illness might or might not be. Gram-negative bacteria stain pink; gram-positive bacteria stain dark violet. This artificial coloring of bacteria is used to facilitate examination under the microscope. Gram-negative bacteria include *Bordetella, Brucella, Escherichia, Hemophilus, Klebsiella, Legionella, Neisseria, Proteus, Pseudomonas, Salmonella, Shigella, Vibrio,* and *Yersinia* species. The chief gram-positive bacteria are *Bacillus, Clostridium, Corynebacterium, Diplococcus, Gardnerella, Sarcina, Staphylococcus,* and *Streptococcus* species.

granulocyte   A type of white blood cell (LEUKOCYTE) that includes NEUTROPHILS, EOSINOPHILS, and BASOPHILS. Granulocytes contain granules of toxins that are used to fight microorganisms in the body.

granulocyte colony stimulating factor (G-CSF)   A synthetic HORMONE that stimulates growth of the GRANULOCYTE, a specific type of WHITE BLOOD CELL. Synthetic G-CSF is the same as a cytokine glycoprotein that occurs in the body. It is used to alleviate the NEUTROPENIA caused by certain drugs and conditions. Side effects of this treatment can be nausea, rash, and bone pain. (Trade name is Neupogen.)

granulocyte-macrophage colony stimulating factor (GM-CSF)   A naturally occurring CYTOKINE GLYCOPROTEIN that stimulates production of NEUTROPHILS, MONOCYTES, and MACROPHAGES. Synthetically produced GM-CSF is effective in treating BONE MARROW deficiency after chemotherapy, bone marrow transplantation, or use of some certain drugs. It is synthetically produced but exactly the same as cytokines produced in every human's body. GM-CSF's generic name is *sargvamostim.* Side effects can include bone pain, edema, and eosinophilia. (Trade names are Leukine and Prokine.)

granulocytopenia   A condition resulting from having a low number of granulocytes. It is common in late HIV disease. It leads to an unusually high risk of bacterial infection. Treatment with GANCICLOVIR and some sulfa drugs can lead to granulocytopenia as a side effect in some instances. It can be treated sometimes with G-CSF.

granuloma   A granular tumor or growth, usually of lymphoid and epithelial cells. It occurs in various infectious diseases such as TUBERCULOSIS (TB), leishmaniasis, and *MYCOBACTERIUM AVIUM* COMPLEX (MAC).

granuloma inguinale   A very rare sexually transmitted disease most often affecting the groin, genitals, or perianal area. It less commonly affects the CERVIX, UTERUS, BLADDER, and RECTUM in females. The infection is caused by a microbacillus known as *Donovania granulomatis,* and the condition is also known as donovanosis. First symptoms occur about one to four weeks after exposure and include swelling, usually in the groin. The swollen area ruptures, and chronic painful ulcers with an unpleasant odor form. New lesions continue to appear, and the disease may eventually cover the reproductive organs, lower abdomen, and buttocks. Massive swelling of the genitals (elephantiasis) is a possible complication. Treatment includes ANTIBIOTICS such as streptomycin, and improvements are usually noted within a few weeks. Recurrences are common.

grapefruit juice   A study in the 1980s showed that a glass of grapefruit juice can help the body absorb several common medicines including sedatives and blood pressure medications. Grapefruit juice decreases the amount of an enzyme present in the small intestine to allow higher body intake. It has been shown in studies to increase the amount of SAQUINAVIR taken in by the body by 50 percent of the usual amount. However, studies have also shown that increasing the level of PROTEASE INHIBITORS in the body is not always beneficial because side effects may increase. Grapefruit juice has also been shown to decrease absorption of other drugs as a result of its high acid content. *Do not* use grapefruit juice to take INDINAVIR (Crixivan) or NELFINAVIR (Viracept) as these drugs break down in the high acid content of the juice and less is absorbed into the body. Talk with a physician about drinking of grapefruit juice with use of these drugs.

gray area The intermediate area or room between a HOT ZONE, an area that contains lethal, infectious organisms, and the normal world; a place where the two worlds meet. Also called gray zone.

green barley leaf extract (GBLE) The dried leaves of young barley, widely used in Japan and other countries as a nutritional supplement. Green barley leaf extract is reported to contain high levels of superoxide dismutase, a potent ANTIOXIDANT. Studies of GBLE, almost all of which have been conducted in Japan, suggest possible in vitro anti-inflammatory and antileukemic activity, as well as reduced healing time of ulcerous lesions in rats. Other studies have reported antioxidative, anti-inflammatory, antiallergic, anticarcinogenic, antiulcer, and antiviral properties. It has been suggested that GBLE may increase production of INTERLEUKIN-2 when added to cell cultures. Some researchers have suggested that there may be an anti-HIV substance in green barley leaf extract, but as yet there has been no proof for this found in research studies.

green juices Barley extracts and other "green juices" are used by many HIV-positive individuals as nutritional supplements.

GRID See GAY-RELATED IMMUNE DEFICIENCY.

grief Grief is an involuntary, complicated, emotional, and psychological response to loss or extreme TRAUMA. It is a process of movement through the pain of loss and simultaneously of healing and learning. Grief is the process that allows us to let go of intense emotional attachments and carry on with our lives.

The experience of grief is personal and subjective. With regard to AIDS, those who have HIV or AIDS will frequently be experiencing loss of health, jobs, homes, friends, finances, and independence and are having to face in the near future the loss of their lives. Their family members will be grieving for them and for the loss of their own future expectations. Medical personnel grieve their loss as well, along with the failure of *their* expectations of themselves—their inability to cure, "letting another person die."

Grief produces both emotional and physical manifestations. The initial reaction may include somatic symptoms such as easy fatigability, hollow or empty feeling in the chest and abdomen, sighing, hyperventilation, anorexia, insomnia, and the feeling of having a lump in the throat, and psychological symptoms beginning with shock and disbelief and an awareness of mental discomfort, sorrow, and regret, followed by tears, sobbing, and other more active expressions of pain. Duration of this initial reaction varies, but in the longer run the process generally includes these stages: denial, anger, bargaining, depression, acceptance, and hope. However, stages do not generally occur in neat, orderly progression. They are confused, frequently happening several at a time, repeated, and over time, assimilated. When the process becomes mired or interrupted, it is referred to as "complicated grief." If the process is not allowed to follow its normal course, it will go underground, so to speak, and fester, causing a variety of psychosomatic illnesses and more misery than the original loss.

Helping a person through grief requires receptiveness, physical presence, tolerance, and permissive listening, as well as a resolve to help him or her keep contact with the ordinary, mundane details of daily life.

Anticipatory grief makes the final grieving less intense and helps toward a more rapid healing. It is healthy and should not be met by family, friends, or providers with condemnation, but with encouragement and understanding. Anticipatory grief helps bring eventual closure. By giving us the chance to project into the future and see the loss before the fact, we are granted time to be "real" with the dying person, to say the things we always meant to and, perhaps, to share on a deeper level than previously.

grief work Helping a person through GRIEF, which, while largely an individual experience, often needs social facilitation and accommodation by others who can provide a nurturing, safe atmosphere. In general, the people near a person in grief play a passive supportive role in the process. With a terminal patient, though, one active moment is often required of the rest of us at some existential point: giving the patient permission to die. Without that permission, it is extremely difficult for the person with AIDS to make it to the stages of acceptance and hope.

griseofulvin An antibiotic commonly used to treat superficial fungal infections.

group M See HIV-1 GROUP M.

group N See HIV-1 GROUP N.

group O See HIV-1 GROUP O.

group sex Sexual activities by a group of people, either heterosexual, homosexual, or a combination of the two, at the same place, involving exchange of partners, variations of types of sexual intercourse, and observation of each other.

group-specific complement Any of a series of enzymatic proteins in normal serum that, in the presence of a sensitizer (a substance that makes the susceptible individual react to the same or other irritants) specific for a given group, destroys bacteria and other cells. The complement is important in maintaining a normal state of health.

group therapy A form of psychotherapy involving two or more patients and one or more psychotherapists for the purpose of treating each patient simultaneously through group discussion and interaction.

growth factor One of many intercellular regulatory molecules that regulate cell proliferation (rapid and repeated reproduction), function, and differentiation. Different growth factors elicit different responses from different cell types, such as stimulating growth, enhancing survival, initiating migration, and stimulating the secretion of tissue-specific hormones.

G-6-PD deficiency See GLUCOSE-6-PHOSPHATE DEHYDROGENASE DEFICIENCY.

guanine One of the four nitrogenous bases that, together with a phosphate molecule and a sugar (deoxyribose), make up the NUCLEOTIDES, or subunits, of DNA. In constructing DNA guanine always pairs with CYTOSINE in building the DNA helix. It is also one of the constituent bases of NUCLEIC ACIDS and NUCLEOSIDES.

guanosine A nucleoside made by the fusion of GUANINE and RIBOSE. It is a major component of RIBONUCLEIC ACID (RNA) and also found in DNA. Guanosine has been the focus of many HIV drugs because it serves as a link between virus and human cells. Abacavir is a carbocyclic guanosine analog. Mycophenylate is a guanosine suppressor that is being studied for use in combination with abacavir.

guardian See SURROGATE.

guardianship See SURROGACY.

guerrilla clinic Any of a group of for-profit facilities established during the AIDS epidemic for the purpose of dispensing black-market drugs or providing treatments or therapies not approved in traditional medical channels.

guided imagery One of many visualization therapies that uses a variety of visual techniques to treat disease. Visualization therapies are based on inducing relaxation in patients and having them visualize their medical problems, literally willing them away. Positive results have been documented with patients suffering loss due to disease, altered body image, or the threat of death. Positive results have also been documented when a total cure may be out of the question. Guided imagery exercises also are used to help patients cope with stress. In these therapies, people imagine themselves in an environment they associate with relaxing—a peaceful beach, a lake, or a favorite mountain. Closing their eyes and taking a few deep, easy breaths, they remember the details of the setting—the sights, smells, and sounds—and focus on feeling peaceful and relaxed.

guidelines In medical cases clinical practice recommendations formulated by experts or based on a literature review by a panel of experts and consumers. Their purpose is to educate health care providers, improve the care provided to individuals with specified conditions, and, when possible, enhance the cost-effectiveness of health care. Guidelines are distinct from "standards of care," which providers are required to meet.

gummatous syphilis   Late benign SYPHILIS.

GVH reaction   See GRAFT-VERSUS-HOST REACTION.

GW420867X   A nonnucleoside reverse transcriptase inhibitor (NNRTI) made by Glaxo-SmithKline. Despite early successes with this medication and phase III trials, all work was stopped on the drug in 2002. Research studies showed the drug caused protease inhibitor levels to drop significantly in the body.

GW-433908   Also known as VX-175. A protease inhibitor jointly under development by Glaxo Welcome and Vertex. It is water-soluble and therefore is processed in the body by the kidneys and not the liver. It is related to the drug amprenavir, another drug from these two companies.

gynecological disorder   A disturbance in any of the female reproductive organs, including the BREASTS.

Gynecological problems are common early symptoms of immunocompromise in HIV-positive women. These may include gynecological infections (most commonly VAGINAL CANDIDIASIS, BACTERIAL VAGINOSIS, TRICHOMONIASIS), as well as GENITAL ULCERS, VAGINITIS, simple urinary tract infections, POSTPARTUM endometritis, and PELVIC INFLAMMATORY DISEASE and cervical neoplasia. These problems may become chronic, less responsive to conventional therapies, and tend to progress as immunocompromise worsens. Specific protocols are needed for the treatment of gynecological problems in HIV-positive women that are appropriate to the degree of immunocompromise. Women who receive gynecological services in the same primary care clinics where they receive care for HIV infection are less likely to be lost to follow-up, and treatment plans can be initiated earlier.

Sexually transmitted infections and genital lesions are likely to facilitate viral transmission. These include GENITAL ULCER diseases (GUD), SYPHILITIC CHANCRES, HERPES GENITALIS, CHANCROID, and, rarely, LYMPHOGRANULOMA VENEREUM (LVG), and GRANULOMA INGUINALE (donovanosis). Other genital lesions that may accompany HIV infection include GENITAL WARTS and MOLLUSCUM CONTAGIOSUM. Chronic vaginitis may predispose women to HIV transmission and to other STDs.

Considerations for the management of gynecological infections include taking an appropriate sexual history, asking about symptoms, performing a speculum and bimanual examination, and obtaining relevant laboratory specimens. It is also important to consider the woman's overall state of health and the degree of immunocompromise. Clients with lowered T4 CELL COUNTS are often pancytopenic, increasing their susceptibility to infection and complicating response to treatment. These women may not mount an elevated white blood count in response to systemic infection, rendering an important diagnostic test less useful. ERYTHROCYTE SEDIMENTATION RATES (ESR) are often elevated in chronic illness and thus become a less useful clue in the diagnostic workup for acute infection. It has been observed that immunocompromised women with acute pelvic inflammatory disease (PID) are less symptomatic than their immunocompetent counterparts, even with marked disease. Consideration of the stage of HIV illness is a useful tool in planning follow-up. All sexually transmitted diseases must be treated by CDC guidelines, and tests of cures obtained. Treatment of sexual partners, where appropriate, should be arranged.

gynecological services   Medical examination, care (including preventive care), and treatment for GYNECOLOGICAL DISORDERS. Gynecological services include taking comprehensive menstrual, sexual, and reproductive histories; performing comprehensive gynecological examinations and evaluations; referrals to prenatal and obstetric care and abortion services; regular screening and other services. Gynecological histories often bring up difficult and unpredictable topics such as early sexual abuse, current domestic violence, sexually transmitted infections, or concerns about sexual functioning. In

HIV-positive women, concerns about fertility, menstrual problems, pelvic pain, and unprotected sex often surface during such an interview. (Gynecological examination often poses the risk of some blood exposure to the examiner, as do so many other simple medical procedures. Universal precautions include wearing gloves and disinfecting spills.)

HIV-positive women who are essentially asymptomatic, with CD4 counts greater than 400, who are not sexually active and who have no new gynecological complaints can be followed with gynecological screening and PAP SMEARS annually. Symptomatic women, women with AIDS, and sexually active women should be scheduled for gynecological evaluations, Pap smears, and STD screening every six months. Interval assessment should occur whenever a woman presents with low abdominal pain; vaginal or rectal discharge; abdominal bloating; genital sores; new onset of swollen or painful inguinal nodes; dysuria, hesi-tancy, frequency, or urgency; new onset amenorrhea; intermenstrual bleeding or any change in menstrual pattern; dyspareunia; or bleeding following sexual activity. Periodic assessments generally include an interval sexual history, careful inspection of external genitalia, speculum examination, GONORRHEA and chlamydia cultures, bimanual pelvic examination, microscopic wet mount, and VDRL. Tests are ordered as needed. Appropriate treatment plans are developed as needed. Client education is geared to the reasons for particular visits, but safe sex counseling should be reintroduced each time.

gynecology   The study of the female reproductive organs, including the BREASTS; the branch of medicine concerned with GYNECOLOGICAL DISORDERS.

Gyne-Lotrimin   See CLOTRIMAZOLE.

HAART See HIGHLY ACTIVE ANTIRETROVIRAL THERAPY.

hair pie Slang term for VULVA, with reference to CUNNILINGUS. See ORAL SEX.

hairy leukoplakia A white lesion seen in the oral cavity of HIV-infected individuals, most commonly on the lateral margins of the tongue. It may be flat or raised with vertical corrugations and is not removable. Acyclovir is an antimicrobial, antiviral agent used to treat hairy leukoplakia as well as Herpes simplex virus, Varicella-zoster virus, and Epstein-Barr virus. (Trade name is Zovirax.)

Haiti A nation in the Caribbean on the island of Hispaniola. Early in the HIV epidemic, the high incidence of AIDS in Haitians living in the United States and in parts of Haiti puzzled clinicians. Haitians were first thought to make up a group at special risk for HIV infection. A variety of proposed theories attempted to implicate Haitians in the introduction of HIV into the United States. Additional study of the HIV infection in Haiti, however, found that the pattern of infection there closely paralleled that found in the heterosexual population in the United States. Although researchers originally thought the high incidence of the virus might lead to a discovery of its origin, this did not happen. After extensive analysis of data it seems that HIV was more likely brought to Haiti by tourists from the United States or by Haitian immigrants in the United States returning to their homes for visits. Study of blood samples of Haitians who went to Central Africa and the United States for political reasons in the 1960s showed no trace of the virus when tested retrospectively.

The clustering of HIV cases in the Carrefour district of Port-au-Prince, the capital, that is the major area for male and female prostitution in Haiti, supported well-established risk factors as the explanation for HIV infection in Haiti. However, during the early years of the epidemic, the 4 H's were often referred to as HIV risk groups: hemophilia, homosexuality, heroin, and Haitians. This led to outright discrimination against Haitians in many parts of the United States. Despite being one of the initial locales for the spread of HIV, Haiti now ranks behind several countries in the Western Hemisphere in cases per capita of HIV.

half-life In biology and pharmacology, the time required by the body tissue or organ to metabolize, inactivate, and eliminate half the amount of a substance (such as a drug) taken in.

hand job Slang term for MASTURBATION, especially of a partner.

handshake See TRANSMISSION.

haploid number Half the usual number of chromosomes found in the cells of a species. Characteristic of the gametes of the species (human = 23).

haplotype A haploid genotype. Pertaining to a single set of chromosomes, haploids are an organism or group of cells having only one complete set of chromosomes—ordinarily half the normal diploid number.

hapten A small molecule that is incapable of inducing an antibody response by itself but can, when bound to a protein carrier, act as an epitope. DINITROCHLOROBENZENE molecules are haptens.

harm reduction The harm reduction model of public health action against contagion was developed in Merseyside, England, during the mid-1980s as a specific response to HIV/AIDS and the increasingly harmful consequences caused by the use of prohibited drugs. Fundamental principles underlying this approach are that HIV/AIDS prevention takes priority over prevention of drug use because it presents a greater threat to drug users, public health, and the national economy; that abstinence from drug use should not be the only objective of services to drug users because it excludes those who will not or cannot abstain; that those who will not or cannot abstain from drug use may still be helped by minimizing the harmful consequences of their behavior, for them, the community, and society as a whole; that the quality of the lives of drug users can be improved and enhanced while they still use drugs; and that HIV infection is not inevitable for drug users. Harm reduction emphasizes needle exchange programs, safer drug use, proper injection techniques, alternative ways of taking drugs, and drug maintenance.

hashish A more or less purified extract prepared from the flowers, stalks, and leaves of the hemp plant *Cannabis sativa*. The gummy substance is smoked or chewed for its euphoric effects.

Hassal's corpuscles Spherical or oval bodies present in the medulla of the thymus, consisting of central areas of degenerated cells surrounded by concentrically arranged flattened or polygonal cells.

HBV Hepatitis B virus. See HEPATITIS.

HCW See HEALTH CARE WORKER.

HDL See HIGH-DENSITY LIPOPROTEIN.

HE 2000 An experimental immune system modulator from Hollis-Eden Pharmaceuticals. HE 2000 is in PHASE I/II trials in the United States. It is unclear exactly how the drug works, but it seems to stimulate the CD4 cells and other enzymes. It currently is being tested as an intramuscular injection that is given for five days, followed by a four-week rest, then another five days of drug.

healing touch Healing touch is believed by some to accelerate wound healing, relieve pain, promote relaxation, prevent illness, and ease the dying process. The practitioner uses light touch or works with his or her hands near the client's body in an effort to restore the client's energy system.

health advocate A person trained in assisting patients to resolve complaints about and problems with health care services. Health advocacy is concerned with the description, trends, patterns, analysis, causes, and resolutions of patient and client complaints and problems. Health legislation specialists, client advocates, and patient representatives are all health advocates and practitioners of health advocacy.

health care Treatment of disease or disability; the provision of services to promote or restore mental and physical well-being. The quality, amount, and expense of available health care varies according to numerous factors—social class, income, eligibility for public programs, amount and type of insurance, type of service required, geography, public funding levels, and of course intangible differences among individual providers and institutions. Anyone seeking health care is well advised to be as well informed as possible, actively willing to make choices and protect his or her interests. This is even more crucial for HIV-infected patients than it is for others.

health care facility A place where HEALTH CARE is provided, usually operated by an institution or small organization. The settings in which health care is provided are, in broad terms, two: outpatient facilities and inpatient facilities. Outpatient facilities are individual physicians' offices, clinics staffed by physicians who practice as a group, HEALTH MAINTENANCE ORGANIZATIONS, and public health department clinics. Inpatient facilities, primarily hospitals and nursing homes, are generally used by persons who need more intensive care.

health care professional An individual who has received special training or education in a health-related discipline concerned with the direct provision of care (medicine, dentistry, medical technology, dental hygiene, physical therapy, and occupational therapy), health care administration, or ancillary services and who is licensed, certified, or registered by a professional organization or government agency to provide health services in his or her field. A health care professional may be an independent practitioner or an employee in a health facility or program.

health care provider One who treats the sick and disabled or provides services to promote or restore mental and physical well-being. The category includes physicians, physicians' assistants, and nurses as well as others who are not licensed professional medical personnel. See HEALTH CARE WORKER.

health care proxy A legal document that authorizes one person to make medical decisions for another in the event he or she cannot make them him- or herself. This document also gives the person named visitation rights in the hospital and access to the patient's medical records. Under normal circumstances, an individual's next-of-kin would have these powers automatically. A health care proxy is suggested if a nonfamily member is preferred. People are generally advised to sign a medical directive in conjunction with a health care proxy as the best guarantee of realizing their wishes for treatment under particular circumstances. See MEDICAL DIRECTIVE.

health care worker (HCW) Anyone employed in the treatment of illness or disability or the provision of services to promote or restore mental and physical well-being. The category includes medical professionals, laboratory personnel, technicians, physical facility staff, and others. See HEALTH CARE PROVIDER.

health insurance A generic term for all forms of insurance and prepayment plans that reimburse (in whole or in part) an individual or organization for the costs of hospital and medical care. Health insurance plans may also reimburse an individual, again in whole or in part, against loss from disease or accidental bodily injury. Health insurance is usually divided into two types: individual (individually purchased) and group (purchased through employment or by reason of association with a defined group or organization).

Health insurance is available under such names as accident and health insurance, accident insurance, sickness insurance, disability insurance, service benefit plan, prepaid health plan, preferred provider plan, health maintenance plan, foundation medical plan, hospital insurance, and dental plan.

health maintenance organization (HMO) An organization that provides comprehensive health care services to members for a nominal fee in addition to an annual charge. A component of MANAGED CARE, an HMO is an alternative to traditional fee-for-service care based on a relationship with an individual doctor.

HMOs provide comprehensive services for a fixed, prepaid fee. When you join a group plan offered by an HMO, you pay a flat fee for all your health care bills, regardless of how much health care you actually get. HMOs finance nearly all medical care. Unlike commercial insurance companies, HMOs allow little choice in physicians and hospitals. Because competition among HMOs for employer contracts is fierce, costs must be kept low. Consequently, the HMO must carefully regulate hospital admissions, expensive drugs, and expensive procedures and must preapprove any consultation or procedure done outside the resources of the HMO.

Health Omnibus Programs Extension of 1988 The Public Health Services Act required development of research and education programs, counseling, testing, and health care for AIDS patients. It also required the FDA to develop a registry of experimental AIDS drugs.

heart disease Term used to describe any pathological condition of the heart. From a variety of studies it is known that certain conditions and lifestyle variations are more likely to be present in people with ischemic heart disease than in the general population. These may be divided into those that are not reversible, aging, male sex, and genetic factors; those that are reversible, use of tobacco, hypertension, obesity, sedentary lifestyle, and stress; and others that may not be reversible; hyperlipidemia, hyperglycemia, diabetes mellitus, decreased levels of high-density lipoproteins, and behavior patterns. In the late 1990s, reports noting an increase in the incidence of heart attacks, angina, or other cardiovascular symptoms in people with HIV began to surface. Associations with PROTEASE INHIBITORS were made, and concerns were expressed about the long-term effects of the high blood lipid levels also observed in those on protease inhibitors.

A tendency increased heart attack risk in people with HIV was noted long before protease inhibitors. In actual fact, there are a variety of factors that contribute to accelerated heart disease in people with HIV. These range from aspects of the infection, to lifestyle factors such as smoking, to the various medications patients may be taking. Within this overall picture, protease inhibitors may magnify the risk through their effect on blood lipids. Protease inhibitors are connected with disorders of lipid metabolism. People who receive protease inhibitors have elevations in triglyceride and cholesterol levels, but they do not seem to have much elevation of the level of high-density lipoprotein (HDL), which is the kind of cholesterol associated with lower cardiovascular disease risk. People who are on protease inhibitors do indeed have these risks for cardiovascular disease.

Other factors that add to the heart disease risk for HIV patients include the fact that many people with HIV infection receive androgenic and anabolic steroids. Androgenic steroids are known to increase the red blood cell mass; people become polycythemic (having too many red blood cells). The reason for this is that the red blood cell mass increases the blood viscosity. The blood becomes more sludgy, and that characteristic can definitely contribute to myocardial infarction. With plaque and other risk factors, steroids just increase clotting.

Note that AIDS itself causes disorders of lipid metabolism. Low cholesterol level used to be totally characteristic of this disease, and low HDL level was just a very early manifestation of HIV infection.

heartburn A burning sensation in the substernal area due to reflux of acid contents of the stomach in the lower esophagus.

heat cautery The use of heat to destroy tissue, especially for curative purposes. Method used for removing genital warts.

helminthic infestation Infestation with intestinal parasites or worms. Helminths are wormlike animals.

Helms Amendment In 1987 Congress enacted a law, commonly known after its Senate sponsor as the Helms Amendment, requiring the exclusion from the United States of HIV-infected aliens as carriers of a "dangerous contagious disease." As a result of this classification, all immigrants were tested for HIV, and those who tested positive were refused entry, including applicants seeking adjustment of status to permanent residency, applicants for amnesty, and refugees. Although the United States has not routinely tested nonimmigrants such as tourists, students, and other travelers to the United States, those whom immigration officials learned were HIV-positive were subject to exclusion as well. The Helms Amendment provoked a torrent of criticism from scientific and human rights authorities. The restriction placed on international travel and temporary residency sparked particularly vehement opposition. Critics were quick to point out that the United States is much more an exporter than an importer of HIV and that casual, everyday contact with HIV-positive travelers posed no public health threat to U.S. residents. The virtually unanimous outcry by public health and human rights authorities against the HIV exclusion led Congress to repeal the Helms Amendment in 1990. As part of the Immigration Act of 1990, Congress directed the secretary of HEALTH AND HUMAN SERVICES to draw up a new list of diseases that would be grounds for excluding aliens. Seeking to remove politics and prejudice from the selection process, Congress specifically admonished Health and Human Services that the list should contain only "communicable disease[s] of public health significance."

Helper T cells Also known as T helper cells, helper cells, and helper t lymphocytes. Helper T cells are T LYMPHOCYTES that belong to the CD4+ subclass. There are two different types of helper T cells, the Th1 and Th2 varieties. Th1 class helpers are involved in CELL-MEDIATED IMMUNITY. They can bind to cells that display antigens and cause other responses such as the arrival of LYMPHOCYTES or LEUKOCYTES. Th2 class helpers provide assistance to B CELLS and are therefore part of the ANTIBODY-MEDIATED IMMUNITY.

In HIV, helper T cells are infected when the virus binds to the CD4 molecule and then is able to enter the T cells. The virus then eventually causes cell death and the infected person's T cell count drops below the norm of around 1,000 per microliter of blood. The lack of T helpers in part causes the body's inability to fight infections.

hemarthrosis   Bleeding into a joint.

hematocrit   The volume of red blood cells expressed as a percentage of the total volume of blood. The volume of red blood cells is obtained by separating the cells from other blood components by means of a centrifuge.

hematopoietic system   All tissues responsible for production of the cellular elements of peripheral blood. This term usually excludes strictly lymphocytopoietic tissue such as LYMPH NODES.

hematuria   Red blood cells in the urine.

hemiparesis   Paralysis on one side of the body.

hemodialysis   A method for artificially performing the function of the kidneys (removing wastes or toxins from the blood) by circulating the blood through a series of tubes made of semipermeable membranes that are bathed in solutions that selectively remove undesirable elements.

hemodialyzer   An apparatus used in performing HEMODIALYSIS.

hemoglobin   The oxygen-carrying pigment of the red blood cells; the iron-containing pigment of the ERYTHROCYTES. It is formed by the developing erythrocyte in BONE MARROW and serves to transport oxygen from the lungs to the tissues.

hemolysis   Destruction of blood cells.

hemophilia   A hereditary bleeding disorder caused by a deficiency or abnormality of a protein known as FACTOR VIII, which is essential to blood coagulation. The blood fails to clot and hemorrhage occurs. Hemophilia is inherited through the mother and mainly affects men. HEMOPHILIACS bleed easily, even with a minor cut. Many have severe hemorrhaging into the joints and eventually get joint disease. Hemophilia has two forms, hemophilia A and hemophilia B. Each form lacks a different clotting protein, called a clotting factor. Hemophilia A (classic hemophilia), results from factor VIII deficiency and hemophilia B, from FACTOR IX deficiency.

Hemophilia is treated by lifelong injections of a synthetic version of the clotting factor the blood lacks. The commercial clotting factor is extracted chemically from blood donated by hundreds or thousands of people. As a result, hemophiliacs are exposed to the blood of thousands of blood donors. Between 1978 and 1985 at least 80 percent of the hemophiliacs in the United States who repeatedly infused factor VIII concentrates became infected with HIV. During that period, the internal bleeding that occurs in persons with hemophilia was treated with pooled blood products that contained impurities, including HIV.

In 1985, heat-treated intermediate-purity factor concentrates became generally available. These products were free of HIV but contained other viruses and proteins. In 1989, a new generation of high-purity concentrates was approved by the FOOD AND DRUG ADMINISTRATION (FDA). These products are purified using MONOCLONAL ANTIBODIES and contain substantially fewer contaminants. In December 1992, the FDA approved a second type of high-purity product, which is manufactured through recombinant technology. The higher-purity products are significantly more expensive than the earlier concentrates.

Since 1985, the risk of being exposed to HIV through clotting factors has dropped to practically nil. One reason is that donated blood is now screened for HIV. Another reason is that clotting factors are heated and purified by detergents and biochemicals that kill HIV. The CENTERS FOR DISEASE

CONTROL found that between 1985 and 1988, only 18 hemophiliacs acquired HIV, an annual rate of under one per thousand.

hemophiliac One afflicted with HEMOPHILIA.

hemophiliac sexual partners Men with HEMO-PHILIA and HIV are faced with a double challenge: the treatment and management of both hemophilia and HIV/AIDS. They and their partners have to deal with medical and social problems that others do not have to face. Living with hemophilia means spending time and energy negotiating the health care system as well as identifying specialized resources and sources of support. Living with hemophilia and HIV means spending more time and energy doing both.

hemoptysis The coughing up of blood from the lungs; may be a symptom of TUBERCULOSIS.

hemorrhage Abnormal, severe internal or external discharge of blood. May be venous, arterial, or capillary, from blood vessels into tissues, into or from the body. Venous blood is dark red and the flow is continuous. Arterial blood is bright red and flows in spurts. Capillary blood is of a reddish color and exudes from tissue. Very small hemorrhages are classified as *petechiae,* those up to one centimeter as PURPURA, and larger ones as *ecchymoses.*

hemorrhagic Pertaining to or marked by HEMORRHAGE.

Heparin This is an anticoagulant drug. It is a complex sugar formed from the mucosal lining of the intestines of cows or pigs. It is used to decrease the clotting ability of the blood and is sometimes referred to as a blood thinner, though it does not in reality thin the blood. Heparin cannot break up blood clots that have already formed, but it can prevent them from enlarging. It is used in the treatment of some heart, lung, and blood vessel conditions and during surgery involving the heart and dialysis. It is also used by people who have had PIC lines or other type of catheters for injectable medicine installed so that the blood does not clog around the PIC line.

hepatic Pertaining to the liver.

hepatic steatosis See STEATOSIS.

hepatitis Hepatitis is an irritation or inflammation of the liver with a variety of causes, including viral infections, bacterial infections, autoimmune diseases, and chemical and medication toxicities. The leading worldwide cause of inflammation of the liver—or hepatitis—is viral in origin. A common misperception is that one virus causes hepatitis; actually there is a diverse group of hepatitis viruses lettered *A* through *G,* except the letter *F:* hepatitis A (HAV), hepatitis B (HBV), hepatitis C (HCV), hepatitis D (HDV), hepatitis E (HEV), and hepatitis G (HGV-C). All of the hepatitis viruses have different size, genetic structure, routes of transmission, and ability to produce chronic infection. Despite these differences, hepatitis viruses have the propensity to produce acute symptoms of fatigue, loss of appetite, intermittent nausea, abdominal pain, fever, jaundice, dark-colored urine, chills, and liver enlargement. Several of the hepatitis viruses can evade the elaborate defenses of the immune system and sustain chronic infections that may last indefinitely. *Chronic infections* are defined as sustained infections of a duration of more than six months. Usually, chronic hepatitis infections do not produce any symptoms, but they may have clinical effects years to decades into the future—from liver failure to cancer. Chronic hepatitis infections are stabilized by a complex arrangement of the immune system, but HIV can disrupt this system. Additionally, not only can chronic viral hepatitis infections cause liver disease, but the incessant ingestion of alcohol, and its direct toxic effects, can also produce liver disease. The importance of liver disease in HIV-positive patients has been recognized.

Viral hepatitis gained tremendous media attention in the late 1990s and into the 21st century as a disease that can have an impact on national health. Within the HIV/AIDS community worldwide, it has also gained tremendous clinical attention. Today, as more people with HIV are living longer, coinfection with hepatitis, and particularly with hepatitis B and C, has emerged as a significant concern. It is important that everyone with HIV be tested for viral hepatitis so that measures can be taken to prevent development of the disease. Overviews of selected clinically relevant hepatitis viruses follow, including discussion of transmission, symptoms, diagnosis, prevention, and treatment.

Hepatitis A Virus

A self-limiting virus-induced liver disease, hepatitis A is acquired through ingesting fecally contaminated water or food or engaging in sexual practices involving anal contact. Injection drug users who share unclean needles also are at risk. It is an RNA enterovirus. Its symptoms include fever, jaundice, nausea, diarrhea, fatigue, abdominal pain, dark urine, vomiting, and loss of appetite. It has no chronic disease state. Diagnosis is by immunoglobulin M (IgM) antibody testing. HAV can be prevented with a vaccination, by good personal hygiene, and by practicing of SAFE SEX. Immune globulins (IGs) are sometimes used to prevent HAV, but they are only effective for about three to six months, depending on the dose. IG is also used as a postexposure prophylaxis, for people who have not been vaccinated but have been exposed to HAV. There is no treatment for HAV; plenty of rest and a low-protein diet can help. People normally contract hepatitis A only once in their lifetime. Rarely, people infected with HAV have a severe form of hepatitis, fulminant hepatitis, which, left untreated, can be fatal. Persons who suspect that they may have HAV should see a physician or health care professional. All who are infected with HIV should be tested for HAV. If they have not been exposed to the virus, they should receive the HAV vaccine. Note that in persons with HIV, the vaccine's effectiveness depends on the individual's CD4 count.

Hepatitis B Virus

A virus-induced liver disease that usually lasts no more than six months but becomes chronic and life-threatening in 10 percent of cases. HBV is a hepadnavirus, meaning that it contains DNA. Although it infects liver cells in both humans and animals, HBV is a noncytopathic virus, meaning that is does not permanently damage the liver cells it infects. The highly contagious hepatitis B virus can be transmitted through many of the same activities as HIV, including unprotected sex (including oral sex); sharing of unsterile needles, accidental puncture by contaminated needles, broken glass, or other sharps; contact between broken or damaged skin and infected body fluids; and blood transfusions. Hepatitis B can also be transmitted from mother to infant either before or during delivery. Note that HBV is easier to contract than HIV because it is more than 100 times more concentrated in an infected person's blood and can exist on surfaces outside the body. Indeed, it is a hardy virus that can exist on almost any surface for up to one month. Many people with HIV are coinfected with HBV. Practicing safe sex and not sharing drug injection equipment provide protection against both HIV and HBV.

HBV causes an initial acute illness very much like hepatitis A. Symptoms include fever, jaundice, and severe fatigue. The illness usually lasts for a week or up to a month. In about 10 percent of HBV cases chronic infection develops. Not only can individuals transmit the virus to others, but they are at risk for development of serious chronic liver disease. People infected with HIV have a greater chance of development of chronic HBV. There are two general types of chronic HBV. Persistent chronic HBV does not produce major symptoms. Chronic, active HBV is a very aggressive infection that can cause cirrhosis and liver cancer. Note that chronic hepatitis B is faster in its progression than chronic hepatitis C. In people with chronic HBV infection, cirrhosis can occur in as little as four to five years, with a significant risk of cancer occurrence within 10 years after infection. Whether aggressive or not, people with chronic HBV can transmit the virus to others.

The HBV surface antigen is detected in serum and is usually the first indication of acute HBV infection. Antibody to HBV core protein does not develop during acute infection; the presence of HBV surface antigen in the absence of core antibody indicates chronic infection. Antibodies to the surface antigen develop after clinical recovery or vaccination and usually persist throughout life. Their presence and detection indicate past infection and immunity. An assay has been developed to detect HBV DNA. Existence of HBV DNA indicates viral proliferation and a chronic disease state. A liver biopsy is necessary to ascertain the degree of liver damage.

HBV can be prevented by practicing safe sex, avoiding contact with the blood of someone who is infected, not sharing drug injection equipment, and receiving a vaccination. All who are infected with HIV should be treated for HBV. If they have not been exposed to the virus, they should receive an HBV vaccine. Currently there are three FDA approved treatments for Hepatitis B. INTERFERON ALPHA, LAMIVUDINE, and, most recently ADEFOVIR. Interferon alpha is successful in eliminating the virus in up to 40 percent of people that take the drug. It is less successful in HIV positive patients. It is an intramuscular injection that is given daily for 16 weeks. Side effects are similar to a person suffering the flu. Muscle aches and pains are reported as constant in almost all patients. Exhaustion, headache, and upset stomach have also been widely reported. Depression is also common, and the drug is not recommended in patients that have suffered from severe depressive episodes in the past. Lamivudine is given as a once daily pill for hepatitis B infection. It can significantly reduce the viral load of hepatitis B in many patients. Some patients have also cleared the chronic virus through treatment with lamivudine, but this is not common. Sometimes resistance to lamivudine can build up over the course of hepatitis B treatment. Adefovir was approved in late 2002 for the treatment of hepatitis B. Originally tested as an HIV drug, adefovir was taken in high doses and was toxic in many people. For hepatitis B treatment, adefovir is taken at much lower doses and has tested safe in several trials. Adefovir has shown to bring significant reduction in HBV viral load, even in cases where the virus has become lamivudine resistant. Statistically significant improvement in the degree of liver fibrosis (scarring) was observed in the patients who received adefovir, in addition to reduction of swelling. It can be used instead of or in addition to treatment with lamivudine. The stopping of any hepatitis treatment has shown to cause aggravated hepatitis in up to 25 percent of patients stopping a treatment. Monitoring of someone stopping treatment should be done on a regular basis. The HIV medication TENOFOVIR has also proven effective in the reduction of HBV viral load in ongoing studies. It has not yet been approved by the FDA for this treatment but is becoming available for compassionate usage by the drug company for such uses. Anyone who is chronically infected should visit a health care professional regularly. Every HIV-positive person should be tested for past infection with hepatitis B and receive the hepatitis B vaccine; if he or she has not been exposed to hepatitis B.

Complete recovery from acute hepatitis B infection depends on the ability of the immune system to control the virus. If it is successful, HBV antigens—proteins produced by the virus, such as HBsAg and HBeAg—eventually become undetectable in the bloodstream and are replaced by specific antibodies produced by the immune system: anti-HBs and anti-HBe. Once these antibodies appear, the virus can no longer be detected in the body, and the liver eventually normalizes. Note that a third antigen, HbcAg (the "core" antigen) can only be detected in liver cells and always results in the production of anti-HBc core antibodies, which are detectable in the blood.

Until recently there have been little information and very little research regarding the effects and treatment of HBV in HIV-positive people. Before the advent of combination antiretroviral therapy, HIV-associated deaths were most commonly tied to "classic" AIDS-related complications rather than chronic HBV disease. Today, however, fewer people are dying of typical AIDS diseases, such as MAC or PCP. Many are now living long enough to see HBV become a major health concern. Several observations have been made. Although only a small percentage of otherwise healthy adults infected with HBV go on to experience chronic hepatitis B, this in not true of HIV-positive adults: in roughly 25 percent of HIV/HBV-coinfected patients chronic infection develops. A number of reports have also suggested that as HIV disease progresses, the immune response to HBV gradually decreases and is sometimes lost. Some patients experience a relapse of infection, marked by the loss of anti-HBs and the return of HbsAg positivity. Other coinfected patients experience gradual decline in anti-HBs activity, sometimes at the expense of increased hepatitis B viral load and HBeAg levels. To date, the impact of HIV on the severity of chronic HBV infection is not entirely understood. There have been a number of reports demonstrating that patients infected with both viruses have higher HBV viral loads and more cirrhosis, regardless of immune system status. There are also data from studies suggesting that HIV-positive people with chronic hepatitis B are more than twice as likely as their HIV-negative counterparts to experience liver failure, thus requiring liver transplantation.

Hepatitis C Virus

A virus-induced liver disease, hepatitis C is a very serious, potentially life-threatening infection. It appears to be more common among heterosexuals and injection drug users than hepatitis B. It is more likely than hepatitis B to become chronic and lead to liver degeneration (cirrhosis). In people with chronic HCV infection, it can take up to 20 years for cirrhosis of the liver to occur and more than 30 years for more serious complications, such as liver cancer, to develop. Unlike HBC, which contains DNA and is a hepadnavirus, HCV contains RNA and belongs to the flavivirus family, which includes a few viruses known to cause some tropical infections, most notably dengue and yellow fever. HCV is a cytopathic virus, which means that it causes direct damage to liver cells. More difficult to transmit than HBV, HCV is almost always spread by direct blood-to-blood contact. In other words, transmission happens when the blood from an infected person's body directly enters another person's body. HCV is tiny and can live in blood for weeks outside the body. Most new infections result from the use of shared injection equipment—cookers, cotton, water, and syringes. Since July 1992, the U.S. blood supply has been screened for HCV, but anyone who received a blood transfusion or used blood products such as clotting factor before that time may have been infected with HCV. Sexual transmission of HCV, though rare, is possible. Unprotected sexual acts that involve blood can increase the risk of HCV infection. The risk of mother-to-child transmission of HCV during labor and delivery is about 6 percent, although the risk can be as high as 25 percent if the mother also has HIV. Sharing tattooing needles and ink wells, using unsterilized piercing equipment, and, less commonly, sharing straws used to sniff drugs and personal care implements such as toothbrushes, manicuring equipment, and razors can result in HCV infection. Health care workers who have had occupational exposure to blood are at risk for HCV.

The initial symptoms of HCV are very similar to those of other viral hepatitis infections, though they tend to be milder. They include fever, fatigue, muscle and joint pain, nausea and vomiting, and jaundice. Only about a quarter of the people who are infected with HCV show any initial symptoms. Nonetheless, HCV is a much more serious disease than either HAV or HBV, especially for people coinfected with HIV. Hepatitis C occurs in approximately 1.8 percent of the general population and has been reported to occur in 12 percent to 90 percent of HIV-infected individuals. Individuals exposed to HIV through injecting drugs are much more likely to contract the disease. The progression of hepatitis C to cirrhosis is more rapid in HIV-infected people who drink alcohol. Active hepatitis B or A infection speeds the progression of cirrhosis in individuals who have hepatitis C. Serum tests for HCV antibodies became available in 1989 and have since improved in specificity. HCV antibodies may take several months to appear in serum after infection. Qualitative POLMERASE CHAIN REACTION PCR tests for actual virus may detect infection during this period. PCR testing can also rule out chronic infection for those who have HCV antibodies but have cleared the virus. PCR assays for HCV viral load are also more accurate than serum antibody tests in HIV-infected persons.

People with hepatitis C should be vaccinated against hepatitis A and B, if they have not already been exposed to it. As HBV can, HCV can become chronic; indeed, most HCV is chronic. Unlike for HAV and HBV, there is no vaccine against HCV. In order to prevent transmission of this potentially fatal virus, people should practice safe sex and should not share drug injection equipment. As HIV does, HCV evolves and develops resistance very quickly, making treatment a difficult challenge. Most physicians prescribe a combination of drugs, which may include one or more types of interferons coupled with ribavirin. Several studies are being done in an effort to find a better treatment for HCV. Several tests are available that help individuals monitor HCV disease progression and make treatment decisions, including liver function testing and genotypic testing. An individual's immune health is also a predictor of treatment response. Ultrasound testing can also provide information about the condition of the liver; liver biopsy remains the most accurate way to identify the extent and cause(s) of liver damage.

HCV disease may progress more rapidly in people with HIV. Studies conducted before the use of HAART showed that HIV could speed HCV disease progression. But HAART's boost to the immune system may help to slow HCV-related liver damage. Coinfected people usually have higher HCV viral loads than people with HCV alone, but much controversy remains about HCV disease progression in coinfection. Further research is needed to confirm whether HCV does make HIV disease worse.

In 1999, HCV was categorized as an OPPORTUNISTIC INFECTION because of the potentially serious health consequences of living with two chronic viral infections. Because of the overlap in modes of transmission between the two viruses, it is recommended that people with HIV undergo HCV antibody testing. In most people who have been infected with HCV antibodies develop within three months. For those with a positive antibody test result, a viral load test can diagnose current HCV infection.

Hepatitis D Virus

A serious and often progressive disorder manifested by an unusually aggressive course, HDV can replicate only in the presence of HBV and occurs either as a coinfection with HBV or as a superinfection in established HBV carriers.

Hepatitis E

Hepatitis E is a virus similar in structure hepatitis A. It is an acute infection instead of a chronic infection. It is not typically found in the United States but has caused wide outbreaks in Asia and South America. Direct contact with human feces or indirect fecal contamination of food, water supply, raw shellfish, or cooking and eating utensils may result in sufficient amounts of the virus entering the mouth to cause an infection.

Hepatitis F

Hepatitis F is nonexistent. It was mistakenly "discovered" and named, but subsequent attempts to repeat the "discovery" have failed.

Hepatitis G Virus

A blood-borne virus that does not seem to cause liver disease or have any effect on hepatitis C. Although its long-term effects are unknown, the hepatitis G virus (HGV, also known as GB virus) is commonly found in people coinfected with HIV and hepatitis C. GB is a member of the Flaviviridae virus family with genetic similarities to HCV. It is transmitted by contaminated blood and shared needles, as well as from mother to fetus. Low levels of sexual transmission are likely. Studies have shown an association between HGV infection and slower HIV disease progression, and there has been some speculation that HGV infection is an independent predictor of better survival rate and slower disease progression. However, it is not known whether it is HGV that is causing the slower HIV disease progression or whether people with HGV have something else in common. If HGV does slow HIV disease, it is not known how it does this—is it acting as an antiviral or is it stimulating the immune system to respond better to HIV? In vitro results would seem to indicate that HGV is somehow able to inhibit HIV replication, but more research is needed to find the answer.

hepatitis A   See HEPATITIS.

hepatitis B   See HEPATITIS.

hepatitis C   See HEPATITIS.

hepatitis D   See HEPATITIS.

hepatitis E   See HEPATITIS.

hepatitis F   See HEPATITIS.

hepatitis G   See HEPATITIS.

hepatobiliary symptoms   Any perceptible change in the liver, bile, or biliary ducts, including disease.

hepatoma   A tumor of the liver.

hepatomegaly   Enlargement of the liver.

hepatotoxicity   Toxicity to the liver.

Hepsera   See ADEFOVIR.

herbalism   An ancient form of healing still widely used in much of the world, herbalism uses natural plants or plant-based substances to treat a range of illnesses and to enhance the functioning of the body's system. Though herbalism is not a licensed professional modality in the United States, herbs are "prescribed" by a range of practitioners, from holistic M.D.s to acupuncturists to naturopaths.

herbs A flowering plant whose stem above ground does not become woody and persistent. Today more and more facts are being reported in prestigious medical journals about their preventative and healing benefits. The exact reasons for the positive effect herbs exert on the human body is not always known. It is evident, however, that the nutrient and nonnutrient chemicals stored within a plant's cellular structure are in forms that are easily metabolized by the gastric juices, enzymes, and hormones of the body. The therapeutic action of herbs comes from alkaloids, organic nitrogenous compounds that cause certain chemical reactions within the body. Herbs may also contain minerals, vitamins, and salts that help the body resist disease, strengthen tissues, and improve the nervous system.

Herbs can be prepared in a variety of ways, including decoction, fomentation, infusion, oil, ointment, poultice, syrup, and tincture. It is believed in order to receive the full beneficial effects that can be obtained from herbs, most must be consumed regularly for long periods of time. However, there are several exceptions like goldenseal, which if taken too long can retrogress the illness. Instructions on the labels should be followed. Additionally, because of vast differences amongst individual metabolisms, if an herb is not agreeable or if adverse effects are experienced, usage of the herb should be discontinued and a more agreeable herb substituted. Herbs can be potent, and moderation is generally recommended. Adverse side effects are possible with many herbs. Medicinal amounts of any herb should not be taken without first consulting a physician. Herbs can be obtained from health food stores, herbalists, homeopathic pharmacies, and some food markets. They should be kept in airtight containers away from heat, light, and dampness to prevent deterioration of their active ingredients.

The use of herbs is often suggested as a possible additional aid in keeping HIV dormant. Herbal remedies should not be used as the only treatment for HIV or AIDS.

heroin A narcotic morphine derivative that appears as a white crystalline powder. Because of its highly addictive nature, importation, sale, and use are illegal in the United States. Its chemical name is *diacetylmorphine*.

herpes A general term for viral infections of HERPES SIMPLEX I or II. These infections cause the eruption of painful blisters, usually in the oral or genital area, and can be sexually transmitted. All can be OPPORTUNISTIC INFECTIONS of AIDS.

Herpes is a family of large viruses that contain a large amount of DNA. Besides HERPES SIMPLEX I (HSV-1) and HERPES SIMPLEX II (HSV-2), it contains CYTOMEGALOVIRUS (CMV), EPSTEIN-BARR VIRUS (EBV), VARICELLA ZOSTER VIRUS (VZV), and HUMAN HERPES VIRUS-6 (HHV-6).

herpes encephalitis Encephalitis due to infection with herpes simplex virus. Though rare, it is frequently fatal. It has been successfully treated with an antiviral agent.

herpes genitalis Infection of the genital and anorectal skin and mucosa with HERPES SIMPLEX VIRUS type 2. It is usually spread by sexual contact and is classed as a sexually transmitted disease. Itching and soreness are usually present before a small patch of erythema develops. Then a vesicle that erodes appears. These are usually painful and heal in about 10 days. They may occur in any part of the genitalia. Although genital herpes lesions usually occur in limited areas (such as the CERVIX), as HIV infection progresses, the herpes may involve more widespread anatomical areas and be resistant to topical therapy. ACYCLOVIR has been of considerable benefit in treating the initial infection.

Genital herpes is one of the gynecological problems that Social Security Disability Determination Service (DDS) specialists consider when assessing the degree to which the disease affects a woman's ability to function.

herpes simplex An acute disease caused by HERPES SIMPLEX VIRUSES, types 1 or 2. Groups of watery blisters, often painful, form on the skin and mucous membranes, especially the borders of the lips (cold sores) or the mucous surface of the genitals. The cold sores usually heal themselves after a while. Type 1 infections generally do not involve genital areas of the body; type 2 infections do. ACYCLOVIR applied locally has been an effective form of treatment, with ANTIBIOTICS often used to treat secondary infections. In persons with AIDS, herpes simplex sores require the intervention of other drugs to heal. Herpes simplex virus persists indefinitely in the body after initial infection and reactivates unpredictably. There is no known cure.

Herpes simplex type 1, caused by the herpes simplex virus 1 (HIV-1), commonly produces oral herpes, characterized by cold sores or fever blisters on the lips, in the mouth, or around the eyes.

Herpes simplex type 2, caused by the herpes simplex virus 2 (HSV-2), is a sexually transmitted herpes virus that causes painful sores in the anus or the genital area. Lesions usually appear two to twelve days after infection. In people with weakened immune systems, lesions may persist for a long period, are more extensive, and can result in severe ulcerations. Physicians use acyclovir to treat outbreaks of HSV-2 and as preventive therapy for people with deficient immune systems. FOSCARNET has been used to treat people with acyclovir-resistant herpes simplex infection.

Genital herpes may be chronic and recurring, and no known cure exists. It has been associated with an increased risk of acquiring HIV. Case reports suggest that persons with immunodeficiency have a more severe clinical course of anogenital herpes than do immunocompetent patients. Genital herpes can present as painful coalescing ulcerations requiring prophylactic maintenance therapy.

Genital ulcers should be considered in the differential diagnosis of any painful ulcerative genital lesion. Ulcerations from this disorder may increase the risk of transmission in women who are HIV-negative. Repeated or persistent treatment may be necessary to control symptoms; symptoms often recur when medication is discontinued.

Herpes simplex virus in the HIV-positive woman is often more persistent and requires higher doses of acyclovir than in the HIV-negative woman. Systematic acyclovir treatment provides partial control of the symptoms and signs of herpes episodes and accelerates healing. It does not eradicate the infection or affect the subsequent risk, frequency, or severity of recurrences after the drug is discontinued. Safety and efficacy have been documented among persons receiving daily acyclovir therapy for up to three years. Most episodes of recurrence do not benefit from therapy with acyclovir.

HIV infection should be considered a possibility in all women with recurrent or persistent herpes simplex. HIV-infected women have herpes simplex more often than women without HIV infection.

herpes varicella zoster (VZV) See HERPES ZOSTER.

herpes virus See HERPES.

herpes zoster An acute infectious disease caused by the varicella zoster virus (VZV), characterized by inflammation of the sensory ganglia. Severe neuralgic pain and lesions, or vesicular eruptions on the skin (presented as patches of red spots), occur along the affected nerve. Herpes zoster generally affects or occurs on only one side and is self-limited. It is the reactivation of latent varicella zoster virus in individuals who have previously had chicken pox and were rendered partially immune. SHINGLES is the more common name for herpes zoster.

het In the gay subculture, a pejorative term for heterosexual.

heterologous challenge Injection of a vaccinated animal with a viral strain similar to the one used to make the vaccine. See HOMOLOGOUS CHALLENGE.

heterosexual Pertaining to a sexual orientation to persons of the opposite sex; one having such sexual orientation. The opposite of homosexual. Often referred to as "straight."

heterosexual intercourse See HETEROSEXUAL SEX.

heterosexual sex Sexual activity that takes place between people of the opposite sex.

heterosexual transmission See TRANSMISSION.

heterosexuality   Sexual orientation toward persons of the opposite sex.

HHV-1, HHV-2   See HERPES SIMPLEX VIRUS.

HHV-3   See VARICELLA-ZOSTER VIRUS.

HHV-4   See EPSTEIN-BARR VIRUS.

HHV-5   See CYTOMEGALOVIRUS.

HHV-6   See HUMAN HERPESVIRUS 6.

HHV-7   See HUMAN HERPESVIRUS 7.

HHV-8 (KSHV, Kaposi's sarcoma [KS] herpesvirus)   A herpesvirus thought to trigger the development of Kaposi's sarcoma lesions. HHV-8's mode of transmission has not been determined. See KAPOSI'S SARCOMA.

Hickman catheter   People who require long courses of drugs that must be regularly and slowly introduced into the body and cannot be taken orally will often have a flexible tube called a Hickman catheter, through which drugs can be injected, surgically inserted into a large vein in the chest and left in place for a long period of time. See CATHETER.

high risk   In the context of AIDS, a term applied to patterns of behavior that place individuals at risk of contracting the HIV virus; any behavior that puts the bloodstream in contact with any of the bodily fluids of another person that can transmit the AIDS virus. High-risk behavior includes sharing needles when injecting intravenous drugs and having unprotected vaginal, anal, or oral sex or sex with an IV drug user. The mode of transmission may influence the likelihood that an exposed individual will become infected. There appears to be a continuum of risk for HIV/AIDS. The risk of HIV infection has been categorized as no risk, low risk, medium risk, and high risk.

high-density lipoprotein   A lipoprotein that contains more protein than fat; often called "good cholesterol."

high-grade squamous intraepithelial lesion (HSIL)   Abnormalities in the cells on the surface of the CERVIX. They cause an aberration that can be discovered by Pap tests. There is unanimous agreement that tissue classified as HSIL should be removed. See ATYPICAL SQUAMOUS CELLS OF UNDETERMINED SIGNIFICANCE; LOW-GRADE SQUAMOUS INTRAEPITHELIAL LESION.

highly active antiretroviral therapy (HAART)   The term used to describe the combination of pills taken by HIV-positive patients to fight the virus. It generally refers to a regimen of three different drugs involving at least one PROTEASE INHIBITOR. The term *mega-HAART* refers to a regimen of four or more drugs taken for the same purpose. These potent HAART combinations have been successful in reducing the viral load in a majority of patients that take the drugs properly. HAART works in situations that involve someone with advanced virus or in people who have recently become infected. There is no particular group or combination of NNRTIs, NRTIs, and protease inhibitors that make up the term *HAART*. An HIV patient may take several different combinations over the course of the illness. HAART does not kill the virus and does not completely stop the replication of the virus in the bloodstream. Small amounts of the virus continue to live despite the drug therapy. As the patient continues to take the drugs, the virus can and will develop immunity to the drug combination, and another grouping of medications will be prescribed. Patients may also be allergic or unable to abide the side effects of particular drug combinations, which will lead to changes in the combination that makes up a patient's HAART. A patient's inability to take the medications as prescribed can lead to HAART failure. As the research community has developed newer medications, they have done so with the attempt to make the dosing easier and less burdensome on the patient, hopefully creating better adherence and results for the patient.

high-risk behavior   See HIGH RISK.

high-risk group/population A group or population sharing a common behavior or characteristic placing it at high risk for HIV infection compared to the population as a whole. Our understanding of, and belief in, the existence of high-risk groups and populations has evolved since the beginning of the epidemic. In the earliest stages of the AIDS epidemic in both the United States and Europe, homosexual and bisexual men accounted for upward of 90 percent of all cases. INTRAVENOUS drug users were a small minority of all cases, limited to only a few geographic areas, and heterosexual cases were distinctly unusual outside of Africa. The epidemic in Africa, more widespread than elsewhere, was almost exclusively in heterosexuals.

Over the first decade of AIDS in the industrial world, it was believed that the virus moved across groups, gaining access to new groups where they overlap. HIV first appeared in the developed world in the male homosexual population and at one point was thought to be a disease exclusively of homosexuals. Bisexual men and male homosexual drug users, who could be categorized in more than one group, formed a ready bridge from this affected group to others. Female partners of bisexual men were exposed to HIV through these sexual relationships. Because of the common practice among intravenous drug users of sharing needles and syringes, infected homosexual users passed HIV on to nonhomosexual men and women with whom they shared them. A large portion of female prostitutes also inject drugs; they introduced HIV among men who neither injected drugs nor were homosexuals, and through them to their wives and other sex partners. Before 1985 anyone from a group at risk for HIV infection could donate blood for medical purposes; thus HIV-infected blood transmitted the virus to those not belonging to such groups. Anyone receiving a blood transfusion or any type of blood product before 1985 was at risk for infection regardless of behavior. Parents especially mothers exposed to HIV by any of these means, passed the virus to their children and fetuses.

Today, research shows that HIV does not discriminate and that no group or population is immune to HIV/AIDS. The research focus has shifted from groups or populations to behaviors, and education to control or limit those behaviors.

high-risk person A person who engages in HIGH-RISK behavior.

high-risk sex Unsafe sex practices with high risk of HIV transmission include having numerous sex partners; unprotected anal-receptive sex with an infected partner; unprotected anal penetration with the hand ("fisting"); anal douching in combination with anal sex; oral-anal contact; and vaginal intercourse without a condom with an infected partner.

Hill-Burton Reconstruction Act The Hill-Burton Reconstruction Act (Hospital Survey and Construction Act of 1946) was a postwar measure designed to create employment and provide better health care through hospital construction grants. In return for grant funds, the private hospitals were expected to provide services for some indigent patients. This quid pro quo was conveniently ignored by hospitals throughout the 1950s and 1960s. In the 1970s, however, litigation about the act developed a right to health care for indigent people at Hill-Burton facilities. In response to these cases, the Department of Health and Human Services promulgated new regulations requiring Hill-Burton hospitals to render a certain amount of uncompensated care to indigent patients each year.

Not all hospitals have Hill-Burton—only those which have received federal construction help are required to participate. However, all publicly owned or operated hospitals, even some private, noncharity hospitals, have some patients who meet income (and, sometimes, asset) guidelines. In addition, a variety of federal, state, local, and private philanthropic health agencies finance free or reduced-fee health clinics, which are typically run by local health departments or nonprofit agencies. Generally those with income below the federal poverty level are fully eligible, with partial bill reductions sometimes available on a sliding scale as income rises above that level. Income and asset levels vary from state to state, locality to locality, and even health program to health program. All Hill-Burton facilities give free care to those with incomes up to the poverty level; many, however, also take the federally offered option of also giving free care to those with incomes up to twice the poverty level. For those becoming eligible for Medicaid via a "spend down," Hill-Burton and hospital charity bill write-offs can cover the portion of a hospital's bill that would otherwise be the patient's liability. Services are available to all needy residents, not just to those found "disabled." Hill-Burton programs have no assets eligibility level and no income disregards; other programs' assets and income disregard policies vary. Hill-Burton hospital and charity programs, as well as many local low-income clinics, require an applicant to apply for and follow through on Medicaid or other public medical assistance. Eligibility is then granted only to those found ineligible for complete Medicaid coverage of their bills. Benefits vary from facility to facility, although all Hill-Burton hospitals and clinics must comply with certain Hill-Burton rules. Details pertaining to how and where to apply also vary from facility to facility.

histamine   A major vasoactive amine (released from mast cell and basophil granules) that exerts a pharmacological action when released from injured cells. Functions of histamine include increasing gastric secretion, dilation of capillaries, and contraction of bronchial smooth muscle responsible for itching/sneezing during allergy.

histocompatibility   The quality of living tissue of one individual of being immunologically compatible with the tissue of another. Histocompatible tissues have ANTIGENS of the same HUMAN LEUKOCYTE ANTIGEN (HLA) complex, and therefore will not cause an immunologic response and will continue to function following transplantation from one individual to another.

histocompatibility complex   The cluster or family of genes that control immune reactions, genes that contain the coding information necessary for the synthesis of ANTIGENS, the specific proteins found on the surface of cells. There is some evidence of an HLA-linked genetic factor in AIDS patients that is not present in non-AIDS individuals.

histocompatibility genes   The genes (comprising the HUMAN LEUKOCYTE ANTIGEN [HLA] complex) that determine the histocompatibility antigenic

markers on all nucleated cells. These genes create the antigens by which the immune system recognizes "self" and, therefore, are important in determining the success of transplanted organs and tissues. Many different forms of one particular histocompatibility gene are found at the seven sites on chromosome 6.

histocompatibility testing   A method of matching the self-antigens on the tissues of a transplant donor with those of a recipient. The closer the match, the better the chance that the transplant will not be rejected.

histoincompatibility   The quality of living tissue of one individual not being immunologically compatible with the tissue of another, and therefore unsuitable for transplantation. See HISTOCOMPATIBILITY.

histopathology   The study of the microscopic structure of diseased tissues.

Histoplasma capsulatum   A fungus present in soil and dust, widespread in the south-central United States and in Latin America. It is the causative agent of HISTOPLASMOSIS.

histoplasmosis   *Histoplasma capsulatum* is a fungus found in the droppings of birds and bats in the Ohio and Mississippi Valley region, the Caribbean islands, and Central and South America. It can then be spread through the air—in spore form—when disturbed. It is spread through breathing the air that contains the spores. People with reduced immune functioning, such as with HIV infection, are susceptible to the illness, which can be disseminated throughout the body via the blood. The symptoms of histoplasmosis are reflective of the diffuse invasive nature of the infection. Fever, weight loss, skin lesions, adenopathy, respiratory complaints, and cough are common. Meningitis and cerebritis are rarely seen. Identification of the fungus in tissue specimens or in culture provides the definitive diagnosis. Bone marrow, blood, lymph nodes, lungs, and skin are all commonly infected tissues that should be examined and biopsied. Serologic tests for histoplasmosis are available. Complement fixation tests are reliable when positive, but may be negative in up to 30 percent of infected people. A new radioimmunoassay for the detection of a histopolysaccharide antigen may be more sensitive. Maintenance or suppressive therapy is then required. Patients with disseminated histoplasmosis disease require intensive induction treatment with amphotericin. Good results have been found with itraconazole and this drug is often used as maintenance therapy.

historical control A group of participants in a clinical trial that did not take the experimental drug being tested, used as a comparison in a later clinical trial.

history taking Systematically recording past medical events as they relate to a person or group of people.

hit early An approach to the treatment of HIV infection that consists of early, aggressive antiretroviral therapy. This approach is compared and contrasted with more cautious, patient-focused, long-term approaches. The hit early approach focuses on the immediate suppression of VIREMIA. Patients must take medications correctly, as prescribed, for potent regimens to be successful. The need for excellent adherence is one of the major limitations of any HIV therapy.

Widespread use of early, aggressive therapy was adopted in the mid-1990s, on the basis of several assumptions about the effect of such treatment on HIV pathogenesis. One key assumption that supported early use of therapy was that ongoing HIV replication caused irreversible damage to the immune system. However, several more recent studies have shown that potent HAART treatment often reverses much of the damage over a period of time and that naïve CD4+ T-lymphocyte counts usually increase, even in patients with advanced HIV infection.

Another key assumption supporting the use of early aggressive therapy is that a given regimen will completely suppress HIV replication. The hope of viral suppression is an idea that many patients and physicians still work toward. Experience and studies have shown current potent regimens do not completely inhibit HIV replication in most patients. Still another assumption that underlies

early use of treatment is that potent therapy will prevent the emergence of drug-resistant strains of HIV. However, resistance has been shown to develop during ongoing viral replication even in the presence of anti-HIV drugs. This leads to still further confusion as to whether the hit early or postpone strategy works best.

U.S. government directives for HIV treatment changed in the late 1990s to delay treatment until a patients CD4+ counts dropped below 350. This is due to the cost of the treatments, the possible side effects of HAART, and the ability of the immune system to reconstitute itself, even after HIV causes depletion of the system. Currently there are studies to evaluate the long-term consequences and effectiveness of both strategies, hit early and delayed treatment. See SMART.

HIV See HUMAN IMMUNODEFICIENCY VIRUS.

HIV-1b A viral subtype of HIV that is most common in the United States.

HIV-1e A viral subtype of HIV that is most common in parts of Asia and Africa, where 90 percent of HIV cases are attributed to heterosexual contact.

HIV-2 HUMAN IMMUNODEFICIENCY VIRUS type 2. HIV-2 is found mostly in western Africa. Like HIV-1, HIV-2 induces AIDS, albeit at a much slower rate, and with less transmissibility. Researchers have found that HIV-2 infection can protect individuals from subsequent infection with HIV-1. Investigators, supported by the National Institute of Allergy and Infectious Disease (NIAID), however, note that the use of HIV-2 as a live attenuated vaccine against HIV-1 infection probably has risks that far outweigh the potential benefits.

HIV antibody (HIV-Ab) The antibody to HIV, which usually appears within six weeks after infection. Antibody testing early in the infection process may not produce accurate results, since some recently infected people have not yet begun producing antibodies and test negative even though they are infected. Thus, a single negative antibody test result is not a guarantee of freedom from infection. The change from HIV-negative to HIV-positive status is called SEROCONVERSION.

HIV antibody negativity Absence of antibodies in the blood directed against HIV. The absence of these antibodies indicates either absence of infection or that infection is too recent to have generated detectable antibodies.

HIV antibody positivity The presence of antibodies in the blood directed against HIV, detected by any of several diagnostic tests (see ELISA; WESTERN BLOT TEST). Synonymous with HIV infection.

HIV antibody test A blood test that shows whether or not a person has antibodies to the virus that causes AIDS. The test indicates only whether a person has at some time been infected with HIV. It cannot determine if a person has AIDS or will develop AIDS in the future. See ELISA; HIV ANTIBODY TESTING; WESTERN BLOT TEST.

HIV antibody testing HIV antibody testing is one of three means of diagnosing HIV infection. This method detects the presence of the virus through the body's response to it. The most common response is the production of antibodies. Tests that detect these antibodies are inexpensive and readily available to all medical laboratories. The other two methods to diagnose HIV infection are by the isolation of virus in the laboratory from blood or other infected fluids and tissues and to infer infection from the presence of characteristic symptoms. This last technique was used before the wide availability of antibody diagnostic kits, and it remains a frequent method of diagnosis where access to these kits is limited.

HIV counseling Information provided to an individual before and after HIV testing regarding the implications and impact of testing, HIV infection care, and prevention of HIV transmission. Pretest counseling may include questions and discussion about past sexual activity, drug use, and medical history. Individuals may also be asked if they think their test will be positive or how they will react if their test is positive. This enables counselors to identify people who need additional counseling or whose tests are more likely than those of others to be positive for HIV. The counselor will then give the individual the opportunity to ask any questions she or he may have about HIV, AIDS, or the test. Post-test counseling includes discussion of the test results (negative, positive, or inconclusive) and may introduce issues pertaining to living with AIDS (treatment, management, prevention).

HIV dementia See HIV ENCEPHALOPATHY.

HIV encephalitis See HIV ENCEPHALOPATHY.

HIV encephalopathy The term for the actions of HIV on the central nervous system. It is known that HIV infects the brain early in the course of disease. Typically it does not produce symptoms until later in the disease process. In some instances, people with early HIV infection may suffer some problems that can be related to HIV activity such as lack of concentration or a drop in short-term memory abilities. As HIV disease progresses, its effect on the nervous system becomes more evident in some people. These early problems may worsen, with significant changes in feelings, behavior, and ability to function. It is unclear still what causes some people to suffer from these central nervous system (CNS) problems whereas other people do not.

HIV encephalopathy was formerly called AIDS dementia complex (ADC) and is still sometimes referred to as HIV encephalomyelopathy. HIV encephalopathy was relatively common in the late stages of HIV disease when HIV first appeared. In the past few years a decrease in the incidence of this illness has led medical doctors and researchers to believe that the PROTEASE INHIBITORS are to some extent crossing the BLOOD-BRAIN BARRIER and working to decrease this result of the virus.

HIV infects the MACROPHAGES of the brain, also called the MICROGLIAL CELLS. It is suspected that the altered cytokines that are excreted by the microglial cells after infection change the neurons of the brain. The frequency of HIV encephalopathy does increase with advancing HIV disease. HIV encephalopathy affects not only the survival of people with HIV disease, but their quality of life as well. The course of HIV encephalopathy is slowly progressive if left untreated, as is any opportunistic infection. Some 30 percent of people with HIV disease experience minor cognitive impairment, and 20 percent have a serious deficit, affecting their ability to function in social or occupational settings. Because the primary involvement of the illness is seen in subcortical regions of the brain, some people refer to this as white matter disease. Nearly 80 percent of HIV patients who have autopsy of the brain after death show evidence of some CNS disease process. The action of the illness is similar to the involvement profile seen in Parkinson's disease and Huntington's disease, and not like that seen in Alzheimer's disease. The major difference between Alzheimer's disease and HIV encephalopathy is that HIV patients typically remain well oriented in their day-to-day lives. If patients show sudden changes of orientation or display quick deterioration, this may be the result of drug reactions or other illnesses such as CRYPTOCOCCOSIS, TOXOPLASMOSIS, CYTOMEGALOVIRUS INFECTION, drug toxicity, ANEMIA, dehydration, substance abuse involvement, hypoxemia (low blood oxygen) from lung disease, and significant kidney or liver problems. (See DELIRIUM.)

Typically a test called a mental status examination can be performed to test the functioning of a patient; the test is designed to reveal problems such as short- or long-term memory loss, disorientation, lack of concentration, and mood swings. CT scans, MRI scans, and single photon emission computed tomography (SPECT) scans are also helpful in the detection of HIV encephalopathy. CT scans usually show signs of atrophy of brain tissue. However, it must be noted that this CT scan result does not always correlate with impairment in the patient. MRI is a sensitive but very expensive brain scan used when CT findings are inconclusive. MRIs usually detect white matter disease in the brain. SPECT scans use a radioactive material to measure blood flow in the brain and may be useful to detect early HIV dementia. They can also follow the response of the senses to antiviral therapy by determining whether the therapy has improved the blood flow in the brain. SPECT scans are still not used much in this field. These tests can also help differentiate HIV encephalopathy from other brain disorders such as CRYPTOCOCCAL MENINGITIS, TOXOPLASMOSIS, lymphoma, or PML. There is no one conclusive test for diagnosis of HIV encephalopathy; more often it involves an elimi-nation of all other possible causes of the patient's condition.

People suffering from HIV encephalopathy have an increased reaction to antipsychotic drug side effects. If these medications are used at all in treatment of symptoms, close watch should be kept on the patient for excessive side effects. There are also complications that arise from involvement of all of the CNS, including the spinal cord. See MYELOPATHY.

HIV genome   The entire genetic information present in a cell. See GENOME.

HIV guidelines   See UNIVERSAL PRECAUTIONS.

HIV incidence   See INCIDENCE.

HIV infection   Infection with the HUMAN IMMUNODEFICIENCY VIRUS, at any stage from the early asymptomatic to the late stages of AIDS.

HIV integrase   See INTEGRASE.

HIV latency   See LATENCY.

HIV measurement   In 1995, two new tests for the measurement of HIV in a patient came into widespread use in laboratories. Dr. David Ho, director of the Aaron Diamond AIDS Research Laboratory in Manhattan, pioneered their use in the analysis of HIV disease. These tests allow the rapid and easy measurement of the amount of HIV genetic code, or RNA, in a sample of blood. This is what patients commonly refer to as VIRAL LOAD. Until 1995, diagnostic tools to monitor levels of HIV in patients' blood were not precise enough to indicate which drugs might be the most useful for a patient.

Much has been learned about the virus's activities using these new tools. Every day in people infected with HIV, including individuals who are otherwise healthy, 10 billion copies of the virus circulate in the body. Every five hours and 45 minutes about one billion new copies enter the bloodstream, a million of which infect CD4 cells of the immune system. Those cells become factories for viral production, spewing out another 10 billion copies over the next 24 hours. In the process, the CD4 cells die but are rapidly replaced. This scenario is ongoing in each patient. This constant creation and death of viral particles can lead to change in the virus structure quite easily. By measuring the amount of HIV in the blood, or the body, researchers have hoped to better treat patients both early and late in their infection stages. See BRANCHED DNA; NASPA; PCR; VIRAL LOAD ASSAY; VIRAL SUPPRESSION.

HIV Network for Prevention Trials (HIVNET)

A group funded by The National Institute of Allergy and Infectious Diseases (NIAID) that conducts domestic and international multicenter trials to evaluate promising interventions to prevent the transmission of HIV. Interventions studied include HIV vaccines, topical microbicides, sexually transmitted disease treatment, prophylaxis to prevent vertical transmission, and behavioral risk reduction strategies.

HIV, origin of It is now known that HIV is a descendant of the SIMIAN IMMUNODEFICIENCY VIRUS (SIV) that is present in several varieties of monkeys in Africa. It is a retrovirus and a member of the lentivirus family along with several other animal viruses. There are two varieties of SIV that bear a resemblance to the two varieties of HIV that are in the world (HIV-1 and HIV-2). HIV-1 closely resembles an SIV found in chimpanzees in west central Africa. HIV-2 is very similar to a SIV found in the sooty mangabey, a monkey sometimes called the green monkey found in West Africa, where that type of HIV is the predominant type.

It has been known for a long time that some viruses can pass from animals to humans; this process is referred to as zoonosis. The first case of a human with HIV or AIDS that has been confirmed was that of a Bantu citizen of the Republic of Congo (Zaire). Several stored plasma samples from research done in Africa were tested in the late 1990s; those samples showed that this particular subject tested positive for HIV-1. In addition, a Norwegian sailor and his family became ill in the late 1960s. Blood taken from them at that time indicated they were all HIV-positive. They all died in 1976, from what was then listed as unknown causes. A Saint Louis teenager, who was admitted to the city hospital in 1968, showed signs of what is now known as HIV infection. His blood was

stored and tested positive. This case is unusual in that he is said not to have traveled outside the United States; he was known, as indicated in hospital records, as a worker in the sex industry.

In western Africa eating of monkey meat is part of the culture. Many green monkeys are killed for this purpose. In addition their abandoned or orphaned young are often taken home as pets in this region. So it is not difficult to see that a pet could have bitten a person or that while cleaning the monkey for eating someone got blood on a cut and was infected in that manner. It is assumed that HIV-1 was spread in the same manner in west central Africa. Scientists believe that given the rate of change of HIV, it was probably introduced into the human population after the 1930s. It is interesting to note, and is yet unexplained, how HIV could transfer from two different types of monkeys to humans twice in the 20th century after thousands of years of not transferring to the human population. Some researchers believe that the greater transportation available into the rain forests, the growing populations migrating from the forests to the cities, and the growing vaccination movement, which has reused needles in Africa could be explanations for the sudden quick spread of the virus.

It was simply a matter of time, once the virus began spreading, before it reached the attention of the medical field in some form of epidemic. In 1978 reports began to trickle in from large American cities and Tanzania and Uganda in East Africa of people with immune deficiencies. Initially in the United States, people of Haitian descent were thought to be susceptible. This has proved incorrect over time. The Haitians who immigrated to the United States or to Central Africa for political reasons in the 1960s had no sign of HIV in blood samples taken at those times. However, many Haitians did work in and around popular gay resorts that were created in Haiti in the 1970s. The people in Haiti who first became ill with HIV were found to have engaged in sex with American gay tourists.

Another theory that has proved incorrect was that HIV was introduced into the human population through polio vaccine research and production. Growth of the vaccine was accomplished in monkey kidneys. So it was suggested that this was the way the virus moved so quickly and extensively into humans. However, in 2001, samples of tissues used in the production of this form of polio virus were found in a lab in the United States. Tests of these materials showed no sign of HIV, so this theory was proved incorrect.

The movement of this virus has drawn attention to the fact that viruses do spread, at times easily, from one species to another. Although it may never be completely shown where and how it was first transferred to humans, HIV has been shown to resemble so closely varieties of SIV that this explanation has become the accepted history of the virus.

HIV pathogenesis   The origin and development of HIV.

HIV RNA   The genetic material of HIV. Many people believe that changes in the level of HIV RNA are good indicators of drug effectiveness; this has not been proved. A new technology that detects blood levels of HIV RNA has been suggested as a promising way for clinicians to gauge the effectiveness of therapy and predict when the disease might get worse. A National Institute of Allergy and Infectious Disease multicenter study began in 1995 to determine if monitoring levels of HIV in the blood can keep patients healthier longer by helping doctors make better treatment decisions. See RNA.

HIV screening   Epidemiologic surveillance of HIV/AIDS in a given population. Such surveillance generally involves an assessment of the existing distribution and scope of infection and its likely spread in the population. Generally such surveillance is an important first step in responding to a disease. Screening is most often associated with compulsory and mass HIV testing, which targets either certain demographic or occupational groups or captive populations (aliens entering the country, military personnel, police officers, drug users, commercial sex workers, prisoners, people with hemophilia, and so forth). Prohibitive cost and complex logistics, as well as human rights considerations, lack of safeguards for confidentiality in testing, and for avoiding discrimination against persons who are found to be infected, have contributed to a decrease in the use and effectiveness of HIV screening programs.

HIV seroprevalence   The prevalence of HIV infection. HIV seroprevalence is an important indication of the scope of the disease and its related problems. With multiple seroprevalence surveys that are based on sample blood specimens, organizations like the CENTERS FOR DISEASE CONTROL AND PREVENTION collect data on HIV infection from several subpopulations. The data collected provide information on the prevalence and incidence of infection in selected populations, provide early warning of the emergence of infection in new populations, and target intervention programs and other resources.

HIV setpoint   The level at which an individual's viral load eventually plateaus. Several studies suggest that the HIV setpoint predicts the rate at which that person will progress to AIDS. If antiviral therapy can help to lower the viral load setpoint so that there is a more stable equilibrium with the immune system, it might slow disease progression.

HIV status   The term "HIV status" often connotes a division between HIV infected and uninfected people. The word "status" implies both a rigid social or moral hierarchy, like caste, and a state of being that is mutable, like a status report. HIV-positive individuals are often portrayed as threatening "others." HIV-negative status is often portrayed as better than—rather than merely different from—an HIV-positive status. When HIV-negative individuals think about the possibility of becoming HIV-positive, they realize their HIV status is something that can change. Their negative status is both precarious and valuable—something they want to protect.

HIV suppressors   A substance that halts the growth of HIV in cell cultures. See CELL ACTIVATED FACTOR (CAF); CHEMOKINES; IL-16.

HIV testing   The use of blood tests that detect the presence or absence of antibodies directed against HIV. The question of involuntary testing emerged early and forcefully in the AIDS pandemic, and testing remains at the center of controversies relating to AIDS prevention and control, including issues of privacy, selectiveness of testing, fear of stigmatization, notification of others, and nondiscrimination. See HIV SCREENING.

HIV type 2 See HUMAN IMMUNODEFICIENCY VIRUS 2.

HIV transmission See TRANSMISSION.

HIV wasting syndrome See WASTING SYNDROME.

HIV-associated adipose redistribution syndrome (HARS) A general term referring to the variety of body fat composition changes associated with anti-retroviral therapy. The natural history and cause (or causes) is not clearly understood. There are a number of different theories about how HARS might evolve. There are a large number of pharmaceutical treatments for high cholesterol level and other lipid disorders; however, there is concern about using some of these drugs for people on HAART because there is a potential for drug interactions since many share the same metabolic pathway as many antiretrovirals. Strategies to ameliorate the signs and symptoms of HARS continue to be studied. See LIPODYSTROPHY.

HIV-contaminated blood HIV-contaminated blood contains blood from donors who have or had AIDS or who are or were HIV antibody positive, and are thus at high risk for AIDS. As of 1987, approximately half of the recipients of seropositive blood were seropositive, and significant percentages of these persons had developed symptoms of HIV infection or AIDS. Routine serological testing of donated blood did not begin until March 1985 in the United States. See BLOOD SUPPLY PROTECTION.

hives see URTICARIA.

HIV-infected Infected with the human immunodeficiency virus. See HIV INFECTION.

HIV-negative Having no detectable HIV antibodies in the blood. A negative test result does not guarantee that an individual is virus-free or cannot transmit the virus to someone else. Case reports have shown that the period between initial HIV infection and the production of detectable antibodies (that is, between infection and SEROCONVERSION) is most often between one and six months. (Uncommon cases have occurred in which more than six months elapsed before antibody was produced. How often this occurs and how to find the virus when infection is suspected but tests are negative, are matters of controversy.) If an individual is tested during this period after being infected but before producing antibodies, the test result will be negative. See ELISA; HIV-POSITIVE; WESTERN BLOT TEST.

HIV-positive Having HIV antibodies present in the blood. The presence of the antibodies confirms the presence of the HIV virus. Inaccurate test results are possible. Antibodies elicited by other substances in the blood may be similar to antibodies directed against HIV and may crossreact in the ELISA, the most commonly used test, falsely indicating the presence of HIV. In all cases of a positive test result, a second blood test must be performed to confirm the results of the first. The WESTERN BLOT TEST is run as a confirmatory test.

Being HIV-positive means that at some point exposure to the virus and infection with HIV have occurred. It does not mean that an individual now has AIDS or will definitely develop AIDS in the future. Being HIV-positive does not mean that an individual is immune to the virus. Being HIV-positive does not mean that an individual can no longer have sex. It does mean, however, a major change in the way an individual lives his or her life. See HIV-NEGATIVE.

Hivid See DIDEOXYCYTIDINE.

HIV-IG An antibody preparation taken from people who produce high levels of HIV antibodies. HIV-IG is under study as a treatment for children with HIV disease and as a therapy to prevent vertical transmission (from mothers to newborns). Side effects include headache, low-grade fever, allergic reaction, and transient rash. HIV-IG differs from passive immunotherapies in which blood from an HIV-positive person with high levels of antibodies is given to an HIV-positive person with low levels of antibodies. See PASSIVE IMMUNOTHERAPY.

HL See HAIRY LEUKEMIA.

HLA See HUMAN LEUKOCYTE ANTIGEN.

HLA I See HUMAN LEUKOCYTE ANTIGENS.

HLA II See HUMAN LEUKOCYTE ANTIGENS.

ho See PROSTITUTE.

Hodgkin's disease A chronic progressive disease of unknown ETIOLOGY that is characterized by inflammatory enlargement of the LYMPH NODES, SPLEEN, and often LIVER and KIDNEYS. Other symptoms may include anemia, anorexia, fever, night sweats, severe itching, and weight loss. It may appear as acute, localized, or latent with relapsing fever or as lymphogranulomatosis and SPLENOMEGALY. Treatment includes radiation and CHEMOTHERAPY.

holistic (wholistic) Various systems of health protection and restoration, both traditional and modern, that are based on the body's reputed "natural healing powers," the various ways the different tissues affect each other, and the influence of the external environment.

home care A continuum of outpatient and home- and community-based services given by family members, nurses (nurse practitioners, licensed practical nurses, RNs), health care providers, home care agencies, technicians, home attendants, social workers, and case managers. A physician is in overall charge of care, but the people who actually deliver the care are removed from his or her immediate supervision. Home care can be a more comfortable, patient-centered, flexible form of care that is also somewhat cheaper than hospital care, and the trend has been to extend it to sicker and sicker patients. But it can also be fragmented, erratic, poorly administered and supervised, and literally out of control. Successful home care must carry into the home setting the team approach that characterizes hospital care, in which case the family and other caregivers must be part of the team in a way that they are not in an institution.

home health care See HOME CARE.

home health services Health services, given to a patient in his own home, that can be provided only by a licensed professional such as a registered nurse or a physical, speech, or occupational therapist. Unskilled care such as housekeeping, feeding, and grooming assistance, comes under this heading only when it is necessary to accomplish the core health service rendered by a professional. Home health services are covered by MEDICARE, MEDICAID, and many private health insurance plans. See HOME CARE.

home- and community-based services Under MEDICAID's 2176 waiver program, these are home health care, home chore aid, personal attendant, outpatient hospice, visiting nurse, and even board-and-care-home services, which are offered as an alternative to more expensive hospitalization or nursing home care.

home-based HIV testing kits Food and Drug Administration approved over-the-counter test kits available in pharmacies and by mail order. The kit is not actually used for home-testing, but, rather, for home collection of samples. Purchasers send a small blood sample to the manufacturer for HIV testing and then phone anonymously for their test results.

homeopathy An approach to healing that is popular in Europe and has many followers in the United States. Its followers believe that a substance which produces a certain set of symptoms in a healthy person has the power to cure a sick person manifesting those same symptoms. Homeopathy has been used by people living with HIV because treatments are unlike conventional scientific medicine, which attacks disease head-on with drugs meant to kill specific bacteria. Homeopathic approaches try to treat "like with like." Once a homeopath has diagnosed a disorder in a patient, a diluted solution to treat the problem is prescribed. This is done by matching or "proving" symptoms with the one substance that most closely reproduces these symptoms in a normal person. Substances may include chemicals, minerals, plant extracts, dilute preparations of animal and insect venom, disease-causing germs, and some standard drugs. Matching the patient's symptoms with the substance that most closely reproduces them is crucial because homeopaths assert that a single dose of that substance, highly diluted and properly prepared, has the capacity to cure the ailing patient. Many people living with HIV report significant reduction of their symptoms using homeopathic remedies.

To date, there have not been an extensive number of controlled clinical studies evaluating the effectiveness of homeopathic treatments. The American Medical Association does not recognize homeopathic medicine because they believe the approach is not based on scientific principles. Currently, only several states license homeopaths. As a result, homeopathic practitioners are often licensed under other accepted forms of medicine, such as a medical doctor, acupuncturist, osteopath, or chiropractor.

homeostasis The state in which the internal environment of the body remains relatively stable by responding appropriately to changes.

homing receptors Cell surface molecules that direct the cell to specific locations in other organs or tissues.

homo Derisive slang term for homosexual.

homocysteine A sulfur-containing amino acid. High levels of homocysteine in the blood have been linked to increased risk of coronary artery disease and stroke.

homologous Similar in appearance, structure, and usually function. For HIV, the same strain of the virus.

homologous challenge Injection of a vaccinated animal with a viral strain similar to the one used to make the virus. See HETEROLOGOUS CHALLENGE.

homophobia The intense fear and/or hatred of homosexuals or of anything having to do with homosexuality. Although the term is of recent origin, homophobia (or heterosexism) as a compo-

nent of our culture has long historical roots, going back at least to early Christian condemnation of sex except for procreation. Like all prejudices, it is based on social myths and stereotyping. Some of the common myths and stereotypes that perpetuate homophobia are that gays are easy to spot—gay men are "swishy," and lesbians are "butch"; that most gays are attracted to certain jobs, e.g., hairdressers, florists, decorators; that gay men are all promiscuous and prone to abuse children; that gay male and lesbian couples have rigid gender roles, with one being the "man" and one the "woman"; that gay men and lesbians have no parental instincts; and that gay parents or teachers can influence children to be gay or lesbian.

Homophobia is manifested in many ways. Gays and lesbians may legally be denied their civil rights, jobs, housing, marriage, parenthood, be taunted and insulted publicly (antigay speech is still tolerated in a way that other prejudiced speech is not), and at times be physically assaulted and even murdered because of their sexual orientation. Homophobia as a response to the AIDS crisis is based entirely on prejudice and misrepresentation. It is inappropriate and destructive.

homosexual Pertaining to same-sex sexual orientation; one sexually attracted to persons of the same sex. Generally, a homosexual woman is called a lesbian. Homosexual men and women are also called gay.

homosexual intercourse See HOMOSEXUAL SEX.

homosexual sex Sexual activity between members of the same sex.

homosexual transmission See TRANSMISSION.

homosexual/bisexual transmission See TRANSMISSION.

homosexuality Sexual attraction toward persons of the same sex.

hooker A slang term for a prostitute.

horizontal transmission See TRANSMISSION.

hormone An active chemical substance secreted by an organ or gland into the blood, which carries it to specific target cells/organs by whose response they bring about a specific and adaptive physiological response (e.g., stimulation or suppression of cell or tissue activity). Hormones tend to be either water-soluble peptides and proteins or lipid-soluble steroids, retinoids, thyroid hormones, and vitamin D3. Examples of hormones include adrenaline, ecdysone, gastrin, thyroxine, insulin, testosterone, and estrogen.

horny Slang term for being sexually aroused.

hospice A facility that provides palliative and supportive services for the terminally ill. Hospice care is an interdisciplinary approach to providing for the terminally ill. The hospice concept emphasizes alleviating a patient's discomfort and supporting the family in the grieving process. Supportive care may include financial, physical, social, and spiritual services. Covered by MEDICARE, MEDICAID, and some private health insurance plans, hospice care may be provided at a hospice facility, at a patient's home, or both. Care is generally provided by a team of health care professionals.

host An organism on which another organism lives and from which the second organism derives nourishment.

host factors Factors intrinsic to the HIV-infected individual that influence the rate at which HIV replicates in the person's body and how rapidly the patient will develop AIDS. These factors include the specific immune response to the virus, nonspecific factors, and the individual's genetic makeup. Such factors are as important, or in some cases even more important, to the HIV disease process than the intrinsic virulence of the virus itself. Host factors, together with viral factors, determine the pathogenesis of HIV disease, the complex events which lead to the destruction of an HIV-infected person's immune system.

hot In sexual terms, slang for sexually arousing. It may be used of a person, image, activity, or thing. In epidemiological terms, slang for actively infective. "Hot" may also mean radioactive.

hot agent Extremely lethal virus that is potentially air-borne.

hot line Telephone service providing crisis intervention to individuals experiencing severe problems. Hot lines are usually staffed continuously by paraprofessionals or professionals in the medical or social sciences. HIV/AIDS–related hot lines typically provide answers to questions about the disease and offer referrals to local service providers.

hot zone An area that contains lethal, infectious organisms. Also hot area or hot side.

housebound Incapacitated and unable to leave home, medical facility, or community residence without assistance. The term is sometimes used in MEDICAID and other social service programs. In military pension programs of the Department of Veterans Affairs, housebound disabled veterans are entitled to a higher pension income eligibility level.

housing People with HIV/AIDS face difficulties in obtaining and maintaining housing. They may have difficulty renting or buying in the private market and may be evicted from current rental agreements. The Fair Housing Act, adopted by Congress in 1968, prohibits discrimination in the sale or rental of housing and in advertising, financing, and the provision of brokerage services. Congress amended the law in 1988 to prohibit discrimination because of "handicap." The Fair Housing Act defines "handicap" as a "physical or mental impairment which substantially limits . . . major life activities." This definition was taken from Section 504 of the Rehabilitation Act of 1973, which courts have unanimously interpreted to include HIV. People subjected to discrimination in violation of the Fair Housing Act may file a complaint with HUD and may bring a lawsuit to federal court. The attorney general may also bring actions in court to prohibit "a pattern or practice" that violates the Fair Housing Act. Today, many states have their own laws prohibiting discrimination in housing on the basis of handicap, some including HIV infection. Several cities have also adopted ordinances prohibiting discrimination in housing against people with HIV. State and local laws have also been used to oppose discrimination by landlords against agencies and professionals providing services to people with HIV/AIDS.

One of the realities people with HIV/AIDS may face is the possibility of losing their homes because of inability to make rent or mortgage payments. Some people with full-blown AIDS may need specialized care facilities or group housing. Many people with HIV become homeless and require housing assistance. The law provides very little support for general claims that the government must provide shelter to those who need it. But people with HIV have redress under the Fair Housing Act and local antidiscrimination laws when they are refused admission to or are evicted from group housing, such as homeless shelters and publicly owned housing, because of their condition.

In the long run, most litigation is likely to concern special-care facilities and group homes for people with HIV. Organized community opposition to group homes or care facilities is a common barrier. These facilities generally must meet state and local health and fire codes. Usually, efforts to prevent homes from opening focus on zoning restrictions. Discriminatory use of zoning restrictions is subject to challenge under both the United States Constitution and the Fair Housing Act. Some cases have also applied the equal protection clause of the federal Constitution to invalidate zoning restrictions and decisions that discrimination against group homes for special populations, such as people with HIV/AIDS.

While much has been done for people with HIV to eliminate discrimination in housing, much remains to be done in meeting their housing needs. People with HIV/AIDS must cope with pressing income as well as health needs. Funding for housing is crucial, a fact Congress recognized in the 1990 Cranston-Gonzalez National Affordable Housing Act, which includes a block grant program designed to encourage state and local governments to provide housing for people with HIV/AIDS. Additionally, the United States social welfare system offers a variety of financial and health care benefit programs for people, including SOCIAL SECURITY, welfare, MEDICAID, MEDICARE, FOOD STAMPS, drugs, and housing. With federal funding, many state, city, or county housing departments run a variety of housing programs for low-income persons, with special projects or units set aside for the aged and the disabled. Persons with HIV/AIDS who need access to housing must identify the programs that are available, find out what benefits are offered, and determine and assess their eligibility before applying and, if necessary, appealing.

HPA-23 See ANTIMONIOTUNGSTATE.

HPMPC See CIDOFOVIR.

HPV See HUMAN PAPILLOMAVIRUS.

HTLV See HUMAN T CELL LYMPHOTROPIC VIRUS.

HTLV-II See HUMAN T CELL LYMPHOTROPIC VIRUS.

HTLV-III See HUMAN IMMUNODEFICIENCY VIRUS (HIV).

HTLV-III/LAV See HUMAN T-LYMPHOTROPIC VIRUS TYPE III.

HTLV-IV See HUMAN T-LYMPHOTROPIC VIRUS TYPE IV.

HU See HYDROXYUREA.

HUD See DEPARTMENT OF HOUSING AND URBAN DEVELOPMENT.

HUD voucher A document that eligible low-income recipients can present to landlords in lieu of rent payment; landlords, in turn, redeem the vouchers for cash from HUD, in a housing counterpart to the food stamps program. Not all landlords participate in this program.

human chorionic gonadotropin (HCG) A naturally occurring hormone that is produced by women during pregnancy. HCG inhibits the mother's immune system from rejecting the fetus as foreign tissue. It is an approved therapy for treating infertility in women and cryptorchidism failure

(failure of the testicles to descend) in boys. Interest in HCG was stimulated by anecdotes of KAPOSI'S SARCOMA regression in two pregnant women. In the first human trial with HCG, intralesional injection of a formulation of HCG was shown to reduce the size and occasionally lead to complete regression of the treated KS lesions. Investigators observed that the active material is not the normal HCG molecule, but something that accompanies it in the crude material, in the pregnant woman's urine. Whatever the active component, it appears to induce apoptosis (a form of cell suicide) in the lesion. Several studies were conducted using the hormone in Kaposi's sarcoma treatment in the mid-1990s, but the results were not clearly positive enough to warrant further work using HCG.

human gene therapy   Treatment of human disease by gene transfer. Most approved gene therapy trials involve use of retroviral vectors for gene transfer into cultured human cells that would be administered to patients. Retroviral vectors are RETROVIRUSES lacking all functional viral genes, so no viral protein is produced in infected cells. Viral replication is achieved using "packaging cells" that produce all the viral proteins without the infective virus. This results in efficient and stable targeting of cells. The main drawback though, is the inability of the vectors to infect non-dividing cells. Proposals for human gene therapy have to pass several levels of review to ensure safety.

human growth hormone (HGH)   Human growth hormone is a peptide hormone secreted by the pituitary gland in the brain that enhances tissue growth by stimulating protein formation. A synthetic recombinant human growth hormone called Serostim is available to HIV positive people who have HIV wasting syndrome. Naturally occurring HGH is secreted most heavily by the body during adolescence. It gradually decreases over the course of a lifetime, though it never is completely absent from the body. Having too much or too little as a child can lead to various growth abnormalities.

HGH has shown it is possible to replace the lean muscle mass that wasting includes. The variety used to treat wasting syndrome is manufactured by one company and is very expensive. Other drug and herbal companies manufacture a variety of synthetic and recombinant HGH. These are sold both through prescription and over the counter formulas. It can come in injectable or pill forms. HGH does not cure the underlying causes of wasting in HIV positives. It does, however, force the body to create more lean muscle mass through rebuilding protein in the body.

Human growth hormone has also been used successfully in the treatment of BODY FAT REDISTRIBUTION SYNDROME. Buffalo hump as well as truncal obesity due to fat redistribution have resolved themselves in a few weeks or months of treatment with HGH. Daily subcutaneous injections are used in the treatment. Treatment can result also in abnormal breast growth in men. Treatment results may reverse themselves somewhat in people who have body fat abnormalities prior to taking HAART.

human herpesvirus 1, 2   See HERPES SIMPLEX VIRUS.

human herpesvirus 3   See VARICELLA-ZOSTER VIRUS.

human herpesvirus 4   See EPSTEIN-BARR VIRUS.

human herpesvirus 5   See CYTOMEGALOVIRUS.

human herpesvirus 6   Herpesvirus that infects lymphocytes, including CD4 cells. HHV-6 infection generally occurs early in life and may cause fever and exanthem (roseola, a red skin rash) in infants. HHV-6 is associated with neuropathology, chronic fatigue syndrome, multiple sclerosis, and certain autoimmune diseases.

human herpesvirus 7   Herpesvirus that infects human T cells but is not known to cause disease.

human herpesvirus 8   See KAPOSI'S SARCOMA–ASSOCIATED HERPESVIRUS.

human immune deficiency virus   See HUMAN IMMUNODEFICIENCY VIRUS.

human immunodeficiency virus (HIV)   One of a large group of IMMUNODEFICIENCY virus (IVs) widely spread among primates and other mammals. SIMIAN IMMUNODEFICIENCY VIRUS (SIV) is the closest relative of HIV. HIV is believed to be the causative agent of AIDS in humans. HIV is not an oncogenic virus like HTLV-I (HUMAN T CELL LYMPHOTROPIC VIRUS TYPE I), but rather the first human LENTIVIRUS to be discovered. IVs form a subgroup of the RETROVIRUSES—whose life is shared with the genomic elements called retrotransposons. Each virion has a protein core surrounding the genome and an enclosed enzyme (REVERSE TRANSCRIPTASE), the whole encapsulated by a segment of host cell membrane in which viral glycoproteins are located. This GLYCOPROTEIN (GP120) recognizes and binds to the accessory molecule CD4, so HIV infects any CD4+ cell, including T-HELPER CELLS. Once bound, the membranes of HIV and the host cell fuse, releasing the infective virus core within the host cell.

HIV's genome comprises an RNA molecule, housing at least three genes (GAG, encoding core proteins; POL-encoding viral enzymes; and ENV, encoding envelope GLYCOPROTEINS). On entry into the host cell, viral reverse transcriptase creates a DNA copy of the RNA genome, which is then converted into double-stranded DNA capable of inserting into the human genome and existing as a PROVIRUS for long periods. However, there is no evidence that HIV integrates into the germ line. Eventually, productive virus synthesis occurs and new HIV particles leave the host cell encapsulated in its modified membrane. T CELLS producing HIV no longer divide, and eventually die. Also, because of the gp120-CD4 binding, HIV-infected cells bind to uninfected CD4+ cells to produce syncytia, at which point the uninfected T cells lose their immune capacity and die. Immunodeficiency results.

There are numerous strains of HIV that cross-react minimally or not at all with neutralizing antibodies targeting other strains and it is not known how many strains would be needed in a vaccine providing broad anti-HIV protection.

human immunodeficiency virus 2   A retrovirus closely related to the simian immunodeficiency virus (SIV) and less closely related to HIV-1. HIV-2 is found primarily in West Africa. HIV-1 and HIV-2 are similar in their viral structure and modes of transmission. Symptoms caused by HIV-2 are similar to those caused by HIV-1 but are typically milder and slower to develop. There are five known types of HIV-2 (A through E).

human leukocyte antigens (HLA)   The major HISTOCOMPATIBILITY genetic region in humans. Specifically, they are the antigens on white blood cells that are representative of the antigens present on all the cells of the individual. Class I MHC are HLA-A, B, C, and the class II MHC are HLA-DP, DQ, DR.

human papilloma virus (HPV)   HPV refers to a group of more than 60 viruses that cause warts. Warts of all kinds, from those that occur on your hand to those that occur in the genital region. More than 80 percent of all people in the world have been exposed and carry some variety of HPV. Not everyone that has been exposed to the virus and carries it with them shows the clinical result, the warts. Up to 70 percent of people exposed to HPV are believed to exhibit no sign of the virus. There is no known cure for HPV, though the warts themselves can be treated and removed.

Most people refer to genital warts when they use the term *HPV.* There are a variety of HPV that cause genital warts, and a few of these types have been linked to cancer of the cervix, anus, and penis. The types numbered 16, 18, 31, 33, and 35 have been linked to changes in the body's tissue, also called dysplasia, and, when this continues, to cancer. The tissue that makes up the cervix is the same type of tissue that makes up the anus. It has been established that HPV types that can cause cervical cancer can also cause anal cancer. Types of dysplasia that can be a sign of possible cancer are called cervical intraepithelial neoplasia (CIN) and anal intraepithelial neoplasia (AIN). All women and men with anogenital warts should have an annual Pap smear of both the cervical and anal regions. This procedure can show development of dysplasias that may cause problems later.

People with HIV are more prone to developing complications with HPV. Women show an increased risk of cervical dysplasias and cancer than women in the general population. Women who show an increased risk for CIN also show an increased risk of AIN. A patient does not have to have had a wart in a particular area to be affected by neoplasia in that region. What this means is that, despite not having genital warts in a particular area, it is still possible to develop CIN or AIN.

The clinical course of HPV and anogenital neoplasia is accelerated in HIV-positive patients. HPV infection and neoplasia in HIV-infected patients are often persistent and recurrent, extend to adjacent areas of skin and mucous membranes, resist conventional therapy, and can progress to invasive cancer. Whether women with both HIV and HPV infection will have an accelerated rate of progression to invasive genital tract cancer cannot be predicted. HIV-infected women have a significant increase in cervical abnormalities and a higher prevalence of (CIN). HIV-positive men have higher incidences of AIN and anal cancers than their HIV-negative counterparts. In HIV-positive patients dysplasia and cancerous lesions occur at a younger age, are frequently multifocal, and occur at multiple sites. Annual PAP smears can prevent any dysplasias from developing unnoticed. Biopsy of warts or dysplasias may also be suggested by medical personnel to keep watch of concerned patients.

The effect of genital wart treatment on HPV transmission and the natural history of HPV is uncertain. Warts and other HPV-related lesions are common and difficult to eradicate, often requiring prophylactic therapy because of their persistence and recurrence. Therefore, the goal of treatment is removal of warts and control of signs and symptoms, not eradication of HPV. In most clinical situations, cryotherapy with liquid nitrogen or cryoprobe is the treatment of choice for external genital and perianal warts. For patients with cervical warts, dysplasia must be excluded before treatment is begun.

human rights AIDS is the first worldwide epidemic to occur in the modern era of human rights. Public health practitioners face a dual standard in the design and implementation of public health programs in order to prevent HIV transmission. Programs must be effective in public health terms and must respect and respond to human rights norms. National and international attention to the human rights aspects of HIV/AIDS prevention and care have ebbed and flowed over the course of the epidemic, often in direct response to the rise of discrimination and a lack of protection of human rights and dignity.

The relationship between HIV/AIDS prevention and care and human rights can be considered in two ways. First, there are possible pressures and problems related to human rights that are created by the choice or manner of implementation of public health measures. This is the more traditional arena in which public health and human rights issues have been negotiated. Second, during the first decade of the epidemic it became clear that a discriminatory social environment was counterproductive for HIV information/education and prevention programs. Because societal discrimination in all its forms creates increased vulnerability to HIV infection, efforts to protect human rights and to promote human dignity are extremely important for protecting public health in the AIDS pandemic. As understanding of the pandemic evolved, the relationship between societal discrimination and the risk of becoming HIV infected became more evident. Being excluded from the mainstream of society, or being discriminated against on grounds of race/ethnicity, national origin, religion, gender, or sexual preference led to an increase in HIV infection. Thus, during the first decade of work against AIDS, the positive contribution that improving protection of human rights could have for public health became evident.

The ways in which many national authorities have responded to the AIDS epidemic have created a wide range of human rights problems by imposing coercive or restrictive AIDS control measures. Virtually every measure of disease control has human rights implications: public health surveillance may seek and record the personal identity of infected persons, and people identified as carriers may be subjected to isolation and quarantine. Even how a disease is classified may lead to compulsory medical examination or hospitalization, depending on local or national disease control legislation. Public health laws specify what individuals must do and what they must not do by defining offenses against public health (including the transmission of infectious diseases). Whether it is AIDS or any other epidemic, the bulk of public health measures identify affected groups and individuals and safeguard against further spread of disease.

To date, no worldwide review of AIDS-related human rights problems has yet been made to indicate what acts constitute human rights violations. Nonetheless, there are patterns of human rights problems. Problems have surfaced with regard to national laws, policies and practices, HIV testing, targets of mass testing, notification, counterproductiveness of compulsory testing, discrimination, and AIDS-related violence.

human T cell leukemia   The first human RETROVIRUS. In published reports of its finding in 1980, Robert C. Gallo of the National Cancer Institute labeled it as "human T-cell leukemia/lymphoma virus" (HTLV). The virus principally targets T4 helper cells.

human T cell leukemia virus   See HUMAN T CELL LYMPHOTROPIC VIRUS.

human T cell leukemia virus III (HTLV-III)   See HUMAN IMMUNODEFICIENCY VIRUS.

human T cell lymphotropic virus (HTLV)   A family of retroviruses that are lymphocytotropic and particularly partial to T lymphocytes of the inducer/helper subset. Also called human T cell leukemia virus. This is the family of viruses to which HIV belongs.

human T cell lymphotropic virus I (HTLV-I)   A virus associated with adult T cell leukemia. It is found more often in Japan than in the United States.

human T cell lymphotropic virus II (HTLV-II)   A virus associated with hairy cell leukemia.

human T cell lymphotropic virus III (HTLV-III)   A slow-acting virus that causes HUMAN IMMUNODEFICIENCY SYNDROME (AIDS). For a more complete discussion of the naming and renaming of the virus, see ACQUIRED IMMUNODEFICIENCY VIRUS.

human T cell lymphotropic virus variant III   Chronicles of the isolation and discovery of the AIDS virus invariably include discussion of the confusion over the virus's name. Luc Montagnier,

head of the Viral Oncology Unit of the Institut Pasteur in Paris, and his colleagues first isolated the virus later shown to be the cause of AIDS in May 1983. They named the virus LYMPHADENOPATHY-ASSOCIATED VIRUS (LAV) because they had isolated it from one of the swollen lymph nodes of a patient with LYMPHADENOPATHY SYNDROME. A second isolate identified by the same group was called immunodeficiency-associated virus, or IDAV.

In May 1984, workers in Robert Gallo's laboratory at the National Cancer Institute (NCI) reported that they had identified a line of cancerous T CELLS that had two important characteristics: 1) susceptibility to infection with the new virus, and 2) the ability to resist the killing effects that had destroyed other infected T-cell cultures. The NCI researchers reported that they had isolated the new virus, which they designated HTLV-III, from 48 patients. The meaning of HTLV was changed from "human T-cell leukemia/lymphoma virus" to "human T-cell lymphotropic virus" to reflect the fact that all known human retroviruses shared an attraction to T lymphocytes. Another virus isolate was described in August 1984 by Jay Levy and his coworkers from the University of California at San Francisco. They named their virus AIDS-ASSOCIATED RETROVIRUS or ARV.

Scientific journals in the United States and Europe adopted one of two compound names, HTLV-III/LAV or LAV/HTLV-III. The compound names afforded recognition to the two principal groups involved in the discovery of the AIDS virus. But, the names were unwieldy and failed to address an issue even more important than who had discovered the virus: how the new virus related to other known human and animal retroviruses. Early studies showed that although the new human retrovirus resembled HTLV-I and HTLV-II in its preference for T-cells, it acted on these cells in a very different way: HTLV-I and HTLV-II caused uncontrolled proliferation of the T-cells, whereas the AIDS virus killed them. The two human T-cell leukemia viruses share many features with the animal ONCOVIRUSes, but the structure and function of the AIDS virus are more akin to those of the LENTIVIRUSes.

Several events in late 1985 and early 1986 increased the urgency of resolving the name issue. First, researchers identified a monkey virus that appeared very similar to the human AIDS virus. Researchers named this virus STLV-III (simian T-lymphotropic virus type III). Several months later, United States and French research teams announced that they had discovered two new human retroviruses in people in West Africa; the United States group called their virus HTLV-IV, while the French group called theirs LAV-2. Subsequent studies showed that the populations studied by the two groups were infected with variants of the same virus and that the new virus was more closely related to the monkey virus than to the original AIDS virus in humans.

Finally, in May 1984, a subcommittee of the International Committee on the Taxonomy of Viruses proposed a new system for naming all AIDS retroviruses in humans and subhuman primates. The human viruses were to be called HUMAN IMMUNODEFICIENCY VIRUSes (HIVs). The monkey virus was renamed SIMIAN IMMUNODEFICIENCY VIRUS, or SIV.

Today, HIV-1 is used to refer to all isolates of HTLV-III, LAV, and ARV. HIV-2 is the official designation for LAV-2 and all related isolates.

human t-lymphocyte virus type III (HTLV-III)
The organism believed to cause the body to lose its immunity. The name HTLV-III came about because the suspected virus is the third member of a family of viruses that are known to cause lymph disorders such as leukemia and other cancers of T lymphocyte cells. These are the same white blood cells that contribute to the body's immunity by producing antibodies against disease. Because the virus is thought to be of the RETROVIRUS family (different virus families have unique physical and growth characteristics), some doctors call the HTLV-III virus the AIDS-ASSOCIATED VIRUS. And yet another term for the virus is LYMPHADENOPATHY-ASSOCIATED VIRUS (LAV). Any one, or a combination, of these terms may be used for the AIDS antibody test. While there are some doctors who feel all three viruses may be identical, there are others who feel the African swine fever virus (a species from a different family of viruses called IRIDOVIRUSES) is the real cause of AIDS. Tests to reveal these antibodies are under investigation. There are also those who feel AIDS may come from several different viruses rather than just one as a means of explaining the variation of signs and symptoms in different patients.

human t-lymphotropic virus type III/lymphadenopathy-associated virus In medical literature, the virus responsible for AIDS is called by different names, including this one. The nomenclature of the virus continues to be debated. Human T cell lymphotropic virus-Type III and lymphadenopathy-associated virus are the same virus or closely similar. Members of the retrovirus family, they are considered a primary cause of AIDS. See HUMAN IMMUNODEFICIENCY VIRUS.

human t-lymphotropic virus type IV This variant was reported in mid-1986. It is believed to be closely related to SIMIAN T-CELL LYMPHOTROPIC VIRUS (STLV, SIV), which causes AIDS in certain species of monkeys in Africa but has not been linked with the disease in humans.

humoral Pertaining to molecules in solution in a body fluid, particularly antibody and complement.

humoral abnormality A deficiency or deviation from the norm in body fluids (the antibody limb of protection).

humoral immunity Immunity that results from the activity of antibodies dissolved in BLOOD, LYMPH, and other body fluids that bind to the ANTIGEN and trigger a response to it. Also called ANTIBODY-MEDIATED IMMUNITY. See TH2 RESPONSE.

hydrocortisone The CORTICOSTEROID hormone produced by the adrenal cortex and produced synthetically. It is essential in maintaining life, sustaining blood pressure, and providing mineralocorticoid activity. Used in the treatment of various ailments, e.g., allergies, collagen abnormalities, inflammations, and certain neoplasms. Many people with advanced HIV disease have decreased adrenal gland function. Hydrocortisone is often used by them as replacement therapy to correct the low natural level. Hydrocortisone is available in a number of formulations. Skin creams containing 0.5 percent to 1.0 percent hydrocortisone are available over the counter. More concentrated preparations are available in various forms by prescription. For most uses, hydrocortisone is applied topically. The side effects of topically administered hydrocortisone are generally mild and may include burning, itching, irritation, dryness, thinning of the skin, slow growth of skin, or secondary infection. The side effects of oral or injectable forms of the drug include dizziness, increased appetite, increased sweating, restlessness, sleep disorders, or weight gain. Serious but rare, side effects include abdominal enlargement, acne, bone or muscle pain, blurred vision, black or tarry stools, convulsions, eye pain, fever, sore throat, headache, slow wound healing, mental depression, mood changes, muscle wasting, nightmares, unusual bleeding, and growth impairment in children.

hydrogen peroxide A colorless syrupy liquid with an irritating odor and acrid taste, which decomposes readily, liberating oxygen. Light is particularly effective in decomposing hydrogen peroxide, so it should be stored in tightly sealed glass jars in a dark place. Hydrogen peroxide is used as a commercial bleaching, oxidizing, and reducing agent. In a 3 percent aqueous solution, it is used as a mild antiseptic, germicide, and cleansing agent. A solution of hydrogen peroxide has value as a cleansing agent for suppurating wounds and inflamed mucous membranes.

hydroxyurea (hydrea, HU) An approved oral drug for some cancers and sickle-cell anemia. It has been tested as an anti-HIV treatment. Hydroxyurea blocks the action of the cellular enzyme ribonucleotide reductase, which helps produce the nucleotides needed for DNA formation. By reducing the amount of the nucleotides that HIV uses for reproduction it takes the false nucleotides made by the HAART medications that the patient is taking. Hydroxyurea has been found to work well with ddI (didanosine) in lab tests. However, in research studies, hydroxyurea was at best marginally effective in adding to the effectiveness of a patient's current HAART regime. Adverse events primarily involving bone marrow suppression and pancreatitis have put a damper on much use currently in HIV infection or drug trials. The side effects were not statistically significant according to the trials

but may increase problems already seen with various HIV medicines.

hygiene The practice of keeping the body clean and in conditions that promote health.

hymen A membrane that partially covers the opening of the vagina. It is broken or greatly stretched after first coitus.

hypercapnia The condition of having an excess amount of carbon dioxide in the blood.

hypercholesterolemia High levels of cholesterol in the blood.

hypergammaglobulinemia Excessive amount of gamma globulin in the blood.

hyperglycemia An increased amount of sugar in the blood resulting in a condition that may lower resistance to infection and may precede diabetic coma.

hypericin A highly concentrated extract of the flowering tops of the St. John's wort plant. It has been used throughout history in many locales for any number of reasons, most applications without any proven efficacy. The same warnings that apply to taking St. John's wort apply to hypericin. It should not be mixed with PROTEASE INHIBITORS, nor taken with other antidepressants. Hypericin causes significant phototoxicity (allergic reactions to light) and has shown no antiretroviral activity in studies conducted with HIV positive patients.

hyperimmunoglobulinemia Abnormally high levels of antibodies in the system. A condition often seen at the outset of HIV infection as the body tries to fight the virus. It was initially not known why this occurred, because patients did not become ill immediately, often for years. As tests to determine the virus in the body became available and easier to use, it became clear that the immune system was engaged in a constant battle with the virus from day one of infection and that the hyperimmunoglobulinemia was part of the body's fight.

hyperkalemia Excessive amount of potassium in the blood, generally caused by defective renal excretion.

hyperkaliemia See HYPERKALEMIA.

hyperlipidemia High levels of blood lipids.

hyperpathia Hypersensitivity to sensory stimuli.

hyperplasia Excessive proliferation of normal cells in a tissue or organ.

hyperreactivity A state of increased reactivity to a provoking stimulus, for instance bronchial hyperreactivity in asthma. Specifically, a greater-than-normal magnitude of response to a given concentration of stimulus.

hypersensitivity An abnormally exaggerated immune response to an agent, such as a drug or an antigen.

hypertension The condition of having higher blood pressure than normal or safe.

hyperthermia Unusually high body temperature. Also, an experimental procedure based on the theory that this temperature kills free HIV and HIV-containing cells—that involves temporarily raising a patient's body temperature to an abnormal height in order to treat HIV disease. Public attention first focused on this therapy in 1990. At that time, Kenneth Alonso, M.D., and William Logan, M.D., of Atlanta, Georgia, announced that they had at least temporarily cured a patient of AIDS-related KAPOSI'S SARCOMA (KS) while raising his CD4 count from 50 to 330 by elevating his body temperature to 42 degrees C (108 degrees F) for one hour.

Since then, whole body hyperthermia has had peaks of public attention from time to time, fed by Italian reports of successful treatment of people with HIV. Dr. Alonso and a team from Rome's European Hospital published the results of single hyperthermia treatments in 31 patients with disseminated KS, but these treatments by no means amounted to a care-fully controlled study with precisely defined eligibility criteria. One of the Italian group's patients, Chuck DeMarco, was so impressed by the results of his 1991 hyperthermia treatment—he recounted not only the disappearance of his KS lesions but eventual remission of his HIV infection as well—that he formed an organization known as HEAT INFO to promote further study of the therapy. Mr. DeMarco's major accomplishment was pressuring the FOOD AND DRUG ADMINISTRATION (FDA) to allow a U.S. study of hyperthermia. This test was inconclusive, although it did indicate that the hyperthermia technique was safe.

In December 1994, the FDA allowed a larger trial. The data from this trial were much more rigorously collected than the essentially anecdotal information provided by Dr. Alonso and the Italian group. The trial took place with people who were on stable anti-HIV drug therapy and had an average CD4 count of 120. The results did not bear out previous claims. However, some clinics outside the United States still offer this treatment for HIV positives.

Another use of the term hyperthermia refers to the removal and heating of a person's blood before returning it to circulation in the body. This, too, is believed to kill the virus in the blood. However in this method, virus would remain in other tissues of the body, such as the lymph system or brain.

hypertriglyceridemia High levels of triglycerides in the blood.

hypertrophy The enlargement or growth of an organ or structure, not involving tumor formation, due to an increase in the size of its constituent cells.

hypnotherapy A range of techniques that ostensibly allow practitioners to bypass the conscious mind and access the subconscious, where suppressed memories and repressed emotions may remain recorded. Hypnosis may facilitate behavioral, emotional, or attitudinal changes. Often used to help people lose weight or stop smoking, it is also used in the treatment of phobias, stress, and as an adjunct in the treatment of illness.

hypodermic Under or inserted under the skin, as a hypodermic injection. It may be given subcutaneously (under the skin), intracutaneously (into the skin), intramuscularly (into a muscle), intraspinally (into the spinal canal), or intravascularly (into a vein or artery). It is given to secure prompt action of a drug when the drug cannot be taken by mouth, when it may not be readily absorbed in the stomach or intestines, when it might be changed by action of the gastric secretions, or to act as a local anesthetic.

hypogammaglobulinemia (agammaglobulinemia) Decreased gammaglobulins in the blood, resulting in a state of immunodeficiency. Acquired hypogammaglobulinemia has its onset in early childhood. Congenital hypogammaglobulinemia is an inherited form of hypogammaglobulinemia in which all immunoglobulins are decreased; this usually manifests as immunodeficiency at six months of age, by which time the maternal immunoglobulins have disappeared.

hypoglycemia Deficiency of sugar in the blood. This condition may result in shakiness, cold sweat, fatigue, hypothermia, headache, and malaise, accompanied by confusion, irritability, and weakness. Hypoglycemia may ultimately result in seizures, coma, and possibly death.

hypogonadism Defective internal secretion of the gonads, resulting in slowed growth and sexual development or, in adults, impairment of normal sexual function.

hypokalemia Extreme potassium depletion in the circulating blood, commonly resulting in episodes of muscular weakness or paralysis, tetany, postural hypotension, renal disease, and gastrointestinal dysfunction. Loss of potassium may occur through renal secretion or through expulsion via the gastrointestinal tract (diarrhea or vomiting).

hypopharynx The lowermost portion of the pharynx, which leads to the larynx and esophagus.

hypotension Decrease of systolic and diastolic blood pressure below normal. Hypotension occurs in shock, hemorrhages, infections, fevers, cancer, anemia, neurasthenia, Addison's disease, debilitating or wasting disease, and approaching death.

hypothermia The condition of having a body temperature below normal. Also a technique of lowering body temperature, usually to between 78 and 90 degrees F, to reduce oxygen need during surgery and in hypoxia, to reduce blood pressure, and to alleviate hyperpyrexia.

hypothesis A specific statement or proposition, stated in testable (researchable) form, predicting a particular relationship among multiple variables.

hypovolemia Diminished blood volume.

hypoxemia Insufficient oxygenation of the blood.

hypoxia Deficiency of oxygen in the blood; also decreased concentration of oxygen in inspired air.

IAS Guidelines The International AIDS Society (IAS) was founded as a nonprofit organization in connection with the fourth International AIDS Conference in Stockholm in 1988. Members from each of five geographic regions, North America, Europe, Africa, Latin America/Caribbean, and Asia and the Pacific, sit on the governing board. It's membership consists of AIDS agencies and alliances from around the world as well as individual members. It is a nongovernmental, nonreligious organization that claims to represent a purely scientific view and point of reason. It lists the following as its purposes:

1. To contribute to the control and management of HIV infection and AIDS throughout the world in co-operation with national and regional AIDS Societies, with UNAIDS and other international organizations including non-governmental organizations.
2. To serve as an international forum for scientific interest groups and caucuses on HIV and AIDS. To initiate, coordinate and evaluate activities to control HIV and AIDS.
3. To organize international conferences and sub-specialty conferences on HIV infection and AIDS, in particular the series of biennial International AIDS Conferences and Conferences on HIV Pathogenicity and Clinical Care in the intervening years.
4. To organize training courses related to HIV infection and AIDS, particularly the Educational Program on Clinical Management and Prevention of HIV Infection (SHARE).
5. To represent the scientific community as a voice of reason in AIDS controversies, to counteract discrimination and promote the ethical aspects of research and interventions.
6. To advocate for adequate resources for research and training as well as for controlling the epidemic and alleviating its consequences.
7. To solicit and receive funds in support for the IAS activities against HIV and AIDS.
8. To serve as a central registry of individuals professionally involved in AIDS research and activities to treat and prevent HIV infection.
9. The IAS is not organized nor is it to be operated for profit.

The IAS has issued guidelines on the treatment of HIV/AIDS, which are often used as the basis of individual country or health agency treatment guidelines. Regarding treatment guidelines the IAS says:

Emerging data indicate that despite limitations, resistance testing should be incorporated into patient management in some settings. Resistance testing is recommended to help guide the choice of new regimens after treatment failure and for guiding therapy for pregnant women. It should be considered in treatment-naive patients with established infection, but cannot be firmly recommended in this setting. Testing also should be considered prior to initiating therapy in patients with acute HIV infection, although therapy should not be delayed pending the results. Expert interpretation is recommended given the complexity of results and assay limitations. Optimal care requires individualized management and ongoing attention to relevant scientific and clinical information in the field. Physicians and patients must weigh the risks and benefits of starting antiretroviral therapy and make individualized informed decisions. When to initiate therapy and what regimen to choose are crucial decisions; otherwise, future options may be severely compromised. Ultimate long-term success may also be a function of the aggregate effectiveness of sequential therapies.

The IAS Guidelines have changed over the years and are periodically updated in major medical publications. They have generated some controversy among activists, who characterize them as out of date and not applicable for all people. Physicians have pointed out that guidelines are typically outdated as a result of the generalities they contain and the need to distribute such material widely. They stress the importance of absolute surety in statements in the guidelines.

iatrogenic   Resulting from the activities of a physician.

ibuprofen   A nonsteroidal anti-inflammatory agent available with or without a prescription. (Trade names are Advil, Motrin, and Nuprin.)

IC   See INHIBITORY CONCENTRATION.

ichthyosis   A noninflammatory condition in which the skin is dry and scaly. Depending on the stage and degree of the condition, it has been described as alligator skin, crocodile skin, or fish skin. Ichthyosis is a hereditary disorder.

ICOD   The immediate cause of death; one of two separate designations for the cause of death distinguished by autopsy pathologists.

icterus   See JAUNDICE.

ICU   See INTENSIVE CARE UNIT.

idiopathic inflammatory pulmonary disease   A pathological condition of unknown origin causing inflammation of the lungs. It is not a result of any other disease.

idiopathic thrombocytopenic purpura (ITP) Also called immune thrombocytopenic purpura. *Idiopathic* means having a cause that is unknown. *Thrombocytopenic* describes blood that does not have enough platelets. *Purpura* means excessive bruising. ITP is a bleeding disorder characterized by low platelet numbers resulting from platelet destruction by the immune system. The disease occurs when immune system cells called LYMPHOCYTES produce ANTIBODIES against PLATELETS. The presence of antibodies on platelets leads to destruction in the spleen. Swollen lymph nodes can occur, and the spleen may also swell as it is predominantly lymph tissue. Skin hemorrhage, easy bruising, abnormal menstrual bleeding, or sudden and severe loss of blood from the gastrointestinal tract may occur. Usually, no other abnormal findings are present. In children, the disease is sometimes preceded by a viral infection and runs its course without treatment. In adults, it is usually a chronic disease and rarely follows a viral infection. ITP in HIV often resolves itself. There is no sex difference in children. Risk factors are unknown. Common in people with HIV, ITP often resolves as immune deficiency worsens. HIV-related ITP usually does not have serious consequences. Its cause has not been definitively determined. Treatment with HAART also frequently alleviates the condition. The most likely hypothesis is that the decrease of platelets is caused by HIV and antibody destruction by the virus causes this problem.

idiotype   The molecular arrangement of amino acids unique to the antigen-binding site of a particular antibody.

IDU   See INJECTION DRUG USER.

IFN   See INTERFERON.

Ig A, D, E, G, M   See IMMUNOGLOBULIN.

IGF   See INSULINLIKE GROWTH FACTOR.

IL   See INTERLEUKIN.

IL-1, -2, -3, -4, -5, -6, -12 and -16   See INTERLEUKIN.

imagery   One of a number of treatment techniques that are alternatives and/or adjuncts to traditional American medical therapeutics. Imagery is one of many mental disciplines which serves to direct our thoughts in order to utilize mental energies to augment the healing process and to combat the debilitating effects of stress. Others include biofeedback, color and sound, meditation, and yoga. The technique is easy and accessible. With eyes closed, one relaxes by envisioning a soothing image. For example, by visualizing walking down a shaded stairway, one might become more and more relaxed as he/she descends into comforting darkness. Once relaxed, an image is brought to mind that may represent a desired change. Some people simply see themselves as being completely healthy. Others imagine the healing white blood cells as white knights charging forth, conquering the invading infections and visualizing the "bad guys" in full retreat. For those who may have trouble focusing clearly on an image, it is suggested to draw the desired image on paper to give it more substance and reality. In addition to visual imagery there are other types of mental imagery. Mental imagery may also be auditory (mental image of sounds that can be recalled); odorous (mental concept of odor sensations previously experienced); tactile (mental image of the feeling of an object); or oral (mental concept of taste sensations previously experienced).

Tapes, books, and even classes on visualization and imagery are available through local metaphysical bookstores. See VISUALIZATION.

immediate hypersensitivity   An antibody-mediated immunological sensitivity that manifests itself in tissue reactions within minutes after an ANTIGEN combines with its appropriate ANTIBODY. Typical reactions involve wheezing, hives, and difficulty in breathing. People require an immediate injection of epinephrine to restore some balance to their system, if the reaction is severe enough. Penicillin is a drug that can cause such an allergic reaction in some people.

immigration   The act of entering a country of which one is not a native, usually for permanent residence. With the spread of AIDS during the past decade, countries all over the world have set up barriers against those with AIDS to "protect" their citizens from the spread of the disease, despite the constant admonitions of the WORLD HEALTH ORGANIZATION (WHO). Some have imposed restrictions on all aliens who have tested positive for HIV; other nations have imposed testing requirements as conditions of entry, denying entry to those who test positive for the virus. Whereas the WHO stresses the importance of cooperation in fighting the pandemic, these countries, including the United States, continue to exclude immigrants and aliens who are infected with HIV. Many countries, however, have heeded the WHO. Some have altered their restrictive travel and immigration laws to allow the entry of HIV-positive aliens. Several countries require HIV testing, not as a condition for exclusion, but as an alert to domestic health care facilities or other care givers within the country. Still others explicitly admit HIV-positive aliens within their borders, following WHO's spirit of global solidarity.

Despite internal opposition from the American public and external opposition from the WHO, the U.S. has continued to maintain restrictive policies toward HIV-positive aliens. These restrictions, although ratified by Congress, were opposed by the former president, Bill Clinton, and modified, in emergency situations, by the U.S. courts.

Before the Immigration Act of 1990, immigrants could be excluded on 33 grounds, including affliction "with a dangerous contagious disease." In June 1987 the Public Health Service (PHS) added acquired immune deficiency syndrome to the list of such diseases. Soon thereafter, despite considerable opposition from AIDS and immigration advocates, doctors, and public interest organizations, the PHS replaced AIDS on the list with human immunodeficiency virus (HIV) infection, dramatically expanding the definition of persons considered to be afflicted with a contagious disease. On July 8, 1987, the Immigration and Naturalization Service (INS) and the U.S. State Department began testing aliens seeking admission to the United States for AIDS.

The Immigration Act of 1990 completely revised the grounds of exclusion. It also permitted, for the first time, a waiver of exclusions on health-related grounds for permanent resident and immigration visa applicants. Early in 1993, shortly after President Clinton indicated that he was prepared to remove HIV from the exclusion list, the PHS drafted new regulations to that effect. In reaction, Congress passed the National Institutes of Health Revitalization Act of 1993, which specifically codified HIV infection as a ground of exclusion. The

United States, therefore, now has a statutory ban on the admission of aliens with HIV.

Aliens of 15 years of age or older are required to undergo serologic testing for HIV if they are applying for immigrant visas, or nonimmigrant visas such as student or refugee or if they are adjusting their status. No testing is required if the alien is below age 15 unless there is "reason to suspect infection." The testing is done by a physician, called a medical examiner designated by the director of the CENTERS FOR DISEASE CONTROL AND PREVENTION. Once the requisite testing has been completed, the medical examiner must submit a document to INS certifying the presence or absence of HIV infection or any other "communicable disease of public health significance."

An alien who tests positive for HIV can request a reexamination from the director of the Centers for Disease Control. The board that reexamines the alien must be composed of "three medical officers, at least one of whom is experienced in the diagnosis and treatment of HIV infections." The final report comprises the majority decision of the board.

A formal reexamination includes a review of all records and laboratory studies. It may also include an independent physical examination performed by the board if the board so requires. The alien has the right to offer information and witnesses and may cross-examine any witnesses called by the examining board. He or she is also free to have an attorney or be assisted by the board in the presentation of his or her case. The board must report its findings to the INS and give prompt notice to the alien. The INS then makes the final decision as to admissibility on the basis of the board's findings. The alien may request reconsideration only once in connection with the current application. In 1998 the U.S. added the following section to the policy: "In view of humanitarian and family unity concerns, the law also provides waivers of inadmissibility, which are discretionary and granted on a case-by-case basis."

In 1998 the INS also added two waivers to the U.S. law on nonimmigrant admissibility to the country. The "Routine HIV Waiver Policy" states, "Nonimmigrants may be granted a waiver for admission to the United States for 30 days or less to attend conferences, receive medical treatment, visit close family members, or conduct business." People admitted under this policy must provide proof of insurance so the government does not absorb the cost of an individual's becoming ill. The "Designated Event Policy" states, "This policy facilitates the admission of HIV-positive persons to attend certain 'designated events,' which are considered to be in the public interest, such as academic and educational conferences and international sports events." For the latter policy the U.S. attorney general must receive written information about the event and then may declare a blanket waiver for the particular event.

immigration restrictions   See IMMIGRATION.

immortalized cells   Typically cancer cells, which are capable of endless divisions.

immune   See IMMUNITY.

immune activation   Activation of the immune system by stimulus from any microbe. The normal activation of the immune system in response to microbes results in a transient increase in CD4 cell production. It is these activated CD4 cells that are then infected by HIV. Since there are more CD4 cells in the body, there is the chance there will be more infection during such an illness. It is thought that the chronic immune activation (the cumulative effect of immune activation against HIV and bursts of activity for other illnesses) contributes to the progression of HIV disease. Therapies directed at the microbes that contribute to a state of chronic and persistent immune activation may have a role in the treatment of HIV-infected people, as may drugs that can be used at certain times to dampen immune activation.

immune boosters   Medicines that strengthen the body's natural defensive response to infections or foreign particles. In HIV interleukin-2 raises the CD4 levels in people, but the long-term boost is not known. Other drugs are also under study in this area.

immune boosting   A drug treatment that repairs or reconstitutes an impaired immune system. See IMMUNE BOOSTERS.

immune complex An aggregate of antibody and antigen that may induce a hypersensitivity response, often by stimulating the complement cascade. When antibodies bind to antigen nine, interacting serum proteins (beta globulins, C1–C9) are activated in a coordinated way. Complement activation causes an amplifying cascade of reactions as the complement proteins are activated sequentially. Immune complexes circulate in the blood and may eventually attach to the walls of blood vessels, producing a local inflammatory response. Immune complexes form in type III hypersensitivity reactions and are involved in the development of glomerulonephritis, serum sickness, arthritis, and vasculitis. In HIV a common immune complex are COTTON WOOL SPOTS seen in HIV retinopathy.

immune deficiency A breakdown or inability of certain parts of the immune system to function, thus making a person susceptible to certain diseases that they would not have contracted with a healthy immune system. Immune deficiencies may be temporary or permanent. In AIDS, the immune deficit is caused by infection with HIV.

immune globulin A preparation used to prevent or treat some illnesses when the body does not produce enough immunity on its own. Hepatitis A vaccine consists of immune globulin that can boost the body's immune response in the event of contact with that antigen. Rabies is another disease whose treatment involves immune globulin. It can be given intramuscularly, as in the preceding two cases, or INTRAVENOUSLY in patients with some IMMUNODEFICIENCY syndromes and in immunosuppressed recipients of BONE MARROW transplants.

immune modulators Agents that restore certain immune responses that are diminished or lost in HIV infection. See INTERLEUKIN.

immune reconstitution It is now obvious to researchers, doctors, and people with AIDS that antiretroviral therapies such as HAART restore a person's immune system to a functioning level. Therapies that may completely restore immunity in people with damaged immune systems hold much interest. However, reconstitution of the immune system depends on a complete understanding of the immune system and of immunology, the branch of medicine that studies the immune system, which is still an infant science. Although progress has been made, still little is actually known about all the elements that regulate and control the normal functioning of the human immune system. See MITOCHONDRIA; THYMUS.

immune reconstitution inflammatory syndrome (IRIS) A syndrome marked by fever, diminished oxygen to the body's organs, and flaring of OPPORTUNISTIC ILLNESSES, such as *Mycobacteria*, PNEUMOCYSTIS CARINII, cryptococcus, and others. It occurs during the course of immune reconstitution, after initiation of highly active antiretroviral therapy (HAART). This reaction is sometimes too severe to continue HAART, and the flaring illness must be treated. Corticosteroid is often required to control the reaction. It is currently difficult to diagnose and treat this reaction. IRIS is just beginning to receive attention and research to fully understand all the causes and problems relating to the syndrome.

immune response The reaction of the body to foreign ANTIGENs so that they are neutralized or eliminated, preventing damage. It requires that the body recognize the antigen as "nonself" or foreign. There are four major types of immune response: cell-mediated immune response, humoral immune response, nonspecific immune response, and specific immune response.

Cell-mediated immune response involves the production of LYMPHOCYTEs by the thymus (T CELLS) in response to exposure to an antigen. This reaction is important in delayed hypersensitivity, rejection of tissue transplants, response to malignant growths, and in some infections.

Humoral immunity response involves production of plasma lymphocytes (B CELLS) in response to antigen exposure with subsequent antibody formulation. This response can produce immunity or hypersensitivity.

Nonspecific immune response is the response of the body's tissues and cells to injury from any source, e.g., trauma, organisms, chemicals, ischemia. The initial response of the immune system to any threat, it involves vascular, chemical, and white blood cell activities.

Specific immune response is required when inflammation is inadequate to cope with injury or invasion of an organism. It is directed and controlled by T and B lymphocytes.

"Cellular immunity" is used to refer to the T lymphocyte response. "Humoral immunity" is the term previously used to refer to the T lymphocyte response.

immune response genes   Genes that control the ability of LYMPHOCYTES to respond to specific ANTIGENS.

immune suppression   See IMMUNOSUPPRESSION.

immune suppressive therapies   See IMMUNOSUPPRESSION.

immune surveillance   A theory that holds that the immune system destroys tumor cells, which are constantly arising during the life of an individual.

immune system   In the body, complex group of components that form a defense network for the body against ANTIGENS, or foreign substances, that enter it. It consists of organs, specialized cells, proteins, and a system of circulation separate from the blood vessels.

The immune system is involved in five major activities in the body. It defends the body against foreign substances, such as viruses and bacteria. It identifies and rids the body of abnormal cells to prevent their growth into tumors. It also eliminates old and deteriorating cells and rejects cells from other organisms that might enter the body. Finally it is sometimes involved in inappropriate responses to harmless substances, which lead to allergies, and, if it attacks itself, it results in an autoimmune disease.

The organs of the immune system are called lymphoid organs. Located in different areas of the body, they are the SPLEEN, THYMUS, tonsils, and Peyer's patches, which are located in the intestine, appendix, adenoids, and bone marrow. These tissues allow for quick interception of various antigens because of their diverse locations. The lymphatic vessels and lymph nodes are part of the circulatory system that moves white blood cells (WBCs) and antibodies around the body to fight infection.

The immune system activity centers around the activity of WBCs, or LEUKOCYTES. Leukocytes are divided into two main types, PHAGOCYTES and LYMPHOCYTES. Phagocytes are responsible for "swallowing" pathogens and old and worn-out cells. Phagocytes are then divided into two types also. There are monocytes/macrophages and GRANULOCYTES. MONOCYTES are immature macrophages. Macrophages are responsible for moving and destroying foreign particles and diseased cells. They display pieces of a destroyed antigen on their surface, allowing lymphocytes to become activated and begin further immune system attacks on the foreign cells. There are different types of macrophages, which have individual names: Langerhans cells are located in the skin, and Kupffer cells are located in the liver.

There are three types of granulocytes: EOSINOPHILS, BASOPHILS, and NEUTROPHILS. They are known as granulocytes because they contain toxic granules that destroy invading pathogens. They travel in the blood and lymph system. When they are located in tissues of the body, they are called mast cells. Eosinophils are involved in allergic responses and make up approximately 2 percent of leukocytes. Basophils are only about 1 percent of granulocytes and are involved in immediate response to antigens, as in asthma. Neutrophils are the predominant type of leukocytes, making up approximately 55 percent–70 percent.

Lymphocytes consist of several different types of cells. There are T lymphocytes, of which there are three types. HELPER T CELLS inform the immune system of the presence of antigens and activate other cells in the immune system. They have a protein on their outer surface called CD4, so they are often called T4 cells or CD4 cells. Inducer T cells also carry the CD4 protein. They recognize antigen on the surface of macrophages and secrete what are called LYMPHOKINES, which attract further intervention from phagocytes. Then there are cytotoxic T cells. These cells carry the protein CD8 and are often referred to as CD8 or T8 cells. These cells help eliminate infected cells by attaching themselves to the antigen cells and inducing apoptosis.

There are also B lymphocytes. They are activated by antigen from T4 cells and are also sensitive to antigen. They produce antibodies known as immunoglobulins that are responsible for binding to antigen and interfering with the antigen's role before encouraging phagocytes to enter the area. MEMORY CELLS are T cells and B cells that are held in "storage" by the body to attack antigen that has already entered. They recognize and recall the antigen and induce a quick response to it.

There are also SUPPRESSOR T CELLS. They are used to shut off the immune system when the antigen has been eliminated from the body. Their role is not fully understood. The final lymphocyte is the NATURAL KILLER (NK) cell. NK cells recognize foreign cells of multiple antigen types. They are not relegated to being informed of a specific antigen but may attack quickly by recognizing many types of foreign cells.

immune system abnormality A deviation in the normal functioning of the immune system.

immune thrombocytopenic purpura See IDIO-PATHIC THROMBOCYTOPENIC PURPURA.

immune tolerance Acquired inability to react to particular self- or non-self-antigens. Both B cells and T cells display tolerance, generally to their specific antigen classes. The concentration of antigen required to induce tolerance in neonatal B cells is 100-fold less than for adult B cells.

immune-based therapies Treatments intended to have their effect by enhancing the general activity of the immune system or by specifically modulating the activity of some of its components. They may be used to help restore a person's general immune responsiveness, suppress specific viral infections, or counteract the bone marrow toxicity of some of the drugs used for HIV-related conditions. Hope is placed in these substances because they promise to reduce the pill burden of HIV patients. Drugs used in such therapies include preparations of antibodies and drugs that stimulate production of red and white blood cells, cytokines, and other immune modulators. Vaccines are also immune therapy drugs. Specific drugs used in immune-based therapies include cyclosporine, cytomegalovirus immune globulin, hepatitis B immunoglobulin, interleukin-2 (IL-2 or Proleukin), HIV-1 immunogen (Salk Vaccine or

Remune), epoetin alpha (Procrit), interferon, and GM-CSF. There is also a hope that gene-based therapy may also hold promise for HIV patients. Researchers are studying the possibility of inserting anti-HIV genes that would make a person's T cells immune to destruction by HIV. It would ideally assist the individual with keeping the virus at bay. Many different immune-based therapies are being studied to find potential therapies for HIV. To date no studies have shown these immune-based therapies to increase a person's life expectancy nor to work effectively and safely to decrease HIV in the body.

immunity The state of being resistant to or protected from a disease. Immunity is usually induced by exposure to the antigenic marker on an organism that invades the body or by administration of a vaccine that has the capability of stimulating production of specific antibodies (immunization). Immunity is also the response of the body and its tissues to a variety of antigens, including pollens, red cells, transplanted tissues, or the individual's own cells.

Acquired immunity is also called specific or adaptive immunity. This is the type of immunity that is learned immunity. The body learns how to respond to certain antigens by being exposed to them and it develops the best way to respond to these antigens and remembers it. Acquired immunity can be divided into two parts: cell-mediated, resulting from activation of sensitized T lymphocytes that are created in the bone marrow but mature in the THYMUS, and humoral immunity, mediated by B lymphocytes that mature in the bone marrow and the SPLEEN.

Acquired immunity is contrasted with natural or innate immunity, a more or less permanent immunity to disease with which an individual is born, the result of natural factors. Natural immunity may be due to the natural presence of immune bodies, but other factors such as diet, metabolism, temperature, or adaptive features of infectious organisms may be involved. Congenital immunity is natural immunity present at birth and may be natural or acquired; the latter results from antibodies received from the blood of the mother. This system is made up of WHITE BLOOD CELLS called MACROPHAGES, EOSINOPHILS, BASOPHILS, and

MONOCYTES. These cells work to engulf and destroy the cell. They also inform the body of the antigen to the acquired immunity system so the proper lymphocytes can respond to the antigen.

Some texts refer to active and passive immunity. Active immunity results from the development within the body of antibodies or sensitized T lymphocytes that neutralize or destroy the infectious agent. This mechanism results from the immune response to an invading antigen. It can also come about by a vaccine designed to spur an immune response. Passive immunity, on the other hand, is immunity acquired by the introduction of preformed antibodies into an unprotected individual. This can occur through injection of immune globulin as in hepatitis A.

A last type of immunity is local immunity, which is immunity in a specific part of the body. HIV vaccine developers consider local immunity an important focus for vaccine research in HIV, for example, a focus on the mucous membranes. If immunity on the mucous membranes could be generated to HIV then 90 percent of all cases could be prevented since HIV mainly enters the body through the mucous membranes.

immunization The process of creating immunity to a specific disease in an individual, usually by the administration of a vaccine consisting of antigenic components of an infectious agent (a weakened form of a disease that cannot cause sickness). These components, in turn, stimulate a protective response and induce the body to form antibodies against the disease. The immune response may be induced naturally or artificially. The immunizations necessary for travelers with HIV vary according to the destination. Travel to developing nations generally requires immunizations. Some immunizations are considered safe for HIV-infected persons (vaccines for killed typhoid, influenza, diphtheria, tetanus, pneumococcus, and hepatitis B, for example); others are generally not recommended for HIV-infected individuals (measles, yellow fever); others are not appropriate for patients with HIV (the live oral polio and typhoid vaccines). In developing world areas the measles vaccine is often given anyway because the death rate is much higher than the possible rate of infection from the virus that is part of the vaccine. Similarly, if an HIV-positive individual in good health is traveling to an area where yellow fever is endemic, a vaccination may be worthwhile, in comparison to the live virus in the vaccine. See VACCINATION.

immunoassay A test to measure the protein and protein-bound molecules that are concerned with the reaction of an ANTIGEN with its specific ANTIBODY.

immunocompetent Capable of developing a normal protective response when confronted with invading microbes or cancer.

immunocompromise The condition that exists when the body's immune system defenses are lowered and the ability to resist infections and tumors weakens.

immunodeficient See IMMUNODEFICIENCY.

immunodeficiency A breakdown or inability of certain parts of the immune system to function, rendering the body susceptible to certain diseases that it would ordinarily be able to resist. Immunodeficiency is classified as an antibody, cellular, combined deficiency, or phagocytic dysfunction disorder.

immunoenhancer Anything that increases the body's ability to fight off infection and disease.

immunofluorescence antibody (IFA) A serologic assay using antibody tagged by a fluorescent molecule. It is used predominantly as a confirmatory test for syphilis and for legionella virus.

immunogen A substance that, when introduced into an animal, stimulates the immune response. The term *immunogen* may also denote a substance that is capable of stimulating an immune response, in contrast to a substance that can only combine with antibody, that is, an ANTIGEN.

immunogenetics The study of the immune system using genetic analysis to gather information in the formation of antibody creation and responses.

immunogenicity The quality of producing an effective or measurable immune response.

immunoglobulin (Ig) An ANTIBODY-rich preparation administered to reduce the likelihood of development of infection after exposure to certain infectious agents. It is a protein produced by plasma cells derived from B LYMPHOCYTES and found in the blood and other body tissues. All antibodies are immunoglobulins, but researchers have not yet determined whether all immunoglobulins have antibody functions. There are five classes: IgA, IgD, IgE, IgG, and IgM. Increased levels of two types of immunoglobulins, IgA and IgG, are usually seen in patients with HIV infection and are related to the HIV-induced activation of B lymphocytes. Immunoglobulin G is found in the serum and does not cross the placenta.

Immunoglobulin A (IgA): a class of antibodies, present in saliva, tears, and other secretions, that render viruses ineffective and prevent bacteria from attaching to mucous membranes. It is an example of local immunity.

Immunoglobulin D (IgD): antibodies, receptors on most cell surfaces, that remove foreign substances from the bloodstream and hold them for further destruction.

Immunoglobulin E (IgE): antibodies, abundant in tissue spaces, that activate histamines and leukotrienes as an allergic reaction to foreign particles.

Immunoglobulin G (IgG): class of antibodies, produced by memory cells and blood plasma cells, that circulate in the bloodstream and impart long-term immunity against previously encountered viruses, bacteria, and so forth. It is B lymphocytes in the form of plasma cells.

Immunoglobulin M (IgM): antibodies that exist for a short time as aggregates of other antibody molecules. They seek out and attach themselves to viruses in the circulatory system and along the internal walls. They are produced early in an infection.

immunoglobulin class A subdivision of immunoglobulin molecules based on unique antigenic determinants in the Fc region of the H chains. In humans there are 5 classes of immunoglobulins designated IgA, IgD, IgE, IgG, and IgM.

immunoglobulin class switch The process in which a B-cell precursor expressing IgM and IgG receptors differentiates into a B-cell producing IgA, IgE, or IgG antibodies without change in specificity for the antigenic determinant.

immunoglobulin subclass A subdivision of the classes of immunoglobulins based on structural and antigenic differences in the H chains. For example, for human IgG (a class of monomeric immunoglobulin proteins), there are 4 subclasses IgGI-4, accounting for at least 70 percent of human immunoglobulin titre.

immunoglobulin superfamily A large GLYCOPROTEIN superfamily including antibodies and their membrane-bound isotypes; T cell receptors, lymphocyte Fc receptors, the CD2, CD4, and CD8 accessory molecules, and MHC molecules.

immunoglobulin supergene family A structurally related group of genes that encode immunoglobulins, T cell receptors, beta-two microglobulin, and others.

immunologic markers Components of the immune system, including different types of cells, such as T4 and T8 cells, as well as proteins secreted by the immune system cells, like neopterin and beta-2 microglobulin. Immunologic markers are used as laboratory measurements of biological activity within the body that indirectly indicate the effect of treatment on disease state. See SURROGATE MARKER.

immunological markers See IMMUNOLOGIC MARKERS.

immunological memory The ability of the body to defend itself against specific invading agents it has encountered in the past because a second encounter with the same agent prompts a rapid and vigorous response. In the first attack on the body by an invading organism, the body has only a few cells able to recognize the invader. This is known as the PRIMARY RESPONSE. During this process many thousands of MEMORY CELLS are created; if and when the attacker returns the body recognizes the invader and is able to mount a quick and deadly attack on the ANTIGEN. This is known as the SECONDARY RESPONSE. See MEMORY CELLS.

immunology The branch of medical science dealing with the study of immunity.

immunomodulation The effect of various chemical mediators, hormones, and drugs on the IMMUNE SYSTEM. Effects might include the restoration or the enhancement of the immune system.

immunomodulator A substance capable of modifying one or more functions of the IMMUNE SYSTEM. Also called an immunostimulator or an immunoregulator. So far immunomodulators have not been found to be very effective in modifying the course of AIDS.

immunopathogenesis A process in which the course of a disease is affected or altered by an immune response or by the products of an immune response.

immunopathology The study of tissue alterations that result from immune or allergic reactions.

immunoregulator See IMMUNOMODULATOR.

immunostimulant See IMMUNOMODULATOR.

immunosuppression The suppression of, or interference with, the body's IMMUNE SYSTEM and its ability to fight infection or disease, by means of drugs or or other medical techniques, or through infection or disease. Powerful immunosuppressive drugs can inhibit the production of white blood cells or interfere with their actions in the immune system. For example, STEROIDS suppress LYMPHOCYTE function, and the drug CYCLOSPORINE holds down the production of INTERLEUKIN-2, which is needed for T CELL growth. Immunosuppression may be used during organ or BONE MARROW transplantation to prevent the body's own immune system from rejecting the foreign organ or bone marrow. Until their immune systems are functioning normally, immunosuppressed per-

sons are at a much higher risk of infections and developing LYMPHOMAS.

Immunosuppression results from HIV infection as well as from some antiviral or anticancer treatments, of which it is a side effect. In its earlier stages, though, HIV infection is associated with chronic stimulation of the immune system. Hyperactive immune responses in people with HIV include overproduction by B CELLS of ANTIBODIES (also called IMMUNOGLOBULINS or Igs); abnormal levels of CYTOKINES, such as TUMOR NECROSIS FACTOR (TNF) alpha and interferon alpha; and increased activation of T cells. Markers of this increased immune activity, such as elevated Igs, can predict CD4 cell count declines and progression of disease. Some scientists believe these overactive immune responses contribute to HIV reproduction, illness, wasting, or the loss of normal immune function. If so, some hypothesize, suppressing such responses early on might slow progression.

immunosuppressive A drug that significantly impairs (suppresses) the functions of the body's immune system. In some cases, IMMUNOSUPPRESSION is an intended drug effect. In other cases, it is an unwanted side effect, as in the long term use of cortisone-like drugs suppressing the immune system sufficiently to permit reactivation of a dormant tuberculosis. Immunosuppressant drugs are being used to treat several chronic disorders that are thought to be autoimmune diseases.

immunosuppressive drugs Drugs which induce IMMUNOSUPPRESSION.

immunotherapy Treatment aimed at reconstituting an impaired immune system. Examples of experimental immunotherapies for AIDS include passive hyperimmune therapy (PHT), IL-2, and therapeutic vaccines. See BIOLOGICAL THERAPY.

impairment Damage or disability; in Social Security Administration parlance, a particular disease or condition that may render the afflicted patient too disabled to perform substantial gainful activity (SGA) and therefore possibly eligible for assistance. Patients can and do have multiple impairments.

impetigo A contagious, inflammatory skin disease caused by direct inoculation of group A streptococci or staphylococcus aureus into superficial cutaneous abrasions or compromised skin. It is marked by isolated pustules that rupture to discharge an amber-colored fluid (composed of serum and pus) that dries to form a thick yellowish crust. The pustules may spread peripherally, but they are usually found around the nose and the mouth.

impotence Weakness; the inability of the male to achieve or maintain an erection.

imreg A natural LEUKOCYTE-derived, polypeptide IMMUNOMODULATOR that has been shown to enhance production of certain lymphokines in the laboratory.

Imreg 1 is an immune modulator to treat AIDS patients that is derived from natural substances produced by white blood cells. It enhances the production of IL-2 and gamma interferon by lymphocytes from patients with symptomatic HIV infection.

Imuran See AZATHIOPRINE.

imuthiol An organic compound that contains sulfur and facilitates the development of T lymphocytes. It has been shown to have anti-HIV activity in vitro. See T CELL.

in utero transmission See TRANSMISSION.

in vitro Literally, "in glass"; the phrase refers to a biological process or reaction that takes place in an artificial environment, usually a test tube or culture plate in a laboratory, rather than in the body. In vitro studies are usually the first step in the development of new treatments of diseases.

in vitro cultivation The propagation of living organisms in an artificial environment such as a Petri dish or test tube.

in vitro fertilization A procedure in which an egg is fertilized outside the womb, in a test tube or Petri dish. The fertilized egg is then surgically implanted in the prospective mother's, or a surrogate mother's, uterus—not necessarily the biological mother. The technique is most often used to help women who cannot conceive naturally.

in vivo Literally, within a living body. The term refers to experiments or testing in animals or humans in a living, natural environment. In AIDS research, in vivo studies are conducted in clinical trials.

inactivation The rendering ineffective of an agent or substance, such as the HIV virus, through the destruction or negation of its activity or effects.

inactivation agent An agent used to destroy biological activity, as of an enzyme, microorganism, or virus.

incapacitated parent See INCAPACITY.

incapacity An incompetence or inability to function. In social services jargon, disability, which can be less severe or less long lasting than that required for SSDI/SSI, used to qualify a parent and thus (even in a two-parent family) an entire low-income family, for AFDC and MEDICAID; sometimes used in GENERAL ASSISTANCE programs, too.

incidence The frequency of a phenomenon; in epidemiology, the frequency of occurrence of a disease over a period of time in relation to the population within which it occurs. Incidence is usually reported in terms of the number of cases per 100,000 population per year. HIV/AIDS is now found on every inhabited continent.

incidence rate See INCIDENCE.

inclusion criteria The medical or social standards by which researchers decide whether to include potential participants in a clinical or research trial. For example, some trials may include only men and others may only include women; other trials may include only persons with a lowered T cell count. Inclusion criteria are generally health factors whose presence in a test subject would be undesirable or inappropriate. Often these are established for reasons of safety. For instance, doctors may know or fear that a new drug may cause a certain disorder to worsen. It would thus be wrong to allow individuals who have the condition to participate in the clinical trial or study and take that risk. See EXCLUSION CRITERIA.

income level Amount specified in needs-based programs, usually on a monthly basis, to determine eligibility for benefits; those with income below the level are eligible, but those with income above it are not.

income maintenance A generic term for welfare, including GA, AFDC, and SSPS; used in New York and several other states.

inconclusive Not determinable definitely one way or another. In medicine, the term usually refers to test results, for instance, a blood test from whose results the presence of the AIDS virus cannot be inferred.

incontinence The inability to control excretory functions (defecation and urination). Also, generally, the absence of restraint; habitual immoderation or excess.

incubation 1. The interval between exposure to a pathogen and the appearance of the first clinical symptom in the development of an infectious disease. See INCUBATION PERIOD. 2. The development of bacteria culture under controlled conditions. 3. The development of a fertilized egg. 4. The care of a premature infant in a controlled environment to promote development and survival.

incubation period The interval between initial infection with a microbe and appearance of the first symptom or sign of disease. For influenza and the common cold, the incubation period is usually several days; for measles, chicken pox, mumps, and infections caused by many other viruses, the incubation period is two to three weeks. The incubation period of HIV falls somewhere between two weeks and six months before people undergo the initial viral conversion. It is why when people test for HIV they are generally told to return in six months to test again to find out whether they have

seroconverted in the intervening time. The time to the first signs of a deteriorating immune system, or what might be called AIDS, is somewhere around 10 years. This time frame varies also with the strain of the virus, whether the virus is treated with medication, and the general health and well-being of the individual.

IND See INVESTIGATIONAL NEW DRUG.

independent review A second or repeated view, a reexamination, a retrospective survey, a looking over again, as a review of one's studies or a review of one's life. Also, an examination with a view to amendment or improvement; revision; as, an author's review of his or her works. Additionally, a critical examination of a publication, with remarks; a criticism; a critique. May also refer to a periodical containing critical essays on matters of interest, such as new productions in literature or art.

independent variable See VARIABLE.

index case The initial individual whose condition led to an investigation of a hereditary disorder.

indication The purpose for which a drug is prescribed. FOOD AND DRUG ADMINISTRATION–approved indications for a drug appear on a printed insert in the drug's packaging.

indicator disease One of a group of infections and diseases, established by the CENTERS FOR DISEASE CONTROL AND PREVENTION, whose presence indicates HIV infection. These diseases are among the criteria used to diagnose a person as having full-blown AIDS.

indigent Impoverished; poor and without resources. In hospital jargon, a poor person without HEALTH CARE coverage.

indigent care coordinator Financial counselor who works with indigent care programs (state, local, or hospital free medical care programs for the poor). They are increasingly used for public subsidies or rate allowances to compensate hospitals for bad debts of indigents, rather than for a patient-oriented entitlement program.

indigent care program Any free state, local, or hospital medical care program for the poor. The term increasingly designates a program of public subsidies or rate allowances to reimburse hospitals for indigent care, rather than a patient-oriented entitlement program.

indinavir Indinavir is a PROTEASE INHIBITOR class anti-HIV drug. It must be taken on an empty or mostly empty stomach. Fat in food interferes with the absorption of indinavir into the body. Kidney stone formation is a fairly common side effect of this drug. This is the reason it is particularly important to drink large amounts of water or liquids while taking this medication. It cannot be taken at the same time as DIDANOSINE because of interactions. Astemizole, an antihistamine available only outside the United States, can be life-threatening if given with indinavir. This drug was one of the first protease inhibitors and also one of the first drugs to be implicated in the METABOLIC TOXICITY seen in some people on HAART. When taken with another protease inhibitor, RITONAVIR, indinavir can be taken with food and taken only twice a day because of increases in the amount of the drug that the combination causes. (Trade name is Crixivan.)

individual treatment IND A program established by the FOOD AND DRUG ADMINISTRATION in which a patient may receive an experimental drug free of charge from the pharmaceutical manufacturer, with the assistance of his or her personal physician. Admission to this program is granted on an individual basis by the Food and Drug Administration. See INVESTIGATIONAL NEW DRUG.

Individuals with Disabilities Education Act (IDEA) Originally entitled the Education for All Handicapped Children Act, this federal legislation sets out requirements for the public education of children with disabilities including AIDS, and allocates federal money to states that meet these requirements. Prior to the act's passage by Congress in 1975, half of the more than 8 million children with disabilities in the United States did not receive appropriate educational services. One million were entirely excluded from the public school systems. State and local authorities generally rationalized this situation as being due to a lack of funding for special programs. As a result, wealthy parents often paid out of pocket for special services that allowed their children to benefit educationally. The children of those who could not afford to pay were left out. Congress stepped in and passed the IDEA to ensure that disabled children would have access to a free, appropriate education and related services designed to meet their special needs. The act applies to children with a variety of disabilities, including mental retardation; impaired hearing, sight, or speech; serious emotional disturbances; impairments that prevent physical movement; and other chronic health problems that negatively affect a child's strength, vitality, or alertness.

induced immunosuppression The prevention or diminution of an immune response by artificial means. See IMMUNOSUPPRESSION.

induction therapy The initial phase of treatment of an illness with a high dose of medication to bring the illness under control. The purpose is to induce a remission then to work on eliminating the virus or bacterium. An example would be the use of ganciclovir for treating CMV. See MAINTENANCE THERAPY.

indurate To harden. For example, pressure and heat indurate the rock. Induration may also be an abnormal hardening of an area of the body.

infant A child from birth through one year of age. See NEONATE.

infected blood Blood contaminated by a virus, which can be passed to anyone whose bloodstream it enters, as in a transfusion.

infection The state or condition in which the body or part of it is invaded by MICROORGANISMS. The microorganisms will multiply under conditions favorable to them, producing injurious results. If the body's defense mechanisms are effective, the infection will remain localized. If the body's defense mechanisms are not capable of staving off the invasion and multiplication, the local infection may persist and spread. Infections occur more readily when the BONE MARROW's ability to produce white blood cells is decreased and the IMMUNE SYSTEM response is lowered. Symptoms of an infection include fever, chills, sweating (especially at night), loose bowels, a burning feeling when urinating, a severe cough, and/or a sore throat. An infection with bacteria that invade the bloodstream is referred to as bacteremia. Bacteria that release by-products into the bloodstream may cause septicemia, which may progress to shock. Infection with viruses in the bloodstream is known as viremia. Fungus in the blood is known as fungemia.

Today it is recognized that viral and most opportunistic infections in AIDS are intracellular. Intracellular and extracellular pathogens have different means of expressing their presence, leading to the interpretation that CD8+ and CD4+ T CELLS have a division of tasks: CD8+ CYTOTOXIC T cells (CTL) control intracellular pathogens, and CD4+ helper T cells help to eradicate extracellular PATHOGENS by cooperation with B cells and by release of cytotoxins.

infectious Pertaining to a disease due to a MICROORGANISM; capable of being transmitted with or without contact; producing infection. See CONTAGIOUS.

infectious agent An organism that produces infection or is capable of being transmitted with or without contact.

infectious disease Any disease caused by growth of PATHOGENIC MICROORGANISMS in the body. An infectious disease may or may not be contagious.

infectious mononucleosis An acute infectious disease that primarily affects lymphoid tissue and is characterized by enlarged LYMPH NODES and SPLEEN with an increase in abnormal mononuclear LEUKOCYTES in the blood. An abnormal functioning liver will be found in about 90 percent of cases. Clinical manifestations are highly variable. The disease is caused by the Epstein-Barr virus, a herpes virus. The incubation period may be as long as four to seven weeks. There is no specific treatment, but for

serious complications (for example hemolytic anemia, pharyngeal swelling interfering with swallowing), cortisone is used.

infertility Inability to become pregnant or bear children.

infibulation The process of fastening, as in the joining of lips of wounds by clasps; also the sewing together of the labia of females or the foreskin of males to prevent sexual intercourse.

inflammation The body's response to tissue injury or infection that occurs in the affected tissue and adjacent blood vessels. The blood vessels' permeability is increased, and the area becomes heavily populated with white blood cells. Signs of inflammation are redness, swelling, pain, and sometimes loss of function. Not all of these signs are necessarily present in any given case.

inflammatory bowel disease A general term that denotes inflammatory bowel diseases of unknown origin. Ulcerative colitis, Crohn's disease, and regional enteritis are examples of such diseases.

inflammatory neuropathy Inflammation of the PERIPHERAL NERVOUS SYSTEM, causing abnormal function.

influenza vaccine A sterile suspension of killed influenza virus types A and B, either individually or combined. Commonly known as a "flu shot."

The influenza vaccine varies in its effectiveness, depending on whether the strain of the virus in the vaccine is related to the virus that is causing the influenza. The effectiveness of the vaccine changes annually with every flu season, since the prevalent types of flu are different each year. In most years, however, the vaccine probably prevents illness in about 70 percent of the people who receive it, and those who become infected despite having been vaccinated usually have less severe symptoms. Influenza does not seem to be unusually common or severe in people with HIV infection. The only problem specific to people with HIV infection is that the symptoms of influenza can be confused with the symptoms of other disorders, such as

PNEUMOCYSTIS CARINII PNEUMONIA. The CENTERS FOR DISEASE CONTROL AND PREVENTION's Advisory Committee on Immunization Practices recommends that people with HIV infection be vaccinated every year. (Trade names are Fluax and Fluogen.)

information campaign Advertising program that is limited to the provision of information. For example, the Centers for Disease Control and Prevention's "America Responds to AIDS" information campaign produced and distributed a brochure to assist parents in discussing HIV and AIDS-related issues with their children. Effective information campaigns are composed of culturally and linguistically appropriate messages; are targeted toward a particular population, such as adolescents, blood donors, IV drug users; and choose persons who maintain credibility with the targeted population to deliver their messages. While print-based materials are an integral component of more effective information campaigns, print information alone cannot be relied on to produce behavioral change. Audiovisuals, multimedia, and the Internet can also be used to disseminate information and promote ideas, as can lectures and discussions; skills training; individual and group counseling education; peer- and professionally-led counseling groups; and empowerment messages.

informed consent Consent given for a course of treatment, surgical procedure, or diagnostic test after being informed fully about its possible benefits and risks. Consent is a legal requirement, and a patient must be given enough information so that he or she can make an informed decision. In an investigational drug trial, individuals considering participation must be informed of the risks and possible benefits of the proposed experimental treatment. A participant must sign a written document attesting that he or she understands the nature, purposes, and risks of the study. Specifically, the consent form contains an explanation of why the research is being done; what researchers want to accomplish; what will be done and for how long; what risks are involved; what benefits can be expected; other treatments available; and a statement confirming a participant's right to leave the trial at any time.

Generally, an HIV test requires a patient to sign an informed consent form.

infusion The introduction of a fluid other than blood into a vein. Infusions are often used when the digestive system does not absorb appreciable quantities of a drug that is also too bulky or too toxic to be given by quick INJECTION.

inguinal lymph nodes Small round masses of tissue located in the groin that drain fluids from the body.

inhalant A prescription, volatile drug, chemical, or other substance inhaled for the effect of its vapor. The device used by asthmatics to inhale medicine is called an inhaler, or bronchodilator. The device used to inhale medicines in a more concentrated form, a procedure that involves usually going to a doctor's office or hospital, is called a nebulizer. There is a tube connected from a patient's nose to the substance with an aerosol or other spray mechanism. Patients inhale as the tube delivers a concentrated medicine that has been "nebulized." Dry or moist air, vapor, gases such as oxygen, or anesthetics are among the substances introduced into the lungs for therapeutic purposes.

Inhalants are also subject to abuse. In the context of AIDS, the word *inhalants* generally refers to "poppers," nitrite inhalants that have been used in the gay community as a sexual enhancer. See POPPERS.

inhibitor A chemical or other substance that inhibits or blocks a biological process in the body from taking place.

inhibitory concentration (IC) The amount of a particular drug in the blood needed to suppress the reproduction of a microbe to a certain limit. This amount is often listed in numerical form. IC50 for an anti-HIV drug means the amount of the drug necessary to reduce the HIV activity in a cell culture by 50 percent, or half. The higher the IC50, the more resistant the microbe is to that drug.

injection drug user (IDU) A person who uses a hypodermic needle to inject drugs, including illegal drugs such as heroin, steroids, or cocaine, into his or her body, for a purpose that deviates from the drug's intended use. IDUs frequently share such drug paraphernalia as needles and syringes, thereby providing opportunities to transmit viruses via their infected contents. Viruses are transmitted through blood that remains in the needle or syringe after injection, not through the injected drug itself. Intravenous drug users are a crucial link in the spread of HIV to wider circles of the population. Other illnesses that can spread in this manner include hepatitis A, hepatitis B, and leishmaniasis.

innate immunity   Various host defenses that are present from birth and do not depend on immunologic memory.

inoculation   The introduction of an ANTIGEN or antiserum into humans and other animals to confer immunity.

inoculum size   The number of MICROBES necessary to cause an INFECTION. In HIV infection, the number is not known. What is known is that the probability of transmitting HIV with the transfusion of one unit (or 500 milliliters) of infected blood is 80 to 90 percent. The probability of transmitting HIV with a needlestick injury, which injects only a fraction of a milliliter of blood, is 0.4 percent. This difference in the probabilities of transmission is most likely due to inoculum size.

inoculum threshold   The minimum dose of a substance introduced by inoculation (generally an ANTIGEN, antiserum, or antitoxin injected to produce immunity to a specific disease) that will produce an effect on a patient.

insect bites   There is no evidence that HIV is spread in any way other than exposure through blood, blood products, perinatal contact between mother and child, or sexual contact. These types of exposure may occur without knowledge that an exposure is taking place. Biting insects may seem likely candidates to transmit HIV, but if that were so, household AIDS cases that were unrelated to known transmission routes would appear. In addition, young children, other than those in risk groups, are frequently bitten by insects, and some

should be infected if transmission takes place in this way. There are no reported cases that clearly fit either of these situations.

Researchers have created laboratory circumstances to determine whether insects carry HIV. They have isolated HIV genetic material from bedbugs and mosquitoes one hour after feeding the insects blood, contaminated with HIV, and the virus did not grow in the insects' cells. In addition, bugs that feed on blood do not inject blood from one person into another. After feeding on blood, mosquitoes and other blood-sucking insects generally must digest the meal before biting someone else. The very low levels of HIV in blood, the tiny volumes ingested by insects, and the absence of field data implicating spread of HIV by insects make this form of transmission impossible.

One way in which mosquitoes have affected HIV-positive people is that after testing positive, HIV-positive people report that their reactions to mosquito bites increase. Bite marks are larger, are bright red, and itch a great deal more than compared to pre-virus-exposure mosquito bites. Researchers are unsure of the reasons for this phenomenon.

insertive anal intercourse   See ANAL INTERCOURSE.

insomnia   The inability to sleep, or to get enough sleep. The difficulty may be either in falling asleep or remaining asleep, or both. This sleep disorder may be primary or secondary to some other illness, condition, or circumstance. Primary insomnia exists when there are no signs or symptoms of a mental or physical condition that would account for the disorder. Secondary insomnia is usually readily explained by the existence of a condition that causes anxiety, stress, or pain or by the use of a drug that interferes with sleep. The causes of insomnia may be mental or physical. A great variety of drugs are available for primary insomnia, including over-the-counter medications. Their use on a short-term basis might be advisable, but all prescription drugs may have undesired side effects, such as overdose, habituation, tolerance, addiction, daytime drowsiness, lethargy, or amnesia. In secondary insomnia, treatment consists of determining the condition causing the insomnia and then treating that disorder. Self-help measures are also recommended to induce sleep.

institutional review board (IRB)   A committee that is formally designated by an institution to review and approve biomedical research that involves humans as subjects. Such committees are mandated and governed by the Department of Health and Human Services (see *Federal Register,* 46(17) (Jan. 27, 1981:8,942–8,980). The overriding purpose of institutional review boards is to protect the human subjects of research done in or under the direction of the institution that the board serves. This protection is provided mainly through the board's approval only of certain kinds of research proposals, and through requirements that the informed consent of all participants be obtained. Research proposals should be approved only if the following conditions, established by federal regulations, are met: the risks to which subjects will be exposed are minimized; the risks to subjects are reasonable in relation to the anticipated benefits, if any, to those subjects, and the importance of the knowledge that may be expected to result; the selection of research subjects is equitable; the informed consent of all participants is sought from each prospective participant or his or her legal representative; the informed consent is appropriately documented; there are adequate provisions to protect the privacy of subjects and to maintain the confidentiality of data; and there are additional safeguards to protect the rights and welfare of subjects who are likely to be vulnerable to coercion or undue influence. Ensuring that the informed consent of research subjects is obtained is done by reviewing and approving informed consent statements that describe the purposes and procedures of the clinical investigation in which the subject will participate.

insulin   Insulin is a HORMONE that is secreted by the PANCREAS in response to high blood sugar levels. Insulin allows the body to metabolize and make use of glucose. The inability of the body to secrete the right amount of insulin or resistance of the body to insulin is the cause of DIABETES. Insulin is found in humans and in other vertebrates. Animal insulin has for many years served as the treatment that diabetics use to treat their inability to produce or use insulin. In recent years genetically produced human insulin has been gaining in use.

insulinlike growth factor   A naturally produced substance in the body that has many of the same effects as GROWTH FACTOR but resembles insulin in structure. There are two types, referred to as IGF-1 and IGF-2. A genetically created form of IGF-1 has been studied but not approved for treatment of AIDS-RELATED WASTING.

insulin resistance   Insulin is a hormone that regulates the transport of sugar in the blood to the cells to be used as energy. Insulin resistance occurs when the insulin is less active than it is supposed to be in a normal situation, or when cells are unable to respond to the insulin that is provided. This leads to an increased level of sugar in the blood. That condition can cause diabetes and several other health problems.

Insulin resistance has been seen in increased numbers in HIV-positive people who are on PROTEASE INHIBITORS. Some researchers have linked the insulin resistance to LIPODYSTROPHY. Diabetes is diagnosed by blood sugar (glucose) tests. Patients fast overnight for this test. If the result is higher than 140 milligrams (mg) per deciliter (dL) of blood, it is termed *impaired glucose tolerance.* Results of this test that are regularly at that level (greater than 140 mg/dL) determine that a person has diabetes. Common symptoms of diabetes include thirst, excessive urination, and weight loss.

Doctors and other medical personnel often use different terms to refer of the same issues. The incidence of diabetes is actually low in HIV patients: less, than 3 percent. The term *impaired glucose tolerance* is fairly commonly used to refer to occasional test results above the level of 140 mg/dL of blood sugar. Insulin resistance can be seen in a range of HIV patients on protease inhibitors. Some researchers think that when blood fat levels are high, glucose metabolism is slowed and glucose is stored temporarily in the blood. High-fat meals may cause fat to be present in the blood, and researchers think numbers of fat molecules may increase when patients are taking protease inhibitors. Other researchers directly link the decrease in insulin production as the cause.

Tests have shown that healthy non-HIV-positive people taking certain protease inhibitors immediately experience cessation of production of most insulin, leading to insulin resistance.

Insulin resistance can be managed by regular exercise and dietary changes. A person should avoid high-sugar, high-fat, and low-fiber foods. Large amounts of high-fiber foods should be eaten. Eating several smaller meals rather than three large meals has also been helpful.

insurance The act, system, or business of insuring property, life, one's person, etc., against loss or harm arising from specified contingencies, in return for payment. As the insurance industry grew increasingly aware of the financial consequences of the AIDS phenomenon, it sought ways to escape from responsibility for health care costs; as affected populations and political decision makers became increasingly aware of the potential for costs that neither was prepared to bear, insurance soared in importance as a legal issue.

In the earliest stages of the AIDS chronology, insurers rather freely admitted to trying to screen out applications from single men in the nation's largest cities, as approximately 80 percent of the AIDS cases at that time occurred in this group. They were also denying life insurance coverage to those already diagnosed with AIDS. Denying coverage to those already diagnosed with a preexisting condition that was then considered to be a terminal illness is a different thing from denying coverage to those who were considered at high risk for the disease. The insurers, however, seemed unable—or unwilling—to see the difference.

Since those early days, the insurance industry's practices relating to HIV disease have come under increasing government regulation. Lawyers and others who work with AIDS patients have long asserted that insurance companies across the country are using unfair and devious tactics to avoid paying claims for AIDS-related medical problems. Suits are being filed about insurers' testing applicants without their consent. Other cases have focused on the possibility of a preexisting condition. An objection sometimes raised by insurers is that treatments performed or sought are experimental—many health policies do not cover exper-

imental treatments. There is a continuing series of cases in which discrimination is the issue. And there is increasing attention being paid to employers' practice of trying to limit their expenses by changing their coverage from outside insurers to self-insured plans, especially once one or more employees file HIV-related claims. Self-insured plans are allowed under the federal Employee Retirement Income Security Act, known as ERISA. Because they are authorized by federal law, these plans generally escape regulation by states, whose laws and regulations are often those most heavily relied on by employees with HIV disease.

Nationally, the way was paved for a more responsible and sensible direction on AIDS and insurance issues by the National Association of Insurance Commissioners (NAIC) in December 1986, when it adopted guidelines recommended by its Advisory Committee on AIDS. These guidelines include the prohibition of discrimination on the basis of sexual orientation. NAIC, however, is merely an association of state insurance regulators, and it has no authority to issue actual regulations in any jurisdiction.

intake The administrative and assessment process for admitting a person to a health care program or facility.

integrase One of three HIV enzymes used for reproduction and survival of the virus. The other two are reverse transcriptase and protease. Integrase is the enzyme used by the virus to insert it's DNA into the host cell's chromosomes. Literally, the integrase cuts and trims the host's DNA, attaches the viral DNA, and the result is a functioning factory for producing virus in the body. Hope is that a drug will be located that blocks the integrase thereby stopping the infection and production of viruses before it starts.

integrase inhibitor Integrase is one of the three enzymes that HIV uses to reproduce after it is in the human bloodstream. The other two are, of course, protease and reverse transcriptase. Integrase is the enzyme that is used to insert the HIV into the DNA of the cell. Both reverse transcriptase and protease are similar structurally to many other enzymes in the human and animal world. Integrase is relatively unique in humans and dissimilar to enzymes in animals. Researchers hope, therefore, that inhibiting this enzyme might have few repercussions in the human body. By using a drug to inhibit this enzyme, similar enzymes will not be affected, and this will result in fewer or no side effects. The drug will work only on the integrase enzyme and not other enzymes similar to it located it elsewhere in the body. Finding these integrase inhibitors has been more difficult than researchers first thought. Several drug companies have held tests and Phase I trials of different integrase inhibitors, but most have not worked well. It is such a potent source of a drug, however, that many companies continue looking for such a chemical.

intensive care Service provided by skilled medical personnel to seriously ill patients with life-threatening conditions requiring special equipment, complex treatment and constant care, and/or monitoring. It is usually provided in a specialized area of a care facility known as an INTENSIVE CARE UNIT (ICU).

Some intensive care units, such as those for coronary, surgical, or newborn intensive care, limit their services to certain types of patients.

intensive care unit (ICU) See INTENSIVE CARE.

intent-to-treat analysis A type of CLINICAL STUDY analysis that looks at data from all participants in that study, whether they completed the study or not. Sometimes people drop out of studies as a result of illness or do not show up for regularly scheduled appointments. These people would be included in the results reported for an intent-to-treat analysis. For instance, if a drug causes severe side effects in some patients so that those patients have to withdraw from the study, the patients completing treatment with the drug appear to be healthier than the CONTROL GROUP even if the drug has no benefit whatever, since only the healthy subjects are left in the study. See AS-TREATED ANALYSIS.

interaction See DRUG INTERACTION.

intercourse Interaction; the most common euphemism for coitus (SEXUAL INTERCOURSE). The term covers both heterosexual and homosexual coitus. Types of intercourse include ANAL INTERCOURSE (both insertive and receptive anal intercourse) and VAGINAL INTERCOURSE.

interfemoral Between the thighs; e.g., interfemoral intercourse (rubbing the penis between a partner's thighs).

interferon (IFN) One of a number of antiviral proteins that modulate the immune response. Interferons serve multiple roles as antiviral, antitumor, and immunity-stimulating agents. Studied since the 1960s, interferon was the first CYTOKINE discovered. Interferons are obtained in two ways: they are made naturally by the body when cells are stimulated by a virus as well as by several other agents or are produced by genetically engineered microorganisms.

There are three major groups of interferons—alpha interferon, beta interferon, and gamma interferon. These major classes have been synthesized, and each is being studied in various applications for the treatment of HIV. Alpha and beta interferons appear to be made by virtually all white blood cells, whereas gamma interferon is made only by T cells and large granulocytes. Gamma interferon is much more potent in its effect on the immune system than alpha or beta interferon. Interferons are important in immune function, have antitumor activity, and can repress the growth of nonviral parasites within the cells.

In November 1988, the U.S. FOOD AND DRUG ADMINISTRATION (FDA) approved interferon as a treatment for KAPOSI'S SARCOMA; it had previously been used to treat hairy cell leukemia and genital warts. The interferon is injected directly into small KS lesions only, to try to reduce their size. The drug is normally given by injection because it is believed that if it were taken orally, digestive processes would destroy it. Alpha interferon (IFN-α) is secreted by a virally infected cell and strengthens the defenses of nearby uninfected cells.

Alpha interferon has been available as a prescription drug in the United States since 1986. There are more than 20 varieties of alpha interferon that have been found in the human body. Beta interferon is also more than one protein and has several varieties. Gamma interferon is just one protein so there is only one variety known. A manufactured version of alpha interferon is an FDA-approved treatment for KS, hepatitis B virus, and hepatitis C virus; trade names are Roferon and Intron A. A version of interferon called PEGYLATED INTERFERON is regular interferon attached to a substance called polyethylene glycol (PEG); it results in longer-lasting, sustained activity of the interferon in the body. This allows someone to only take one injection of interferon a week instead of three or four.

Trade names are Pegasys and PEG-intron. Interferon alpha-2 (IFN-α-2) is a variety of alpha interferon that with beta interferon has been used as an experimental treatment for PROGRESSIVE MULTIFOCAL LEUKOENCEPHALOPATHY (PML).

Beta interferon (IFN-β) is an antiviral that may work in the same way as alpha interferon but has fewer side effects. Early clinical trials tested beta interferon and low-dose AZT on patients who could not tolerate full-dose AZT. Beta interferon with interferon-alpha-2 has been used as an experimental treatment for PROGRESSIVE MULTIFOCAL LEUKOENCEPHALOPATHY (PML). As there are of alpha interferon, there are a variety of beta interferons.

Gamma interferon (IFN-γ) is synthesized by immune system cells (NK CELLS and CD4 CELLS). It activates MACROPHAGES and helps orient the immune system to a mode that promotes cellular immunity (TH1 response).

interim analysis　An intermediary analysis of clinical trial data, performed at a point at which enough data have been gathered to derive preliminary, but not necessarily complete, conclusions. Interim analyses are performed to determine whether continuation of a clinical trial is warranted. A Data Safety Monitoring Board (DSMB) is responsible for doing interim analysis of a study's data.

interleukin (IL)　Interleukin is the generic name for a group of CYTOKINES that are produced by LEUKOCYTES and other immune cell types. They have a broad spectrum of functional processes that regulate the activities and capabilities of a wide variety of cell types. They are particularly important in regulating inflammatory and immune responses. There are a variety of types known and probably more that will be found. Research on several interleukins has possible implications for future treatment of HIV.

Interleukin-1 (IL-1 or hematopoietin-1) is a protein produced by a variety of cells in the body, including the NATURAL KILLER CELLS, T CELLS, and B CELLS. IL-1 triggers a range of processes involved in inflammation, a localized immune reaction. It activates T cells and stimulates BONE MARROW growth.

Interleukin-2 (IL-2) is a protein produced by activated T cells in the body. It plays a central role in the regulation of immune responses against infection or cancerous cells. In people living with HIV, IL-2 levels are abnormally low. It is thought that this deficiency contributes to the overall deterioration of the immune system in HIV disease. IL-2 was discovered in 1976 at the National Cancer Institute and was originally called T cell growth factor. IL-2 stimulates the growth and activities of a range of cells, including CYTOTOXIC T LYMPHOCYTES (CTLs), LYMPHOKINE-activated killer cells (LAK cells), and tumor-infiltrating lymphocytes (TIL cells). As HIV disease progresses, levels of IL-2 are reduced. As alpha interferon has been, IL-2 has been synthesized and is approved for treatment of kidney cancer in several countries. In addition, it is under development as a treatment for other diseases, including HIV. It is known that IL-2 induces the multiplication of CD4 (T-helper) cells in the body. In particular, people who had a T-cell count greater than 300 showed increases in CD4s after treatment. It is not known whether this effect will prolong the life of anyone who has taken IL-2. There is also evidence suggesting that HIV is controlled in the body during the early period of infection by a strong response by the cell-mediated arm of the immune system (chiefly suppressor and cytotoxic CD8 T cells activated by IL-2 released by CD4 cells). The cells involved in this response gradually lose their ability to respond effectively to HIV and other pathogens, possibly as a result of a decline in IL-2 production by CD4 cells. IL-2 has serious dose-limiting toxicities. It produces side effects. Because it increases the T cells, it also simultaneously increases the opportunities for HIV to increase because HIV infects T cells. For this reason IL-2 is not given to people with HIV unless they are also receiving HAART therapy. Typically IL-2 causes nausea, muscle aches, and fever. It can also cause mouth ulcers, diarrhea, and abdominal pain. In rare cases it can cause hypothyroidism and elevated liver enzyme levels. Blood tests need to be performed while taking IL-2 to monitor any changes in liver enzyme, mineral, or electrolyte levels. IL-2 is given in subcutaneous (under the skin) injections. Some swelling is also reported at the site of the injection; ice can reduce its duration. Tylenol and ibuprofen are generally also given to IL-2 patients to reduce the fever and flulike symptoms.

Interleukin-3 (IL-3 or multicolony stimulating factor) is produced by activated T cells. It stimulates the proliferation of precursors in all bone marrow cells (red cells, GRANULOCYTES, MACROPHAGES, and LYMPHOCYTES).

Interleukin-4 (IL-4 or B-cell stimulatory factor-1), another immune-system messenger naturally present in the body, has been tested as an anti-KS treatment. Synthetic versions are produced in the laboratory by genetic engineering. Early results of the IL-4 study showed the drug had no apparent effect on KS progression but appeared to have some anti-HIV activity. IL-4 enhances B-cell growth and antibody production and stimulates production of other immune system cells.

Interleukin-5 (IL-5 or eosinophil colony stimulating factor) stimulates the growth of the blood cells known as EOSINOPHILS, which kill bacteria.

Interleukin-6 (IL-6 or B-cell stimulatory factor-2) stimulates B-cell growth.

Interleukin-7 (IL-7) is a T-cell growth and activation factor and a macrophage activation factor.

Interleukin-8 (IL-8) is produced by most cells of the body, especially macrophages and endothelial cells. It enhances inflammation, by enabling immune cells to migrate into tissue, and is a powerful inducer of chemotaxis for neutrophil cells.

Interleukin-9 (IL-9) up-regulates Th1 responses (enhancing inflammation) by inhibiting T-cell apoptosis.

Interleukin-10 (IL-10) down-regulates antiviral responses by inhibiting the production of interferon-gamma (IFN-γ), antigen presentation, and macrophage production of IL-1, IL-6, and TNF-α. IL-10 is also very important in B-cell activation. IL-10 may decrease fibrosis in tissues and is in clinical trials for treatment use in chronic hepatitis.

Interleukin-11 (IL-11) is produced by bone marrow stromal cells. It stimulates megakaryocytopoiesis.

Interleukin-12 (IL-12) triggers maturation of Th1 CD4 cells and specific cytotoxic T-lymphocyte

responses and an increase in the activity of NK cells. It is under study as an immunotherapy in HIV infection, since it stimulates production of the very cells that AIDS destroys, thereby boosting immune cells directly.

Interleukin-13 (IL-13) has structural and functional similarities to IL-4 and promotes B-cell differentiation.

Interleukin-14 (IL-14) is a cytokine produced by T cells that enhances proliferation of activated B cells and inhibits immunoglobulin synthesis.

Interleukin-15 (IL-15) is produced by the epithelial cells and monocytes. It has many of the same functions as IL-2 but has more importance in the development of natural killer (NK) cells.

Interleukin-16 (IL-16) is another naturally occurring variety of interleukin. The way it works is unknown, but it is known to bind to the CD4 receptor and may inhibit CD4 cell activation. Investigators have found that a factor isolated from the CD8 cells of African green monkeys that suppresses SIV, the monkey virus similar to HIV, is virtually identical to human IL-16 but has a more dramatic HIV-suppressive effect than pure IL-16. Other scientists suggest that IL-16 may be working together with other suppressive factors. At the doses used by the investigators, IL-16 was not toxic to cells and so perhaps has some therapeutic potential. However, as with other cytokines that have shown anti-HIV activity in the lab, it may also concurrently stimulate the production of inflammatory cytokines when administered in people, undermining whatever direct anti-HIV activity it might have. And generally administration of the HIV-suppressor cytokines has been associated with many side effects.

Interleukin-17 (IL-17) is T-cell-derived and mimics proinflammatory actions of TUMOR NECROSIS FACTOR and lymphotoxin; its in vivo function is unknown.

Interleukin-18 (IL-18) induces interferon-gamma (IFN-γ) production. See CHEMOKINES; HIV SUPPRESSORS.

intermammary Between the breasts; e.g., intermammary intercourse or rubbing the penis between a partner's breasts.

intermediate care facility (ICF) A facility that provides health-related care and services to individuals who do not require the degree of care and treatment standard nursing facilities (SNFs) provide. The bulk of nursing home patients need ICF-rather than SNF-level care. MEDICAID and cash payments are the sole sources of financing for this level of care. It is not covered by MEDICARE or HEALTH INSURANCE.

international unit (IU) The internationally accepted quantity of a substance. This type of measure is used for the fat-soluble vitamins (such as vitamins A, D, and E) and certain hormones, enzymes, and vaccines. International units are officially defined by the International Conference for Unification of Formulae.

interstitial pneumonia See INTERSTITIAL PNEUMONITIS.

interstitial pneumonitis A localized acute inflammation of the lung. A definite diagnosis of interstitial pneumonia in a child under 13 years of age is indicative of AIDS unless another cause is identified or tests for HIV are negative.

intertriginous infection An inflammation or superficial dermatitis occurring in the folds of the skin, such as the creases in the neck, between the toes, or in the groin. It is characterized by redness, maceration, burning, itching, and occasionally ulceration and erosion.

intertrigo labialis See PERLECHE.

intervention In health care economics and clinical practice, intervention refers to an action that interrupts or changes events in progress; in behavior modification research, to those techniques or devices by which one behavior is interrupted and another, presumably healthier, behavior is instituted. Within the context of HIV/AIDS, many intervention efforts of the first decade were designed and implemented quickly in response to a new health problem that in some areas took on characteristics of a crisis. Today, many researchers and program planners believe that the time has come to view behavioral intervention from a more long-term perspective. Today's challenge is to develop effective intervention strategies that sustain healthy behavioral patterns in individuals who are not currently at risk and facilitate change among individuals who are at risk. Efforts of the first decade bear witness to the fact that, to be effective, intervention efforts must be well-designed, carefully implemented, and thoughtfully evaluated.

Intervention models vary considerably, ranging from individual intervention efforts to community-level intervention efforts that are designed to reach a critical mass of individuals with information, motivation, and skills training. There are information interventions that utilize lectures, videotapes, and support groups; social interventions, such as safer sex parties; and media interventions, such as the multimedia public service campaign utilized in the second year of the Centers for Disease Control and Prevention's "America Responds to AIDS" media campaign. This latter campaign included television and radio announcements, print advertisements, and public transit posters.

intestinal malabsorption A condition in which nutrients found in food are not properly absorbed by the body and can lead to malnutrition and weight loss at a result.

intolerance In medicine, inability to take a drug, or a food substance, because of an extreme sensitivity—an allergic reaction or side effect.

intracranial disorder Any pathological liver condition within the skull.

intrahepatic disease Any pathological liver condition that produces a group of clinical symptoms peculiar to it and that sets it apart as abnormal.

intralesional Inside or into a lesion; e.g., an intralesional injection.

intramuscular Inside or into muscle; e.g., an intramuscular injection.

intraocular Inside or into the eye; e.g., an intraocular injection.

intraocular implant A tiny device (about half the size of a peppercorn) surgically placed directly into the eye. It is designed to deliver a steady, concentrated dose of a drug directly to the infected area for an extended period of time. Intraocular implants are used to deliver GANCICLOVIR to the area of the eye infected by CMV.

intrapartum   During childbirth or delivery.

intrapartum transmission   Transmission that occurs during childbirth or delivery. It more commonly occurs than IN UTERO TRANSMISSION, which occurs during pregnancy. To date, there are few data concerning the impact of certain obstetrical practices on the transmission of HIV. It is thought that events during delivery that expose the baby to maternal blood or cervicovaginal secretions might promote transmission. Minimal use of invasive procedures involving the fetus may decrease the risk of transmission, but optimal treatment of the fetus should take priority. Delivery by cesarean section has not been proved to protect the fetus better than normal spontaneous delivery. Allowing women to deliver in a more comfortable position does not compromise the use of UNIVERSAL PRECAUTIONS for blood and body fluids.

Intrapartum care includes the use of universal precautions; managing labor to optimize outcomes for both mother and infant; utilizing the method of delivery indicated by obstetrical conditions. HIV infection is not currently a contraindication to the use of any analgesia or method of anesthesia. See ANTEPARTUM PERIOD; POSTPARTUM PERIOD; TRANSMISSION.

intrathecal   In or into the fluid surrounding the spinal cord.

intrathoracic adenopathy   Swelling of the glands or lymph nodes within the chest.

intrauterine device (IUD)   Any of several small plastic devices that may be fitted into a woman's uterus as a barrier to prevent pregnancy. The use of an IUD is considered an effective method of contraception; the failure rate is said to be about 3 percent. For almost 100 percent effectiveness, the simultaneous use of contraceptive cream, jelly or foam, and condoms, is recommended. Using IUDs increases a woman's chances of developing PELVIC INFLAMMATORY DISEASE (PID) and consequent infertility, and are a poor choice for woman at risk of developing a SEXUALLY TRANSMITTED DISEASE (STD). IUDs alone offer no protection against STDs or HIV.

intravenous (IV)   In or into a vein; e.g., an intravenous injection or feeding tube.

intravenous drug abuser (IVDA)   See INJECTION DRUG USER.

intravenous drug user   See INJECTION DRUG USER.

intravenous drugs   Drugs, such as heroin, that are administered by injection into a vein, directly into the bloodstream.

intravenous immunoglobulin (IVIG)   A sterile solution of concentrated antibodies extracted from the blood of healthy people, injected into a vein or muscle to prevent bacterial infections in people with low or inappropriate ANTIBODY production. It is used particularly for children who have IDIOPATHIC THROMBOCYTOPENIC PURPURA.

intravitreal   In or into the eye's vitreous humor, between the lens and the retina.

intromission   The introduction of the penis into a partner's body; i.e., vaginal intromission, anal intromission, or oral intromission.

introns   Noncoding regions of DNA interspersed among the EXONS.

intubation   The insertion of a tube into a body canal or into any hollow organ, such as the trachea or larynx, to permit the entrance of air; to dilate a structure. Endotracheal intubation refers to the insertion of a tube through the nose or mouth into the trachea. Nasotracheal intubation refers to insertion of a tube through the nose into the trachea.

invasive nutritional substitute   Any nutrient administered intravenously as an alternative to solid food ingested orally.

invasive procedure   Any technique involving the insertion of foreign matter into the body. The term covers procedures ranging from simple injection to intubation to major surgery.

investigational new drug (IND)   IND is the status the federal government gives a drug that a company or researcher wants to investigate for treatment of humans. If the status is granted, an IND number is assigned to the drug for further reference if needed. According to the FDA, "Federal law requires that a drug be the subject of an approved marketing application before it is transported or distributed across state lines." Because a sponsor will probably want to ship the investigational drug to clinical investigators in many states, it must seek an exemption from that legal requirement. The IND is the means through which the sponsor obtains this exemption from the FDA. The applicant must submit all data about the drug, from how it is derived to tests performed in the laboratory to tests performed in animal models. The FDA has 30 days to review materials before an IND number can be granted

There are three types of IND; An investigational IND is submitted for research into a new product or a new use of an already existing product. An emergency use IND allows the FDA to approve the drug for use in an emergency that does not allow time for a full application. A treatment IND is submitted for drugs showing promise in clinical testing for serious and immediately life-threatening conditions while the final clinical tests continue.

invirase   See FORTOVASE.

iodoquinol   An antiamebic agent appearing as a yellowish to tan crystalline powder used in the treatment of AMEBIASIS. Also called diiodohydroxyquin and Diodoquin. (The trade name is Yodoxin.)

IRB   See INSTITUTIONAL REVIEW BOARD.

irrevocable beneficiary   A beneficiary designation on a life insurance policy that cannot be changed without the beneficiary's consent.

Iscador   See MISTLETOE.

ischemia   Local deficiency of blood supply due to functional constriction or actual obstruction of a blood vessel.

ischemic   Pertaining to or affected with ISCHEMIA.

isobutyl nitrite inhaler   Also known as "poppers." Nitrite inhalants, originally made for treating certain heart conditions, which came to be used as sexual stimulants in the gay community. Following research reports that these chemicals might be contributing to immune problems in AIDS or to the development of KAPOSI'S SARCOMA, they were banned in the United States in 1988. Section 8 of the Consumer Product Safety Act bans the manufacture for sale, distribution in commerce, or importation of various forms of "butyl nitrite." In 1990, Congress amended the law to also ban "volatile alkyl nitrites that can be used for inhaling or otherwise introducing volatile alkyl nitrites into the human body for euphoric or physical effects." The amendment specifies a broader class of nitrites, not just the chemical named in the 1988 law. But manufacturers found a way around the ban by substituting different kinds of nitrites. These chemicals were then sold in adult bookstores, sex clubs, and bars. The result was that, unknown chemicals, never tested for human consumption, came into widespread use with no regulatory or public-health oversight. It is noted that the issue of poppers in the gay community first surfaced in 1981. Some observers suspected that poppers themselves might cause AIDS. Later, those theories were largely dismissed, but confusion occurred because some people thought the issue was finished. Remaining concerns are that poppers might be a cofactor in the development of AIDS, could lead to relapses to unsafe sex, may make HIV infection more likely by causing changes in blood vessels, or could possibly cause poisoning if unknown chemicals are substituted in an effort to evade the law. Additionally, some of the chemicals are known to degrade over time allowing harmful by-products. Some researchers also suspect that the body may metabolize the nitrites into the strongly carcinogenic nitrosamines While there are many medical journal articles on poppers, most of them reporting evidence of health risks, poppers have not been conclusively proven to be harmful. It is generally felt that we may never fully understand the health hazards of poppers. Evidence does strongly suggest that poppers are certainly not safe and probably do cause damage to health, especially to persons with HIV.

isolate   See SUBTYPE.

isolation   In medical institutions, procedure that keeps patients with contagious infections separated from others who are sick but do not have the same disease. Specifically, it is the limitation of movement and social contacts of a patient suffering from or a known carrier of a communicable disease. QUARANTINE, by contrast, limits the movements only of exposed or contact persons. There is no value in isolating AIDS patients, since the HIV associated with AIDS is not airborne or spread by casual contact. UNIVERSAL PRECAUTIONS suggest blood and body fluid precautions and a private room if personal hygiene habits are poor.

isoniazid (INH)   An ANTIMICROBIAL agent that has activity against *Mycobacterium tuberculosis,* the MICROORGANISM that causes TUBERCULOSIS. Isoniazid is an odorless compound appearing as colorless or white crystals or as a white crystalline powder. Isoniazid is usually recommended for persons with HIV infection who have tuberculosis or have had a positive tuberculosis skin test result. It may be administered orally or intramuscularly. Isoniazid is always given in conjunction with pyridoxine (VITAMIN B_6) to alleviate the peripheral neuropathy that often accompanies the use of the drug. It is also used in the prevention of TB in HIV-positive people who show positive exposure to the virus through a skin test. Aluminum-containing antacids can decrease the absorption of INH and reduce its effect. On the other hand, INH can inhibit liver enzymes that metabolize certain drugs, leading to increased blood levels of some medications. Liver function tests are typically run on people taking isoniazid to monitor any changes in various drug levels. (Trade names include Cotinazin, Dinacrin, and Nydrazid.)

Isoprinosine (inosine pranobex)   An antiviral drug used to treat subacute sclerosing panencephalitis in some countries. It is not approved for use in the United States. In the early history of AIDS this drug was marketed as an anti-HIV drug that stimulated the immune system. It was shown in clinical studies to have no effect on HIV or on the immune system.

Isospora belli   A species of coccidian protozoan that causes self-limiting diarrhea in healthy individuals and a severe chronic disease of the gastrointestinal tract in immune-compromised individuals. It is common in tropical areas but rarely seen outside those areas. See COCCIDIOSIS.

isosporiasis   Infection by any member of the protozoan family isospora. See COCCIDIOSIS.

itch   Any irritation of the skin, inducing the desire to scratch; any of a variety of skin disorders characterized by itching; scabies.

ITP   See IDIOPATHIC THROMBOCYTOPENIC PURPURA.

itraconazole   An oral antifungal drug used for a number of AIDS-related fungal infections. It is the drug of choice for HISTOPLASMOSIS, blastomycosis, ASPERGILLOSIS, onychomycosis (toenail fungus), and oral and esophageal CANDIDA (thrush), all of which are infections due to various fungi. It is also being tested as a treatment for CRYPTOCOCCAL MENINGITIS in people with HIV. Itraconazole concentrates in the skin, and concentrations there may be 3 to ten times higher than in the blood. Possible side effects include digestive upset, loss of potassium, headache, and liver toxicity. Liver enzyme tests must be conducted often and their results monitored regularly. (The trade name is Sporanox.)

IUD   See INTRAUTERINE DEVICE.

IV   See INTRAVENOUS.

IVDU   See INJECTION DRUG USER.

jack-off party A group sex event in which people masturbate either themselves or each other. It can be a safe-sex technique.

jaundice A condition characterized by yellowness of skin, whites of eyes, mucous membranes, and body fluids that is due to deposition of bile pigment that results from excess bilirubin in the blood. It may be caused by obstruction of bile passageways, excess destruction of red blood cells, or disturbances in functioning of liver cells. Jaundice is typically seen in late-stage HEPATITIS and is often a sign of cirrhosis of the liver. Noninvasive procedures such as ultrasonography, MRI, and computed tomography, as well as clinical laboratory studies, may be used to determine the cause of jaundice. Invasive studies may also be used, including biopsy of the bile ducts or liver.

JC virus Named after the initials of the patient from whom the virus was isolated in 1970. JC virus is a polyomavirus, in the same family of viruses, Papovaviridae, as HUMAN PAPILLOMA VIRUS. JC virus is spread throughout the human population. Approximately 70 percent of HIV-negative individuals have antibodies to the virus. It is believed to be acquired during childhood and is not known to cause any symptoms on infection. In healthy individuals primary infection with JC virus causes no known disease; the virus assumes a latent state in the kidney and perhaps other organ sites as well. However, with decreased immunity, JC virus can cause persistent urinary tract infections. It has also been shown to be the cause of PROGRESSIVE MULTIFOCAL LEUKOENCEPHALOPATHY (PML) through its infection of GLIAL cells, particularly OLIGODENDROCYTES, in patients. JC virus has also been theorized as a cause of several types of tumors in humans; however, this relationship has not been confirmed in research studies. JC virus is unusual because its genes are astoundingly resistant to mutation, a distinctly uncommon trait in a virus. Seven major types of JC virus are known to exist, and scientists have used these virus types to trace human migration through thousands of years. Native American Navajos carry the same form of the virus as residents of Tokyo, Japan. Chamorros in Guam carry the same form as some people from New Guinea. Europeans, Africans, and Asians all carry different varieties, which indicate different human migration patterns.

jilling off A women's slang term for female masturbation.

jockstrap A piece of underwear that holds and supports a man's penis and scrotum.

john Slang for a prostitute's customer.

joint See PENIS. Also a slang term for marijuana cigarette.

judgment-proof Beyond the legal reach of creditors; immune from legal compulsion to pay debt. A person with no assets and no income (except from public entitlements) may be said to be judgment proof.

junkie A slang term for a heroin addict.

K cell   Killer cell. A type of nonspecific LYMPHO-CYTE that seeks out, binds to, and kills any cell coated in antibodies. K cells contain Fc receptors on their surface that recognize and bind themselves to the antibodies, which are bound to the virus. This process is known as ANTIBODY-DEPEND-ENT CELL-MEDIATED CYTOTOXICITY (ADCC). K cells make up about 1.5 percent to 2.5 percent of the lymphocyte population in human blood.

Kaletra   Abbott Laboratories' PROTEASE INHIBITOR contains a fixed formulation of two protease inhibitors, lopinavir and ritonavir. It is available as either a capsule or oral solution. In a dose-ranging study, the most common adverse effects were diarrhea and asthenia. Because ritonavir inhibits CYP3A4, coadministration of lopinavir and ritonavir can complicate lopinavir's interaction with other drugs metabolized by this hepatic enzyme. Kaletra's resistance profile is not yet fully understood, causing a great deal of concern among researchers and health care providers. Without this information it is difficult to determine which protease inhibitor people can switch to if they start therapy with Kaletra and eventually the drug fails.

Kaplan-Meier curve   Also known as the product-limit curve or method, the curve is common method of graphing patient progress over time. The Kaplan-Meier method is especially well suited to situations that involve censored data, such as those encountered in blind clinical trials, in which patients are enrolled over a period and followed for a specific period. The curves generated by the Kaplan-Meier technique provide the cumulative probability of that an event (e.g., opportunistic infection or death) will not occur as a function of time. Plotting the curves for a trial's different treat-ment arms on the same chart yields a comparison of the various regimens. The chart allows researchers to compare people who enter a study at different times.

Kaposi's sarcoma (KS)   KS is an overproduction of cells that make up the walls of small blood vessels. Sarcomas are malignancies that arise in muscle, connective tissue, and bone. Sarcomas also occur in the liver, lungs, spleen, kidneys, bladder, and tissues that make up the blood vessels. KS remains the most commonly diagnosed malignancy in HIV-positive people, despite the decline of its incidence in developed countries since the introduction of HIGHLY ACTIVE ANTIRETROVIRAL THER-APY (HAART). KS was one of the first signs that foreshadowed the failing immune systems of gay men in the early 1980s and led to the discovery of HIV. It was often seen as an expected illness, for gay men that were positive at that time.

KS was first described by Moritz Kaposi in 1877 as a cancer of the muscle and skin. Characteristic signs of early KS are bruises and birthmark-like lesions on the skin, especially on the lower legs and feet. KS was described as a slow-growing tumor found primarily in elderly Mediterranean men (mainly Italians) and Ashkenazi Jews. Classic KS has a variable prognosis, is usually slow to develop, and causes little pain. Indeed in these regions it pre-existed HIV in people with suppressed immune systems. Patient survival in the United States ranges from eight to 13 years, with some reported cases of survival for up to 50 years. Symptoms of classic KS are ulcerative skin lesions, swelling of the legs, and secondary infection of the skin lesions. It is called Classic Kaposi's now.

Endemic KS is found in the equatorial regions of Africa. It is diagnosed in 9 percent of men who have cancer in Uganda. KS assumes a different form in equatorial Africa. It is a more aggressive disease in Africa and in younger people and is not associated with HIV. It can occur in children, affecting their lymph nodes and spreading quickly. In other words, an individual could have KS and not have HIV.

Transplant associated KS is also seen. It occurs 150 to 200 times more often in transplant patients than in the general population. This is because people who have had transplants must take immunosuppressive drugs that lower the response of their immune system so that the transplanted organ will not be rejected. This type of KS will improve when people stop taking their immuno-suppressive drugs.

The AIDS epidemic has brought a more virulent and progressive form of KS. KS skin lesions usually present as red to purple (bruise-colored) patches or nodules that may appear in or on several parts of the body simultaneously. The patches can progress to become nodules, sometimes with associated edema, or large, painful, raised patches called plaques, particularly when located on the thighs or feet. KS can develop in HIV-positive people before they experience other OPPORTUNISTIC INFECTIONS. KS can also progress to involve internal organs, where it may be life-threatening. In rare cases, KS can affect organs without involving the skin.

KS in AIDS patients can come on swiftly. KS can have enormous psychological impact on people, particularly if the lesions occur on exposed areas. Some of the most painful KS targets include the soles of the feet, the nose, and the oral cavity. Lesions on the lower extremities or on the feet are often associated with the collection of fluid and swelling, causing not only severe pain but difficulty putting on shoes and walking. Swelling can be complicated by bacterial cellulitis, ulceration, and skin breakdown, often with infections. Lesions on the face may be accompanied by swelling around the eyes that can sometimes progress to the point where the eyes cannot open. Oral lesions can be painful and make eating and speaking problematic. Loss of appetite due to mouth sores or pain from swallowing can be caused by KS as well as by candidiasis, herpes infection, or other infections. KS involvement of the gastrointestinal tract occurs in 40 percent of cases at diagnosis and up to 80

percent at autopsy but is frequently asymptomatic. Pulmonary involvement, which often occurs late in the disease, may cause severe respiratory symptoms and is associated with a poor prognosis.

In Western countries, HIV-associated KS is the most common malignancy in men with AIDS. It occurs about 20 times more frequently in homosexual and bisexual men than in hemophiliacs and male injection drug users with AIDS, and 50 to 100 times more often in men than in women. It is extremely rare in children, a phenomenon that may partially be explained by the fact that human herpesvirus type 8 (HHV-8), the virus associated with Kaposi's sarcoma, is not usually found in children in the United States. Indeed, the incidence of lymphomas and sarcomas that do occur in children is much lower than it is in adults with HIV disease. Finally it is noted that whites are more frequently affected than blacks.

This distribution of the disease has led epidemiologists to believe that KS is caused by a sexually transmitted virus other than HIV. Recent research linked a sexually transmitted human herpesvirus, the Kaposi's sarcoma–associated herpesvirus (KSHV, later called human herpesvirus 8, or HHV-8), in the development of KS. It is now known that HHV-8 is present in all KS lesions, both in patients infected with HIV and those with no HIV. While HHV-8 is a necessary factor for the development of KS lesions, other factors, such as immunosuppression, are also required.

KS cases have dropped 70 percent since the advent of HAART. Most people that take HAART will be able to suppress KS and the lesions will even disappear over time. KS diagnosis is done visually and with biopsy to confirm, if necessary. If the patient is reporting other body problems then chest X rays and endoscopy may also be performed to determine the spread through the body. Lesions can be removed when small, if this desired. Incisions will leave a small scar, but the lesion will be gone. Treatment can also be started when various radiotherapy or chemotherapy. Neither of these options proved long lasting in the pre-HAART era in HIV positive patients. Chemotherapy for skin lesions is typically injected directly into the lesion.

kava kava An herb made from the ground root of a Pacific Islands plant in the pepper family. It is also sold in many health food stores under the name kava. It is used by naturopaths as a treatment for anxiety, nervousness, insomnia, pain, and muscle tension. The U.S. FOOD AND DRUG ADMINISTRATION issued a warning in 2002 that the use of this supplement has led to liver failure in people that previously had reported no problems with liver function. Liver abnormalities in patients were also noted in several other countries that issued warnings regarding the herb. It is not known whether excessive amounts of the substance caused the problem, or interactions with other herbs or medications. Potential problems overshadow any beneficial usage of this supplement at this time, the warnings indicate.

Karnofsky index (or scale) Clinical estimate of a patient's physical state, performance, and prognosis. The scale is from 100 (perfectly well) to 0 (zero, dead). It is used in studying cancer and chronic illness. Clinical trial studies often require a Karnofsky rating of at least 60 to qualify for participation in the study.

Kegels A series of exercises to strengthen the pubococcygeal (P.C.) muscles, which aid in the enjoyment of sex and ease in reaching orgasm. Kegel exercises also help women prepare for childbirth. Also called elevator exercises.

kemron An oral form of ALPHA INTERFERON given in doses more than 100,000 times lower than in conventional subcutaneous administration. At one point Kenyan researchers reported dramatic improvements, including HIV seroreversions (that is, conversion from HIV-POSITIVE to HIV-negative), with the drug. Subsequent studies have failed both to replicate these results and to find any benefit to Kemron at all.

Kennedy-Cranston Amendment In 1987, Senator Jesse Helms sponsored legislation forbidding the use of federal funds to "promote or encourage, directly, homosexual sexual activities," and requiring instead that all sex education materials "emphasize" sexual abstinence outside of heterosexual marriage and complete abstinence from drug use. The Helms Amendment was replaced,

after one year in effect, by a compromise engineered by Senators Edward M. Kennedy and Alan Cranston. The Kennedy-Cranston Amendment forbade use of federal funds only for materials "designed to promote or encourage, directly" IV drug abuse or homosexual or heterosexual activity. When it passed the Kennedy-Cranston Amendment in 1988, Congress also stipulated that federally funded HIV education "contain material, and be presented in a manner, that is specifically directed toward the group for which such materials are intended." It ordered that the prohibition on promoting or encouraging homosexuality and drug abuse "may not be continued to restrict . . . accurate information about various means to reduce an individual's risk . . . provided that any informational materials used are not obscene." This satisfied proponents of HIV education, who took the position that even the most explicit messages were "designed to promote" risk reduction.

ketoconazole An antifungal medication, available in pill, cream, and liquid forms, that is effective against a variety of fungal infection such as oral, vaginal, and esophageal thrush and CRYPTO-COCCOSIS. Ketoconazole requires acid in the stomach to be absorbed into the system, if taken orally. Other medicines that neutralize stomach acids should therefore not be taken until at least two hours after taking ketoconazole. It is not currently prescribed as frequently as it was in the past for HIV patients. It is used predominantly in its cream form and in over-the-counter shampoos. Possible side effects, when it is taken orally, include nausea, vomiting, hormonal problems (menstrual problems and reduced sex drive), rash, headaches, and liver damage. (The brand name is Nizoral.)

ketotifen In the United States, a prescription ophthalmic solution that is used for temporary prevention of itching of the eye caused by a condition known as allergic conjunctivitis. It works by acting on certain cells, called mast cells, to prevent them from releasing substances that cause the allergic reaction. In Canada and Europe the drug has been approved as an antihistamine, to be used in the treatment of asthma-related allergies. Early in the HIV epidemic ketotifen was thought to contain some TUMOR NECROSIS FACTOR-alpha (TNFα) inhibitor properties that might be useful in the treatment of AIDS-related wasting. Clinical studies have not confirmed any effect of ketotifen on these conditions.

kidney stone Known medically as nephrolithiasis or renal calculius. A kidney stone is a solid lump that can vary from the size of a grain of sand, up to as large as a tennis ball. Kidney stones are made up of crystals that separate from urine and build up on the inner surfaces of the urine-collecting tubes outside the kidney. Of all kidney stones 80 percent occur in men. People of European ancestry have more kidney stones than people of African descent. People who have had kidney stones are likely to have recurrences; the stones can cause permanent damage to the kidney or urinary tract if not treated. They are known as one of the most painful conditions humans can suffer. They generally require some form of painkiller. In HIV patients, 20 percent of all people taking the PROTEASE INHIBITOR indinavir experience kidney stones. The indinavir separates from the urine and mixes with calcium to form the stone. People who take indinavir as part of a HAART regimen may even see crystals of the drug in their urine. People may also notice blood in their urine before passing a stone. Treatment for kidney stones involves excess hydration, either by drinking lots of water, or if necessary, intravenously. The stone most often passes after a few days of this method. If the kidney stone is too large or does not pass the body via the urinary tract, a STENT may be inserted in a kidney bladder tube to hold it open and ideally allow the stone to pass. Surgical removal of the stone or lithotripsy, shock waves aimed at the back, generally while the patient is sitting in a tub of water, may be required. Surgical removal is generally no longer performed.

kidneys The organs that remove poisons and other harmful waste from the body in the form of urine. They are located in the small of the back on each side of the spine.

killer cell A general name for immune cells that kill cancerous and virus-infected cells. Among the killer cells are killer T CELLS (cytotoxic T-lymphocytes), NK (natural killer) cells, and K CELLS.

kinins A group of vasoactive mediators formed in body tissues and produced following tissue injury. Kinins are capable of influencing smooth muscle contraction, inducing hypotension, increasing the blood flow and permeability of small blood capillaries, and inciting pain.

kinky In slang, pertaining to any unconventional sexual behavior or desire.

kiss A touch or contact with the lips. Kisses may be light and gentle or passionate, dry ("social" kisses) or wet (French kisses). They may be tokens of affection, greeting, or reverence.

kissing French kissing is considered to be a practice with a low risk of HIV transmission and dry kissing is considered to have almost no risk of HIV transmission. Given that the AIDS virus has been found in saliva, although only in low concentrations, French kissing, also called deep kissing or tongue kissing, cannot be considered completely safe. An infection through very long and intimate deep kisses is, however, not very likely. If one of the partners carries the virus and the other suffers from bleeding gums or other, even slight, injuries inside the mouth, there could be danger. Dry kissing, and social kissing, on the other hand, do not involve an exchange of saliva or any other body fluid. This is also true of kissing any other part of the body, except, of course, the anus, the vaginal opening and the tip of the penis. Any other part of the body may be kissed without any fear of infection as long as the skin is intact.

Klebsiella Bacteria found in the feces that can cause cystitis.

knowledge and ignorance The literature on AIDS has attempted, and attempts, to teach us the "facts" about this disease, or to provide a narrative account of scientific discovery and developing public health policy. In addition to precipitating a crisis that is medical, political, financial, and social, AIDS has precipitated a crisis of signification. The "meaning" of AIDS continues to be hotly contested. That there is a powerful cultural narrative surrounding AIDS (as there is around every cultural phenomenon) goes without saying; analysis of this narrative reveals that AIDS has given rise to a semantic as well as a pathological epidemic.

An analysis of AIDS discourse by author Paula Treichler reveals that "no clear line can be drawn between the facticity of scientific and nonscientific (mis)conceptions." Treichler observes that AIDS is both a material and a linguistic reality and notes that in speaking, writing, and thinking about AIDS, "the facts" change less often than the way in which they are used to construct the AIDS "text," or cultural narrative, and the meanings we are allowed, or able, to read from that text. Treichler focuses on one particular aspect of this linguistic reality—that it is constructed around a series of discursive oppositions fundamental and apparently natural. "Knowledge and ignorance" is one of these. In terms of this opposition, cultural analysts ask us to question: What is knowledge and what is ignorance? Is science knowledge and not-science ignorance? Who has access to knowledge and who is denied access to knowledge? Are scientists and other health care providers privy to knowledge that is "off-limits," or otherwise unaccessible to persons with HIV/AIDS? Cultural analysts and activists advise us to resist the luxury of listening to the thousands of language tapes playing in our heads that tell us in plain English, in black and white, what AIDS "really means." Within the context of this example, each of us is encouraged to use what science (or knowledge) offers us in ways that are selective, self-conscious, and pragmatic. Each of us is also encouraged to question whether, or to what extent, scientific discourse can be privileged.

Other discursive oppositions are: self and not-self; homosexual and heterosexual; active and passive; guilty and innocent; perpetrator and victim; vice and virtue; us and them; anus and vagina; sins of the parent and innocence of the child; love and death; sex and death; sex and money; death and money; science and not-science; doctor and patient; expert and patient; doctor and expert; addiction and abstention; contamination and cleanliness; life and death; injection and reception; instrument and receptacle; normal and abnormal; natural and alien; prostitute and paragon; whore and wife; safe sex and bad sex; safe sex and good sex. If we are to understand the AIDS text, to (re)read or (re)write the narrative more clearly and perceptively, then we must see how these discursive oppositions structure our thinking. We must *deconstruct* the text, in other words, so we can evaluate what goes into it and revise our thinking with less unrecognized conceptual bias.

kombucha The kombucha (or "Manchurian mushroom," among other nicknames) is a substance that is said to have anti-AIDS effects. It is one of a number of organic "miracle" treatments that come and go with the seasons. The distributor of kombucha states that according to "folklore," it is a super immune booster that can fight a list of ailments: AIDS, cancer, arthritis, and numerous other maladies. The kombucha is not really a mushroom at all but a yeast culture. It is not eaten, it is placed in a large glass bowl with a solution of water, tea, and sugar. The culture grows there at room temperature for seven to 10 days. During this time, the solution ferments to produce a "tonic" or tea that is drunk for its therapeutic properties. There are safety concerns with kombucha, focusing on the storage of the mushroom and the fermentation process. The seven- to 10-day period in which the solution ferments may permit the contamination and growth of other organisms. According to mycologists, the mold that sometimes grows on the kombucha may contain a fungus of the *Aspergillus* species, which is also known to contaminate moldy marijuana. ASPERGILLOSIS is a fungal infection that attacks the brain and may be fatal in persons with weakened immune systems. Since Kombucha purportedly contains naturally occurring antibiotics, the long-term use of this substance raises concerns about development of bacterial strains that can resist standard, approved antibiotic drugs. Furthermore, ketoconazole, ddI, and other drugs whose absorption depends on sensitive pH levels (base versus acid) of the stomach may be poorly absorbed in the presence of the acidic kombucha tea. References to kombucha in the standard medical literature are, to date, few. Most of what has been written has appeared in articles in health food and alternative medicine newsletters and magazines.

KS See KAPOSI'S SARCOMA.

KS-OI Kaposi's sarcoma and opportunistic infections, an early designation for AIDS used by CDC officials when it was first reported in 1981.

K-Y The brand name of a water-based lubricant. Unlike petroleum-based lubricants like Vaseline, it does not degrade latex and is therefore suitable for use with gloves in medical examinations and with condoms.

K-Y jelly See K-Y.

L

L. acidophilus See LACTOBACILLUS ACIDOPHILUS.

L. bulgaricus See LACTOBACILLUS BULGARICUS.

labeled uses Uses of a drug currently included in Food and Drug Administration approved labeling.

labia Scientific term for lips of the vagina, usually used to denote the genital labia minora and labia majora.

labia majora Large folds of skin-covered fatty tissue protecting the vagina and urethral openings.

labia minora Small folds of mucous membrane inside the labia majora.

laboratory testing Testing that is done in a room or building equipped for scientific experimentation, research, testing, or clinical studies of materials, fluids, or tissues obtained from patients.

labyrinthitis Inflammation of the labyrinth (the internal ear consisting of osseous and membranous labyrinths). It can cause loss of balance or dizziness. It is caused by primary infection, trauma, complication of influenza, otitis media, or meningitis.

lactic acid A product of normal human metabolism. Lactic acid is formed during everyday or strenuous activity. During exercise, pyruvate is formed from the breakdown of glucose, blood sugar. Lactic acid is produced when there is not enough oxygen in the blood to break down the pyruvate. It enters the surrounding muscle cells,

tissue, and blood, which in turn break down the lactic acid to fuel (adenosine triphosphate) for immediate cellular use or use in the creation of glycogen. The glycogen then remains in the cells until the next time energy is required.

lactic acidosis A buildup of lactic acid (a by-product of carbohydrate metabolism) in bodily tissues. See MITOCHONDRIAL TOXICITY.

Lactobacillus Bacteria common in normal vaginal flora.

Lactobacillus acidophilus A group of several *Lactobacillus* species that inhabit a wide range of habitats and serve many different functions. Some inhabit the gastrointestinal (GI) tract and others are in milk, meat, and plants. None serves the same function, and it is unclear what function many serve. Health activists believe that by eating milk products, particularly yogurt, a person is increasing their good bacteria in the GI tract. This is largely a myth and the *Lactobacillus* in the GI tract are greatly different from that in yogurt. Current genomics projects are examining the variety of *Lactobacillus* to learn more about the variety and purpose of the bacteria.

Lactobacillus bulgaricus A bacillus found in fermented milk. Milk fermented with this organism is known as Bulgarian milk.

lactose intolerance The inability to digest milk products, owing to the absence or low activity of the enzyme lactase, which breaks down milk sugar. Lactose intolerance can lead to painful gas and diarrhea in people.

LAI   A group of closely related HIV isolates that is used in vaccine development and includes the LAV, IIIB, and BRU strains of HIV. LAI belongs to clade B, the clade to which most HIV-1 found in America and Europe belongs. See CLADE.

LAK cells   Lymphocytes transformed in the laboratory into lymphokine-activated killer (LAK) cells that attack tumor cells.

Lambda Legal Defense and Education Fund   National organization committed to achieving full recognition of the civil rights of lesbians, gay men, and people with HIV/AIDS through impact litigation, education, and public policy work. Founded in 1973, Lambda is not-for-profit and tax-exempt. *The Lambda Update* is the tri-annual newsletter of the Lambda Legal Defense and Education Fund. It contains docket listings and articles about crucial cases and legal issues of relevance to lesbians, gay men, and people with HIV/AIDS. The *Update* includes an AIDS docket. Lambda has addressed a broad spectrum of AIDS-related challenges, cases, and issues in areas such as employment, standards of care, prisons/confidentiality and the right to privacy, and criminal and family law.

Lamisil   See TERBINAFINE.

lamivudine   A NUCLEOSIDE REVERSE TRANSCRIPTASE INHIBITOR (NRTI) from GlaxoSmithKline. It is used in the treatment of HIV and hepatitis B. It was the first drug to be approved for the treatment of hepatitis B. It has been one of the longest used drugs against HIV and has proved durable for many people. It is used in the combination pills COMBIVIR and TRIZIVIR. 3TC works well in combination with AZT and has shown to decrease mutations causing resistance that can arise in taking AZT. It is available in both a liquid and a pill formulation. It is taken twice daily. The most common side effects are nausea, vomiting, fatigue, and headaches. 3TC does not work well with ZALCITABINE. (Also known as 3TC and Epivir.)

lamotrigine   Antiseizure medication in studies for treatment of peripheral neuropathy. (The trade name is Lamictal.)

lancinating   Characterized by piercing or stabbing sensations.

Langerhans cells   Antigen-presenting cells, found primarily in the skin, that emigrate to local LYMPH NODES to become DENDRITIC CELLS; they are very active in presenting antigen to T CELLS.

laparoscopy   A procedure in which a lighted tube and telescope are inserted into the abdominal cavity to view, biopsy, or remove the various organs in the region. Organs that can be viewed or operated upon through this procedure include the gallbladder, uterus, fallopian tubes, appendix, and stomach.

large granular lymphocytes (LGLs)   A group of morphologically defined LYMPHOCYTES containing the majority of K CELL and NK CELL activity. They have both lymphocyte and MONOCYTE/MACROPHAGE markers.

large simple trial (LST)   A type of expanded access mechanism allowing patients to take an experimental drug, or drug combination, not yet approved by the United States Food and Drug Administration and available for general prescription use. Large simple trials are used to measure with certainty whether a particular treatment has an effect on survival. The "simple" in large simple trial refers to simplifying the study design so that researchers do not have to collect much information. Additionally, the paper work required to enroll a patient in these trials is greatly reduced. The methodology for these trials was developed by Dr. Richard Peto of Oxford University.

In the mid-1990s, the LST approach was proposed by New York's Treatment Action Group (TAG) to answer questions pertaining to PROTEASE INHIBITORS, such as How are we to determine when and how well they work? and How easily can HIV evolve to overcome this new therapeutic challenge? TAG proposed a large two-year clinical efficacy trial comparing various protease inhibitors to a placebo in a sample of approximately 18,000 people with HIV. As proposed, this LST would go beyond previous parallel track or expanded access programs that have allowed people failing standard therapies to receive experimental drugs even before FDA approval. It was proposed that the phase II/III LST efficacy trial commence immediately after the preliminary phase I safety trials were completed. The trial would be open to nearly anyone with HIV, and participants could take any drugs they desired in addition to the protease inhibitor.

The proposed trial would offer access to the experimental protease inhibitor, one-third of the trial participants would receive placebo rather than protease inhibitor in blinded fashion, i.e., neither the doctors nor participants would know who was in the placebo arm. But TAG also proposed a nonplacebo trial comparing different doses of protease inhibitors for people who have CD4 counts of less than 50, who cannot tolerate any of the NUCLEOSIDE ANALOGS, or who have reached advanced disease in the large simple trial.

As proposed, the large simple trial concept is one that has a number of attractive features. The data collected in the LST would be much more extensive than that previously gathered from expanded access participants. The information on clinical outcome (incidence of opportunistic infections, death, etc.) would be recorded by people's usual physicians and would reflect the effects that a certain drug or combination of drugs has during actual use by the public. Finally, LSTs lend themselves to subset analysis, in which particular subgroups are monitored for the predictive power of laboratory tests, drug-drug interactions, and specific toxic reactions that might normally go unobserved.

The LST concept also has a number of immediate drawbacks. Conducting a large trial as proposed would consume huge amounts of resources in terms of research dollars, risk to human beings exposed to an experimental drug, and attention diverted from other potential therapies inching their way through the pipeline. Additionally, cooperation between industry, government agencies, patients from diverse communities, and primary care providers, essential in completing these trials, does not have a long history. One often-heard criticism of LST designs is the belief that participants might have to remain on one treatment, excluding all others for the duration of the trial. The criticism is countered by the argument that, if that were the case, then a lot of the polemics about "body counts" determining trials analysis would have

more validity. Those in favor of LSTs believe that treatment restrictions are not only unnecessary, they are undesirable.

LAS   See LYMPHADENOPATHY SYNDROME.

laser surgery   See LASER THERAPY.

laser therapy   The use of extremely narrow, intense and controlled light beams in the diagnosis and treatment of some forms of cancer. A laser beam can sever, fuse, or eliminate body tissue. The first working laser (light amplification by stimulated emission of radiation) was developed in 1960. Lasers were first medically used in 1961 to treat skin discoloration and to repair detached retinas. Laser therapy has several advantages over traditional surgical treatment: it is more precise than a scalpel; the heat produced by the laser sterilizes the surgery site; there is less chance for infection; less operating time may be required; healing time is frequently reduced; there is less bleeding, swelling, and scarring; and more procedures can be done on an outpatient basis. The major disadvantages associated with laser treatment are the relatively small number of trained surgeons, the high cost of the equipment, and the fact that strict safety precautions must be observed.

Lassa fever   A viral disease with a relatively high mortality rate in Africa. Lassa fever is caused by an arenavirus. The common carrier is a native African rat species. Acute high fever, abdominal and chest pain, headache, dizziness, cough, nausea, diarrhea, and vomiting are among the symptoms. The skin and membranes may begin to hemorrhage. It is not related to HIV.

last observation carried forward   A type of data analysis in clinical trials in which the last results before a subject drops out of the trial are counted as if they occurred at the end of the trial. It is used when data are missing as a result of loss to follow-up.

late breaker   A presentation at a scientific conference that was submitted too late to be included in the original program but that was deemed to merit inclusion in the conference.

latency   The period between the initiation of a stimulus, or contracting of a disease, and the response or clinical manifestation of the disease. Clinical latency is an asymptomatic period in the early years of HIV infection. The period of latency is characterized in the peripheral blood by near-normal CD4 counts and HIV levels. Cellular latency is the period after HIV has integrated its GENOME into a cell's DNA but has not yet begun to replicate. One of several widely held myths about AIDS in conventional medicine before 1992 was that HIV remains dormant, or latent, for up to 10 years before initiating immune damage. HIV replication starts immediately after infection at high levels in the lymphoid organs. Because the lymphoid organs are the major reservoirs of virus and sites of viral replication, peripheral blood measurements (measurements of P24 ANTIGEN, NEOPTERIN levels, and CD4 cells) do not always accurately reflect the total body burden of HIV infection. By the time of the onset of HIV symptoms, the lymphoid organs will have become massive generators of virus. These findings suggest the importance of the widespread use of the POLYMERASE TECHNOLOGY that measures blood viral load.

Latency may also refer to the state of being concealed, hidden, inactive, or inapparent; for example, a MICROBE is said to be latent when it is in the body but not actively reproducing, invading tissues, or causing symptoms. Once in the body, these microbes remain in the body. PNEUMOCYSTIS CARINII, TOXOPLASMA GONDII, HERPES SIMPLEX VIRUS, and CYTOMEGALOVIRUS are microbes that are latent or dormant in most healthy people. They remain so until something disorders the immune system and permits them to become active.

latent period (reaction time)   Time between application of a stimulus and first detectable response in an irritable tissue. See LATENCY.

latex   A natural or synthetic rubbery substance used to make flexible, sterile nonporous barrier materials like condoms and surgical gloves.

latex agglutination test   A medical test to see if antigens of a known condition have already caused a defensive (antibody) reaction against that condition. If antibodies are present and clump with the known antigen, the test response is positive. In a latex agglutination test, antigens are exposed to latex particles (antigens clump better when exposed to latex particles). Agglutination occurs as a reaction against various diseases, primarily infections. Whenever the body is exposed to bacteria, viruses, fungi, or toxins containing antigens, the body reacts by producing antibodies. These antibodies then attempt to fight off the specific organism that has invaded the body. Antibodies found in the patient's blood indicate that the patient has already been exposed to a particular infection. The exposure may have occurred many years previously, or it may be of very recent origin.

latex allergy   Allergy to the fluid or sap produced by some plants. People with this allergy could be allergic to such simple things as balloons, doctors' gloves or condoms made out of latex. This is a potential problem for doctors, fast-food workers, toll takers, janitors, police officers, and especially health care workers who routinely wear latex gloves as protection against AIDS. Mild sensitivity can produce a skin rash. Extreme sensitivity can include symptoms similar to hay fever or asthma. Severe allergic reactions to latex can include anaphylactic shock and death. Medical and dental personnel should ask every patient about the possibility of latex allergy, especially those scheduled for surgery. Patients who have had multiple surgeries are at high risk. Also at high risk are those allergic to bananas, chestnuts, avocados, and some tropical fruits. Potential sexual partners should also be queried about latex allergy. The government has yet to set standards on safer alternatives.

Latin America   Latin America consists of the countries south of the United States border with Mexico, other than the Guyanas and Belize, which are considered a part of the CARIBBEAN. There are 1.5 million people living with HIV there according to UNAIDS. There are 330,000 orphans in Latin America whose parents' death resulted from HIV disease, the majority of them in Brazil. Infection rates for the virus top 1 percent of the population in Guatemala, Honduras, and Panama. Brazil has an HIV-positive population of more than 600,000 people.

The spread of HIV in Latin America is one of contrasts. The main route of transmission has differed in different countries. That would tend to indicate that the virus is just beginning to make inroads in these countries and there may be time to prevent high rates of infection as seen in Africa or the Caribbean. However, despite knowledge of these statistics, there are still countries in the region that do not have any method of tracking or testing HIV in their citizenry, even anonymously, nationwide. Neither Venezuela nor Nicaragua has made HIV testing or tracking part of their public health plans. Data in these two countries are very sketchy and several years old. Although some countries state that transmission is predominantly male to female sex, the cultural mores of the region may indicate that other transmission routes are available. Latin America has a code of machismo. Latin American men do not generally identify as gay and do not consider some homosexual activities they engage in even as men's having sex with men. Women indicate that it is not unusual for men to brag about the amount of sex they are having and the number of people they are having it with at the time. If these reports of cultural mores are accurate, then the region may have more HIV cases if the behavior is not coupled with the use of condoms.

In Costa Rica and Mexico HIV has been spread predominantly via men who have sex with men (MSM). The virus has not been found to a significant extent in the rest of the population—at least until recently. 2001 UNAIDS studies show female sex workers' HIV rates topping 1 percent in major cities and U.S. border regions. Mexico also shows a high rate of infection among people who go to health clinics for treatment of sexually transmitted diseases (STDs). In Costa Rica, testing of sex workers continues to show very low rates. In 1997 and 1993 rates of less than 0.0025 percent were registered for this population. The rates in the MSM population, however, register between 10 percent and 16 percent. Both Mexico and Costa Rica have well-established market economies that have a relatively greater degree of wealth and opportunity, among their population than have many other Latin American nations. These conditions have led to a greater degree of gay organizing and a higher rate of HIV prevalence.

In other Central American nations the spread is predominantly heterosexual. Honduras, which has collected information on HIV in a thorough manner for several years, has the best available data. Four of five cases in that country are spread in heterosexual activities. Although 10 percent of men did report MSM activities, they had a HIV rate of just 1 percent, whereas female sex workers averaged a rate of 10 percent HIV-positive. It is believed that between 1 percent and 2 percent of 15- to 19-year-old women in Honduras are HIV-positive and this possibility is of future concern for this nation. In Panama, Guatemala, and El Salvador the rates are highest among female sex workers. Rates range from 5 percent to 10 percent across the country in Guatemala to 2 percent in El Salvador.

Brazil leads the countries of the region in numbers of HIV-positives. It also leads the region in its approach to the virus. The second leading cause of death among men and women 20–50 remains AIDS. Initially the virus was transmitted predominantly through MSM sex. It has changed to a virus passed through heterosexual sex and IDU activities. Brazil has spent an enormous amount of money on education for their citizens, and HIV awareness in this country may be the best in Latin America. Brazil was the first country that ignored pharmaceutical conglomerates' patents and began making the generic forms of the HAART medications. After initially suing the government of Brazil, the drug companies have dropped their cases for the time being.

Brazil has also made a law that guarantees citizens are provided with HAART as part of the course of the treatment. More than 100,000 people in Brazil are now provided HAART for HIV disease. This number is the highest outside the United States and Western Europe. Brazil has seen the number of nongovernmental AIDS organizations triple in the last five years, through 2002. The people have also responded to public education programs advocating condom usage. Although some money has been provided by the World Bank, other funds have been generated through savings the government has realized by making generic drugs. In 1996 Brazil spent $200 million on drugs for HIV disease and served 20,000 patients. In 2000

Brazil spent twice that amount but served four times the people by using generics.

Concern is also great in Argentina, Uruguay, and Chile, where IDU activity has become a recent fad among some parts of the citizenry. This leads those countries to expect a high rate of HIV in the next few years, predominantly because of the number of people testing positive in those countries as a result of IDU. Outside the IDU-positive people in those countries there is very little HIV in the populace, even among sex workers in the cities. In the Andean region, the numbers are similar, though Peru has somewhat higher numbers of HIV-positive individuals than Bolivia or Ecuador. Colombia has both extensive testing and measuring programs and a large education program. The country shows a relatively low rate of infection. In Nicaragua and Venezuela no recent data are available, so it is unknown whether there is an ongoing epidemic in those countries. Extrapolating numbers from neighboring areas indicates that both nations may have burgeoning problems that are not being addressed. Although Argentina also guarantees the HAART medications to people with HIV disease, the country has at times been unable to provide citizenry with the medications. This inability is probably due to financial difficulties of the government and could prove disastrous if the virus were able to mutate while the people waited for medications.

In El Salvador people report that they are not tested because of restrictive laws. These laws require that HIV-positive people divulge all sexual partners so they may be notified they may be at risk. It is also legal in El Salvador for employers to fire or refuse to hire people who are HIV-positive. Some reports from the country indicate that the question is included in employment applications. This would indicate a greater problem than the 0.6 percent HIV-positive rate that is available currently from the government.

LAV See LYMPHADENOPATHY-ASSOCIATED VIRUS.

lavage The process of washing out an internal organ or cavity for treatment or for obtaining of a sample.

L-carnitine A naturally occurring cell constituent that modulates fat metabolism, in particular the mitochondrial intake of lipid derivatives. L-carnitine has been proposed as a treatment for AIDS-related wasting and the myopathy associated with AZT.

LD-50 Median lethal dose of a substance that will kill 50 percent of the animals receiving that dosage. Dosage is usually calculated on amount of material given per gram or kilogram of body weight or the amount per unit of body surface area.

LDL cholesterol See LOW-DENSITY LIPOPROTEIN CHOLESTEROL.

lean body mass The body's muscle and organ tissue.

lecithin A fatty substance of the group called phospholipids (phosphoglycerides), found in blood, bile, brain, egg yolk, nerves, and other animal tissues. It yields stearic acid, glycerol, phosphoric acid, and choline on hydrolysis.

lecithinized superoxide dismutase (PC-SOD) A synthetic version of superoxide dismutase (SOD), one of the more potent antioxidants produced by the body.

lectin One of several plant proteins that stimulate lymphocytes to proliferate. Lectins are commonly MITOGENS as well.

Legionella pneumophila A species of GRAM-NEGATIVE bacterium that causes Legionnaires' disease and Pontiac fever. It is responsible for pneumonia in immunosuppressed people. *Legionella* has been isolated from numerous locations where standing water gathers, such as water cooling towers, and from aerosolized droplets from inside heat-exchange systems.

leishmaniases A group of diseases caused by a flagellate protozoon that belongs to the genus *Leishmania*. It is spread through the bite of a blood-feeding female sandfly. There are more than 30 varieties of biting sandflies that can carry this disease between dogs, rats, opossums, humans, and other mammals. There are four forms of leishmaniasis that occur in humans. Visceral leishmaniasis, also known as kala azar, is a very severe form of the disease. It causes bouts of fever, weight loss, swelling of the spleen and liver, and anemia. It is almost 100 percent fatal if untreated. Ninety percent of the cases of this form occur in Bangladesh, Brazil, India, Nepal, and Sudan. Annually 500,000 new cases are reported.

Mucocutaneous leishmaniasis, also known as espundia, causes disfiguring lesions of the mucous membranes of the nose, mouth, and throat that can destroy the mucous membranes. Ninety percent of all cases of this form occur in Bolivia, Brazil, and Peru. It typically creates marked disfigurement.

Cutaneous leishmaniasis produces large numbers of skin ulcers on exposed body parts such as the face, arms, and legs. It can cause disabilities and leave scars for life. Ninety percent of cases of this form occur in Afghanistan, Brazil, Iran, Peru, Saudi Arabia, and Syria. There are between 1 and 1.5 million new cases a year reported. Most cases of cutaneous leishmaniasis heal without drug treatment and leave the person immune to further infection.

Diffuse cutaneous leishmaniasis never heals spontaneously and tends to recur after treatment. It also causes skin ulcers on exposed parts of the body.

Leishmaniases are endemic in 88 countries and five continents, and this incidence is increasing. Only Australia does not currently have cases of leishmaniasis. Many people who are bitten by sandflies do not contract the disease. However, in immunocompromised people cases can quickly become severe and life-threatening. Developed countries such as Spain and Italy have large problems with leishmaniasis and HIV coinfection, as do other countries such as India and Brazil.

When the sandfly injects the leishmania under the human skin the macrophages arrive and attack the antigen by swallowing it. Once inside the macrophage the leishmania protozoon transforms itself into a slightly different form and reproduces in the macrophage, killing the macrophage and spreading to other tissues. Those tissues most predominantly affected are the lymph tissues of the bone marrow, spleen, and lymph nodes. Leishmaniasis infects and kills many of the same disease-fighting cells that HIV infects and kills, making the disease doubly dangerous in HIV-positive people. People who have cutaneous leishmaniases usually

have a skin lesion within two weeks or so. People with visceral or systemic leishmaniasis usually have signs of infection within several months of when they were bitten. Very rarely does the time extend beyond these limits.

It has become such a problem in some countries that the United Nations has established a specific unit of the WORLD HEALTH ORGANIZATION (WHO) to work on the problem. Leishmaniases may also be spread by people sharing needles in INJECTION DRUG USE. Visceral leishmaniasis has increased in the HIV epidemic, spreading it to new areas, whereas it typically occurred only in the region of Sudan, Eritrea, and Ethiopia in the past.

Blood test results often to not reveal the protozoa, especially among coinfected people. Tests to determine whether someone is infected include bone marrow biopsy, lymph node biopsy, liver biopsy, and spleen biopsy. Treatment of leishmaniases generally involves a long course of pentavalent antimony drugs. They are made from the heavy metal antimony. Two drugs, meglumine antimonite (Glucamtine) and sodium stibogluconate (Pentostam), have been most effective in treatments. Secondary drugs that have been used include pentamidine and amphotericin B. Cure rates are high with antimony compounds, and lower with the other drugs. A drug called miltefosine is a new oral drug being tested by WHO for leishmaniases and has performed well. On some occasions G-CSF and interferon-gamma are used to boost the effects of antimony drugs. Side effects of antimony drugs include heart irregularities, kidney enzyme irregularities, and various anemias.

lentivirus A subfamily of RETROVIRUSES that until recently was known to include only the VISNA viruses in sheep, the equine infectious anemia virus in horses, and the caprine arthritis-encephalitis virus in goats. Newly recognized members of the family include the HUMAN IMMUNODEFICIENCY VIRUS (HIV), the SIMIAN IMMUNODEFICIENCY VIRUS (SIV), the feline immunodeficiency virus (FIV), and the bovine immunodeficiency virus (BIV). The original ungulate lentiviruses produce chronic diseases in their natural hosts. Visna viruses cause a chronic interstitial pneumonitis similar to that seen in AIDS and young children. All cause ENCEPHALITIS. The diseases are characterized by erratic relapses and remissions. The chronic carrier state, in which infected animals themselves do not get sick but can transmit the virus to other animals, is common.

Lentiviruses persist in the body by evading natural defense mechanisms. Lentiviruses can cross the blood-brain barrier, destroy brain tissue, and remain in the body in a chronic subclinical state (period before appearance of typical symptoms of a disease) for long periods. HIV is a lentivirus that causes forms of mental incapacity in an estimated 70 percent to 80 percent of patients and end-stage dementia in many.

leprosy   A chronic infectious disease caused by MYCOBACTERIUM LEPRAE. It progresses slowly and may manifest itself in various clinical forms. The two principal, or polar, forms are lepromatous and tuberculoid. The lepromatous form is characterized by the development of lesions in the skin and symmetrical involvement of the peripheral nerves, yielding skin anesthesia, muscle weakness, and paralysis. The lepromatous form tends to involve the skin, respiratory tract, and testes. In the tuberculoid forms, skin anesthesia occurs early and the nerve lesions are symmetrical; this form is usually benign. Lepromatous leprosy is much more contagious and malignant. Two other types of leprosy include borderline and indeterminant leprosy. Borderline leprosy possesses clinical and bacteriological features representing a combination of the two polar forms. Indeterminant types of leprosy present fewer skin lesions and less abundant bacteria in the lesions.

lesbian   A woman sexually and emotionally attracted predominantly to other women and who identifies herself voluntarily as such.

The myths that lesbians are at low risk for AIDS, that lesbians don't and can't get AIDS, that AIDS has nothing to do with lesbians, persisted well into the first decade of the epidemic. That lesbians suffered through the negligence and bias of HIV researchers early in the epidemic and beyond is unquestionable. The lack of research or documentation on female-to-female TRANSMISSION clearly helped fuel the myths, as did the CENTERS FOR DISEASE CONTROL AND PREVENTION's initial "stance" that there was no female-to-female transmission.

Today, however, cases of AIDS transmitted between lesbians have been reported. The following factors are also likely to put lesbians at higher risk: sharing needles or other IV drug paraphernalia; having or having had repeated vaginal or anal intercourse with men who have been actively gay or bisexual since 1979, with people whose sexual history is unknown, with women who use IV drugs, or with HEMOPHILIACS or others who received blood transfusions between 1979 and 1985; having received blood transfusions or blood products between 1979 and 1985; and having used semen for donor insemination from a donor in a high-risk group who is known to be ANTIBODY-POSITIVE, or whose risk status is unknown. Another potential risk is the unsafe use of needles for piercing and tattooing.

Another myth about lesbians is that if they are not exposed to high-risk factors or high-risk groups, they do not have to be concerned about AIDS. Although they are likely to be at lower risk for AIDS medically, lesbians are still at high risk for discrimination by virtue of their HOMOSEXUALITY. The public often perceives lesbians to be in the same high-risk category as gay men, and as a result vulnerable to the same discrimination and hostility and the same AIDS hysteria as their gay male counterparts. Fear of AIDS has become synonymous with fear of homosexuality, a phenomenon that potentially threatens the rights of gay men and lesbians relevant to employment, housing, and freedom to travel. Legislative measures generated during the AIDS crisis affect lesbians as well as their gay male counterparts, and discriminatory practices by insurance companies affect gay males and lesbians and heterosexuals as well.

Many lesbians have been personally affected by AIDS-related deaths or illnesses of people close to them. The AIDS epidemic raises the need to address problems of substance abuse, and especially IV drug abuse, in the lesbian community. Insemination choices and coparenting options have been limited by AIDS. Many lesbians are involved in AIDS-related work as volunteers and paid workers. Lesbian contributions have strengthened and enriched the entire gay and lesbian community and furthered the fight against AIDS.

For lesbians who would like to make sex safer—if they are unsure of their own or their partners'

HIV/STD status, or if they or their partners are HIV-POSITIVE—several guidelines are suggested to reduce the risk of transmission. Avoid contact where either partner's blood or vaginal fluids can get into the other partner's body through the mouth, vagina, anus, or a cut in the skin. Use non-powdered surgical gloves for digital penetration and fisting. Surgical gloves can be found at most drugstores. Finger cots can also be used for digital penetration. Change gloves between vaginal and anal insertion, or use one hand for vaginal and the other for anal sex. Use latex or plastic barriers for oral sex and rimming. Special care should be taken if either partner is menstruating. Several products can be used as barriers, such as unlubricated latex condoms (which can be cut into flat barriers by cutting off the tips and cutting through one edge before unrolling), dental dams, or plastic wrap.

Other guidelines advise the use of water-based lubricant, which makes safe sex not only more comfortable and enjoyable but safer. Activities to avoid include sharing sex toys without putting a fresh condom on between uses or washing thoroughly with soap and warm water; S&M activities that draw blood when the blood may get in eyes or open cuts; and sharing IV needles without cleaning them with bleach.

Today there are lesbian-sensitive AIDS-related resources; there are services for lesbian inmates and ex-offenders who are HIV-positive. There are programs that affirm the lives of lesbians living with AIDS by recognizing and responding to the fact that lesbians with HIV are in many ways a unique group. Their clinical symptoms can differ from those of men and they have different psychosocial concerns and needs than their heterosexual or bisexual female peers. Data are being collected about lesbians and are being used to shape service delivery, education, prevention, and transmission messages.

lesbianism   Homosexual practice between women.

lesion   Any pathological or traumatic damage to tissue, which may cause a loss of function of the affected or surrounding tissue.

lesser AIDS   See AIDS-RELATED CONDITION.

leucovorin   A vitamin, also called FOLINIC ACID or citrovorum factor, long used to counteract the effects of the anticancer drug METHOTREXATE. While that is still its primary use, it is now also used by people with HIV to counteract the toxicity of drugs used for OPPORTUNISTIC INFECTIONS. These drugs include PYRIMETHAMINE, and TRIMETREXATE.

FOLIC ACID is a B vitamin essential for a wide variety of biochemical reactions in the body, including the synthesis of components of proteins, DNA, and RNA. A number of ANTIBIOTICS and anti-cancer drugs, called folic-acid antagonists, interfere with the body's ability to use folic acid. When that happens, serious side effects, including life-threatening anemia, can occur. Leucovorin is a water-soluble B vitamin that counteracts the effects of folic-acid antagonists. It is available in tablet form or as a sterile powder for intravenous or intramuscular injection. The injectable form is used primarily when the digestive tract is not functioning well enough to absorb the oral drug, a condition that often occurs during anticancer chemotherapy. Leucovorin may increase the toxicity of the anticancer drug FLUOROURACIL. Leucovorin in high doses may counteract the antiseizure effect of epilepsy drugs and increase the frequency of seizures in children. (Trade name is Wellcovorin.)

leukemia   A chronic or acute disorder of the blood-forming elements characterized by the unrestrained growth of LEUKOCYTES and their precursors in the blood and BONE MARROW. Types of leukemia are classified on the basis of the dominant cell type involved.

leukemia inhibitory factor   A cytokine related to interleukin-6 that is produced during pregnancy and has been shown to inhibit HIV transmission from mother to child. It is found in the placenta, the organ that connects the mother to the child through the umbilical cord. The level of leukemia inhibitory factor was significantly higher in the placentas of women who did not pass the virus to their babies than in women whose infants contracted the infection. Researchers are looking at ways to increase the level of LIF in the mother to prevent transmission. One way to do this is through increasing the progesterone levels of the mother. Research is also being done to test microbicides that have LIF as the main ingredient, for prevention of HIV transmission during sex.

leukocyte A white blood cell essential to the body's defenses against infection. Leukocytes may be classified into two main groups: granulocytes and agranulocytes (nongranular). Granulocytes possess granules in their cytoplasm and include neutrophils (cells that gobble up microbes), eosinophils, and basophils. Agranulocytes do not possess granules in their cytoplasm and include monocytes and LYMPHOCYTES (cells that recognize foreign material). The normal leukocyte count is 4,000 to 8,000 per milliliter of blood. In people with certain infections, especially bacterial infections, leukocyte count is high (this condition is called *leukocytosis*). In people with viral infections, including HIV infection, leukocyte count is low *(leukopenia).* See LYMPHOCYTE; LYMPHOPENIA; NEUTROPENIA.

leukocyte functional antigen (LFA) One of a group of three molecules that mediate intercellular adhesion between LEUKOCYTES and other cells in an ANTIGEN-nonspecific fashion.

leukocytosis A condition of the blood in which there is an abnormally large number of LEUKOCYTES (white blood cells), a condition that may occur in acute infection.

leukoencephalopathy Any of a group of diseases affecting the white matter of the brain.

leukopenia A condition of the blood in which there is an abnormally a low number of LEUKOCYTES (white blood cells). The condition may occur in viral infections, including HIV infection. Leukopenia may also be caused by drugs or BONE MARROW failure.

leukoplakia Formation of white spots or patches on the MUCOUS MEMBRANE of the tongue or cheek. The spots are smooth, irregular in size and shape, hard, and occasionally fissured. Leukoplakia caused by HPV or occasionally other illnesses may

become malignant. Hairy leukoplakia patches can not become malignant.

leukotrienes A collection of metabolites of arachidonic acid, which have powerful pharmacological effects.

levamisole hydrochloride An anthelminthic drug used originally in veterinary medicine. It is now used as adjuvant therapy in treating metastatic colorectal cancer. (Trade name is Tramisol.)

lexipafant A platelet-activating factor antagonist that is being studied for the treatment of HIV-encephalopathy.

LFA See LEUKOCYTE FUNCTIONAL ANTIGEN.

LGV See LYMPHOGRANULOMA VENEREUM.

liarozole An experimental drug that stimulates the production of retinoic acid that is being studied as a treatment for KAPOSI'S SARCOMA.

libido In psychoanalysis, a Freudian term for sexual instinct, drive, or psychic energy.

licorice A dried root of the licorice plant, glycyrrhiza glabra, used as a flavoring agent, demulcent, and mild expectorant. Ingestion of large amounts of licorice can cause salt retention, excess potassium loss in the urine, and elevated blood pressure.

lidocaine A local anesthetic drug. (Trade name is Xylocaine.)

life and death One of the oppositions that structures and determines the discourse of AIDS. Author Paula A. Treichler notes that AIDS is no different from other linguistic constructions thought to transmit preexisting ideas and represent real-world entities but, in fact, do neither. Oppositions such as "life and death" help construct the disease and make it intelligible. We can think about AIDS in terms of life or death, as the possible loss of life, in terms of our mortality, and as a life-and-death struggle.

life cycle   The series of changes in form undergone by any developing organism from its earliest stage to the recurrence of that same stage in the subsequent generation.

life expectancy   The expected remaining average number of years of life for a group of persons of a given age according to a mortality table. The data from which such tables are constructed may be obtained as much as two decades or more prior to their date of publication. This is particularly true for data used for insurance purposes.

life insurance   Insurance that provides for the payment of a specific amount to a designated beneficiary in the event of the death of the insured. Most insurance companies in the United States do not offer life insurance policies to people that are HIV positive. Insurance companies cannot cancel such policies that are already purchased if you have continued to pay for them. Many companies contend that the underlying principle is the same for anyone with any other serious, life-threatening disease. So they have denied life insurance to many HIV positive people.

Viatical settlements involve the sale of an already existing life insurance policy. If a person has a terminal illness, he or she may consider selling his or her insurance policy to a viatical settlement company. In a viatical settlement transaction, a person with terminal illnesses assigns his or her life insurance policies to viatical settlement companies in exchange for a percentage of the policy's value. The viatical settlement company, in turn, may sell the policy to a third-party investor. The viatical settlement company or the investor becomes the beneficiary to the policy, pays the premiums, and collects the face value of the policy after the original policyholder dies. The person that is ill will receive regular payments for the policy or a one-time payment, called a lump sum.

ligand   Any molecule that binds to the surface of another molecule, such as an immune cell receptor. For examples of receptors, see CCR5; CXCR-4; CD4.

limit of detection   The sensitivity of a quantitative diagnostic test, such as the viral load assay. The limit of detection is the level below which the test can no longer accurately measure the amount of a substance, such as HIV RNA. If a person has an "undetectable" viral load, it does not mean that HIV is no longer present, but, that the test is not sensitive enough to measure the amount. It is also called the LIMIT OF QUANTIFICATION.

limit of quantification   See LIMIT OF DETECTION.

lipid abnormalities   Metabolic abnormalities. HAART regimens are now known to be associated with profound lipid abnormalities. PROTEASE INHIBITORS are associated with increases in total cholesterol, low-density lipoprotein cholesterol, and triglyceride levels and with lipoprotein abnormalities such as increases in apolipoprotein B and lipoprotein ($\overline{a}$) levels. The nonnucleoside reverse transcriptase inhibitors (i.e., efavirensz and nevirapine) often used in lieu of protease inhibitors are known to increase levels of total cholesterol but are associated with an increase in the level of high-density lipoprotein (HDL) cholesterol. Insulin resistance is another metabolic consequence of protease inhibitor therapy, although progression to diabetes mellitus is not common. Truncal/visceral adiposity is also becoming a common consequence in the HAART era of treatment. Hypertension and hypercoagulability/impaired fibrinolysis may also appear in excess HAART-treated patients with insulin cross-resistance. Note too that HIV LIPODYSTROPHY, a heterogenous syndrome observed in patients who respond to antiretroviral therapy, and fasting hyperinsulinemia and insulin resistance, which are common among patients taking protease inhibitors as part of their HAART regimen.

Therapeutic approaches include the use of atorvastatin, gemfibrozil, and pravastatin to lower cholesterol and tribyceride levels. Management approaches currently under study to correct metabolic abnormalities associated with HAART include studies of statins, fibrates, and niacin, and "switch" studies (studies in which patients are switched from protease inhibitors to nonnucleoside reverse transcriptase inhibitor or other agents) of the treatment of dyslipidemia and the use of thiazolidinediones and metformin in the management of insulin resistance.

Data show that ritonavir is the worst offender with regard to lipid changes. The data are variable for the other protease inhibitors. Note that cholesterol levels usually reverse within weeks of drug discontinuation.

lipoatrophy   Lipoatrophy is abnormal fat loss, often seen especially in the face, arms, and legs. At the same time, other fat in the abdomen may increase while the fat under the skin continues to be lost. It is thought that lipoatrophy is caused by antiretrovirals, although there are different views on whether it is PROTEASE INHIBITORS, nucleoside analogs, or the combination of both that is most responsible. It has been noted that the lost fat is not quickly regained even if the antiretrovirals are stopped. See NUCLEOSIDE REVERSE TRANSCRIPTASE.

lipodystrophy   A disturbance in the way the body produces, uses, and distributes fat. Lipodystrophy is also referred to as "buffalo hump," "protease paunch," or "Crix belly." The cause is unknown; the condition may be a result of HIV infection and/or antiretroviral therapy, especially protease inhibitor therapy. How PROTEASE INHIBITORS may cause or trigger lipodystrophy is not yet known. Lipodystrophy symptoms involve loss of the thin layer of fat under the skin, making veins seem to protrude; wasting of the face and limbs; and accumulation of fat on the abdomen (both under the skin and within the abdominal cavity) or between the shoulder blades. Women may also experience narrowing of the hips and enlargement of the breasts.

lipomas   Tumors consisting of fat cells.

lipomatosis   A disorder characterized by deposits of fat beneath the skin of the neck, upper body, arms, and legs. The origin is uncertain, but the condition is thought to be genetic. Lipomatosis often occurs in conjunction with alcoholic liver disease, macrocytic anemia, and peripheral neuropathy. It usually affects men and is most common in the Mediterranean.

lipopolysaccharide (LPS)   A product of some GRAM-NEGATIVE bacterial cell walls, which can act as a polyclonal B-CELL mitogen.

lipoprotein   A chemical compound made of fat and protein. Lipoproteins are found in the blood, where they carry cholesterol.

liposomal amphotericin B   Liposomal amphotericins are "high-tech" versions of standard amphotericin (used to treat such life-threatening fungal infections as CRYPTOCOCCAL MENINGITIS as well as other fungal infections that are resistant to other antifungal drugs), in which the drug is encapsulated in tiny fat globules known as liposomes. Liposomal amphotericin must be administered through INTRAVENOUS infusion like the standard drug, but it is hypothesized that the liposomes will be preferentially absorbed at the sites of infection and avoid most of amphotericin's side effects. Toxic effects of amphotericin can include fever, chills, muscle pain, phlebitis, vomiting, potassium loss, kidney dysfunction, and anemia. The amphotericin must be released from the liposome to be active, and depending on the packaging, this may not occur readily. Also, laboratory comparisons have shown that to be effective, doses of liposomal amphotericin B need to be significantly higher than doses of the standard amphotericin.

liposomal chemotherapy   Liposomal chemotherapy involves the use of chemotherapeutic agents encapsulated within LIPOSOMES (tiny fat globules that regulate the passage of the entrapped drug from the blood stream to specific sites). These agents have been successfully used in patients with AIDS-related KAPOSI'S SARCOMA. Liposomal chemotherapy drugs include liposomal daunorubicin and liposomal doxorubicin.

liposome   The sealed concentric shell formed by certain lipid substances in an aqueous solution. As it forms, the liposome entraps a portion of the solution in the shell. Liposomes may be found inside a cell or in the bloodstream. Liposomes may be manufactured and filled with a variety of medications. These have been used to deliver substances to particular organs. These drugs may be more effective and less toxic than drugs given by other means.

liposuction   A surgical procedure in which fat deposits are suctioned from specific parts of the body (e.g., the abdomen, buttocks, hips, thighs, or back). Liposuction is sometimes used to treat truncal adiposity or buffalo hump, although its effectiveness varies.

lipoxgenase   See LIPOXIDASE.

lipoxidase   An enzyme that catalyzes the oxidation of the double bonds of an unsaturated fatty acid.

liquid nitrogen   A substance used in the process of removing genital warts.

Listeria monocytogenes   A type of GRAM-POSITIVE BACTERIA. In humans, it produces such disorders as MENINGITIS and perinatal septicemia. It is a food poisoning that causes prolonged illness unless treated properly.

listing of impairments   A comprehensive listing, in SSDI and SSI regulations, of the most common diseases and medical conditions, including standards of diagnosis, medical proof, and evaluation to determine disability.

lithium carbonate   A drug that is particularly useful in treating the manic phase of manic-depressive illness. Given orally, it is readily absorbed and eliminated at a fast rate for five to six hours and eliminated at a much slower rate over the next 24 hours. It is essential to monitor the blood level of the drug in patients on this therapy. Side effects including fatigue, weakness, fine tremor of the hands, nausea and vomiting, thirst, and polyuria (the passing of an excessive quantity of urine) may be noticed in the first week of therapy. If these are mild, most will disappear, but the thirst, polyuria, and tremor tend to persist. (Trade names are Eskalith, Lithane, Lithonate, and Litho-tabs.)

live recombinant vector vaccine   Vaccine that uses a nondisease-causing virus—an avirulent virus—other than HIV in which certain genes from HIV have been inserted through recombinant DNA technology. The avirulent virus serves merely as a vehicle, or vector, that carries the HIV genes, along with its own, into the body cells. There, the avirulent virus replicates harmlessly but produces both its own proteins and those encoded by the HIV genes. In theory, all the viral proteins should elicit an immune response, including a response against HIV proteins. Vaccinia and canarypox viruses are examples of the several live recombinant vector HIV vaccines that have undergone development and early testing.

live-attenuated vaccine   A vaccine composed of a live virus chemically or procedurally weakened so that it is incapable of causing disease.

lived-in home   A residence owned and actually dwelled in by an applicant for or recipient of assistance; generally, it is the only kind of real estate whose ownership is permitted by welfare programs.

liver   The largest organ in the body, the liver is situated on the right side of the human body beneath the diaphragm. The liver secretes bile and is the site of a great many metabolic functions (see LIVER FUNCTION). Disorders of the liver and the associated bile ducts and gallbladder can have serious complications involving many organs in the body, all of which depend on the liver's products to support their activity.

Liver problems are frequent causes of illness and death in people with HIV infection, even in those previously considered healthy. Both physicians and patients should be aware of the symptoms, methods of diagnosis, and available treatments (and drug toxicities) for HIV-related liver conditions. Symptoms such as pain on the right side of the stomach, enlarged liver (hepatomegaly), jaundice (yellowing of eyes or skin), fever of unknown origin, fatigue, malaise, itching, and abnormal liver function tests (LFTs) deserve early and complete evaluation.

The majority of liver diseases in patients with HIV are caused by viruses (especially HEPATITIS B and HEPATITIS C), or OPPORTUNISTIC INFECTIONS (MAC, CRYPTOSPORIDIOSIS, CMV). As early as 1990, studies suggested that the liver is an important site of HIV replication, too. There have been well-documented cases of liver inflammation during primary HIV infection, the initial flulike syndrome that often precedes SEROCONVERSION, and this is a strong indication that HIV attacks liver cells directly.

Liver cancer is not commonly found in any population, but it is increased in HIV positive people. Particularly with the advent of HAART, people are living longer and they must also handle the infections that can lead to liver cancer, such as hepatitis B or hepatitis C. Up to one-third of people with KAPOSI'S SARCOMA will have some involvement in the liver, but this generally remains asymptomatic, being found only at autopsy. In lymphoma, the GASTROINTESTINAL TRACT and liver are the most common sites of involvement outside of the lymph nodes. Since the liver processes toxic compounds absorbed by the body, its cells are particularly sensitive to the side effects of medications. Many drugs used in AIDS therapy induce changes in liver enzymes or cause other impairments of liver function. Some common ones that may cause hepatotoxicity are Bactrim, Efavirenz, tuberculosis drugs, NNRTIs, and protease inhibitors.

Naturopaths recommend taking milk thistle, N-acetyl Cysteine (NAC), and other food supplements, to reduce liver toxicity. Although benefits of these are not established, it has been established that milk thistle is not toxic to patients and does not interfere with HAART. NAC is used in medical therapy to reduce toxicities seen in overdoses of acetaminophen, so it too may be helpful in reducing liver toxicity.

liver function   The liver has many critical functions, including filtering blood, eliminating toxins, secreting bile (a fluid that helps absorb and digest fat), and making clotting factors. It also converts sugar into triglycerides (lipids) and glycogen (a carbohydrate) to be stored for energy and, between meals, converts triglycerides, glycogen, and amino acids into blood sugar to meet the body's immediate energy needs. The work of the liver is particularly critical to the brain and central nervous system. These tissues receive their energy supply only from sugar, and so are extremely vulnerable to liver failure.

Various tests are available for liver disorders. These include tests for liver function and viral hepatitis. COMPUTERIZED AXIAL TOMOGRAPHY (the familiar CAT, or CT, scan) and ultrasound sonograms may also frequently be useful. Liver chemistry tests are an initial means for measuring the liver's condition. High blood levels of two common liver enzymes involved in amino acid breakdown (AST and ALT, also designated as serum glutamic-oxaloacetic transaminase [SGOT] and serum glutamic pyruvic transaminase [SGPT] in lab reports) are a sign of acute liver cell injury. Such damage to cell integrity allows these chemicals to escape from the cells and is associated with viral hepatitis and the toxic effects of drugs and poisons.

Some specialists recommend a liver BIOPSY for HIV-positive patients with unexplained fever or abnormal liver tests. In this procedure, a segment of tissue is removed with a needle inserted through the skin. The tissue is then examined microscopically.

liver function tests   This is a group (a panel) of blood tests that indicates some component of liver function. Several are listed below, as well as the reasoning for taking them.

Alanine aminotransferase (ALT): ALT is an enzyme produced within the cells of the liver. Any form of liver damage can result in an elevation in the ALT. The ALT level may or may not correlate with the degree of damage or inflammation. ALT is the most sensitive and commonly used marker for liver cell damage.

Aspartate aminotransferase (AST): AST is not as specific for liver function as the ALT; ratios between ALT and AST are useful to physicians in assessing the possible cause of liver enzyme abnormalities.

Gamma glutamic transpeptidase (GGT): Certain GGT levels, as an isolated finding, reflect rare forms of liver disease. Medications commonly cause GGT to be elevated. It is an enzyme that is also produced by the bile ducts, so it may reflect problems there.

Alkaline phosphatase: This is an enzyme that is associated with the biliary tract. If the alkaline phosphatase is elevated, biliary tract damage and inflammation should be considered.

Bilirubin: Bilirubin is a major breakdown product of hemoglobin. As the liver becomes irritated, the total bilirubin may rise. If the direct bilirubin is low, while the total bilirubin is high, this can show liver cell damage or bile duct damage within the liver.

Albumin: Albumin is the major protein present within the blood. It is created by the liver. As such, it represents a major synthetic protein and is a marker for the ability of the liver to synthesize proteins. Low albumin would indicate a problem in the liver creating these proteins.

Prothrombin time (PT): Another measure of liver synthesizing function is the prothrombin time. Particularly, these proteins are associated with changing of vitamin K into a protein. This addition allows normal clotting of blood. So when patients have prolonged prothrombin times, liver disease may be present.

Platelet count: Platelets are cells that are the base of clotting in the blood. While the collection of platelets is a normal function for the spleen, in liver disease it becomes concentrated because of the enlarged spleen. The result is that the platelet count may become diminished.

liver Lactobacillus casei factor   See FOLIC ACID.

live-vector vaccine   A vaccine that uses a non-disease causing organism (virus or bacterium) to transport HIV, or other foreign genes, into the body, thereby stimulating an effective immune response to the foreign products. This type of vaccine is important because it is especially capable of inducing cytotoxic T-lymphocyte (CTL) activity. Examples of organisms used as live vectors in HIV vaccines are the viruses canarypox and vaccinia.

living will   A document detailing a person's wishes regarding artificial life support in the event of impending death. Living wills are not legally binding in all states. See POWER OF ATTORNEY; MEDICAL DIRECTIVE; NO CODE.

local nerve block   Infiltration of a local anesthetic around a peripheral nerve to produce anesthesia in the area supplied by the nerve.

locus   A location or a place. In genetics, the specific site of a gene on a chromosome.

Lodenosine   A NRTI that is also known as F-ddA. It was under study by U.S. Bioscience as a possible HIV treatment. It was studied in humans up to PHASE II studies where drug trials were stopped after 12 weeks. Studies were stopped due to a high incidence of liver toxicity.

log (logarithm)   Formally, the number of times 10 must be multiplied by itself to equal a certain number. For example, log 5 is 100,000 ($10 \times 10 \times 10 \times 10 \times 10$). Viral load is often reported in terms of log. In addition, logs are used to measure changes in viral load. For example, a reduction in viral load from 100,000 to 1,000 copies/mL is a two log (or 99 percent) reduction (100,000 divided by 100 [i.e., 2 log or 10×10] equals 1,000). Note that whereas a one log reduction is a 10-fold difference, a half log change is not a fivefold difference but a change of 3.16-fold (the square root of 10) because $10^{0.5}$ or $10\frac{1}{2} = 3.6$. In medicine, a log is in base 10. In mathematics a log can be in any number base.

logarithm   See LOG.

long terminal repeat (LTR) sequence   The genetic material at each end of the HIV genome. When the HIV genome is integrated into a cell genome, the LTR interacts with cellular and viral factors to trigger the transcription of the HIV-integrated HIV DNA genes into an RNA form that is packaged in new virus particles. Activation of LTR is a major step in triggering HIV replication.

longitudinal study   A research design in which the same sample of subjects is examined repeatedly over an extended span of time, typically to investigate problems of developmental psychology.

long-term care   Care, usually for more than 30 days, in a mental hospital, specialized rehabilitative hospital, skilled nursing facility, intermediate care facility, board-and-care home, or, sometimes, hospice.

long-term nonprogressor   HIV-infected individuals who show very low and steady levels of HIV in their blood and normal or nearly normal CD4 cell counts for more than 10–15 years. Long-term nonprogressors make up 5 percent to 7 percent of all HIV-infected individuals. Animals that remain immunologically intact despite being infected by HIV are also called long-term nonprogressors. Note the distinction between long-term nonprogressors and slow progressors, HIV-infected individuals who at more than 10 years after infection have few or no symptoms of HIV disease and only a small, slow drop in CD4 lymphocyte numbers. Fewer than 5 percent of people who are HIV-positive are slow progressors.

long-term survivor An individual infected with HIV for at least seven to 12 years (different researchers and authors use different time spans) who yet retains a CD4 CELL count within normal range. It has been found that the good health of long-term survivors probably is due to multiple factors, which may vary from individual to individual. Multiple immune system factors, genetic and other host factors, and viral factors contribute to the clinical profiles of these patients, who usually have preserved immune function and low levels of HIV in their bodies.

Recently there was some speculation that heterozygosity for a defective gene for CC chemokine receptor 5 (CCR5) is the sole determinant for the immunologic and virologic phenotype of HIV-infected long-term survivors. However, investigators found that long-term survivors with one copy of the mutant CCR5 gene were indistinguishable from long-term survivors with two normal copies of the gene with regard to all immunologic and virologic parameters they measured, including CD4+ T cell counts and viral load in the bloodstream and lymph nodes. Investigators reported that although an HIV-infected individual who carries one copy of the mutant CCR5 gene has an increased chance of becoming a long-term survivor, other factors in the complex interaction between HIV and the body allow individuals with normal copies of the gene to maintain similar immunologic status. The epidemiological data that show that many people with the CCR5 gene mutation in cohorts of long-term survivors is explained as follows. Around the time of initial infection with HIV, people with the specific mutation in the CCR5

gene have lower levels of virus in their blood and a smaller initial decline in CD4+ T cells, as compared to other patients. The lower "set point" probably has an important influence on the subsequent rate of disease progression.

Studies of long-term survivors have contributed greatly to our understanding of the HIV disease process, and provide perhaps the best evidence that protective immunity may exist in HIV infection. Also called a long-term nonprogressor.

look-back program In HIV/AIDS terminology, a program that attempts to identify recipients of blood from a donor who is later found to be HIV ANTIBODY positive.

loop See INTRAUTERINE DEVICE.

loperamide A drug used to treat the symptoms of diarrhea. In people with HIV, it is often used to treat diarrhea caused by intestinal infections or that is a side effect of other drugs. Loperamide is available by prescription and over the counter as a liquid and in tablet form for oral administration. The prescription form of the drug should be used only under the guidance of a physician. At over-the-counter and prescribed doses, loperamide is generally well tolerated. Reported side effects include allergic reactions, abdominal pain or discomfort, nausea, vomiting, constipation, tiredness, drowsiness or dizziness, and dry mouth.

lopinavir/ritonavir See KALETRA.

lost to follow-up A patient who can no longer be followed for the outcome of interest, for example, a patient who is unwilling or unable to return to the clinic for follow-up examinations in the case of a clinical trial using an outcome measured at the clinic, or a patient who cannot be located for subsequent follow-up in the case of a trial involving mortality or some other outcome that can be measured outside the clinical setting.

lotrimin See CLOTRIMAZOLE.

lovastatin A cholesterol level–lowering drug. See STATINS.

loviride An NNRTI that progressed through PHASE III trials in the United States before being discontinued by the drug's manufacturer, Janssen Pharmaceuticals. Studies showed no benefit of this drug over other NNRTIs currently used. Usage in combination with 3TC showed no significant patient improvement over use of 3TC alone. Development was stopped at this point.

low-density lipoprotein (LDL) cholesterol A lipoprotein that contains more fat than protein, often called "bad cholesterol."

low-dose oral alpha interferon (LDAI) Low-dose alpha interferon, including Kemron and other similar products, attracted a great deal of attention in the late 1980s and early 1990s when Dr. Davy Koech of Kenya announced a stunning reversal of the AIDS disease process in patients who let lozenges containing the substance dissolve in their mouths. Dr. Koech also claimed a series of controversial "serodeconversions," in which HIV-POSITIVE patients became HIV ANTIBODY-NEGATIVE after Kemron therapy. These results received widespread publicity, creating a significant demand. In 1992, however, the National Institute of Allergy and Infectious Diseases reviewed thirteen different LDAI studies in the United States and abroad and concluded that the initial claims made on behalf of Kemron have not been confirmed. In 1993 a study sponsored by the World Health Organization found no difference between Kemron and a placebo. There was no evidence of any effect on CD4 CELLS, viral load, disease progression, survival, or "quality-of-life" indicators. And more recent scientific evidence also shows that LDAI products give no benefit in fighting HIV or in improving the immune system of persons with HIV infection.

Nonetheless, LDAI keeps reappearing, as evidenced by calls for more trials. Many observers have reported that LDAI is being kept alive by political pressure, especially from medical clinics connected with the Nation of Islam, which has helped popularize LDAI in the African-American community. But LDAI has also received support from the National Medical Association, the well-established organization of African-American physicians in the United States. Other observers note that LDAI keeps reappearing precisely because the medical establishment has nothing really effective to offer people with HIV, especially those in disenfranchised and poor communities, who have the least access to care and promising therapies.

lower limit of normal The bottom of the normal range for a particular laboratory; a value that helps assure between-lab compatibility.

low-grade squamous intraepithelial lesion (LSIL) Abnormalities in the cells on the surface of the cervix; an aberration that turns up on Pap tests. LSILs have a slightly higher degree of abnormality than do atypical squamous cells of undetermined significance (ASCUS). Three approaches to managing this abnormality include colposcopy (a procedure in which the clinician examines the cervix through a lighted, binocular-like magnifying instrument and biopsies abnormal areas), "watchful waiting" (repeating the Pap test every six months), and testing the cells in the smear for the strains of human papilloma virus (HPV). See ATYPICAL SQUAMOUS CELLS OF UNDETERMINED SIGNIFICANCE and HIGH-GRADE SQUAMOUS INTRAEPITHELIAL LESION.

low-risk group/individual A group or individual whose behavior does not put them at risk for exposure to the virus that causes AIDS. AIDS research to date indicates that low-risk groups include those who have not used intravenous drugs, those who have not been sexual partners of IV drug users or individuals who had or later developed AIDS, those with only one sex partner, and those who have not received blood transfusions.

low-risk sex Low-risk practices with some risk of HIV transmission include ANAL or VAGINAL SEX with proper use of an intact CONDOM; WET KISSING; and FELLATIO interruptus (contact with male genitals without ejaculation).

LPS See LYPOPOLYSACCHARIDE.

lube See LUBRICANT.

lubricant An agent, either artificial or natural, that reduces friction between parts that brush against each other as they move. In sexual activity, lubricants are used to lessen friction and add moisture during intercourse. Lubrication aids the insertion of penis, dildo, or fingers into an orifice.

Lubricants may be oil based or water based, and may or may not be made for the specific purpose. Oil-based lubricants include petroleum jelly, mineral oil, most hand creams, massage oil, baby oil, butter, and Crisco. Oil-based lubricants weaken latex and natural membrane fibers, so should not be used with condoms. Many condoms come with their own lubricant, a water-based gel or silicone, along with a spermicide.

lumbar puncture   A procedure in which a needle is inserted into the lumbar region of the spinal canal to obtain a sample of CEREBROSPINAL FLUID for examination. Also known as a SPINAL TAP.

lumbosacral polyradiculopathy   Any of a group of diseases affecting the nerve roots in the lumbar vertebrae and the sacrum (low back region).

lung inflammation   Pneumonia.

lupus anticoagulant   An acquired coagulation inhibitor first noticed in patients with systemic lupus erythematosus but since found in association with other immune disorders, including HIV. It is typically silent, meaning it does not effect illnesses at all, but it may on occasion, paradoxically, cause excessive clotting.

luteinizing hormone   A hormone, secreted by the anterior lobe of the hypophysis (the pituitary gland), that stimulates the development of the corpus luteum (the temporary endocrine gland formed from an ovarian follicle that has released an ovum; secretes progesterone and estrogen).

lymph   A clear fluid containing LYMPHOCYTES, or white blood cells (including CD4 CELLS), which are a part of the immune system. It differs from blood in that red blood corpuscles are absent and the protein content is lower. It also travels through the body in its own system of vessels. Osmotic pressure is slightly higher than in blood plasma; viscosity slightly less. Lymph may vary considerably in different parts of the body. Lymph is manufactured in the LYMPH GLANDS.

lymph gland   A clump of lymphatic tissue. Lymph glands are distributed widely throughout the body and are responsible for manufacturing lymph. Lymph glands near the surface of the skin can be felt as bumps below the skin's surface. The back of the neck, below the jaw, under the armpits, and the groin are the usual locations where lymph glands can be felt. Many infections involve the lymph glands, which are commonly swollen and sometimes painful and tender when infected. In HIV infection, swollen lymph glands are likely to occur in three circumstances: with persistent generalized LYMPHADENOPATHY, in which many lymph glands are swollen for months; with infection of the lymph glands by certain opportunistic diseases; and with LYMPHOMAS, which are tumors of the lymphatic system seen more frequently in people with HIV infection than in the general population. Swollen lymph glands may require diagnostic tests. The usual test is a biopsy of the lymph gland or removal of the whole gland to permit microscopic examination of the lymphatic tissue.

lymph nodule   A small, compact, densely staining mass of cells, each containing a lighter-staining central area in which lymphocytes are formed. They constitute the structural unit of lymphatic tissue. May occur singly, in groups (as in Peyer's patches) or in encapsulated organs as lymph nodes.

lymphadenopathy   A chronic condition of the lymph nodes and glands due to infection or cancer, in which the nodes enlarge, grow, and swell and may be palpable or visible from outside the body. Swollen LYMPH GLANDS, most common at the back of the neck, along the jaw, in the armpits, and in the groin, may feel like rubbery, discrete pea-sized nodules that are rarely tender to touch. Swollen glands occur in everyone, in conditions unrelated to HIV infection. However, lymphadenopathy is sometimes thought to be an early sign of infection with the virus associated with AIDS. If lymph glands are swollen to abnormal size for longer than a month in at least two different areas, they constitute persistent generalized lymphadenopathy.

lymphadenopathy syndrome (LAS) Also known as generalized lymphadenopathy syndrome, a condition characterized by persistent, generalized, enlarged LYMPH NODES (sometimes accompanied by signs of minor illness, such as fever and weight loss) and that apparently represents a milder reaction to infection with HTLV-III than full-blown AIDS. BIOPSY reveals nonspecific lymphoid hyperplasia. Some patients with LAS have gone on to develop full-blown AIDS. In others, LAS represents the height of clinical illness in reaction to infection with HTLV-III.

lymphadenopathy-associated virus (LAV) The name given by French researchers to the first reported isolate of the retrovirus now known to cause AIDS. This retrovirus was recovered from a person with lymphadenopathy (enlarged lymph nodes) who also was in a group at high risk for AIDS.

The French classified LAV as a lentivirus, a subgroup of slow-acting viruses that cause disease in horses, goats, and sheep but was not previously known to cause disease in humans and other primates. See HIV.

lymphatic system A circulatory system of vessels, spaces, and LYMPH NODES that fight infection.

lymphatic vessel One of a bodywide network of channels, similar to the blood vessels, that transports LYMPH to the LYMPHOID TISSUE and into the bloodstream.

lymphoblast An immature cell that gives rise to a LYMPHOCYTE.

lymphocyte A white blood cell that matures and resides in the lymphoid organs and is responsible for the acquired immune response. The two major types of lymphocytes are T CELLS and B CELLS. The acquired immune response is achieved by means of HUMORAL IMMUNITY produced by B cells and CELL-MEDIATED IMMUNITY produced by T cells. Lymphocytes originate in the BONE MARROW, pass through

the bloodstream and enter other organs, where they become modified to B or T lymphocytes. During infections B lymphocytes (bursa dependent) are transformed into plasma cells that produce antibodies to specific pathogens. This transformation occurs through interactions with various types of T cells and other components of the immune system. T lymphocytes (thymus dependent) are derived from the thymus and participate in a variety of cell-mediated immune reactions. Three fundamentally different types of T cells are recognized: helper, killer, and suppressor.

lymphocytic interstitial pneumonitis (LIP) An inflammation within the lungs that develops gradually and is characterized by infiltration of the lungs by LYMPHOCYTES, LYMPHOBLASTS, and PLASMA CELLS. LIP affects 35 percent to 40 percent of children with AIDS and causes hardening of the lung membranes involved in absorbing oxygen. LIP is an AIDS-defining illness in children. The cause is unknown, but it is often associated with a compromised immune system. Also called LYMPHOID INTERSTITIAL PNEUMONIA.

lymphogranuloma venereum (LGV) A tropical STD caused by the chlamydia trachomatis bacterium. Its most common presentation is inguinal lymphadenopathy.

lymphoid interstitial pneumonia See LYMPHOCYTIC INTERSTITIAL PNEUMONITIS.

lymphoid tissue The organs of the lymph system throughout the body, including the BONE MARROW, THYMUS, LYMPH NODES, SPLEEN, tonsils, PEYER'S PATCHES, and the lymphocyte aggregates on mucosal surfaces.

lymphokine One of a number of substances that act as mediators of cellular immunity, released by sensitized LYMPHOCYTES when they contact specific ANTIGENS. Lymphokines help to produce cellular immunity by stimulating MACROPHAGES and MONOCYTES. Included in this group of materials are INTERLEUKINS 1, 2, and 3; INTERFERON-GAMMA; TUMOR NECROSIS FACTOR; COLONY STIMULATING FACTOR; B-

CELL growth factor; LYMPHOTOXIN; migration inhibition factor; leukocyte migration inhibition factor; macrophage chemotactic factor; macrophage activating factor; lymphocyte mitogenic factor; soluble immune response suppressor; and T-CELL replacement factor.

lymphoma   A cancer of the cells responsible for normal immune function. Lymphoma occurs most frequently in people without HIV infection, but people with weakened immune systems, including those with HIV infection, have lymphomas about 40 times more frequently than normal. About one to three percent of people with AIDS have lymphomas, which are classified as opportunistic tumors. There are many types of lymphomas. Some progress extremely slowly, cause few symptoms, and require minimal treatment. Some are more severe, and symptoms may include LYMPH NODE swelling, weight loss, and fever. People with AIDS generally have lymphomas called NON-HODGKIN'S LYMPHOMAS, of B CELL origin. These lymphomas tend to be severe, and they also tend to involve unusual areas of the body like the brain, intestines, kidneys, and lungs. The diagnosis is usually established with a biopsy. Treatment is variable and often requires chemotherapy or radiation.

lymphopenia   Deficiency of LYMPHOCYTES in the blood.

lymphoproliferative disease   See LYMPHOPROLIFERATIVE DISORDER.

lymphoproliferative disorder   Any of a group of malignant neoplasms that involve LYMPHORETICULAR CELLS. Hodgkin's disease, lymphocytic lymphomas, multiple myeloma, and the histiocytic, lymphocytic, and monocytic lymphomas are included. Also called *lymphoproliferative disease* and *lymphoproliferative syndrome*.

lymphoproliferative response   A specific immune response that entails rapid T CELL replication. Standard ANTIGENS, such as tetanus toxoid, that elicit this response are used in lab tests of immune competence.

lymphoproliferative syndrome   See LYMPHOPROLIFERATIVE DISORDER.

lymphoreticular cell   Any reticuloendothelial cell of the lymph node.

lymphotoxin (LT or TNF-B)   A LYMPHOKINE that causes direct cytoloysis following its release from stimulated LYMPHOCYTES.

lymphotrophic   Having an affinity for lymphatic tissue. HUMAN IMMUNODEFICIENCY VIRUS and human T CELL leukemia virus are lymphotropic for CD4+ LYMPHOCYTES and EPSTEIN-BARR VIRUS is lymphotropic for B LYMPHOCYTES.

lysine   An amino acid that is a hydrolytic cleavage product of digested protein. It is essential for growth and repair of tissues.

lysis   The splitting and dissolution of cellular or viral material by chemical action.

lytic infection   Infection of a cell by a virus that results in the death of the cell. HIV infection of the T-helper lymphocytes is a lytic process.

MA See MEDICAL ASSISTANCE.

MAC See MYCOBACTERIUM AVIUM COMPLEX.

MAC disease See MYCOBACTERIUM AVIUM COMPLEX.

macaque A family of monkey species (i.e., rhesus, pigtail, and cynomolgus) often used in scientific research. Macaques can be infected with SIMIAN IMMUNODEFICIENCY VIRUS (SIV) and are used as an animal model for AIDS.

macrobiotics A way of life according to the macroscopic, or largest possible, view. Translated literally, *macro* is Greek for "large" or "great," and *bios* is the word for "life." The practice of macrobiotics involves understanding and applying this universal order of change to one's lifestyle, including the selection, preparation, and manner of eating food. The first principle in the selection and preparation of food is to eat unrefined cereal grains and cooked vegetables as the main foods. A second principle is to eat in accordance with the immediate environment, specifically the climatic conditions in which one lives. Within a particular climate, various seasonal changes are experienced, and diet should vary accordingly, primarily using foods that are either naturally available during a particular season or can be naturally stored. The fourth principle of macrobiotic eating is modifying the diet to suit individual differences.

A macrobiotic diet is also based on the belief that there is a yin/yang quality of all foods. For example, it is believed that animal foods exert a yang, or contractive, influence and vegetables produce a more yin, or expansive, influence. External factors, such as pressure, fire, salt, and time (aging), produce a more contractive influence, whereas less pressure,

water, oil, and freshness (less time) result in expansion. For example, within the vegetable kingdom, a vegetable's size, direction of growth, color, juiciness, firmness, and chemical composition affect its yin/yang. Indeed, all foods, not only vegetables, can be classified into yin/yang. In order to reflect the over-all order of biological evolution in eating, as well as to maintain a proper yin/yang balance, the macrobiotic diet calls for approximately 50 percent of one's daily food to be unrefined cereal grains. In fact, following the macrobiotic regime to its highest level has been interpreted to mean eating a 100-percent cereal diet.

A macrobiotic diet is a radical departure from the dietary customs of the Western world. Proponents of this lifestyle argue that such a diet of natural foods, cooked in accordance with macrobiotic principles, can promote health and minimize disease. Some supporters claim that a macrobiotic diet is an effective primary treatment for cancer. Others claim that it can be effective when combined with other forms of treatment. Critics caution that macrobiotic diets are hazardous because they are both nutritionally unbalanced and restrictive, excluding nearly everything but grains. The American Medical Association, the Food and Drug Administration, and many nutrition experts say that a macrobiotic diet can be harmful. The National Cancer Institute and the American Cancer Society believe that strict adherence to it poses a serious health hazard and that it is not effective in preventing or treating cancer. They further claim that there is no scientific evidence supporting its use, either alone or combined with standard cancer treatment.

macrocytic anemia Anemia marked by abnormally large erythrocytes. There are multiple causes for large red blood cells. For reasons unknown AZT produces larger than normal red blood cells; D4T produces the same phenomenon.

macrophage   A WHITE BLOOD CELL that internalizes, swallows up, ANTIGENS and attempts to destroy them. If destruction of the antigen is not possible, then macrophages process the antigen and present it to the CD4 CELLS that will normally kill it. There are different types of macrophages in different parts of the body. Examples of macrophages include MICROGLIAL cells, which are located in the brain; LANGERHANS cells, which are located in the skin, and Kupffer cells, which are located in the liver. Precursor cells that grow into macrophages are found in the blood and are called MONOCYTES.

Macrophages generally do not live long. There are new ones being created almost continuously from the bone marrow and the blood. They migrate to the various tissues and typically do not divide and replicate themselves. They live a few weeks and then die. Microglial cells are an exception, often living for extended periods instead of merely a few weeks. Scientists are still unsure if some may live, in the brain, the entire life of the human. The job they serve is to move about the tissues and collect cellular waste, antigens, and other cellular debris. They also clean up dying red blood cells in parts of the body that these reside.

Once the macrophage has encountered an antigen, in this case an HIV VIRION, it will secrete CYTOKINES that signal B and T CELLS to come to that location and fight the particular antigen. They can also secrete proteins that stimulate fever to reduce growth of various bacteria or other healing responses that encourage new cellular growth.

When a patient takes HAART, the typical reaction in cells is that the virus is killed, because it cannot reproduce, and the CD4 cells kill the remaining virus. In macrophages this does not seem to happen. The virus seems to use the macrophage as a place to rest until the opportunity arises to begin infecting cells again. This is what is referred to as viral RESERVOIRS. Because macrophages travel across the body's systems and tissues, macrophages are now known to be the way the virus transports itself to places such as the brain and liver. This makes them very effective transporters of HIV and other viruses.

HIV is now known to require both CD4 antigen and coreceptors CXCR4 or CCR5 for entry into cells. Both of these chemokine receptors are found on macrophages, as well as T cells. Macrophages also display the CD4 antigen. The CD4 proteins bind to the virus and complete binding when the coreceptors are present. This allows the macrophages to quickly become infected and allows the virus to begin inserting it's RNA into cellular DNA. Researchers are looking extensively into finding agents that will block this initial entry into the cell. These agents are called ENTRY INHIBITORS.

Macrophages are also a fundamental cause of atherosclerotic plaque. It is now believed by researchers that inflammation of any type, even simple cell death causes the macrophages and other blood cells to congregate. These cells then secrete many healing proteins, causing inflammation and eventually building up tissue to repair the injury. In turn, a cycle of inflammation, destruction, and repair goes on, allowing small buildups of fat and tissue. This then allows cholesterol and other cells to attach themselves—causing blockages. Agents such as aspirin reduce the inflammation that, in turn, keeps the macrophages away and the cholesterol and platelets from building up in the veins and arteries. This is a simplified description, and science is just beginning to understand this process.

macrophage inflammatory protein-1 alpha and beta (MIP-1a and MIP-1b)   These proteins are chemokines that bind to the CCR5 receptor site and interfere with HIV's fusion with uninfected cells.

macrophage-tropic (M-tropic)   Characteristic of strains of HIV that have an affinity for infecting macrophages as well as CD4 cells. When entering new cells, M-tropic HIV usually binds to the CCR5 receptor in addition to the CD4 receptor. This type of HIV is generally a non-syncytia-inducing (NSI) virus; it is the type of HIV that is transmitted sexually and is generally predominant until late-stage disease.

MACS   See MULTICENTER AIDS COHORT STUDY.

macula   The pigmented central area or "yellow spot" of the retina, adjacent to the optic nerve. It is the most sensitive area of the retina and contains the fovea, the region responsible for detailed central vision.

magic bullet   A hypothetical, hoped-for single drug that can knock out a particular malignancy or other disorder without toxicity.

magnetic resonance imaging (MRI)   A noninvasive, non-X-ray diagnostic technique that produces images of the interior of the body using powerful electromagnets, radio waves, and a computer; formerly known as nuclear magnetic resonance, MRI is used, along with other procedures, in the diagnosis and evaluation of disease and disorder and to monitor for their recurrence. MRI may be done in conjunction with a CT (computerized tomography) SCAN and/or ultrasound. It can produce clear three-dimensional images of blood vessels, blood flow, cartilage, BONE MARROW, muscles, ligaments, cerebrospinal fluid and the spinal cord. MRI is somewhat different from a CT scan. The person undergoing MRI is placed inside a large tubular structure and remains motionless for a lengthy period of time (approximately 30 minutes to an hour). During that time, her body is bathed in a magnetic field, which causes the atoms in different tissues to give off tiny radio signals. The signals are different depending on the kind of tissue.

An MRI is better than a CT scan at detecting diseases of the brain and spinal cord. An expensive technique, MRI is painless, harmless, and does not involve exposure to ionizing radiation. Nor is there a need, as in radiological (X-ray) imaging, to inject a radiopaque contrast medium such as barium sulfate to provide a visual contrast between the tissue or organ being filmed and the surrounding tissue. MRI may not be suitable for people with heart pacemakers, joint pins, surgical metal clips, artificial heart valves, IUDs, shrapnel, or any other electronic or metal implants.

MRIs may induce feelings of claustrophobia; if such occurs, a minor tranquilizer such as an antianxiety drug may be prescribed to help calm an individual before the procedure.

MAI   See MYCOBACTERIUM AVIUM COMPLEX.

MAI infections   See MYCOBACTERIUM AVIUM COMPLEX.

mail-order pharmacies   A source for filling prescriptions by mail to reduce costs. Mail-order pharmacies are high-volume operations which can locate where costs are low and can negotiate good prices from suppliers. They compete with each other primarily on price because location doesn't matter, whereas traditional corner drugstores have a captive market. They usually, but not always, have the lowest prices available. Shopping around is therefore recommended. Patients can get price and other information over the phone.

If patients can pay by credit card or if the prescription is fully paid by insurance, physicians usually can call in the prescriptions, avoiding the need to wait for the mail. Most drugs are sent by two-day express, unless overnight delivery is necessary. Drugs which need to be refrigerated are shipped overnight in insulated containers. Delivery can be to a separate address, so that nobody needs to stay home to receive the medicines. The pharmacies generally bill insurance directly and handle the paperwork. Some mail-order pharmacies require full payment from the patient, with the insurance company reimbursing the patient for the percentage it pays—a process which can take months. Filling prescriptions is usually a solitary or personal activity, one which patients seldom talk about. For some people, ordering prescriptions by mail meets important needs of privacy and convenience. Local pharmacies, unlike mail-order pharmacies, provide both a place where individuals can develop a working relationship with their pharmacist or physician, and a place for in-person discussion of drugs and drug interactions.

Mail-order pharmacies exist serving both regional and national audiences. Some mail-order pharmacies specialize in serving HIV-infected people and offer supplementary educational materials. Some accept 80 percent payment from insurers as "payment in full" and sell other products at a discount.

mainstream treatment/therapy   Use of drugs that are standard therapy for a given condition, typically those that have been approved by the Food and Drug Administration (FDA) and are prescribed by doctors for a specific indication.

maintenance therapy   Extended drug therapy, usually at a diminished dose, administered after a disease has been brought under control; also called *continuation therapy.* Maintenance therapy is utilized when a complete cure is not possible and the disease is likely to recur if therapy is halted. Maintenance therapy is generally given for a fixed amount of time and then stopped.

major histocompatibility complex (MHC)   A group of genes that code for Human Leukocyte Antigens (HLA) (markers on the surface of cells for the differentiation of self from nonself). MHC consists of either of two classes of molecules on cell surfaces. MHC class I molecules exist on all cells and hold and present foreign ANTIGENS to CD8 CYTOTOXIC T-LYMPHOCYTES if the cell is infected by a virus or other microbe. MHC class II molecules are found on the immune system's antigen presenting cells and display antigen to activate CD4 T-HELPER CELLS.

major medical insurance   Insurance that covers expenses for most serious medical conditions, up to a maximum limit, usually after deductible and coinsurance provisions have been met. These policies usually complement hospital-medical-surgical coverages.

malabsorption   Faulty or incomplete absorption of nutrients in the intestines.
   Cells in the gastrointestinal (GI) tract are particularly prone to damage during HIV infection, and this results in reduced absorption of nutrients. The HIV virus itself, intestinal parasites, and COLITIS induced by CYTOMEGALOVIRUS (CMV) are the main sources of tissue damage. The diarrhea connected with these conditions may also result in malabsorption. Fat, carbohydrate, protein, and micronutrient (vitamin and mineral) malabsorption can occur. Malabsorption may also be present before infection with HIV. Infection by intestinal parasites triggers diarrhea and malabsorption in persons with AIDS by causing atrophy of the villi, the small threadlike projections (on the interior of the small intestines) that absorb nutrients when working properly. The protozoan CRYPTOSPORIDIUM *parvum,* the most commonly identified parasite in people with AIDS, causes massive secretory diarrhea.

MICROSPORIDIA (*Enterocytozoon bieneusi* or *Septata intestinalis*) is a second common GI parasite in people with AIDS. Infection can cause diarrhea and decreased intestinal absorption.

malabsorption syndrome   Decreased intestinal absorption resulting in loss of appetite, muscle pain, and weight loss.

malaise   A vague feeling of discomfort or uneasiness, often the result of infection or a drug's side effects.

malaria   One of the most widespread infectious diseases in the world, malaria is an acute and sometimes chronic disorder caused by the presence of protozoan parasites within the red blood cells. Malaria is transmitted to the human by the bite of an infected female Anopheles mosquito. The mosquito becomes infected by ingesting the blood of a human infected with malaria. Chloroquine and mefloquine, the medications that prevent malaria, do not interact with medications commonly prescribed for HIV-related indications. Despite prophylaxis, certain forms of malaria can occur weeks to months after an individual has left a malaria-infested area. Fever is the prominent symptom, and a simple blood test determines the diagnosis. Chloroquine phosphate is prescribed for all types of malaria except those due to drug-resistant *Plasmodium falciparum.* In drug-resistant *P. falciparum,* treatment with combinations of quinine, pyrimethamine, and a sulfonamide is indicated. Malaria due to other species should be treated with both chloroquine and primaquine. Severe malaria due to *P. falciparum* with evidence of cerebral involvement may be treated with continuous infusion of quinidine gluconate and exchange transfusion.
   Similarities and differences between malaria and HIV bear noting. Like HIV, malaria kills millions of people each year and is a scourge of developing nations in Africa, India, Southeast Asia, and South America. Most people who contract malaria or HIV are poor. Whereas HIV is pandemic, spread from person to person by sexual contact in an increasingly mobile world, malaria is endemic, dependent on a local symbiosis between infected

anopheline mosquitoes and humans. The severe symptoms of malaria caused by *P. falciparum* appear within days and cause the death of about 15 percent to 25 percent of those stricken when great quantities of infected red blood cells are destroyed in a single burst. HIV infection is a slow, insidious process that can take years to deplete immunologically crucial white blood cells. AIDS results in death for nearly all patients. Both diseases can be transmitted by contaminated blood. In the 1980s, some partially blamed the initial spread of HIV in Africa on the transfusion of infected blood to treat malaria-associated anemia. The infection rates of both diseases can be reduced by behavior changes, barrier protection (condoms or bed nets), and medical prophylaxis. Vaccine development for both diseases has been slow. But malaria can often be treated and cured with an inexpensive week-long course of drugs, whereas current HIV treatment is a lifelong process of daily medication at costs that have so far limited their use in developing countries.

Because of shared geographic and demographic characteristics, coinfection is common, yet to date few obvious clinical associations between HIV and malaria are reported. Studies are contradictory about the frequency and severity of malaria in HIV-infected people. Malaria does not appear to act as a classic opportunist in immune-compromised hosts. People who have grown up in endemic regions often retain partial immunity to malaria, and there is no solid evidence to date that this immunity is lost as HIV disease progresses.

The two diseases critically intersect in the bodies of pregnant women. In parts of Africa, severe anemia during pregnancy can be caused by nutritional deficits, hookworm, malaria, or HIV disease. Asymptomatic malaria can exacerbate the common mild anemia of pregnancy, and recrudescence of malaria may be more frequent because of the immune suppression normally experienced by pregnant women. Falciparum malaria episodes are associated with low birth weight, fetal distress, premature labor, and an increased number of stillbirths, miscarriages, and neonatal deaths. Placental malaria may be associated with an increased frequency of mother-to-child HIV transmission. Acute falciparum malaria during pregnancy is a particularly dangerous condition, since any underlying anemia can be dramatically amplified by red

blood cell destruction. More commonly, however, malaria is asymptomatic during pregnancy and not always easily diagnosed. Research has shown that even such subacute malaria can contribute to anemia and placental infection; the role of HIV in this complex has been documented. A heightened risk of HIV transmission with placental malaria could be the result of one or more factors. There may be a disruption of the placental cellular architecture that allows an intermingling of maternal and fetal blood. Another mechanism might be that placental malaria stimulates a local increase of HIV-infected macrophages and other lymphocytes, and these increase the risk of viral transmission. Or placental malaria may simply be a consequence of advanced HIV infection and higher viral load, which is itself associated with mother-to-child transmission.

To summarize, findings suggest that women with HIV are at greater risk of contracting malaria during pregnancy—a condition that increases the risk of the baby's contracting malaria or of passing HIV to the child. Prophylactic treatment lowers the incidence of subacute and placental malaria. It can improve the health of the mother and child and reduce the risk of placental transmission of both malaria and HIV.

The degree to which first- and second-line malaria treatments affect HIV has not yet been definitively established. Similarly, the mechanisms used by the immune system to fight malaria are not fully understood, although it is clear that both humoral immunity and cell-mediated immunity are involved and that various T-cell subsets are important for regulating the immune response. HIV too has an intricate relationship with the immune system, and it appears that there may be several points of intersection between the pathogenesis and the response to each disease. Some have suggested that the malarial antigens and pigments released during the burst of red blood cells stimulate cytokines that can activate HIV replication. A connection between HIV and malaria may exist in the way the immune system responds to certain similar molecular features on their structural proteins. With regard to the immunological connection between the two diseases, some have proposed that the immune response to malaria can increase the pool of lymphocytes available for HIV infection, resulting in accelerated progression to AIDS. Whether this actually occurs is, to date, not known.

male homosexual   A man whose primary erotic and emotional interests are in other men.

male-to-female transmission   See TRANSMISSION.

male-to-male transmission   See TRANSMISSION.

malignancy   A cancerous tumor or neoplasm.

malignant   Evil, malicious; in medicine, life-threatening. When used in a medical setting, it means "cancerous" and commonly refers to a cancerous tumor, as distinct from a benign tumor. The main characteristic of a malignant tumor is that it is likely to penetrate the tissues or organ in which it originated as well as move to other sites (metastasize), eventually causing death.

malnutrition   Any disorder of nutrition; specifically, either the deficit of efficient or substantive food substances in the body or the inability of the body to properly absorb food substances. Physical signs of malnutrition and deficiency state in adolescents and adults include nasolabial sebaceous plugs; sores at the corners of the mouth; Vincent's angina; red, swollen lingual papillae; glossitis; papillary atrophy of tongue; stomatitis; spongy, bleeding gums; muscle tenderness in extremities; poor muscle tone; loss of vibratory sensation; increase or decrease of tendon reflexes; hyperesthesia of skin; bilateral symmetrical dermatitis; purpura; dermatitis; thickening and pigmentation of skin over bony prominences; nonspecific vaginitis; follicular hyperkeratosis of extensor surfaces of extremities; rachitic chest deformity; anemia not responding to iron; fatigue of visual accommodation; vascularization of cornea; and conjunctival changes.

The word *malnutrition* often conjures up images of emaciated people who do not have regular meals. However, the medical application of the word is more subtle. Most people with HIV disease do not know they are malnourished, since malnutrition is specific to the absence of vitamins and minerals essential to healthy body function. Research has shown that nutrient deficiencies begin very early in HIV infection and have a significant influence on how well the immune system functions and how quickly HIV disease progresses.

Malnutrition in AIDS can result from many different factors. Inability to take in a proper amount of nutrients can be the result of impaired swallowing and taste due to infections in the mouth or the esophagus, AIDS medications that have anorexia, nausea, and vomiting as side effects, or limited financial resources that make three meals a day difficult to manage. Diarrhea and changes in absorption caused by bacteria, viruses, or parasites may impair nutritional intake. Some medications, particularly antibiotics, may change the normal bacterial composition of the intestine and interfere with breakdown of food. Finally, an increase in metabolism often occurs in many people with HIV and leads to an increased need for nutrients. The presence of HIV itself as well as some of its associated infections can increase the metabolic rate. These three factors—diminished intake, malabsorption, and hypermetabolism—usually occur simultaneously to deplete the body of nutrients.

It has long been known that malnourished individuals are at higher risk for infectious disease as a result of their inadequate immune response. Infection then leads to inflammation and worsening nutritional status, which further compromises the immune system. This has been called the "vicious cycle." The outcomes of certain infectious diseases, including HIV and tuberculosis, are worse when the host is malnourished. Protein-calorie malnutrition has a significant negative effect on various components of the immune system. Studies have shown decreased function of organs (thymus, spleen, lymph nodes) of the immune system in malnourished humans. The branch of the immune system that produces antibodies is depressed in malnutrition: specifically, the number of circulating B cells and antibody responses decrease. Malnourished humans also exhibit decreased CD4+ and CD8+ T-cell counts, and the cells have less ability to multiply or respond to infectious organisms such as viruses that live inside them. Other mechanisms that kill infectious organisms are also depressed in malnutrition. The function of CYTOKINES, chemicals that act as cell messengers, is altered in malnourished individuals. Replenishment of calories and protein is difficult but essential intervention for people living with HIV/AIDS to mount the most effective immune response possible to fight OPPORTUNISTIC INFECTIONS.

In addition to a balanced diet, vitamin therapy and vitamin and mineral megadosing have been used to treat malnutrition. Multivitamins are generally preferred over individual vitamins because of lower cost and lower risk of toxicity, and because single-nutrient deficiencies are unusual. Despite the high cost and time involved, megadosing has been effective for many people; studies have demonstrated heightened immune function when supplements are given at several times the United States Recommended Daily Allowance (RDA). Caution should be exercised since toxic effects are possible when vitamins and minerals are used improperly. Generally, people with HIV/AIDS are advised to consult with a trained professional and a doctor before changing treatment regimens and to inform all health care providers when making significant alterations in their diets. It is also important to note that not all trained nutritionists subscribe to various regimens.

malpractice   Incorrect or negligent treatment of a patient by professionals responsible for health care, such as dentists, nurses, or physicians.

MALT   See MUCOSA-ASSOCIATED LYMPHOID TISSUE.

mammography   The use of radiography to diagnose breast cancer. This technique has increased the rate of early detection. Mammography is capable of detecting 85 percent to 90 percent of existing breast cancers.

The American Cancer Society (ACS) and the National Cancer Institute (NCI) delivered their recommendations on mammography for women in their 40s, even though the National Institutes of Health Consensus Development Panel abstained from doing so. Both advise regular mammograms for women in this age group (the ACS, annually; the NCI, every one to two years). Women who are in this age group and who have decided to have regular mammograms are advised to have an annual screening. Breast cancer tends to develop more rapidly in younger women, and having a mammography every year increases the likelihood of catching early-stage tumors. Use of mammography as a diagnostic tool does not mean that careful, periodic clinical (physical) examinations should be omitted. Similarly, use of mammography as a diagnostic tool does not mean that self-examination should be omitted. The benefits to the self exam include its convenience, cost (it is free) and the fact that it is without physical risk. There is another benefit to the self exam. A women is likely to have more time for a careful examination than her clinician does. Given the limitations of the office visit under MANAGED CARE, many clinicians simply cannot devote several minutes to a routine breast examination. A woman who has examined her own breasts for years is likely to have a better idea of what is abnormal for her as each monthly exam gives her more information about the structure of her breasts.

Note that gynecologic problems are common among HIV-positive women and are frequently present at the time of initial evaluation and care. Some gynecologic issues are unrelated to the patient's serologic status, whereas others are directly related to HIV disease and associated with immunosuppression. Still others are associated epidemiologically with HIV because of common risk factors, such as sexual behavior or substance abuse. To date, breast cancer has not been related to HIV disease, associated with immunosuppression, or associated epidemiologically with HIV. Nonetheless, along with routine gynecologic evaluations, Pap smears, STD screening, and sigmoidoscopy/colonoscopy, routine mammography is one of the core components of a sound health maintenance program for women.

managed care   The goal of containing costs by coordinating care through a gatekeeper, or general practitioner who decides on all referrals. Employers increasingly are choosing managed care plans to cut costs even though such plans have traditionally been reluctant to cover "high risk" groups such as people with HIV. HIV-positive beneficiaries should educate themselves on the services provided by each plan. Some features that are left out may be important in managing HIV infection, including mental health and substance abuse coverage. It is also advisable to ascertain which medications, nutritional supports, and alternative treatments are in the plan's formulary, as some therapies have been "carved out" from the program, and to determine the HIV expertise of the network or health maintenance organization physicians. A plan's complaint and grievance procedures also are important should needed services be denied.

Patients insured under the MEDICAID or MEDICARE programs also are experiencing a growing shift toward mandatory managed care plans, although many state Medicaid programs have little experience providing HIV care under this new type of system. Managed care presents particular problems for both HIV specialists and HIV/AIDS care. First, most persons with HIV/AIDS, even if they are treated initially by a primary care physician, eventually become the patients of an AIDS specialist. Studies have demonstrated that experience of primary care physicians in the management of AIDS is significantly associated with survival of their patients. One of the hallmarks of managed care is the gatekeeping function of the primary care physician; referrals to specialists are closely monitored and often reluctantly granted. The supply of primary care physicians is inadequate, and many of those already in practice are not trained in state-of-the-art HIV/AIDS management. Limiting the choice of primary health care providers to doctors who have agreed with health maintenance organizations to charge less but who have little or no experience treating AIDS patients may decrease quality of care. Furthermore, state-of-the-art AIDS care must include the treatment to many different groups of people, types of conditions, and co-morbidities, such as substance abuse, tuberculosis, sexually transmitted diseases, and others.

A second issue, somewhat related to the first, is that the HIV specialist is being squeezed by managed care. Often, the HIV specialist is not considered as primary care so that patients can be kept out of health plans. HIV specialists have long recognized that delivering comprehensive, coordinated high-quality care costs more up front but saves on big ticket items, including hospitals and emergency room services.

A third issue arises in the access to investigational protocols or alternative therapies, including natural and alternative medicines. Payer con-

straints severely and adversely influence what treatments are possible for their patients. Managed care organizations are not the ideal environments to support or accept either investigational protocols or alternative therapies. They are not even ideally suited to adapt rapidly to changing standards of care, which happen frequently in AIDS care. Yet, there are forms of care that are important to patients and physicians. The earliest gains in speeding up the drug approval process and in broadening the inclusion criteria for clinical trials may have little effect in a managed care setting that reacts slowly and cautiously to change, especially to financial change.

Fourth, managed care plans may limit, contractually or in practice, access to beneficial but expensive treatments, or to such relatively routine decisions as emergency hospital admission. The appeal process may be slow or unresponsive, while the patient's needs are urgent. Providers may have financial disincentives to offer such care, and real incentives, such as bonuses, to deny it.

Fifth, and in a related vein, managed care plans may limit, contractually or in practice, reimbursement for "offlabel" prescriptions. Managed care has prior authorization and restricted formularies. HIV/AIDS specialists often prescribe drugs for indications that are not officially approved, mostly for treatment and prevention of opportunistic infections. Although such usage frequently reflects the standard of care, third-party payers often deny reimbursement for these prescriptions. When faced with such obstacles, many patients will receive less effective, albeit covered, therapies or be hospitalized to gain access to the preferred therapy.

management trials Part of the drug development process that integrates multiple trials, such as the MAPS (Master Antiretroviral Protocol Strategy) proposal from the COMMUNITY PROGRAMS FOR CLINICAL RESEARCH ON AIDS (CPCRA) or the SMART (Standardized Master Antiretroviral Trial) concept from CPCRA. In contrast to the prevailing trial methods, with restraints on eligibility, concomitant medications, and clinical management, management trials cultivate diversity of clinical management. Management trials incorporate the heterogeneity of the HIV population and ask "What is the effect of starting this treatment now, rather than another time—or never?" They do not presume that people can be assigned to a treatment or placebo and remain on it like lab rats.

mandatory reporting A legal requirement for a physician to inform health authorities when a specified illness is diagnosed. Reporting of AIDS is mandatory in all 50 states, and it has been proposed that the requirement be extended to HIV infection.

mandatory testing Medical testing that is legally required. In the case of AIDS, some government agencies do have mandatory testing policies. For example, before enrollment in the Job Corps, the Peace Corps, or the military, applicants are required to take a blood test. The Immigration and Naturalization Service, which regulates immigration and the entry of noncitizens into the United States, requires all potential immigrants to take a blood test. An infected person wishing to visit the United States may receive a waiver that allows him or her to travel here for 30 days.

mange A skin disease in mammals characterized by itching, lesions, scabs, and loss of hair caused by parasitic mites. Mange is a communicable disease occurring in various animals, including dogs, cats, cattle, horses, sheep, rabbits, rats, and some birds. The causative agent is any of several mange mites, including *Chorioptes, Demodex, Psoroptes,* and *Sarcoptes.* In humans, this condition is known as scabies.

mange mite Any of the various mites that cause mange.

mania Any mental disorder, especially when characterized by violent, unrestrained behavior. When used as a suffix, a morbid preference for or an irrepressible impulse to behave in a certain way. The term also refers to one of the two major forms of manic depressive illness. The manic form of manic-depressive psychosis is characterized by an elated or euphoric, although unstable, mood; increased psychomotor activity, restlessness, agitation, etc.; and increase in number of ideas and speed of thinking and speaking, in which in more severe forms proceed to flight of ideas (rapid shift-

ing from one topic to another), often with a grandiose trend. In mania, the following disturbances in the ideational sphere may be present: overproductivity, flight of ideas, distractibility, leveling of ideas (essentially all topics have about the same value to the patient), ideas of importance and/or grandiose ideas (the patient expressing delusions of greatness perhaps in all fields), and feelings of well-being in the sphere of physical excellence. In mania, the following may be present in the emotional field: exaggerated feelings of gaiety, well-being, and extreme happiness—in consonance with the ideas expressed.

manicure A cosmetic treatment of the hands or fingernails, especially the cleaning, trimming, and polishing of the nails and the removal of cuticle. Because HIV is transmitted via blood, manicurists and their clients constitute a group at potential risk for HIV infection. Exposure to small cuts and abrasions that may develop during a manicure, or that existed before, may lead to HIV infection. However, the risk is not considered high. See TRANSMISSION.

manifestation An outward sign that an illness is present—a symptom or condition.

man-to-man transmission See TRANSMISSION.

Mantoux method An old test for tuberculosis (after Charles Mantoux, a French physician, 1877–1947); also called the Mantoux test. It consists of an intracutaneous injection of one-tenth ml of intermediate strength PURIFIED PROTEIN DERIVATIVE (PPD).

man-to-woman transmission See TRANSMISSION.

manual-vaginal intercourse See VAGINAL-MANUAL INTERCOURSE.

MAO inhibitors See MONOAMINE OXIDASE INHIBITORS.

MAOI See MONOAMINE OXIDASE INHIBITORS.

MAP-30 See BITTER MELON.

Marburg virus   A disease caused by a virus classed as a member of the family Filoviridae. Clinically, it is identical to that caused by the EBOLA VIRUS.

marijuana   The dried flowering tops and leaves of the hemp plant *(Cannabis sativa)*. Marijuana may be consumed by eating or smoking; smoked, it is an intoxicant—possibly the most widely used, after alcohol—and an illegal drug. Marijuana and its constituents or derivatives may be useful in the treatment of acute glaucoma and control of the severe nausea and vomiting caused by cancer chemotherapy. The psychoactive constituent of marijuana is DELTA-9-TETRAHYDROCANNABINOL (THC). Synthetic THC, DRONABINOL, is approved for use as an antiemetic in treating cancer. Many people with AIDS contend that smoking marijuana is more convenient and useful than swallowing dronabinol. In addition, studies have reported that cannabidiol, the precursor of THC and one of the noripsychoactive components of marijuana, reduces blood levels of the immune modulators TNF and IL-1, and that this effect may moderate the basic wasting process.

Health risks related to the use of medical marijuana, excluding risks related to smoking, include both short- and long-term effects of marijuana. Acute marijuana use diminishes psychomotor performance; therefore, for example, driving a car is not advisable while under the influence. There may also be short immunosuppressive effects. For many persons, chronic THC use may involve psychological dependence. Risk factors include antisocial personality and conduct disorders, which are risk factors for other forms of substance abuse as well. Finally, smoking in general is associated with abnormal changes in respiratory cells and tissue and with increased risk for cancer, lung disease, and poor pregnancy outcome.

In 1999, the Institute of Medicine completed its review of evidence concerning marijuana's potential benefits and risks for medical use. Its report was published in the aftermath of voter referenda that supported the legalization of marijuana as medicine in California and Arizona and five other states. The institute's conclusions marked another step forward in marijuana's acceptance for such uses as suppression of nausea, relief from pain, and stimulation of appetite in people with HIV or AIDS.

The 250-page report, "Marijuana and Medicine: Assessing the Science Base," can be ordered over the Internet at www.nap.edu, the National Academy Press website.

Marinol   See DRONABINOL.

masochism   The deriving of pleasure from receiving physical and/or psychological pain.

mass media disease   Many hold that AIDS is the first international mass media disease. Throughout the world, more people have learned about AIDS from radio, television, and the press than from personal contacts with health professionals. Although there has been considerable criticism of the media's coverage of AIDS, virtually every treatment of AIDS in the mass media has in fact been a first. Although other sexually transmitted diseases remain relatively taboo as mass media topics, AIDS has been discussed extensively.

News coverage of AIDS has concentrated on new information released by scientists, on human interest stories, and on controversies rather than prevention. Journalists tend to focus on coverage that attracts large audiences. As different media compete to release information that appears to be new or controversial, relatively little press and broadcast space is devoted to detailed analysis or to the natural history of the disease, and even less on education and prevention specific strategies. Many countries have organized national information/education campaigns on AIDS, because efforts to curb the epidemic cannot rely solely on news media, whose coverage of AIDS has been slow, erratic, and focused on new and unusual events. Today it is safe to say that the mass media are gradually becoming more effective channels for AIDS education. At the same time, however, government resources and political motivation for mass media education campaigns are becoming constrained.

massage   Manipulation, methodical pressure, friction, and kneading of the body. Types of massage include introductory (massage consisting of centripetal strokings around the affected part), local (massage confined to particular parts), tremolo (a type of mechanical massage), vapor (treatment of a cavity by a medicated and nebulized vapor under interrupted pressure), or vibratory (massage by rapidly repeated tapping of the affected surface by means of a vibrating hammer or sound). Caressing and stroking of the body may also be done for sensual enjoyment or relaxation. Touching, massaging, hugging, and stroking are considered to be practices with probably no risk of HIV transmission.

massage therapy   This is a general term for a range of therapeutic approaches with roots in both Eastern and Western cultures. It involves the practice of kneading or otherwise manipulating a person's muscles and other soft tissue with the intent of improving a person's well-being or health.

mast cell   A cell resident in connective tissue just below epithelial surfaces, serous cavities, and around blood vessels, including those in bone marrow. They synthesize and store histamines. When stimulated, they release mediators of inflammation. They are also important in producing the signs and symptoms of immediate hypersensitivity reactions (e.g., drug anaphylaxis, urticaria, insect stings, allergic reactions, and certain forms of asthma).

mastitis   Inflammation or infection of the breast or mammary gland. It is most common in women during lactation but may occur at any age.

mastoiditis   Inflammation or infection of the air cells of the nipple-shaped portion of the temporal bone (mastoid process), located behind the ear.

masturbation   The purposeful stimulation of one's genitals, or other erogenous zones, to produce sexual pleasure, sexual excitement, and/or orgasm. It is usually thought of as an activity one practices alone, but it can be done to a partner or to oneself in the presence of others. Self-masturbation and masturbation of a partner (if there are no cuts on the hands of either partner) are considered to be practices with probably no risk of HIV transmission.

matching placebo   A pill (capsule or tablet) that is designed to resemble in shape, texture, size, taste,

and other characteristic, a therapeutically active drug and that is used as the control treatment.

maternofetal transmission   See TRANSMISSION.

maximum tolerated dose   The largest dose of a drug a patient can consume without unacceptable adverse side effects.

MDMA   Also known as ecstasy or X. It's chemical name is 3, 4-methylenedioxymethamphetamine. It is an illegal psychoactive drug that has both hallucinogenic and stimulant properties. It is known to interact with several PROTEASE INHIBITORS, causing an increase of MDMA in the body. This increase can quickly cause overdoses, which could lead to death. MDMA is taken orally, usually in tablet or capsule form, and its effects last approximately four to six hours. Users of the drug say that it produces profoundly positive feelings, empathy for others, elimination of anxiety, and extreme relaxation. MDMA is also said to suppress the need to eat, drink, or sleep, enabling users to endure two- to three-day parties. Consequently, MDMA use sometimes results in severe dehydration or exhaustion. MDMA users also report aftereffects of anxiety, paranoia, and depression. An MDMA overdose is characterized by high blood pressure, faintness, panic attacks, and, in more severe cases, loss of consciousness, seizures, and a drastic rise (or fall) in body temperature. Since MDMA is only made and sold illegally, some manufacturers sell substances other than MDMA that are easier to make since their chemical precursors are not illegal to possess.

MDMA was unsuccessfully developed as a weight-loss pill by a German drug company in 1912. The drug remained obscure and forgotten until its psychedelic properties were rediscovered in the 1960s. MDMA emerged fully into public view in the late 1970s and early 1980s when a group of psychotherapists openly advocated its use as an adjunct to therapy, and underground chemists began producing it for recreational users. Its possession, distribution, and manufacture were criminalized in 1985 by the Drug Enforcement Agency (DEA). The DEA classifies ecstasy as a Schedule I drug, which means that it has no medical use and a high potential for abuse.

MDR-TB   See MULTIDRUG-RESISTANT TUBERCULOSIS.

mean   The arithmetic average or the sum of all the values divided by the number of values.

"me too" drug   An informal term used to describe a drug that offers little or no benefit over a similar drug that has already been approved by the U.S. FOOD AND DRUG ADMINISTRATION (FDA).

measles   A highly communicable disease caused by the rubeola virus and characterized by fever, general malaise, sneezing, nasal congestion, brassy cough, conjunctivitis, spots on the buccal mucosa, and a maculopapular eruption over the entire body. It is most common in school-age children. An attack of measles almost invariably confers permanent immunity. Active immunization can be produced by administration of measles vaccine. Passive immunization is afforded by administration of GAMMA GLOBULIN. Pregnant women who are not immune to German measles are advised to avoid exposure. If they are exposed in the first 16 weeks of pregnancy and if they get the disease, chances are high that the fetus will have problems. At this point, they will have to make a decision about whether or not to continue their pregnancy. A blood test will determine if they have or have had German measles.

Studies in Africa have shown that when children become infected with measles they show inhibited HIV viral replication. Children were monitored after they had caught the virus. The children showed increases in CD-8 killer T-cells during their infection. HIV replication increased again after recovery from the measles virus. Whether this discovery leads to any advances in HIV treatment is unknown at this time.

mechanical ventilation   The process of exchanging air between the lungs and surrounding atmosphere by artificial, extrinsic means (i.e., a respirator).

median   The midpoint value in a series; the median is not necessarily the same as the mean.

Medicaid   Medicaid, one of our country's two major government-run health insurance programs (the other is MEDICARE), is a federally aided but state-operated and -administered program that provides medical benefits to eligible low-income persons. Authorized by TITLE XIX of the SOCIAL SECURITY ACT OF 1965 , it is basically for the poor, but it doesn't cover all of the poor. Rather, Medicaid is only for those who are members of one of the categories of people who may also be covered under welfare cash payment programs—the aged, blind, disabled, and members of individual families and dependent children in which one parent is absent, incapacitated, or unemployed.

Medicaid is operated by state health or welfare agencies under the rules of the Health Care Financing Administration of the United States DEPARTMENT OF HEALTH AND HUMAN SERVICES. Subject to broad federal guidelines, states determine eligibility, coverage, rates of payment for providers, and methods of administration. Eligibility varies from state to state, but generally, persons whose incomes and assets are below state-set poverty levels, or (in most states) whose incomes fall to those poverty levels through incurred (but not necessarily paid) medical expenses are eligible. In most states, Social Security's decision that an individual is eligible for SSI also makes them eligible for Medicaid coverage. Others covered are those in AFDC-eligible families, those who meet the SSI/SSDI medical definition of blindness or disability, pregnant women, those under age seven or over age 65, and some or all persons (depending on the state) between ages seven and 21.

Programs vary widely from state to state, but Medicaid generally covers these services: care in skilled and intermediate nursing homes; inpatient hospital services; outpatient hospital services; clinic health services; laboratory and X-ray services; hospice services (in about half the states); home health services of registered nurses or other medical professionals; physician services; M.D. psychiatrist services (some states also cover services of licensed psychologists and psychiatric social workers); premiums, coinsurance, and deductibles for poor, disabled, and aged people also on Medicare; ambulance service; mass-transit charges, taxi vouchers, and handicapped van services to get to medical care (in some states); outpatient prescription drugs (with some exceptions); personal home care attendants when ordered in writing by a doctor; and home- and community-based services. Medicaid recipients are also eligible for social services such as counseling, "meals on wheels," home chore aid, and transportation through the "adult services" sections of the state welfare agencies. There is a broad right of appeal for unfavorable agency decisions.

Medicaid recipients are given plastic or paper cards with which to purchase covered services from participating providers. Cards are used similarly to credit cards. However, cash outlays by patients are never reimbursed.

In recent years, much has been written about mounting drug expenditures and runaway health care costs and the impact of both on Medicaid. Shrinking state and federal budgets have put Medicaid programs under tremendous pressure to hold down costs. Laws designed to contain state or consumer drug expenditures have been passed in a number of states, and a number of experiments in tighter administration of public drug spending are under way. Additionally, unable to sustain ballooning Medicaid drug budgets, several states have told pharmaceutical makers either to lower prices or to face banishment to a list of medications that require third-party approval in order to be prescribed. Note that in a highly competitive market, prior approval is a steep hurdle that effectively means that a competitor's drug gets Medicaid's lucrative business. Experience has shown that prior approval can create hurdles for patients as well. While the pharmaceutical industry has responded with lawsuits and public outcry, a variety of cost-containing experiments are nonetheless currently under way. Many legitimate consumer organizations are alarmed about the potential impact of these plans on the country's most vulnerable citizens: the elderly, the disabled, and people with complicated treatment needs, including those with HIV. See PRIOR APPROVAL; PRIOR AUTHORIZATION.

medical assistance (MA) A generic term for MEDICAID, GENERAL MEDICAL ASSISTANCE (GMA), and other health care programs for the poor.

medical care The range of services provided by physicians for the maintenance of health, the prevention of illness, and the treatment of illness and injury.

medical consultation A physician's review of a patient's history, examination of a patient, or recommendations for treatment, given to another physician at the request of the first.

medical directive A document detailing a patient's wishes concerning kinds of treatment he or she does not wish to have administered under particular circumstances in the future. A patient can request, for example, that he or she not be kept alive on a respirator if his or her medical condition is irreversible. Individuals have a much better chance of realizing their wishes if they express them in writing in advance. The best guarantee is to sign a medical directive in conjunction with a HEALTH CARE PROXY in which a sympathetic person is named as a health care agent. See CODE STATUS; POWER OF ATTORNEY; LIVING WILL; NO CODE.

medical history The portion of a patient's life history that is important in diagnosing and caring for the medical or surgical condition or conditions present. Ancestry and social, occupational, and medical information are all components of a complete medical history. This information is recorded in the patient's permanent record.

medical waste Infectious or physically dangerous medical or biological waste material, including discarded blood and blood products; pathology lab waste; contaminated animal carcasses and body parts; contaminated bedding; sharps (medical articles such as hypodermic needles that may cause punctures or cuts to those handling them); and discarded preparations made from genetically altered living organisms and their products. In 1985, the CENTERS FOR DISEASE CONTROL AND PREVENTION (CDC) developed the strategy of "universal blood and body fluid precautions" to address concerns regarding transmission of HIV and other infectious illnesses in the health care setting. See UNIVERSAL PRECAUTIONS.

medically needy In MEDICAID parlance, persons who share qualifications with AFDC or SSI recipients, but who have incomes above AFDC, SSI, or SSI/SSP eligibility levels. At state option, medically needy people can receive Medicaid when their income is below (or falls below through "spend-down") a state-set level between the AFDC level and an amount one-third higher.

Medicare One of our country's two major government-run health insurance programs (the other is MEDICAID), Medicare is a nationwide health insurance program for people aged 65 years and over, persons eligible for Social Security disability payments for at least two years, and certain workers who need kidney transplantation or dialysis. Medical health insurance protection is available to eligible persons without regard to their income. Medicare consists of two separate programs: hospital insurance (Part A) and supplementary medical insurance (Part B). The programs are financed from payroll taxes and premiums paid by beneficiaries. Medicare monies are deposited in special trust funds for use in meeting the expenses incurred by the insured. The program was enacted on July 30, 1965, as TITLE XVIII of the SOCIAL SECURITY ACT, "Health Insurance for the Aged," and became effective on July 1, 1966.

Eligibility for Medicare is fairly straightforward—anyone who has been entitled to SOCIAL SECURITY DISABILITY INSURANCE (SSDI) benefits for two years, or who is over 65, or who experiences permanent kidney failure, is eligible. Allowable benefits vary, depending on whether an individual has hospital or medical insurance. There are certain charges and services Medicare will not cover, such as charges billed at amounts above those in the Medicare allowable fee schedule; services provided by organizations or individuals not Medicare-approved and participating; intermediate nursing home care; custodial care in any setting; care that is not reasonable or necessary; and services or supplies not generally accepted. Hospice benefits have no deductibles and cover inpatient care, home health care, "significant other" counseling and support services, and almost all charges for drugs.

The Hospital Insurance Program, Part A, is compulsory for everyone. Part A automatically enrolls all persons aged 65 and over who are entitled to benefits under the Old Age, Survivors, Disability and Health Insurance Program or the railroad retirement program; persons under age 65 who have been eligible for disability for more than two years; and insured workers (and their dependents)

requiring renal dialysis or kidney transplantation. The Supplementary Medical Insurance Program, Part B, is the voluntary portion of Medicare. It covers physician and other individual provider services for all persons entitled to Part A who enroll and pay a monthly premium.

Those receiving Social Security Disability Insurance benefits will automatically be enrolled when the two-year waiting period is over. Others may apply at the local Social Security office. A fairly broad range of appeal rights exists.

medication Treatment with (drug) remedies; administration of medicine.

meditation According to Dr. Bernie Siegel is "an active process of focusing the mind into a state of relaxed awareness. There are many ways of doing this. Some teachers recommend focusing attention on a symbolic sound or word (a mantra) or on a single image, such as a candle flame or mandala. Others teach people to focus on the sound and flowing of the breath. The result of all meditation methods is ultimately the same: to induce a restful trance which strengthens the mind by freeing it from its accustomed turmoil." In the last 25+ years, a considerable body of research has demonstrated how meditation benefits health. For example, blood chemistry reports have shown a lessening of lactate in the blood. Also, electroencephalograms have shown an increase in alpha brain wave activity. Meditation tends to lower or normalize blood pressure, pulse rate, and the levels of stress hormones in the blood. It also lowers abnormally high cholesterol levels and reduces mild hypertension. There is also evidence that with regular practice over a period of time, meditation may increase concentration, memory, intelligence, and creativity.

medroxyprogesterone Female sex hormones; progestins used to initiate and regulate menstruation and to correct abnormal patterns of menstrual bleeding caused by hormonal imbalance. Medroxyprogesterone works by inducing and maintaining a lining in the uterus that resembles pregnancy. This drug can prevent uterine bleeding until it is withdrawn. By suppressing the release of the pituitary gland hormone that induces ovulation and by stimulating the secretion of mucus by the uterine cervix, this drug can prevent pregnancy. Possible risks include thrombophlebitis (rare), pulmonary embolism (rare), liver reaction with jaundice (rare), and drug-induced birth defects.

medulla   The inner portion of an organ.

Megace   See MEGESTROL.

megadose   A very large dose of a nontoxic substance, usually a vitamin.

mega-HAART   The use of six or more antiretrovirals, typically some or all of which have been used previously, to treat HIV.

megaloblast   An abnormally large red blood corpuscle, oval and slightly irregular in shape, from 11 to 20 microns in diameter. Megaloblasts are classified as basophilic, orthochromatic, and polychromatic, and are found in the blood in cases of pernicious anemia.

megaloblastic anemia   Anemia characterized by the presence of MEGALOBLASTS in the blood and BONE MARROW.

megestrol   A synthetic derivative of the female sex hormone progesterone, megestrol is an appetite stimulant. It has also been used for the treatment of breast and endometrial cancers. Megestrol is available in two different forms. The oral liquid is prescribed for the treatment of anorexia and unexplained weight loss in people with HIV. The tablets are prescribed for treatment of symptoms of breast or endometrial cancer. Megestrol does not affect the course of breast cancer, endometrial cancer, or HIV; it simply alleviates the symptoms. Patients on megace, the brand name for megestrol, tend to gain fat, according to studies. Patients should notice a return of appetite and some weight gain within the first six weeks.

Megestrol should not be used by pregnant women, because it causes birth defects. To prevent possible birth defects, women taking megestrol are encouraged to use effective contraception. Note that HIV can be passed from a women to her child through breast milk. In areas where nutritionally sound alternatives are readily available, breast-feeding is discouraged for HIV-positive women. Megestrol passes through breast milk, and although it has not been shown to cause problems in nursing infants, women should consider alternatives to breast-feeding while taking the drug. Note, too, that Megestrol has been shown to decrease testosterone levels; therefore, people taking the drug may want to have their testosterone levels monitored and utilize testosterone replacement therapy as appropriate.

melanin   The dark, protective pigment of the skin. Exposure to sunlight stimulates melanin production. It can be prepared chemically. MELANOMA, the most serious type of skin cancer, originates in the cells that produce melanin.

melanoma   A malignant, darkly pigmented mole or tumor of the skin.

membrane   A thin sheet or layer of pliable tissue serving as a covering.

membrane attack complex (MAC)   The terminal complement components that, when activated, cause lysis of target cells.

membrane fluidizers   Nutritional substances made from egg and soy lecithin, believed to extract cholesterol from the cell walls of viral lipid coatings and the cell membranes of T CELLS. It was theorized that the cholesterol produces structural rigidity essential for binding of a virus to the target host cells, so that causing a fluidity of interaction between virus and host would reduce infectivity. Prior to the advent of reverse transcriptase-inhibiting drugs, many people reported some degree of success using these products as a treatment for HIV.

memorial quilt   See QUILT.

memory   The mental registration, retention, and recall of past experience, knowledge, ideas, sensations, and thoughts. Memory defects are a symptom of many diseases. Recall may fail because memories have been obliterated or suppressed psychologically, because there has been organic brain damage by drugs, disease (or age), or because of a temporary interference with normal brain function by drugs or disease. See HIV ENCEPHALOPATHY.

memory cell   A cell that remains after the body mounts an immune response to an antigen and is capable of an immediate response to the reappearance of the same antigen. Memory cells can include certain subsets of T cells (CD4 and CD8) and some B cells.

memory T cell   A T cell that bears receptors for a specific foreign antigen encountered during a prior infection or vaccination. After an infection or a vaccination, some of the T cells that participated in the response remain as memory T cells, which rapidly mobilize and clone themselves should the same antigen be reencountered during a second infection at a later time. See IMMUNITY.

men who have sex with men (MSM)   A term created to define MSM who do not identify as gay or bisexual.

meninges   The three membranes that ensheathe the brain and spinal cord: the pia mater (internal), the arachnoid (middle), and the dura mater (external).

meningitis   An infection of the MENINGES, the membranes that envelope the brain and the spinal cord. Cryptococcosis is the most common cause of meningitis in people who have AIDS. It is caused by the yeast *Cryptococcus neoformans.* Development of cryptococcosis usually requires significant impairment of the immune system and generally does not occur until the CD4 count drops below 100 cells per millimeter. Symptoms of cryptococcus include headache, fever, lethargy, nausea, and vomiting. Patients often experience intermittent symptomatic and asymptomatic periods. The infection can occur in the brain itself; there it can mimic the appearance of a brain tumor in diagnostic images produced by computed tomography (CT) and magnetic resonance imaging (MRI). Other

sites of infection include the lungs, liver, heart, skin, lymph nodes, adrenal glands, and genitourinary tract. Diagnosis of cryptococcal meningitis is important because early treatment of the disease can be very effective. Note that there are also other causes of meningitis in HIV-infected patients. These include the bacterium that causes TB and possibly HIV itself.

meningoencephalitis   Inflammation or infection of the brain and its MENINGES. The usual cause is a bacterial infection, but HIV can also cause meningoencephalitis.

menopause   The period during which menstruation ends permanently; the end of a woman's period of fertility. Diagnosis of menopause is indicated by the absence of menses accompanied by symptomatology and strengthened when serum LH and FSH are found to be elevated, indicating failure of the ovaries to produce estrogen in the presence of adequate hypothalamic/pituitary stimulation. Definitive diagnosis is indicated by the completion of 12 months without menses. Women generally develop some signs of estrogen depletion prior to the cessation of periods. Until the periods have stopped for 12 months, conception is still possible and contraceptive measures should be taken. Menopause usually occurs naturally between ages 45 and 55. It may also be surgically induced, or occur prematurely. Early onset of menopause is not uncommon in HIV-positive women. Compounding a possible association with HIV are factors such as anemia, chronic illness, weight loss, tobacco use, use of street drugs (particularly heroin), and possible effects of antiretrovirals such as AZT or ddI.

Estrogen replacement therapy is generally offered to menopausal women to reduce bothersome or debilitating symptoms (hot flashes, insomnia, decreased sexual functioning, decreased appetite, night sweats, weight loss, fatigue, vaginitis, dysuria, etc.), to prevent demineralization of bones (leading to osteoporosis), and to offset changes in lipid metabolism related to heart disease. Estrogen is supplemented with progestin to offset the documented increase in endometrial cancer and potential increased risk of breast cancer in women with unopposed estrogenic stimulation. The use of exogenous hormones in HIV-positive women presents incalculable risks, including unknown drug interactions with HIV medications and uncertain effects on immune response.

menses See MENSTRUATION.

menstrual blood Blood that is shed from a woman's uterus during her menstrual period.

menstrual cycle The periodically recurrent series of changes in the uterus and associated sex organs (ovaries, cervix, and vagina) associated with menstruation and the intermenstrual period. Many women with HIV infection experience an abnormal or changing menstrual cycle, and clinicians experienced in the care of women with HIV infection often feel that a higher than expected percentage of women in their care have menstrual problems. Whether the absence of a menstrual period (amenorrhea) or lighter than normal menstrual bleeding (oligomenorrhea) has an HIV-related cause is not known. Gonadal (ovarian) failure in women could be manifested as a menstrual cycle disturbance. Heavy bleeding (menorrhagia) and painful periods (dysmenorrhea) could be explained by low platelet levels (thrombocytopenia) associated with HIV infection or a complication of severe pelvic inflammatory disease, both conditions frequently associated with HIV disease.

Optimal care of HIV-infected women requires a good understanding of the clinical manifestations of gynecological disease. However, in HIV-infected women, little is known about menstruation and abnormal vaginal bleeding, despite the importance of the menstrual history in evaluating ovarian function and detecting gynecologic disorders. Virtually nothing is known about any potential effects of newer antiretroviral therapies on hormonal levels and menstrual cycles of women.

Evaluation of HIV-related effects on the menstrual cycle is complicated by the fact that substance abuse, chronic disease, and significant weight loss can result in disregulation of the hypothalamus and affect menstruation.

HIV-infected women with abnormal or dramatically changed menstrual bleeding should have the full investigation accorded HIV-negative women to determine the cause of the abnormality. Heavy bleeding can cause anemia, a problem already prominent among women with advanced HIV infection, and can be a symptom of an underlying problem such as a fibroid tumor, blood clotting problems, or infection. Amenorrhea can be a symptom of pregnancy, ovarian cyst, ovarian failure, or menopause. Missing of two periods (if pregnancy is ruled out) requires investigation by pelvic exam and blood tests to determine whether the problem lies within the reproductive tract. In the course of identifying the cause of menstrual irregularities, women should report to their providers any change in drug therapy, use of recreational drugs, weight, and all related symptoms.

menstruation The cyclic discharge of blood and mucosal tissues from the UTERUS through the VAGINA; also called menses. It is brought on by reduced production of ovarian HORMONES and in healthy women occurs at approximately four-week intervals, except during pregnancy, throughout the reproductive period of a woman's life (from puberty to MENOPAUSE). It is the culmination of the menstrual cycle.

Menstrual disorders often accompany chronic illness. Specific menstrual disorders encountered by HIV-positive women may be exacerbated by anemia, weight loss, medications, street drugs and psychogenic factors, particularly depression. In addition, women with HIV infection also experience the usual range of menstrual difficulties that afflict non-HIV-positive women. HIV-positive women frequently complain of changes in their menstrual cycles such as irregular periods, abnormally heavy or light periods, or an increase in premenstrual symptoms such as breast pain, cramping, fluid retention, anxiety, or depression. These changes may be due to HIV itself or to specific medications, particularly AZT. Other variables include the use of prescribed medications, the use of street drugs (particularly heroin), and weight loss. The immune system and the endocrine system interact with one another in ways that are not entirely understood. We cannot be certain of the effects of exogenous hormones in an immuno-compromised individual.

Current standards of care for HIV-positive women neither approve nor forbid the use of hormone therapies or oral contraceptives for birth control or menstrual regulation. There is no present information that would alter treatment strategies for AMENORRHEA, DYSMENORRHEA, premature or natural menopause, or premenstrual syndrome in immunocompromised clients. Research into the etiology as well as the effect of absent menstruation on the immune and endocrine health of women is needed.

Menstrual problems can adversely affect a woman's health during HIV illness. Blood loss from heavy periods can predispose to or exacerbate anemia. Irregular or absent periods may signal significant systemic illness. Intermenstrual bleeding and amenorrhea should be investigated in all women, even if it is a long-standing complaint.

mental health   The capacity of an individual to form harmonious relationships with others; to participate in or contribute constructively to changes in one's social and physical environment; and to achieve a harmonious and balanced satisfaction of one's own potentially conflicting drives. Mental health is a highly variable concept influenced by both biological and cultural factors. It is often defined as the absence of any identifiable or significant mental disorder, or it may simply refer to mental status.

mental health professionals   Persons who work with the behavioral, social, and emotional problems of the emotionally or mentally disturbed. Mental health professionals treat symptomatic and causative elements affecting clients' ability to respond appropriately to their environment.

mental health services   Examination, treatment, and care of emotional and mental disorders and accompanying conditions.

mental status   The psychological or psychiatric state of an individual. The assessment of mental status based on a case review or examination may include consideration of behavior, appearance, responsiveness to stimuli of all kinds, speech, memory, and judgment.

meta-analysis   A quantitative method for combining the results of many studies into one set of conclusions. Meta-analyses are attempted when previous studies were too small individually to achieve meaningful or statistically significant results. Because combining data from disparate groups is problematic, meta-analyses usually are considered more suggestive than definitive.

metabolic acidosis   A disturbance that results in excessive acid in body fluids due to an increase in acids other than carbonic acid. It may be caused by such conditions as severe infection, dehydration, shock, diarrhea, renal dysfunction, or hepatic dysfunction.

metabolic encephalopathy   Neuropsychiatric disturbance caused by metabolic brain disease. It may be the result of disease in other organs, such as the lungs or kidneys, or it may be caused directly by low blood sugar (hypoglycemia), low oxygenation (hypoxia), or decreased blood flow (ischemia).

metabolic toxicity   A collection of conditions seen in long-term HIV patients who have used several antiretroviral medicines. It is unknown how great a role different medications play in various conditions but the role is theorized to be important. Some researchers believe some of the conditions are a result of the HIV itself, and the situation is developing now because in the past HIV-positive people did not survive as long as they do now.

LIPOATROPHY is the loss of subcutaneous fat from the face and/or upper arms. This condition has proved very disturbing for many people, who appear "wasted" as a result. Some studies have linked this condition to d4T and other NRTIs and PROTEASE INHIBITORS. Other factors that may be associated with this condition are sex, age, insulin resistance, smoking, viral load, and CD4 nadir. Some HIV-positive individuals have had plastic surgery for facial implants to restore shape to the face. Some researchers believe that protease inhibitors cause the condition.

Lipodystrophy is the formation of fat deposits, more properly a fat redistribution, in parts of the body, most usually the back of the neck (buffalo hump), the stomach (protease paunch, Crix belly), and the chest. It can be seen at the same time the arms and legs have lost fat. It can also appear in conjunction with HYPERLIPIDEMIA, that is, abnormal levels of blood cholesterol and/or triglycerides. It also involves INSULIN RESISTANCE, or inability of the body to move the blood sugar to the cells, where it can be processed for energy.

Some studies are under way to test the theory that perhaps STRUCTURED TREATMENT INTERRUPTIONS may lessen the side effects of antiretroviral medications. Others are trying to determine whether it is solely the PIs or NRTIs, or a combination of both, that causes these problems.

PERIPHERAL NEUROPATHY is another condition that has been at times associated with *metabolic toxicity*. This is the degeneration of the nerves in the extremities, the arms and legs, which is described as numbness and a sensation of pins and needles, or a constant humming of the feet and legs.

There are no current medical case definitions for metabolic toxicity nor for lipoatrophy or lipodystrophy. This lack complicates collecting data as different researchers and doctors label different symptoms as different problems according to their own definitions of each condition. See MITOCHONDRIAL TOXICITY; SMART.

metastasis Transfer or spread of a disease, especially cancer, or its manifestations from one organ or part to another not directly connected with it; change in location of bacteria or body cells from one part of the body to another.

metastasize To spread to other parts of the body by METASTASIS; to form new foci of disease in distant parts of the body by metastasis.

metformin (glucophage) A drug used to treat high blood sugar level. Metformin helps to reduce the amount of glucose produced by the liver, thereby generally leading to reduced amounts of insulin and glucose in the bloodstream. Metformin helps antagonize the insulin resistance characteristic of type 2 diabetes mellitus. It is being tested for treatment of LIPODYSTROPHY and high blood sugar level in HIV disease, since PROTEASE INHIBITORS, corticosteroids, and Megace all increase insulin resistance. There is some concern about whether it could

contribute to lactic acidosis, but so far it appears not to do so. The jury is still out as to whether metformin holds a great deal of promise for HIV-positive people who have insulin resistance.

methadone hydrochloride An inexpensive long-acting strong narcotic used for the control of withdrawal symptoms from addictive morphinelike drugs, particularly heroin. Methadone hydrochloride is also used for pain control in disorders such as AIDS, cancer, and chronic pain syndrome. Side effects are those shared by all morphinelike drugs that depress the CENTRAL NERVOUS SYSTEM: dizziness, mental clouding, depression, and sedation. Although used to assist addicts kick their drug dependence, methadone like all opiates, may itself cause physical dependence. Stopping it abruptly after prolonged and regular use can cause withdrawal symptoms. Methadone can be given orally or injected intravenously. Methadone maintenance is permitted only in programs approved by the FOOD AND DRUG ADMINISTRATION and the designated state authority for narcotic addiction. (Trade names are Dolophine Hydrochloride and Methadose.)

methadone maintenance clinics Clinics which dispense methadone for treatment of drug dependence due to use of opium derivatives. These clinics may be community-based or hospital-based. Because methadone is a habit-forming agent, its use should be carefully supervised. The major goal of methadone maintenance is for the client to stop using illicit drugs, develop a productive life, and become a valued member of society. HIV/AIDS is an additional assault to these clients' self-esteem and is often a new reason to resume taking nonprescribed drugs. It is safe to say that the onset of HIV/AIDS has had an enormous impact on the clinics and staff involved in methadone maintenance as a drug treatment modality.

Most methadone maintenance clinics are managed by a medical director, and staffed by a number of mental health providers, including counselors. Often, some of these counselors are former IV drug users. Clinics function to provide access to medical care and counseling. Clinic services include seeing people every day, providing psycho-social support for them, and dispensing methadone and/or other "meds." Effective treatment is composed of first forming a working relationship with people who are often very resistant. The staff must convey understanding, respect and commitment, as well as insight in order to develop a therapeutic alliance.

Clients on methadone are generally not people who have a history of tolerating intrapsychic stress: their primary way of coping has been use of drugs. With the onset of HIV/AIDS, their social and health problems have increased dramatically. Very often they have been using drugs intravenously for many years before beginning to take methadone. In many cases, they continue to use illicit drugs or abuse alcohol even while on methadone. Patients on methadone frequently struggle with issues of poverty, homelessness, and crack. Many patients face all of these issues simultaneously on a daily basis. These people do not usually trust either the health care establishment or drug treatment professionals since most often they are not treated with respect, care, or gentleness.

Today, most urban methadone maintenance programs are experienced with working with clients whose lives are impacted by HIV/AIDS. These programs provide an alternative to the rejection many clients experience from their families and friends. They provide one safe place for their clients to discuss fears and concerns. The challenges the clients present to staff are enormous, but by not rejecting them the staff make a significant difference in their clients' lives. Somewhat ironically, one further problem confronts people with HIV/AIDS who want methadone or another form of treatment for their drug addiction—a current shortage of methadone maintenance clinics.

Current law in the United States dictates that methadone maintenance clinics try to get people off methadone; many, however, believe that long-term methadone maintenance is the best health strategy for some individuals.

methaqualone hydrochloride A hypnotic sedative that has become a drug of abuse. Because of the illegal abuse of this drug, it is no longer distributed in the United States.

methotrexate (MTX) An immunosuppressive drug that like cyclophosphamide (CY), is used at high doses as a cancer chemotherapy. At lower doses, MTX suppresses inflammation in immune disorders such as Wegener's granulomatosis, rheumatoid arthritis, and psoriasis. At low doses, MTX has anti-inflammatory effects, and can reduce levels of various markers of immune activity, particularly serum antibodies and rheumatoid factor, a component of immune complexes characteristic of rheumatoid arthritis. Numerous side effects are associated with MTX treatment. BONE MARROW SUPPRESSION has been seen but is infrequent at the lower doses used for arthritis. The most common side effects of lower doses of MTX are GASTROINTESTINAL (nausea, diarrhea, anorexia, oral ulcers). Such toxicities appear to be lessened by coadministration of folic acid. Even at the low doses used in autoimmune disease, though, MTX treatment for periods of more than three months is associated with development of opportunistic infections, especially PNEUMOCYSTIS CARINII PNEUMONIA and varicella zoster. Previously used name was amethopterin. (Trade names are Mexate and Folex.)

methylphenidate A stimulant used primarily to treat narcolepsy (recurrent spells of uncontrollable drowsiness and sleep) and attention-deficit disorders in children. Additional uses include the treatment of mild to moderate depression, and the management of mild dementia, apathy, and withdrawal states in HIV encephalopathy and in the elderly. Nervousness and insomnia are two possible side effects. (Trade names are Ritalin and Ritalin-SR.)

meticorten See PREDNISONE.

metronidazole An antibacterial and antiprotozoal drug. It is used to treat amebiasis and giardiasis. It can also be used against trichomoniasis, bacterial vaginosis, and other non-HIV related illness. The drug interferes with the DNA in susceptible organisms, preventing them from multiplying. It has also been used as an ointment to successfully treat rosacea on the skin. It is available as tablets and as a gel for topical use. Treatment can run from five to 10 days depending on the fungi or protozoa involved. The most common side effect is nausea; nausea may be accompanied by headache, loss of appetite, vomiting, diarrhea, heartburn, constipation, or cramping. Alcohol should be avoided while using metronidazole and for one day after stopping its use because it will cause vomiting. It will increase greatly the amount of lithium in the body and is not recommended for those taking lithium. Over-the-counter cimetidine (Tagamet) will seriously lower the amount of metronidazole and cause it not to work. (Trade names include Flagyl, Metryl, Protostat, Satric, and Neo-Tric.)

MHC   See MAJOR HISTOCOMPATIBILITY COMPLEX.

microbe   A microscopic one-celled organism—bacterium fungus, protozoan, or virus—not distinguishable as vegetable or animal. Microbes cause infectious diseases and may be carried from one host to another by human and animal sources, air, contact infection, food, fomites (inanimate objects) such as linens, books, cooking utensils and clothing, insects and soil. The microbes that most commonly cause the OPPORTUNISTIC INFECTIONS associated with HIV infection are: bacteria—MYCOBACTERIUM AVIUM-INTRACELLULARE, MYCOBACTERIUM TUBERCULOSIS, SALMONELLA, NOCARDIA; fungi—CRYPTOCOCCUS, HISTOPLASMA, CANDIDA ALBICANS; parasites—TOXO-PLASMA GONDII, PNEUMOCYSTIS CARINII, CRYPTOSPORID-IUM, *Isospora;* and viruses—CYTOMEGALOVIRUS, HERPES SIMPLEX, HERPES ZOSTER, MOLLUSCUM CONTA-GIOSUM. HIV is itself a virus.

microbicide   An agent that kills MICROBES. Applied in the vagina or rectum, these compounds, in different formulations, act in various ways to reduce the transmission of STDs including HIV. Although such products are also needed by women and men who have anal sex, virtually all the microbicide research now under way focuses on vaginal use. Similarly to birth control products that have been sold over the counter for decades, microbicides are produced in many forms: suppositories, films, gels or creams inserted with a disposable or reusable applicator, and even sponges or rings inserted into the vagina that release a microbicidal compound slowly over time. Some are formulated as contraceptive agents; for those wanting pregnancy without fear of infection, noncontraceptive forms are available.

There are various theories as to how microbicides work. Some work by boosting the body's natural defense systems, others introduce new substances to destroy pathogens or chemically block their entry into human cells, and still others create a type of physical barrier. The most promising products probably combine several of these approaches. The basic idea behind the various microbicides under development is that they will be, like condoms, convenient, simple to use, inexpensive, available without a prescription, and appropriate for distribution in stores, clinics, and kiosks, and peer health educators. It is important to note that microbicides are not expected to be as effective against some infections as internal ("female") and external ("male") condoms, given that it is always safer to prevent viruses or bacteria from entering the body than to try to disable those that enter. For those for whom consistent condom use is not an option, an effective microbicide is much safer than unprotected sex. Couples already using condoms will also benefit from microbicides as a supplement to be used with a condom for added protection. In the future, some microbicides may also be developed in other formulations such as a mouth rinse for protection during oral sex, a vaginal wash that can be used by HIV-positive women before childbirth as a low-cost way of reducing risk of perinatal transmission, and applications for postcoital use to reduce risk of infection after forced sex or condom failure. As better microbicides are developed, they will be designed to be "bidirectional": in other words, use of a vaginal microbicide will inactivate HIV present in the vaginal secretions, thus protecting her partner as well as protecting a woman from HIV in her partner's semen.

microbiology   Science that deals with the study of microorganisms, including bacteria, fungi, and viruses.

microcytic   Anemia characterized by abnormally small erythrocytes.

microencapsulated   Surrounded by a thin layer of biodegradable substance referred to as a microsphere. Microencapsulation is means of protecting a drug or vaccine antigen from rapid breakdown. It may also enhance an antigen's absorption and the immune response to that antigen.

microhemagglutination assay for *Treponema pallidum* (MATP)   One of two types of confirmatory (or "treponemal") tests for syphilis; the other is FTA-ABS. The two tests are equivalent. In testing for syphilis, a nontreponemal test is done first to screen. If the finding is positive, a treponemal test is used for confirmation; this method is analogous to the HIV ELISA and WESTERN BLOT testing process. The treponemal variety of syphilis tests look for *T. pallidum,* the corkscrew-shaped organism that causes the disease.

micronutrient   An essential nutrient, as a trace mineral, that is required in minute amounts. Micronutrients are essential to the body in small amounts because they either are components of enzymes or act as coenzymes in managing chemical reactions. Micronutrient supplementation has been found to strengthen immune defenses; however, some studies have found that the genetic makeup of the virus plays a role in whether or not micronutrients actually strengthen the immune system, in effect countering years of reports concerning micronutrient deficiencies in people living with HIV.

microorganism   An organism of microscopic scale, not perceptible to the naked eye; a MICROBE.

Microspora   An order of parasitic protozoa; also called Enidosporidia and Microsporidia.

It is conjectured that there are many different species and classes of microspora, which can cause a variety of problems in people with HIV. However, these are very difficult to detect by the current available diagnostic tests. Although best known as a cause of diarrhea, microspora can also cause infections of the eye, kidney, liver, muscles, brain, and several other tissues. See MICROSPORIDIOSIS.

Microsporidia   An order of parasitic protozoa. Also called Enidosporidia and Microsporidia. See MICROSPORIDIOSIS.

microsporidiosis   An intestinal infection that causes diarrhea and wasting in people with AIDS.

It is caused by two different species of MICROSPORA (or MICROSPORIDIA) an order of protozoal parasites. Although difficult to detect, a variety of microspora is widespread in animals and humans. The most common type is called *Enterocytozon bieneusi*, which invades the small intestine and seems to cause severe chronic diarrhea. Prior to the HIV/AIDS epidemic, only eleven cases of microsporidiosis had been reported in world medical literature.

The mode of transmission of microsporidiosis is unknown, although many patients with it have a history of extensive foreign travel or residence. Other suspected forms of transmission include unprotected sexual activity and eating food contaminated with microsporidia. Symptoms such as diarrhea, abdominal cramps, fever, and weight loss do not always occur immediately after exposure.

Small obscure microsporans are thought to exist in the intestine, liver, muscles, cornea, and other tissues. They rarely show up with routine methods of detection and in fact often evoke little or no response. Examining stool with an electron microscope may be the only means to recognize or classify microspora. However, because there is not yet an accepted standard technique to detect microsporans in human stool, diagnosis of intestinal microsporidiosis is usually done by small bowel BIOPSY. It is noted that there is beginning to be some success with detecting spores in stool by light microscopy.

Diagnostic confirmation still requires biopsy.

To date, there is no known effective therapy for microsporidiosis. A few scattered anecdotal reports have indicated partial success with various antiparasitic agents; these have not been confirmed by controlled trials. Diarrhea almost always abates if anti-HIV therapy can produce a significant increase in CD4 cells.

Middle East and North Africa   There are 500,000 people in this region living with HIV. Nearly one-fifth of that number have tested positive in 2001 according to UNAIDS. Sexual activities appear to be the main route of transmission, though increases in the number of members of the IDU population who test positive have been recorded since 1999. Two exceptions to this are Yemen and the Sudan, where IDUs have always been the main route of transmission. It is believed by UNAIDS that unless this issue is addressed soon, HIV will quickly spread into the heterosexual population. Countries experiencing large increases in HIV-positive numbers in the late 1990s include Libya and Iran. Both countries have seen large increases in IDU HIV-positive rates in the last couple of years. Iran had approximately 2 percent of its prison population testing positive in the 2001 past year. Algeria has seen a marked increase in the percentage of HIV-positive expectant mothers since 2000. The proportion has reached 1 percent among women in the southern part of Algeria. In Morocco, the HIV rate has not increased greatly but other STD infection rates have, so it is thought this area is ripe for HIV infection if education is not begun now.

As is true in much of Asia and the Caribbean, a large mobile population has caused extensive outbreaks in some countries. Sudan and Djibouti have large numbers of HIV-positive people. Both countries have political instability and large differences in economic resources among their people. There is also the double disease burden in these countries of tuberculosis (TB) and HIV. Rates of infection among TB patients in the Sudan are 8 percent; in Iran, 4 percent; in Oman, 5 percent; and in Pakistan, 2 percent.

Culturally this is a relatively conservative region of the world. Men hold most prominent positions in local and national roles. In some parts of this region polygamy is still practiced. In southern Iran, the area called Baluchistan has a large rate of heterosexually transmitted HIV. Officials fear that it is due to polygamy, as one man has contracted the virus and then spread it to several of his wives. This area is also rife with smuggling of heroin from Afghanistan, which has created a large number of IDUs in the region.

Morocco for many years has run a sex tourist business. It is not often discussed because of religious mores, but it is there. Moroccan officials are very concerned, given the rate of STD infections, that HIV will quickly become a national problem. However, some politicians refuse to allow discussion of condoms, believing that it "would encourage sexual promiscuity." This conservative attitude is similar to that often expressed in the United States, which has the highest rate of HIV infection

in the industrialized world. The rate of HIV infection rose four times in 2001.

In Turkey, officials were not able to institute blood scanning for virus across all of the country, and this inability led to an unusually large number of HIV infections caused by tainted blood as late as the late 1990s. As a result, several rural areas of Turkey experienced outbreaks of HIV infection, which normally occur in urban areas before they reach country areas. The bad news in much of this region is that medical care is poor.

That Turkey, a relatively Westernized and wealthy country, does not screen blood indicates the possibilities for infection in this area, where activities that generally encourage HIV spread are available.

The good news in this region is that the rates of Infection are still low. No country other than Sudan has a rate above 1 percent of the population. Several still have rates below 0.001 percent. So there is time for education if the governments are able to provide the funding for it. But in countries where medical care is not provided, hoping for education or prevention discussion may be unrealistic.

milk thistle   See SILYMARIN.

miltefosine   This drug was originally developed for possible anticancer treatment. It has become, however, the first oral drug used for the treatment of visceral LEISHMANIASES. It has recently been registered in India, and pharmaceutical companies have already begun production of generic formulations for consumption around the world. It is taken orally for 28 days. Cure rates have been at a level of about 98 percent. This rate is quite high and better than that of current medications that have been available. The drug is an ether-lipid (alkylphospholipid) analog. It has the effect of limiting the proliferation of the protozoon and attacking it in all the phases of its life cycle. For these reasons it has also been used in anticancer treatment. (Trade name is Miltex.)

mind-body therapies   Alternative and holistic therapies that focus on the mind, body, and spirit; includes meditation, image/visualization, biofeedback, hypnosis, expressive therapies (music, art, dance/movement), therapeutic healing, touch, and spiritual healing. Many believe such therapies enhance immunity in people with HIV/AIDS. A person living with HIV can learn about these approaches from a variety of practitioners and then integrate them with standard medical care in collaboration with an HIV-experienced physician. See ALTERNATIVE MEDICINE; ALTERNATIVE TREATMENT.

mineralocorticoid The hormones secreted by the adrenal cortex that affect fluid-ELECTROLYTE balance; aldosterone is the major hormone in this group. See CORTICOSTEROIDS.

minimal dose The smallest dose of a medication that produces an effect.

minimum effective dose (MED-50) The lowest dosage of a drug required to produce the desired effect in 50 percent of subjects.

minimum inhibitory concentration The smallest amount of a substance, when diluted, that kills pathogens or prevents them from reproducing.

miscarriage Termination of pregnancy at any time before the fetus has attained extrauterine viability. HIV-infected women are three times more likely to experience a miscarriage than healthy women. Researchers have suggested four possible factors that alone or in combination contribute to fetal demise in HIV-infected women: direct toxic effects of HIV on the fetus; fetal thymic dysfunction; placental changes; and elevated uterine levels of the inflammatory CYTOKINES IL-4, IL-6, and TNF.

mistletoe An extract of European mistletoe (*Viscum album*) has been used since the 1960s in Europe as an anticancer agent. It is purported to possess both antitumor and immunostimulatory properties. Lung and ovarian cancers have been treated with mistletoe. Mistletoe should be used only under the supervision of a physician. (Trade name is Iscador.)

mite Any arthropod of the order Acarina except the ticks. Mites are minute arachnids related to the spiders. Some are parasitic and are causative agents of such conditions as mange or scabies.

Others serve as intermediate hosts and carry causative organisms of disease from infected to noninfected individuals.

mitochondria Membrane-enclosed cellular compartments existing in the cell cytoplasm (not the nucleus) that are the major source of a cell's energy. Mitochondria accomplish this by oxidizing the products of carbohydrate and lipid metabolism. Mitochondria are also involved in protein synthesis and lipid metabolism. Mitochondria contain some independent DNA genes and are reproduced as needed by the cell in which they reside.

mitochondrial toxicity A term used to define a group of conditions that are believed to be caused by treatment of HIV disease with various antiretroviral medications. In particular it refers to the altering of the mitochondria of the body. The mitochondria are located in each cell. Their job is to break down the oxygen, fats, and sugars in the cell and turn them into energy for the cell. The mitochondria produce adenosine triphosphate (ATP), which is stored until the cell needs the energy and uses the ATP to provide it. Different cells have different amounts of mitochondria living in them. Cells in the liver, nerves, and muscles have more mitochondria than other cells in the body.

A unique feature of mitochondria is that even though they reside in the cell, they reproduce independently of it. To reproduce mitochondria do not use the nuclear DNA that the cell uses. Unlike nuclear cells, mitochondria are not able to correct defective reproduction of themselves. So over the course of a person's life, dysfunctional mitochondria build up in the body. Many researchers believe that mitochondria are a key to aging. If the mitochondria are dysfunctional and are not producing enough energy, the cell can malfunction and/or die. It is thought that after happening millions of times this process can create an aging nonworking body. As the nonfunctioning mitochondria reproduce, eventually the body becomes loaded with nonworking mitochondria. When this happens, many illnesses can occur. Among these are LACTIC ACIDOSIS, NEUROPATHY, muscle WASTING, ANEMIA, STEATOSIS, and PANCREATITIS.

Mitochondria use an enzyme called polymerase gamma, which is similar to REVERSE TRANSCRIPTASE, to reproduce in the cell. The reverse transcriptase that HIV antiretrovirals inhibit is so similar that the antiretrovirals seem to inhibit the polymerase gamma as well. When this happens, fewer mitochondria are produced in the body's cells. It is believed that the NRTIs are all toxic and cause mitochondrial toxicity to some degree. It is not known whether one is worse in these regard than another.

One sign of mitochondrial toxicity is muscle weakness (myopathy). Because muscles have more mitochondria than other parts of the body, they require a great deal of cell energy. If they do not get this cell energy (from oxygen, fat, and sugars), then they need to create their energy without oxygen. This process is called anaerobic production. When anaerobic energy production happens in the body, a "waste" product called lactic acid is created. Some people who have been on NRTIs for a long time or who react poorly to NRTIs have a large amount of lactic acid in their blood. This condition is LACTIC ACIDOSIS, a potentially fatal syndrome that can be reversed if caught early enough. A milder form of the condition is called SYMPTOMATIC HYPERLACTATEMIA.

A test to determine levels of mitochondrial DNA circulating in the bloodstream is currently being examined. Low levels of circulating DNA correlate to mitochondrial toxicity in patients. It may be used in the future treatment of HIV patients to determine when or whether to stop particular drugs in people that show low levels of mitochondrial DNA.

mitogen A protein substance derived from plants that is used in the laboratory to stimulate cells to divide (mitosis). Frequently used IN VITRO, q.v. to study the proliferation of lymphocytes from blood drawn during a research study.

mixed lymphocyte reaction/mixed lymphocyte culture (MLR/MLC) An assay system for T-CELL recognition of allogenic cells in which response is measured by proliferation in the presence of the stimulating cells.

mixed opioid agonist antagonist A compound that has an affinity for two or more types of opioid receptors and blocks opioid effects on one receptor type while producing opioid effects on a second receptor type.

MN An HIV-1 strain belonging to CLADE B, the clade to which most HIV-1 found in North America and Europe belong. MN is used in vaccine development.

mobilization The making movable of a fixed or ankylosed part; restoration of motion to a joint; making an organ free or movable; the freeing, or making available, of substances held in reserve, such as glycogen or fat.

mode In statistics, the value or item of the class that occurs most frequently in a series of variables.

mode of transmission See TRANSMISSION.

molecular biology The field of biology in which biological systems are analyzed in terms of the physics and chemistry of their molecular components.

molecular mimicry Immunological cross-reactivity between determinants on an environmental antigen, such as a virus and a self-antigen, a notion that has been proposed to explain autoimmunity.

molluscum See MOLLUSCUM CONTAGIOSUM.

molluscum contagiosum A common skin disease that is persistent and sometimes disfiguring in HIV-infected individuals and others with weakened immune systems. Molluscum contagiosum can appear on the epithelium of the genitals or other areas of the skin and is caused by a poxvirus infection. Spread by skin-to-skin contact, it is considered to be benign, but may cause itching and rapid spreading. The virus causes small dome-shaped (3 to 5 millimeters in diameter) bumps called papules. In people with healthy immune systems, the papules are usually few in number and generally resolve spontaneously within a few months. Treatment, when needed, is usually akin to that used for warts: freezing, treatment with caustic agents, removal with a sharp instrument, or electrocautery. In people with HIV infection, molluscum contagiosum is often a progressive disease resistant to treatment. In HIV-infected individuals with relatively intact immune systems, MCV papules are usually few in number, localized to the groin or face. Once an individual's CD4+ T cell count falls below 200 cells per cubic millimeter of blood, the lesions tend to proliferate and spread. At this stage of HIV disease, a person may have more than 100 papules on the face (including the eyelids), trunk, and groin. Lesions sometimes coalesce to form giant lesions that measure 1.5 centimeters in diameter. In patients with CD4+ T cell counts lower than 50/mm the lesions may extend onto mucosal surfaces of the lips or conjunctiva. MCV is one of only two poxviruses known to specifically infect people. The other human poxvirus is a distant relative: variola virus, which causes smallpox. Whereas smallpox is a sudden and severe infection that either the immune system quickly controls or death results, molluscum contagiosum is a slow disease that evokes a minimal immune response.

Antiretroviral therapy alone may prevent infection with the poxvirus, since this normally minor viral infection tends to develop in severely immunocompromised people. Destructive methods such as cryotherapy and curettage are the treatments of choice when lesions arise. Topical imiquimod and cidofovir have also been used for refractory cases. Clinicians have also treated recalcitrant lesions with topical cidofovir.

monitoring boundaries Statistical phrase referring to the set of values formed by a line or set of lines (curves), usually specified before or shortly after the start of patient recruitment for a clinical trial, which, if exceeded, indicates the existence of a test-controlled treatment difference that satisfies certain statistical properties for example, a value of p less than a certain size. The boundaries are used as a basis for stopping the trial when developed in conjunction with a sequential design, but not necessarily when used in conjunction with a fixed sample size design. Z values larger in absolute values are declared statistically significant. Boundaries are designed to control the overall type I error.

monoamine oxidase inhibitors (MAO inhibitors; MAOI) A class of antidepressants that increase levels of neurotransmitters in the brain by interfering with an enzyme—monoamine oxidase—that breaks them down.

Depression is thought to be caused by a reduction in the level of certain chemicals, neurotransmitters, in the brain. MAO inhibitors increase the levels of these chemicals in the spaces (synapses) between nerve cells in the brain. Monoamine oxidase inhibitors differ from the other classes of antidepressants, the tricyclics and serotonin reuptake inhibitors, which prevent cells from absorbing certain neurotransmitters and thus increase their levels in the synapses.

MAO inhibitors are potentially toxic and must be used with caution because they deactivate enzymes in the body that break down chemicals found in many foods such as meat, cheese, yeast extracts, and red wine. Eating these foods while taking an MAO inhibitor can cause a dramatic rise in blood pressure (hypertension).

monoclonal Derived from a single clone. See MONOCLONAL ANTIBODY.

monoclonal antibody An antibody produced in the lab for a specific ANTIGEN by a hybidoma (a clone resulting from the division of a hybrid cell produced from artificial fusion of a normal antibody-producing B cell with a B cell tumor cell). Chemically and immunologically homogenous, their exceptional purity and specificity make them useful as laboratory reagents in various tests, such as the ELISA test. They are also used experimentally in cancer immunotherapy.

Monoclonal antibodies have two properties that lead scientists to believe they may be useful therapeutically. In some cases, they are directly cytotoxic: monoclonal antibodies, on their own, may destroy unwanted cells. In other cases, the monoclonal antibodies have no destructive effects themselves but can carry toxins or radioactive particles directly to target cells or tissues. Monoclonal antibody therapy has been used to treat HODGKIN'S DISEASE (HD) and NON-HODGKIN'S LYMPHOMA (NHL).

monocyte A mononuclear phagocyte (white blood cell) derived from the MYELOID stem cells. Monocytes are formed in the BONE MARROW, and are short-lived, with a half-life of approximately one day. They circulate in the bloodstream, from which they move into tissues, where they mature into long-lived MACROPHAGES. Monocytes produce INTERLEUKIN-1, a substance that activates T LYMPHOCYTES in the presence of ANTIGEN.

Monocytes and macrophages form one of the first lines of defense in the inflammatory process. This network of fixed and mobile phagocytes that engulf foreign antigens and cell debris is commonly called the RETICULOENDOTHELIAL SYSTEM.

monogamous In a long-term sexual relationship with only one partner. See MONOGAMY.

monogamy Literally, the practice of being married to one person at a time. In contemporary usage the term also refers to the practice of maintaining unmarried relationships between two people in which the partners have sexual relations only with each other. Monogamous relationships have become more widespread among single adults in the 1980s and 1990s as the AIDS epidemic has spread.

monokine A type of cytotone (chemical mediator) released by MONOCYTES and MACROPHAGES during the immune response. Monokines affect the growth and activity of other white blood cells. INTERLEUKIN-1 is the most important monokine.

monolaurin A saturated fatty acid with a mode of action believed to be similar to that of lecithin extracts. It is a chemical constituent of mother's milk, known to confer immunity on nursing infants until their development of independent immunity. It is known to be safe and is licensed by the USDA as a food additive for the purpose of preventing the growth of bacteria and viruses in food products. It has demonstrated antiviral activity against lipid viruses in the test tube. Its use in alternative medicine has been based on theoretical anti-CMV activity. It has been used in conjunction with BHT as a putative CMV prophylaxis.

mononeuritis multiplex (MM) Inflammation of nerves in separate body areas. MM tends to occur

during the asymptomatic early period of HIV infection, but a more severe type, attributed to CMV infection, has been observed in people with advanced AIDS.

mononuclear phagocyte system Mononuclear cells found primarily in the reticular connective tissue of lymphoid and other organs that are prominent in chronic inflammatory states.

mononucleosis A condition characterized by the presence of an abnormally large quantity of mononuclear LEUKOCYTES (monocytes) in the blood. INFECTIOUS MONONUCLEOSIS is an acute infectious disease that primarily affects lymphoid tissue, and is due to EPSTEIN BARR VIRUS.

monotherapy Medical treatment consisting of a single drug, such as AZT or DIDANOSINE (ddI)administered alone (as contrasted to COMBINATION THERAPY with one or more drugs, such as AZT and ddC or AZT and ddI). See ANTIRETROVIRAL THERAPY.

monovalent vaccine A vaccine that contains only one antigen.

morbidity The condition of being diseased. More specifically, having significant symptoms or disabilities due to a disease. The morbidity rate is the frequency of disease occurrence in proportion to the population.

morning-after pill Phrase now used for a regimen administered as a morning-after treatment to prevent AIDS infection after a possible exposure to HIV.

The popular name for a drug taken the morning after an unprotected act of sexual intercourse to expel any ovum that may have been fertilized. The drug, diethylstilbestrol (DES), is used orally. In the 1960s, the drug was associated with cancer in daughters of pregnant women, who used it to ameliorate morning sickness. Despite the lack of studies supporting the use of the morning-after pill, some doctors are using it for patients who have engaged in high-risk sex. The use of expensive AIDS drugs as a morning-after remedy raises troubling questions about who has access to such treatment. While affluent Americans may soon be able to drop by their doctors' offices to get the miracle pills, AIDS sufferers in the developing world receive woefully inadequate medical care and die much sooner than they might have had they received proper medication. Physicians and researchers are concerned that if the public perceives morning-after pills together with condoms, as part of a new, improved "safe sex" package, the result may be reinforcement of the potentially dangerous idea that any form of sex with anybody at any time is indeed safe. If people know there is a morning-after remedy, they may do things the night before that they might otherwise have avoided, and whose dire consequences the treatment may not ultimately prove capable of preventing.

mortality The number of deaths in proportion to the population, over a specified time. Also, the state of being mortal.

mortality tables Actuarial tables used by the insurance industry to predict the survival and death rates of large groups of people.

mother's milk HIV has been isolated from the breast milk of infected women. The epidemiologic data suggest that HIV is transmissible through the milk of an infected mother to her breast-fed child. Physicians estimate the risk of transmission via breast milk at 29 percent for mothers who are postnatally infected. The risk is even higher, as high as 43 percent for women who are infected prenatally, in addition to the risk of transmission IN UTERO or during delivery.

The World Health Organization (WHO) recommends bottle feeding for HIV-infected mothers who reside in the United States or Europe. Formula feeding in many developing countries is not considered as safe; after reviewing the various risks for the two alternatives, WHO judged that breast-feeding is preferable to the risk of bottle-feeding in these areas, irrespective of the presence of HIV in the mother. See BREAST-FEEDING; TRANSMISSION.

mother-to-child transmission See TRANSMISSION.

mother-to-fetus transmission See TRANSMISSION.

motor dysfunction Abnormal, disturbed, or impaired functioning of a muscle, nerve, or center that effects or produces movement.

motor function impairment See MOTOR DYSFUNCTION.

Motrin See IBUPROFEN.

Mozenavir An experimental PROTEASE INHIBITOR also known as DMP-450. Studies have been discontinued because of heart arrhythmias in animal test models. Interest in its potential arose from its property of being metabolized by the kidney and not interacting or interfering with the liver's cytochrome P450 enzyme.

MRI See MAGNETIC RESONANCE IMAGING.

MSM See MEN WHO HAVE SEX WITH MEN.

MTCT (mother to child transmission) See VERTICAL TRANSMISSION; WOMEN.

mucocutaneous infection The invasion by and multiplication of a pathogenic agent in a mucous membrane or the skin.

mucopurulent cervicitis Infection of the CERVIX, that may be due to STDs, such as chlamydia or gonorrhea.

M-tropic See MACROPHAGE-TROPIC.

mucocutaneous Concerning or pertaining to mucous membranes and the skin, as in the mouth, eyes, vagina, lips, or anal area.

mucosa A mucous membrane; the epithelial lining of a body cavity (mouth, vagina, rectum, or urethra) that opens to the environment.

mucosa-associated lymphoid tissue (MALT) Generic term for LYMPHOID tissue associated with the GASTROINTESTINAL TRACT, bronchial tree, and other MUCOSA. This tissue produces a unique immunoglobulin (secretory IGA) and T-CELL immunity for these mucosal surfaces.

mucosal homing The ability of immunologically competent cells that arise from mucosal follicles to travel back to mucosal areas.

mucosal immunity Resistance to infection across the mucous membranes. Mucosal immunity depends on immune cells and antibodies present in the linings of the reproductive tract, gastrointestinal tract, and other moist surfaces of the body exposed to the outside world.

mucositis Inflammation of a mucous membrane. Oral mucositis is a common complication of chemotherapy and radiation therapy.

mucous membrane The surface tissue lining various tubular structures of the body that communicate with air, such as the mouth, nose, nipples, urethra, anus, vulva, and tip of the penis. It consists of a surface layer of EPITHELIUM, a basement membrane, and an underlying layer of connective tissue. Mucous membranes are kept moist by the secretions of mucus-producing glands.

mucous membrane exposure Exposure to infection via the mucous membranes such as the lining of the mouth, vagina, or rectum.

mucus The thick fluid secreted by mucous membranes or mucous glands.

multiagent therapy Treatment with more than one drug. See MONOTHERAPY.

Multicenter AIDS Cohort Study (MACS) The Multicenter AIDS Cohort Study is one of the largest prospective HIV studies in the world. MACS enrolled its first participants in 1984. Data to 1995 are significant because they are pre-HAART. Of the 5,579 men who entered the study, 2,191 were infected with HIV. During the study, 488 men have become HIV infected. MACS clinical sites are located in Baltimore (Johns Hopkins), Los Angeles (UCLA), Pittsburgh (University of Pittsburgh), and Chicago (the Howard Brown Memorial Clinic/Northwestern University). The men come to the clinical sites twice a year for exams and laboratory testing as well as to answer questions about any preventive and treatment medications they take. From enrollment through March 30, 1995, 1,362 men have developed AIDS, of whom 1,158 died. Another 101 HIV-infected men died before they developed AIDS. At enrollment, MACS men were 83.1 percent white, 10.1 percent African American and 5.3 percent Hispanic, while the rest were from other or unknown racial groups. The men ranged in age from 18 to 70, and more than half had college degrees when they entered the study.

By studying the outcome of various medications in real clinical practice, MACS provides an observational database that indicates the unsuspected value of available therapies. Important MACS accomplishments and findings: the identification of more than 60 HIV-infected men who are LONG-TERM NONPROGRESSORS, many of whom have served as critical sources of information on this phenomenon in studies conducted at several United States laboratories; the discovery that prevention of PNEU-MOCYSTIS CARINII PNEUMONIA can delay the first AIDS-defining illness by six to 12 months; the discovery that response of CD4+ T CELLS to AZT predicts AIDS-free time and survival among HIV-infected patients; the finding that risk factors for HIV encephalopathy include anemia, lower body mass, older age, and the presence of such symptoms as fever, fatigue, diarrhea, or thrush before an AIDS diagnosis; and the finding that symptoms of depression do not independently predict poorer outcomes to HIV infection. MACS collaborations with the National Cancer Institute, a component of the National Institutes of Health, and the Agency for Health Care Policy and Research (AHCPR), an agency of the United States PUBLIC HEALTH SERVICE, part of the United States DEPARTMENT OF HEALTH AND HUMAN SERVICES, have supported studies on HIV-related cancers and the impact of treatments on patients' use of health services.

multidrug-resistant tuberculosis (MDR-TB) See MULTIPLE DRUG-RESISTANT TUBERCULOSIS.

multifocal giant-cell encephalitis See HIV ENCEPHALOPATHY.

multiple allergic reactions Increased number of reactions (fever, rash, swelling, itching) to insect bites or common medications such as sulfa or penicillin.

multiple drug-resistant tuberculosis (MDR-TB) A strain of TB that does not respond to two or more standard TB drugs. MDR-TB usually occurs when treatment is interrupted, thus allowing drug-resist MUTATIONS to occur in the organism. Outbreaks (the rapid spread from one person to another) have occurred, such as that in the New York City area in the early 1990s and that currently overwhelming Russian prisons. MDR-TB is more difficult to treat when there is resistance to the two strongest antituberculosis drugs, isoniazid and rifampin.

The prevalence of MDR-TB may be increased in coinfected individuals. Every HIV-positive patient with *Mycobacterium tuberculosis* should have his or her isolate tested for drug susceptibility. The results should provide the basis for clinical therapeutic decisions.

Inadequate treatment is the primary cause of MDR-TB. Multiple levels of resistance are likely to compound when single drugs are added to a failing regimen. When initiating treatment in patients with confirmed MDR-TB, both the treatment history and the in vitro susceptibilities of the patient's strain should be evaluated. The patient should be hospitalized, and the selected regimen should include between four and seven drugs. Drugs with potential utility in a retreatment regimen include pyrazinamide, ethambutol, streptomycin, ofloxacin, ciprofloxacin, ethionamide, cycloserine, capreomycin, and PAS. In cases where chemotherapy is unsuccessful, adjunctive treatment with resectional surgery may be considered.

Note, too, that there are indications that multidrug resistance in HIV-positive people can also result from reinfection with resistant strains of *M. tuberculosis*. Reinfection can occur during or after therapy for drug-sensitive tuberculosis.

multiple outcomes A term used to refer to the fact that a trial involves several different outcome measures, each of which is used or is to be used to make treatment comparisons.

multivariate analysis A statistical analysis technique in which multiple variables are analyzed separately to determine the contribution made by each variable to an observed result.

mushrooms Any of various fleshy fungi, including the toadstools, puffballs, coral fungi, and morels. The subject of immune potentiators and antivirals from medicinal fungi is, as one might expect, very large. Within the context of HIV/AIDS, commercial product literature and reports have been published that discuss both the potential of different varieties of mushrooms as immune modulation agents and their mechanisms.

Shiitake is an edible mushroom traditionally cultivated in Japan and now used as a delicacy in cooking throughout the world. Traditionally, shiitake has been used as a folk remedy in Japan. Lentinan, a substance found in shiitake, has important effects on the immune system, and is well accepted by physicians in Japan to increase T-CELLS for cancer treatment. Japanese scientists have found that the drug can be used orally and that it has very little toxicity. It has immune potentiating effects and may also be antiviral against HIV.

It is not known how much lentinan is in the mushrooms. Too much can result with the opposite of the intended effect. Due to the possibility of toxicity, it has been used every other day or every fourth day. Traditional cooking recipes have most often been used by persons with HIV as a guide to deciding how much of the mushroom to use and how to prepare it. More studies are needed to determine if lentinan is an effective therapy for delaying or preventing the development of AIDS in persons at early stages of illness.

mutagen An agent that has a tendency to increase mutations.

mutation A change in the genetic material of a virus or a cell that may lead to a change in the structure of functioning of an organism; a change in the genetic material of a gene that is transmissible to offspring.

mutually monogamous sexual relationship A relationship in which each partner agrees to be MONOGAMOUS.

myalgia Tenderness or pain in a muscle or muscles.

Mycelex G See CLOTRIMAZOLE.

mycobacteriosis An infection caused by any mycobacterium.

Mycobacterium A genus of acid-fast organisms of the Mycobacteriaceae family, which includes the causative organisms of TUBERCULOSIS, LEPROSY, and MAC. The term *acid-fast* refers to a property of mycobacteria on staining done in microbiology labs, namely, that these bacteria do not decolorize when dilute acid is applied to the slide.

Mycobacterium avium **complex (MAC)** A serious bacterial infection that causes systemic infection in immunosuppressed persons and lung disease in persons with underlying chronic lung disease. Of unprecedented frequency in persons with AIDS, MAC is the most common bacterial OPPORTUNISTIC INFECTION of people who have advanced HIV disease. It is also one of the last opportunistic infections to develop.

MAC is caused by two species of bacteria, *Mycobacterium avium* and *Mycobacterium intracellulare,* which are collectively referred to as *Mycobacterium avium* complex. Both *M. avium* and *M. intracellulare* are closely related to *M. tuberculosis,* the bacterium that causes TB. MAC bacteria are found commonly in nature and probably enter the body by inhalation of dust and during the consumption of food and water. The infection is not transmitted from person to person, so MAC patients need not be isolated as HIV-infected patients with active TB must. MAC infection is thought to begin in the intestines. The bacteria then spread from there to the lymph nodes, blood, and other organs of the body. Generally, infection becomes apparent when the CD4 lymphocyte count drops below 50 cells/mm, and cell counts as low as 10 cells/mm are common at the time of MAC diagnosis.

The bacteria responsible for MAC are commonly found in food, water, and the environment. To date, there are no recommendations for avoiding exposure.

Symptoms of MAC include fever, malaise, weight loss, chronic diarrhea, and abdominal pain. The infection can interfere with the absorption of food and nutrients from the intestines, thereby contributing to malnutrition and wasting during late-stage disease.

MAC can be localized (limited to a specific organ or area of the body) or disseminated throughout the body. Disseminated MAC infection affects a variety of organs, including the lungs, liver, spleen, lymph nodes, bone marrow, intestines, and blood. MAC infection is found almost exclusively in people with HIV disease; it rarely occurs in people who are immune-suppressed for other reasons. Note that as children live longer with HIV disease, MAC occurs with increasing frequency. It is an indicator of markedly advanced disease and requires treatment with multiple drugs.

The development of highly effective MAC prophylaxis has been a major advance in the treatment of HIV infection. New therapies offer promise for both prevention and treatment. At present, the drug azithromycin is preferred for prophylaxis, and the related drug clarithromycin for treatment of MAC illness. Individuals who cannot tolerate azithromycin or clarithromycin can take rifabutin. Prophylaxis is generally given when the CD4 lymphocyte count drops below 50 cells/mm and stopped if CD4 count rises and remains above 50–100 cells/mm. Therapy generally includes clarithromycin (without which treatment is much less effective), ethambutol, and one other drug (usually rifabutin or ciprofloxacin). Alternatives for prophylaxis are clarithromycin and rifabutin. MAC may become resistant to therapy if patients do not take the full doses of the anti-MAC drugs. Studies are needed to ascertain potential drug interactions and toxicities.

The presence of disseminated MAC should be ruled out before prophylaxis is started. If disease is present, multidrug therapy is used to treat it, whereas prophylaxis requires only one drug. If only one drug is given to treat the disease, drug resistance may develop. Similarly, TB should be ruled out in individuals who are receiving rifabutin for MAC, as resistance to rifabutin can result in cross-resistance to rifampin and make treatment of TB much more difficult.

People may be colonized with MAC in the lungs or intestinal tract. The dividing of MAC on sputum cultures done to rule out TB is frequent in patients with counts less than 100 CD4 cells/mm. On acid-fast staining (the preliminary step the lab takes to look for TB), MAC is indistinguishable from TB. Although MAC is in the same family as TB, it is not contagious and its treatment differs from that of TB. Note too that the term *TB* refers only to *Mycobacterim tuberculosis* or the disease it causes, not to all mycobacteria or acid-fast bacilli. MAC is intrinsically much less virulent than TB and basically does not cause disease in a healthy person. However, in AIDS, the infection can reach enormous proportions and there may be such large numbers of bacteria in the bloodstream that the condition may become untreatable.

Mycobacterium avium-intracellulare (MAI) See MYCOBACTERIUM AVIUM COMPLEX.

Mycobacterium kansasii A microbacterium that causes a TUBERCULOSIS-like pulmonary disease in humans, and occasionally disseminated infection in AIDS.

Mycobacterium leprae The causative agent of LEPROSY in humans.

Mycobacterium tuberculosis The microorganism that causes tuberculosis in mammals.

mycophenolic acid Also known as mycophenolate, mycophenolic acid is a compound that inhibits the creation of guanosine nucleotides. It is currently used in organ transplantation. Guanosine nucleotides are necessary enzymes for DNA and RNA synthesis. Blocking of the creation of these guanosine nucleotides stops cell reproduction. Ribavirin is another such chemical.

Some testing in patients of ribavirin and mycophenolic acid has shown enhancement of anti-HIV activity when they are used along with NRTIs. Furthermore, some drug researchers claim that very little negative effect on mitochondrial

DNA was seen in those patients using this drug (see MITOCHONDRIAL TOXICITY). The possible toxicity warrants further study to eliminate the risk of severe problems, as were seen with HYDROXYUREA. Until further testing is completed, this drug may just be the source of another false hope in anti-HIV drug development. (The trade name is Cell Cept.)

mycoplasma One of a group of very small organisms in which the ability to form a cell wall has been lost. There are more than 70 organisms in this group, including 12 species that infect humans.

Human mycoplasma infections are usually pulmonary, cervical, and pelvic. Although it was once postulated that mycoplasma was a necessary cofactor in HIV-related disease progression, research to date has shown that the presence of mycoplasma DNA in the blood of HIV-infected patients is transient and not prognostic.

mycosis Any disease caused by a fungus.

Mycostatin See NYSTATIN.

myelin sheath Many layers of membrane of Schwann cell (in peripheral nerves) or of oligodendrocyte (central nervous system) wrapped in a tight spiral around a nerve axon forming a sheath that prevents leakage of current across all of the surrounded axon membrane except at the nodes of Ranvier.

myelitis Inflammation of the BONE MARROW or the SPINAL CORD.

myeloma A LYMPHOMA produced from cells of the B-cell lineage. Usually called multiple myeloma, it may occur somewhat more frequently in persons with HIV than in the general population. However, it is a rare disease, even in persons with AIDS.

myelopathy A general term denoting any pathological condition of the spinal cord or BONE MARROW. The term is used to refer to nonspecific lesions, as opposed to inflammatory lesions, which are termed MYELITIS.

myelosuppression Suppression of the bone marrow activity, causing decreased production of red blood cells (ANEMIA), white blood cells (LEUKOPE-NIA), or platelets (THROMBOCYTOPENIA). Myelosuppression is an effect of some drugs. It is common in late HIV disease, even in the absence of infection or myelotoxic drugs. A number of drugs used in HIV may have myelotoxicity, most commonly AZT, ganciclovir, and most cancer chemotherapy drugs.

myelosuppressive   Concerning inhibition of BONE MARROW function.

myelotoxic   Destructive to BONE MARROW.

myocardial   Concerning the heart's muscle mass.

myocardial dysfunction   Abnormal, disturbed, or impaired functioning of the muscular walls of the heart; MYOCARDIOPATHY. HIV may cause cardiomyopathy, most often in children. Also called cardiomyopathy.

myocardiopathy   See MYOCARDIAL DYSFUNCTION.

myocarditis   Inflammation of the MYOCARDIUM.

myocardium   The middle layer of the walls of the heart, composed of cardiac muscle.

myofascial pain   A large group of muscle disorders characterized by the presence of hypersensitive points, called trigger points, within one or more muscles and/or the investing connective tissue together with a syndrome of pain, muscle spasm, tenderness, stiffness, limitation of motion, weakness, and occasionally autonomic dysfunction.

myometrium   The muscular layer of the uterus.

myopathy   Inflammation of muscle tissue due to infection or adverse reaction to a medication. Myopathy may arise as a toxic reaction to AZT or as a consequence of HIV infection itself.

myositis   Inflammation of a muscle, especially a voluntary muscle.

N-9 See NONOXYNOL 9.

NAC See *N*-ACETYL CYSTEINE.

***N*-acetyl cysteine** A natural substance that is metabolized by the body into the amino acid CYSTEINE. Cysteine is one of the three components of the important ANTIOXIDANT GLUTATHIONE. People who have HIV infection have severely decreased levels of glutathione. Many physicians and natural health practitioners recommend taking NAC supplements, which have been shown to increase gluathione levels. NAC is the standard medical treatment for people suffering from liver stress brought on by an overdose of acetaminophen (Tylenol). Although glutathione aids in the protection of all cells and membranes, some studies have shown that glutathione is especially effective in enhancing immune system cells, protecting against damage from radiation and helping to reduce the side effects of chemotherapy, irradiation, and use of alcohol. It is unknown whether NAC helps protect against liver damage from HAART medication, but many HIV patients use the supplement. NAC has been shown to inhibit the replication of HIV in the test tube. In one double-blind study patients with HIV who supplemented their diet with 800 mg/day of NAC had a slowing of the rate of decline in immune function. NAC also has been shown in vitro to inhibit TUMOR NECROSIS FACTOR, which is present in high levels in HIV patients.

nadir The lowest point. Used to describe a blood count that has reached a low point and then returned to a more normal level. If used to describe drugs, it refers to the lowest concentration of a drug in the body.

naive T cell A T cell that arises from the immune system's production of fresh cells in the THYMUS. Naive T cells are cells that have not yet encountered any antigen of any kind. They respond to PATHOGENS containing ANTIGENS the immune system has not encountered before. The naive T cells' activation and proliferation create an acquired immune response to the newly encountered pathogenic agent. After the antigen is eradicated, a portion of the now-activated T cells is stored in the body as MEMORY CELLS for the next time a similar antigen appears in the body. Naive T cells make up about half of the T cells in an average human. In HIV they may constitute only 20 percent of the T-cell population. Memory cell production increases when someone begins HAART therapy. After a period of use of the drugs, new naive T cells begin production. Because HIV attacks naive T cells, the OPPORTUNISTIC INFECTIONS have easier access to the body because the body is overloaded with memory that cannot fight an unknown antigen. By overstimulating the immune system HIV causes normally naive T cells to mature into memory cells, leaving fewer naive T cells to fight new infections.

naked DNA A vaccine strategy that uses a piece of a bacterium called a plasmid to hold foreign genetic material; also called a gene vaccine or genetic immunization.

Naprosyn See NAPROXEN.

naproxen A nonsteroidal, anti-inflammatory drug used for the treatment of a number of inflammatory diseases, including osteoarthritis and rheumatoid arthritis, and for the relief of mild-to-moderate pain. Naproxen is quickly absorbed into the bloodstream. Pain relief is usually evident within an hour after the first dose, but its maximum effect on arthritis or other inflammatory disorders may not be observed for up to a month of continual dosing. (Trade names are Anaprox and Aleve.)

narcotic Producing stupor or sleep; loosely, anything that soothes, relieves, or lulls; a drug that in moderate doses depresses the CENTRAL NERVOUS SYSTEM, thus relieving pain and producing sleep, but that in excessive doses produces unconsciousness, stupor, coma, and possibly death. Most are habit-forming. Examples include opium, morphine, codeine, papaverine, heroin, and many synthetics.

nasal ulcer An open sore or lesion of the nose, accompanied by sloughing of inflamed necrotic tissue.

NASBA See NUCLEIC ACID SEQUENCE-BASED AMPLIFICATION.

nasopharynx The part of the pharynx above the soft palate.

National Cancer Institute (NCI) One of the institutes of the NATIONAL INSTITUTES OF HEALTH, with a mission of coordinating research, training, and dissemination of information about the causes, diagnosis, and treatment of cancers. NCI also holds the responsibility for these functions for HIV-related cancers.

National Institute of Allergy and Infectious Diseases (NIAID) NIAID is the U.S. government agency that provides major support for scientists conducting research aimed at developing better ways to diagnose, treat, and prevent infectious, immunologic, and allergic diseases that afflict people worldwide. It is a division of the NATIONAL INSTITUTES OF HEALTH. It is responsible for the national basic research program in AIDS, which is managed through the DIVISION OF AIDS. The institute supports basic research, epidemiology, vaccine development, drug discovery and development, and treatment studies. It administers the ADULT AIDS CLINICAL TRIALS GROUP (AACTG), the PEDIATRIC AIDS CLINICAL TRIAL GROUP (PATCG), and the COMMUNITY PROGRAMS FOR CLINICAL RESEARCH ON AIDS (CPCRA). Its Internet address is http://www.niaid.nih.gov.

National Institute of Child Health and Human Development (NICHD) An institute of the NATIONAL INSTITUTES OF HEALTH. The NICHD supports and conducts research on reproductive biology and population issues; on prenatal development as well as maternal, child, and family health; and on medical rehabilitation. NICHD research is also directed to restoring or maximizing individual health, when disease, injury, or a chronic disorder intervenes in the developmental process. Its Internet site is http://www.nichd.nih.gov.

National Institutes of Health (NIH) A division of the U.S. Department of Health and Human Services composed of several agencies involved in health research. It conducts and manages research in its own laboratories, universities, medical schools, hospitals, and institutions around the United States. Its Internet address is http://www.nih.gov.

natural and alien An apparently fundamental conceptual opposition within AIDS discourse; like the opposition normal/abnormal, it distinguishes self from nonself. The AIDS virus is linguistically identified with that which is alien, or unnatural. See KNOWLEDGE AND IGNORANCE.

natural history studies Studies that observe the course of a disease. Concerning women and HIV, for example, much attention has been given to natural history studies designed to answer the question, Are there gender differences in HIV disease? At the VIII International Conference on AIDS (Amsterdam, July 1992), data was presented that compared men and women with HIV disease who were similar in a number of ways, including disease progression, age, and mode of transmission.

natural killer cell (NK cell) A type of large LYMPHOCYTE that performs surveillance against bacteria, viruses, and cancer cells and attacks and destroys foreign, infected, and cancerous cells. NK cells kill on contact by binding to the target cells and releasing a lethal burst of chemicals. Normal cells are not affected by NK cells. NK cells are thought to play a major role in cancer prevention by destroying abnormal cells before they have a chance to pose a real threat. NK cells are not targeted at specific ANTIGENS the way CYTOTOXIC T-CELL LYMPHOCYTES are. While they are not B or T lymphocytes, they are thought to be precursors of T-suppressor cells.

naturopathic medicine   A specialty of alternative medicine; a combination of natural therapies that includes nutritional therapy, herbal medicine, HOMEOPATHY, spinal manipulation, exercise therapy, hydrotherapy, electrotherapy, stress reduction, and natural cures. Naturopathic medicine assumes that the body is always striving for good health. Disease is viewed as a result of a healing effort of nature. If an illness develops, the symptoms accompanying it are the result of the organism's intrinsic attempt to defend and heal itself. A naturopathic physician focuses on aiding the body in its effort to regain its natural health instead of initiating a treatment that might interfere with this process. Naturopathic doctors prefer nontoxic and noninvasive treatments that minimize the risks of harmful side effects. They are trained to distinguish which patients they can treat safely and which need referral to other health care practitioners. Naturopaths currently are licensed to practice in nearly all the states in the United States. Naturopathic physicians who have attended an accredited four-year program are trained in most of the same scientific disciplines taught in conventional medical schools. Consequently, most naturopaths use medical tests for diagnosis. Many naturopaths may use modern medicine for certain crisis situations. During the first visit, a naturopath uses history-taking, physical examination, laboratory tests, and other standard diagnostic procedures to learn as much as possible about the patient. Diet, environment, exercise, stress, and other aspects of lifestyle also are evaluated. Once a good understanding of the patient's health and disease is established, doctor and patient work together to establish a treatment and health-promoting program.

nausea   Unpleasant sensation in the stomach, usually including the urge to vomit. It is present in seasickness, early pregnancy, diseases of the CENTRAL NERVOUS SYSTEM, neurasthenia, and hysteria. It may be provoked by the sight or odor or mental images of obnoxious matter or conditions. It may be present, without vomiting, in certain gallbladder disturbances and in carsickness and other types of motion sickness.

Although not all CHEMOTHERAPY patients experience nausea and vomiting, they are the most common side effects of chemotherapy. They may also result from other strong medications, RADIATION therapy to the gastrointestinal tract, liver, or brain, or from an illness or cancer itself. Nausea is one of the most dreaded side effects of such treatments and can have a psychological as well as physical impact on a patient. Nausea and vomiting can lead to nutrition depletion and a general deterioration of the patient's physical condition. It could also lead a patient to quit a potentially curative or useful treatment as well as to neglect self-care and reduce functional ability. Antiemetic drugs are the greatest defense against nausea and vomiting; other methods include hypnosis, acupuncture, distraction, relaxation techniques, and imagery.

NCI   See NATIONAL CANCER INSTITUTE.

NDA   See DRUG APPROVAL PROCESS.

nebulized pentamidine   See PENTAMIDINE.

nebulizer   An apparatus for producing a fine spray or mist. This may be done by rapidly passing air through a liquid or by vibrating a liquid at a high frequency so that the particles produced are extremely small.

necropsy   An examination of a dead body to determine cause of death or pathological condition; an AUTOPSY.

necrosis   The death of areas of tissue or bone surrounded by healthy parts; the constellation of morphological changes indicative of cell death and caused by the progressive degenerative action of various enzymes. Necrosis may be caused by a variety of factors: insufficient blood supply; physical agents such as trauma and radiant energy; or chemical agents acting locally, acting internally following absorption, or placed into the wrong tissue.

needle access   Increasing access to sterile injection equipment, including needles and syringes, has been the primary HARM REDUCTION strategy by governments to reduce TRANSMISSION of HIV among INJECTION DRUG USERS (IDUs).

A variety of programs has been implemented to accomplish this end, including lifting restrictions on sales; pharmacy-based interventions; vending machines; and equipment exchanges. Different types of service may be used by different subpopulations; for example, recreational or occasional drug users may prefer the "normality" of the pharmacy and gay users may prefer programs targeted to their particular group by nongovernmental organizations. The overall impact of increased access, however, has been difficult to assess. Moreover, in the United States there has been substantial public disagreement about the propriety of allowing protected access to needles and syringes, even while the possession of some such equipment remains illegal in many jurisdictions. See DRUG ABUSE; DRUG PARAPHERNALIA LAWS; NEEDLE EXCHANGE PROGRAM; NEEDLE-PRESCRIPTION LAW.

needle exchange program   Any HARM REDUCTION in which INJECTION DRUG USERS may exchange used needles and syringes for sterile ones. Such programs have been created in an effort to remove contaminated works from this community and reduce the spread of HIV via this route of transmission. The concept is controversial. Those who oppose needle exchange programs believe that they encourage an illegal, destructive, and undesirable activity—drug addiction. Those who support such programs believe that AIDS prevention measures, to be effective, must deal practically with the world as it is, and that moralizing about drug abuse will only make it harder to reach the very people who are at the greatest risk and who pose the greatest danger to the larger community. The AMERICAN FOUNDATION FOR AIDS RESEARCH (AMFAR)

was the first foundation willing to take a stand on this issue and fund an AIDS prevention program aimed at a group of people often considered to be expendable. Exchanges are generally conducted by outreach workers in a variety of settings—in vehicles and health care clinics, on the streets, or in visits to addicts' homes. Usually materials are provided free of charge, and each exchange involves an encounter between a drug user and a program staff member. Programs have taken various forms: some distribute needles, others sell needles and syringes as well as exchange them, and still others conduct a strict exchange of one used for each new needle or syringe.

Exchange programs have been initiated by governmental and nongovernmental agencies. In some areas, exchange has been organized by drug users themselves. In the United States, most of the operating exchange programs began in defiance of drug paraphernalia laws, in effect as acts of civil disobedience. Some are still illegal or unsanctioned, although there are some government-sponsored programs.

Needle exchange programs have several advantages. They remove financial barriers to low-income drug users' obtaining sterile equipment. They allow exchange personnel to deliver prevention messages, incorporate high-risk users into a helping system, and reduce biowaste. Disadvantages are the high cost of materials, staff, and implementation, and that they provide less coverage of the injection drug-using population than do other NEEDLE ACCESS programs.

needle-prescription law   Drug paraphernalia laws do not prohibit or regulate the sale of hypodermic needles and syringes if the seller has no reason to believe that the equipment will be used for injection of illicit drugs. Accordingly, over-the-counter sales of hypodermic syringes and needles are permitted in most states. Pharmacists are not obliged to question buyers' intentions in purchasing the equipment, and wide variations in sales practices exist. Some states, however, significantly restrict over-the-counter sales. These jurisdictions prohibit the sale, distribution, or possession of hypodermic needles or syringes without a valid medical prescription. Needle-prescription laws are more onerous than drug paraphernalia laws because they do not require criminal intent. Under needle-prescription laws, physicians may write prescriptions for hypodermic needles and syringes for patients under their care only if there is a legitimate medical purpose for them to do so. A wholesale druggist or surgical supplier must keep careful records of the sale of this equipment. People charged with illegal possession have the burden of proving that they have sufficient authority or license.

Proposals for statutory reform consistent with public health objectives call for narrowing the focus of drug paraphernalia laws and repealing needle-prescription laws. It is argued that this repeal would be less controversial than needle distribution programs because the state would not be directly involved in the distribution of drug injection equipment. Repeal of these laws would have no revenue impact for state legislatures. It would simply remove the state as an affirmative obstacle to providing IV drug users with sterile equipment necessary to protect their health. Repeal of needle-prescription legislation is already supported by numerous public health and bar associations. Additionally, experience in jurisdictions that already permit over-the-counter sales of hypodermic needles and syringes shows that they are better able to control the needle-borne spread of HIV and that allowing over-the-counter sales does not result in greater drug use. See DRUG PARAPHERNALIA LAWS.

needle sharing The act or practice of using a hypodermic syringe in common with another person or persons. Generally the term refers to the reuse of needles by drug addicts, without sterilization, after they have been used by others.

People who use needles to inject drugs can get the HIV virus by sharing works with other users who have the virus in their blood. INJECTION DRUG USERS can reduce their chances of infection if they do not share works (needles, syringes, or cookers), or rent or buy works that have been used by someone else. They can also reduce their chances of infection if they clean their works with either ethyl alcohol or household bleach before and after use.

needlestick The unintentional puncture of the skin with a hypodermic needle. When this occurs in medical personnel, the CDC recommends post-exposure prophylaxis of HAART in some cases. If the person the needle had been used for is HIV-negative or extremely low-risk, then another decision can be made. See UNIVERSAL PRECAUTIONS.

nef One of the regulatory genes of HIV. HIV that appears without nef seems to reproduce poorly, so its function is thought to increase the virus's toxicity. Nef seems to block HIV-infected cells from expressing CD4 and MAJOR HISTOCOMPATIBILITY COMPLEX 1 (MHC-1) on their surfaces. This effect reduces the immune system's ability to recognize and kill these infected cells. As a result the virus can reproduce more of itself before it is killed. The term *nef* also refers to the nef protein produced by the gene. The nef protein protects its infected host and simultaneously destroys the neighboring uninfected cells of the immune system in a process known as APOPTOSIS. Research has shown that nef does this by binding to and inhibiting a protein called ASK1, a key player in apoptosis. Researchers believe that if they can block the effectiveness of the nef protein, they may be able to short circuit HIV, preventing it from causing much harm to the body and from reproducing in the body.

nef-deleted vaccine A live-attenuated HIV vaccine composed of HIV with NEF, a key component of the virus, deleted to lessen its ability to replicate or reproduce.

nef gene The gene in the HUMAN IMMUNODEFICIENCY VIRUS that encodes the NEF protein and affects virus replication by decreasing production.

negligence In forensic medicine, the failure to act as a reasonably prudent person with the same knowledge, experience, and background would under similar circumstances, causing injury or damage to a person. There are four elements of negligence: duty owed, breach of duty or standard of care, proximate cause or causal connection, and damages or injuries. Nurses are legally liable for their own negligence, as well as the negligence of others of which they have knowledge but do not report. In law, the failure to exercise a reasonable degree of care, especially for the protection of other persons. Negligence may be an act of omission or commission, characterized by intention, recklessness, inadvertence, thoughtlessness, or wantonness. In health care, negligence resulting in legal liability is the failure to exercise that degree of care and skill ordinarily practiced by other professionals of similar skill and training under similar circumstances. The failure to exercise ordinary professional care must have caused an injury to the patient in order for there to have been a negligent act.

negotiated safety   A term coined by researchers in Australia to denote the practice of HIV-negative gay couples who have decided to forgo the use of condoms because they believe that if neither partner is infected, the virus cannot be transmitted between them. The question of negotiated safety forces partners to weigh their trust in each other against the consequences of betrayal, and to do so amidst homophobia, gay men's freewheeling sexual culture, and the epidemic itself. The subtext of negotiated safety is that gay couples can be strong and trustworthy, and should be. Despite considerable criticism from researchers and public health officials, Australian prevention workers have launched prevention campaigns to educate couples on how to responsibly forgo condoms. They insist that the issue is not whether people will contract HIV through negotiated safety, but rather whether fewer people will contract HIV through clarified negotiation.

Prevention researchers point out that making this strategy work requires honest communication about emotionally volatile subjects. They worry that negotiated safety could elevate unprotected intercourse to the ultimate test of true love. They offer an alternative term—"negotiated danger." Those who support teaching negotiated safety counter that current prevention campaigns already mystify sex by prescribing a simple dogmatic truth, rather than presenting a complex and honest discussion. Critics point out that even if promulgated in counseling sessions or other controlled settings, the negotiated safety regimen may be too demanding for most couples. Others note that the complex dynamics of negotiated safety may be most difficult

for those most at risk. Public health officials urge counselors to emphasize the use of condoms with every partner, and remain wary of muddying the condom message.

The crucial prevention question is can HIV-negative couples abandon condoms and still be safe? Is it a "reasonable decision" for HIV-negative couples to have unprotected sex? Should AIDS workers offer such guidance?

Studies show that men in relationships in which both partners have the same HIV status are much more likely to have unprotected anal sex than men in sero-discordant couples or men who don't know whether their partner is infected. Research consistently indicates that gay men are far more likely to forgo condoms when having sex with a lover than with a casual partner. It is clear that the dynamics of a long-term relationship increase the likelihood of sexual risk-taking. The risk for HIV-positive couples is mutual reinfection, although this remains the subject of much debate. By exchanging semen, HIV-positive men might also contract other sexually transmitted diseases, thus weakening their immune systems. But clearly, the stakes are lower for these couples than for partners who are negative.

Neisseria gonorrhoea   A type of GRAM-NEGATIVE BACTERIA, belonging to the genus *Neisseria*, that causes gonorrhea.

nelfinavir   Agouron Pharmaceuticals' PROTEASE INHIBITOR. Nelfinavir is commonly recommended as a first-line protease inhibitor as it is known to be less effective for people who have taken protease inhibitors previously. Nelfinavir has been reported to increase the level of Viagra in the body.

The dosage of nelfinavir has been difficult for some people. It requires either three pills three times a day or five pills twice a day. The drug should be taken with some food as it is better absorbed if digested with stomach acids. The main side effect that many seem to suffer is diarrhea. This can be controlled generally with LOPERAMIDE. Other methods of control that have been used are Metamucil or 500 mg twice daily of calcium, which was clinically shown to control the diarrhea in many people. Other side effects include headache and nausea.

As all protease inhibitors, it seems to create METABOLIC TOXICITY to a certain degree. Researchers have yet to determine which drug or drugs or whether HIV itself is the root of these problems. It is also available in a children's formula. There has been a government warning about protease inhibitors' causing high blood sugar level and diabetes. Symptoms to watch for include increased thirst and hunger, unexplained weight loss, increased urination, fatigue, and dry, itchy skin. (Trade name is Viracept.)

neonate   Newly born; a newborn infant.

neoplasm   An abnormal growth of tissue in which the expansion is uncontrolled, progressive, and serves no useful function. Neoplasms may be benign (not spreading by METASTASIS or infiltration of tissue) or malignant (infiltrating tissue, metastasizing, often recurring after attempts at surgical removal). Other kinds of neoplasms include histoid (in which the structure resembles the tissues and elements that surround it); mixed (composed of tissues from two of the germinal layers); organoid (similar to some organ of the body); multicentric (arising from a number of distinct groups of cells); and unicentric (having origin in one group of cells).

neoplastic   Pertaining to, or of the nature of, a NEOPLASM (new, abnormal tissue formation).

neopterin   A molecule produced by MACROPHAGES in response to GAMMA INTERFERON and found in serum, urine, and CEREBROSPINAL FLUID. Neopterin levels have been used to predict HIV disease progression much in the same way as BETA-2 MICROGLOBULIN. The neopterin level is approximately 5.4 nanomoles per liter of blood (nmol/l). Elevated neopterin levels have been reported in individuals in all phases of HIV disease. According to some studies, high neopterin levels are associated with a poor prognosis; low levels correlate with a better prognosis. Serum neopterin levels are measured in some studies as an additional SURROGATE MARKER for HIV disease.

nephropathy   Any disease of the kidney. The term covers inflammatory (nephritis), degenera-tive (nephrosis), and sclerotic (arteriosclerotic) lesions of the kidney.

nephrotoxicity   The quality of being toxic or destructive to kidney cells.

nerve cell   See NEURON.

nerve growth factor (NGF)   A naturally produced substance that has many roles in the maintenance of nerves and nerve cells, especially sensory ones. Synthetic, recombinant NGF is a proposed therapy for HIV- and drug-associated neuropathies.

neurologic, neurological   Relating to the nervous system, including the brain and spinal cord.

neurologic assessment   Assessment of diseases of the nervous system.

neurologic complication   A disease or abnormality of the nervous system that is superimposed upon another disease without being specifically related to it, yet affecting or modifying the prognosis of the original disease.

neurological disease   There are several neurological diseases that can affect people with HIV disease. Some are OPPORTUNISTIC INFECTIONS, and others are effects of the virus itself. HIV ENCEPHALOPATHY is one of the more common problems in late-stage HIV. HAART has led to a decrease in incidence of HIV encephalopathy, but it still occurs in some form in approximately 30 percent of all HIV-positive people. Symptoms include decrease in short-term memory, inability to keep track of conversations or appointments, and motor impairment such as changes in gait and problems with handwriting or keyboarding. Occasionally a patient's partner reports a decrease in emotions or social withdrawal and apathy.

Other problems in HIV encephalopathy include vascular MYELOPATHY, a degeneration of the spinal cord that leads to leg weakness, stiffness, sensory loss, imbalance, and sphincter dysfunction. Small holes, or vacuoles, develop in the middle part of the spinal cord, which controls the lower part of the body, and become larger over time. MYELIN, the protective coating around nerve fibers, is slowly destroyed. As more and more fibers die, the brain's signals are short-circuited, thereby blocking communication with the lower body. Myelopathy can occur at any time in HIV disease and up to 55 percent of HIV-positive people at autopsy show some degree of myelopathy.

Also connected is HIV NEUROPATHY, which also affects up to a third of HIV-positive people. Patients initially report a numb or tingling feeling in their feet that may later spread to other extremities. Others report painful sensations when they stand or apply pressure on the feet. A decrease in foot and ankle reflexes accompanies this problem. This can be caused both by the progress of the disease and by some of the medicines that HIV-positive people take; ddI, ddC, and d4T have been linked to these problems.

About 3 percent of all people with HIV have an opportunistic infection called PROGRESSIVE MULTIFO-CAL LEUKOENCEPHALOPATHY. The JC VIRUS is reactivated in immune dysfunction and leads to walking problems, visual difficulties, cognitive problems, and eventually death. The brain shows many lesions when MRI is performed.

Primary central nervous system (CNS) lymphoma occurs in about 2 percent of HIV disease patients. CNS lymphoma is a tumor of a form of white blood cells called LYMPHOCYTES. Lymphomas can occur anywhere in the lymph system and often spread to the nervous system. *Primary CNS lymphoma* refers to a form of lymphoma that is confined to the brain, spinal cord, their lining, and/or the inside of the eye. Irradiation is sometimes successful as treatment. It has been shown to increase in effectiveness when combined with the drug methotrexate.

TOXOPLASMOSIS is a disease caused by a parasite called *Toxoplasma gondii*. It is found in many animals and humans. It generally is kept under control but in immune suppressed people can cause a range of neurological problems. It can be spread in the feces of animals, particularly cats. Once exposed, however, cats generally only are infectious for one or two weeks. The combination of two drugs, pyrimethamine and sulfadiazine, is used to treat the disease. Diagnosis is through tests for the parasite in the blood and CT or MRI. Typi-cally the parasite can cause a form of encephalitis that is very dangerous. Symptoms include fever, confusion, headache, disorientation, personality changes, tremor, and seizures.

CYTOMEGALOVIRUS causes another infection that a majority of people in the United States already have in their body but that a healthy immune system can keep in check. The most common illness caused by CMV is retinitis. This is the death of cells in the retinas, leading to blindness. Advanced cases can spread to many parts of the body and cause problems. This does not occur until late-stage HIV disease. HAART has brought most cases of CMV under control, and CMV infection has dropped in occurrence.

neurologic dysfunction   Abnormal, disturbed, or impaired functioning of the nervous system.

neurology   The branch of medical science dealing with the study of the nervous system and its disorders.

neurolytic block   The injection of ethyl alcohol or another chemical around a group of nerves to provide long-lasting relief from pain that has not been controlled successfully with medication. Alcohol or phenol damages the nerves, which will therefore give longer pain-relieving ability than topical or injection medications. After the nerves have been damaged, they try to repair themselves over the next several years; greater pain than was originally experienced may result. Therefore, these blocks are usually only performed for the treatment of pain as terminal illnesses such as cancer. Neurolytic blocks can often have unintended side effects of damaging nerves not intended to be blocked.

neuromuscular therapy   Physical therapy that emphasizes the role of the brain, spine, and nerves in muscular pain. One goal of the therapy is to relieve tender congested spots in muscle tissue and compress nerves that may radiate pain to other areas of the body.

neuron   Major cell of nervous tissue; the structural and functional unit of the nervous system, specialized for transmission of information in the form of patterns of impulses. The brain cells influence neurons by secreting neurotransmitters that alter the affected cell by physically contracting it. Alternatively, a neuron may release neurohormones into the bloodstream. The nucleus and its surrounding cytoplasm comprise the cell body, or perikaryon, which may be the site of multiple synaptic connections with other nerve fibers. In non-receptor cells, numerous projections from the cell body, or dendrites, provide a large surface area for synaptic connections with other neurons. One or more regions of the cell body (axon hillocks) extend into long thin axons and carry impulses away from the cell body to other neurons and to effectors, making contacts via synapses through the secretion of neurotransmitters. There are many different types of neurons: some distinguished by function, others by process, and still others by location.

neuronal cell death   The death of a NEURON or nerve cell.

neuropathic pain   Pain caused by damage, injury, or change in ability to function of one or more nerves. It is the type of pain experienced in NEUROPATHY, shingles, and any number of nerve-related or nerve-involved illnesses such as cancer that can constrict or interrupt nerve function. This type of pain responds best to treatment by prescribed antidepressants or antiseizure medications.

neuropathology   The branch of medicine that deals with the study of diseases of the nervous system, as well as microscopic and macroscopic structural and functional changes occurring in them.

neuropathy   An abnormal, degenerative, or inflammatory condition of the PERIPHERAL NERVOUS SYSTEM. Nerves are responsible for, among other functions, the movement of muscles and the sensation of touch, including the sensation of pain. The symptoms of neuropathy can therefore be weakness of a muscle or pain and tingling. In people with HIV infection, the most frequent symptoms of neuropathy are painful feet and legs. Often, individuals experience numbness or tingling in the hands and feet; weakness in the legs, arms, and hands; or a burning pain in the soles of the feet and

the ends of the fingers and toes. The pain can be severe and, depending on where it occurs, may interfere with walking or using the hands. Neuropathy may be a neurological complication of HIV infection itself, and certain drugs, including alcohol, ddC, d4T, ddI, ISONIAZID, and VINCRISTINE can cause it. Ascending neuropathy is a pathological condition of the nervous system that rises from the lower body to the upper. Another term, *peripheral neuropathy,* describes damage to, or disruption of, the cells of the peripheral nervous system, which consists of the nerves outside the brain or spinal cord.

Treatment can include a variety of different drugs, usually intended to relieve pain, as there is not much that can be done to rebuild diseased or atrophied nerves. If the cause is thought to be a particular drug, then removing the drug from the regimen is the first step. Once the drug is discontinued, the pain often slows and eventually stops over a period of six to nine months. If this does not work or is not the principal cause, then the first line of treatment is currently an antiseizure medication such as Neurontin or Dilantin. If this is not effective, then the next line of treatment is a class of antidepressants such as amitriptyline or nortriptyline. Treatment can progress to use of narcotic medications. Typically they are used as a last choice because of the disadvantages of their use, such as sleepiness and potential addiction. They can include OxyContin and similar medications.

neuropsychiatric complication   A nervous or mental disease or difficulty superimposed upon another disease without being specifically related to it, yet affecting or modifying the prognosis of the original disease.

neuropsychiatry   The branch of medicine concerned with the study of nervous and mental disorders.

neuropsychological defect   An alteration in behavior that is related to a central nervous system illness and interferes with the ability to function in an age-normative fashion.

neuropsychological test   A test designed to measure certain aspects of brain function, such as memory, concentration, attention, and visual-motor skills.

neurosyphilis   A form of advanced syphilis in which the infection has spread to the central nervous system. The treatment of syphilis in HIV-infected patients is controversial. Although there is some evidence to the contrary, there has been documentation of an increased incidence of treatment failures and a more rapid progression to neurosyphilis in HIV-infected individuals who have syphilis. Patients with syphilis should be tested for HIV infection, and HIV-infected individuals should receive testing for syphilis. Altered mental status, facial palsy, herniplegia or herniparesis, ocular symptoms, and hearing loss may occur in neurosyphilis. Recent exposure or reexposure to syphilis is also a concern in central nervous system disorders and HIV. The antibiotic penicillin is used to treat neurosyphilis; Ceftriaxone is used if the patient is allergic to penicillin. Patients who have documented neurosyphilis should have repeat cerebrospinal fluid (CSF) examinations after six and 12 months.

neurotoxicity   Having the capability of harming nerve tissue.

neurotransmitter   A chemical that transmits information across the junction that separates one nerve cell from another nerve cell or a muscle. When an electrical impulse traveling along the nerve reaches the junction, the neurotransmitter is released and travels across the synapse, either causing or stopping continued electrical impulses along the nerve. Abnormalities in the production or functioning of certain neurotransmitters have been implicated in a number of disorders, including Parkinson's disease, amyotrophic lateral sclerosis, and clinical depression. There are more than 300 chemicals in the brain and nerve cells that can serve as neurotransmitters/norepinephrine, endorphins, acetylcholine, and serotonin. Each transmitter has its own receptor, which it matches up with on the nerves. The pain-regulating endorphins, for example, are similar in structure to heroin and codeine, which fill endorphin receptors to accomplish their effects. The alertness that follows caffeine consumption is the result of its blocking of the effects of adenosine, a neurotransmitter that inhibits brain activity. Medications and drugs can both inhibit and stimulate neurotransmitters, causing unwanted or unknown effects on occasion.

neutralization   1. The opposing of one force or condition with an opposite force or condition to such a degree as to cause counteraction, which permits neither to dominate. 2. In chemistry the process of destroying the peculiar properties or effects of a substance (e.g., the neutralization of an acid with a base). 3. In medicine, the process of checking or counteracting the effects of any agent that produces a morbid effect (e.g., the process by which ANTIBODY or antibody plus complement neutralizes the infectivity of MICROORGANISMS, particularly viruses).

neutralizing antibody   A protein produced by B CELLS, that can directly inactivate an invading MICROORGANISM, such as a VIRUS or BACTERIUM.

neutralizing domain   A section of the HIV ENVELOPE PROTEIN gp120 that elicits antibodies with a neutralizing activity.

neutrexin   See TRIMETREXATE.

neutropenia   An abnormal decrease in the number of NEUTROPHIL cells in the blood. The neutrophil is the most common WHITE BLOOD CELL in the body. Neutropenia can be a result of HIV infection or of drug reaction. Someone is considered to have neutropenia if his or her absolute polymorphonuclear (PMN) count is less than 1,000. It typically is not treated until the count falls below 500 PMN. This is a fairly common problem in HIV disease.

neutrophil   The most common WHITE BLOOD CELL in the body. It is considered a polymorphonuclear leukocyte, which is a type of white blood cell filled with granules of toxic chemicals that enable it to digest microorganisms. Because neutrophils "swallow" the antigen and destroy it, they are also called PHAGOCYTES. Other cells in this group include EOSINOPHILS and BASOPHILS. These cells are formed in the bone marrow and migrate out to the bloodstream and beyond. Unlike other immune system cells these cells often move into the tissue under attack by an antigen to do their work. Neutrophils are the main line of defense against bacterial infections. Typically when an infection occurs the body produces more neutrophils to fight it. This is why people have a high white blood cell count during an infection. The pus seen at the site of an infection is made up predominantly of neutrophils that have completed their job of destroying the foreign substance. An overactivity of neutrophils in the absence of antigens can cause problems such as rheumatoid arthritis, whereas a lack of them (NEUTROPENIA) can make the body vulnerable to illnesses caused by antigens that are not stopped.

nevirapine A NONNUCLEOSIDE REVERSE TRANSCRIPTASE INHIBITOR (NNRTI). It was the first NNRTI on the market in the United States. Reverse transcriptase is a part of HIV required to infect cells in the body and make more viruses. NNRTIs prevent the reverse transcriptase from working properly. Nevirapine has been approved for use in treating HIV in combination with other NNRTIs as well as with PROTEASE INHIBITORS and NRTIs. HIV becomes resistant to nevirapine fairly quickly if taken alone, so it should always be used as part of a multidrug combination. Resistance to nevirapine may also indicate that the HIV is resistant to several other NNRTIs. The main side effect of nevirapine is a rash, which occurred in 22 percent of people in studies. If nevirapine causes a severe rash that prevents patients from taking the drug, it is advisable that it not be used again, because resumed use may cause a worse reaction the second time. Many people get a mild rash and physicians may choose to treat through the rash to develop tolerance to the drug. Patients may also choose to build up to the desired dosage of nevirapine over the first two weeks of treatment. Studies have shown that taking an antihistamine during start-up of this drug can prevent the rash. Other side effects can be elevated liver function test results, fever, and muscle soreness. Nevirapine has been associated with severe liver toxicity in some cases, and the FDA has issued a warning regarding this activity. Liver function should be closely monitored when a person is taking nevirapine, particularly during the first 12 weeks of treatment. Nevirapine is a cytochrome P450 (CYP) inducer, which means it increases the metabolic activity of the drug and drugs taken at the same time because it is absorbed well. This effect can increase the various dosing levels and interactions that may occur while taking nevirapine. Nevirapine is under investigation as a single-drug treatment to prevent transmission of the virus from a mother to the baby she is carrying. It has been approved for this use in some countries, such as South Africa. (Trade name is Viramune.)

new drug application (NDA) See DRUG APPROVAL PROCESS.

newborn screening The testing of human infants less than one month old to determine the presence of a particular disease (i.e., HIV/AIDS), or of certain risk factors known to be associated with that disease. Today, AIDS testing and screening of large groups of people remain controversial issues; whether or not HIV testing provides a net benefit both to the public health and to persons infected with HIV is still debated. One heavily debated issue concerns screening programs for all pregnant women and newborns. Advocates argue that such a program would be reasonable, given the accuracy of new confirmatory tests and the fact that perinatally acquired HIV infection is less common than congenital syphilis or phenylketonuria (both are tested for routinely). Infected women, it is further argued, could make more informed choices about family planning, and infected newborns could be treated earlier.

Opponents argue that testing newborns for the presence of HIV antibodies is medically ineffective and inconclusive. They argue that with an increase in screening, discrimination arises once a person (or an infant) is known to be infected. They characterize newborn screening as counter-productive and coercive, as it does not confront the difficult reality of treating newborns with HIV/AIDS. They argue that only when those with HIV infection are assured of receiving all the medical care they need, can we pursue the basic elements of infection control more resolutely and thus spare others the tragedy of this disease. See TRANSMISSION.

NGO See NONGOVERNMENTAL ORGANIZATION.

NGU See URETHRITIS.

NIAID See NATIONAL INSTITUTE OF ALLERGY AND INFECTIOUS DISEASES.

NICHD See NATIONAL INSTITUTE OF CHILD HEALTH AND HUMAN DEVELOPMENT.

night sweats Profuse sweating during sleep at night, often an early sign of disease, especially if accompanied by intermittent fever. Night sweats are considered a symptom of HIV only when the body is drenched. Slight to moderate sweating is not a symptom. In addition to being an early sign of HIV disease, severe night sweats may also be a symptom of several HIV-related conditions, including TUBERCULOSIS.

NIH See NATIONAL INSTITUTES OF HEALTH.

nimodipine A calcium channel blocker used primarily to improve nerve damage caused by stroke. It works by slowing the amount of calcium that enters cells, resulting in blood vessels opening wider, allowing more blood to flow through them. (Most calcium channel blockers are used to treat heart conditions.) It is also occasionally used for the treatment of migraine headaches. In people infected with HIV, nimodipine is sometimes used as a treatment for neurological damage caused by HIV, especially PERIPHERAL NEUROPATHY.

nipple The structure on the breast through which milk is exuded (in women). In men it is vestigial. Also a source of erotic enjoyment.

nitazoxanide An ANTHELMINTHIC drug used to control tapeworm and liver fluke parasites in many countries of the world. It has shown to be effective and controlling CRYPTOSPORIDIOSIS in HIV disease. It also stops the pervasive diarrhea that accompanies cryptosporidiosis. Other research shows that it has broad effectiveness against many protozoa and helminths. It has not been approved for sale in the United States yet but is available through the Food and Drug Administration compassionate use program. Many people who live near the Mexican border transport the drug over to the U.S. border and it is often available in border states. (The trade name in Mexico is Cryptaz.)

nizoral See KETOCONAZOLE.

NK cells See NATURAL KILLER CELLS.

NMRI See MAGNETIC RESONANCE IMAGING.

NNRTI See nonnucleoside reverse transcriptase inhibitor.

no code An indication on a terminally ill patient's chart that he or she does not want heroic, lifesaving measures or artificial life support when death is imminent. Also called no code blue or no code blue status. See POWER OF ATTORNEY, MEDICAL DIRECTIVE, and LIVING WILL.

no code blue See NO CODE.

no code blue status See NO CODE.

Nocardia A genus of GRAM-POSITIVE aerobic bacteria. Some species are ACID-FAST and thus when stained may be confused with the causative organism for TUBERCULOSIS. The species pathogenic for humans causes the disease NOCARDIOSIS.

nocardiosis An acute or chronic pathological condition caused by infection from any species of NOCARDIA. It may occur as a pulmonary infection but has a marked tendency to spread to any organ of the body, especially the brain. It results in abscesses in the lungs, brain, skin, or other areas.

nociceptive pain Pain derived from bone breaks, bruises, muscle strain, burns, or arthritic inflammation. Nociceptors are the nerves that sense and respond to parts of the body that are damaged. This type of pain is typically localized or centralized and has an aching or throbbing quality. It responds to typical over-the-counter pain medication or prescribed painkillers.

node A knot, knob, protuberance, or swelling; a small mass of tissue in the form of a knot or swelling. Also used to refer to an aggregate of lymph tissue in the body. Lymph nodes are present in several places in the body, most notably along the neck, underarm, and groin regions.

nodular lesion A circumscribed area of pathologically altered tissue that possesses the characteristics of a NODULE.

nodule A small knot or protuberance that can be detected by touch.

Nolahist See PHENINDAMINE.

nonadherent In HIV or other medical terminology it refers to a patient who does not take prescribed medication. Many HIV patients are nonadherent because of the side effects of the medications or the dosing regimens that the drugs require. Others are nonadherent as a result of inability to remember to take the medications. Some people simply do not expect them to be effective and therefore do not take them. Studies do show a longer life span among those who adhere to their medication requirements.

non-communicable disease A disease that cannot be directly or indirectly transmitted from host to host.

noncompliant See NONADHERENT.

nondirective counseling A type of counseling in which the counselor supplies information and helps the client to arrive at a decision that reflects the client's needs and wishes.

nongonococcal urethritis See URETHRITIS.

nongovernmental organization (NGO) Any private nonprofit voluntary organization or institu-

tion that provides health; rescue; human rights; charitable, financial, economic development; or other aid and services wherever they are needed, but mainly in poorer countries. Nongovernmental organizations have been at the forefront of the response to AIDS in most countries of the world. In economic terms, NGOs focus on social needs that cannot be met otherwise, for economic or political reasons. Politically, NGOs provide public good to groups of people too small or marginalized to be served by the state. Most observers agree that NGOs working in AIDS typically offer the advantages of being cost-effective and responsive to new needs and of having access to target communities. For volunteers and activists involved in NGOs, the chief strength of the organizations would almost certainly be seen as their ability to represent effectively the needs and values of a particular constituency. Although they have recognized weaknesses, NGOs clearly serve certain functions well and can effectively complement and improve governmental response. NGOs encompass a wide variety of organizational styles and missions, and their role in response to AIDS has varied accordingly. Today, short- and long-term financial issues are a major concern of both governmental and nongovernmental AIDS programs.

non-Hodgkin's lymphoma (NHL) A LYMPHOMA (cancer of the lymphatic system), other than Hodgkin's disease, that is prevalent among AIDS patients. NHL is one of the AIDS-defining OPPORTUNISTIC INFECTIONS the U.S. government recognizes. Lymphoma is a disease that involves the uncontrolled multiplication of dysfunctional LYMPHOCYTES (a type of white blood cell), the B cells. There are typically two types of non-Hodgkin's lymphoma that strike people with HIV disease: primary central nervous system (CNS) lymphoma and systemic lymphoma.

Primary CNS lymphoma is a cancer of the brain and/or spinal cord and nervous system. It is called *primary* because it has started in the brain and not moved there from other regions of the body. *Systemic* means the cancer has spread throughout the body, though it started in the lymph glands. Non-Hodgkin's lymphoma is the most common lymphoma that affects people with HIV/AIDS. It involves the uncontrolled proliferation of abnormal B CELLS (lymphocytes responsible for ANTIBODY production) and appears first as nodular tumors, then as diffuse tumors in extranodal tissues. Other lymphomas such as Hodgkin's disease occasionally affect people with HIV/AIDS. They are more prevalent in HIV-positive people, but less common than NHL.

The major difference between Hodgkin's disease and non-Hodgkin's lymphoma is that the former always includes a specific type of cell called the Reed–Sternberg cell (a large cell of unknown origin with an unusual bilobed nucleus). Hodgkin's disease also starts out as localized nodular tumors, which disseminate as the disease progresses. One of the first signs of NHL is the presence of what are called B symptoms, which include fever, night sweats, and loss of greater than 10 percent of body weight. Many other AIDS-related complications have similar symptoms. Another symptom of lymphoma may be enlarged and asymmetrical lymph nodes. It has been reported that NHL can occur at practically any site on the body. The most common extranodal sites are the CENTRAL NERVOUS SYSTEM (brain and spinal cord), GASTROINTESTINAL TRACT, BONE MARROW, and LIVER. NHL also has appeared in such unusual sites as the anus, rectum, mouth, muscle, and other soft tissue.

A definitive diagnosis of lymphoma can be made only through a surgical BIOPSY of the involved tissue. If lymphoma is found, it is graded on the basis of how rapidly the cancerous cells are growing. It is designated high-, intermediate-, or low-grade. The lymphoma is also staged (I through IV), on the basis of the extent of tissue involvement. HIV disease patients almost always have stage 3 or 4 NHL, because the symptoms are similar to other HIV symptoms. Stage I indicates very limited involvement at only one site, whereas stage IV indicates very extensive involvement in multiple sites. NHL becomes much more common the longer someone lives with HIV. Primary CNS lymphoma almost always occurs in people who have a T-cell count lower than 200. Systemic lymphoma can occur at any time in the HIV disease process.

Whether a person can survive NHL depends on a variety of factors. Low CD4 CELL count (less than 100), central nervous system involvement, previous opportunistic infections, stage IV disease, and

low ability to perform daily activities have been reported to be associated with poor survival rate. Patients who have higher CD4 cell units (greater than 199), no extranodal disease, no previous opportunistic infections, and near-normal ability to perform daily activities have a greater survival rate and potential for cure. Exactly what causes NHL is not completely understood. Most researchers agree that it may be a combination of factors such as EPSTEIN-BARR VIRUS (EBV) infection, gene mutations, and CYTOKINE [TNF], dysregulation (IL-1, IL-4, IL-6, IL-10, and TUMOR NECROSIS FACTOR coupled with the underlying immune suppression in AIDS. EBV cells appear in CNS lymphoma, but there is no link yet established between this or other viruses and various lymphomas. People who have had EBV exposure are thought to be at a higher risk for the disease.

Treatment usually involves some type of chemotherapy, and in the case of brain involvement it may include radiation therapy. Since chemotherapy, because of its bone marrow toxicity, has a significant impact on decreasing white blood cell count, it increases the risk of bacterial infections. Administration of COLONY STIMULATING FACTORS such as G-CSF (Neupogen) or GM-CSF (Leukine) can increase white blood cell production and reduce risk. Chemotherapy may also cause anemia by reducing red blood cell counts and causing spontaneous bleeding that is due to low platelet counts. Infusions of synthetic erythropoeitin (Epogen) can stimulate red blood cell production, and the cytokine IL-3 has proved of value in reversing both low white blood cell and platelet counts in AIDS patients on chemotherapy. Treatment of NHL in HIV-positive people has not been very successful because of the late-stage diagnosis, the involvement of multiple sites in the body, and the low functioning of the immune system.

nonlytic infection Infection of a cell by a virus that results in production of virus, but survival of the cell. Most retroviruses normally create nonlytic infections. HIV infection of macrophages is nonlytic.

nonnucleoside reverse transcriptase inhibitor (NNRTI) A member of a class of compounds, including delavirdine, efavirenz, and nevirapine, that act directly to combine with and block the action of HIV'S REVERSE TRANSCRIPTASE. In early clinical trials of these drugs, it was found that HIV developed resistance in as little as two to seven weeks when the drugs were used alone. Therefore, NNRTIs are used only in conjunction with other types of HIV drugs. They are considered a first line of therapy in HIV treatment. The nonnucleoside drugs are similar to NUCLEOSIDE ANALOGS: they both change the function of REVERSE TRANSCRIPTASE (RI), an enzyme that HIV needs to replicate. However, the nonnucleoside drugs do not have to be activated by cellular enzymes. Whereas inhibitory mechanisms of nucleoside analogs include tricking reverse transcriptase into making faulty DNA copies from strains of RNA, the nonnucleosides disarm reverse transcriptase by binding directly to it. They do not allow the reverse transcriptase to bind as it normally would. Their role in HIV therapy has always been uncertain because HIV rapidly develops resistance when exposed to the current members of the class, particularly when these drugs are taken alone. NNRTIs can be used as part of a combination with nucleoside analogs (AZT, 3TC) or with PROTEASE INHIBITORS (nelfinavir, indinavir). NNRTIs can often cause a rash at the beginning of use. Many doctors now prescribe an antihistamine such as Benadryl to prevent the rash. If the rash forces a patient to stop taking the drug, he or she should *not* start using the drug again unless a doctor is absolutely sure that no further reaction will occur. See EFAVIRENZ; DELAVIRDINE; NEVIRAPINE.

non-nuke   See NONNUCLEOSIDE REVERSE TRANSCRIPTASE INHIBITOR (NNRTI).

nonoxynol 9   A detergent chemical agent used in some spermicides and lubricants that may reduce the risk of infection with HIV. It has been shown to kill HIV in the test tube. It is generally used in the lubricant that is employed for prelubricating condoms. There is some evidence that it might irritate or disrupt cells in the vaginal area and in the anal area, making women and men more vulnerable to infection. It was tested as a spermicide among female sex workers and showed no effectiveness in

preventing the spread of HIV. It is therefore unclear whether this agent has any benefit on the condoms or in lubricant.

nonprogressor   A person with HIV whose infection has not progressed to successive stages in the usual amount of time. Long-term nonprogressors are defined as individuals infected with HIV for 10 years or more who have stable CD4+ T-CELL COUNTS of 600 or more cells per cubic millimeter of blood, no HIV-related diseases, and no previous ANTIRETROVIRAL THERAPY. They may have low levels of virus in their blood and LYMPH NODES although HIV replication persists. A National Institute of Allergy and Infectious Diseases study has also found that the internal structure of these individuals' lymph nodes, unlike that of most people who have HIV infection, appears essentially undamaged, and that their immune function remains virtually unimpaired. Long-term nonprogressors also have higher levels of neutralizing antibodies than patients with progressive disease, and the blood of each long-term nonprogressor tested has had the ability to kill HIV-infected cells. Higher-level HIV-specific cytotoxic immune responses indicate that both antibody and cell-mediated responses are preserved in long-term nonprogressors, suggesting that these individuals are constantly exposed to HIV antigens, yet somehow control the infection. Researchers believe that it is likely that long-term nonprogressors are a heterogeneous group: some may be infected with a weakened virus, and others may illustrate that host factors such as the immune system can, in some circumstances, contain HIV disease.

nonresponder   A mammal unable to respond to an ANTIGEN, usually because of genetic factors.

nonself versus self   A specific immune response that is triggered when a foreign substance (nonself), such as another person's cells or tissues, enters a body (self). Graft rejection works by this mechanism.

nonsteroidal anti-inflammatory drug (NSAID)   Well-tolerated, widely-used pain medication that is sold over the counter at pharmacies or by prescription from a doctor. It is also used to reduce fevers. NSAIDs do not suppress the immune system as steroids do, hence the name they are given. Aspirin is a commonly known NSAID. Other common NSAIDs are ibuprofen (Advil) and naproxen (Aleve). Acetaminophen is not a NSAID but a nonopioid ANALGESIC. NSAIDs work by blocking the enzyme cyclooxygenase (COX), which helps the body form chemicals called prostaglandins. There are two types of COX in the body. The first, COX-1, is a chemical that lines the stomach. When this chemical is blocked by an NSAID, people may sometimes experience stomach upset after taking a NSAID. COX-2 is the chemical responsible for prostaglandins that lead to inflammation, pain, and fever. Some prescribed NSAIDs block only COX-2 formation. COX-2 pain relievers mainly include prescription drugs such as Celebrex and Vioxx. NSAIDs and COX inhibitors have been reported to have a protective effect against colon cancer and Alzheimer's disease. Future uses of NSAIDs may involve these illnesses as well as pain relief.

non-syncytium-inducing (NSI) virus NSI virus is a virus that does not cause syncytia (see SYNCYTIUM), the fusion of infected cells into large multicelled infectious and noninfectious molecules. These multicelled molecules die and also destroy healthy cells in the process. Syncytium-inducing virus is much more trauma-inducing to the immune system. It is found in all end-stage patients who have HIV.

Researchers have learned that more than one RECEPTOR site is required in order for HIV to infect cells in the immune system. Typically the virus uses a receptor site on the CD4 molecule, which is found on the surface of T4 CELLS, MACROPHAGES, and some other immune cells. There are about 10,000 CD4 molecules on each macrophage and T4 cell. They are the "locks" that HIV uses to insert its "key" to attach itself to the cell. Studies have shown that to infect the cell, HIV must have coreceptors that allow the virus to "twist" itself in the "lock" and achieve entry to the cell. These coreceptors then are essential to allowing the virus to enter the cell and reproduce itself.

There are a few coreceptors. The CXCR-4, also known as FUSIN, is located on T4 cells. The CCR5 coreceptor is located on both macrophages and T4 cells. The CCR3 coreceptor is a recently discovered coreceptor involved in the transfer of the virus to the CENTRAL NERVOUS SYSTEM. Both types of HIV use different coreceptors. The NSI virus or "macrophage-tropic" virus uses the CCR5 coreceptor. NSI virus is less virulent and is typically found at the initial stages of HIV disease.

normal 1. In medicine normal connotes standard, natural, regular; performing proper functions. 2. In biology, it indicates unaffected by experimental treatment; occurring naturally and not because of disease or experimentation. 3. In psychology, it means free from mental disorder, or of average development or intelligence. 4. In chemistry, it is a term for a solution so made that 1 liter contains 1 gram equivalent of the solute.

Norplant See PROGESTERONE IMPLANT.

North America The United States and Canada have by the nature of the similarities of the population and the border they share had very similar AIDS epidemics. HIV-positive people account for between 0.006 percent and (0.008 percent) of the total U.S. population. The United States has 900,000 people who are HIV-positive and Canada has around 60,000 HIV-positive people. HIV-positive individuals account for 0.003 percent of the total population in Canada. These countries were among the first to record HIV disease cases in the early 1980s. There are believed to be over 300,000 orphans as a result of the epidemic in North America, the majority of those in the United States. There have been nearly 500,000 deaths due to the virus during the epidemic in North America.

The epidemic began to appear in homosexual men and quickly spread to the IDU population and people who used blood products, before rates of new infections began to level off in the mid-1990s. The people who had been exposed by blood products were first brought under viral control, when the CDC required screening of blood and blood products in the mid-1980s. Very few cases due to blood products or TRANSPLANTATION have been reported since this step occurred. The virus was also seen early among people of Haitian descent, but this incidence was later linked to the phenomenon that these people were working in the United States away from family. Usually in such cases an increase in both sexual activity and drug use occurs. This type of transmission pattern has also been seen in South and Southeast Asia, as well as Africa. Also, at the time the virus may have transferred to humans from simians, Haitians were playing a large role in the workforce of the former Belgian Congo, again as migrant workers. So there are any number of reasons why Haitians appeared more susceptible than others initially.

The virus then began to appear in heterosexual women and their children, and a pattern was recognized. In the years of the virus in North America, the numbers infected by HIV have changed from nearly 80 percent gay men in the early years to more than 50 percent heterosexuals in the past few years. In the United States in particular there is a change in the epidemic related to social class: poor people have become more likely to experience the epidemic than middle- or upper-class people. This prevalence is due to several factors. As opposed to many developed countries the United States government does not provide medical care for its citizens. This is a privatized function in U.S. society. Therefore, people who do not have jobs that include health insurance as a benefit may not have medical insurance. This leaves them unable to afford medicines and also less likely to seek medical care. The United States also incarcerates a greater percentage of its people than other Western nations, and HIV has proved especially difficult to handle in prison populations, among whom MSM and IDU activities may be more predominant than in other settings. So in the United States the epidemic has come to represent the underclass and therefore minority populations. This has made it far more difficult to educate and inform the population as the government is slow to provide funding for either medical care or educational material that discusses the behavior that can cause the virus to flourish and transmit itself between people. For these reasons the United States has the highest rate of HIV-positive people of any developed nation.

Since 2000 the United States has seen a rise in the number of new cases after a drop in this total for several years. This increase has been attributed to an increase in sexual activity of young people who are unfamiliar with the terrible scenes of the disease in the 1980s or to an increase of unsafe sexual activity among gay men. It has been suggested that both groups may believe that the HAART drugs now available to people are cures for the disease. This is not true. The number of cases transmitted through heterosexual activity has increased each year in the past several years. In 1995 AIDS was the leading cause of death of people aged 25–44 in the United States. It is now in 2002, the fifth leading cause. It is still the leading cause of death of people who are incarcerated in the United States.

So after 20 years of HIV epidemic, HIV is still a cause of much suffering in North America, but it has been tempered by some education and some medication. It has not been conquered yet, and North America has a higher rate of infection than many industrialized nations. The United States in particular may need to provide further money for education, given recent numbers, to stem the tide of another HIV disease increase. See CARIBBEAN and LATIN AMERICA.

northern blot technique   A procedure for separating and identifying RNA fragments. Fragments are separated by electrophoresis on an agarose gel, blotted onto a nitrocellulose or nylon membrane and hybridized with labeled nucleic acid probes.

nortriptyline hydrochloride   An antidepressant drug of the tricyclic class. (Trade names are Aventyl Hydrochloride and Pamelor.)

norvir   See RITONAVIR.

Norwegian scabies   A rare, severe form of scabies, characterized by an extremely heavy infestation of mites, that occurs in immunosuppressed patients. It is highly contagious and may involve all family and close contacts who are taking prophylaxis. Typically a person who is affected has 10–15 mites on the body. In Norwegian scabies there are thousands, causing thickened crusty skin that flakes off and therefore makes the spread much easier than in typical scabies.

nosocomial infection   An infection acquired in a hospital or other health-care institution.

notifiable disease   A disease whose occurrence must, by law, be reported to health authorities.

Among the diseases that the laws of various states require to be reported are all communicable or contagious diseases, such as scarlet fever and diphtheria; enteric fevers, such as typhoid; epidemics of acute diarrheal disease; cholera; typhus; meningococcal meningitis; AIDS; acute anterior poliomyelitis; polioencephalitis; encephalitis lethargica; tuberculosis; rubella; chicken pox; gonorrhea; and syphilis.

notification of partners See PARTNER NOTIFICATION.

NRTI See NUCLEOSIDE REVERSE TRANSCRIPTASE INHIBITOR.

NSAID See NONSTEROIDAL ANTI-INFLAMMATORY DRUGS.

NSI virus See NON-SYNCYTIUM-INDUCING (NSI) VIRUS.

NtRTI See NUCLEOTIDE REVERSE TRANSCRIPTASE INHIBITOR.

NTZ See NITAZOXANIDE.

nuclear magnetic resonance imaging (NMRI) See MAGNETIC RESONANCE IMAGING.

nucleic acid A compound that carries genetic information, found in all viruses and living organisms. DNA and RNA are the two principal forms.

nucleic acid sequence-based amplification (NASBA) An ASSAY used to detect HIV VIRAL LOAD in blood PLASMA. It is one of three assays used for the process. See bDNA ASSAY; PCR.

nucleoside A combination of one of five single- or double-ringed "bases" and a sugar (ribose for RNA or deoxyribose for DNA). These molecular units are the building blocks of DNA and RNA, the genetic material found in living organisms. Before joining a DNA or RNA sequence, nucleosides must have a phosphate group added. See PHOSPHORYLATION.

nucleoside analog See NUCLEOSIDE REVERSE TRANSCRIPTASE INHIBITOR.

nucleoside analog therapy Anti-HIV therapy with nucleoside analog reverse-transcriptase inhibitors.

nucleoside reverse transcriptase inhibitor (NRTI) A class of antiretroviral drugs used in the treatment of HIV disease. The drugs used are ZIDOVUDINE, DIDANOSINE, ZALCITABINE, LAMIVUDINE, STAVUDINE, and ABACAVIR. This was the first class of drugs that became available in the treatment of HIV in the late 1980s and early 1990s. Nucleoside analogs take the place of the natural nucleosides, blocking the completion of a viral DNA chain during infection of a new cell by HIV. The HIV enzyme REVERSE TRANSCRIPTASE is more likely to incorporate nucleoside analogs in the DNA it is constructing than is the DNA polymerase normally used for DNA creation in cell nuclei. By preventing reverse transcription, NRTIs successfully interfere with one of the steps of the HIV life cycle and prevent the virus from reproducing and establishing itself in the patient's body. The NRTIs are used in a variety of HAART combinations, which often include two NRTIs and one PROTEASE INHIBITOR.

A set of serious side effects of NRTI drugs is now being called METABOLIC TOXICITY. This set of side effects is probably the result of MITOCHONDRIAL TOXICITY. MITOCHONDRIA are the cell's power organs that supply the energy needed for normal cell growth. Anti-HIV nucleoside analogs impair the production and function of mitochondria in the body, in many cases altering the mitochondria. This impairment can lead to increased acid levels in the blood and an enlarged, fatty liver. Clinical features that can usually be seen in patients with genetic mutations of mitochondrial DNA, such as polyneuropathy, myopathy, cardiomyopathy, fatty liver, lactic acidosis, pancreatitis, vomiting, pancytopenia (low blood counts), and renal proximal tubular dysfunction, also occur in NRTI-related toxicities. Thus some have hypothesized that all adverse effects of NRTIs can be attributed to mitochondrial toxicity. However, why toxicity related to NRTIs develops differently in different patients has not been completely explained; it may be due to differences in accumulation of drugs in various tissues and differences in metabolic properties of individuals' tissues.

nucleotide   A glycoside (any of a group of sugar derivatives that, when combined with water, yields a sugar and one or more other substances) formed by the combination of a sugar (pentose) and a purine or pyrimide base.

nucleotide analog   See NUCLEOTIDE REVERSE TRANSCRIPTASE INHIBITOR.

nucleotide reverse transcriptase inhibitor (NtRTI)   Sometimes called a nucleotide analog, it is a synthetic molecule that is structurally similar to a specific nucleotide. As do NRTIs, nucleotide analog drugs interfere with reverse transcriptase, the viral enzyme that normally allows HIV to translate its genetic material (in the form of RNA) into DNA. The presence of defective synthetic nucleotides (the basic structural units of nucleic acids, such as RNA and DNA) causes premature termination of the viral DNA chain, thus preventing successful replication. Nucleotide analogs are believed to be more potent than NUCLEOSIDE ANALOGS because they are incorporated directly into a DNA chain more readily than nucleoside analogs, which must undergo several chemical reactions before becoming active. The term for these reactions is *phosphorylation* because it involves the adding of a phosphate atom to the molecule. See ADEFOVIR; TENOFOVIR.

nucleus   The usually round protoplasmic structure within a cell that contains the cell's hereditary material. It is involved in growth, metabolism, and reproduction. The nucleus is surrounded by a double membrane and serves as the principal site of DNA and RNA synthesis.

nuke   See NUCLEOSIDE REVERSE TRANSCRIPTASE INHIBITOR.

null cell   A white blood cell that is a lymphocyte but lacks the specific identifying surface markers for either T or B LYMPHOCYTES.

Nuprin   See IBUPROFEN.

nurse   An individual who provides health care. The extent of nursing care varies from simple patient-care tasks to the most complex medical techniques necessary in acute life-threatening situations. The roles of nurses constantly change in response to the growth of biomedical knowledge, changes in patterns of demand for health services, and the evolution of professional, relationships among nurses, physicians, and other health care professionals.

Also, to nurse is to feed an infant at the breast; to perform the duties of caring for an invalid; or to care for a young child.

nursing home   An extended-care facility for persons who need medical attention and general care too taxing to be done at home but not requiring hospitalization.

nutrient   Any substance that supplies the body with elements necessary for metabolism. Carbohydrates, fats, proteins, and alcohol are nutrients that provide energy. Water, electrolytes, minerals, and vitamins are nutrients that are essential to the metabolic process. Nutrients containing carbon are organic food nutrients.

nutrient deficiency   There are many causes of nutrient deficiency in people living with HIV, including malabsorption because of damage to the intestines (by HIV or other infections); the high demand for antioxidants; the increased metabolism that begins in the earliest disease stages; and decreased intake of food because of mouth or throat problems, loss of appetite, loss of taste, fever, nausea, and vomiting. The resulting serious deficiency of nutrients critical for supporting immune function, and malnutrition, are common among people with HIV and frequently contribute to the development of OPPORTUNISTIC INFECTIONS and general deterioration that are the immediate causes of death.

Recent research has made it clear that HIV-associated nutrient deficiencies and malnutrition are not just late-stage occurrences. Many nutrient deficiencies begin in early disease stages when patients appear to be well and free of symptoms and have CD4+ counts upwards of 400. Because nutrients seldom work alone in the body, a deficiency of one nutrient may cause other nutrients to work improperly. Research has shown that people living with HIV need to consume much more than the standard recommended daily allowances (RDA) of nutrients to maintain normal levels—diet is far more important in treating HIV disease than most people realize. But even the most nutritious diet may not be sufficient to fully meet the needs of people living with HIV disease.

nutrient supplementation   An optimal approach to managing HIV disease includes a rational nutrition program encompassing both sound dietary choices and nutrient supplementation. The goal is to provide optimal levels of nutrients in order to help prevent damage, manage symptoms related to HIV, and boost the body's capacity to heal. Multiple vitamin and mineral supplements that supply the basic level of nutrients most important to body functions are a common type of nutrient supplementation. Because of the serious deficiencies and the increased need for a number of nutrients, many nutritionists believe that it is necessary to take additional supplements such as ANTIOXIDANTS, essential fatty acids, carnitine, acidophilus, and digestive aids such as pancreatic enzymes or hydrochloric acid supplements, both to increase dosage levels and to include nutrients not usually found in multiple supplements. Studies have also shown that some nutritional supplements like zinc, selenium, and vitamins C, A, E, and B together with AZT may increase AZT's antiviral effect while at the same time strengthening the immune system. Additionally, there is increasing evidence for an autoimmune aspect of HIV infection that may be treated with antioxidants and other nutrients, like GLUTATHIONE, COENZYME Q10, VITAMINS C, E, and A, SELENIUM, and ZINC, that protect cell membranes and dampen the inflammatory response of the body to the infection. Maintaining a good supplementation program helps prevent deficiencies and loss of immune function. In addition, symptoms that result from deficiencies can often be eliminated with an appropriate supplement program. Symptoms that may be related to nutrient deficiencies and may be reversible with appropriate supplementation include serious fatigue, memory loss or other cognitive dysfunction, skin problems, neuropathy, weight loss, loss of the senses of smell or taste, appetite loss, muscle pain or cramps, digestive problems, night blindness, canker sores, constipation, depression, anxiety, menstrual cramps, and menopausal problems.

nutrition   All the processes involved in the taking in and utilization of food substances by which growth, repair, and maintenance of activities in the body as a whole or in any of its parts are accomplished. Nutrition includes ingestion, digestion, absorption, and metabolism. Some nutrients are capable of being stored in the body in various forms and drawn upon when food intake is not sufficient. Today medical practitioners are increasingly aware that good nutrition is a fundamental component of the care of people with HIV/AIDS. Specially designed nutritional programs, including NUTRIENT SUPPLEMENTATION, have been shown to boost immune function, increase the efficacy of medical treatments, and improve energy levels and general quality of life. Conversely, malnutrition may contribute to the development of OPPORTUNISTIC INFECTIONS and physical deterioration that may be the immediate cause of death. In the early years of the epidemic, AIDS-related wasting was of high concern to researchers focusing on nutrition and HIV infection. In more recent years the emphasis has shifted; today, the researchers' attention has been redirected to such areas as LIPODYSTROPHY, fat redistribution problems, the impact of dietary fat on the development of elevated blood lipids levels, and the metabolic complications of HIGHLY ACTIVE ANTIRETROVIRAL THERAPY (HAART). MICRONUTRIENTS have also taken center stage. Examples of core questions under study include whether or not patients given aggressive nutritional support and hormone replacement therapy do better than those given standard care, and whether or not there is more to nutrient supplementation than strengthening of immune defenses.

Registered dieticians and naturopaths may know more about general nutrition than medical doctors, since they have much more extensive training in the area. Many are also especially knowledgeable about nutrition of people with HIV. See MALNUTRITION; NUTRIENT DEFICIENCY; PARENTERAL NUTRITION; WASTING.

nutritional deficiency   See NUTRIENT DEFICIENCY.

nutritional supplement   See NUTRIENT SUPPLE-MENTATION.

Nydrazid   See ISONIAZID.

nystatin   An antifungal used in the treatment of cutaneous, intestinal, oral, or vaginal candidal infections (thrush). Nystatin may be administered orally or topically. It works by interfering with the ability of fungi to build their cell walls. It is also available as an oral suspension that is swished in the mouth or gargled before being swallowed. Nystatin rarely causes side effects, although nausea and irritation of the mouth and vagina are occasionally reported. Large oral doses may cause diarrhea, stomach upset, vomiting, or rashes. (Trade names are Mycostatin, O-V Statin, and Mykinac.)

OASDI See OLD AGE, SURVIVORS, AND DISABILITY INSURANCE.

obscene Defined by *Merriam-Webster's Collegiate Dictionary* as "disgusting . . . abhorrent to morality or virtue," the term is commonly used to apply to offensive depictions of sexual activity. It is used in this sense as a legal term.

Although everyone seems to know what the word means, obscenity is notoriously difficult to identify, since what offends one person or group may not offend others. Accusations of obscenity are therefore routinely countered with accusations of censorship and defenses of freedom of speech, and no legal determination of obscenity has ever been generally accepted as proper.

observational study A study that does not involve randomization but available data are nonetheless analyzed to make treatment comparisons. Observational studies are subject to bias, which may render their conclusions less reliable than those obtained by well-controlled randomized clinical trials. Still, they may be useful for hypothesis generation and definition of the natural history of disease.

obstetrics The branch of medicine concerned with the care of women during pregnancy, childbirth, and the puerperium.

occupational exposure The risk of exposure to a communicable disease through the normal procedures associated with a specific profession (e.g., a NEEDLESTICK during a surgical procedure). In June 1996, the Public Health Service published guidelines for treating occupational exposure to HIV (Centers for Disease Control and Prevention.

MMWR 1996; 45: 486–472). According to these recommendations, doctors, nurses, and other health care workers who are accidentally exposed to HIV-tainted blood should promptly receive antiretroviral therapy. The guidelines address type of exposure (percutaneous, mucous membrane, and skin), source material (blood, fluid containing visible blood, other potentially infectious fluid), antiretroviral prophylaxis, and antiretroviral regimen. The recommendations specify two- or three-drug treatment regimens depending on the degree of risk associated with the exposure. If possible, treatment should begin within one to two hours of exposure. It is recommended that therapy be administered for four weeks, if tolerated, although optimal duration of treatment is also unknown.

Oceania Oceania comprises the island nations of the Pacific Ocean along with Australia and New Zealand. HIV infection rate for the most part remains low in this region, in 2001 the lowest in the world. There are just two countries where HIV has managed to reach a greater than .1 percent rate of infection. Both Papua New Guinea and East Timor, which share parts of islands with Indonesian provinces, have rates around .7 percent of their people who are now believed to be HIV-positive. With approximately 4000 cases outside those countries one might think there is nothing to worry about. However, that number is five and one-half times higher than it was five years ago (1996).

After Australia and New Zealand began to detect cases of HIV in the early 1980s they both began large programs of public education. They also began treating patients immediately. The result of these programs is that both countries saw the rate of infection drop or remain steady every year until 2001. In 2002 these two countries experienced an increase, as did the United States and Western Europe. Unsafe sexual behavior is believed to be increasing among the young and among men who have sex with men. Whether the reason is that the young do not remember the 1980s or the advent of HAART has made people believe that the epidemic is over remains to be seen. It will be a challenge for these nations to make their rate drop again. Australia has just 12,000 cases of HIV, fewer than its northern neighbor Papua New Guinea, yet it has more than four times the population of Papua New Guinea, which has four million residents. New Zealand has just 1,200 cases.

In addition there are six countries or territories in the Pacific Islands that have yet to see any cases of HIV infection: American Samoa, Cook Islands, Pitcairn, Niue, Tokelau, and Vanuatu. However, a reluctance to report cases of illness is nothing new for governments. Nor is it unusual that many have not been tested for fear of knowing results. It is difficult to believe statistics of zero cases for particular countries, given the travel possible and migration patterns of people in the 21st century. The majority of these locales are fairly small. The population of five of the six countries totals only 70,000 people. Vanuatu, however, has a population of 186,000 people. Many of the other microstates of the Pacific have case numbers in the one or two digits. Five of the 23 countries in the Pacific (excluding New Zealand and Australia) have managed to hold the number of cases of HIV below 100 people. East Timor and Papua New Guinea have rates at .6 percent and .7 percent of their population. The other three locations of the five countries are Guam, French Polynesia, and New Caledonia. What is probably unsurprising about these three locales is that they are all territories of Western nations that have had HIV infections for a long time. Travel between the parent nation and the territory is believed to have introduced the virus to these locales.

The high rates of prevalence in East Timor and Papua New Guinea have some common denominators. Both countries share an island with a province of Indonesia. Both countries have a low level of literacy and a relatively large rural popula-

tion. East Timor is the newest independent country. For many years all communication in or out of the country was nonexistent. Indonesia blocked all phone lines and kept all reporters out of the country for the most part. The result was a population that was a probably mostly ignorant of the disease until after independence balloting in 1999. The East Timor health minister said recently that all the necessary ingredients for a large problem were present. He said that poverty, street children, unemployment, and prostitution were all rampant. In Papua New Guinea the health minister stated that education is difficult because the country has a low literacy rate and more than 800 languages are spoken in the country.

octoxynol A nonionic surfactant mixture that varies in the number of repeating ethoxy (oxy-1,2-ethanediyl) groups. It is used as a detergent, emulsifier, wetting agent, defoaming agent, and in other applications. Octoxynol-9, the compound with nine repeating ethoxy groups, is a spermaticide.

octreotide An antidiarrheal used for refractory secretory diarrhea. Side effects may include pain or burning at the injection site, abdominal cramps and pain, diarrhea or loose stools, nausea/vomiting, and postprandial hyperglycemia. (Trade name is Sandostatin.)

ocular Relating to the eye.

ocular herpes A HERPES simplex infection of the eye, usually caused by touching an infected area of the body and then touching the eye.

odds ratio A statistical measure of the likelihood of development of a disease or condition with exposure to a certain factor or pathogen.

odynophagia Pain upon swallowing.

off-label An "off-label" drug is one approved by the FOOD AND DRUG ADMINISTRATION for some uses, but prescribed for another use for which it has not been approved. Drug therapy administered to people with AIDS often involves off-label use of medications. Frequently, off-label use of a drug merely anticipates Food and Drug Administration approval for that use. Obtaining insurance reimbursement for off-label prescriptions may be problematic. Patients who do not have insurance or who are members of health maintenance organizations (HMOs) often have less chance of receiving off-label therapies.

ofloxacin A broad spectrum antibiotic used in the control of tuberculosis, gonorrhea, cervicitis, and urethritis, among other bacterial illnesses. It is one of the quinolone drugs. Side effects can occur, particularly if a patient has had side effects from other quinolone drugs. (The trade name is Floxin.)

OI See OPPORTUNISTIC INFECTION.

oil-based lubricant See LUBRICANT.

Old Age, Survivors, and Disability Insurance (OASDI) Collectively, the range of worker-based income insurance programs operated by the Social Security Administration for the insured aged, disabled, and their families. The term is no longer used.

onanism The practice of withdrawing during coitus to ejaculate. The term is often used incorrectly to mean masturbation.

oncogene A gene associated with cancer. Oncogenes are of either viral or mammalian origin and are found widely in the living world, including in human cells. When oncogenes are "turned off" their function is unknown. When they are "turned on" they begin to form products that may transform the host cells into cancer cells.

oncology The branch of medicine dealing with tumors.

oncovirus One of a subfamily of retroviruses that includes tumor-causing agents such as the Rous sarcoma virus, the BOVINE LEUKEMIA VIRUS, and HTLV.

oocyst The encysted form of a fertilized egg occurring in certain sporozoa and parasites, such as isospora and toxoplasmosis.

"Opal" trials Trials conducted in Australia, Austria, Belgium, Denmark, France, Finland, Germany, Iceland, Italy, Luxembourg, the Netherlands, Norway, Spain, Sweden, and the United Kingdom to determine the best time to start treatment of HIV infection based on the presence or absence of clinical symptoms. See CONCORDE.

open-label study See OPEN-LABEL TRIAL.

open-label trial A study in which both researchers and participants know what drug participants are taking and at what doses.

ophthalmoscopy Examination of the interior of the eye.

opiate Any drug containing or derived from opium.

opiate antagonist An agent (e.g., naltrexone) that binds to the body's opiate receptors, thereby blocking the activity of opioid drugs (e.g., heroin) and endorphins.

opiate receptor Molecular structure on the cell that responds to or is influenced by opiate and endorphin molecules. Opiate receptors are found on certain types of cells in the brain, lungs, pancreas, endocrine glands, and other organs and tissues.

opioid A class of drug (e.g., heroin, codeine, methadone) that is derived from the opium poppy plant, contain opium, or is produced synthetically and has opiumlike effects. Opioid drugs relieve pain, dull the senses, and induce sleep.

opioid agonist Any morphinelike compound that produces bodily effects including pain relief, sedation, constipation, and respiratory depression.

opioid partial agonist A compound that has an affinity for and stimulates physiologic activity at the same cell receptors as opioid agonists but that produces only a partial (i.e., submaximal) bodily response.

opium, tincture of An antidiarrheal analgesic commonly used to treat diarrhea refractory to other agents. Side effects may include constipation, drowsiness, hypotension, nausea/vomiting, sweating, and dizziness. Anticholinergics may add to the effects of tincture of opium. Central nervous system depressants can have an increased effect. Tolerance to antidiarrheal effects may develop with repeated use.

opportunistic Of a pathogen, usually able to produce disease only in an immunologically compromised host.

opportunistic infection Infection that arises when the immune system is suppressed or otherwise compromised. The primary effect of HIV on the body is the gradual destruction of key immune-system cells, particularly helper T lymphocytes. Helper T cells, also known as CD4 lymphocytes, play a key role in initiating and coordinating immune responses. The loss of CD4 lymphocytes and other cells with the CD4 receptor, especially monocytes/macrophages, causes a progressive weakening of the immune system. This in turn gives microbes that are normally kept in check by the immune system an opportunity to flourish and cause disease. For this reason, the diseases induced by these microbes are known as opportunistic infections.

Opportunistic infections are responsible for up to 90 percent of all AIDS-related deaths. They develop primarily from two sources. Some, such as TOXOPLASMOSIS, occur through the reactivation of an infection acquired by many people earlier in life, often during childhood. An infection such as this is kept under control and harmless by a fully functional immune system. As the immune system becomes progressively dysfunctional during HIV disease, the infection then redevelops and causes disease.

Other opportunistic infections represent pathogens that are newly acquired from the environment. Many arrive in the body when inhaled into the lungs as either free spores or spores associated with dust and dirt; others are ingested with water or raw foods. Again, a normal immune system prevents them from causing disease, but the damaged immune system of people who have advanced HIV disease is no match for them. MYCOBACTERIUM AVIUM is a microbe acquired from the environment that is dangerous only to people with profound immune impairment.

Some microbes, such as the fungi responsible for athlete's foot and CANDIDIASIS, are so common in both the environment and the human body that they are simply considered always present from birth. They cause serious disease only in cases of immune impairment. In the case of *Pneumocystis carinii*, scientists now believe the pneumonia (PCP) it causes in people with HIV disease results mainly from newly acquired *Pneumocystis carinii* infections.

Opportunistic infections also occur in people whose immune system is severely depressed after organ transplantation or chemotherapy for some types of cancer (chemotherapeutic drugs damage cells in the bone marrow that give rise to immune-system cells). Additionally, perhaps as a corollary to their increased prevalence, or because of heightened physician awareness, opportunistic infections seem to be occurring more frequently in the elderly, who may be rendered vulnerable by age-related declines in immunity. Research on the prevention of opportunistic infections in people with HIV disease is helping to prevent opportunistic infections in other immune-suppressed patients as well.

Opportunistic infections can be caused by any of four types of microbial life: bacteria, viruses, fungi, or protozoan parasites. Bacteria are the most primitive of cells, and they are capable of independent life in the environment. Bacterial infections are usually treated with antibiotics. Viruses are capable of independent life but must be inside cells in order to reproduce or replicate. Viral infections are usually unaffected by antibiotics and must be treated, if available, with antiviral drugs. Fungi are primitive plantlike organisms. In people with HIV disease, fungal infections can occur on the surface of the skin, as in athlete's foot or ringworm; on mucous membranes of the mouth, throat, and vagina, as in candidiasis; or as an infection that spreads throughout the body, as in disseminated COCCIDIOIDOMYCOSIS. Systemic fungal infections tend to be more resistant to treatment than are bacterial infections, and a longer course of treatment is often necessary. Note that yeasts are also fungi. Protozoan parasites are one-cell animals that invade human cells and live in them as parasites. Many of these organisms also enter the body during a sporelike phase in their life cycle. CRYPTOSPORIDIOSIS and toxoplasmosis are examples of protozoan infections.

New opportunistic infections are now being diagnosed because the pool of people who contract them is so much larger, and, in addition, new techniques for identifying the causative elements have been developed. However, because most of the infections considered opportunistic are not reportable, lack of information interferes with a clear-cut count of their growing numbers. Although opportunistic infections are still not commonplace, they are no longer considered rare; their prevalence in the United States has been well documented. Note that whereas more than 100 microorganisms can cause disease in individuals with T4-CELL counts below 200 cells/mm, only a fraction of these are included in the current surveillance definition for clinical AIDS.

Although a broad range of infections is known to arise in people with HIV disease, it is very unlikely that any one person will experience all the opportunistic infections possible. The kinds of infections that do arise can vary in different parts of the country and the world because the organisms that cause them are found more abundantly in some areas than in others. Whenever possible it is essential to prevent opportunistic infections. A strong immune system is the first line of defense against them. Thus the early use of combination antiretroviral therapy can help preserve immune function and prevent opportunistic infection. Diet and rest are also important in helping to maintain the health of the immune system.

The management of opportunistic infection is divided into three phases: PRIMARY PROPHYLAXIS, treatment of active infection, and SECONDARY PROPHYLAXIS. Primary prophylaxis, or prevention of an initial infection, is important whenever possible because once the disease arises, the drugs used to treat it usually do not eliminate the disease-causing organism from the body. This means that when treatment stops, there is a good chance the infection will return. CD4 counts determine when primary prophylaxis should begin. Secondary prophylaxis is used to prevent an infection from recurring, and it must usually be taken for life. It is

also known as suppressive, or maintenance, therapy. With the advent of HAART therapy, many HIV positive people have stopped taking prophylaxis for certain opportunistic infections. Their immune systems have rebuilt enough strength to prevent some of these illnesses from occurring.

Drug prophylaxis against opportunistic infections has become a cornerstone of treatment for AIDS patients. However, it is important to note that as HIV infection progresses to advanced and late-stage disease, there may be cases in which the advantages and disadvantages of prophylactic or suppressive drugs for some opportunistic infections should be discussed with a physician. The advantages of prophylactic therapy include prevention of disease, decreased severity of disease, decreased risk of and necessity for hospitalization, probable decrease in the number of sick days and lost wages, potential psychological benefits, and preservation of health insurance benefits by staying healthier. The disadvantages of prophylactic or suppressive therapy for some infections can include the following: additional drug side effects; the risk of harmful drug interactions, which becomes a growing consideration as the number of drugs taken increases; the possibility that use of the drug will produce drug-resistant forms of the pathogen, which is of particular concern with fungal infections; the psychological effect on the patient of adding another drug to those already being taken, which may discourage the patient from following his or her prescribed antiretroviral treatment; and the cost of the therapy. The fact that viruses and organisms that cause opportunistic infections become resistant to the drugs over time is one of the primary reasons researchers are looking for ways in which to boost an immunosuppressed patient's immune system.

The most common opportunistic infections that can occur during HIV disease include, in alphabetical order: bacillary angiomatosis, candidiasis (oral, esophageal, vaginal), coccidioidomycosis, CRYTOCOCCOSIS, CRYPTOSPORIDIOSIS, CYTOMEGALOVIRUS (retinitis, esophagitis, colitis), HERPES SIMPLEX infection, HISTOPLASMOSIS, KAPOSI'S SARCOMA, MICROSPORIDIOSIS, *MYCOBACTERIUM AVIUM* COMPLEX, ORAL HAIRY LEUKOPLAKIA, *PNEUMOCYSTIS CARINII* PNEUMONIA, SHINGLES, toxoplasmosis, and TUBERCULOSIS. Today, an array of drugs can be used in strategies to prevent or delay nearly all the major oppor-

tunistic infections; this was not the case in the early 1990s.

The time elapsed since the discovery of HIV infection can be divided into two distinct periods: a pre-HAART era (before 1995) and the current era of HAART. The United States Public Health Service and the Infectious Diseases Society of America have guidelines that discuss standards for prevention and treatment of opportunistic infections in HIV-positive individuals. Since 1995, key amendments to the guidelines concern the management of patients who have responded to HAART. Current guidelines can be found at the Centers for Disease Control website at http://www.aidsinfo.nih.gov/guidelines/op_infections/html_oi_11-28-02.html. HAART reduces the risk of opportunistic infections more than any previous intervention available, and starting patients on HAART is clearly the most important therapy clinicians can offer to alter the natural history of infection and risk of opportunistic diseases. A critical question for patients who start HAART regimens and have rises in their T4 counts above thresholds for initiating prophylaxis has been whether prophylaxis can be stopped. The safety of discontinuing prophylaxis in patients whose T4 cell counts have risen to levels above 200 and for starting preventive therapy has now been established. The guidelines recognize this information and make specific recommendations regarding stopping prophylaxis.

Note that it is now clear that sustained viral suppression is not feasible in all patients receiving HAART. Failure of HAART or rebound in HIV RNA levels after initial response has been amply documented. Although the risk of clinical progression of the disease, despite viral rebound, has been low thus far, the long-term outcome of these patients remains uncertain.

opsonization   A process by which PHAGOCYTOSIS is facilitated by the deposition of opsonins (e.g., ANTIBODY and C3b) on the ANTIGEN.

optimal health   The highest state of well-being attainable at a particular time of life. Although the optimal health for an HIV-infected person may be different from that of someone who is HIV-negative, optimal health, defined in terms of the individual patient, should still be the goal for care of an HIV-infected individual.

oral candidiasis   See CANDIDIASIS.

oral contraceptive   A method of birth control (known as "the pill") in which a synthetic HORMONE pill is taken regularly by mouth to prevent conception. The pill interferes with ovulation, fertilization, and implantation of a fertilized egg in the uterus. Oral contraceptives were first made available and became popular during the early 1960s. The formulation has changed since its introduction, and newer versions provide a significantly lower dose of hormones than the original. The major advantages of oral contraceptives are their effectiveness, ease of use, ease of discontinuing use, and regulation of effects of the menstrual cycle. Many women cannot take them, however, because they have conditions that contraindicate their use, including known or suspected breast cancer or tumor; genital bleeding of unknown origin; circulatory disorders; cerebral-vascular or coronary-artery disorders; severely impaired liver function; cystic fibrosis; sickle-cell disease; or a past history of these disorders.

oral eroticism   A psychoanalytic term for pleasure derived from activities involving the mouth, including oral-genital contact, kissing, sucking, eating, biting, chewing, thumbsucking or smoking. Some of these activities are considered unsafe sex practices with high risk of HIV transmission (oral-anal contact). Others are considered possibly unsafe practices with unclear risk of HIV transmission (fellatio, cunnilingus). Other activities, such as wet kissing, are considered low-risk practices with some risk of HIV transmission. See ORAL SEX.

oral hairy leukoplakia (OHL)   The symptoms of oral hairy leukoplakia are white lesions or patches on the tongue and elsewhere in the mouth; the lesion appears raised with a corrugated, or "hairy" surface. These patches produce no symptoms. It is often the first opportunistic infection that appears in HIV-positive people. Generally, OHL is caused by the EPSTEIN BARR VIRUS (EBV), which causes INFECTIOUS MONONUCLEOSIS. The patches often appear similar to those of thrush. Oral hairy leukoplakia occurs mainly in people with declining immunity. It is usually not treated with drugs, as there does not seem to be anything that works to control it. Acyclovir in heavy doses can be used to remove it initially, but it will return if the drug is stopped. Heavy doses of acyclovir can be dangerous over a long period. OHL is more common in people who smoke.

oral herpes Another name for Herpes simplex virus type 1 that causes cold sores or fever blisters. Cold sores occur when the virus reactivates after being dormant. A person's initial expression of the virus does not take the form of cold sores so many people do not relate these to the virus. The initial effect of the virus is a sore mouth, inflamed lips, then a series of grayish mouth ulcers that blister then heal themselves.

oral HIV test An HIV test which uses mouth secretions. It is believed that the new test will encourage more people at risk of AIDS, particularly minorities, to get tested, because it does not involve a needle and can be given easily outside of a clinic. Patients take the oral test by placing a flat, inchlong cotton swab, attached to a stick, between their gums and their cheeks for two minutes. The swab, treated with a salt solution, draws fluid from the mucous membrane. The fluid contains HIV antibodies in people infected with the virus.

oral lesion A circumscribed area of pathologically altered tissue or skin in the mouth.

oral sex Sexual activity in which the genitals and anus are stimulated with the tongue and/or mouth. Contact between the mouth and the genitals is probably the most common form of oral sex (FELLATIO is the oral stimulation of the penis; CUNNILINGUS is the oral stimulation of the clitoris). Oral sexual activities may include kissing, biting, sucking, licking, exploring the partner's body including erogenous zones and genitals with the tongue and lips, and tasting and swallowing the partner's sexual secretions. Oral sex, particularly oral-anal sex, is considered high-risk—many SEXUALLY TRANSMITTED DISEASES (particularly AIDS, SYPHILIS, GONORRHEA, and HERPES) can be transmitted through it—but because individuals who engage in it rarely

do so to the exclusion of other forms of sexual contact, it is difficult to attribute transmission in any particular case to oral sex rather than to other types of sexual activity. The role of oral sex as a route of transmission of HIV is, at best, poorly studied in populations other than homosexual men.

Slang terms include blow job, eating out, giving head, going down, pussy licking, and ass licking.

oral-anal sex See ORAL SEX.

oral-genital contact See ORAL SEX.

oral-genital sex See ORAL SEX.

Orasone See PREDNISONE.

OraSure See ORAL HIV TEST.

organ A body structure with specific functions; made of two or more tissues.

organ donation The transplantation of an organ from a donor to a recipient. Organ transplants have become a routine medical practice that has dramatically improved and—sometimes—saved lives. Successful transplantation is increased by matching donors and recipients of the same racial and ethnic groups. The organ recovery process may involve several steps, including obtaining medical examiner approval, obtaining next-of-kin consent, reviewing medical and social history for organ safety, and testing blood to lower the risk of spreading infectious diseases. Once a recovery team surgically removes the organs without disfiguring the body, the organs are evaluated for transplant. People who receive organs are generally selected according to the United Network for Organ Sharing guidelines. There is no cost to the donor family for any organ presentation or donation procedures. Donor cards are legal documents under the Uniform Anatomical Gift Act. Signing a donor card signifies a donor's commitment to make a gift of any needed organs and/or tissues for the purpose of transplant, medical study, or education. The transplant takes effect after the donor's death.

organ system   A group of related organs that work together to perform specific functions (i.e., the digestive system, the reproductive system). The immune system is the organ system that fights disease.

organ transplantation   More than 50,000 people receive organ transplantations each year. When people first became ill with HIV all options for organ transplantation were stopped. The medical establishment and the insurance corporations did not consider it worth the cost or the effort to secure organs for transplantation into HIV-positive people. In the late 1990s this attitude began to change within the medical community.

As HAART has proved very successful in keeping people healthy PWAs have begun to die of problems that were not faced in the era of OPPORTUNISTIC INFECTION. For many HIV disease patients that may mean end-stage liver or kidney disease. Then transplantation may be the only option for survival. Liver failure can result from complications of hepatitis B or C and renal problems can result from neuropathy or diabetes related to HAART. HIV-positive individuals who are nevertheless healthy have begun to explore possible transplantation. The United Network for Organ Sharing (UNOS) which maintains all waiting lists for organs around the United States, considers this is a possibility. UNOS has never forbidden HIV-positive individuals to add their names to waiting lists. (They still do not allow HIV-positive persons, among other restrictions, to sign up to donate organs.) Early studies of end results of transplants into HIV-positive people have been promising. The problem may be that medical personnel at transplant centers and insurance corporations will not agree to perform the procedures as a result of ignorance.

Reviews of transplantations that have been done in HIV-positive people show that if a person is in good relative health and maintains a high stable CD4 count, then he or she should do as well as usual organ transplant patients. Approximately 20 percent of people receiving transplants do not survive. Currently there are 14 transplant centers in the United States that are involved in developing a study to measure results of transplantation of organs in HIV-positive people. Experience at both the University of Pittsburgh and the University of California—San Francisco has led physicians there to believe that it is possible to perform successful kidney and liver transplantation without endangering patients more than they would be otherwise endangered by transplantation were they HIV-negative. Doctors in those studies caution that monitoring an HIV-positive person's HAART medications is important because several of these drugs can cause interactions with the immunosuppressive drugs required after a transplantation.

In late 2001 the well-known author Larry Kramer had liver transplantation at the University of Pittsburgh. He had reached end-stage liver disease caused by hepatitis B. He was still alive in May 2003. Mr. Kramer has spoken about his attempts to get on hospital waiting lists so that if a liver became available he could have the operation at that particular hospital. He indicated that he felt both homophobia and AIDS phobia during his search. He eventually moved to Pittsburgh to await a possible liver. His operation unleashed a torrent of complaints about his receiving the liver on talk radio in the United States.

organelle   One of the specialized small organs of a living cell (e.g., mitochondria).

organic   A chemical compound that contains carbonhydrogen covalent bonds; includes carbohydrates, lipids, proteins, and nucleic acids.

organic brain damage   Physiological harm to the brain cells, causing impairment of brain function. HIV infection of the central nervous system can cause such damage.

orgasm   A state of physical and emotional excitement, especially that which occurs at the climax of sexual intercourse. It is the third stage of the sexual response cycle, after the excitement and plateau phases. In the male, it is accompanied by the ejaculation of semen. In the female, tension is released in a series of involuntary and often pleasurable muscular contractions that expel blood from the pelvic tissue. Women may feel contractions in the vagina, uterus, and rectum. Some women describe orgasm without contractions.

Orgasm can be mild, like a hiccup, a sneeze, a ripple; it can be a sensuous experience; it can be intense or ecstatic. Today, it is generally understood by sexologists and researchers that all orgasms are not physiologically the same. No one is sure as to how many types of orgasms there are and which kind is better, stronger, or more satisfying. Slang terms include the "big O."

orgy An event consisting of uninhibited excessive group indulgence in a variety of pleasurable activities, including sex, drinking, singing, or dancing.

orogenital contact See ORAL SEX.

orphan See AIDS ORPHAN.

orphan diseases Rare, debilitating illnesses that strike small numbers of people. See ORPHAN DRUG; ORPHAN DRUG ACT.

orphan drug Drugs that are effective for certain ORPHAN DISEASES but, for a variety of reasons, are not profitable for manufactures to produce. See ORPHAN DRUG ACT.

Orphan Drug Act The U.S. FOOD AND DRUG ADMINISTRATION (FDA)–sponsored Orphan Drug Act of 1983 was passed to encourage development of drugs that possibly could not be patented and for which there would be only a limited market due to the small number of people with a particular disease that the drug would work to heal. Orphan status is granted before FDA approval, and afterward the manufacturer is allowed tax benefits and seven years of marketing exclusivity. Some critics have claimed that drug companies use this act to gain tax credits for all newly developed drugs, whether they are "orphan" drugs or not. They also claim that drug companies use this act to bypass long testing periods for new medications, which the act allows. Others have encouraged continued funding and expanded funding of the act because they claim it has been successful in encouraging research and development that would otherwise be avoided in a pure capitalistic market. These forces have introduced several expansions of the original bill in the 2001–2002 session of Congress.

orphan drug status See ORPHAN DRUG ACT.

orphanage One of today's challenges (and tomorrow's problems) is the impact of AIDS-related deaths on both the lives of community members and the individual lives of children and adolescents. To deal with this growing problem, some advocate that the institution of orphanages be revived. Today, the term conjures up images from Dickens—starving children abused by heartless masters. It is true that child care practices in some institutions in the past, especially during the 19th century, seem punitive and rigid by contemporary standards. But some orphanages in the United States today provide good care. An example is transition homes for HIV-infected orphaned babies. These have been successful in providing appropriate health care as well as emotional nurturing. They were created to offer an out-of-hospital environment for such babies until longer-term placement can be arranged. Those who support the return of the orphanage as an institution call for creating small-scale institutions that can offer children nurturing and care as well as shelter. They hold that congregate care is both a useful and temporary option and that orphanages are the only answer to the failure of families or foster care. On the other hand, the primacy of family life has been stressed repeatedly in the 1990s. The jury is still out with respect to institutional child care settings. A rigorous, unemotional analysis of the appropriate role of congregate care, and the services that are needed to make it work in the interests of children, is essential.

osteoporosis Loss of bone density caused by depletion of calcium and bone protein. In HIV-positive people, women especially, this can be worsened by the virus and possibly HAART. Persons with osteoporosis are at high risk for bone fractures, due to the loss of bone mass. Bone density can be measured by an exam called bone densitometry. This can determine the loss of bone in patients and whether treatment is required. It can often be reduced through calcium intake and hormone treatments. Weight-bearing, high-impact exercise can also be prescribed, as this encourages bone formation and strengthens muscles attached to the bones.

otitis An inflammation of the ear, differentiated as externa (inflammation of the external auditory canal), media (inflammation of the middle ear), and interna (inflammation of the labyrinth of the ear).

otopharyngeal Concerning the ear and pharynx.

otopharyngeal tube The passage between the tympanic cavity and the pharynx.

ototoxic Having a detrimental effect on the eighth nerve or the organs of hearing.

outcome variable An observation recorded for patients in a trial at one or more time points after enrollment for the purpose of assessing the effects of the study treatments.

outercourse A term originating in the anti-AIDS, safe-sex movement, designating forms of sexual expression, such as massage, hugging, caressing, mutual masturbation, and rubbing bodies together that do not involve the exchange of body fluids. These forms of sexual expression are considered practices with no risk of HIV transmission.

outlier Any value, reading, or measurement that is far outside established limits or the central range of the data and, for this reason, is questioned or considered to be in error.

outreach worker A professional or paraprofessional health or social services worker who actively seeks out patients in their own environments and communities and provides education and medical services.

O-V Statin See NYSTATIN.

ovarian cancer Cancer of the ovaries, the female reproductive organs in which the ova, or eggs, are formed and estrogen is produced.

The cause of ovarian cancer is not known, although a number of factors have been associated with its occurrence. It appears that HORMONES play a role in the development of ovarian cancer. Expo-sure to high levels of radiation may also cause ovarian cancer. The most common type of ovarian cancer is the EPITHELIAL carcinoma in the ovary's outer layer. Frequently there are no symptoms in the early stages of ovarian cancer, making it difficult to obtain an early diagnosis, when there is the greatest chance for effective treatment. An ovarian tumor can grow for some time before pressure or pain can be felt or other problems are noticed. When symptoms do occur, they may include abdominal swelling or bloating, discomfort in the lower part of the abdomen, a full feeling after a light meal, lack of appetite, nausea, vomiting, gas, indigestion, weight loss, constant need to urinate, diarrhea, or constipation, and nonmenstrual bleeding. Procedures used in the diagnosis and evaluation of ovarian cancer may include an internal exam of the uterus, vagina, ovaries, fallopian tubes, bladder, and rectum, a PAP SMEAR, ultrasound, blood and urine tests, and X rays. Additional procedures that may be done are a CT SCAN, lymphangiography, IVP, lower GI series, exploratory laparotomy, and biopsies.

Treatment depends on the stage of the disease at the time of diagnosis, the type of cells that make up the tumor, and how fast the cancer is growing. Current medical options for treating ovarian cancer include surgery, chemotherapy, and/or radiation. Biological therapies are also now available. These therapies are evolving as a result of research, which continues to offer hope for improving the outcome of treatment for women with ovarian cancer.

ovary The major female reproductive organ that produces eggs (ova) and the female sex hormone estrogen. There are two ovaries, one on either side of the uterus.

overdose A dose of a drug sufficient to cause an acute reaction, such as mania, hysteria, coma, or even death. While an overdose is often one that clearly exceeds the normal dosage range recommended by the manufacturer, the optimal dose of many drugs varies from person to person. What may be an average dose for most people may be an overdose for some and an underdose for others. Numerous factors such as age, body size, nutritional status, and liver and kidney function have significant influence on dosage requirements. An overdose may be accidental or deliberate and may result from accumulation of prescribed daily doses.

over-the-counter (OTC) drugs   Drug products that can be purchased without prescription, for example aspirin. Like the more potent drug products sold only on prescription, they are chemicals that are capable of a wide variety of actions on biological systems. Within the last 30 years, many OTC drugs have assumed greater importance because of their ability to interact favorably with widely used prescription drugs. Serious problems in drug management can arise when the patient fails to tell the physician of the OTC drug(s) he or she is taking and when the physician fails to note the inclusion of OTC drugs when asking the patient about what medicines the patient currently uses. During any course of treatment, whether medical or surgical, the patient should consult with the physician regarding any OTC drug that the patient wishes to take. The major classes of OTC drugs for internal use include allergy medicines, antacids, antiworm medicines, aspirin and aspirin combinations, aspirin substitutes, asthma aids, cold medicines, diarrhea remedies, digestion aids, diuretics, iron preparations, laxatives, menstrual aids, motion sickness remedies, pain relievers, reducing aids, salt substitutes, sedatives and tranquilizers, sleeping pills, stimulants, sugar substitutes, tonics, and vitamins.

oviduct   The tube through which the egg passes from the ovary to the uterus.

ovine-caprine lentivirus   Any lentivirus associated with sheep or goats.

ovulation   Release of the egg from the ovary, generally 14 days after the end of a woman's last menstrual period.

oxandrolone   A synthetic form of an anabolic steroid used to treat deficiencies in testosterone that result in weight loss, reduced sex drive, and loss of energy. Weight loss is a common symptom in people with HIV that has many possible causes and solutions. Anabolic steroids are derivatives of testosterone, the natural male hormone produced primarily by the testes. Women also produce testosterone, but in smaller amounts than men do. Testosterone is responsible for the masculinizing and tissue-building (anabolic) changes that occur in males during adolescence, including the growth of the reproductive tract and the development of secondary sexual characteristics. Approximately half of the HIV-positive men with CD4+ counts below 200 have testosterone deficiencies, probably caused by HIV suppression of normal endocrine-gland function or by drugs (such as ketoconazole) used to treat opportunistic infections. These deficiencies are associated with the weakness and loss of lean tissue mass in HIV-related weight loss.

For treatment of HIV-related weight loss, anabolic steroids are probably most effective for people with abnormally low testosterone levels. Consequently, before initiating treatment, physicians usually measure their patients' testosterone levels. Oral and injectable forms of testosterone have long been available to treat testosterone deficiencies. Synthetic forms, such as oxandrolone, are also available. Oxandrolone is not potent enough to be used as testosterone replacement therapy. Unlike most other anabolic agents, however, which have not been approved by the Food and Drug Administration for treating HIV-related weight loss, Oxandrolone is approved for treating weight loss when the cause of the weight loss is unknown (e.g., not associated with low testosterone or an infectious agent, such as parasites, for example). HIV-associated weight loss falls into this category. Oxandrolone is available as tablets for oral administration. The advantages of synthetic steroids include lower risk of liver toxicity and fewer of the "masculinizing" side effects common when injectable testosterone is used. Anabolic agents should not be used by anyone with a known allergy to them: Men with known or suspected breast or prostate cancer should avoid them. Because of the risk of serious side effects, people with heart, kidney, or liver disease should use anabolic steroids with extreme caution. Oxandrolone has been studied in women and shown to have some masculinizing affects, although far less than what is commonly seen with testosterone therapy. In small studies, some women reported irregular menstrual cycles and vaginal bleeding. If women are using anabolic agents and begin to show mild signs of virilization (e.g., facial hair growth, deepening of the voice), they should discontinue anabolic therapy as these side effects can become permanent. (The trade name is Oxandrin.)

oxidation A chemical reaction resulting from exposure to oxygen or other electron-donating atom or molecule. On the cellular level, oxidative reactions are the source of energy, but free radicals and other oxidizing agents can damage cellular components such as membranes and interfere with cells' regulatory systems.

oxidative stress Increased levels of free radicals and other oxidation-promoting molecules associated with disease, immune response, and aging. When the production of prooxidants exceeds the cellular supply of antioxidants, harmful effects may result, including cell membrane damage, cell death, and damage to genetic material (DNA and RNA) that results in mutations. Oxidative stress is thought to promote HIV replication.

oxymetholone An anabolic-androgenic steroid used to treat anemia. (Its trade name is Anadrol.)

P1 lab facility   A basic laboratory such as could be found lining the hallways of university science departments, found within the CENTERS FOR DISEASE CONTROL AND PREVENTION's high-security laboratories.

P2 lab facility   A laboratory within the CENTERS FOR DISEASE CONTROL AND PREVENTION's high-security laboratories. Entry is limited to trained, authorized personnel who perform research work under hoods that suck air away from the experiment, up a ventilator duct, and past scrubbers that disinfect the air with ultraviolet light and microscopically gridded fibers.

P-3 biosafety level   Applicable to clinical, teaching, research, or production facilities in which work is done with agents that may cause serious or potentially lethal reactions as a result of exposure by inhalation. Special airflows and filters and an antechamber with a sink, must be installed. Protective garments must always be worn, and nothing may be taken out of the room without being sterilized. See P1 LAB FACILITY; P2 LAB FACILITY; P3 LAB FACILITY.

P3 lab facility   A lab within the CENTERS FOR DISEASE CONTROL AND PREVENTION's high-security laboratories in which scientists perform high-security research. Researchers are generally required to pass through a series of guarded locked doors, presenting their security pass for entry. All personnel shower before and after entry with disinfectant soap and wear head-to-toe protective clothing, a gauze face mask, double latex gloves, and a radiation badge that monitors levels of exposure to isotopes used in research. One enters the inner core of the facility after passing through two or more double air-locked doors lined with microbe-killing ultraviolet lights. Rooms in the inner core of the facility are generally kept under pressure and direct all air—and all microbes—toward special ventilators in which the microbes are destroyed by ultraviolet lights. The remaining air is filtered through several layers of sheets that strain out anything bigger than a large molecule.

p24   A protein ANTIGEN from HIV's core. The p24 level can be measured in blood and other body fluids; this level has been used to monitor viral activity. This is not considered a very accurate method, however, due to the existence of p24 ANTIBODY that binds with the antigen and makes it undetectable.

p24 antigen test   A laboratory test (also called the p24 antigen capture assay) that detects the presence of HIV in the blood. p24 is one of the several proteins that make up HIV; its presence therefore indicates the presence of HIV. This test is not especially sensitive, and most people with HIV infection test negative.

Levels of p24 are highest early and late in the disease. The number of HIV viruses is likewise highest at those times. Some physicians therefore suggest that the p24 antigen test might help track the course of the disease in people with HIV infection. It might identify people with HIV infection who are likely to develop symptoms and who are most likely to transmit the virus to others. It might also help evaluate response to antiviral drugs.

P450 enzyme system   This is the system of enzymes, located in the liver and the intestines, responsible for the processing in the body of chemicals, medicines, steroids, pollutants, and pesticides. Other types of chemicals as yet undetermined may also be metabolized by this enzyme system.

Drugs themselves can have the ability to increase or decrease the metabolizing of other drugs, by affecting the function of the P450 system. Foods can also have the same ability to increase or decrease the metabolizing action. Grapefruit juice is known to increase the amount of some protease inhibitors in the body, thereby increasing doses of the medicine to more than recommended dosage. St. John's wort has also been responsible for interactions with HAART medications.

P450 inhibitors generally increase concentrations of other drugs. P450 inducers generally decrease concentrations of other drugs. P450 enzymes are classified using Roman numerals and letters. Almost half of all human drugs use P450 3A4; another 30 percent use P450 2D6. Foods and other chemicals use these same enzymes. HIV medicines comprise both groups. Rifabutin, efavirenz, and nevirapine are P450 inducers. Delaviridine, indinavir, nelfinavir, ritonavir, and saquinavir are P450 inhibitors.

This is one reason why doctors need to know what medications a person is taking before they prescribe new medications: to reduce interactions while maintaining the correct amount of drug in the body. Many recreational drugs and alcohol also are metabolized by the enzyme system and can also cause interactions. Severe interactions have occurred in usage of some recreational drugs and HAART medicines. Several websites provide information on the P450 enzymes and their inhibition or inducement by recreational drugs, for those that insist on using such substances.

p **value** A probability value that is reported in experiments such as clinical trials. The *p* value indicates how likely it is that the result obtained by the experiment is due to chance alone. The lower the *p* value, the more likely it is that the results are not due to chance. A *p* value of less than 0.05 is considered statistically significant, that is, not likely to be due to chance alone.

package insert A printed information sheet from a drug manufacturer approved by the FOOD AND DRUG ADMINISTRATION for a prescription drug product, which accompanies the product in its packaging. The insert is usually not enclosed by a pharmacist with a dispensed prescription. Intended mainly for the use of prescribing professionals, principally physicians, the insert gives the recommended uses, mode of administration, dosage, and contraindications to use of the drug, with appropriate warnings.

pain Physical suffering, typically from injury or illness. Pain is a common companion of persons living with HIV and AIDS. Pain occurs at all points on the HIV/AIDS continuum and is the most common reason for people with AIDS to be hospitalized. It appears that as people with AIDS survive longer, pain is becoming an increasingly severe complaint. Pain in HIV/AIDS can be traced to HIV infection and its complications, medical treatments, or causes independent of HIV. Pain is often complicated by multiple concurrent diagnoses as well as chemical dependency and encephalopathy. It is crucial that medical practitioners understand the sources of pain in people with AIDS as well as the pharmacological factors affecting use of pain relievers in this population. Active pain management is fundamental to the provision of care.

Pacific Islands See OCEANIA.

pain management Active management of pain, which seeks to ensure the greatest comfort and functioning with minimal medication-related side effects is key to relieving the effects of AIDS. Since multiple illnesses often coexist in PWAs, the importance of identifying and appropriately treating underlying causes of pain is primary. Treating the disease may eradicate the pain all by itself. While the cause of pain is being determined, pain management with appropriate analgesics should be initiated. There is much that can be done to ameliorate pain, but drug therapy is the mainstay of any treatment program.

The WORLD HEALTH ORGANIZATION has developed a four-step ladder approach to the treatment of cancer pain, and this has been adapted for the treatment of HIV-related pain. The first step is to use acetaminophen or other nonsteroidal anti-inflammatory drugs, such as ibuprofen, sulindac, or aspirin. If these measures do not provide adequate relief, then a weak opiate, such as codeine or oxycodone, is added. If this is inadequate, a stronger opiate, such as morphine, hydromorphone, fentanyl, or levorphanol, is used. The fourth step, which can be incorporated at any point in the process, is to add adjuvants, such as hydroxyzine, that boost the effectiveness of pain medications.

Alternate routes of administration of drugs is an important element in pain management. Dehydration, malnourishment, and ELECTROLYTE imbalance due to vomiting, diarrhea, and anorexia impede the effectiveness of oral medication. In the case of vomiting, rectal or topical routes are advised. For difficulties with swallowing, liquid or rectal preparations are suggested. Few people with AIDS require injected opiates if the appropriate analgesics are prescribed in adequate doses via the most suitable route. However, skin patches releasing fentanyl, designed to last up to 72 hours, are a convenient way to administer topical pain relief.

Other interventions include general comfort measures, radiation or chemotherapy, nerve blocks, and complementary therapy believed by some to offer relief, such as aromatherapy, therapeutic touch, and relaxation and imagery techniques. Massage, acupuncture, physical therapy, heat, ice, music, and topical mentholated products may also provide additional comfort.

pain threshold The extent of neurological or emotional stimulation required to produce the sensation of pain.

paleopathology The study of diseases in ancient remains of bodies and fossils.

palinavir A PROTEASE INHIBITOR introduced in 1995, characterized as having excellent antiviral activity, good bioavailability, and an acceptable safety profile in animals. Palinavir has some of the same problems as other protease inhibitors in development: it is a complex molecule and will probably be difficult to manufacture. It also binds to alpha acid glycoprotein, the naturally occurring blood protein that was found in 1994 to bind to and inactivate another protease inhibitor. Unlike

that compound, however, plasma levels of the drug should still be high enough to suppress HIV—assuming that palinavir is absorbed well by the intestines. HIV does become resistant to the compound in lab cultures. One mutation occurs that makes the virus slightly less susceptible to palinavir, but a second mutation is required to develop substantial resistance. One of these mutations is unique to palinavir while the other is also seen in lab cultures treated with the drug AG1343. The mutant virus is not cross-resistant with saquinavir, but there does appear to be some decreased susceptibility to the Merck protease inhibitor.

palliative Offering comfort or relief of symptoms without ameliorating the underlying disease process; also a treatment or device that has such an effect.

Pancoast's tumor Tumor originating from the superior sulcus of the lung that invades all or a portion of the brachial plexus.

pancreas A compound acinotubular gland situated behind the stomach in front of the first and second lumbar vertebrae in a horizontal position, with its head attached to the duodenum and its tail reaching to the spleen. The pancreas produces both an external and an internal secretion. The external secretion, called pancreatic juice, passes through the pancreatic ducts into the duodenum, where it plays an important role in the digestion of all classes of foods. The internal secretion, elaborated by the beta cells of the islets of Langerhans, includes the HORMONES insulin and glucagon secreted by the alpha cells. These hormones, in conjunction with hormones from other endocrine glands, play a primary role in the regulation of carbohydrate metabolism.

pancreatic enzyme One type of pancreas-produced protein that aids digestion of fats, carbohydrates, and proteins.

pancreatitis Inflamed condition of the pancreas. An occasional side effect of ddI, pancreatitis can result in severe abdominal pain and death. Its onset can be predicted by rises in blood levels of the pancreatic enzyme AMYLASE.

pancytopenia   Low levels of all types of blood cells.

pandemic   An epidemic over a wide geographic area, usually worldwide, affecting large numbers of people at the same time.

Pap smear   See PAPANICOLAOU (PAP) SMEAR.

Pap smear screening   The need for rigorous surveillance in HIV infection has given rise to the argument for routine Pap smear screening in HIV-positive women. At the time of screening, it is equally important to examine the vulva and vagina, culture the cervix for STDS (gonorrhea and chlamydia), and diagnose and treat any vaginitis present, including atrophic vaginitis. Management strategies also include liberal referrals for colposcopic evaluation, particularly for vulvar and vaginal lesions that cannot be definitively diagnosed, so that colposcopically directed biopsies can be obtained.

Most clinicians feel that Pap smear screening should be performed every six months for the majority of HIV-positive women. It is equally important to utilize a cytology laboratory that is consistently accurate and that uses the 1988 Bethesda system for reporting. Using this system, all Pap smears with recurrent atypias, CERVICAL INTRAEPITHELIAL NEOPLASIAS of all grades, and carcinoma-in-situ should be referred for colposcopic evaluation within six weeks. See PAPANICOLAOU (PAP) SMEAR.

Pap test   See PAPANICOLAOU (PAP) SMEAR.

Papanicolaou (Pap) smear   A test for detecting cancer in women in its early stages. It is a standard component of routine gynecological examinations. It involves removal of a smear of loose cells from the surface of the cervix and examining them under a microscope. Cells are graded from class I (no abnormalities) to class V (cancer cells observed). The Pap test usually does not detect uterine lining cancer (endometrial cancer). The accuracy of Pap smears, long considered the standard method for detecting abnormalities that might develop into cervical cancer, has been called into question, particularly in the case of women with HIV. Studies have shown that Pap smear screening does not always uncover cytological abnormalities that were evident from colposcopically directed biopsies obtained at the same time. Moreover, HIV-positive women frequently have lower genital tract infections that may obscure Pap results.

HIV-positive women are found to have approximately a tenfold increase in abnormal cervical cytology. Abnormal findings include inflammatory changes, vaginal pathogens, cellular atypia, CERVICAL INTRAEPITHELIAL NEOPLASIA (CIN) of all grades, and cervical cancer. The severity of the abnormality is believed to correlate with the degree of immunosuppression. The entire lower tract may be affected and at risk of development of squamous cell cancers. In immunocompromised women, this type of disease tends to persist, recur, and extend, even with conventional treatment. It is accepted that the vast majority of squamous cell abnormalities in the genital tract are associated with HUMAN PAPILLOMA VIRUS (HPV) infection and specifically with particular strains of HPV. It is also known that immunocompromise accelerates the progress from viral infection to neoplasias in both renal transplant patients (on immunosuppressive therapy) and in HIV-positive women with lowered CD4 counts.

Risa Denenberg, a family nurse practitioner in the AIDS Clinic at New York's Bronx Lebanon Hospital cautions that the accuracy of Pap smears can vary greatly from one clinical setting to another. She advises that patients and clinicians remember the following: The best smears are obtained mid-cycle; smears taken during a period or when bleeding for any other reason are unacceptable; patients should not douche, use tampons, or have sexual intercourse for 48 hours before a Pap smear; Pap smears require two tissue samples; lubricants interfere with obtaining proper tissue samples; as a preservative measure, it is necessary to apply fixative within ten seconds after spreading samples on microscope slides; proper labeling of slides is the clinician's responsibility; and patients and clinicians should only accept Pap smear results from a lab that uses the standardized Bethesda system to report results.

papillary tumor A neoplasm composed of or resembling enlarged papillae.

papilloma An EPITHELIAL tumor of skin or mucous membrane consisting of hypertrophied papillae covered by a layer of epithelium. Papillomas are often found in the genital area. Included in this group are warts, condylomas, and polyps. Most are caused by a strain of the HUMAN PAPILLOMA VIRUS (HPV). There are more than 40 types of HPV infections. Certain viral strains predispose women to and indeed probably cause cervical, vaginal, and vulval cancer. Women known to have HPV infections need to be monitored carefully with PAP SMEARS and at times COLPOSCOPY and BIOPSY. Cryosurgery or laser surgery may be necessary if precancerous changes occur. Male partners of women with HPV infections should be evaluated by a physician familiar with this problem, as HPV infections can be invisible to the naked eye and require special staining techniques and/or colposcopy to evaluate.

papillomavirus A virus that causes papillomas or warts in humans and animals. Papillomaviruses belong to the papovavirus family or group.

papovavirus One of a group of viruses important in viral carcinogenesis. Included are polyoma virus, simian virus 40, and papillomaviruses.

papule A red elevated area on the skin, solid and circumscribed. Papules often precede vesicular or pustular formation and may appear in erythema multiforme, eczema papulosum, prurigo, syphilis, measles, and smallpox. They may develop after use of bromides, iodides, or coal tar preparation.

paracrine Effects of a HORMONE that are only local.

parallel track A FOOD AND DRUG ADMINISTRATION–approved program to allow patients who are not in trials, but who meet certain criteria, to take an experimental drug. In the program, doctors monitor patients' response and report data to the pharmaceutical company sponsoring the drug and the program.

paralysis Temporary or permanent loss of function, especially loss of sensation or voluntary motion. Paralyses are divided into two groups: spastic, when due to lesion of upper motor neuron, and flaccid, when due to lesion of lower motor neuron.

Temporary paralysis can also result from a psychological disorder. Psychic inhibition of motor function occurs most characteristically in hysteria. Evidence of organic disease is always lacking in hysterical paralysis.

parasite An organism whose survival depends on food from a host organism. A parasite does not necessarily cause disease.

parenteral Introduced into the body by a route other than through the GASTROINTESTINAL TRACT; the term usually refers to intravenous or intramuscular administration of substances such as therapeutic drugs or nutritive solutions. See PARENTERAL NUTRITION; CATHETER.

parenteral nutrition The INTRAVENOUS administration of liquid nutrients to patients who are unable to eat or to absorb nutrients normally. It is most often used for patients suffering moderate to severe WASTING associated with cancer or HIV/AIDS. The nutrient solution generally contains protein, carbohydrates, vitamins, minerals, and electrolytes, with the formula adjusted for individual patient's needs. An infusion pump is generally required; infusions can take from 12 to 14 hours a day. No definitive studies have been published on the side effects of parenteral nutrition.

PARTIAL PARENTERAL NUTRITION (PPN) may be used in combination with solid food to treat moderate wasting. TOTAL PARENTERAL NUTRITION (TPN) is used in cases of severe wasting, to provide patient's entire nutritional needs. In addition to the nutrient mix described above, TPN also supplies essential fats.

Studies indicate that patients receiving TPN gain significant amounts of body cell mass and weight if they are free of systemic infections. Other studies have shown that administering TPN during secondary infection can increase weight gain and improve quality of life by improving the ability to fight infection. TPN has also been shown to have favorable effects on immune cell responsiveness.

In a home care environment, TPN is expensive. It is usually used to support someone through a limited period of acute illness but may be required for more lengthy periods.

Adequate and balanced nutrition is the key to maintaining lean body mass in people with HIV. Vitamins and nutrient supplements may be appropriate at all stages of HIV disease. OPPORTUNISTIC INFECTIONS of the intestines should be treated aggressively to prevent malabsorption. Appetite stimulants such as megestrol or dronabinol may be appropriate to treat symptomatic loss of appetite. Wasting may also be treated with hormone therapy or cytokine manipulation, both experimental procedures.

paresthesia Abnormal sensations such as burning or tingling. Paresthesia may constitute the first symptoms of PERIPHERAL NEUROPATHY, or it may be a limited drug side effect that does not worsen with time.

paromomycin sulfate An antibiotic used in treating intestinal AMEBIASIS and various tapeworms, CRYPTOSPORIDIOSIS in particular. (It should be noted that there is no standard treatment for cryptosporidiosis.) It is not effective against extraintestinal infections with amoebae. Paromomycin is an antibiotic of the aminoglycoside class, similar in action to neomycin, streptomycin, erythromycin, and others. It is poorly absorbed into the bloodstream, so high concentrations stay in the gut where many parasites that cause diarrhea multiply. Paromomycin is available in tablet form. Paromomycin generally causes few side effects, but among possible side effects are nausea, abdominal cramps, and diarrhea. (Trade name is Humatin. Other names are Aminosidine; AMS.)

parotitis Inflammation of the parotid gland.

paroxetine An antidepressant of the class known as serotonin reuptake inhibitors. It is primarily used for the treatment of depression but is also used for obsessive-compulsive disorder. It has become widely used because it is effective and tends to have fewer side effects than older antidepressants. It is available in tablets. (Trade name is Paxil.)

paroxysm A sudden, periodic attack or recurrence of symptoms of a disease; a sudden spasm or convulsion of any kind. It also pertains to a sudden emotional state, as fear, grief, or joy.

Part A See MEDICARE.

Part B See MEDICARE.

partial parenteral nutrition See PARENTERAL NUTRITION.

partialism Erotic responsiveness to a part of the body, for example a foot partialism.

partially blinded clinical trial A clinical trial in which some, but not all, of the study treatments are administered in a single- or double-blinded fashion. Also refers to a clinical trial in which some, but not all, of the staff in a clinic are blinded to treatment assignment.

partner negotiation Negotiation of the terms of a sexual encounter; the primary strategy for living by safe-sex guidelines. The first step is becoming clear in one's own mind about what one is and is not willing to do, would like to do, or might be talked into doing. The second step is negotiating an agreement about it with one's partner. Negotiation involves finding out about the partner's background and other sexual relationships, past and present. It involves finding out whether he or she is easy to talk to, comfortable discussing sexual details, flexible in his or her sexual habits, caring, imaginative, and creative.

Negotiating safer sex may not be easy for many reasons. Many people don't like to change their habits. Others may assume that safer sex will be too complicated, not worth the effort, unromantic, a poor substitute for the real thing, or a compromise. Still others may be embarrassed to do some of the things that are safe. Buying condoms or spermicides may be uncomfortable for some persons. Often, individuals don't know how to bring up the subject with someone they've just met. Others may fear they will offend or lose their partners by suggesting safer sex. Some persons resent all the advance planning required by safer sex, and just want to follow their feelings. Today, books about sexual management include advice on living by the guidelines and negotiating safer sex.

partner notification The process of informing sex or needle-sharing partners of an HIV-infected person that they have been or are at risk of contracting HIV. Notification may be done by the HIV-infected person, a HEALTH CARE PROVIDER, or a PUBLIC HEALTH worker.

Partner notification for STDS (including HIV) encompasses two distinct approaches: patient referral and provider referral. All partner notification activities within STD/HIV prevention programs are based on some combination of these. With patient referral, the HIV-infected person is encouraged to inform partners of their risk for infection, so that partners can seek appropriate medical services. Provider referral (previously called CONTACT TRACING) is a voluntary, confidential process in which health professionals obtain partner names and identifying information from an infected person, then notify the partners and help them to seek or obtain appropriate services. Partner notification has been considered an essential component of sexually transmitted disease control programs in North America and Europe for more than 40 years.

With no curative therapy for HIV infection, partner notification for HIV control has been controversial. Concerns about the potential for discrimination against patients and identified partners have to be weighed against the rights of exposed individuals to be informed of their risk. Although the development of antiviral treatment and prophylactic antimicrobials has provided clear benefits for the early detection and treatment of HIV infection, thereby reducing opposition to partner outreach, many countries lack the resources to provide these costly therapies and long-term care. The debate worldwide has continued to center on the role partner notification should play in HIV prevention programs relative to other preventive interventions.

The ability of any country to develop a formal HIV partner notification program is influenced by a number of factors, including the organization and strength of services for STD diagnosis and treatment, the epidemiology of HIV infection in that country, the attitude of HEALTH CARE PROFESSIONALS who must carry out partner notification in conjunction with other health care services, and the government structure for setting health policy. In many countries only a small proportion of STD cases—and presumably HIV cases—are seen in STD or other health clinics. Treatment services are often fragmented and delivered by a variety of health care providers with limited skills in provider referral. Clinicians responsible for STD treatment and partner management, in general, have had little support from organized HIV prevention programs and receive no special training for carrying out complex partner notification activities. See PRIVACY.

passive hyperimmune therapy (pht) An experimental treatment for HIV infection that involves monthly infusions of p24 antibody-rich plasma (hyperimmune plasma) from asymptomatic healthy HIV-positive donors to patients with advanced HIV disease.

passive immunity Protection against infection achieved in a nonimmune host by introduction of preformed ANTIBODY or immune cells from another person. Passive immunity usually lasts only a short time.

passive immunotherapy (PIT) Passive immunotherapy for HIV involves the transfer of plasma (the fluid portion of the blood without the cells) from asymptomatic HIV-infected donors with high HIV ANTIBODY levels to individuals with advanced HIV infection or AIDS and low levels of HIV antibodies. The hope is that the HIV antibodies in the transferred plasma will help preserve the recipient's health. PIT's originator and chief promoter, Abraham Karpas, Sc.D., an AIDS researcher at the University of Cambridge in England, published his first paper on PIT in 1988. Challenges facing PIT researchers have included the lack of a well-funded backer, the high cost of the technique, and the difficulty of finding enough eligible plasma donors.

Pasteurella multocida A small nonmotile GRAM-NEGATIVE coccobacillus that can cause cellulitis, abscesses, osteomyelitis, pneumonia, peritonitis, or meningitis.

patent The exclusive right granted to an inventor to manufacture or sell an invention for a specified number of years; also an invention or process protected by this right. Patent reform activists have become particularly vocal in recent years in response to the fact that, increasingly, HIV/AIDS patients are squeezed by soaring drug prices—a phenomenon that is also driving Medicaid woes. Many patent reform advocates see excessive terms of market exclusivity as the culprit. Some have called for cutting back patent protection from 20 years to as little as three years before lower-cost generic drugs are allowed to compete. The strength of patent rights may also be conditional on the source of drugs that are subsequently developed by industry and then sold back to government programs at monopoly prices. In effect, taxpayers are paying twice for these medications. Many patent reform advocates are pressing the administration to apply an existing law that could compel drug companies with products derived from federally funded research to sell them at reasonable prices. This legislation, part of the Bayh-Dole Act, was passed in 1980, but its provisions have never been exercised. Other efforts to lower drug prices in the United States today span the gamut of a national discount card for seniors to state government initiatives to hold down costs. See DRUG PATENTS AND PRICING.

pathogen A disease-causing MICROORGANISM. There are four types of pathogens: bacteria, fungi, protozoa, and viruses.

pathogenesis The development of morbid conditions or disease; more specifically, the cellular events and reactions and other biological processes occurring in the development of disease.

pathogenic Productive of disease. See PATHO-GENESIS.

pathological Diseased, or due to a disease; concerning pathology.

pathology A condition produced by disease; also, the study of the nature and cause of disease.

pathophysiology The study of how normal physiological processes are altered by disease.

patient One who receives HEALTH CARE services from a health care practitioner and who gives consent for the practitioner to provide that care.

patient advocate A person in an institutional setting responsible for meeting the personal and social needs of patients, with a special concern for high quality patient care, and for responding to patient inquiries and concerns about the care given by a practitioner or by a hospital or other health care facility. The patient advocate speaks and acts on behalf of patients, investigates the patients' problems and complaints, and mediates between the patients and the hospital or other health care facility. The patient advocate is also called a PATIENT REPRESENTATIVE or *ombudsperson*.

patient close-out The process of separating patients from a clinical trial at the end of treatment and follow-up.

patient close-out stage The stage of a trial in which patients leave a trial: the end of treatment and follow-up.

patient pay See SPEND DOWN.

patient recruitment The process of identifying suitable patients for enrollment in a clinical trial.

patient recruitment goal The number of patients scheduled to be enrolled in a trial. Usually it is set before the trial starts, or shortly thereafter, via a sample size calculation or via practical considerations.

patient referral See PARTNER NOTIFICATION.

patient representative See PATIENT ADVOCATE.

Patients' Bill of Rights   A HEALTH CARE provider or facility–adopted document that defines the rights of patients or clients. The American Hospital Association House of Delegates approved a document entitled, "Statement of a Patients' Bill of Rights" in 1973. The statement has become a standard for advocacy on behalf of patients' and families' rights. Many hospitals make the Patients' Bill of Rights available to patients through a patient information booklet.

Patients have rights that all medical care organizations and HEALTH CARE providers should honor as a matter of routine. In times of critical medical emergencies, it becomes even more important to ensure patients' rights: to ask questions and to have them answered completely; to have all medical procedures explained completely; to refuse any test, procedure, or medication; to go to another health care provider or get a second opinion; and to be assured of the confidentiality of their medical records and especially their HIV test results.

PBMC   See PERIPHERAL BLOOD MONONUCLEAR CELL.

PCA   Self-administration of analgesics by a patient instructed in doing so; usually refers to self-dosing with an intravenous opioid (e.g., morphine) administered by means of a programmable pump.

PCM-4   PCM-4 is a product combining two components purported to have immunomodulating effects. The two components are an extract (the polypeptide, or *P*) from the porcine spleen and a highly concentrated form of Siberian ginseng. The oral dosage of these two extracts was developed in 1987. The pill was developed after initial studies done with Siberian ginseng suggested that the combination might be capable of increasing T CELLS. Studies have shown that patients with cancer of the stomach who experienced immune suppression had general improvement with the use of the porcine spleen extract. To date, there are reports of some studies in HIV-infected people being conducted, but these studies are either incomplete or have not been published.

PCM-4 is available at health food stores in drops, tablets, and capsules. No toxicities from PCM-4 have been reported, but it is suggested that the compound not be used by those with high blood pressure.

PCOD   The proximate cause of death, one of two separate designations for the cause of death distinguished by AUTOPSY pathologists. See ICOD.

PCP   See *PNEUMOCYSTIS CARINII* PNEUMONIA.

PCP prophylaxis   See *PNEUMOCYSTIS CARINII* PNEUMONIA PROPHYLAXIS.

PCR test   See POLYMERASE CHAIN REACTION TEST.

peak level   The highest concentration of a drug in blood plasma, which occurs soon after it is administered. Sometimes abbreviated as CMAX. Peak levels that are too high cause excess side effects without necessarily enhancing the antimicrobial effects of the drug. See TROUGH LEVEL.

pediatric   Concerning the treatment of children.

pediatric HIV/AIDS   Pediatric AIDS refers to infants and young children who became infected through perinatal transmission or to HIV-infected school-age children, the majority of whom contracted HIV through blood transfusions (mostly hemophiliacs). Global estimates of children living with HIV infection have increased in recent years, with sub-Saharan Africa and South and Southeast Asia having the greatest number of HIV-infected children. Global estimates of AIDS deaths in children have also increased, with the greatest number of children's deaths occurring in sub-Saharan Africa and in South and Southeast Asia. It is estimated that for each pediatric AIDS case reported, there are three to four other HIV-infected children who have not been reported. Studies show children of color account for a higher percentage of pediatric AIDS cases than their Caucasian counterparts. Note, too, the existence of so-called AIDS ORPHANS. This phenomenon presents an illustration of the far-reaching effects of the HIV and AIDS epidemic. The numbers of orphaned children due to HIV infection and AIDS have stressed families, social systems, and governments, particularly in Africa.

The CENTERS FOR DISEASE CONTROL AND PREVENTION uses four categories of increasing disease severity for classifying children with HIV disease. The category in which a child is placed depends on the degree of immune suppression and the kinds of complications and infections the child has developed. Asymptomatic children (CDC Category 'N') show no signs or symptoms of HIV infection or show only one of the conditions for category 'A.' Mildly symptomatic (CDC Category 'A') children have two or more symptoms, such as swollen lymph nodes, enlarged liver or spleen, dermatitis, or recurrent or persistent respiratory tract infections, sinus infections, or middle-ear infections. Moderately symptomatic (CDC Category 'B') children develop conditions considered to be of intermediate severity. These include oral CANDIDIASIS that persists for more than two months, bacterial meningitis, pneumonia, recurrent or chronic diarrhea, and LYMPHOID INTERSTITIAL PNEUMONITIS. Finally, severely symptomatic (CDC Category 'C') children have OPPORTUNISTIC INFECTIONS, cancers, or other conditions characteristic of advanced disease. These include serious bacterial infections such as SEPTICEMIA or pneumonia (two or more in a two-year period), PCP, bone or joint infections, abscesses of an internal organ or body cavity, ENCEPHALOPATHY, crypotcoccal disease, CRYPTOSPORIDIOSIS, esophageal or pulmonary candidiasis, TUBERCULOSIS, or LYMPHOMA.

Pediatric clinical signs and symptoms as well as disease progression are different in children than in adults. For children who become HIV-infected during gestation, clinical symptoms usually develop within six months after birth. Few children infected as fetuses live beyond two years, and survival beyond three years used to be rare. With the use of anti-HIV drugs and therapy for opportunistic diseases, some children born with HIV are still alive at five, 10, and 15 years of age.

The clinical course of rapid HIV disease progression in infants diagnosed with AIDS is marked by failure to thrive, persistent lymphadenopathy, chronic or recurrent oral candidiasis, persistent diarrhea, enlarged liver and spleen, and chronic pneumonia. Bacterial infections are common and can be life-threatening. An excess of gamma globulin and depressed cell-mediated immunity and T cell infection are frequently encountered. See CHILDREN; PREGNANCY; TRANSMISSION; and WOMEN.

peer review organization (PRO) A nonprofit organization, usually an arm of a state medical society, which reviews appropriateness of care and length of stay under MEDICAID and MEDICARE.

pegylated alfa interferon A modified form of the drug alfa interferon that allows for less frequent dosing. It is currently in studies for the treatment of hepatitis C. (Trade names are Pegasys and PEG Intron.) See PEGYLATION.

pegylated interferon Interferon that is attached to polyethylene glycol (PEG). Pegylation allows the interferon to last longer, thereby requiring less frequent administration. See PEGYLATION.

pegylation Advances in the treatment for hepatitis C include new drugs that have been developed by using pegylation. This means that a moiety of polyethilene glycol (PEG) is added to the molecules of interferon alpha.

PEG is a neutral, water-soluble, nontoxic polymer. When PEG is dissolved in water it becomes heavily hydrated; all of the molecules soak up the water (meaning the water molecules are bound to them). When this happens, the PEG begins to move quite rapidly. As the PEG moves swiftly around the body, it sweeps out a large area, known as its exclusion volume. As the PEG sweeps out its exclusion volume, it stops other molecules from approaching.

The body is not really aware of what's going on; PEG is very difficult for the biological system to detect. If anything, the cells in the body perceive the PEG as bound water molecules that are moving quickly through the system. In fact, PEG itself is actually nonimmunogenic—it does not provoke a response from the immune system. If the immune system does not know it is there, it does not send messages through the body or send an army of cells out to fight it. If it were a virus, the immune system would kick into action to try and get rid of it.

The PEG itself is not a treatment. It does not kill off the hepatitis C virus, and on its own it does not do anything significant at all to the body.

Nowadays the treatment of hepatitis C predominantly involves two drugs: ribavirin, which is a tablet or capsule, and interferon. Using a combination of interferon and ribavirin to treat the virus has already been shown to be more beneficial than using just one or the other alone (monotherapy). However, there have been problems with interferon. It is a subcutaneous injection (into the skin)—usually self-administered. Basically, the person with hepatitis C has to inject himself or herself (usually in the stomach or thighs) every other day. The reason for the frequent injections is that interferon actually clears from the body rather quickly. Interferon has a very short half-life—approximately six hours—and it spreads rapidly around the body and is very quickly cleared by the kidneys. There were two options—more frequent injections to ensure a high level of interferon in the body at all times or a way to make it last longer and at a sustained level. The latter is basically what pegylation achieves.

A typical treatment regimen for hepatitis C is now pegylated interferon with ribavirin. Pegylating the interferon is a bit like putting a protective coating on it, making the drug last far longer in the body and at a much steadier level, rather than in the peaks and troughs that were resulting from nonpegylated interferon. The pegylation results in a sustained absorption, altered distribution, and delayed clearance. Pegylated interferon only needs to be injected once a week, for many patients a welcome improvement on the three times a week initially required for nonpegylated (or standard) interferon.

PEG can be linear or branched. Linear pegylation is a single-strand molecular structure; branched pegylation has more than one strand branching off in various directions. PEG can be attached to the base substance (interferon alpha, for example) by different types of protein linkages. These links or bonds may alter the stability of the PEG protein and may also affect its activity. The larger or branched PEGs lead to a longer, sustained absorption period. They also have a reduced clearance by the kidney. (Clearance is measured as liters or volume per hour per kilogram of body weight.) These larger/branched PEGs are removed from the underlying interferon in the liver, whereas smaller and linear PEGs have a less sustained and shorter absorption period. Branched PEGs have greater clearance by the kidney and are removed from the underlying interferon in the kidney, not the liver. Research has shown that

there is a trade-off between increased PEG size and reduced specific activity.

Overall, PEG attachment to interferon alpha leads to longer half-life of the interferon. This results from decreased clearance by the kidney and reduced proteolysis (slower breakdown of protein). In addition, PEG attachment to interferon leads to lowered antigenicity of interferon: this means less probability that the immune system will make antibodies against the interferon, as can occur among those who use non-pegylated interferon alpha. PEG attachment also leads to increased chemical and thermal (heat) stability of the "base" substance interferon.

The best described drug is the PEG interferon alpha 2-a (Pegasys), in development by Hoffmman La-Roche. Initial data about Pegasys indicate about 40 percent sustained response six months after drug is stopped. The data on PEG in combination with ribavirin (RBV) are pending but suggest cure rate above 50 percent. The side effects of PEG are similar to the ones during monotherapy but less severe. The drug is much better tolerated and dropout rate is lower.

peliosis hepatis The presence of blood-filled lakes in the body of the liver. The condition may be associated with use of ORAL CONTRACEPTIVES or ANABOLIC STEROIDS. It has also been reported in patients with HUMAN IMMUNODEFICIENCY VIRUS infection.

pelvic examination Physical examination of the VAGINA and adjacent organs by palpation. One hand is placed intravaginally and the other on the abdominal wall, and tissues between the fingers of the two hands are palpated. This is called a bimanual examination. Visual examination of the vagina and CERVIX is made with the use of a speculum inserted intravaginally.

pelvic infection Any infection involving any of the pelvic structures (endometrium, ovaries, tubes) or extending beyond the peritoneum, as in the perihepatitis known as FITZ-HUGH-CURTIS SYNDROME. There may be an acute initial episode following infection by a sexually transmitted pathogen, most commonly GONORRHEA or CHLAMYDIA, less frequently a MYCOPLASMA. Later it may become a chronic and recurrent syndrome. When sexually transmitted PATHOGENS ascend from the vagina into the upper pelvic organs, the resulting infection is generally polymicrobial in nature. At this point, cervical and vaginal cultures are not useful in determining therapy. Often the outcome of a pelvic infection, or PELVIC INFLAMMATORY DISEASE, is recurrent infections, tubal infertility, formation of tubo-ovarian abscesses, and chronic pelvic pain syndrome.

pelvic inflammatory disease (PID)   Any serious inflammatory disorder of the upper genital tract in women. PID is difficult to diagnose and has not received much attention in the United States. PID takes different courses in different women, but can cause abscesses and constant, severe pain almost anywhere in the genital tract. PID may include endometritis, salpingitis, tubo-ovarian abscess, and pelvic peritonitis. Sexually transmitted organisms may also cause PID. Clinically, physicians report that PID seems to occur more frequently in HIV-infected women than in those who are HIV-negative, and is often more severe, requiring longer hospitalizations and more frequent surgery for treatment of abscesses.

A woman's pelvic region, including the cervix, uterus, fallopian tubes, abdominal cavity, and ovaries, may be infected by a SEXUALLY TRANSMITTED DISEASE such as GONORRHEA. The infection may spread more rapidly if an INTRAUTERINE DEVICE (IUD) is used. The condition may lead to infertility and cause such symptoms as low abdominal pain, pelvic tenderness upon palpation, cervical manipulation tenderness, adnexal tenderness or suspicion of pelvic mass, nausea, fever, and irregular menstrual cycles. These are usually accompanied by temperature above 100.5°F, elevated white blood count, elevated erythrocyte sedimentation rate, positive gram stain, wet mount loaded with white blood cells, mucopurulent cervicitis, positive culture for gonorrhea or CHLAMYDIA or pelvic mass. In persons who are immunocompromised due to HIV infection, bacterial infections are often recurrent, chronic, and extensive. In these cases PID may fail to yield the usual signs. Failure to mount an immune response may cause the inflammation and pain by which a diagnosis may be made.

PID diagnosis can most easily be made by examining the abdomen with a laparoscope. Because there exists no suitable diagnostic test and LAPAROSCOPY is not always available, a diagnosis of PID is often based on imprecise clinical findings and culture or ANTIGEN detection tests of specimens of the lower genital tract. Detection of PID in HIV-infected women may be extremely difficult. In some, particularly those infected with HIV, there may be resistance to therapy. Pelvic inflammatory disease is one of the gynecological problems Social Security Disability Determination Service specialists consider when assessing the degree to which disease affects a woman's ability to function.

Consideration is usually given to hospitalization of HIV-positive women with clinical evidence of PID. Some considerations that favor immediate hospitalization are suspicion of tubo-ovarian abscesses, suspicion of ectopic pregnancy, upper peritoneal signs, uncertain diagnosis with signs of acute abdomen, inability to tolerate or comply with outpatient regimen, and failure to improve within 48 hours on oral antibiotics and bed rest.

The outpatient regimen for oral antibiotics in PID recommended by the CENTERS FOR DISEASE CONTROL AND PREVENTION is the same as in the treatment for CHLAMYDIA. Bed rest and abstention from sexual activity are also part of the standard treatment regimen. Failure to improve in 48 to 72 hours is an indication for immediate hospitalization and for IV antibiotics. Many experts recommend that all patients with PID be treated with PARENTERAL ANTIBIOTICS.

Since most PID is caused by sexually transmitted diseases that are not detected, it is important for all women to have regular gynecological exams and PAP SMEARS. HIV-positive women should get Pap smears every six months.

pelvic mass   Routine pelvic examination will occasionally find a pelvic mass with or without significant symptomatology. Further examination is necessary to identify it; possibilities include an ovarian cyst, PELVIC INFLAMMATORY DISEASE, a tubo-ovarian abscess, fibroid tumor, normal or ECTOPIC PREGNANCY, malignant tumor, genital tuberculosis, and lymphoma.

The initial workup is intended to rule out pregnancy. A thorough history and careful pelvic exam will help to focus the remainder of the workup in the appropriate direction. It is logical to obtain a pelvic sonogram, if it can be done promptly. A diagnosis must be definitive and may require exploratory surgery.

penicillin   One of a group of antibiotics biosynthesized by several species of molds. Penicillin is antibacterial, inhibiting the growth of most GRAM-POSITIVE BACTERIA and certain GRAM-NEGATIVE forms. It is also effective against certain molds, spirochetes, and rickettsiae. It is also used to treat SYPHILIS. There are many different penicillins, including synthetic ones, and their effectiveness varies for different organisms.

Penicillin was one of the first antibiotics to be discovered and used. It interferes with a bacterium's ability to build cell walls, thus preventing it from multiplying. Penicillin is available in tablet form and solutions for oral and INTRAVENOUS administration. The most common reactions to penicillin include nausea, vomiting, stomach upset, diarrhea, and black, hairy tongue. Allergic skin reactions and anaphylactic shock occur less frequently. (Trade names include Bicillin, Wycillin, Ledercillin, Pen-Vee, and Veetids.)

Penicillium   A genus of molds belonging to the class Ascomycetes. These are the blue molds that grow on fruit, bread, and cheese. A number of species are sources of penicillin. Occasionally in humans they produce infections of the external ear, skin, or respiratory passageways. They are common allergens.

penis   A male's external sex organ. It contains the urethra, the tube through which urine and semen flow. Slang terms include cock, dick, joint, joy stick, prick, and rod.

peno-vaginal intercourse   Sexual activity with the penis inside the vagina; COITUS.

pension   A generic term for any public or employer retirement or disability income benefit.

pentafuside   See T-20.

pentamidine   An antiprotozoal agent; used to treat or prevent PNEUMOCYSTIS CARINII PNEUMONIA

(PCP). It can be administered INTRAVENOUSLY or delivered directly into the lungs as an aerosol, using a breathing machine. Common side effects of intravenous pentamidine are low blood pressure, low blood sugar, high blood sugar, kidney failure, liver disease, low blood counts, or inflammation of the pancreas. Because it doesn't go directly into the bloodstream, aerosol, or nebulized, pentamidine rarely causes severe side effects (the most frequent are coughing and tightening of the chest that interferes with breathing). Fatigue, metallic taste in the mouth, decreased appetite, dizziness, rashes, nausea, irritation of mouth or nasal cavities, congestion, night sweats, chills, and vomiting also occur. It does not, however, affect PCP in parts of the body other than the lungs, so intravenous treatment is usually preferred for advanced PCP infections. Generally it is felt that pentamidine should be dispensed with caution if given with other drugs that can damage the kidneys. In addition, other substances that cause pancreatic damage, such as alcohol, ddI, and RIFAMPIN, may be dangerous if taken concurrently with pentamidine. (Trade names include NebuPent, Pentam, and Pentacarinat.)

pentoxifylline   A blood flow agent, xanthine, that reduces levels of TUMOR NECROSIS FACTOR (TNF). Pentoxifylline is a FOOD AND DRUG ADMINISTRATION–approved treatment for a circulation disorder called intermittent claudication, caused by a narrowing of the arteries. For this condition it is essentially used to thin the blood. Pentoxifylline has had variable results in AIDS patients in attempting to halt weight loss which may be caused by tumor necrosis factor. The drug once was thought to hold promise for HIV-infected people but trial data have shown otherwise. Possible side effects include nausea and other digestive upset, dizziness, and headache (Brand name is Trental.)

people living with AIDS (PLWA)   At the October 1987 March on Washington for Lesbian and Gay Rights, persons with AIDS from all over the United States took the naming of their condition one step further, announcing that they are "people living with AIDS." As with "PEOPLE WITH AIDS," the insistence here upon naming as a key to identity, though partially aimed at the press, the public, the government, and the medical profession, is primarily an act of self-acclaim.

People With AIDS The People With AIDS movement started from support and counseling networks and has had a complex and often turbulent relationship with the mainstream AIDS organizations. In the early 1980s, new political perspectives developed; people with the AIDS virus began to acknowledge that they could use insights gained from their personal struggles with AIDS to contribute to the larger political battle against the disease. Groups exclusively containing people infected with the virus, developed in New York, San Francisco, and other cities. At the 1983 AIDS Forum in Denver, some of these groups consolidated under the name People With AIDS (a name attributed to Mark Feldman) and together claimed the right to be included in the leadership of all AIDS organizations. The following year, an attempt was made to establish a national association of people with AIDS with its own hot line and newsletter, the latter of which began appearing in June 1985.

"People" With AIDS remind us that they are more than "victims" or "patients" with AIDS. Primarily as an act of self-acclaim, the naming demonstrates how they should be viewed by others:

> We do not see ourselves as victims. We will not be victimized. We have the right to be treated with respect, dignity, compassion, and understanding. We have the right to live fulfilling, productive lives—to live and die with dignity and compassion . . . We are born of and inextricably bound to the historical struggle for rights—civil, feminist, disability, lesbian and gay, and human. We will not be denied our rights!
>
> (National Association of People with AIDS, "Statement of Purpose," September 1986)

In several cities People With AIDS has been a key organization in the AIDS movement and has been involved in supportive, educational and lobbying work. Since 1983, members of People With AIDS have been prominent figures in Gay Pride marches across the country, often including many members who march with great physical and emotional pain and difficulty. The expertise of those who have experienced the disease offers a new perspective to our understanding of AIDS not usually discussed by academic science and medicine.

Today, People With AIDS furnishes a broad variety of support services to the rising numbers of AIDS sufferers, and continues to campaign for the acceleration of availability of experimental drug therapies.

People With AIDS Coalition (PWA) Founded in 1985, this New York City–based nonmembership organization provides local support networks for persons afflicted with AIDS. Programs include: public forums, a drop-in lounge, liaisons with social service agencies, a meal program, and an apartment referral service. PWA also operates a speakers' bureau and maintains a library.

PEP See POSTEXPOSURE PROPHYLAXIS.

peptide One of a class of amino acids compounds. Because some peptides function as the active portions of many HORMONES, growth factors, and neurotransmitters, they play important roles in digestion, immunity, and emotion. These peptide components interact with key cells in the responsive organs by means of receptor molecules located on the cells' surfaces.

peptide T A synthetic amino acid compound created in 1986 at the National Institute of Mental Health (NIMH). It was one of the first drugs to be designed specifically as an AIDS therapy. The drug's developers suggest that peptide T can slow or reverse the neurological and cognitive effects of HIV, including HIV ENCEPHALOPATHY, fatigue, and pain, although an NIMH study shows no such benefit.

Peptide T is designed to mimic the attachment sequence in GP120, the protein on the outer surface of the HIV virus, to CD4 receptor sites, taking its place and preventing HIV from interfering with brain function. However, the process leading to HIV-associated nerve tissue damage is extremely varied from one individual to another. The inflammatory process that arises in response to the presence of HIV in the brain can disrupt the operation of neurons and their support cells, which form a complex and delicate interactive network. Another important factor is the opening up of the calcium channels on neuron membranes; too much calcium can poison cells. In addition, other HIV proteins, besides gp120, seem to be toxic to cells in neural tissue. Moreover, many researchers suspect that when gp120 links up with the CD4 sites on the immune system's T-HELPER CELLS it leads to a cascade of events fatal to these cells.

Peptide T has been found to reduce levels of TUMOR NECROSIS FACTOR-alpha (TNF-α). Release of this CYTOKINE has been associated with HIV disease progression. Excess TNF-α is widely alleged to contribute to WASTING syndrome, increased replication of HIV, immune cell dysfunction, nerve cell damage, and death. Peptide T is very similar to the active section of vasoactive intestinal peptide (VIP), a naturally occurring regulator of digestion that may have growth-promoting functions in the CENTRAL NERVOUS SYSTEM. VIP seems to interact with the CD4 immune system cells, too, leading some researchers to suggest that peptide T can supplement VIP in promoting general mental and physical health.

Despite the lack of clinical evidence for action against the neurological and cognitive damage caused by HIV/AIDS, peptide T is one of the top sellers of the AIDS underground. Its status is fueled by widespread anecdotal accounts of increases in quality-of-life variables and relief from HIV ENCEPHALOPATHY, cognitive impairment, and the pain of PERIPHERAL NEUROPATHY.

Reported side effects of peptide T have been relatively minor. Potentially troubling side effects include hormonal and emotional changes.

percutaneous   Through the skin. The term refers to the application of a medicated ointment by friction, or the removal or injection of a fluid by needle.

pericarditis   Inflammation of the pericardium.

pericardium   The double membraned fibroserous sac enclosing the heart and the origins of the great blood vessels. It is composed of an inner serous layer and an outer fibrous layer. The space between the two constitute the pericardial cavity, which is normally filled with a small amount of serous fluid.

perinatal   Near the time of birth, and specifically the period beginning after the 28th week of pregnancy through the 28 days following birth.

perinatal transmission   See TRANSMISSION.

perineum   The area between the anus and the scrotum (in men) or the vulva (in women).

period   See MENSTRUATION.

periodontal disease   Disease of supporting structures of the teeth, the periodontium, including the alveolar bone to which the teeth are anchored. The most common symptom is bleeding gums, but loosening of the teeth, receding gums and teeth, and necrotizing ulcerative gingivitis may be present as the process continues. Proper dental hygiene will help to prevent periodontal disease.

In the early stages of the disease, curettage of the irritating material from the crown and root surfaces of the teeth may be the only treatment required. In more advanced stages, procedures such as gingivectomy, gingivoplasty, and correction of the bony architecture of the teeth may be required. Adjustment of the occlusion of the teeth and orthodontic treatment may be used in order to prevent recurrences.

peripheral blood mononuclear cell (PBMC)   Circulating white blood cell with one round nucleus (e.g., lymphocytes and monocytes). Usually, the majority of circulating PBMCs are lymphocytes. See MONONUCLEAR CELL.

peripheral lymphoid organs   Those lymphoid organs not essential to the development of immune responses, such as the SPLEEN, LYMPH NODES, tonsils, and PEYER'S PATCHES.

peripheral nervous system   That portion of the nervous system outside the CENTRAL NERVOUS SYSTEM. Included are the 12 pairs of cranial nerves, 31 pairs of spinal nerves, and their branches to the entire body. Also included are the sensory nerves, the sympathetic and the parasympathetic nerves.

peripheral neuropathy Any functional disturbance and/or change in the PERIPHERAL NERVOUS SYSTEM, characterized by sensory loss, pain, muscle weakness, and wasting of muscle in the hands, legs, or feet. It may start with burning or tingling sensation or numbness in the toes and fingers. In severe cases, paralysis may result. Peripheral neuropathy may arise from an HIV-related condition or as a side effect of certain drugs, some of the NUCLEOSIDE ANALOGS in particular. Two types of peripheral neuropathy are most common to HIV infection: inflammatory demyelinating polyneuropathy (IDP), which arises in the early stages of infection, and sensory axonal polyneuropathy, a late-stage complication.

IDP morbidity stems from the progressive breakdown of the fatty envelope around the neurons—the myelin sheet—which impairs conduction of signals to and from the brain. In most cases, this complication appears even before susceptibility to opportunistic PATHOGENS and is thought to be an autoimmune disease. Patients experience mild sensory problems, decreased clinical reflexes, and chronic progressive weakness, similar to Guillain-Barré syndrome in HIV-negative patients. Symptoms can be managed with CORTICOSTEROIDS.

The major symptom of sensory axonal polyneuropathy is painful tingling or burning sensations. AZT is ineffective in treating this; tricyclic antidepressants have been found useful, particularly low-dose AMITRIPTYLINE. Brief bursts of pain can be treated with the anticonvulsants phenytoin or carbamazepine. Topical capsaicin has also been tried. ACUPUNCTURE is now under evaluation, alone or in combination with amitriptyline.

peripherally inserted central catheter (PICC) line
A catheter inserted into an arm vein and used for periods of up to three months. This catheter does not need to be surgically implanted and can be inserted at home by a trained nurse.

peritoneal cavity A space between layers of the parietal and visceral peritoneum, containing a small amount of fluid. The fluid minimizes friction as the viscera move against each other or the wall of the abdominal cavity.

peritoneal dialysis Dialysis (passing solute through a membrane) in which the lining of the peritoneal cavity is used as the dialysis membrane. Dialyzing fluid introduced into the peritoneal cavity is allowed to remain there for one or two hours and is then removed. The procedure may be repeated as often as indicated. The use of strictly sterile instruments helps prevent the development of peritonitis. Three related types of dialysis are intermittent peritoneal dialysis (performed using automated equipment), continuous cyclic peritoneal (treatments are performed every night with fluid remaining in the cavity until the next night), and continuous ambulatory peritoneal dialysis (a type of maintenance dialysis that uses an implanted peritoneal catheter).

peritoneum The thin, strong lining of the abdomen. The serous membrane reflected over the viscera and lining the abdominal cavity.

peritonitis Inflammation of the peritoneum, the membrane lining the abdominal cavity and investing the viscera.

perleche A disorder marked by fissures and EPITHELIAL desquamation (shedding of the epidermis) of corners of the mouth, usually seen in children. It may be due to oral CANDIDIASIS or may be a symptom of dietary deficiency, especially of riboflavin.

perphenazine Used to treat acute and chronic psychotic disorders; may be used as a tranquilizer to help agitated and disruptive behavior in the absence of true psychosis; sometimes used to treat severe nausea and vomiting. By inhibiting dopamine, perphenazine acts to correct an imbalance of nerve impulse transmissions thought to be responsible for mental disorders. Perphenazine belongs to a class of psychoactive drugs called phenothiazines, which have potent effects on the CENTRAL NERVOUS SYSTEM and other organs. They can reduce blood pressure, stop seizures, control nausea and vomiting, and control the symptoms of psychosis. Perphenazine is available as tablets, oral concentrate, and solution for injection. It is also available in a number of combination products with the tricyclic antidepressant AMITRIPTYLINE.

Drowsiness, stuffy nose, dizziness, blurred vision, tremors, and constipation are common side effects. (Brand names are APO-Perphenazine, PMS-Perphenazine, Elavil Plus, Entrafon, Etrafen, Etrafon-A, Etrafon Forte, Phenazine, PMS-Levazine, PMS-Perphenazine, Triavil, and Trilafon.)

Persantine   See DIPYRIDAMOLE.

persistent generalized lymphadenopathy (PGL) A disorder of the LYMPH GLANDS. PGL is diagnosed when the lymph glands are swollen for at least a month at two different sites, not counting the groin area, and in the absence of any current illness or drug use known to cause such symptoms. PGL often occurs early in HIV infection and is generally of little consequence.

person living with AIDS (PLWA)   See PEOPLE LIVING WITH AIDS.

person with AIDS (PWA)   See PEOPLE WITH AIDS.

person with AIDS-related complex (PWARC) An individual exhibiting signs and symptoms indicative of the AIDS-RELATED COMPLEX (e.g., fever, PERSISTENT GENERALIZED LYMPHADENOPATHY, and weight loss accompanied by the presence of HUMAN IMMUNODEFICIENCY VIRUS antibodies). It is noted that AIDS-related complex was originally used in cases of HIV-infected individuals not diagnosed with AIDS but with compromised immune systems and decreased T-CELL counts. The term is now widely considered to be obsolete. Similarly, the term *person with AIDS–related complex* is also now widely considered to be obsolete. See AIDS-RELATED COMPLEX.

personal care service   Assistance with activities of daily living, such as dressing, walking, getting up and down, preparing food, eating, and taking medication.

personal needs allowance   The amount long-term hospital patients and nursing home and board care residents are permitted to retain for "spending money," with the balance of their incomes applied to the cost of care; the monthly and SSI benefit paid to institutionalized MEDICAID patients with no other income.

PET   See POSITRON EMISSION TOMOGRAPHY.

petting   Sexual activity including fondling, hugging, kissing, and mutual masturbation, but not COITUS.

Peyer's patches   Collections of lymphoid tissue in the submucosa (the layer of connective tissue below the mucosa) of the small intestine that contain LYMPHOCYTES, plasma cells' germinal centers, and T-cell-dependent areas.

PGL   See PERSISTENT GENERALIZED LYMPHADENOPATHY.

P-glycoprotein   A phosphorylated and glycosylated plasma membrane protein belonging to a family of plasma membrane proteins encoded by the multidrug resistant (MDR) gene(s) that are well conserved in nature. P-glycoprotein (P-gp) functions as a membrane-localized drug transport mechanism that has the ability to pump out all currently prescribed HIV PROTEASE INHIBITORS (PIs) from the intracellular cytoplasm. This effect may result in limited oral bioavailability of the PIs as well as decreased ability of the drugs to cross the blood–brain barrier (BBB), the blood–testis barrier (BTB), and the maternofetal barrier (MFB). MDR-encoded P-gp has also been implicated in the cytotoxicity process and the induction of immune responses during HIV infection. It also plays a role in oxidative and inflammatory processes and may be involved in lipid transport and metabolism.

pH   A formula for measuring acidity and alkalinity, expressed as a number on the pH scale. This measurement is a diagnostic tool used on vaginal discharges.

phagocyte   A cell in blood or tissue that binds to, engulfs, and destroys MICROORGANISMS, damaged cells, and foreign particles.

phagocytosis The process by which PHAGOCYTES engulf material and enclose it within a vacuole (phagosome) in the cytoplasm.

phallus The PENIS.

pharmaceutical industry The drug industry.

pharmacokinetic boosting The coadministration of a PROTEASE INHIBITOR (PI) in combination with a low dose of ritonavir to enhance or boost exposure to the PI. In recent years, pharmacokinetic (PK) boosting has begun to offer an exciting new dimension to the management of HIV infection. Drug boosting results in improved efficacy and reduced toxicity and allows more convenient dosing. Ritonavir boosts other PIs by affecting the CYP3A4 system by using a dual mechanism, which consists of increasing the peak of drug absorption and simultaneously delaying the half-life to allow longer exposures to the PIs. The goals for boosted PIs are better PK in terms of potency, durability, and resistance; decreased number of pills; decreased frequency of dosing; fewer food restrictions; and lower treatment costs. The key is to achieve drug boosting without affecting drug tolerability. The key determinants of durable antiviral effect are drug potency and adherence to treatment regimens. Therefore, the optimal goal is to develop simplified potent regimens. Indeed, once-daily regimens are recommended for patients who have a poor history of adherence, patients who are substance abusers, those who suffer from psychiatric illnesses, homeless individuals, as well as those patients who have hectic lifestyles.

pharmacokinetics The study of how drug levels change over time in the body.

pharmacology The branch of medical science that deals with the study of the action of drugs on living systems.

pharyngeal gonorrhea GONORRHEA in the throat.

phase I See CLINICAL TRIAL.

phase II See CLINICAL TRIAL.

phase III See CLINICAL TRIAL.

phase IV See CLINICAL TRIAL.

phenindamine An antihistamine used to temporarily relieve runny nose, sneezing, itching of the nose or throat, and itchy, watery eyes due to hay fever or other upper respiratory allergies. In people with HIV, the drug is also used to reduce certain drug-induced allergic side effects, including skin rashes, swelling, hives, and breathing difficulties. Drowsiness is the most common side effect; less often, dry mouth, nervousness, insomnia, and increased irritability or excitement may occur. Available over the counter in tablets. (Trade name is Nolahist.)

phenotype An organism's functional capabilities and outward appearance. It is the physical expression of the genotype. Also the trait or behavior that results from changes in genotype, for example, the ability of the virus to replicate in the presence of a drug, compared with a drug-sensitive control virus or wild-type nonmutant HIV. See GENOTYPE.

phenotypic assay A virus culture–drug test that measures some aspect of an organism's functions, for example, the amount of a certain drug needed to inhibit the growth of an HIV isolate in a test tube culture. If HIV has developed resistance to a certain drug, higher than normally administered amounts of that drug are necessary to inhibit viral activity. Resistance is characterized as high-level, intermediate-, or low-level. Note that interpretation is not standard and that the standard deviation is considerable on both this and genotypic assay resistance testing. Phenosense and Antivirogram are commercially available in the United States. Phenotype testing is very expensive; because of this and the time element (about two to five weeks for results), such testing is not readily available. Thus, patients rely on the cheaper and faster (one week) genotypic testing. Most third-party payers do not cover these tests. See GENOTYPIC ASSAY.

phone zap A technique used by AIDS activists and others to bring pressure on a corporation, organization, or government agency to take a certain action. It consists of a systematic mass campaign of telephone calls to the selected target over a period of time.

phosphorylate   To introduce the trivalent group =P=O into an organic compound; phosphorylase is any enzyme that in the presence of an inorganic phosphate catalyzes the conversion of glycogen into sugar phosphate. Within the context of HIV/AIDS, it is noted that factors other than viral cross-resistance, such as pharmacological mechanisms, may also be important considerations when planning a long-term strategy. For example, the nucleoside analogs are actually prodrugs that must be converted into their active, triphosperate form by cellular enzymes in the human body. In the late 1990s, research described problems with this process that limit AZT's clinical efficacy. Interest increased in the intracellular phosphorylation of AZT. Two key unknowns at the time were of particular interest: (1) whether not the rate of phosphorylation decreases after prolonged exposure to a particular drug over time and (2) whether prior use of one compound affects the subsequent ability of the cell to phosphorylate new drugs.

phosphorylation   The addition of a phosphate group (phosphorous plus four oxygen atoms) to an organic molecule.

photophoresis   A process by which a light-sensitive drug called psoralen is used to treat various autoimmune diseases. The drug is injected into the body; after an interval blood containing psoralen is removed from the body and exposed to ultraviolet light, thus activating the drug in white blood cells. Finally, the blood is returned to the body by reinfusion. The whole procedure is usually performed on two consecutive days at monthly intervals and takes about four hours per session. Photophoresis is an approved therapy for a skin cancer called cutaneous T-CELL LYMPHOMA. In the test tube, it has been shown to work to inhibit viruses that involve RNA and DNA including HIV.

photosensitivity   Heightened skin response to sunlight or ultraviolet light (rapid burning when exposed to the sun).

PHS   See PUBLIC HEALTH SERVICE.

physical dependence   See ADDICTION.

physical modalities   Therapeutic interventions that use physical methods, such as heat, cold, massage, or exercise, to relieve pain.

physician-assisted suicide   The question of whether physicians should be allowed actively to assist competent, terminally ill patients who wish to end their intolerable suffering is currently the subject of widespread debate. (This is a separate question from that of merely forgoing or withholding treatment, which is legal in some circumstances.) Although the activities of Dr. Jack Kevorkian have dominated public discussion, the issue is by no means limited to his highly controversial methods. Those who favor the practice argue that the obligation to relieve suffering and to respect patients' wishes for their own treatment makes it ethical. Those who oppose it feel that it is never right for a physician to cause or bring about a death. To date, none of Dr. Kevorkian's cases has involved an AIDS patient, but several studies have shown that AIDS patients kill themselves at a much higher rate than people with other serious diseases. See SUICIDE.

physiologic   Related to the functions of the body. When used in the phrase *physiologic age* it refers to an age assigned by general health, as opposed to calendar age.

physiological leukorrhea   A normal but persistent whitish vaginal discharge that is not a symptom of infection. Usually white or yellow mucous discharge from the cervical canal or the vagina. It may constantly be present but somewhat increased preceding and following menstruation, and during sexual excitement. Leukorrhea may be abnormal if it is increased in amount, has a change of color, is malodorous, or contains blood.

phytohemagglutinin   A plant chemical used to stimulate the multiplication (proliferation) of T lymphocytes in laboratory tests.

PI   See PRINCIPAL INVESTIGATOR.

PICC line See PERIPHERALLY INSERTED CENTRAL CATHETER (PICC) LINE.

PID See PELVIC INFLAMMATORY DISEASE.

piercing The practice of placing rings or bars through the body for adornment and/or sexual excitement. Since the needle(s) used for piercing do come into contact with blood, it is possible to become infected with HIV if the needle(s) was (were) previously used on an HIV-infected person and not properly cleaned or sterilized.

pill burden The number and size of pills required for a particular treatment.

pilot trial A feasibility study intended to gain preliminary information about efficacy, safety, or a particular research hypothesis. Pilot trials are used to work out the details of further clinical trials.

pinocytosis The process by which cells absorb or ingest nutrients and fluid. A hollowed-out portion of the cell membrane is filled with liquid, and the area closes to form a small sac or vacuole. The nutrient, now inside, is available for use in the cell's metabolism.

pioglitazone A drug used to lower blood triglyceride levels. See GLITAZONE.

piss Slang for URINE.

Pitresin See VASOPRESSIN.

PK boosting See PHARMACOKINETIC BOOSTING.

placebo A pharmacologically inactive substance designed to look like and taste like a new drug. It is often used in studies as a control with which to measure clinical responses to pharmacologically active substance. Also called "sugar pills."

placebo effect A positive or therapeutic benefit resulting from the administration of a placebo to someone who believes the treatment is real.

placebo-controlled study/trial See CLINICAL TRIAL.

placenta The blood-filled organ that connects the fetus by the umbilical cord to the uterine wall. It is the source of blood exchange between the mother and the developing fetus during pregnancy.

placenta barrier A membrane that encloses the embryo. It is a composite of several structures. At the center of the concave side is attached the umbilical cord through which the umbilical vessels pass to the fetus. Maternal blood enters the intervillous spaces of the placenta through spiral arteries, branches of the uterine arteries. It bathes the chorionic villi and flows peripherally to the marginal sinus, which leads to uterine veins. Food substances, oxygen, and antibodies pass into fetal blood of the villi. Metabolic waste products pass from fetal blood into the mother's blood. In general, there is no admixture of fetal and maternal blood.

While it is known that HIV may be transmitted from mother to fetus during pregnancy or from mother to child through childbirth or BREAST-FEEDING, at present it is unclear when the TRANSMISSION of HIV to the child occurs. The virus has been isolated from the placenta, the amniotic fluid, and the fetal tissue. Infection may occur prenatally, at delivery, or through breast-feeding. Present research suggests that mother-to-fetus transmission is most likely to occur during the birth process itself, generally through exposure to infected blood and mucus in the birth canal.

plague A word once used to describe any widespread contagious disease associated with a high death rate. Now it is also applied specifically to a highly fatal disease caused by *Yersinia pestis* infection. High fever, restlessness, staggering gait, mental confusion, prostration, delirium, shock, and coma are some of the symptoms. Plague exists in different forms: bubonic, with acutely inflamed lymph nodes; septicemic, with absence of such nodes; and primary pneumonic, characterized by pulmonary symptoms. The pneumonic form may spread from person to person. Treatment is with streptomycin, tetracyclines, and choramphenicol. The first suspected cases of plague occurred in the

11th century B.C. A plague from 1347 to 1352 killed 25 million people, estimated to have been one-third of Europe's population.

Other major recorded pandemics (global) and epidemics (regional) that have devastated large populations in history include measles, cholera, tuberculosis, malaria, scarlet fever, polio, typhus, influenza, smallpox, gonorrhea, yellow fever, and HIV/AIDS. The historical time line on first suspected cases of these diseases is as follows: measles, from 430 B.C.; cholera, 1781; tuberculosis, 451 B.C.; malaria, 1748; scarlet fever, 1735; polio, 1894; typhus, 1083; influenza, 1580; smallpox, 429 B.C.; gonorrhea, 1768; yellow fever, 1647; HIV/AIDS, United States, 1970s; Africa, 1959. Richard Holbrooke, the former U.S. ambassador to the United Nations, compares Africa's AIDS crisis to the Black Death or bubonic plague that annihilated a quarter of Europe in the 14th century.

plasma   The liquid part of the lymph and of the blood. In the blood, corpuscles (blood cells) and platelets are suspended in plasma. The plasma consists of serum, protein, and chemical substances in aqueous solution. The aqueous solution also contains solids and dissolved gases, among which are electrolytes; glucose; proteins, including enzymes and hormones; fats, bile pigments, and BILIRUBIN. Plasma serves as the medium for transporting these substances to the body's structures, as well as transporting waste products from them to sites of clearance, that is, the lungs, liver, kidneys, and spleen. Different constituents of plasma have specific functions within the blood. Normal plasma is thin and colorless when free from corpuscles and has a faint yellow tinge when seen in thick layers. See BLOOD.

plasma cell   A fully differentiated antibody-synthesizing cell that is derived from B lymphocytes.

plasma viremia   Presence of viruses in the plasma (the liquid part of the lymph and of the blood). Currently the most reliable virologic marker to monitor the effect of ANTIRETROVIRAL THERAPY, plasma viremia is a valid indicator of virus replication in the lymphoid organs. Its down regulation may reflect a systemic decrease in virus replication.

plasmacytosis   An excess of plasma cells in the blood.

plasmapheresis   Removing blood from the body and centrifuging it in order to separate the cellular elements from the plasma. The red cells then are suspended in a physiological solution. They may be reinjected into the donor or injected into a patient who requires red cells rather than whole blood. After blood is drawn, it is tested for ABO group (blood type) and Rh type (positive or negative), as well as for any unexpected red blood cell antibodies that may cause problems in the recipient. Screening tests are also performed for evidence of donor infection with hepatitis viruses B and C, HIV 1 and 2, human T-lymphotropic viruses (HTLV) I and II, and syphilis.

plasmid   A piece of genetic material that exists outside the chromosomes in the nucleus of a cell. Genetically engineered plasmids are often used in biotechnology.

Plasmodium   A genus of protozoa belonging to subphylum Sporozoa, class Telosporidia. This group includes causative agents of malaria in humans and lower animals.

Plasmodium falciparum   The organism that is the causative agent for malignant tertian malaria.

platelet   One of three cellular components of the blood that plays an important part in clotting. Platelets are also involved in immune response, especially in inflammation. Without platelets any wound could result in death by bleeding. The number of platelets is often low in people with HIV infection—sometimes so extremely low that the person is prone to bleeding. The cause of low platelets may be HIV infection itself, or the drugs used to treat it.

pluripotent stem cell   A hematopoietic cell in the bone marrow that is capable of differentiating into any type of blood cell.

PLWA   See PERSON LIVING WITH AIDS.

PML   See PROGRESSIVE MULTIFOCAL LEUKOEN-CEPHALOPATHY.

PMN (polymorphonuclear) cell See NEUTROPHIL.

PMPA See TENOFOVIR.

pneumocandin One of several experimental antifungal drugs currently being tested against fungal infections resistant to standard treatment, a growing problem for people with HIV.

pneumococcal vaccine A vaccine to immunize against the most common cause of bacterial pneumonia in HIV-negative people, the bacterium *Streptococcus pneumoniae* or pneumococcus. Pneumococcus is also a common cause of pneumonia in people with HIV infection. Pneumococcal vaccine is recommended for anyone who is especially prone to frequent or severe infection by pneumococcus. It is best for those with HIV to take this vaccine relatively early in the course of the disease when the immune system is strong.

pneumococcus An oval-shaped, encapsulated, non-sporeforming, GRAM-POSITIVE bacterium occurring usually in pairs having lancet-shaped ends. There are more than 80 serological types of pneumococci. In addition to causing pneumonia, pneumococci are found to cause infections such as bronchitis, conjunctivitis, keratitis, mastoiditis, meningitis, otitis media, and bloodstream infections. A pneumococcal vaccine is available. Pneumococcal infections are effectively treated with PENICILLIN or with erythromycin in a patient allergic to penicillin.

Pneumocystis carinii A protozoan (or possibly a fungus) that infects the lungs, causing fever, inflammation, and impaired gas exchange in immunocompromised people. Debate over the nomenclature of *P. carinii* has raged since the first description of the organism as a new entity was published in 1912 (Delanoë, P., and Delanoë, M. "Sur les rapports des kystes de Carinii du poumon des rats avec le *Trypanosoma lewisi*." *Comptes rendus de l'Académie des sciences* 1912, no. 155: 658–661). Currently receiving critical consideration is a proposal for a new name (*Pneumocystis jiroveci*, yee row vet zee) for *Pneumocystis* from humans. Note that as of this writing the change of *P. carinii* to *P. jiroveci* is far from final—the organism and infection are unchanged, and the name *P. carinii* continues to serve persons with HIV/AIDS, physicians, health care workers, and scientists well.

Pneumocystis carinii pneumonia (PCP) The most common OPPORTUNISTIC INFECTION in untreated HIV-infected patients in the United States. The onset of pneumocystis pneumonia is insidious with early, nonspecific symptoms of fever, fatigue, weight loss, diarrhea, and malaise. Cough, either nonproductive or productive of scant, thin, clear mucous is variable at the onset but becomes more prominent later in disease. Shortness of breath and dyspnea on exertion are suggestive of PCP. Other organs may be involved, and disseminated pneumocystis has been seen. Tachypnea, fever, cyanosis (in severe PCP), wheezes, crackles, or rales may be present in PCP. Generally, CD4 counts are <200 in patients with PCP. While not excluding PCP, counts >200 suggest other pathogens. It is important to obtain arterial blood gases in individuals with suspected PCP because the arterial blood gas is often markedly abnormal despite a seemingly comfortable patient. Sputum induction, gallium scan, and bronchoscopy are other means of diagnosis.

Current guidelines recommend that adults and adolescents with HIV infection receive chemoprophylaxis against PCP if they have a CD4 cell count below 200 cells/mm, unexplained fever for more than two weeks, or a history of oropharyngeal candidiasis. The treatment of choice for PCP prevention is TRIMETHOPRIM-SULFAMETHOXAZOLE (TMP/SMX) (Bactrim/Septra). It is the standard of care for prophylaxis because it is very effective (failing only in patients whose immune system is extremely compromised) and inexpensive. Several different dosing schedules have been found to be roughly equivalent for PCP prophylaxis. Many patients who are intolerant of sulfa drugs can be successfully desensitized by concurrent antihistamines, by gradual dose escalation, or by rechallenge. Patients who cannot be desensitized may be able to tolerate either dapsone or dapsone/pyrimethamine. Other second-line options include aerosolized pentamidine and atovaquone.

Dapsone or dapsone/pyrimethamine is generally the next choice for PCP prophylaxis for patients who are intolerant of TMP/SMX. Aerosolized pentamidine is recommended as primary or secondary prophylaxis when patients cannot tolerate TMP/SMX or dapsone.

Current guidelines consider discontinuing primary prophylaxis for patients who have sustained CD4 cell counts above 200 cells/mm longer than three to six months. Current guidelines do not recommend halting secondary PCP prophylaxis for patients who have a history of PCP who have had a successful immunological response to HAART. Recent studies suggest that it is possible to discontinue primary PCP prophylaxis when patients have had sustained CD4 cell counts above 200 cells/mm after initiating effective combination anti-HIV therapy.

TMP/SMX is the standard treatment for mild, moderate, or severe PCP. Second-line regimens include pentamidine, TMP/dapsone, clindamycin/primaquine, and trimetrexate with concurrent leucovorin. The usual duration of treatment for acute PCP is 21 days. Longer courses are sometimes necessary. Adjunctive corticosteroid therapy improves survival rate of patients with moderate or severe disease.

Note that bacterial resistance to TMP/SMX has increased among HIV-positive patients. Since SMX is responsible for most intolerance to the regimen, the better-tolerated dapsone is sometimes substituted. Intravenous pentamidine remains the most common alternate drug used to treat PCP in patients who have had adverse reactions or when therapy with TMP/SMX fails. Although pentamidine has been found to be an effective therapy for mild to severe PCP, it has been associated with higher mortality rates than TMP/SMX. A higher incidence of adverse reactions, including anemia, creatinine level elevations, liver function test result elevations, pancreatitis, hyper- or hypoglycemia, and hyponatremia, have been reported with pentamidine.

Clindamycin combined with primaquine appears to be an effective alternative to TMP/SMX for patients with mild to moderate PCP. Trimetrexate/leucovorin has also been shown to be an effective alternative to TMP/SMX or pentamidine for the treatment of PCP in some salvage situations. Atovaquone has been reported to be a slightly less effective but well-tolerated PCP treatment.

pneumonia An inflammation of the lungs usually associated with infection with a MICROORGANISM. The usual symptoms are cough, fever, and shortness of breath. Pneumonia can be caused by viruses, mycoplasmas, cocci, protozoa, bacilli, chlamydia, fungi, and rickettsiae, as well as by oil aspiration, radiation, chemicals, vegetable dusts, infections associated with silo-filler's disease, and chemical irritants. There are more than 50 potential causes.

pneumonitis Inflammation of the lung.

PNU-142721 An experimental NON-NUCLEOSIDE REVERSE TRANSCRIPTASE INHIBITOR (NNRTI) developed by Pharmacia and Upjohn that was dropped when that company decided to leave the AIDS/HIV marketplace. It had similar potency in research trials to the antiviral efavirenz but did not have the same resistance CODONS.

pol One of three genes in HIV responsible for the production of 10 structural proteins. The pol gene produces a POLYPROTEIN that is cleaved by the HIV protease to produce the enzyme REVERSE TRANSCRIPTASE, RNase H, INTEGRASE, and PROTEASE. See POLYPROTEIN.

polio vaccine There are two types of vaccine for the prevention of poliomyelitis, live and inactivated. Both immunize against the three types of polio virus. The live vaccine contains live, attenuated polio viruses and is suitable for both children and adults. It is administered orally. The inactivated vaccine contains inactive viruses and is also suitable for children and adults, although it is preferred for adults because of the slightly high risk of vaccine-associated paralysis. It is administered parenterally.

polycillin T See AMPILLICIN SODIUM.

polyclonal Derived from different cells. Pertaining to cells or cell products derived from several lines of clones.

polycythemic Characterized by high levels of red blood cells.

polymerase An enzyme that catalyzes polymerization of nucleosides to form DNA.

polymerase chain reaction (PCR) A synthetic process that permits making, IN VITRO, unlimited numbers of copies of genes. This is done beginning with a single molecule of genetic material, DNA. One hundred billion similar molecules can be generated within a few hours. The practical importance of this method of investigating genetic material is enormous. The technique can be used in investigating and diagnosing bacterial diseases, viruses associated with cancer, genetic diseases such as diabetes mellitus, pemphigus vulgaris, and various diseases of the muscles and the blood, such as SICKLE-CELL ANEMIA.

polymerase chain reaction test   An extremely sensitive blood test that detects the presence of HIV DNA or RNA in cells and tissue. (DNA and RNA are the gene particles that carry instructions for making more HIV.) The PCR test is able to detect the HIV virus whereas other tests may report false negatives. The test works by amplifying segments of genetic DNA or RNA of known composition with primers in sequential repeated steps. Unlike the standard blood test for HIV infection, which detects antibodies to HIV, the PCR detects HIV itself. The test is very accurate.

The great majority of people who take the standard antibody test for HIV infection need not take the PCR test, which is most useful when the results of the antibody test are ambiguous. It is also useful for early detection of perinatally infected infants. PCR is similar to a culture for HIV but is substantially less expensive.

polymerase technology   Molecular technology that permits the measurement of total body viral load, including activity in the LYMPH NODES and MUCOSA, and that has rendered blood measurements such as P24, NEOPTERIN, and CD4 cell counts increasingly useless. See POLYMERASE CHAIN REACTION TEST.

Polymox   See AMOXICILLIN.

polyneuropathy   Any disorder or affliction of the peripheral nerves. The term is usually restricted to disorders of a noninflammatory nature.

polyomavirus   A virus of the papovavirus family that produces malignancies in some animals, but not in humans.

polyprotein   A string of proteins linked together, polyproteins are produced by a single long messenger ribonucleic acid (mRNA). Later, polyproteins are cleaved by HIV's protease enzyme into the individual working proteins. A protease is an enzyme that cuts other proteins into smaller pieces. Because polyproteins must be processed to obtain working proteins, they are sometimes known as *pre-proteins*. Anti-HIV drugs known as PROTEASE INHIBITORS work by blocking the action of the viral protease enzyme. Three of HIV's genes—the GAG, POL, and ENV genes produce—polyproteins.

The gag polyprotein is produced by a long mRNA that leaves the nucleus unedited by mRNA splicing enzymes; i.e., no introns are eliminated from the mRNA. The mRNA leaves the nucleus and is read by ribosomes. There, the amino-acid chain is constructed with the help of transfer ribonucleic acids (tRNAs). The finished polyprotein contains four final proteins: the p17 matrix protein; the major capsid protein, p24; the nucleic acid-binding protein, p9; and the p7 protein, which is important for virion assembly.

HIV's pol gene carries information for three enzymes: protease, reverse transcriptase, and integrase. The mRNA produced by the pol gene sometimes also includes the information for these enzymes plus the matrix and capsid proteins. This long mRNA travels straight to the ribosome, again without any editing. There, an unusual polyprotein is produced. As a ribosome reads the mRNA, it stops at one point, jumps backward one base, then continues reading the mRNA. This is called frame shifting, which means that the ribosome has paused and shifted over one base and is now "reading" a different set of codons. As a result of frame shifting, the ribosome produces two polyproteins fused together—a gag/pol fusion protein. The fusion protein is also cleaved by the HIV protease. The fusion protein produces the matrix and capsid proteins from the gag gene plus the protease, reverse transcriptase, and integrase enzymes encoded by the pol gene.

The env gene also produces a polyprotein, the gp160 molecule. The gp160 is cleaved by a cellular protease enzyme to produce HIV's envelope proteins, the gp120 and gp41 GLYCOPROTEINS. The gp120 is the molecule in HIV that binds with host cells and begins the process of infection.

There are several possible advantages to HIV producing polyproteins: Because of gene overlapping, a maximum of genetic information is encoded in a minimum of genetic material. Polyproteins reduce the number of viral components that have to be synthesized and targeted to the cell membrane for self-assembly, and, because they are packaged in the form of a nonfunctional polyprotein, viral enzymes such as reverse transcriptase and protease are prevented from becoming active prematurely.

polyvalent vaccine   A vaccine that is produced from multiple viral strains or is made to induce immune responses from multiple viral strains.

poppers   See ISOBUTYL NITRITE INHALERS.

pornography   Writing or pictures that explicitly depict sexual activity, with the purpose of arousing the reader or viewer sexually.

porphyrin   Any of a group of nitrogen-containing organic compounds that occur in protoplasm and form the basis of animal and plant respiratory pigments, obtained from hemoglobin and chlorophyll.

porphyruria   A group of disorders that result from a disturbance in porphyrin metabolism, causing increased formation and excretion of PORPHYRIN or its precursors.

port   See CATHETER.

positive attitude   Attitudes measured or proceeding in a direction assumed as beneficial or progressive. People living with HIV disease frequently attest that the overall attitude a person with HIV takes toward his or her illness makes a difference. They challenge the notion of the person with AIDS as "helpless victim," and stress the importance of persons with AIDS being active participants in their health care.

Michael Callen's book, *Surviving AIDS* (1990), is infused with this attitude. The author presents the stories of 14 long-term survivors illustrating some of the methods and approaches by which some people are living with and indeed surviving AIDS. "Anything is possible. Miracles happen. It's as reasonable to believe that you'll be lucky as it is to believe you are doomed. The worst thing that might happen is

that you'll fail. But then again, you may live just long enough to be around for the cure that community-based research is going to find. Stick around for the celebration. It's gonna be some party." (*Surviving AIDS*, p. 201.) See POSITIVE THINKING.

positive thinking   Negativity and fear were rampant in the beginning of the AIDS epidemic. Today, the new facts about AIDS inspire optimism, not fear, and positive thinking has, for the most, supplanted negativity and fear. A disease once viewed as an automatic death warrant is now in the process of becoming a chronic, potentially long-term treatable illness. Today we know that not everyone who is exposed to HIV becomes infected. We know too that not everyone who is infected with HIV gets AIDS. And, we know that not everyone with AIDS dies from it. Components of positive thinking include having a positive attitude about survival, and feeling one is in charge of one's medical care and the medical knowledge surrounding that health care. Similar to positive attitude, positive thinking has been shown to have a direct immunological and physical effect. Several of the common denominators of long-term survivors of AIDS are examples of positive thinking in action—they gather information about the disease, they talk to people and tell them what is going on, they make a commitment to life and to others who will have AIDS, and they want to make a difference. See POSITIVE ATTITUDE.

positron emission tomography (PET)   A noninvasive technique for scanning the brain that utilizes radiolabeled substances such as glucose to measure some body functions. More recent applications of PET include demonstrations of brain response to hearing, vision, memory applications, and psychological stimuli.

"possibly safe" sex   Once it is recognized that the AIDS virus is transmitted through bodily fluids and that any exchange of these fluids during sex is unsafe, it is possible to consider various ways of reducing the risk. Even some otherwise "unsafe" sexual practices can be made safer. Each person has to decide for him or herself if the risk is worth taking. Still, it is useful to list and think about some of the "possibly safe" sexual practices individually.

The precautions listed below should be considered very seriously and applied conscientiously in order to achieve a reduction of risk. And, of course, the fewer sexual partners one has, the smaller the overall risk. The most important elements that can make otherwise "unsafe" sex somewhat less risky are condoms and certain spermicides and lubricants. Their use does not guarantee complete safety but, in general, condoms and spermicides can and will play an important role in reducing the risk of infection with the AIDS virus. The following practices remain only "possibly safe" or "possibly unsafe."

Condom use is considered only "possibly safe" and not absolutely safe, as they are often used incorrectly. To correctly use a condom, always use new condoms. Keep a ready supply of condoms where they cannot be damaged by moisture or heat. Never test a condom by blowing it up. Put a dab of lubricant into the tip of the condom to increase sensation. Prevent any air bubbles from forming that could cause the condom to break. Put the condom on the fully erect penis and roll it down all the way to the bottom of the shaft. Generally, lubricate the vaginal entrance or the anus before entry. Use only a water-soluble lubricant. Upon withdrawal, hold tightly onto the base of the condom. After use, throw the condom away. Use a lubricant that contains NONOXYNOL-9, a mild detergent that kills not only sperm cells but also all kinds of other organisms, such as amoebas, the HERPES VIRUS, bacteria that could cause gonorrhea and syphilis, as well as the AIDS virus.

Vaginal intercourse should be somewhat safe if the man uses a condom correctly and the woman uses a spermicide containing nonoxynol-9. This double precaution does reduce risk of infection and is strongly recommended whenever partners cannot be completely certain if either of them carries the virus.

Generally speaking, using a condom during anal intercourse does not offer the same level of protection as with vaginal intercourse. Nevertheless, a lubricant containing nonoxynol-9 should still be used as it does further reduce the risk. One should never use the same condom for both anal and vaginal intercourse.

French kissing, also called deep kissing or tongue kissing, is not considered completely safe, even though there has been no known case of HIV transmission in this way. The AIDS virus *has* been found in saliva, albeit in very low concentrations. An infection through kissing therefore is not very likely. If one of the partners carries the virus and the other suffers from bleeding gums or other injuries within the mouth, there could be danger. It seems wise, therefore, to consider long and intimate deep kisses to be somewhat risky.

Oral intercourse with precautions is also considered "possibly safe" (oral intercourse with no precautions is definitely unsafe). Sucking the penis is also considered "possibly safe." One way of reducing the risk of infection is to avoid swallowing semen. One should also avoid swallowing the clear pre-ejaculatory fluid. A better practice is to suck the penis after it has been thoroughly covered with a condom.

Licking the female sex organs is also considered "possibly safe." Using spermicides containing nonoxynol-9 in and around the vaginal opening or licking it through the covering of a dental dam are two safer options.

Playing with urine ("golden showers") is also considered "possibly safe." As long as urine comes in external contact only with unbroken skin, there should be no risk of infection. It is sometimes difficult to be certain that the skin is intact everywhere. Slight cuts, bruises, or pimples are easily overlooked. Therefore persons playing with urine, even if only externally, need to be extremely careful.

post hoc analyses Analyses conducted after results that were not defined before the start of a clinical trial are available. Such analyses are particularly prone to FALSE-POSITIVE claims or type I error.

postexposure prophylaxis (PEP) Administering of drug treatment to prevent disease after an individual has been exposed to an infectious organism. Sometimes referred to as the "morning-after pill" for individuals with unanticipated sexual or injection drug–related exposures to HIV, PEP is a compelling prevention intervention because it may prevent an exposure to HIV from becoming an established infection. Nonetheless, PEP is not as simple as swallowing a pill. The theory underlying the use of PEP is that antiviral treatment instituted immediately after exposure may abort the infection by inhibiting local HIV replication and by allowing the host's immune system to eradicate virus from the inoculum. Information about early HIV infection suggests that HIV can take several days to become established in the lymphoid and other tissues. This creates a window of opportunity during the immediate 24 to 72 hours post exposure when antiviral treatment may possibly head off HIV infection. The CENTERS FOR DISEASE CONTROL AND PREVENTION (CDC) currently recommends the use of antiviral drugs to reduce the risk of HIV transmission from mother to child (vertical transmission) and in health care workers who have been exposed to HIV in the workplace (occupational exposure). Questions have arisen about whether antiviral treatment should be offered to individuals who have been exposed to HIV through sex or sharing of injection drug use equipment (nonoccupational exposure). The issue of PEP after nonoccupational exposure is important because these routes of HIV transmission are far more frequent than is occupational transmission. To date there are no formal efficacy trials in the nonoccupational setting, and the CDC remains reluctant to offer definitive recommendations. A panel of AIDS prevention experts has developed some basic guidelines for implementation of nonoccupational PEP (Lurie P et al. "Postexposure Prophylaxis after Nonoccupational HIV Exposure." *JAMA*. November 25, 280(20) (Nov. 25, 1998): 1,769–1,773). Factors relevant to the assessment of the appropriateness for PEP treatment for nonoccupational exposure include route of exposure (receptive anal intercourse, receptive vaginal intercourse, injection needle sharing, insertive anal sex, insertive vaginal sex), likelihood of transmission, sporadic versus continuing incident, and status of preexisting HIV infection.

Even as debates continue about how best to assess the appropriateness of PEP treatment, concerns have been raised that the availability of PEP may increase so-called high-risk behavior: if PEP is perceived as a morning-after pill that prevents infection, individuals may believe it is no longer necessary to practice safe sex or use clean needles. Proponents argue that PEP is not a replacement strategy for avoiding HIV exposure; nor is it intended to replace adopting and maintaining behavior that guards against exposure to HIV. However, they continue, a person with a recent exposure has already failed primary prevention. In addition, many persons diligently practice safe sex but are accidentally exposed to HIV when a con-

dom breaks or slips off or is not used inadvertently under the influence of drugs or alcohol. Proponents of PEP caution that even if PEP prevents some HIV transmission, a modest increase in the number of unprotected sexual acts could actually lead to an increase in HIV transmission. They contend that for this reason, HIV prevention and risk reduction counseling must be integrated into the PEP treatment program.

post-exposure prophylaxis registry   A prospective surveillance program designed to collect data on utilization, safety, and outcome on the use of antiviral agents in persons who receive postexposure prophylaxis for nonoccupational HIV exposure.

post-infection immunization   See THERAPEUTIC VACCINE.

postmortem examination   See AUTOPSY.

postnatal transmission   See TRANSMISSION.

postpartum period   The period after a woman gives birth. There have been a number of documented cases of HIV transmission through breastfeeding, but the mechanism for transmission is unclear. See TRANSMISSION.

post-sex vaginitis   Vaginitis that appears a few hours after sexual activity, with itching and other symptoms. It often disappears on its own.

postsurgical PID   A condition in which an already-present infection is aggravated and worsens to an acute PELVIC INFLAMMATORY DISEASE (PID) after a surgical procedure.

post-traumatic stress syndrome (PTSD)   A clinical psychological disorder that arises in response to a catastrophic, or traumatic, event. The best-known instances are those of men traumatized in combat, but it also afflicts those who have survived or witnessed other extremely traumatic events. PTSD responses may be acute, chronic, or delayed. Their central feature is that the survivor reexperiences elements of the trauma in dreams, uncontrollable and emotionally distressing intrusive images, and dissociated mental states. There may be a feeling of numbing, loss of normal affect and emotional responsiveness, and loss of interest and involvement in work and personal relationships. Secondary symptoms include startle response, hyperalertness or hypervigilance, memory impairment, depression, survivor's guilt, avoidance of situations associated with the trauma, emotional explosiveness, and loss of capacity for intimacy. Post-traumatic stress syndrome was first defined in the *Diagnostic and Statistical Manual* of the American Psychiatric Association in 1980. In the revised edition of 1987, it was classified as a disorder.

Therapists and health care providers who work with people with HIV and AIDS are exposed to traumatic experiences through their patients. Families and others also experience secondary, or vicarious, trauma from their day-to-day contact with men, women, and children struggling to live with AIDS. Exposed to the emotional and psychological hazards intrinsic to these relationships, these individuals often manifest symptoms of traumatic stress similar to these observed in survivors of catastrophic events.

postural hypotension   A decrease in blood pressure upon assuming an erect posture. To a degree, this is normal, but in some circumstances it may be severe enough to cause fainting, as in persons who stand up after having been lying in bed for several days. A common symptom, along with diarrhea and impotence, of autonomic neuropathy.

potentiation   An increase in activity or efficacy, such as an interaction between drugs that results in a synergistic effect.

poverty level   An amount determined by the United States DEPARTMENT OF HEALTH AND HUMAN SERVICES, based on a calculation of the minimum amount of money necessary for basic living costs. It is used as a standard for MEDICAID and other needs-based programs.

power of attorney   A legal document with which one person gives another the right to act on his or her behalf in legal or financial matters. Powers of attorney may be restricted in various ways or be virtually unqualified. They are most often given by people in poor health who want their interests protected if they become unable to act for themselves.

PPD   See PURIFIED PROTEIN DERIVATIVE.

PPD test   See PURIFIED PROTEIN DERIVATIVE TEST.

pravastatin   A drug that blocks the ability of the body to make the fat called cholesterol. It is currently in studies to see whether it can reduce high cholesterol levels caused by anti-HIV drugs. High cholesterol levels can be a side effect of the anti-HIV drugs called PROTEASE INHIBITORS and the NNRTI drug Sustiva. Side effects include headache, fever, dizziness, skin rash, elevated liver function test results, and muscle damage leading to muscle aches or cramps and weakness. (The trade name is Pravachol.)

preclinical testing   The testing of experimental drugs in the test tube or in animals before CLINICAL TRIALS in humans may be carried out.

prednisone   A synthetic STEROID HORMONE, with the same effects as CORTISONE, that is used to treat a wide variety of conditions, including hormone deficiencies, arthritis, lupus and other rheumatic, autoimmune diseases, connective-tissue disease, certain blood disorders, inflammation of the brain, multiple sclerosis, and as a palliative treatment of certain cancers. Less often, it is used in combination therapy to prevent organ or tissue transplant rejection. In people with HIV, prednisone is commonly used to counteract allergic drug reactions and as part of combination chemotherapy for the treatment of AIDS-related lymphoma. In this population, prednisone is also frequently used to treat people with severe *PNEUMOCYSTIS CARINII* PNEUMONIA and low blood oxygen to reduce lung inflammation and improve oxygenation of the blood. It is available as tablets or as a liquid for oral administration. At low doses, prednisone rarely causes serious side effects. Large doses, taken over prolonged periods, may cause indigestion, mood changes, bone or muscle weakness, fluid retention, acne, diabetes, facial rounding, abnormal hair growth, and high blood pressure (Trade names are Deltasone, Liquid Pred, Meticorten, Orasone, and SK-Prednisone.)

pre-existing condition   Under some state laws, an individual has a preexisting medical condition if, before taking out a health insurance policy, he or she had symptoms of, or sought medical treatment for, such a condition. Most health insurance policies have a preexisting condition clause which states that, for a certain period of time (commonly 12 months) any such condition will not be covered. Most policies do cover such conditions after the expiration of the specified period. In many states, if an individual had been covered by a previous policy within 60 days before the start of the new policy, the new policy must give credit for the time on the old policy. Under federal law, which applies to group self-insured plans, there is no standard definition of a preexisting condition and no limit on the amount of time an individual can be excluded from coverage for such a condition.

preferred Rx   Preferred medical product, including prescription(s); the written direction or order for dispensing and administering drugs. It is signed by a physician, dentist, or other practitioner licensed by law to prescribe such a drug. Today, many people with HIV/AIDS are taking a wide variety of therapies simultaneously—ranging from experimental and approved ANTIVIRALS and PROPHYLAXIS for OPPORTUNISTIC INFECTIONS to complementary approaches and over-the-counter medications. As more drugs have become available to treat HIV and to prevent opportunistic infections and HIV-related malignancies, the potential for drug interactions has become an increasing concern. Not only does every therapy have potential side effects, but how each therapy might augment or diminish the benefit of another must be considered when making treatment decisions. How therapies interact is not always considered and may play a major role in the success of any plan for managing HIV disease. A medication review for safety, appropriateness, compatibility, and instructions for use will help decrease the likelihood of drug interactions.

pregnancy   The condition of carrying a developing embryo(s) in the uterus. Transmission of HIV from mother to child (vertical transmission) has been established. Today, two plus decades into the AIDS pandemic, AIDS research and corollary advances in prevention and treatment have resulted in a significant reduction in the rate of transmission of HIV from mother to child. In many industrialized nations, rates of transmission have dropped substantially, to below 5 percent. Success has been more difficult to achieve in the developing world, where traditional obstacles to care and treatment impede the implementation of sometimes costly and complex interventions aimed at preventing vertical transmission. An understanding of HIV and pregnancy requires awareness of vertically acquired HIV infection, effects of pregnancy on HIV disease, effect of HIV on pregnancy course and outcome, HIV-infected babies, prevention, and the treatment of HIV-infected childbearing-age women.

Vertical Transmission

Children can acquire HIV from their mothers in several ways. There is evidence that transmission can occur during the course of pregnancy, around the time of labor and delivery, or post partum through breast-feeding. Most transmission appears to occur during or close to the intrapartum period, particularly in non-breast-feeding populations.

A pregnant HIV-infected woman can transmit the virus to her fetus in utero (during gestation) as the virus crosses over from the mother into the fetal bloodstream. In utero infections can occur throughout pregnancy; however, it is likely that most arise late in the gestation period, not long before delivery. At least 50 percent of newborn infections occur during delivery through ingestion of blood or other maternal fluids. If breast-fed, the newborn may also become infected from breast milk. In case reports, women who contracted HIV by blood transfusions immediately after birth subsequently infected their newborns via breast-feeding. Other studies suggest that the risk of HIV transmission through breast-feeding is increased if the mother becomes HIV-infected during lactation. The relative efficiency of these three routes of infection is unknown. However, the data on mother's milk add to the urgency of learning more about mucosal transmission. The most likely explanation for HIV transmission through breast-feeding is that the virus penetrates the mucosal lining of the mouth or gastrointestinal tract of infants.

Potential variables in vertical transmission have been identified. These include HIV-related factors, such as HIV RNA level; strain variation (genotype); biologic growth characteristics (phenotype); plasma versus genital tract viral load; genotypic resistance; CD4 cell count; and maternal immune response. Maternal and obstetric factors have also been identified: clinical stage, STDs or other coinfections, vitamin A deficiency, substance abuse, cigarette smoking, antiretroviral agents, sexual behavior, gestational age, duration of membrane rupture, placental disruption-abruption, chorioamnionitis, invasive fetal monitoring, episiotomy, forceps use, and vaginal versus cesarean delivery. Finally, fetal neonatal factors have been identified, including immune system immaturity and genetic susceptibility.

Pregnancy and HIV Disease

Early findings in pregnant women indicated that those with T4-cell counts of less than $300/\mu L$ of blood were more likely to experience HIV-associated illness during pregnancy. Pregnant HIV-infected women exhibit a greater T4-cell count decline during pregnancy than do women without HIV infection. T4-cell counts in the HIV-infected do not return to prepregnancy levels. However, the overall declines in counts of HIV-infected women likely represent declines that would have occurred in the absence of pregnancy and suggest that pregnancy does not accelerate disease progression. Note that most studies to date have not shown significant differences in HIV progression or survival between pregnant women and nonpregnant women with HIV infection. The relationship of common pregnancy complications (e.g., spontaneous abortion, stillbirth, perinatal mortality, infant mortality, intrauterine growth retardation, low birth weight, preeclampsia, gestational diabetes, chorioamnionitis, oligohydramnios, and fetal malformation) to HIV infection has not been definitively established. Note that concerns have been raised that antiretroviral treatment itself may increase the incidence of some pregnancy complications. Note too that both HIV and pregnancy may affect the natural history, presentation, treatment, or significance of certain infections, including vulvovaginal candidiasis, bacterial vaginosis, genital herpes simplex, human papillomavirus, syphilis, cytomegalovirus, toxoplasmosis, hepatitis B, and hepatitis C. These infections may be associated with pregnancy complications or perinatal infection.

HIV-Infected Babies

One challenge in perinatal transmission is determination of which babies are truly HIV-infected as opposed to just carrying the mother's HIV antibodies (which would produce a false-positive test result). HIV transmission can occur during pregnancy (in utero) as well as at the time of delivery (intrapartum) and through breast milk, as noted. HIV transmission is more likely if the virus can be cultured from the mother's blood, or if she has later-stage HIV disease, or if her T4 counts are low; and is more likely to occur in the firstborn than in the secondborn of twins. Note that a baby automatically acquires the mother's antibodies and may carry them for two or more years. Usually by the time the infant is 18 months of age, most of the mother's antibodies are gone. The babies may then begin to show signs of clinical AIDS-related illness. But, even at 18 months, a child cannot be unequivocally diagnosed. The most commonly used HIV antibody test to date is not sufficiently accurate until the child is at least two years old.

The rate of perinatal and breast milk HIV transmission is unknown; however, evidence indicates that more than 90 percent of pediatric AIDS cases result from acquisition of the virus in utero from an HIV-infected mother after the first trimester or during the birth process. Studies have shown that a fetus can become infected as early as the eighth week of gestation.

Reports on the probability of a fetus's becoming HIV-infected when the untreated mother carries the virus vary widely. The most often quoted estimate in the United States is from 30 percent to 50 percent.

Prevention and Treatment

Mother-to-fetus infection can be prevented by preventing pregnancy, but this is possible only in cases when the female is aware of her infection and takes measures to prevent pregnancy (i.e., birth control or tubal ligation). In many cases, pregnancy occurs before the mother knows she is carrying the virus. In other cases, the mother becomes infected after she has become pregnant.

For pregnant women, guidelines for care are generally divided into guidelines for antepartum care, intrapartum care, and postpartum care. In antepartum care, the emphasis is on history and physical examination, fetal surveillance and testing, antiretroviral treatment, opportunistic infection prophylaxis, immunizations, the reduction of secondary risk factors, frequency of visits, counseling, and support. Universal precautions, fetal and maternal monitoring, mode of delivery, intrapartum ARV prophylaxis, antibiotic prophylaxis, and vaginal cleansing are the main foci of intrapartum care. The emphases of postpartum care are infant feeding, assessment of healing, care of the mother and infant, contraception and condom use, and long-term follow-up for both mother and infant.

One of the most important steps forward in the use of antiviral agents has been the discovery that antiretroviral drugs can decrease the rate of perinatal transmission of HIV. It has been established that drug therapy for mother and child does reduce the frequency of vertical transmission of HIV. Today, the mechanism by which AZT and other drugs prevent vertical infection is well understood; with such therapy, the incidence of vertical transmission has been reduced dramatically in nations in which good obstetric care and affordable drugs are available. Indeed, by combining drug therapy with cesarean delivery, which minimizes fetal exposure to maternal blood and secretions, the incidence of vertical infection in infants can be reduced to as low as 2 percent of infants born to HIV-positive women. Moreover, women who become pregnant while receiving HIGHLY ACTIVE ANTIRETROVIRAL THERAPY (HAART) have been shown to transmit virus to their offspring even less often.

A three-part course of AZT treatment (administered before birth orally, during labor with an IV infusion, and to the newborn orally) has become the standard of care in industrialized countries. However, it is not economically feasible in the developing world. Researchers have been evaluating abbreviated courses of treatment overseas that may be more affordable and practical. Researchers have also been evaluating the use of other drugs in decreasing the rate of vertical transmission in developing countries. In addition, efforts to address other risk factors associated with vertical transmission have revealed more information on the roles of breast-feeding, maternal viral load, and elective cesarean sections.

Noting the obstacles to the elimination of breast-feeding among HIV-positive women in developing countries, researchers have identified alternative approaches to preventing transmission. These include providing antiretroviral therapy during breast-feeding, preventing HIV seroconversion in HIV-negative mothers during breast-feeding, treating breast sores and other infections in the mother and mouth sores in the infant, vitamin A supplementation in the mother, and possibly avoidance of mixed feeding.

Viral load, transmission, and HAART have also received attention. Given that maternal viral load is a factor in the risk of vertical transmission, HAART may be a good choice for HIV-positive pregnant women who have access to therapy. Note that HAART achieves the goal of greatly reducing HIV viral load. However, to date, there is limited experience in using these drugs during pregnancy, and their possible benefits must be weighed against the lack of information on potential long-term effects on children exposed to them. For additional considerations for antiretroviral therapy in HIV-infected pregnant women, see "Guidelines for the Use of Antiretroviral Agents in Adults: Updated Recommendations" (2000).

Finally, researchers have looked into the fact that since a large proportion of vertical transmission occurs at or near delivery, intervention at this time might prove beneficial. Elective (nonemergency) cesarean section *before the time the mother's water breaks* can prevent the infant from being exposed to maternal blood and secretions. As a prevention intervention, antiretroviral therapy may be a better option than elective cesarean section, as treatment during pregnancy may prevent transmission in the prenatal period and provide POSTEXPOSURE PROPHYLAXIS to the infant. An elective cesarean section may be beneficial for women who have not taken antivirals during pregnancy, for women with persistent or rising viral loads, and for women with difficulty in adhering to HAART. The U.S. Public Health Service Guidelines do not recommend universal cesarean section for HIV-positive pregnant women. Instead, women should be apprised of all available information, and individualized decisions should be made jointly by the physician and the patient. Since the cesarean section is major surgery, there are associated complications for the mother. Although cesarean sections are generally quite safe in industrialized countries, some studies have found that HIV-positive women have an increased risk of postoperative complications. Furthermore, surgical procedures may not be an option for the majority of women in resource-poor countries with limited health care infrastructures and budgets.

Knowledge of HIV Transmission

A report in the January 2001 issue of *Obstetrics and Gynecology* indicates that although many women in the United States are aware that HIV-infected pregnant women can transmit their infection to their infants, some are not so sure how the virus is actually passed on. Emmanuel Walter of Duke University Medical Center found that almost 40 percent of the 1,400 pregnant women surveyed were not certain whether an HIV-positive woman could transmit the virus to her baby via breast-feeding. About 33 percent thought that babies born to a women with HIV would definitely become infected, and 49 percent were not aware that there are drugs that can help reduce the risk of newborns' contracting HIV. It was noted, however, that about 90 percent of the women questioned had been offered an HIV test during their pregnancy, that most had agreed to the test, and that 60 percent said that routine testing of all pregnant women should be required by law.

It is noted that the U.S. Public Health Service recommendations for HIV counseling and voluntary testing for all pregnant women acknowledge that knowledge of HIV status is important for several reasons. First, women who know their serostatus can gain access to HIV-related care and therapies during pregnancy and post partum as needed. Second, HIV-infected women can be offered zidovudine to block potential maternal–fetal transmission of HIV. Third, an obstetrician would postpone rupture of amniotic membranes and avoid scalp electrodes or other potentially invasive procedures, all of which may be cofactors for enhanced transmission of HIV. Fourth, zidovudine can be offered to infants of HIV-seropositive women who have recently delivered.

Reproductive Rights and Testing

Central to a woman's right to control her body, reproductive rights take on new meaning in HIV-infected pregnancies. Today the choices of becoming pregnant or terminating the pregnancy continue to be disputed. However, as more women become HIV-infected and give birth to HIV-infected children, many fear that childbearing may come under the surveillance of the state. Women of childbearing age may be among the first groups to undergo mandatory testing as part of an attempt to control the birth of HIV-infected newborns. Note that routine HIV counseling and voluntary testing of all pregnant women have been proved to be effective in several communities nationwide. Note too that the state has traditionally expressed an interest in protecting the rights of the fetus. This interest was transcended in the 1973 *Roe v. Wade* decision when the U.S. Supreme Court recognized a woman's right to choose an abortion. The court ruled that a woman's right to privacy must prevail against the state's interest in protecting the future life of the fetus. Some of the ethical issues that have been debated since the decision include whether or not couples have a right to have children when one of the partners is known to be HIV-positive. This issue takes on a different cast if the woman is HIV-positive or if both are HIV-positive. There has been also debate as to whether there is any stage of HIV disease/AIDS when a woman should lose the right to become pregnant. See BREAST-FEEDING; CHILDREN; PEDIATRIC AIDS; TRANSMISSION; WOMEN.

pregnancy counseling   Advising a woman of childbearing age of her options regarding pregnancy. Women who are pregnant or thinking about getting pregnant are advised to consider the risks; to consider taking the AIDS antibody test; and to get help making decisions from their partner, a counselor, a health worker, or an AIDS information agency.

Decisions about pregnancy and AIDS are not easy to make. A woman may decide not to have children if she or her partner is infected. If a woman is pregnant and infected, she needs to decide whether to continue the pregnancy. If a woman wants to have a child, and is infected, it is important for her to get regular medical care from a health worker or doctor who knows about AIDS. It is also important to get emotional support from a counselor or group.

premium   Amount paid periodically by an insured person or employer to secure insurance coverage. Premiums for health insurance are paid either to MEDICARE or a private insurer or health plan.

prenatal   Existing or occurring before birth.

prenatal care   Care of a woman and her fetus during pregnancy. Routine care includes periodic examination for determination of blood pressure, weight, changes in the size of the uterus, and condition of the fetus; urinalysis; instruction in nutritional requirements, preparation for labor and delivery, and care of the newborn; and assistance and support to deal with the discomforts of pregnancy. Examinations at regular intervals offer the opportunity to detect any untoward changes in the condition of a mother or fetus so that necessary treatment can be instituted.

Medical care besides this routine testing and preparation includes screening for hepatitis; serological testing for toxoplasmosis; treating opportunistic infections per standard medical protocols; using aggressive therapy if warranted for syphilis; providing women on methadone increases in dosage if needed; and, to optimize fetal outcome, fetal surveillance through ultrasound and biophysical profiles. For women with HIV, CD4+ count is followed by testing once a trimester at a minimum. For CD4+ counts of less than 200 mm, current National Institutes of Health and CENTERS FOR DISEASE CONTROL AND PREVENTION treatment recommendations are followed; for CD4+ counts between 200 mm and 500 mm, the decision to start medication is left to the patient. See INTRAPARTUM and POSTPARTUM PERIOD.

prenatal testing   See PRENATAL CARE.

prepartum   Before childbirth, during pregnancy.

prerandomization examination   Any examination that is part of the evaluation process of a patient for enrollment into a clinical trial and that is carried out before the randomization examination.

prerandomization visit   Any visit made to a clinic by a potential study patient for the purpose of evaluation for enrollment into a clinical trial that takes place before the randomization visit.

prescription drug   A drug available to the public only upon prescription written by a physician or other practitioner licensed to do so.

preseminal fluid   The milky fluid that escapes from the penis before ejaculation. Also called PRE-CUM.

presumptive diagnosis   A diagnosis by a HEALTH CARE PROFESSIONAL that an infection or disease is present, based on certain signs and symptoms, rather than clinical tests. It cannot be considered definitive.

presumptive disability determination   A preliminary determination by a SOCIAL SECURITY district officer finding that a needy applicant with a specified impairment will likely be found to be disabled by legal standards. This permits SSI payments to begin immediately, meeting urgent expenses and medical care needs while a complete disability determination of the medical records is conducted. Since 1988 a diagnosis of full-blown AIDS allows for presumptive disability determination.

prevalence   The total number of cases of a disease in existence at a particular time in a specified area.

prevalence rate   The frequency of the occurrence of a disease in a population, usually expressed as the number of cases per 100,000 population.

prevention   The basic steps in the prevention of the spread of HIV and AIDS include education of the public about HIV infection; encouragement of condom use, especially among teenagers and young adults; education about the hazards of using shared and unsterile needles; education of heterosexuals, homosexuals, and bisexuals to limit their number of sex partners; screening of donated blood for HIV antibodies; and education of people with AIDS about how to avoid infecting others. Perinatal prevention efforts, or efforts to prevent transmission of

HIV from mother to fetus or to infant, include routine and universal HIV counseling and voluntary testing combined with AZT therapy.

Preveon See ADEFOVIR.

primaquine An antiprotozoal agent used primarily as a treatment for malaria. In people living with HIV, it is sometimes used with CLINDAMYCIN to treat or prevent PNEUMOCYSTIS CARINII PNEUMONIA (PCP). Nausea, vomiting, loss of appetite, and abdominal discomfort are common side effects. Less commonly, blurred vision, allergic skin reactions, dizziness, headache, darkening of the urine, and anemia may occur.

primary brain lymphoma A rare cancer that starts in the brain. It is an OPPORTUNISTIC INFECTION that often kills people with AIDS. See PRIMARY CENTRAL NERVOUS SYSTEM LYMPHOMA.

primary care Basic health care; the point of entry into the health care system for most people. The concept encompasses continuity care, health maintenance, prevention, medical management of acute and chronic illness, immunizations, age-appropriate screening for disease, and referral and follow-up for all problems that are identified. People with HIV infection or AIDS have different primary care needs than those without, in important ways. Similarly, the primary care needs of asymptomatic HIV-positive people are different from the primary care needs of symptomatic HIV-positive people. An initial evaluation of an HIV-positive person may include lab workups, immunizations, tuberculosis testing, a complete physical examination, an ophthalmological evaluation, a dental evaluation, and a psychosocial assessment. Discussion of management strategies and therapy or treatment options for HIV infection and its complications generally follows. See ACQUIRED IMMUNODEFICIENCY SYNDROME; HUMAN IMMUNODEFICIENCY VIRUS.

primary care provider A HEALTH CARE PROVIDER (e.g., physician, physician assistant, NURSE practitioner) who offers basic health care services and coordinates comprehensive patient care.

primary care setting The place where basic and comprehensive care is delivered, such as a physician's office, community health clinic, or a preventive nursing service.

primary central nervous system lymphoma (PCNSL) A cancer of the central nervous system occurring most often as a complication of late-stage AIDS. It takes the form of B-cell tumor growth. B cells' normal task is to produce antibodies selectively when stimulated by CD4+ HELPER T CELLS. Factors that may contribute to their unrestrained proliferation in HIV infection include chronic stimulation, loss of T-cell control mechanisms, and infection by EPSTEIN-BARR VIRUS, which is closely associated with the development of PCNSL. Historically, this lymphoma was thought to affect only a few percent of people with AIDS, but in the MULTICENTER AIDS COHORT STUDY (MACS) survey, it was increasing at a rate faster than HIV-sensory neuropathy, TOXOPLASMOSIS, CRYPTOCOCOCCAL MENINGITIS, and PROGRESSIVE MULTIFOCAL LEUKOENCEPHALOPATHY. Symptoms include focal neurologic signs such as hemiparesis, aphasia, seizures, loss of cranial nerve function, lethargy, confusion, and memory loss. Presumptive diagnosis is established through MRI and CT SCANS, complemented with lumbar puncture and cytologic examination of spinal fluid. It has been suggested that Epstein-Barr virus in spinal fluid is a marker.

Primary CNS lymphoma is unusually aggressive in people with AIDS. Survival time after the onset of PCNSL depends on CD4 count, and even with treatment, averages as little as five or six months in people with advanced symptomatic AIDS. Therapy consists of whole-brain irradiation, sometimes along with short-term administration of STEROIDS to control and shrink tissue swelling and tumors. Relapse is frequent. Use of chemotherapy for PCNSL is under investigation.

primary CNS lymphoma See PRIMARY CENTRAL NERVOUS SYSTEM LYMPHOMA.

primary health care See PRIMARY CARE.

primary HIV infection See PRIMARY INFECTION.

primary immune response Immune responses to the HUMAN IMMUNODEFICIENCY VIRUS during the first weeks of infection. Studies have shown that primary immune response to HIV predicts disease progression. Data suggests that the immunologic factors during this early period of infection are the critical determinants of the ultimate outcome of HIV disease. The growing understanding of the initial interaction between HIV and the immune system, and of immune responses to HIV during primary infection (both favorable and unfavorable), is important to the development of effective HIV vaccines. Once it enters the body, HIV infects a large number of CD4+ T CELLS and replicates rapidly. During this acute, or primary phase of infection, the blood contains many viral particles that spread throughout the body, seeding various organs, particularly the lymphoid organs with the virus. (Up to 70 percent of HIV-infected persons have been known to suffer flu-like symptoms.) The patient's immune system fights back with killer T cells (CD8+ T cells) and B-cell-produced antibodies. One important way in which a person's immune system responds to primary HIV infection is by mobilizing different subsets of certain white blood cells—CD8+ T cells—that can destroy cells that have been infected with HIV. Studies have shown a clear correlation between the patterns of CD8+ T cell expansion during primary infection and how well a patient clinically fared during the subsequent year and 18 months afterward. Regardless of the amount of HIV in the blood during primary infection, patients who mobilized a broad repertoire of CD8+ T cells had slower progression of disease than individuals who showed a pronounced expansion of only a single subset of CD8+ T cells. Scientists currently do not know the reasons for the qualitative differences in the immune responses of different individuals during primary HIV infection, but they probably include factors intrinsic to the HIV-infected person, such as the genes that encode specific markers called HUMAN LEUKOCYTE ANTIGENS (HLAs) on the immune system cells.

primary infection   The acute stage of HIV disease just after transmission. Primary HIV infection usually passes unnoticed. Typical symptoms such as fevers, swollen glands, rashes, and diarrhea are frequently mistaken for the flu or the common cold. If a person undergoing primary infection does seek medical attention, HIV is rarely diagnosed unless

there is good reason to suspect it, such as a known recent exposure. During primary infection, HIV replicates extensively and large quantities of HIV disseminate throughout the body, especially to the lymphoid organs. Viral load levels are extremely high, but this initial burst of viral replication is brought under control within several weeks by CYTOTOXIC T-LYMPHOCYTES (CTLs). The CTLs can reduce virus levels by a thousand-fold or more, a greater reduction than any currently available drug can accomplish. Despite the fact that the body's immune responses following initial infection usually reduce the virus to very low levels, some HIV invariably escapes. One explanation for this escape is that the immune system's best soldiers in the fight against HIV—certain subsets of CD8+ T CELLS, multiply rapidly following initial HIV infection but then exhaust themselves and disappear, allowing HIV to escape and continue replication. In the few weeks that they are detectable, the initially expanded CD8+ T cells that effectively kill HIV-infected cells are found in the blood-stream rather than in the lymph nodes where the virus is replicating. Researchers have found that major, restricted expansion of T cells in primary HIV infection is transient, and that among these expanded cells are CTLs specific for HIV. Note that this is not a term that is unique to HIV/AIDS.

primary isolates   HIV strains obtained from people and not put into laboratory cultures.

primary lymphoid tissue   Lymphoid organs in which LYMPHOCYTES complete their initial maturation steps; they include the fetal liver and the adult BONE MARROW and THYMUS.

primary physician   The physician to whom a family or individual goes initially for basic medical care. See PRIMARY CARE.

primary prophylaxis   A prophylactic medicine or measure (prophylactic treatment) to prevent an initial infection. Primary prophylaxis is important whenever possible because once a disease arises, the drugs used to treat it usually do not eliminate the disease-causing organism from the body. This means that when the treatment stops, there is a good chance that the infection will return. See SEC-ONDARY PROPHYLAXIS.

primary response   The immune response (cellular or humoral) following an initial encounter with a particular ANTIGEN.

prime   The first round in a series of vaccinations.

prime boost   In HIV vaccine research, administration of one type of vaccine, such as a live-vector vaccine, followed by or together with a second type of vaccine, such as a recombinant subunit vaccine. The intent of this combination regimen is to induce different types of immune responses and enhance the overall immune response, a result that might not occur if only one type of vaccine were to be given for all doses.

priming   Giving one vaccine dose(s) first to induce certain immune responses, to be followed by or administered together with a second type of vaccine. The intent of priming is to induce certain immune responses that are to be enhanced by the booster dose(s).

principal investigator (PI)   The lead researcher responsible for organizing and overseeing a CLINICAL TRIAL.

principal neutralizing determinant   The part of an antigen that most reliably induces a protective immune response. The principal neutralizing determinant of HIV is the V3 loop of the envelope glycoprotein gp120.

prior approval   See PRIOR AUTHORIZATION.

prior authorization (PA)   In essence, a treatment authorization request. Born in the private health plan industry as a way to assure that the prescription of superexpensive drugs is justified, it requires an agent of the payer to review a drug prescription and approve its use for that patient before it can be dispensed. PA is supposed to provide a checkpoint between the pharmacy and the consumer to ensure that the rules for dispensing drugs are fol-

lowed. These rules may have their origins in concerns about drug safety, mandates to restrict waste and abuse, and the desire to make drug selections more rational and ultimately hold down costs. Critiques of the process note the increased burden it places on doctors, patients, and pharmacists; some contend that PA schemes put savings ahead of patients' needs.

A PA procedure may look like this: if an individual (plan member) is currently taking one of the restricted medications, his or her doctor may request a review by calling the health maintenance organization's pharmacy benefits manager. If, however, a review is not sought in advance, the prescription is presented to the pharmacy. When the pharmacy submits the prescription to the plan's pharmacy benefits manager, an on-line message tells the pharmacist that authorization is necessary. The pharmacist is provided with the pharmacy benefits manager's phone number to begin the authorization process. The member should ask the prescribing physician to contact the pharmacy benefits manager to discuss the criteria for use and other clinical parameters. Coverage is determined, and patient and physician receive notice of either approval or denial. If coverage is denied, the physician can request an appeal. With an appeal, new information must be provided; for example, the physician may need to specify another reason why the member should be treated as he or she thinks best.

prison   The health problems, including HIV/AIDS, tuberculosis, and sexually transmitted diseases, that increasingly affect correctional inmate populations pose difficult programmatic and fiscal challenges for the administrators and staff of prison and jail systems. Populations continue to increase in both federal and state facilities, but budgets are often frozen or declining for the facilities. In addition, the problems of substance abuse, high risk sexual activity, poverty, homelessness, and poor access to preventive and primary health care in the community cause many more problems than are faced in typical medical settings. Prisons consider themselves as control facilities and not medical facilities. So concern is primarily to control the people there and not to treat them for illness. Prisons have been known to be notoriously slow in offering medical treatment for illness, inefficient in providing prescriptions to the incarcerated, unhelpful in protecting those that are sick, and unable to provide condoms to inmates.

The 2000 national report of HIV/AIDS in correctional facilities, written by the Bureau of Justice Statistics covered the prevalence and deaths of sexually transmitted diseases among inmates. According to the report, HIV SEROPREVALENCE incidence rates are four times higher among inmates than in the total United States population. According to CENTERS FOR DISEASE CONTROL AND PREVENTION reports about .5 percent of Americans are believed to be HIV positive. Two percent of prison inmates are HIV positive. The rate of inmates with AIDS is also four times higher in the prison population. In the general population .13 percent has AIDS; .52 percent of the prison population has AIDS. Seroprevalence and AIDS rates, however, appear to be either stable or declining in most systems. The lone upswing in numbers has been in the female prison population. Seroprevalence is also higher in state prisons among female inmates (3.6 percent) than male inmates (2.2 percent). As in previous reports, there were no documented cases of occupational HIV transmission from inmates to correctional staff. Studies have shown that inmate-to-inmate HIV transmission does occur, but at unknown rates. HIV seroprevalence also remains higher among Latino and African-American inmates than among Caucasian prisoners.

Despite the higher rates of HIV among prisoners, the number of correctional facilities providing inmate HIV education remains low. Only 10 percent of state and 5 percent of federal prisons offer HIV education. In addition, prisons in only two states—Vermont and Mississippi—and in four city jails—Philadelphia, New York City, San Francisco, and Washington, D.C.—allow distribution of condoms. Typically, prisons forbid sexual activity, and these rules allow the prisons to ignore sexual activity that does occur. Assumptions are also made that men do not engage in sexual activity in prison or that prisoners who engage in male-to-male sex aren't worth worrying sufficiently to receive condoms. Other items that prevent the spread of HIV, such as clean needles or bleach to clean needles, are typically illegal in prisons. Despite the evidence that hepatitis C is prevalent and rampant in prison, through statistics taken before and during incarceration that show increases in HCV during incarcer-

ation, officials continue to acknowledge these items would prevent further deterioration of inmate lives. Language issues also make HIV education difficult. Spanish is the predominant language of many prisoners in California, Texas, and New York. Employees of prisons often do not speak languages other than English, making medical and educational conversations particularly difficult.

Most all prisons require HIV testing upon entrance to the facility. Few correctional systems notify correctional officers of inmates' HIV status as a matter of official policy. Actual practice, however, may differ from official directives, and unauthorized disclosure to officers and others remains a problem. Staff and resource shortages have prevented pre-test and post-test counseling. In regards to the housing of inmates with HIV and AIDS, there has been a steady decline in segregation policies. Case-by-case decisions and presumptive general population assignments remain most common. Validation study results reveal the complexity in implementing housing policies in institutions with different security levels and different population characteristics. In most systems, inmates with HIV/AIDS are eligible for all program and work assignments. However, several systems exclude such inmates from kitchen work. This remains a controversial issue, despite strong evidence that HIV is not transmitted through food. Medical care for inmates with HIV/AIDS continues to be uneven in quality. Although the best-known therapeutic drugs for HIV/AIDS are in widespread use, access to experimental drugs and CLINICAL TRIALS remains quite rare in correctional systems. Citing a study of prisons by Abt Associates, several factors such as high medication costs, fear and denial by inmates, uneven medical services, and uneven treatment regimens cause a variety of problems with treatment of HIV. Support groups and other supportive services are not offered as widely as they might be. Most prisons state that they follow one of two methods of prescription dispensing. KOP, or keep on person, allows inmates to hold a week or other set time period of drugs to take when required. DOT, or directly observed therapy, is where doctors or other prison officials dispense and observe each dose being taken. Prison schedules, lockdowns, and unavailable fluids or foods to take with the medicines can be disruptive and dangerous to inmates trying to take medications. Discharge planning and continuity of care for inmates leaving correctional facilities remain areas also in need of significant improvement. Medical personnel in prison facilities are also different than in the community. Many prison physicians are known to not be licensed or to have had their licenses revoked from the regular community practice.

Legal issues raised by inmates with HIV/AIDS include protection from harm by fellow inmates, challenges to mandatory testing, challenges to other testing policies, confidentiality, segregation and housing assignments, access to programs, and adequacy of medical care. Also of legal interest are patterns and trends in the criminal indictment and sentencing of persons with HIV infection. Whether and how the judicial system should consider HIV infection in it's processing of persons accused and/or convicted of crimes remains a challenging question for the nation's criminal and appellate courts. Conflicting rulings appear largely related to the nature of the crime committed and to the nature of the defendant's illness. For example, while in recent years several courts have considered not prosecuting, or commuting the sentences of, defendants with HIV or AIDS who have been charged with or convicted of nonviolent crimes, defendants charged with other crimes, like having unprotected sex with teenagers, are treated quite severely. Lastly, despite evidence that HIV has never demonstrably been transmitted through saliva, over the last several years at least two HIV-infected inmates have been prosecuted and convicted of attempted murder for biting or spitting on a correctional officer. The American Bar Association (ABA) adopted a policy on AIDS and the criminal justice system in 1989. The ABA said that appropriately funded training and education programs regarding HIV should be instituted in all correctional facilities. Further, the ABA recommended that inmates in correctional facilities should be afforded appropriate medical care for the full range of HIV-related infections and should be afforded appropriate counseling as well. The ABA policy further stated that prisoners should not be segregated from the general population of the correctional facility or be placed in other special areas solely because of their known or perceived HIV status. It specified that mass HIV-antibody testing

should not be done for the purpose of segregating inmates in special cells or areas. Information about an inmate's HIV status should not be disclosed except to the warden, key supervisory staff who have a legitimate need for the information, or medical staff for care and treatment purposes. And according to the ABA, parole or temporary release should not be denied to a prisoner, nor should a prisoner be barred from participating in other community release programs solely because of the prisoner's known or perceived HIV status. The National Commission on AIDS has also addressed these concerns. In March 1991 it issued a report on HIV disease in correctional facilities. The report found that prisoners with HIV infection are rapidly acquiring tuberculosis, and many more are at increased risk from the resurgent tuberculosis epidemic in the nation's prisons. It also found that prisoners with HIV are often subject to automatic segregation from the rest of the prison community despite the fact that there is no public health basis for this practice. Third, it found that lack of education of both inmates and staff creates fear and discrimination as well as unjust policies directed toward inmates with HIV. Finally, it found that despite high rates of HIV infection and an ideal opportunity for prevention and education efforts, former prisoners are reentering their communities with little or no added knowledge about HIV and how to prevent it. Inmates continue to be tested without their consent, to be segregated and made subject to other inmates' and staffs ridicule and animosity, and to be denied privileges available to those who are not HIV-infected.

privacy Freedom from unwanted observation or examination, implying, in a medical context, the right of a patient to control the distribution and release of records and information concerning his or her medical history, encompassing all information the patient has provided to health care professionals and any other information contained in medical charts, records, and laboratory data. Specifically, this includes diagnoses of HIV infection, AIDS, or related disorders.

People with AIDS, their families, and others close to them often have to contend with social stigma along with their anger, guilt, grief, and denial. As a result, the right to privacy has been the subject of heated public debate. In the United States legal tradition, issues of HIV testing and dissemination of medical information fit into the portmanteau category of "privacy," which is protected in various ways in state and federal law and constitutions.

The U.S. Constitution and many state constitutions protect personal privacy against government and other institutional intrusion, although in all but a few state constitutions the right to privacy of medical information is not explicitly stated. Instead, it has been derived by the courts from the general tenor and purposes of these fundamental charters. Protection of privacy has been found by courts to be particularly necessary in cases of HIV-related information. Reasons for this include the moral stigma society attaches to the disease and activities associated with it (especially sexual relations and drug use), and the potential for harm in the event of a nonconsensual disclosure and the fact that the consequences of the hysteria surrounding AIDS extends beyond those who have the disease. Even in instances where courts have found release of information to be justified, they have usually been careful to make the allowable disclosure as narrow as possible. The right of privacy also encompasses the freedom to choose or refuse medical care and to decide for oneself when to release sensitive information to others.

Individual privacy is also protected by the Fourth Amendment, which establishes "the right of people to be secure in their persons, houses, papers, and effects, against unreasonable searches and seizures" by government or its agents. This means that a person has a right to expect that the privacy of his or her personal records, including medical information, will be respected and that the revelation of such information through medical testing may not be coerced. The actual degree of protection under the Fourth Amendment, however, depends on the case-by-case application of the rules by the courts. Judges assessing the reasonableness of HIV testing under the Fourth Amendment have reached varying and even contradictory decisions, and is likely that they will continue to do so for some time.

The public health consensus in support of privacy and against coercion led a majority of states to adopt measures in the late 1980s governing HIV testing and confidentiality. By the end of 1991, 36 states had enacted legislation requiring informed consent for HIV testing; virtually every state provided some degree of confidentiality. Some laws address disclosure not only of test results, but of any confidential HIV-related information developed in the course of any health or social service. A second wave of statutes that began to emerge in 1988 generally expanded the range of counseling required and information protected but also set forth more detailed exceptions.

Most confidentiality laws provide that information may be disclosed to health departments and hospital oversight agencies and to the subjects of tests and the physicians who order them. Most also contain exceptions based on the "need to know" (whether such needs are genuine or not has been subject to debate). In addition, many states have mandatory testing and disclosure provisions that override the general policy of voluntariness and nondisclosure. Major exceptions have been won, for example, by funeral directors, insurers, and health care providers. Some states authorize involuntary testing of, and disclosure of information about, people in prisons, mental hospitals, juvenile facilities, and residential centers for the developmentally disabled. Mandatory testing and disclosure is becoming more common in the criminal justice system. Physician warnings to third parties and testing and disclosure by court order remain two of the most debated issues in health policy.

Today it is generally recognized that the protection of privacy is important for an effective public health response to HIV in a just society. History has shown that testing and disclosure programs too often reflect a preoccupation with low but frightening risks, and a preference for identifying people whose exposure is unusual over providing services to the easy-to-identify. The claim that privacy is in conflict with public health too often reflects underlying disdain for those with, or at risk of, HIV; we have simultaneously enacted legal protections of privacy while allowing it to be needlessly compromised on too many occasions. Today those concerned with the treatment and prevention of HIV/AIDS generally agree that anyone who comes into possession of information about HIV-infected individuals or is in a position to do HIV testing must understand and respect the importance of privacy to both individuals and society. It is understood that, occasionally, this respect may bring them into conflict with legal rules and regulations.

privates   A euphemism for genitalia.

PRN   A term used on prescriptions to mean "take as needed," from the Latin phrase *pro re nata.*

PRO   See PEER REVIEW ORGANIZATION.

PRO-542   A FUSION protein that functions similarly to human antibodies. It is in PHASE II development by Progenics, Inc. It appears to be well tolerated and has been shown to work well in children. It works by binding to the gp120 protein of the outer coating of the HIV virus and prohibiting the virus from binding to uninfected cells. See GP120.

PRO 2000   A topical microbicide to be used against HIV, in Phase III trials in the United States.

Pro90   An amino acid that binds protein cyclophilin A (what HIV takes with it when it buds from a cell). The binding of cyclophilin A by Pro90 seems necessary for a viral particle to be infectious. If Pro90 is present in an abnormal form, HIV particles are not infectious, even though they appear normal. Researchers have previously hypothesized that the binding of cyclophilin A to the p24 capsid protein changes the conformation of the protein, thereby enabling the virus to release its genetic contents into a target cell. In recent experiments, Pro90 has been observed to exist in two separate conformations. It is hypothesized that one of these conformations may be necessary for the p24 capsid proteins to assemble, in order to form the viral core. The other conformation would be necessary for the core to disassemble. Pro90 may serve as a molecular switch for capsid assembly or disassembly, with cyclophilin A either flipping the switch or locking it into a particular position.

probate   The process by which an executor, if there is a will, or a court-appointed administrator, if there is not, under court supervision manage and distribute a deceased person's property.

probenecid   A drug that enhances the kidney's excretory functions. Patients who receive cidofovir for CYTOMEGALOVIRUS must take probenecid and intravenous hydration with saline solution in order to protect the kidneys from damage caused by cidofovir buildup within kidney cells. (Trade names include Benemial and Probalan.)

procarbazine hydrochloride   A cytotoxic drug used in treating HODGKIN'S DISEASE and certain other neoplastic diseases. (Trade name is Matulane.)

prochlorperazine   An antiemetic (antinausea) drug. (The trade name is Compazine.)

Procrit   See EPOGEN.

proctitis   Infections of the ANUS and RECTUM.

proctocolitis   An inflamed condition of the COLON and RECTUM.

prodromal stages   Stages of infection that fall short of the onset of a full-blown disease. In cases of HIV infection, stages that do not meet the CDC criteria for a diagnosis of AIDS.

prodrome   A complex of physical and clinical signs and symptoms that may precede the onset of a full-blown disease.

prodrug   A compound that is converted within the body into an active form that has medical effects. Prodrugs are useful when an active drug may be too toxic to administer systemically, is absorbed poorly by the digestive tract, or broken down before it reaches its target.

progesterone   A female hormone produced by the ovaries.

progesterone implant   A surgically implanted contraceptive for women that prevents pregnancy for up to five years. It consists of six match-size flexible rubber capsules, each containing the synthetic progestin levonorgestrel, which is present in some birth control pills. This hormone is released slowly through the walls of the capsules until the capsules are removed. The capsules can be felt and sometimes can be noticed as ridges or bumps. The capsules are implanted beneath the skin of the inner arm just above the elbow. The procedure takes approximately 15 minutes and is performed in a physician's office under a local anesthetic. When the rods are removed, fertility is restored. Possible side effects include amenorrhea, menstrual irregularities, weight change, mood swings, and headache. (Trade name is Norplant.)

progestin A hormone produced by the corpus luteum, placenta, or adrenal cortex (or synthetically manufactured) that has progesteronelike effects. Synthetic progestin is used as a contraceptive.

prognosis A forecast of the probable course and/or outcome of a disease. Currently, scientists believe that all patients who are infected with HIV will progress to the AIDS stage and die. The length of time between infection and death may be brief or many years. The time from infection to clinical signs is, on the average, 10 to 11 years.

progressive multifocal leukoencephalopathy (PML) A central nervous system disease that results in the destruction of brain tissue and the sheath that covers the nerves. PML develops in approximately 4–5 percent of HIV-infected individuals. It should be considered in cases of progressive neurologic disease in HIV-infected patients. PML results in HIV-infected persons due to infection with a virus called the JC VIRUS. It is believed that up to 80 percent of the population contracted this asymptomatic virus of the kidney in childhood. In a person with a weak immune system, the virus is reactivated and spread to the brain by white blood cells from the bone marrow. Once in the brain, the virus infects the brain cells responsible for producing the protective sheath around the nerves. Without this protection on the nerves, nerve cells die and cause lesions in the brain. Neurologic dysfunction may follow quickly.

PML can cause a series of symptoms related to neurological impairment, including confusion, disorientation, lack of energy, loss of balance, weakness in the arms or legs, speech problems, blurred or double vision, and blindness. The onset is gen-erally subacute with slowly progressive neurologic dysfunction. Dementia, visual defects, hemiparesis, ataxia, difficulties with speech and language, abnormal gait, sensory deficits, or other focal deficits may occur. Altered consciousness resulting from brain swelling does not occur. Physically, focal neurologic deficits are apparent. Patients are generally afebrile. Diagnosis is by CT or MRI. These studies reveal focal or diffuse lesions in the white matter typically without mass effect or contrast enhancement. MRI is more sensitive than CT. The white matter lesions observed with PML may be mimicked by those seen with HIV encephalopathy. The definitive diagnosis rests on brain biopsy.

No effective treatment for PML has been identified. PML is usually rapidly progressive and fatal, although rare cases of prolonged survival and remission have been documented. There have been contradictory reports of arrested symptoms and remission of lesions after initiation of protease-containing antiretroviral regimens. Cidofovir, a nucleotide analog approved for the treatment of cytomegalovirus, may be effective against JC virus. Treatment with HAART alone and treatment with cidofovir alone do not seem to combat PML effectively. Various case study reports have observed that whereas one treatment may not be effective, concomitant treatment with cidofovir and HAART may be effective to treat PML. Studies are currently looking at the use of intrathecal cytosine arabinoside (ara-C, cytarabine) for PML; of topotecan, an experimental DNA topoisomerase I inhibitor; and of alpha-interferon treatment, in addition to HAART. Other studies are looking at whether administration of low-dose chlorpromazine and neutralizing antibodies in combination inhibits the spread of the JC virus and essentially halts the progression of PML. Note too that some reports have suggested that HAART may exacerbate PML.

Although rare cases of spontaneous sustained remission have been reported, the prognosis is poor with the mean length of survival <6 months after the onset of neurologic symptoms.

proinflammatory cytokine Soluble chemical messengers produced by white blood cells (leukocytes) that trigger an inflammatory immune response and may, as a side effect, stimulate HIV, which only infects and replicates in activated cells. See TUMOR NECROSIS FACTOR; INTERLEUKIN-2.

project inform   Founded in 1985, a San Francisco–based project that is the nation's leading and most respected community-based AIDS treatment information and advocacy organization. Services include a toll-free Treatment Information Hotline, free publications (*PI Perspective*, a quarterly HIV treatment journal, fact sheets on therapies and diseases, and position papers on complex and timely issues about HIV treatments and research), outreach ("town hall meetings"), and activism. Project Inform's Treatment Action Network (TAN) is a national grassroots network whose members respond to public issues about AIDS research and access to treatments. TAN plays an important role in protecting and increasing federal funding for AIDS research, prevention, care, and housing.

Project Inform is credited for compiling *The HIV Drug Book*, the first comprehensive, user-friendly guide to all the drugs most used by people with HIV/AIDS. Formatted for quick reference and written in nontechnical language, the handbook features an extensive master index. Drug descriptions are categorized by their specific treatments. Drug profiles include antibiotics, anticancer drugs, antidiarrheal drugs, antifungal drugs, antihistamines, antinausea/antivomiting drugs, antiprotozoal drugs, antiseizure drugs, antiulcer drugs, antiviral drugs, antiwasting treatments, corticosteroids, immune-based therapy, neuropathy drugs, pain relievers, psychoactive drugs, and vaccines.

proliferation   Rapid or uncontrolled reproduction or replication.

promiscuity   Characterized by having numerous sexual partners on a casual basis. Because sexual intercourse is one of the principal routes of HIV transmission, the AIDS epidemic has fostered a new etiquette of sex. A woman or man can no longer actively or passively participate in continual one night stands or a freewheeling lifestyle and still secure a healthy future. The AIDS epidemic urges us to change the habitual sexual expectation of unprotected intercourse. Developing new habits with each of our partners is the only way to keep ourselves safe. In practical terms, this means we must scrupulously be careful to practice safer sex in all relationships except those that are long-term and monogamous—and be absolutely trustworthy. The importance of trustworthy monogamy, even among loving, lifelong partnerships, cannot be underestimated. Similarly, the risk of being promiscuous cannot be underestimated. Promiscuity does not accommodate new dating rituals, such as a period of healthy skepticism and information gathering, slower moves toward the bedroom, insistence on intimacy before intercourse, a shift toward monogamous, long-term relationships, and increased acceptance of periodic abstinence and celibacy.

prophylactic   An agent or regimen that contributes to the prevention of infection and disease. Also popular term for a condom. See PROPHYLAXIS.

prophylactic vaccine   See VACCINE.

prophylaxis   Any intervention intended to preserve health and prevent the initial occurrence (PRIMARY PROPHYLAXIS) or the recurrence (SECONDARY PROPHYLAXIS) of a disease. The intervention may be in the form of a drug (such as a vaccine) or other treatment or the use of a device (such as a condom).

propolis   A sticky resin present in the buds and bark of certain trees and plants. It is collected by bees for the purpose of repairing combs, filling cracks, and making the entrance to the hive waterproof. There is anecdotal evidence that propolis may be of benefit in treating certain diseases. Scientific IN VITRO investigations indicate that the material inhibits the reproduction of certain viruses.

prospective study   A study designed to follow the progress of a cohort forward in time, rather than analyzing data from previous research.

prostaglandin   A variety of naturally occurring aliphatic acid (a series of organic chemical compounds characterized by open chains of carbon atoms) with various biological activities, including increasing vascular permeability, smoothing muscle contraction, relieving bronchial constriction, and altering the pain threshold.

prostate gland A muscular gland that surrounds the first inch of the male urethra; secretes an alkaline fluid that becomes part of semen. Its smooth muscle contributes to ejaculation.

prostitute Anyone who agrees to participate in sexual acts for money; a whore. Unmodified, the term generally applies to women. If male prostitutes or prostitution are discussed, they are generally so identified. Slang terms include *call girl, fille de joie, ho,* and *working girl.*

protease A protein enzyme (of the HIV virus) that is crucial to the life cycle of HIV. Protease plays a major role in viral infectivity and replication. It is used by the virus to clip a long HIV protein molecule, known as Gag-Pol, into a number of smaller proteins. Each of these smaller units then assists in the assembly of proteins and genetic material into a mature, and infectious, viral particle. These clips can occur only because, before the process begins, protease is able to cut itself loose from the other components of the larger, inactive viral protein, a process known as autocatalysis.

HIV protease is quite small and makes an ideal target to stop HIV replication. It is a member of the aspartylprotease enzyme family that also includes the major human enzymes renin (which regulates kidney action) and pepsin (which digests protein in the stomach). See PROTEASE INHIBITOR.

protease inhibitors A class of antiretroviral drugs that block the production of infectious HIV virions by inhibiting the action of HIV's protease enzyme, protease inhibitors constitute the second drug class in the history of anti-HIV drug development. They revolutionized antiretroviral therapy when they first appeared.

The viral enzyme protease plays an essential role during the final stages of the viral life cycle. The enzyme, a protein product of HIV replication, is packaged by the new virus particles. As these new particles bud from the host cell, protease cleaves immature polyproteins into smaller, functional proteins that are necessary components of the mature virion. Without these proteins, the budding particles are not infectious. Protease inhibitors (PIs) bind to the enzyme's active site and block its activity. Since these drugs act at a later phase of the viral life cycle, they have no protective effect on cells whose genomes already contain integrated proteins.

Protease inhibitors with potent and selective antiretroviral activity in cell culture were identified in 1988, but the insolubility, poor oral absorption, and rapid liver metabolism of candidate drugs delayed the identification of suitable therapeutic agents until 1992. From the time they were first marketed in 1996, protease inhibitors have been hailed as lifesaving antiretroviral drugs. Word quickly spread that protease inhibitors used alone or in combination with two or three of the nucleoside or nonnucleoside reverse transcriptase drugs dropped viral load counts to unmeasurable or undetectable levels in people with HIV disease and in AIDS patients. Studies also showed that those with significantly lowered viral loads demonstrated surprising recovery—their T4 cells rebounded, in some cases from below 200 to back up to, or approaching, normal. These "AIDS cocktails," as the combination therapies were soon called, gave people with AIDS a new chance at a productive life for the first time since the beginning of the pandemic in the United States in 1981.

A variety of downsides of this gift were identified—ranging from metabolic to psychological concerns, and including the limitation that not all who would benefit from the drug cocktail could afford it. Additionally, for those who have access to these drugs, downsides include guilt, the challenge of reestablishing relationships, the loss of disability pay (after return to work), and the myriad dilemmas of returning to work. There were also treatment downsides: treatment success may create a false sense of security and lead to complacency in prevention efforts. Another downside is that the therapy is not available to 95 percent of the population of HIV-infected people, even in developed countries such as the United States. What of the millions of others living with HIV infected worldwide? Political downsides were also noted: the premature declaration of victory might lead to a weakening of the political will to fight the disease.

Today there is a major rift in the HIV/AIDS community concerning the use of protease inhibitors. On the one hand, protease inhibitors have saved people's lives. On the other hand, their side effects are occasionally fatal, and some have damaged and altered physical appearance. Note that these side effects are not unique to HIV disease: many other illnesses and their treatments produce changes in appearance. Drug cocktails that comprise protease inhibitors—now considered to be the standard treatment for infected patients who are both sick and healthy—have caused many to suffer liver damage, kidney failure, strokes, kidney stones, heart attacks, and other devastating side effects that are deemed inevitable by advocates of the new antiretroviral treatments but called horrific and unnecessary by opponents. The jury is still out as to whether protease inhibitors have helped more people than they have hurt. To date, the people for whom benefit has been proved beyond a doubt are really sick people who would have died without them. Opponents note that the target population for the drug therapy are those who are still healthy and question the extent to which these people will have their lives shortened by these drugs.

Six protease inhibitors have been approved by the Food and Drug Administration as part of a combination antiretroviral regimen: saquinavir (approved December 1995), ritonavir (approved March 1996), indinavir (approved March 1996), nelfinavir (approved March 1997), amprenavir (approved April 1999), and Keletra (lopinavir/ritonavir, approved September 2000). Note that saquinavir is available both as a soft-gel capsule (Fortovase) and as a hard gel capsule (Invirase). All inhibit HIV-1 and HIV-2 protease. Awaiting approval as of this writing is atazanivir.

As a group, protease inhibitors are tolerated fairly well. All approved PIs are metabolized by and also inhibit the CYTOCHROME P450 enzyme system, primarily by isoenzymes from the 3A4 family, and there is potential for pharmcokinetic interactions between it and other drugs metabolized by this system. Drugs that inhibit P450 enzymes increase plasma PI concentrations; drugs that induce P450 enzymes accelerate PI clearance. These changes in plasma PI levels may cause toxicity or resistance. It is also important to be aware of potentially toxic interactions between this drug class and other medications. On the other hand, taking two PIs at the same time has beneficial results. Ritonavir, the most potent P450 enzyme inhibitor to date, dramatically increases plasma levels of other PIs that

are normally difficult to maintain because of their rapid clearance or poor absorption. In general, these drugs must be taken at specific times relative to meals: that is, some must be taken on a full stomach and others on an empty stomach.

It is important to note that all antiretroviral agents have potentially serious toxic and adverse events associated with their use. Without exception, protease inhibitors cause significant side effects. All cause gastrointestinal and metabolic disturbances, particularly LIPODYSTROPHY syndrome (lipoatrophy, central fat accumulation, and increased blood fat-levels). Although similar changes have occurred in HIV-positive individuals who were not taking any anti-HIV medications, the effect appears to be worsened by the use of protease inhibitors. All currently approved protease inhibitors have been associated with this condition. Its clinical significance is unknown. Further study of large numbers of patients for longer periods is needed before any change in antiretroviral therapy or use of lipid level–lowering drugs can be recommended. Additionally, each drug has its own dose-limiting toxicity. A serious side effect of indinavir is nephrolithiasis (kidney stones); nefinavir causes significant diarrhea. Managing PI side effects has become an important component of HIV treatment.

Which protease inhibitor to use in a drug regimen depends on many factors, including the individual patient's medical profile and lifestyle. An individual's prior experience on HIV therapy is also a factor in formulating an antiretroviral regimen. Current guidelines for antiretroviral therapy for adults outline the use of available treatment regimens for individuals with no prior or limited experience on HIV therapy. In accordance with the established goals of HIV therapy, priority is given to regimens in which clinical trial data suggest the following: sustained suppression of HIV plasma RNA (particularly in patients with high baseline viral load), sustained increase of CD4+ T-cell count (in most cases more than 48 weeks), and favorable clinical outcome (i.e., delayed progression to AIDS and death). Particular emphasis is given to regimens that have been compared directly to other regimens that perform sufficiently well with regard to these parameters to be included in the "Strongly Recommend" category. Additional consideration is given to the regimen's PILL BURDEN, dosing frequency, food requirements, convenience, toxicity, and drug interaction profile when compared with other regimens.

Note that the possibility of drug interactions is particularly a problem in persons who are being treated with multiple drugs, and it can influence the choice of drugs to be used in combination. For example, protease inhibitors affect the metabolism of the drug rifampin, which is sometimes given for active tuberculosis. At the same time, rifampin lowers the blood level of protease inhibitors and thus can reduce their therapeutic effectiveness.

Medical complications of advanced HIV disease can also influence the use of combination antiretroviral therapy. Wasting and anorexia can prevent individuals from following the dietary requirements necessary for effective absorption of protease inhibitors. Protease inhibitors may pose a greater risk of liver effects for individuals with HIV-related liver dysfunction. Because of the broad possibilities for detrimental drug interactions, individuals taking antiretroviral therapy should always discuss with the physician any new drugs they may consider taking, including over-the-counter and "alternative" medications.

Although research has established sound principles of HIV treatment, all anti-HIV drugs have advantages and disadvantages, and there is still no standard way of combining and using them. The treatment of HIV disease remains in flux, and the use of HAART is still under study. For this reason, an individual seeking treatment for HIV disease is best advised to rely on a physician experienced in this disease.

protease paunch An informal term used to describe an accumulation of fat in the abdomen. The syndrome is possibly linked to treatment with PROTEASE INHIBITORS. See LIPODYSTROPHY.

protective equipment CDC guidelines *(Guidelines for Prevention of Transmission of Human Immunodeficiency Virus (HIV) and Hepatitis B Virus (HBV) to Health-Care and Public-Safety Workers)* recommend that masks, eyewear, and gowns should be present on all emergency vehicles that respond to medical emergencies or victim rescues and used in accordance with the level of exposure encountered. The guide-lines also recommend that masks and eyewear should be worn together, or a face shield should be used in any situation where splashing of blood or other body fluids to which universal precautions apply are likely to occur. http://www.cdc.gov/epo/mmwr/preview/mmwrhtml/00001450.htm.

protein Large molecule made up of long sequences of amino acids. Some hormones, enzymes, and cellular structures are proteins. Three-fourths of the dry weight of most cells consists of proteins. The HIV protease enzyme is made of a protein with two main moving parts hinged by a flexible sequence of amino acids. The job of the HIV protease is to attach to other HIV precursor proteins and cut them apart between specific amino acid pairs. After the HIV substrate proteins have been cut, they are free to fold themselves into the various structural bits and machinery that make up a new HIV particle. These new proteins may include parts of the inner and outer shells of HIV as well as the HIV enzymes reverse transcriptase, integrase, and protease itself. If HIV protease can be prevented from cutting the HIV substrate protein in the right places, the virus cannot replicate (the function that protease inhibitors are designed to fulfill).

protein binding A process that inactivates some of the drug in the bloodstream and carries it throughout the body.

protein S Protein S is involved in preventing spontaneous formation of clots; a deficiency predisposes to thrombotic (clotting) episodes. It is unclear why some HIV-positive persons have protein S deficiency and are consequently at higher risk of unprovoked thrombotic episodes.

proteinuria The presence of protein in the urine. Proteinuria generally indicates some form of kidney disease.

Proteus A bacteria genus that can cause cystitis; found in feces.

protocol The blueprint or design for an experimental drug trial that describes the trial's rationale, treatment duration, and who and how many may participate.

protozoan   A one-celled organism of the animal kingdom containing many different species. Some protozoa (plural) cause disease in humans, notably TOXOPLASMOSIS and CRYPTOSPORIDIOSIS, especially in the setting of altered immunity.

provider referral   The process by which health care providers find the sex or needle-sharing partners of people found to be infected with HIV (based on information given voluntarily by the infected people), notify them of their exposure to the virus, and refer than for examination or treatment. See PARTNER NOTIFICATION.

provirus   A copy of the genetic information of an animal virus that is integrated into the DNA of an infected cell. Copies of the provirus are passed on to each of the infected cell's daughter cells.

prunellin   The active component of the herb prunella vulgaris *(Prunella vulgaris labiatae),* known as heal-all or self-heal, once used to treat cuts and wounds. Test tube studies have shown that prunellin can block cell-to-cell transmission of HIV. Other in vitro studies suggest that prunellin also inhibits REVERSE TRANSCRIPTASE because of its content of anionic polysaccharides, which are known to inhibit reverse transcriptase in such drugs as HEPARIN.

prurient   Having to do with, or arousing, an "unhealthy" interest in sex; from a Latin root meaning "to itch."

pruritus   Itching, as a symptom. It may be paroxysmal or constant, may be associated with skin lesions or occur independent of any skin lesion.

pseudovirion   A viruslike particle that resembles a virus but does not contain its genetic information and cannot replicate. In some viral diseases pseudovirions can interfere with infection by the real infectious virus.

psittacosis   An infectious disease caused by Chlamydia *psittaci* in parrots and other birds that may be transmitted to humans. TETRACYCLINES, ERYTHROMYCIN, and PENICILLIN are effective in treatment.

psoriasis   A common chronic disease of the skin in which erythematous papules coalesce to form plaques with distinct borders. As the disease progresses, and if left untreated, a silvery yellow-white scale develops. New lesions tend to appear at sites of trauma. They may be in any location, but most frequently are located on the scalp, knees, elbows, umbilicus, and genitalia. Severity and clinical course are variable. The cause of psoriasis is unknown, but a genetic factor is present. Certain conditions, such as infection, some drugs, climate, and perhaps hormonal factors and smoking, may trigger attacks.

psychobiology   The process of interaction between body and mind in the formation and functioning of personality; also the study of such interaction.

psychological dependence   A subjective need for a specific psychoactive substance, either for its positive effects or to avoid negative effects associated with its absence. See ADDICTION.

psychological factors   The psychological or internal challenges a person with HIV/AIDS faces vary from individual to individual. Not everyone will experience all of the emotional responses or stages of the emotional responses described. Each HIV/AIDS situation is as unique as the people involved.

Due to the "terminal" prognosis associated with AIDS, diagnosis can be catastrophic to the individual, who might face catastrophic changes not only in their personal and job relationships, but in their physical bodies and in their self-images and self-esteem as well. Initially, daily routine may be interrupted; income may be disrupted or diminished. Diagnosis could lead to feeling the sense of loss of control of one's life.

Coping with an HIV or AIDS diagnosis involves confronting fear and denial while maintaining hope. After diagnosis the patients may respond with shock or disbelief. After the initial shock and disbelief may come denial, an attempt to ignore or forget the diagnosis. Hiding in denial allows a person time to regroup and become prepared to deal with the challenges ahead. After denial, a bargaining stage often occurs, hopefully followed with an ongoing commitment to work on the challenges at hand and toward recovery. Some persons with AIDS, though, give up and never allow themselves to see beyond the possibility of their own demise.

Several other possible emotional responses are noted. Coping with an HIV or AIDS diagnosis may also involve confronting or reexamining one's sexual identity and the behavioral choices one has made in support of that identity. By associating HIV/AIDS with what society has traditionally considered illicit or immoral, the person with HIV/AIDS is faced with working through his or her feelings so that his or her sexual identity may be reaffirmed in such a way as to allow him or her to feel good about himself or herself. Changing sex habits is part and parcel of living with HIV/AIDS.

In a similar vein, coping with an HIV or AIDS diagnosis may also involve confronting or reexamining one's use of drugs and/or alcohol and the behavioral choices one has made in support of that identity.

Persons with HIV/AIDS are also confronted with other people seeing them as "contagious," which may cause them to feel undesirable. This is another emotion that can cause a person with AIDS to become isolated—emotionally, geographically, or both.

One of the biggest and most destructive stressors is that of feeling isolated. This sense of isolation can stem from many factors, including the withdrawal of support by lovers, family, and friends; the isolation from friends and daily routine due to hospitalization; and the general public's ongoing failure to respond to people with HIV/AIDS as it has to others who are ill. Finally, the sexual and personal precautions persons with HIV/AIDS must take to protect themselves and others certainly underscore the feelings of being "different" and alone.

A second destructive stressor is that of feeling being dependent. In addition to having to rely more heavily on family and friends for emotional support, many people with HIV/AIDS are faced with applying for social services for the first time. The experience of applying for social services is almost always frustrating and demoralizing. Additionally, there is the conflict between continuing to work and remaining self-sufficient or forgoing work in order to be eligible for services. Applying for help is one thing; accepting and using the services is another. There is a final aspect of dependence that is potentially the most frustrating of all: the fear of a protracted illness that will drain family and friends financially as well as emotionally.

The person with HIV/AIDS will likely respond to the experience, and those described above, with a wide variety of emotions: anger, depression, fear, guilt, despair, anxiety, hurt, sadness, and, at times, joy, peace and happiness. These feelings change frequently and, if they become too intense, they can become immobilizing. Or, because it is possible to experience a combination of hopeless lows and hopeful highs at the same time, the person with AIDS can become snared in the emotional confusion and be unable to move ahead with life.

psychological need   Persons with HIV/AIDS generally experience a range of psychological needs. These needs vary with the stage in the illness plus other factors. As with psychological factors, experiences vary from individual to individual. Not everyone will experience all of the needs described below.

At diagnosis, people with HIV/AIDS may have an increased need for physical contact and emotional intimacy. These feelings may be enhanced by emotions that arise in coping with an HIV or AIDS diagnosis. But during this time, due to fear and a sense of helplessness, lovers, family, and friends may withdraw their support. When this happens, the person with AIDS may feel alone and isolated.

The need to remain independent often accompanies and increases with the progression of the illness. Accepting increasing dependency is part and parcel of living with HIV/AIDS. At various stages of the illness, people with HIV/AIDS may have an increased need for different kinds of help: help with understanding the medical aspects of their diagnosis; with coping with the diagnosis; with identifying alternative treatments; with maintaining order as concerns legal and financial matters; with their emotions; and with coping on a day-to-day basis. Asking for help is one thing; accepting and utilizing the help of friends, family members, AIDS service providers, and others is just as important.

psychological services   Because HIV/AIDS effects not only the body, but also emotions and interpersonal relations, and because self-empowerment in the age of AIDS is increasingly important, the role of psychological services is often critical to the well-being of the AIDS-inflicted person. Psychological services are also designed to support AIDS care-givers and those (partners, family, friends) coping with the fear of AIDS. These services often focus on living or on dying. They may include peer counsel-ing or counseling by social workers; support groups (either facilitated or unfacilitated); therapy groups (generally facilitated by a mental health profes-sional); or individual therapy (provided by mental health professionals including psychologists, psy-chiatrists, psychiatric nurses). They may be pro-vided independently, under the auspices of an AIDS service provider, under the auspices of AIDS-advocacy organization, or by another organization. They may be free or fee-based.

In thinking about psychological services, it is important to note that one's religion also offers human and spiritual support. Priests, rabbis, minis-ters, nuns, pastors of all religions give help in a sim-ilar fashion as social workers and psychologists, but they talk particularly to people strictly on a religious level. They offer advice, comfort, and company.

psychoneuroimmunology The study of the interrelationships between psychology, the nerv-ous system, and the immune system.

psychosis Loosely, any mental disorder; more specifically, the term is used to refer to a particular class or group of mental disorders, particularly to differentiate this condition from neurosis, sociopa-thy, character disorder, psychosomatic disorder, and mental retardation. Traditionally, the psychoses are subdivided into organic brain syndromes, func-tional psychoses, schizophrenia, affective psychoses (e.g., manic-depressive psychoses), paranoid states, and psychotic depressive reaction. As a result of conflicting usage over time, there is no single acceptable definition of what psychosis is. In gen-eral, however, the disorders labeled psychoses differ from the other groups of psychiatric disorders in severity, degree of withdrawal, affectivity, intellect, and regression. The psychoses are "major" disorders in that they are more severe, intense, and disrup-tive; they tend to affect all areas of the patient's life.

The psychotic patient is less able to maintain effec-tive object relationships; external, objective reality has less meaning for the patient or is perceived in a distorted way. The emotions are often qualitatively different from the normal, at other times are so exaggerated quantitatively that the constitute the whole existence of the patient. Intellectual func-tions may be directly involved by the psychotic process so that language and thinking are disturbed; judgment often fails; and hallucinations and delu-sions may appear. Finally, there may be generalized failure of functioning and a falling back to very early behavioral levels. Such regression is more than a temporary lapse in maturity and may include a return to early and primitive patterns.

psychosocial Pertaining to the effects on individ-uals and groups of the interaction between social conditions and psychological functioning. In a health care context, the term refers to psychologi-cal support services concerned with such effects, often needed by persons with HIV infection.

psychosocial intervention A therapeutic inter-vention that uses cognitive, cognitive-behavioral, behavioral, and supportive interventions to relieve pain. These include patient education, interven-tions aimed at aiding relaxation, psychotherapy, and structured or peer support.

psychostimulants A class of drugs used to stimu-late the central nervous system. Psychostimulants are sometimes used in the treatment of DEPRESSION and HIV ENCEPHALOPATHY. These medications are very addictive and may activate an addiction to stimulants (amphetamines) in a patient in recov-ery. Side effects include insomnia, loss of appetite, loss of weight, and paranoia.

psychotic disorder See PSYCHOSIS.

psychotropic drug A drug that affects psychic function, behavior, or experience. Many drugs are intended to be psychotropic, but others also may produce undesired psychotropic side effects.

PTSD See POST-TRAUMATIC STRESS SYNDROME.

pubic hair Hair growth around the genitals. Pubic hair first appears during puberty, when adult sexual characteristics develop.

pubic louse (pl. lice) A parasitic insect that may infest the pubic area. See CRAB LOUSE.

pubis Another term for the pubic area.

public accommodation Since the enactment of the Civil Rights Acts of 1964, discrimination on the basis of race, color, religion, and national origin has been unlawful in places of public accommodation. The concept of public accommodation has traditionally encompassed eating establishments, hotels and motels, theaters, and other facilities open to the public. But with the onset of the AIDS epidemic, there have been calls to extend the concept to include a variety of professional services as well. Among the first such services was that provided by the funeral industry. Other professions have been affected as well. Denial of medical and dental services to those infected by HIV has been a particular problem. Institutional settings where health care is given are considered public accommodations under the law and some courts have interpreted this to include doctors' and dentists' offices as well as hospitals and clinics. Standard protective procedures adequately protect health care workers, and the medical as well as legal consensus is that people with AIDS should not be denied treatment.

public aid A generic term for basic state social support services (welfare).

public assistance See PUBLIC AID.

public health The combined medical and social service discipline providing protection and promotion of community health through institutional and collective measures.

Public Health Service (PHS) The federal agency charged by law to promote and assure the highest level of health attainable for every individual and family in the United States and to develop cooperation in health projects with other nations. The major functions of the service are to stimulate and assist states and communities with the development of local health resources and to further the development of education for the health professions; to assist with improvement of the delivery of health services to all Americans; to conduct and support research in the medical and related sciences and to disseminate scientific information; to protect the health of the nation against impure and unsafe foods, drugs, cosmetics, and other potential hazards; and to provide national leadership for the prevention and control of communicable disease and for other public health functions. The PHS has its origin in an act of July 16, 1798, authorizing marine hospitals for the care of U.S. merchant seamen. Subsequent legislation has vastly broadened the scope of its activities. The Public Health Service Act of July 1, 1944, consolidated and revised substantially all existing legislation relating to the Public Health Service. The basic PHS legal responsibilities have been broadened and expanded many times since 1944.

Public Health Service Act Legislation signed by the president July 1, 1944, and administered by the FOOD AND DRUG ADMINISTRATION (FDA). The act gives the FDA authority to ensure safety, purity, and potency of vaccines, blood, serum, and other biological products. It also empowers the FDA to ensure the safety of pasteurized milk and shellfish, as well as the sanitation of food services and sanitary facilities for travelers on buses, trains, and planes. See FOOD AND DRUG ACT OF 1906.

Public Health Service Act, Title VI The section of the PUBLIC HEALTH SERVICE ACT, which, with title XVI of that act, authorizes and sets forth the requirements of the federal HILL-BURTON program.

Public Law 92-603 The 1972 federal statute that created Supplemental Security Income (SSI) and introduced a set of complex state options, some with burdensome antirecipient biases, to the system. Up until 1972, everything was relatively simple: everyone on Aid to Families with Dependent Children (AFDC) and the old state welfare programs for the aged, blind, and disabled got automatic Medicaid cards. About half of the states also covered the "medically needy": AFDC-type families and aged, blind, and disabled people who started out "too rich" for welfare but whose medical bills "spent them down" to the Medicaid level. The changes made by P.L. 92-603, and the wide range of state options exercised under its provisions, introduced what are often described as even more Byzantine complexities into the welfare system. Highlights of 92-603 follow.

As a result of the addition of Title XVI (SSI) to the Social Security Act, states were required to allow Medicaid eligibility for SSI recipients but not necessarily automatically. Section 1634 of the amended act provided for state-SSA contracts for "automatic" Medicaid for SSI recipients, but only at state option. Section 209(B) of the law allowed states to retain some or all of the stricter Medicaid eligibility rules from their pre-SSI welfare programs. This "loophole" was added to save the poorer, less liberal states from the sudden Medicaid budget increases that would result if they had to give Medicaid to all those newly eligible under the more liberal SSI rules. However, Congress provided a "sop" to the recipients in states that take this option: if the state did not already have a "spend down" rule for those "too rich" for Medicaid, it had to allow one if it took this "209(b)" option. Finally, Section 1616 of the amended act allowed states to give higher incomes to their needy aged, blind, and disabled by having the SSA simultaneously pay out "State Supplementary Payments (SSPs)" as part of, and on top of, the SSI payment. Thus, state-financed SSPs could, in effect, "raise" the SSI (and, therefore, the Medicaid) level in those liberal states wishing to be more generous. This feature was made optional for the states.

pulmonary alveolar proteinosis   A disease of unknown cause in which EOSINOPHILIC material is deposited in the alveoli. Principal symptom is DYSPNEA. Death from pulmonary insufficiency may occur, but complete recovery has been observed. There is no specific treatment, but general supportive measures, including ANTIBIOTICS and BRONCHOALVEALOR LAVAGE have helped.

puncture wound   A wound made by piercing with a sharp instrument.

purified protein derivative   A protein-rich material derived from the MICROORGANISM *Mycobacterium tuberculosis* and used as a skin-test reagent to detect current or prior infection with that organism.

purified protein derivative (PPD) test   A simple data test used to detect prior exposure to TUBERCULOSIS. PPD is injected under the skin of the forearm. After 48 to 72 hours, the injection site will exhibit a hard red bump if the subject has been infected with TB.

purine   A white, crystalline compound from which a group of compounds including uric acid, xanthine, and caffeine is derived. Also, one of several purine derivatives, especially the bases adenine and guanine, which are fundamental constituents of nucleic acids.

purpura   A skin rash of purple or brownish red spots resulting from the bleeding into the skin of subcutaneous capillaries.

PWA   The abbreviation for *People With AIDS*. This label was devised to eliminate the moralizing character of the everyday discourse of AIDS, as in terms such as *AIDS patient*, *AIDS victim*, *innocent victim*, *invariably fatal*, and *promiscuous*. PWARC and PWHIV have been used as abbreviations, respectively, for persons with AIDS-related complex (once known as *pre-AIDS*) and persons with HIV infection. See PEOPLE WITH AIDS.

PWARC   See PWA.

pyelonephritis   Inflammation of kidney substance and pelvis, usually due to bacteria that have ascended from the bladder after entering through the urethra. Treatment generally begins with the recognition and removal of the cause substance; and includes measures to increase resistance of patient and bedrest. Alcohol and drugs irritating to the kidney should be avoided. Antipyretic drugs and an appropriate antibiotic are often administered. If there is urinary tract obstruction, surgery may be indicated. See NEPHRITIS.

pyrazinamide   An ANTIBIOTIC used in multidrug combinations to treat TUBERCULOSIS.

pyridoxine hydrochloride One of a group of substances, including pyridoxal and pyridoxamine, that make up vitamin B$_6$. (Trade names are Hexa-Betalin and Seesix.)

pyrimethamine An ANTIBIOTIC used to treat TOX-OPLASMOSIS, usually in combination with a sulfa drug such as SULFADIAZINE or CLINDAMYCIN. The major side effect after prolonged use is ANEMIA. Other side effects include gastric intolerance, allergic reactions, and HEPATITIS, some of which are attributable to the sulfa drug that is taken with it. To avoid anemia, another drug, leucovorin, is given at the same time.

Pyrimethamine is a FOLIC-ACID antagonist that interferes with the uptake of this essential B vitamin in susceptible parasites, including those that cause MALARIA and toxoplasmosis, thus weakening and eventually killing these organisms. Because parasites can rapidly develop resistance to pyrimethamine, the drug is usually used in combination with a sulfa drug. The activity of the combination against parasites greatly exceeds that of either drug used alone. FOLINIC ACID is usually added to protect against BONE-MARROW toxicity. Because both drugs cross the BLOOD-BRAIN BARRIER, the combination is effective against toxoplasmosis encephalitis, a serious and potentially fatal infection of the brain. While the response to therapy is high, the relapse rate is also high when therapy is stopped, so lifelong maintenance is usually necessary. Pyrimethamine is also used alone and in combination with other drugs to prevent malaria or recurrent toxoplasmosis. Pyrimethamine is available for oral administration under the trade name Daraprim. The combination of pyrimethamine and sulfadoxine is sold under the trade name Fansidar.

pyrogen A substance that is released either endogenously from LEUKOCYTES or exogenously; usually from bacteria. It produces fever in susceptible hosts.

pyrogenic Producing fever.

QC-PCR (quantitative competitive PCR assay)
An assay test used to measure viral loads in HIV-positive people. It is a fairly expensive test but has proved reliable in measuring viral load in body fluids other than blood.

In QC-PCR, a known tiny amount of a control sequence, similar to the DNA sequence being tested but able to be distinguished, is added to the sample before the PCR process begins. During the successive doublings, both the target sequence (the one being looked for) and the control sequence are multiplied similarly. Finally, the quantity of the target sequence in the original sample is calculated from its ratio with the control sequence. Because it is a fairly labor-intensive test, its cost is high. It may be used only in clinical trial studies because of its high reliability but high cost.

QD (*quaque die*) Latin phrase that means "daily." Often used in a pharmacist's or doctor's prescription instructions.

q.i.d. (*quater in die*) Latin phrase that translates as "four times a day." The letters *Q.I.D.* often appear in a pharmacist's or doctor's prescription instructions.

QOL See QUALITY OF LIFE.

q.q.h. (*quaque quarta hora*) Latin phrase that translates as "every four hours."

quack One who pretends to have knowledge or skill in medicine. One of the social consequences of the AIDS epidemic has been the rise in quackery in general, hardly a surprise when one considers the exploitative and sensational media coverage of the epidemic, its size and cost, the politics of medical research and funding, and the relationship between money and expertise.

qualitative assay A medical test that determines the presence or absence of a particular substance.

quality of care In social-service terms, the impact of medical, psychological, or social support care on quality of life. Most analyses focus on medical treatment and use scales that measure changes in various indicators of health status (individual comfort, mobility, etc.). Well-known scales include the Karnofsy Index, Sickness Impact Profile, Symptom Distress Scale, Spitzer Quality of Life Index, McMaster Health Index, and Nottingham Health Profiles. Each of these has its own criteria for types of care, health status, and how different aspects of care are compared and weighed.

quality of life A subjective concept that differs for each person and may vary for the same individual as that person's situation changes. The holistic treatment of a patient requires that the health care team assess what is most important to that individual. In persons with certain diseases, it may not be possible to establish and maintain complete freedom from the signs and symptoms of the disease. In these cases, the goal is to have quality of life be as good as possible despite the disease. In persons who have suffered disabilities, the goal is to have perceived quality of life associated with remaining capabilities rather than on what has been lost.

The Medical Outcome Study (MOS) is an example of a reliable quality of life measure for persons with HIV infection and AIDS. The basis for the

MOS analysis is a questionnaire in which patients rate their perception of 20 criteria, including physical, social, and mental functioning; health perceptions; and pain. The scale is especially sensitive to symptoms associated with HIV and AIDS.

quantitative assay A medical test that measures the amount of a particular substance in a specified sample size.

quarantine A state of physical isolation or restriction of movement imposed on carriers or potential carriers to prevent or control the spread of an infectious disease. Also, the period during which such isolation is imposed.

The possibility of quarantine has from time to time been raised by authorities, religious fundamentalists, or others as a way of restricting the spread of AIDS. Quarantine, probably the oldest public health measure, developed from concepts of spiritual uncleanliness. In the Middle Ages it was used against those suffering from either leprosy or the PLAGUE, and quarantine of lepers persisted well into the 20th century. Certain diseases are still regarded as potentially quarantinable, but it is a measure most often used to contain animal diseases. Proposals to quarantine AIDS patients or homosexual establishments such as gay bathhouses and bars have occasionally been put forward. Fear, prejudice, and ignorance about the spread of the disease are generally considered to be at their root.

Those who argue in favor of AIDS quarantine generally focus on what they call "noncompliance," the failure or refusal of those who have the virus to refrain from repeating activity that risks its further spread. The examples most often cited are the PROSTITUTE who knows that he or she is HIV-positive and who won't stop turning tricks; the promiscuous individual who knows that he or she is HIV-positive and who, out of recklessness or viciousness, refuses to stop having unprotected sex; the INJECTION DRUG USER who continues to share needles even after being told of an HIV-positive status and of the consequences of further needle sharing.

Laws and regulations also isolate HIV-positive persons by limiting their interactions with others. In education, quarantine orders have been issued to remove HIV-positive children from public and private schools. Some states mandate hospital isolation of AIDS patients. Some federal employees must be HIV-tested by law; one identified as HIV-positive may be barred from certain jobs. In the military all personnel are HIV-tested twice yearly; HIV-positive persons are not deployed overseas or given sensitive assignments such as the Special Forces.

In prisons and jails, HIV quarantine is now common. Because of sexual violence behind bars, STDs spread like wildfire. Instead of ending the violence, corrections officers often quarantine the known HIV-positive individuals. HIV testing is mandatory for federal prisoners; state and county prisoners can be tested against their will in certain circumstances. Federal law prohibits HIV-positive prisoners from having conjugal visits. Given that most prisoners today are people of color, race weighs heavily in HIV quarantine.

Outside prison walls, probation can impose a de facto quarantine. Judges can—and do—order an individual HIV-positive prostitute to stay off the street. An HIV-positive man or woman can be ordered to stop having unprotected sex or stop having sex altogether.

queer Homosexual. In the early 20th century this was a derogatory term applied to male homosexuals only. In more recent usage it also applies to lesbians. Today, many gay men and lesbians, consciously refusing the implied condemnation, use the term to describe and identify themselves and their community.

The people and communities characterized as "queer" (like all other people and communities) are too diverse politically, economically, and demographically to be described adequately by a single reductive adjective. Nevertheless, in an age of identity politics, *queer* serves as an expedient term to define oneself or one's community in opposition to others, in this case the "straight" or the "mainstream."

quiescent Being in a state of rest; still; not moving. When used in a medical setting, it usually refers to an illness or disease that is currently inactive or in remission.

quilt   At an AIDS rally in San Francisco, protesters placed placards with the names of people who had died of AIDS on the walls of a building. This striking image—in which the whole was gigantic but the individual components were not lost—led the activist Cleve Jones to propose a huge memorial quilt composed of individual panels designed by lovers, family, friends, and others, in honor of one or more persons who died of AIDS-related causes. The colorful panels typically include photos, quotations, and other mementos of the deceased. By 1995, quilt-related activities had raised over $1.5 million for AIDS service organizations. Panels were included in President Bill Clinton's 1993 inaugural parade, the project was nominated for the Nobel Prize in peace in 1989, and the entire phenomenon was the subject of an Academy Award–winning documentary, *Common Threads: Stories from the Quilt*. Other artistic spin-offs have been *The AIDS Quilt Songbook* and *Quilt: A Musical Celebration*. The NAMES Project Foundation, headquartered in San Francisco, includes dozens of local chapters, as well as offering international, display, and direct service grant programs. (For more information on the Project, visit their webpage at http://www.aidsquilt.org). Far beyond anyone's expectations, the AIDS memorial quilt has become perhaps the single most widely recognized symbol of the epidemic. First unfurled on the National Mall in 1987, it has grown to proportions so large—over 50,000 panels covering more than 30 acres as of February 2002, that it can no longer be displayed in its entirety. It is, however, being placed on the World Wide Web at http://www.quilt.org.

For further information on Cleve Jones, see his biography, which also functions as both primer for activism and a complete history of the quilt's early days, *Stitching a Revolution: The Making of an Activist* (San Francisco: HarperCollins, 2000).

quinolone   A type of antibiotic medication used to treat a variety of bacterial illnesses. CIPROFLOXACIN and levofloxacin are two varieties of quinolones.

quinone   Important small hydrophobic components of the electron transport chain. Quinones carry the equivalent amount of electrons of a hydrogen atom. By alternating electron transfer between components that carry or do not carry a proton with the electron, protons can be moved across the membrane, setting up proton gradients. Most quinone molecules are not attached to proteins and diffuse rapidly in the plane of the membrane.

race/ethnicity For much of the first decade of the AIDS epidemic, the source and transmission of AIDS was attributed to black people, and specifically Africans. Later people of other races and ethnicities, such as Haitians and West Indians, were added to this hypothesis. This hypothesis was a form of scapegoating and resembles an earlier hypothesis that emerged when AIDS first appeared among white American homosexuals who became the obvious scapegoat. Given the racist stereotyping of black people as dirty, disease carrying, and sexually promiscuous, it was virtually inevitable that, on the first sighting of the disease among them, they would be associated with its source. Thus the "gay plague" changed overnight to the "Haitian disease." Although the Haitian hypothesis collapsed, the idea of black people as the source of AIDS was not abandoned. Attention shifted to the African continent itself, and medical scientists and journalists escalated their search for the origin of AIDS in Africa. Today our knowledge of the disease makes it clear that preconceptions and prejudices about Africa and Africans, coupled with assumptions about Western conditions and behavior, fueled the widespread, uncritical acceptance of the AIDS-from-Africa hypothesis by the normally skeptical scientific community, the media, and the public at large.

racial differences Today we have a relatively clear definition of the epidemiology of AIDS in most countries of the world. As the picture of AIDS becomes more clearly defined, the numbers continue to grow and change, and patterns emerge. The numbers show that there are widely variant patterns of HIV infection existing in the same population, as well as in different populations. Race may, and most likely does, influence an individual's experience of AIDS, but race in and of itself is not a risk factor for HIV infection or AIDS. On the other hand, the effects of infection on specific racial groups often varies for genetic and social reasons from the effects of infection on other groups.

radiation therapy Treatment of cancer with intense beams of radiation. The radiation actually kills cancer cells (and any cells it must pass through to get to cancer cells). Also, the branch of medicine that utilizes such treatment.

radiation-resistant HIV expression in vivo (R-HEV) A technique used in viral research since the 1960s, but until 1989 had not been previously applied to HIV. It consists of viral cultures on cells that have been treated with radiation. The goal is to measure the HIV expression levels of the patient's virus, following the theory that radiation will suppress cells carrying HIV but not express itself (radiation) in the patient.

Ordinary viral cultures are unreliable as a measure of disease progression. Part of the reason is that the latent virus, which is not causing any immediate problem, can be stimulated to become active by the culturing process itself, causing a positive result that does not reflect disease progression or poor prognosis for the patient.

In the R-HEV test, the radiation treatment causes the cells to die shortly after the time culturing begins. If the virus was latent at the time the blood was drawn from the patient, the cells containing the latent virus die without being able to infect cells in the culture medium. But if the virus was active in the patient, some of the infected cells will transmit the infection to cells in the culture medium. Eight separate wells are cultured for each test; the result reported by the R-HEV test is the percentage of wells which do grow the virus.

When it was announced, the R-HEV test promised to have great importance in speeding CLINICAL TRIALS of new AIDS drugs.

radiography   The making of images of the internal structures of the body through exposure to X radiation that acts on a sensitized film.

radioimmunoassay (RIA)   A very sensitive method of determining the concentration of substances, particularly the protein-bound HORMONES, in blood plasma. The procedure is based on the competitive inhibition or binding of radioactively labeled hormones to a specific ANTIBODY. It can also be used to determine the concentration of any substance that causes the production of a specific antibody or of antibodies themselves.

radioimmunoprecipitation (RIP)   Immunoprecipitation is the formation of a precipitate (a deposit separated from a suspension or solution by the reaction of a reagent that causes the deposit to fall to the bottom or float near the top) when an ANTIGEN and ANTIBODY interact.

radioimmunoprecipitation assay (RIPA)   A technically demanding method of HIV ANTIBODY testing used primarily in research. The virus is detected by the phenomenon of aggregation of sensitized ANTIGEN upon addition of specific antibody to antigen in solution (immunoprecipitation). The precipitate is then washed extensively and disrupted and distributed through a polyacrylamide gel. Antibody-antigen bands are detected by autoradiography. Autoradiography is the use of radiographs formed by radioactive materials present in the tissue or individual in investigating certain diseases. These "autoradiographs" are made possible by injecting radiochemicals into the tissue and then exposing X-ray film by placing the tissue adjacent to the film.

radiotherapy   See RADIATION THERAPY.

random controlled trial   An experimental study for assessing the effects of a particular variable, in which subjects are assigned on a random basis to either of two groups, experimental or control. The experimental group receives the drug or procedure being tested, while the control group does not. Laboratory tests or clinical evaluations are performed on both groups (usually using the double-blind technique) to determine the results.

randomization   In research, a method used to assign subjects to experimental groups. Prior to this step every attempt is made to ensure that the subjects are as equivalent as possible. Then by some random method, each individual in the study is assigned to either a treatment or nontreatment group. The purpose is to prevent inadvertent selection bias in research studies.

randomized   Pertaining to a study in which participants are selected randomly to receive either the treatment being studied or a PLACEBO. See RANDOMIZATION.

randomized controlled trials   See RANDOM CONTROLLED TRIAL.

randomized trial   See RANDOM CONTROLLED TRIAL.

rantes (Regulated-Upon-Activation, Normal T-Expressed and Secreted)   A chemokine protein that binds to the CCR5 receptor site and interferes with HIV's fusion with uninfected cells. Rantes is believed to act in conjunction with two other chemokines, macrophage inflammatory protein-1a and macrophage inflammatory protein-1b.

rape   The coerced or forced participation in sexual acts.

rapid plasma reagin   A nontreponemal serological test for detection of syphilis, the basis of which is agglutination. Unlike treponemal tests that look for *Treponema pallidum*, the corkscrew-shaped organism that causes the disease, nontreponemal tests give passive evidence of the presence of the disease.

rapid screening trial   A pre-trial clinical trial. In 1989, AIDS treatment activists and government and academic statisticians joined forces in order to improve the design of CLINICAL TRIALS. They sought to develop a new kind of eight- to 15-week clinical trial to compare and prioritize new drugs that successfully complete PHASE I (early dosage and toxicity studies). The winners from the rapid screening process would then immediately enter into larger trials designed to lead to drug approval. The impetus for the new system was that dozens of potential AIDS ANTIVIRALS were coming out of laboratories, and there was no way all could receive the full-scale clinical trials required to convince the FOOD AND DRUG ADMINISTRATION that the drugs were good enough for general use. Even if more money were available, it was argued that there were not enough experienced scientists, research nurses, or patients meeting entry criteria, to run so many large trials. The proposed new system was designed to speed the development of brand new therapies by quickly screening all the promising drugs, so that the more successful ones quickly could be moved into larger, definitive trials.

This drug-screening system was designed to test several different drugs at one time. Every approved volunteer randomly was offered one of the currently available drugs to take for a short period of time (about 12 weeks). Improved T-helper counts were the primary measure of efficacy. The drugs then would be compared to pick out those few that stood out from the others. They might then be made available for early access through a system like parallel track. Clinical trials experts reason that most proposed drugs do not work, so they will in effect become the placebo. The trials are kept short, probably two or three months, to avoid exposing participants to ineffective drugs for long. In some cases, a placebo or no-treatment arm might be acceptable in these trials. Since many drugs would be tested, patients would have only a small chance of receiving no treatment. Persons who were not critically ill might be willing to risk entering a no-treatment arm for two or three months.

One of the main concerns about the proposed trials is that some drugs may be valuable but not show benefits early. It is suspected that pharmaceutical companies might be afraid their products will be rejected too early. Designers argue that any drug showing potential will be followed up; the screening trials were designed to help set priori-

ties, not to kill drugs that have other evidence in their favor.

Advantages of the concept include the fact that a screening trial would identify early activity in a high-quality study before PHASE II TRIALS begin. It would provide information to support prioritization decisions for phase II trials, give the earlier definition of a drug's efficacy, and provide much useful information to phase II trial designers. The system would also allow combination therapies to be tested as easily as single drugs. The single study would cost less than multiple small trials. The trials could easily find volunteers, both because of the short time commitment required and because it would be easier to publicize one trial than many separate ones.

Limitations and problems of the new system include the lack of long-term data, the possibility that entry and safety criteria unique to one drug might have to be applied to others to allow randomization, and the fact that the trial only identifies winners according to the criteria of early T-cell count increases, meaning that a better drug that takes longer to be effective might be missed. The question of whether drug companies would be willing to compete with other companies in terms of AIDS-related drug production and to support the program was also raised. Some scientists questioned whether or not there were enough new promising drugs that a screening system was even needed; some researchers even said that they do not know what drugs to test. It was noted that there were many scientifically promising compounds; the problem was in getting them through the pre-clinical development required for the all-important IND (Investigational New Drug approval) and then through the early phase I human test. Overall, the new proposal for screening trials did not solve this problem.

rash A general term applied to any eruption of the skin, especially those associated with communicable diseases. Rashes are usually temporary. They are usually a shade of red, which varies with disease.

raw food Uncooked. Virtually all organisms that might be present in food and that can cause infections are easily killed by even brief exposure to heat, so cooking generally eliminates any danger. Persons whose immune systems are compromised, however (especially if their CD4+ counts are below 150), are particularly advised to follow safety guidelines to avoid food-borne infections, which can cause severe diarrhea and vomiting and can be difficult to treat. Even the commonest, mildest types of "food poisoning" can be dangerous for people with HIV. Because toxic drugs are necessary to treat many infections, everything possible should be done to prevent them in the first place.

Guidelines: avoid red meat, undercooked eggs, and raw seafood, all of which can contain parasites or bacteria, as well as raw egg yolks, which can contain salmonella. Raw fruits or vegetables should be peeled or dipped in boiling water for five seconds. Cheese that has not been pasteurized (aged, ripened cheeses such as Brie, bleu, and feta) should be avoided. Uncooked root vegetables, such as radishes and carrots, that grow in the soil, as well as other salad vegetables, may be used if they are either peeled and rinsed in purified water, steamed for two minutes, or dipped in boiling water for five seconds. Vegetables with thick skins should be peeled and rinsed with purified water. Apples and pears may be eaten raw if peeled and rinsed. Bananas, oranges, and grapefruits are safe when peeled. The bottom line with raw food is: boil it, cook it, peel it, or forget it.

RBC See RED BLOOD CELL.

reactivation The recurrence of a previously latent (inactive) infection to an active, pathogenic state.

reactogenicity The capacity of a vaccine to produce adverse reactions.

reagent A substance used in a chemical reaction to detect, analyze, measure, or produce other substances. In virology, strains of HIV are reagents. The term may also be used to refer to the subject of a psychological experiment, especially one reacting to a stimulus.

rear entry Intromission from behind. See COITUS.

reasonable charge An allowable charge, under a health insurance policy or program, especially MEDICARE and MEDICAID.

rebound As in basketball, when the ball reverses its course and bounces back off the backboard, in medicine a rebound is a reversal of response after withdrawal of the stimulus. With regard to HIV/AIDS, rebound constitutes increases in viral load above a set limit over a period. For example, a person may be rebounding if his or her viral load is less than 400 copies/mL for several months and subsequently more than 400 copies/mL at three consecutive clinic visits. These parameters vary among doctors. "Blips" are transient increases. See VIRAL LOAD BLIPS.

receptive anal intercourse Sexual intercourse in which an individual allows the insertion of a penis into his or her anus. This is a high-risk mode of transmission for the HUMAN IMMUNODEFICIENCY VIRUS. Also called *passive anal intercourse*.

receptor In pharmacology, a cell component that combines with a drug, hormone, or chemical mediator to alter the function of the cell. In neurology, a sensory nerve ending.

rechallenge To administer a substance (drug, pathogen) a second time after an initial adverse result. For example, if someone has an allergic reaction to a drug, he or she may be rechallenged by taking a smaller dose and building up to a normal dose.

recombinant An organism whose genome contains integrated genetic material from a different organism. Also used in relation to compounds produced by laboratory or industrial cultures of genetically engineered living cells. These cells' genes have been altered to give the capability of producing large quantities of the desired compound for use as a medical treatment. Recombinant compounds are often altered versions of naturally occurring substances.

recombinant DNA DNA prepared through laboratory manipulation in which genes from an organism of one species are transplanted or spliced to an organism of another species. When the host's genetic material is reproduced, the transplanted genetic material is also copied. This technique permits isolating and examining the properties and action of specific genes. Studies in this area must be done in a carefully controlled environment. Levels of need for containment have been defined and are designated as P-1 for the lowest level and P-4 for the highest. The P-4 level is for experiments involving animal virus DNA that contains potentially lethal genes. Experiments using DNA from pathogenic organisms, cancer-causing viruses, and viruses associated with certain toxins are prohibited in the United States.

recombinant live vectors   See LIVE RECOMBINANT VECTOR VACCINES.

recombinant subunit vaccines   Vaccines that use viral proteins produced by using recombinant DNA technology. In this case, recombinant DNA technology involves transplanting the genes for certain HIV proteins into bacteria or other microorganisms or into mammalian cells. The host cells then churn out large quantities of the "recombinant" HIV protein. This method of production is a safer and more cost-effective way to obtain large quantities of HIV protein than the alternative which requires growing large amounts of infectious HIV particles. Recombinant GP160 proteins and P24 proteins have been tested in early clinical trials. Their apparent drawback resides in a component of the recombinant product that was subtly different from that of the natural HIV proteins. As a result, the antibodies elicited by the recombinant proteins did not effectively neutralize strains of HIV that are commonly transmitted.

recovery (from addiction)   The process of overcoming physical and psychological dependence on a psychoactive substance. This generally includes a period of abstinence and treatment, the return of physical and emotional health, and a commitment to sobriety. Real recovery requires such a commitment and a willingness to work at it—as the expression goes, "one day at a time."

rectal   Pertaining to the rectum.

rectal douche   A cleansing current or stream of water directed against the rectum. It may or may not be medicated.

rectal mucosa   The mucous membrane that lines the rectum.

rectum   The end of the intestines that is located between the sigmoid flexure (colon) and the anal canal. Bowel movements or stools are passed through the rectum.

recycling drugs   Within the context of HIV/AIDS, redirecting the excess supply of HIV/AIDS drugs, generally from so-called rich countries to developing countries. Proponents argue that exporting surplus drugs has several benefits beyond the lives directly involved: notably it helps improve local professional capacity to prescribe and manage antiretroviral therapy; helps spread knowledge and provide experience; and helps develop local public health infrastructure. Critics say recycling programs are futile since drug donations provide a mere drop in the bucket compared to what is needed in developing countries. They also raise concerns about the likelihood that scarce resources might not be used to the greatest effect and call for standards for accepting clients, ensuring the quality of the drugs, protecting the confidentiality of the clients, and following up to see that drug regimens are effective. They note too that equally important are procedures that provide education for professional development and a system for medical review of cases and outcomes.

red blood cell   See ERYTHROCYTE.

red blood corpuscle   See ERYTHROCYTE.

red ribbons   Among the most common symbols of AIDS since their introduction at the 1991 Tony Awards ceremony by the group Broadway Cares/Equity Fights AIDS as a mark of compassion and support. In the early 1990s, red ribbons figured prominently at the Academy Awards ceremony and at other events in the entertainment industry and soon found their way onto everything from a U.S. postage stamp to Christmas tree ornaments. In the mind of some, overuse of the symbol quickly trivialized it, but the precedent of the red ribbon also led to the adoption of a pink ribbon for breast cancer awareness, and the ribbon remains a familiar image.

red tape   A popular expression for (presumably excessive or silly) bureaucratic routines that must be performed before an official action can be taken. Within the context of AIDS, such routines have been protested as endangering those who are ill by complicating or delaying urgently needed research, health care delivery, and political action.

red tape protest   See RED TAPE.

red-baiting   The practice of attacking as politically radical or Communist. Such attacks are usually made against politically dissenting, nonconformist, or simply unpopular people or groups and are meant to stigmatize or demonize them or distract attention from the substance of their criticism of the social status quo.

reference virus   A "standard" virus used for comparison. For example, in HIV resistance testing the resistance or susceptibility of a patient's virus is compared to that of a reference virus.

referral numbers   Telephone and/or fax numbers that direct a person to someone or for something. Within the context of AIDS, referral may be made to national, state, or local HIV/AIDS prevention, treatment, or information services. Nationwide resource groups can be useful in locating or double-checking state or local resources. Referral numbers may also lead to publications published especially for people living with HIV.

refractory   Severe and resistant to treatment.

regimen   A systematic program, or routine, as in a course of treatment or a diet.

regimen goals   The end(s) to which effort is directed for a particular treatment plan; regimen goals may specify which drugs are used, in what doses, according to what schedule, for how long,

and for which desired outcomes. Regimen goals are generally developed collaboratively by a medical care provider and a patient.

registration trial   A trial designed to provide solid support for a drug's approval by the U.S. FOOD AND DRUG ADMINISTRATION.

regulatory genes   As related to HIV, three regulatory HIV genes (TAT, REV, and NEF) and three so-called auxiliary genes (VIF, VRP, and VPU) contain information for the production of proteins that regulate the virus's ability to infect a cell, produce new copies of itself, or cause disease.

regulatory T cells   T cells that direct other immune cells to perform specific functions. The chief regulatory cell, the CD4 cell or T helper cell, is HIV's chief target.

Rehabilitation Act of 1973   More popularly referred to as Section 504, the Rehabilitation Act of 1973 requires that any program or activity that receives federal monies cannot deny access to a handicapped person. Included in its definition of handicapped are hearing, sight, and speech impairments; cancer; heart disease and diabetes; cerebral palsy; epilepsy; mental illness and retardation; muscular dystrophy; multiple sclerosis; AIDS; and drug addiction and alcoholism. Section 504 has pervasive legal ramifications because almost every aspect of daily life receives some form of federal aid.

reinfection   A possible additional "super" infection with a second strain of HIV some time after initial infection. While there is little evidence to document such a phenomenon, there is evidence that two strains of HIV can circulate simultaneously ("coinfection"). Whether there is a serious risk of reinfection for couples in which both partners are HIV positive is unknown. Aside from HIV, however, such couples have more immediately to worry about other infectious agents with the potential to affect HIV activation and replication.

Reiter's syndrome   A condition in which urethritis, arthritis, and conjunctivitis appear together, for the most part in young men. Urethritis usually appears first, but arthritis constitutes the dominant feature. The syndrome is of unknown origin and generally runs a self-limited but relapsing course.

relapse A return to a previously worse condition of illness, after a period of recovery. In the language of addiction, relapse refers to the return to the use of alcohol or drugs after a period of abstinence or a serious attempt at recovery. A relapse can occur regardless of the length of time someone has been sober. Before returning to alcohol or drugs, the alcoholic or addict will generally exhibit an attitudinal change and emotional deterioration. Some situational changes may also signal a coming relapse. Warning signs of relapse may include: increased arguing with others for no apparent reason; decreasing or stopping 12-STEP PROGRAMS (AA, NA, etc.); returning to high-risk situations, such as socializing in a bar or returning to a drug-using environment; reestablishing contacts with alcohol or drug-using friends; no longer caring about sobriety; increased negativity about life and how things are going; increased moodiness or depression; increased feelings of boredom; sudden feelings of euphoria; strong feelings of anger at oneself or another person; thinking one "deserves" alcohol or drugs after being sober for a period of time; thinking it wouldn't be harmful to substitute one drug for another; thinking that the alcohol/drug problem is "cured" due to period of sobriety.

There are a number of relapse warning signs that can help terminally ill, chemically dependent clients recognize that they are moving toward a chemical relapse and take corrective action. These include the belief that returning to the addictive use of alcohol and other drugs will make the illness more manageable or provide relief from pain; the belief that the use of previous drugs of abuse will be more effective in pain management than the use of prescription drugs; the belief that returning to alcohol or drugs will bring a quick and painless death; the belief that having a terminal illness means that there is nothing left to live for and that, therefore, alcohol and drug use is justified.

Because alcohol and drug use escalate disease progression and add pain and complications to almost any situation, staying sober is especially important to persons with HIV/AIDS. Staying sober increases the length and quality of survival time. Staying sober also gives persons with HIV/AIDS the possibility of death with dignity.

relaxation A lessening of tension or activity; the phase or period in a single muscle-twitch following contraction, in which tension decreases, fibers lengthen, and the muscle returns to resting position. In MAGNETIC RESONANCE IMAGING (MRI), the return of an excited atom to alignment with the applied magnetic field. General relaxation refers to relaxation of the entire body and is distinct from local relaxation, which is limited to a particular muscle group or to a certain part.

remission A period when the signs of a disease have been eliminated through treatment or the immune response. A disease may be in remission without a complete cure having been effected.

Remune A therapeutic VACCINE consisting of killed HIV stripped of its envelope protein and mixed with a mineral oil–based adjuvant known as incomplete Freund's adjuvant (IFA). IFA increases the vaccine's ability to stimulate cell-mediated immunity (cytotoxic lymphocytes.)

Administration of inactivated virus may stimulate cellular immune responses, which may slow the replication of HIV-1 through increased immunologic control over infected cells or other as yet undetermined mechanisms. The use of inactivated virus could theoretically stimulate broader immune responses that are capable of suppressing more diverse strains of HIV than vaccines based on subunits of the virus. It was thought that Remune might work with currently available antiviral drugs (AZT, ddI, ddC, and protease inhibitors) as a complementary treatment for HIV infection. The belief was that whereas antiviral drugs interrupt the reproduction process of HIV within infected cells, Remune stimulates the immune systems to destroy HIV-infected cells.

A phase III trial ended in May 1999 when an independent safety monitoring board decided that the Remune arm in the trial had shown no clinical benefit over placebo and was unlikely to do so. In the course of this trial, many participants switched to HAART from earlier, less effective regimens. Smaller trials continued that included Remune plus HAART. In the summer of 2001, Pfizer, which was codeveloping Remune with Immune Response Corporation, dropped its sponsorship. This left Remune without any substantial funding for further research. The only side effect noted was irritation at the injection site. Other names are HIV-1 immunogen. It is sometimes referred to as the Salk vaccine.

renal   Of or pertaining to the kidneys or the surrounding regions.

renal failure   Failure of the kidneys or the surrounding region. Acute renal failure may be due to trauma; any condition that impairs the flow of blood to the kidneys; certain toxic substances; bacterial toxins; glomerulonephritis; or acute obstruction of the urinary tract. Treatment includes specific therapy for the primary disease and either peritoneal dialysis or hemodialysis.

repertoire   The full range of T and B cells that make up a competent immune system. Each clone of such cells targets a particular antigen. In AIDS, it is thought that when the CD4 cells are depleted to a certain point, entire clones have been lost, reducing the CD4 cell repertoire and making people vulnerable to opportunistic conditions. Increasing CD4 counts through treatment may not produce the full range of cells but just multiply those that are left. Various immune-based therapies are being studied in an attempt to restore the full repertoire.

reporting requirements   See MANDATORY REPORTING; MANDATORY TESTING; PRIVACY.

reproductive counseling   The issue of reproductive choice is a most difficult and ethically charged aspect of HIV testing and counseling of women. For HIV-positive women, SEROSTATUS is only one of many factors that influence reproductive decision-making. Others are individual, community, or religious morality or ethics regarding abortion; a desire to parent; the influence of partner, family, and friends; religious faith/optimism; risk evaluation; access to care; prior experience with HIV; maternal

health concerns; cultural norms; parenting concerns; psychological adaptation to HIV; and non-HIV–related psychological issues. Counseling about reproductive options takes all these into account.

Reproductive counseling usually involves providing up-to-date information about HIV and its impact on infected women and discussing such topics as perinatal transmission, pediatric disease and assessment, and the effects of pregnancy on maternal HIV disease and on prenatal care; care of the child with HIV and plans in the event of worsening disease; and psychological support systems. Optimally, counselors should take into consideration a woman's educational level, primary language, and idiomatic or regional speech patterns. To be effective, counselors must be comfortable with the moral terrain of HIV and reproduction as well as with sexuality and drug abuse. Cultural and social or peer-group belief systems can influence the efficacy of communication.

The appropriateness of various modalities for the reproductive counseling of women also continue to be debated. For both ethical and pragmatic reasons, many care providers working with HIV-positive women espouse the generic nondirective counseling model. Here, the counselor translates medical information into personal calculations in the course of helping women to decide what is right for them and their families.

reproductive decision-making   Until fairly recently, the CENTERS FOR DISEASE CONTROL AND PREVENTION (CDC) and the American College of Obstetricians and Gynecologists (ACOG) officially recommended that HIV-positive women be discouraged from bearing children. Research has shown, however, that HIV-positive women do not differ significantly from HIV-negative women in making personal decisions regarding carrying or aborting a pregnancy. Women with HIV infection who are not overwhelmed by illness generally have the same attitudes and emotions as other women regarding childbearing.

Health care providers are generally advised to be supportive of women's rights and abilities to make informed personal decisions. An important challenge for clinicians is working with couples who wish to have a child. Couples in which only one partner is HIV-positive present an additional challenge. Support and knowledge of referrals for alternative insemination, infertility workups, and adoption agencies can assist a couple in achieving the goal of having children without practicing unsafe sex. Further, the clinician is responsible for discussing birth control choices with clients and providing the gynecological care necessary for their appropriate use.

reproductive rights In December 1985, the CEN-TERS FOR DISEASE CONTROL AND PREVENTION (CDC) officially recommended that women who are HIV-positive or who have AIDS should "be advised to consider delaying pregnancy until more is known about perinatal transmission of the virus." The materials offered by the departments of health in many states go beyond that advice and recommend unequivocally that HIV-positive women should not become pregnant. Nonetheless, many infected women are having babies even when they know they are infected and have been counseled about the risks of perinatal transmission or already have a child with HIV infection or AIDS, or have lost a child to AIDS. It is generally felt that despite its gravity and consequences, HIV infection is only one of a range of conditions that can be passed from mother to fetus and should not be singled out for moral censure and coercive policies. Additionally, it is widely recognized that reproductive decisions are critical to biological and social life, and HIV-positive women must remain free to make choices that are consistent with their cultural, religious, and personal values. Given the current knowledge, there is no way to predict whether an HIV-positive woman will infect her fetus, no reliable way to determine IN UTERO or at birth whether a baby is infected (unless it is born with symptoms), and no way to foretell the likely course of the disease. This array of uncertainties is weighted very differently by public health officials and physicians and by women at risk.

reproductive system The bodily organs and processes employed in reproduction.

Rescriptor See DELAVIRDINE.

rescue therapy See SALVAGE THERAPY.

research Systematic inquiry or investigation into a subject.

research laboratories Places where scientific research is carried on. Usually, these are affiliated with or located in government agencies, large universities, and major hospitals.

research papers Reports that generally include several standard components: the abstract, the background and rationale, a description of the methods used, the actual results, and the discussion—the author's interpretation of the results. Within the context of HIV/AIDS, thousands of papers are published every year, in print and on the Web; some are far more reliable and relevant than others. Deciding which papers to trust is a challenge; key factors influencing this decision are the source (lead author[s], lead author[s] affiliation, sponsor), study design (e.g., prospective versus retrospective), and methods (e.g., eligibility criteria, endpoints, primary hypothesis, secondary objectives, measurements, mathematical methods used to analyze the data).

reservoir A part of the body that may contain HIV and that is not readily penetrated by drugs. Examples include MACROPHAGES, LYMPHOCYTES, the brain, and the testes.

reservoir of virus The longer-lived cells infected with HIV, such as MACROPHAGES and MONOCYTES, which continue to produce virus for weeks, functioning in effect as "reservoirs" of the virus. In contrast, an actively infected CD4 cell dies in two days. Many researchers believe that since currently available drugs do not kill infected cells, they can eliminate all of the virus from the body only if they can keep suppressing HIV replication—even in the face of mutations that confer partial resistance—for a period longer than these cells' lifetimes.

residential care facility A live-in facility for individuals who, because of their physical, mental, or emotional condition, are not able to live independently but whose treatment does not require them to be in an in-patient facility.

residual functional capacity (RFC) In SSA disability determinations, if a patient's medical condition does not explicitly appear in, or clearly equal, any of those in SSA's Listing of Impairments, an RFC criterion is used to assess medically his or her ability to work, taking into account the functional limitations and environmental restrictions imposed by all medically determinable impairments. The RFC method, rather than the listing, must always be used for "ARC-only" claimants. It is also sometimes relied upon for full-blown AIDS cases, as AIDS has not historically appeared in the listing.

residual virus Virus that has been left behind.

resistance In relation to HIV, resistance is the ability of a microorganism to mutate or change its structure to overcome a drug or medication used to treat it. A resistant organism can function and replicate despite a drug's presence. Resistance is the result usually of a genetic mutation. In HIV, such mutations can change the structure of microbial enzymes and proteins so that an antiretroviral drug can no longer bind with them as well as it used to or attack them in the same way.

When AZT is used alone to treat HIV disease, it typically produces an increase in CD4 CELL counts of 30 cells/mm to 50 cells/m, and it decreases the viral load by 60–70 percent. But after a few months, the viral load begins to increase again, and the CD4 count drops. A similar course is seen when any other antiretroviral drugs are used alone (that is, monotherapy). The rebound in viral load and the renewed drop in CD4 cells occur because HIV quickly becomes resistant to single drugs.

There are always errors each time the virus's genetic material is copied. It is generally believed that HIV develops drug resistance so effectively largely because of the high rate at which genetic mutations occur during its replication. These gene mutations occur because reverse transcriptase (RT) is prone to making errors when it copies HIV's RNA genes into DNA. Thus, when an HIV particle enters a cell and produces a provirus, it is the provirus that contains the gene mutations introduced by reverse transcriptase. When that provirus begins producing new virions, those virions will have genetic characteristics that are different from those of the virion that originally infected the cell. Note, too, that most mutations are not successful. They are unable to reproduce at all because of the large number of mutations.

This tendency of RT to make inexact copies of the virus's original RNA genes results in great genetic diversity among the HIV infecting an individual. Thus, a person with HIV is soon infected with many genetically different populations of virions. Some of these populations consist of HIV particles that have relatively unmodified (or "wild-type") genes. These virions are sensitive to antiretroviral drugs and therefore cannot replicate when they are present in the body. Other populations, however, consist of small numbers of HIV particles that, by chance, have mutations that make them resistant to one or more antiretroviral drugs. The growth of these mutated HIV particles is not slowed in the presence of these drugs. In fact, the virions then have an advantage over the wild-type HIV particles. The drug-adapted virions can infect cells and replicate, even as the wild-type virions are prevented from doing so, as long as the patient continues to be treated with those drugs to which the mutated virions are resistant. Some of these virion populations will have mutations that make them resistant to AZT; some will have mutations that make them resistant to ddI; and others will be resistant to the non-nucleoside drugs. Still others might have mutations that confer resistance to the PROTEASE INHIBITORS. Additionally, virus populations do arise that are resistant to multiple drugs. Occasionally, chance produces mutations in HIV that confer resistance to one drug and reverse resistance to another drug.

The number of genetic mutations needed to make a virus resistant to any one drug can be very small. For example, a single mutation that causes a change of one amino acid in the structure of HIV's RT enzyme can produce a virus that is 1,000 times more resistant to the drug 3TC. It would take a dose of 3TC that is a thousand times stronger to block the replication of the mutated virus, a dose that would also be deadly to the individual.

Adherence, drug resistance and antiretroviral therapy have received considerable attention in recent years. Adherence, the taking of drugs according to prescribed directions, plays an important role in preventing or slowing the development of drug resistance. Adherence is important for the effective use of all medications, but it is critical for antiretroviral regimens that are designed to suppress HIV. Skipping doses or reducing a drug's dosage even briefly allows the level of drug in the body to drop, giving an opportunity for resistant mutants to replicate. In the worst case, resistance to one drug can result in cross-resistance to all of the drugs in the same class. Should this happen for protease inhibitors for example, it would make all protease inhibitors ineffective thereafter for that individual. Therefore, it is of the utmost importance to adhere to the requirements of HAART so as to suppress viral replication as completely as possible or prevent or forestall the development of drug resistance. Sometimes side effects or other problems might prevent patients from taking full doses of all their antiretroviral drugs. In such cases, it is better to either stop taking all these drugs together for a time or to try a different combination of drugs than to reduce the dosage. In the absence of any drugs, all virus populations replicate and compete with one other, although the wild-type virions replicate most effectively. The presence of any antiretroviral drug at low levels, however, favors the replication of the mutated drug-adapted, or drug-resistant, virions, which then become the most numerous HIV particles in the body. See ADHERENCE.

resistance assays   Tests that measure resistance. Physicians find resistance testing to be a helpful tool for guiding treatment decisions for patients for whom current HIGHLY ACTIVE ANTI-VIRAL THERAPY (HAART) is failing, as well as for chronically infected naive patients.

Currently, the Department of Health and Human Services' *Guidelines for the use of Antiretroviral Agents in HIV-Infected Adults and Adolescents* (August 13, 2001), available at http://aidsinfo.nih.gov/guidelines/adult/archive/AA_020501%5Cindex.html, propose that resistance testing be used as follows: virologic failure (i.e., failure to achieve a viral load of less than 1,000 copies/mL after more than 16–24 weeks of treatment) and suboptimal suppression of viral load after initiation of treatment (i.e., less than 0.5–0.75 log10 reduction in plasma HIV RNA by four weeks following initiation of therapy or more than 1

log 10 reduction by eight weeks). The *Guidelines* also propose that resistance testing be considered for acute HIV infection and do not recommend testing for chronic HIV infection in treatment of naive patients, after discontinuation of treatment for more than two weeks, and when plasma viral load is less than 1,000 HIV RNA copies/mL. To date, no resistance tests have been approved by the FOOD AND DRUG ADMINISTRATION. There are a number of tests being used, however, and many health insurance plans cover them, including some state AIDS drug assistance programs (ADAPs) and Medicaid programs. These include both GENOTYPE TESTS (TRUEGENE HIV-1 Genotyping Kit, VircoGEN, INNO-LiPA HIV-1 RT, and HIV-1 GentypR) and PHENOTYPE TESTS (PhenoSense, Antivirogram).

Pregnant women are a group of patients in which physicians generally feel genotyping definitely has a niche for ensuring intelligent treatment decisions. Of note, as NNRTI therapy becomes a more common treatment option for HIV+ pregnant women, specifically the use of Viramune (nevirapine), it is anticipated that many women treated with Viramune during pregnancy will eventually develop NNRTI resistance. Repeat resistance testing of these women, if they experience treatment failure, will be important in making treatment decisions. It will also be necessary to genotype these same women during future pregnancies if they have detectable viral loads.

resistance exercise   Forms of exercise, such as weight lifting, that increase lean body mass.

resistance mutation   See RESISTANCE.

resistant   Not susceptible to the effect of a drug. See RESISTANCE.

respirator   A machine that assists a patient to continue breathing by producing either intermittent or continuous positive pressure in the lungs, a process known as artificial respiration.

respiratory alkalosis   A metabolic condition resulting from an excessive loss of carbon dioxide from the lungs.

respiratory burst The process by which NEUTROPHILS and MONOCYTES kill certain microbial PATHOGENS by conversion of oxygen to toxic oxygen products.

respiratory infection An infection in the nose, pharynx, larynx, trachea, bronchi, or lungs.

respiratory syncytial virus A virus that induces formation of syncytial (of the nature of the syncytium, a multinucleated mass of protoplasm such as striated muscle fiber) masses in infected cell cultures. It is a major cause of acute respiratory disease in children.

respite care Patient care provided intermittently in an institution or at home to provide temporary relief to family members providing continuous care.

resting cell One of a large number of nondividing or "quiescent" CD4+ T CELLS, MACROPHAGES, and other nondividing cells that harbor large quantities of HIV virus in a stable, extrachromosomal form, possibly a "primed" state ready for rapid replication upon cell activation. It is believed that these cells are probably important to the PATHOGENESIS of HIV disease.

reticulocytosis An increase in the number of reticulocytes in circulating blood. A reticulocyte is a red blood cell that contains remnants of the ER, an immature stage in red blood cell formation; it indicates active erythropoiesis in red BONE MARROW and occurs after hemorrhage, during acclimatization to high altitude, and following treatment for pernicious anemia.

reticuloendothelial cell A PHAGOCYTE cell of the reticuloendothelial system. These cells are responsible for PHAGOCYTOSIS of damaged or old cells, cellular debris, foreign substances, and PATHOGENS, removing them from the circulation. Found in large concentrations in the spleen, liver, lymph nodes, and alveoli, as well as in other tissues such as the brain, blood vessels, and mucous membranes, they play a major role in the nonspecific immune response.

reticuloendothelial system Former name for the tissue macrophage system, the organs or tissues that contain MACROPHAGES; the liver, spleen and red bone marrow.

reticulosis See RETICULOCYTOSIS.

retina The innermost layer of the eye, which receives images transmitted through the lens and is the immediate instrument of vision.

retinal detachment Separation of the inner sensory layer of the retina from the outer pigment EPITHELIUM, leading to loss of retinal function. It is usually caused by a hole or break in the inner sensory layer that permits fluid from the vitreous humor to leak under the retina and lift off the innermost layer. Blurred vision, flashes of light, vitreous floaters, and loss of visual activity are among the symptoms.

retinitis Inflammation of the retina; it is linked to CYTOMEGALOVIRUS infection in persons with AIDS. Untreated, it can cause blindness.

retinochoroiditis An inflamed condition of the RETINA and the choroid of the eye.

retinoid Resembling a resin.

retroactive Medicaid eligibility date The date, up to three calendar months prior to the month of application, from which an applicant may be found eligible for MEDICAID.

retrospective study A study based on the review of medical records of patients, looking backward at events that happened in the past. Because a retrospective cohort study uses the records of a specific group of patients, it cannot be rigorously designed and risks attributing effects to the wrong causes. See PROSPECTIVE STUDY.

Retrovir See AZIDOTHYMIDINE; ZIDOVUDINE.

retrovirus A type of virus that, when not infecting a cell, stores its genetic information on a single-stranded RNA molecule instead of the more usual double-stranded DNA. HIV is an example of a retrovirus. After a retrovirus penetrates a cell, it constructs a DNA version of its genes using a special enzyme, REVERSE TRANSCRIPTASE. This DNA then becomes part of the cell's genetic material.

There are many different kinds of retroviruses. LENTIVIRUSES and leukoviruses, for instance, are retroviruses. HIV is the most important retrovirus to infect humans.

rev One of the regulatory genes of HIV. Three HIV regulatory genes—NEF, REV, and TAT—and three so-called auxiliary genes—VIF, VPR, and VPU—contain information necessary for the production of proteins that control the virus's ability to infect a cell, produce new copies of itself, or cause disease. Also the protein produced by the gene, which regulates the construction of the structural components of HIV and is necessary for the production of new virus particles.

rev gene The gene in the HUMAN IMMUNODEFICIENCY VIRUS that is required for viral protein RNA processing.

reverse resistance A mechanism through which a mutation that allows HIV to resist one drug makes the virus more susceptible to another drug.

reverse transcriptase A viral enzyme that constructs DNA from an RNA template, an essential step in the life-cycle of a retrovirus such as HIV.

reverse transcriptase inhibitor An agent that deters or prevents RNA-directed DNA POLYMERASE. See REVERSE TRANSCRIPTASE.

Reyataz See ATAZANAVIR.

Reye's syndrome A condition first recognized in 1963, characterized by acute ENCEPHALOPATHY and fatty infiltration of the liver and possibly of the pancreas, heart, kidney, spleen, and lymph nodes. It is seen in children under 15 years of age after an acute viral infection. The mortality rate is variable, depending on severity, but may be as high as 80 percent. Symptoms include upper respiratory infection followed in about six days by pernicious nausea and vomiting and a change in mental status and HEPATOMEGALY without jaundice in 40 percent of cases.

rhesus monkey A small monkey native to India, used frequently for research purposes, especially testing the safety and efficacy of vaccines.

rhNGF Recombinant human (rh) nerve growth factor. It is used in studies for treatment of HIV-associated peripheral neuropathy.

rhu IL-1R Used in experimental treatments for KAPOSI'S SARCOMA (KS), IL-1 is a cytokine produced in response to infection that may contribute to KS, which binds to IL-1.

RIA See RADIOIMMUNOASSAY.

ribavirin A NUCLEOSIDE ANALOG approved as a treatment for RESPIRATORY SYNCYTIAL VIRUS. Ribavirin also has shown activity against hepatitis C disease.

ribonucleic acid (RNA) A nucleic acid, found mostly in the cytoplasm, rather than the nucleus, of cells. RNA, like the structurally similar DNA, is a chain made up of subunits called nucleotides. RNA plays several roles in determining the synthesis of proteins. Messenger RNA replicates the DNA code for a protein and moves to sites in the cell called ribosomes. There, the much shorter transfer RNA (tRNA) assembles amino acids to form the protein specified by the messenger RNA. Most forms of RNA (including messenger and transfer RNA) consist of a single nucleotide strand, but a few forms of viral RNA that function as carriers of genetic information (instead of DNA) are double-stranded. Some viruses, such as HIV, carry RNA instead of the more usual genetic material DNA. Researchers have found that the level of HIV RNA in a person's plasma is a predictor of the risk of disease progression independent of the CD4+ T-cell count. Measurements of CD4+ T cells, the immune cells typically depleted during HIV infection, are routinely used as an indirect or SURROGATE marker of HIV disease progression. See DEOXYRIBONUCLEIC ACID.

ribonucleotide reductase A viral enzyme that cuts ribonucleotides in order to create deoxyribonucleotides, the building blocks of DNA. Ribonucleotide reductase is essential for DNA replication. Drugs such as hydroxyurea, that inhibit ribonucleotide reductase may enhance the activity of nucleoside analog drugs.

ribosome A cell organelle found in the cytoplasm; the site of protein synthesis.

ribozyme A naturally occurring RNA molecule that functions as a catalytic molecular scissors, chopping up RNA strands at selected sites. Ribozymes can be synthesized and targeted against specific RNA sequences, like antisense compounds, and have as much potential against HIV. Moreover, since ribozymes can effectively destroy many targets, according to its proponents, lower levels of drug might be needed than would be the case with antisense, and therapy could be more thorough. To date, however, chemists have not yet figured out how ribozymes can be made to reach and penetrate cells in the body.

Rickettsia A genus of MICROORGANISMS that occupies a position between viruses and bacteria. *Rickettsiae* differ from bacteria in that they are obligate parasites (they cannot survive in the free-living or parasitic mode) requiring living cells for growth, and from viruses in that they are retained by the Berkefeld filter. The Berkefeld Filter is a filter of diatomaceous earth designed to allow virus-size particles to pass through. These parasites are the causative agents of many diseases, including typhus fevers, spotted fevers, and scrub typhus, and are usually transmitted by arthropods (fleas, lice, mites, ticks), which serve as vectors.

rifabutin An oral drug approved by the U.S. FOOD AND DRUG ADMINISTRATION for preventing MYCOBACTERIUM AVIUM COMPLEX (MAC) in people with AIDS and CD4 cell counts of less than 75. Rifabutin is also used in combination with other drugs for the treatment of active MAC infection. Rifabutin seems to have fewer drug interactions than RIFAMPIN, yet like ISONIAZID (INH) can change liver enzyme production and thus alter the metabolism of Coumadin, Dilantin, Tegretol, theophylline, and the benzodiazepines (Atavin, Valium). Other possible side effects include NEUTROPENIA and eye and muscle irritation. (Trade name is Mycobutin.)

rifadin See RIFAMPIN.

rifampicin See RIFAMPIN.

rifampin An ANTIBIOTIC synthesized from RIFAMYCIN B, which is produced by fermentation of *Streptomyces mediterranei*. It is used in treating MYCOBACTERIUM TUBERCULOSIS and carriers of NEISSERIA MENINGITIS. It is administered orally. Rifampin decreases the blood levels of such common drugs as atovaquone, Coumadin, corticosteroids, cyclosporine, dapsone, digoxin, fluconazole, ketoconazole, levothyroxine, oral contraceptives, quinidine, propanolol, and theophylline. It is also called rifampicin. (Trade names are Rimactane and Rifadin.)

rifamycin Any of a group of ANTIBIOTICS biosynthesized by a strain of *Streptomyces mediterranei* and effective against a broad spectrum of bacteria, including GRAM-POSITIVE cocci, MYCOBACTERIUM TUBERCULOSIS, some GRAM-NEGATIVE bacilli, and certain other mycobacteria.

right to know One of the most controversial HIV-related legal issues is the right of medical service providers to know whether their patients or prospective patients are infected with HIV and of patients to know whether their medical service providers or prospective providers are so infected. Complicating the issue are the overlapping issues of confidentiality, testing, and the provision of professional service. Any consideration of the matter should take account of the medical/dental community's reaction to this issue, the validity of the scientific evidence of any alleged transmissions, the professional responsibility established and recommended by the professions' governing bodies, the actual risk of infection, and the role of federal and state licensing and regulatory authorities.

This issue had been simmering for some time during the first decade of the AIDS epidemic and heated up as rumors circulated that the CENTERS FOR DISEASE CONTROL AND PREVENTION (CDC) was investigating a documentable case of transmission from dentist to patient. In July 1990, the CDC confirmed that it was investigating the possibility of a transmission of HIV from a dentist with AIDS to a patient during surgery for extraction of two wisdom teeth. When speculation focused on Florida, state health officials there insisted that a confidentiality requirement prohibited them from warning the dentist's patients. Inferring that the CDC reports were of her case, the infected patient took steps to sue. Next and quite dramatically, the dentist identified himself in an emotional letter released on September 4, 1990, the day after his death. He was Dr. David J. Acer of Stuart, Florida. Less than a week later, the patient, 21-year-old Kimberly Bergalis, went public. Genetic testing later "strongly suggested" that Dr. Acer somehow infected three of his patients. Bergalis settled her claim against the dentist's insurer and against her own insurer, a dental plan that had sent her to Dr. Acer. In early June 1991, the Florida Department of Health and Rehabilitative Services announced that genetic testing by the CDC had linked two more HIV infections of Dr. Acer's patients to him.

In January 1991, the CDC was heading toward requiring mandatory testing for all health care workers. The public, spurred by a dying Kimberly Bergalis, was feverishly pressing policymakers for harsh restrictions. Also in January 1991, the American Medical Association (AMA) and the American Dental Association (ADA) both announced new guidelines for doctors with AIDS advising HIV-infected doctors to avoid high-risk procedures without their patients' consent. In February 1991, various rights groups forced the CDC to hold a national conference to discuss the agency's policy regarding HIV-infected health care workers. A critical mass of medical workers, union leaders, public health officials, and advocates for people with AIDS opposed to mandatory testing and other restrictive policies began to form.

In April 1991, the CDC released draft guidelines recommending that doctors and dentists infected with HIV get permission from local panels of experts before continuing to perform certain operations and invasive procedures (and also that doctors and dentists should test themselves for HIV). The guidelines were less restrictive than those issued by the AMA and the ADA calling for

infected health-care professionals to stop performing surgery or inform their patients.

Focusing on this issue at its annual meeting in June 1991, the American Medical Association rejected a policy endorsing mandatory HIV-antibody testing for health care workers and instead supported voluntary testing of those facing the highest risk. It also reiterated its policy that infected doctors should inform patients or refrain from doing invasive procedures. Within less than three weeks, the Academy of General Dentistry voted at its annual meeting to follow federal recommendations that dentists voluntarily take HIV-antibody tests and that those infected inform their patients. It, too, declined, however, to urge mandatory testing.

The CDC agreed. Just one day before the Academy's recommendations, the CDC released its new guidelines calling for doctors and dentists who perform procedures risking exposure to submit voluntarily to HIV-antibody tests, and that those who test positive refrain from performing such procedures until they notify prospective patients and discuss with a board of experts the conditions, if any, under which they might resume such operations. The CDC concluded that "[t]he current assumption of the risk that infected [health care workers] will transmit HIV . . . to patients during exposure-prone procedures does not support the diversion of resources" that mandatory testing would entail. The CDC then began seeking the advice of various medical groups to develop its list of "exposure-prone procedures."

In November 1991, the CDC floated a draft list containing virtually every standard surgical procedure. If adopted, this list would have effectively written into law the notion that HIV can be easily transmitted in this way—even though 10 years of the epidemic had yet to produce one case. Medical groups and AIDS advocates were invited by the CDC to Atlanta in early November to discuss its proposed list. On November 27, 1991, unable to find any support from the scientific community for its proposal, and with the threat of at least one lawsuit over its head from LAMBDA LEGAL DEFENSE AND EDUCATION FUND, the CDC jettisoned its proposal. As recommended by advocacy groups such as Lambda and public health experts around the country, it began to focus its policy efforts on proper infection control rather than mandatory testing and forced disclosure, with their potential for generating discrimination.

The case for the right of either medical/dental service providers or patients to demand testing of the other is extremely problematic. Consider, for example, the damage likely to be done to the medical/dental practices of those who adhere to the CDC recommended universal precautions, the already inadequate number of practitioners willing to treat HIV-positive patients, and the difficulty of bringing those who may have been exposed to the virus into the testing and treatment process. Many argue that strict enforcement of infection-control measures and implementation of the UNIVERSAL PRECAUTIONS recommended by the CDC would be the far better solution. See CONFIDENTIALITY; NOTIFICATION; PRIVACY.

right-wing backlash The AIDS epidemic in the United States coincided with the politicization of religious fundamentalism that began in the late 1970s and was expressed most clearly in the growth of groups like the Moral Majority and the Christian Coalition. The spread of AIDS was linked to changes in sexual and social behavior, which in turn were part of a general shift in mores that created anxiety among those who saw their traditional values under siege and were attracted to the certainties of the religious right. It is hardly surprising that the spokespersons for the new right, already prone to cite the social acceptability of homosexuality as a sign of moral decay, were quick to seize upon AIDS as fodder for their argument. The right-wing backlash against those who suffer from AIDS and those who seek to help them has included political attacks, social stigmatization, cultural paranoia, the fear of "bad blood," documented breaches of confidentiality, calls for quarantine, discrimination and increased surveillance, and the promotion of a general attitude of moralistic hostility and punitiveness.

Rimactane See RIFAMPIN.

ringworm A popular term for a dermatomycosis caused by various species of fungi belonging to the genera *Microsporum* and *Trichophyton*. Red-ringed patches of vesicles, itching, pain and scaling of the skin are symptoms.

RIPA See RADIOIMMUNOPRECIPITATION ASSAY.

ripoff A theft, cheat, or swindle, also a person who rips off another. Responding to the surge of interest in thymic peptide drugs in the early 1990s, several groups have made various thymic products available through underground channels. Many AIDS BUYERS' CLUBS are ethical and responsible community organizations helping ailing people obtain lifesaving medication. However, there are always some blatant profiteers. Exaggerated claims of efficacy and high prices for any underground drugs are usually indicative of "thymo-ripoffs." To protect against being ripped off when buying an underground drug, find out who is selling the medication, how it has been priced, and who produced it and is ultimately responsible for it.

risk The possibility of developing a disease or experiencing an injury. Attributable risks are those that can be attributed to known risk factors and may be estimated based on studies of factual evidence. Relative risks are those that are likely because of exposure to a PATHOGEN or injury-causing circumstances that would have been unlikely without such exposure.

risk assessment A personal risk assessment for AIDS requires willingness to think and talk about HIV and AIDS honestly and openly. A good start would be to answer a set of questions pertaining to sex, drugs, and other common risks. If a person answers yes to any of these questions, then he or she has some risk of exposure to the HIV virus. The more yes answers, the greater the risk.

- Have you ever had unprotected sex (anal, vaginal, or oral) with anyone you know has AIDS or has tested positive for HIV?
- Have you had unprotected sex (anal, vaginal, or oral) with anyone without knowing about his or her past sexual behavior?
- Have you had unprotected sex (anal, vaginal, or oral) with anyone who has been in prison or jail?
- Have you had multiple sex partners?
- Have you had a sexual partner who has or has had other sexual partners?

- Have you ever given or received sex for money?
- Have you had one or more sexually transmitted diseases?
- Have you had sex with a partner who has had VD more than once?
- Have you ever been talked into doing sexual things you did not want to do?
- Have you had unprotected sex (anal, vaginal, or oral) with anyone who injects or has injected drugs?
- Have you or any of your sexual partners shared needles or works to shoot drugs or for any other purpose?
- Have you ever traded or given sex for drugs?
- Have you ever had sex with a new friend or stranger after doing drugs?
- Have you had sex with someone who has had sex with other people who shoot drugs with needles?
- Have you used needles or syringes that had been used by anyone before?
- Have you ever shared needles with someone who was infected?
- Have you ever had sex with someone who shared needles?
- Have you ever used alcohol or drugs to feel good in or about a social setting?
- Have you used a needle to take drugs?
- Have you used the same needle as a friend, spouse, lover or someone else to inject drugs, take vitamins or medicine, make tattoos, or do ear or body piercing?
- Have you ever shared a needle with anyone who has gotten AIDS or is HIV-positive?
- Did you or any of your sexual partners receive treatment for hemophilia between 1978 and 1985?
- Did you or any of your sexual partners have a blood transfusion or organ transplant between 1978 and 1985?

risk behaviors Activities that may entail the risk of exposure to a PATHOGEN, or an injury. In the case of HIV/AIDs, risk behaviors are generally thought to include receipt of blood products (1978 through 1985); INJECTION DRUG USE (since 1978); homosexual/bisexual activity (since 1978, predominantly males); prostitution (male and female, since 1978); and sex with a partner who participates in any of the above. In the late 1970s and early 1980s, the CENTERS FOR DISEASE CONTROL AND PREVENTION (CDC) and others believed that behaviors associated with "the gay lifestyle" were responsible for bringing people into contact with the virus. Among the factors considered were AMYL NITRATE "poppers," rogue genes, repeated bouts of common sexually transmitted diseases, and too much sex.

risk factor Environmental, chemical, psychological, physiological, or genetic factors thought to create a predisposition to a particular disease or condition. The major risk factors for HIV infection are needle-sharing with INJECTION DRUG USERS and sexual contact with a person who has or may have been exposed to HIV. Another risk factor is having received blood products between 1978, when HIV infection is first known to have existed in the United States, and May 1985, when the blood supply was first screened for HIV. Other risk factors include promiscuous or casual sexual contact without precautions and being born to an HIV-infected woman. A NEEDLESTICK injury in the course of caring for people with HIV infection or AIDS is a minor risk factor. It is possible for people with HIV infection to have no clearly defined risk factor; in such cases the patients may have provided inadequate or suspect information.

risk group An epidemiological concept referring to a group of people sharing a common behavior or characteristic placing them at greater risk for contracting a particular disease or developing a particular condition than the general population. In the case of AIDS, the syndrome was first identified in gay men, leading the CENTERS FOR DISEASE CONTROL AND PREVENTION and others to speculate on the possibility that something they termed the "gay lifestyle" might itself be responsible for the condition. The discovery in late 1981 that Haitians and IV drug users were also affected by the syndrome did not support this theory, and a virus became the main suspect. The risk group concept was useful for public health, preventive purposes in the early years of the epidemic. In the media and in political debate, the epidemiological category of risk group has been used to stereotype and stigmatize people already seen as outside the moral and economic parameters of the "general population."

risk practice   This concept, that has replaced RISK GROUP for all but surveillance purposes by the National Academy of Sciences, shifts the emphasis away from characterizing and stigmatizing people as members of groups.

risk reduction   Process by which an individual changes behavior to decrease the likelihood of acquiring an infection.

Ritalin   See METHYLPHENIDATE.

ritonavir   A PROTEASE INHIBITOR manufactured by Abbott Laboratories and approved for the treatment of HIV disease. The most common adverse effects associated with ritonavir are gastrointestinal: nausea, vomiting, diarrhea, and anorexia. Circumoral and peripheral paresthesias have also been reported. Common laboratory abnormalities include elevated liver enzymes in the blood and elevated cholesterol and triglycerides. Metabolic abnormalities, redistribution of body fat, and diabetes have been associated with regimens containing protease inhibitors. Initial adverse effects associated with ritonavir may be because of high drug concentration in the blood during the first two weeks of therapy. The manufacturer recommends a dose-escalation protocol to increase tolerance. Ritonavir is a potent inhibitor of the CYTOCHROME P450 3A4 isoenzyme, an important metabolic pathway for many common drugs. Other P450 pathways are induced by ritonavir and some drug levels are lowered. Note that all approved protease inhibitors inhibit cytochrome P450 enzymes but that ritonavir is the most potent. Thus, its clinical importance lies more in its ability to improve pharmacokinetic profiles of other protease inhibitors than its efficacy and tolerability as a single protease inhibitor as part of a triple-combination regimen. Current practice favors the use of ritonavir in combination therapy, for example, with nucleoside ana-

log drugs, to prevent the development of drug-resistant virus. Ritonavir enhancement is the use of ritonavir with other drugs, especially with other protease inhibitors, to increase their level in the blood. (The trade name is Norvir.)

RMP-7   A drug that allows substances to cross the blood–brain barrier.

RNA   See RIBONUCLEIC ACID.

Robimycin   See ERYTHROMYCIN.

Robomox   See AMOXICILLIN.

Roferon-A   See ALPHA INTERFERON.

rosiglitazone   A drug used in the treatment of Type II DIABETES (noninsulin-dependent). It is a drug that increases the sensitivity of the body to natural insulin. Insulin is the substance the body produces to control and maintain stable blood sugar levels. Drugs that perform this function are called thiazolidinediones. They also have effects on fat metabolism. This drug had been tested in trials recently in HIV patients that are effected by LIPODYSTROPHY and other metabolic changes due to treatment with HIGHLY ACTIVE ANTI-VIRAL THERAPY (HAART). Results of these studies have been mixed, with some trial results showing no changes in abnormal body composition and other trials showing a better balance of blood sugar in the body and fewer changes in fat distribution. These studies are ongoing and results will determine the use of this type of drug in managing body composition issues in people taking HAART.

route of administration   See ADMINISTRATION.

route of transmission   See TRANSMISSION.

routine testing   Systematic testing of everyone in a particular class (for instance, all pregnant women or all men over age 40) for a given disease or condition.

roxithromycin   A macrolide ANTIBIOTIC, like CLARITHROMYCIN and AZITHROMYCIN, being developed for use against CRYPTOSPORIDIOSIS and other bacterial infections.

rPF4   Recombinant platelet factor 4. A synthetic version of a naturally occurring protein that inhibits blood vessel formation that is being studied for the treatment of KS. New blood vessel formation is believed to be important in the development of KS.

RT-PCR (reverse transcriptase polymerase chain reaction)   A U.S. FOOD AND DRUG ADMINISTRATION-approved test to measure viral load. This test is also known as PCR. See POLYMERASE CHAIN REACTION.

RU-486 (mifepristone)   A progesterone antagonist drug that has abortifacient (abortion-inducing) activity and may inhibit HIV replication.

rubber   See CONDOM.

rubber dam   A thin rubber tissue used by dentists to seal off a tooth from saliva during dental treatment. See DENTAL DAM.

rupture of membranes   The breaking open of the amniotic sac (or "bag of waters") surrounding the fetus in a pregnant woman before the start of labor and delivery.

rush   A strong contraction wave that moves down the small intestine; the first surge of pleasure produced by a drug, especially a narcotic drug. See AMYL NITRITE INHALANT; BUTYL NITRITE INHALANT.

Russia   See EASTERN EUROPE AND CENTRAL ASIA.

Ryan White CARE Act   See RYAN WHITE COMPREHENSIVE AIDS RESOURCES EMERGENCY (CARE) ACT OF 1990.

Ryan White Comprehensive AIDS Resources Emergency (CARE) Act of 1990   An act that amends the Public Health Service Act, the Ryan White Comprehensive AIDS Resources Emergency Act provides emergency assistance to localities that are disproportionately affected by the Human Immunodeficiency Virus epidemic and makes financial assistance available to states and other public or private nonprofit entities to provide for the development, organization, coordination, and operation of more effective and cost-efficient systems for the delivery of essential services to individuals and families with HIV disease.

Ryan White National Fund   Founded in 1986 and named after a young victim of AIDS who died amid great public notice in 1990, this organization seeks to assist seriously ill children, particularly those with AIDS. It provides emergency financial aid, counseling, referral and placement services, promotes research, operates clinics, maintains a speakers' bureau, compiles statistics, and conducts education and awareness programs.

S & M Also written S/M, SM, and S-M, this is a slang term for sadism and masochism, or slave/master. See SADOMASOCHISM.

sadism Sexual behavior in which participants obtain erotic enjoyment from inflicting physical or psychological pain on their partner or partners.

sadomasochism Sexual behavior in which erotic enjoyment is obtained by giving or receiving physical or psychological pain. Alternate terms include S/M, S-M, S & M, B/D, D/S, and English.

sadomasochism safety For people who practice what has been called politically incorrect sex—fantasy and role playing, bondage and discipline, fetishes, alternate gender identities, and especially SADOMASOCHISM (S&M)—there are now safety manuals available. These guides emphasize health and hygiene as well as emotional and psychological safety. Because occasionally physical injuries can arise from "doing scenes," S&M first aid has received particular attention in the age of AIDS. The consequences of anal, rectal, and vaginal injuries; bleeding, abrasion, or bruises; rope burns; fainting, dizziness, and nausea; muscle strains and nerve irritations; and even occasionally worse injuries take on an entirely different dimension when one or both partners are HIV-positive. In addition to safety manuals, local S&M support groups also offer safe sex information. National groups, some of mixed gender, can also be tapped for information or referrals to local support groups. These groups generally encourage practices that are safe, sensible, and consensual.

safe sex Sex practices in which participants protect themselves from viral transmission. Generally, safe sex is sex in which there is no mucous membrane contact or bodily fluid (SEMEN, VAGINAL FLUIDS, blood, etc.) exchange between partners. Safe sex protects from HIV as well as other sexually transmitted diseases such as GONORRHEA, SYPHILIS, and CHLAMYDIA. Unfortunately, protection can never be absolute; the only absolutely safe sexual practices are celibacy and MASTURBATION.

Aside from those activities, the best way to prevent HIV infection is to have only one sex partner, who you know is not infected. Testing negative to HIV twice with six months between tests is generally thought to indicate safety if neither partner has been involved with others in the meantime. It is impossible to create an exhaustive list of sex acts and assign each a relative risk of infection with HIV. It is best to be consistent about following overall safe sex guidelines that combine precautions based on both what is known to be true and what seems reasonable in terms of today's state of knowledge. Some basic principles of safe sex are highlighted in the following.

The use of latex CONDOMS is highly recommended for protection when engaging in any sexual activities that could result in the exchange of body fluids. Lambskin and other natural membrane products have not tested as well as latex or polyurethane condoms for protection and can allow HIV to pass through the condom. The use of spermicidal (sperm-killing) lubricants, especially those with NONOXYNOL-9, may increase protection but has not been proved effective. Spermicides should always be used with a condom and never instead of a condom. Many condoms are prelubricated, some with SPERMICIDES. Condoms should always be used for protection in anal sex and in vaginal sex. Condoms can also be used in oral sex between men and between men and women. They can be purchased with flavored lubricant to reduce the "rubber taste" that can occur when they are used for oral sex.

If neither partner has clinical or laboratory evidence of HIV, each may safely engage in intimate sexual activities with the other, without using condoms, provided that neither has outside sexual partners or other risk factors for HIV. If both or one of the partners has evidence of infection with HIV, effective birth control measures should be employed. Any heterosexual person having casual sexual contacts should always use condoms during vaginal or anal sex. Homosexual men engaging in casual sexual activity should also use condoms for all sexual activities in which ejaculation might lead to semen's contacting the skin or mucosa of the partner. It is also important to realize that a single negative laboratory test result for HIV may provide a false sense of security and that the time required for HIV to progress to possible opportunistic infections may be years.

safe sex and bad sex   See BAD SEX.

safe sex and good sex   See BAD SEX.

safer sex   A term sometimes preferred to *safe sex*, because it does not imply that sexual contact can be made 100 percent safe. The term recognizes the likelihood of human error, the inexactness of human knowledge, and the fact that people will engage in activities that may not be 100 percent safe. Latex, polyurethane, or other plastic barriers for oral and anal–oral sex between lesbians and gay men are often recommended by safer sex educators. These educators note that lesbians are definitely at risk for HIV and other sexually transmitted diseases because exchange of bodily fluids and possibly blood is often involved in lesbian sex. Viruses such as HERPES SIMPLEX and HUMAN PAPILLOMAVIRUS (which causes genital warts) can be transmitted by oral–genital contact, which is considered a medium to low risk on the spectrum of HIV transmission. Several different products can be used by lesbians as barriers for oral sex. Unlubricated latex condoms can be cut into flat barriers by cutting off the tips and cutting through one edge of the condoms before unrolling them. Flavored condoms are also available. DENTAL DAMS are larger then condoms and therefore easier to use as barriers. However, they can be more expensive and are less commonly available. Plastic food wrap can also be used as a barrier, and testing has shown that microwavable and nonmicrowavable wraps are equally protective.

safest sex   The safe sex practices with the least risk of infection with HIV or other sexually transmissible disease. Sexual ABSTINENCE and self-MASTURBATION are the safest sexual practices and the only ones that are 100 percent effective.

Saint John's wort   A popular herbal treatment sold over the counter as a treatment for depression. It was named after Saint John because it blooms around the saint's day, *Wort* is an Old English word for "plant." It has been proved in studies to have many times fewer side effects than prescribed antidepressants. It is not effective when taken in conjunction with selective serotonin reuptake inhibitors (SSRIs), as it works in the same manner that they do. The chemical in Saint John's wort, hypericin, has been shown in vitro to have antiviral activity against a number of viruses. A National Institutes of Health study showed in 2000 that Saint John's wort interferes with the absorption of INDINAVIR, as, well as cyclosporine, an antirejection drug used after organ transplantation, because Saint John's wort is metabolized by the same CYTOCHROME P450 ENZYME SYSTEM that metabolizes many drugs. This action causes PROTEASE INHIBITORS, in particular, to drop to levels that may not suppress HIV, leading to RESISTANCE.

saliva   The clear waterlike fluid found in the mouth, secreted by the salivary and oral mucous glands, that begins the process of digesting food. Test-tube studies have suggested that a protein in saliva called SLPI (SECRETORY LEUKOCYTE PROTEASE INHIBITOR) inhibits HIV.

salivary gland infection   A viral infection of the oral cavity glands that secrete saliva.

Salk HIV-1 vaccine   A vaccine, also known as the Salk immunogen, made from inactivated HIV-1 (minus the gp120 envelope) with Incomplete

Freund's Adjuvant (IFA), a mineral and oil emulsion used to increase the antigenicity of the vaccine. Polio vaccine discoverer, Jonas Salk, first proposed the idea of therapeutic vaccination for HIV-infected people in 1987. His concept involves inoculating with virus particles that have been both killed and stripped of their outer coat. The idea is to stimulate an immune response to HIV's inner protein appearing on the surface of HIV-infected cells. Researchers continue to harbor doubts about therapeutic vaccines, and Salk's colleagues who have continued research since his death have been unable to resolve these doubts.

Salk immunogen   See SALK HIV-1 VACCINE.

Salk polio vaccine   See SALK VACCINE.

Salk vaccine   The first successful poliomyelitis vaccine, it contains three types of formalin-inactivated poliomyelitis viruses and induces immunity against the disease. It was developed by Dr. Jonas Salk and first made available in 1954.

sallowness   Texture and temperature of skin are important signs of underlying causes. Sallowness is generally indicative of cachexia; syphilis; chronic gallbladder disease; arthritis deformans; constipation; some anemias; and gastric, pancreatic, enteric, or hepatic disorders. See SKIN DISORDER; SKIN RASH.

Salmonella   A genus of GRAM-NEGATIVE BACTERIA belonging to the family Enterobacteriaceae. Over 1,400 species have been identified, some of which are pathogenic. The most common manifestation is food poisoning, ranging in severity from mild gastroenteritis to death.

salmonellosis   Any disease caused by infection with bacteria of the genus *Salmonella*. It can be manifested as gastroenteritis, septicemia, or typhoid fever.

salpingitis   Inflammation and infection of the fallopian tubes. Part of the PELVIC INFLAMMATORY DISEASE (PID) syndrome.

salvage drug regimens   See SALVAGE THERAPY.

salvage therapy   Generally, drug regimens used after the initial course of treatment or therapy for HIV has not caused the viral load to drop to minimal levels. There is no standardized definition for the term, so different physicians use it in different ways. Some may use the term for a second or third set of drugs. Others use it to refer to the last known set of drugs available to a patient. Some physicians refuse to use the term because of its negative connotation of junked freighters at the bottom of the ocean. Also called rescue therapy.

same-gender sexual behavior   See HOMOSEXUALITY or LESBIANISM.

sample   In the vocabulary of statistical analysis, a number of individuals selected from a population to test hypotheses about the population or to derive estimates of its characteristics.

sample size   In statistics, a subset of a population. Within the context of scientific research and clinical trials, to decide on a sample size *(N)* for a clinical trial, investigators must first establish standards for the precision of their measurements, then decide how much comparative benefit from the drug would be meaningful or possible to observe. Finally, researchers calculate the number of people who should be enrolled in order to obtain statistically significant results.

San Joaquin Valley fever   See COCCIDIOIDOMYCOSIS.

sanctuary   The inner room of a church; also used to refer to a safe place where someone cannot be harmed. In HIV topics, *sanctuary* refers to a place in the body where the virus "hides" or locates itself and avoids detection by drug therapies and the immune system. Scientists have found that HIV can reside in the CENTRAL NERVOUS SYSTEM and the brain, long after the virus has been eliminated from the blood or other fluids. What this means is that although test results may indicate that someone has low or no VIRAL LOAD, he or she probably still has HIV living in the body somewhere. HAART and other current drug therapies in HIV treatment are currently not very successful in crossing the BLOOD-BRAIN BARRIER, therefore making the brain a sanctuary for the virus.

Sandimmune   See CYCLOSPORINE A.

saquinavir   Saquinavir was the first PROTEASE INHIBITOR approved by the FDA for treatment of HIV. It is currently approved for treatment in combination with NUCLEOSIDE ANALOGS. Saquinavir should be taken after a full meal. The most common side effects, which occur in very few people, are diarrhea, stomach discomfort, and nausea. The initial formulation of saquinavir was called Invirase. Invirase did not have very high anti-HIV activity because of its poor absorption in the intestine and rapid breakdown in the liver. Maintaining sufficient levels of the drug in the blood was difficult. Combining saquinavir with ritonovir increases its blood levels tenfold. Therefore, Invirase is usually used in HAART with ritonovir to create a useful drug regimen. The saquinavir formula has been changed to a gel formula that also increases the availability of the drug in the body. As in other HAART regimens, saquinavir is believed to be one cause of LIPODYSTROPHY. Liver function test results should be monitored regularly. (The trade names are Fortovase and Invirase.)

sarcoma   A malignant tumor of the skin and soft tissue.

scabies   A highly contagious skin disease caused by the itch mite. It is transmitted by close contact and is characterized by the eruption of papules, vesicles, and pustules. Eczema may result from scratching.

scapegoating   A person or group made to bear the blame for others or to suffer in their place. In the first five years of the epidemic, as AIDS virus evidence mounted, fear also erupted; exposure to Americans of the virus was much higher than had previously been suspected. As fears escalated, so did blaming so-called high risk persons or groups associated with HIV/AIDS (e.g., homosexuals, immigrants, injection drug users) for the continuing spread of the disease.

scat   The excrement of an animal or human; also a slang term for sexual fetishes that involve human feces.

scavenger cell   One of a diverse group of white blood cells with the capacity to engulf and destroy foreign material and dead tissue and cells.

Schedule 1 drugs   On the basis of the Controlled Substances Act, which the U.S. Congress passed in 1970, controlled substances are classified into five "schedules." Schedule 1 drugs have a high potential for abuse and no current accepted medical use in the United States or are not safe to use even under medical supervision. It is not legal to possess these substances under any circumstances. Drugs in this class include opium and heroin, hallucinogenic substances (including LSD, marijuana, MDA, MDMA, GHB, mescaline, peyote, and psilocybin), Quaaludes, cocaine (including crack), and a few other substances. Use of these substances has been linked to increased risk for infection with HIV. Pharmacies, other than those in facilities that are registered for investigative or research uses, should not have any Schedule 1 controlled substances in inventory. Further, physicians are not authorized to prescribe Schedule 1 controlled substances unless registered to perform investigations or research under approved research protocols. Most of the controlled substance ANALOGS of drugs in other schedules, sometimes called designer drugs, are classified as Schedule 1 controlled substances.

Schedule 2 drugs   Drugs that have a high potential for abuse, they have a currently accepted medical use in the United States or a currently accepted use with severe restrictions. Abuse may lead to severe psychological or physical dependence. Morphine, amphetamines, and methamphetamine fall into this schedule, as does PCP, which is legally used as a veterinary anesthetic. Other major pain relievers, such as oxycodone (OxyContin, Percocet, Roxicodone), hydromorphone (Dilaudid), and meperidine (Demerol), also fall into this schedule. Methylphenidate (Ritalin), a stimulant in this class, is commonly used to treat attention deficit hyperactivity disorder. Schedule 2 prescription orders must be written and signed by the practitioner. They may not be telephoned into the pharmacy except in an emergency. In addition, a prescription for a Schedule 2 drug may not be refilled; the patient must see the practitioner again in order to obtain more drugs. Schedule 2 drugs are manufactured each year on the basis of the amount used in preceding years. Their manufacture after this enforced limit has been reached is illegal.

Schedule 3 drugs Substances that have less potential for abuse than substances in Schedules 1 and 2. The substances have a currently accepted medical use for treatment in the United States and a moderate or low physical or high psychological dependence potentiation when abused. Ketamine falls into this category. It is used legally as a human and veterinary anesthetic. Anabolic steroids are in this class, as are codeine and some barbiturates. For Schedule 3 drugs, the prescription order may be either written or oral (that is, telephoned to the pharmacy). In addition, the patient may (if authorized by the practitioner) have the prescription refilled up to five times and at any time within six months of the date of the initial dispensing.

Schedule 4 drugs Having low potential for abuse relative to substances in Schedule 3, substances that have a currently accepted use in treatment in the United States and a limited physical or psychological dependence potentiation when abused relative to substances in Schedule 3. FLUNITRAZEPAM (Rohypnol), the "date rape" drug, is in this classification although it cannot be prescribed by American doctors. It is included in this classification as a result of U.S. treaty obligations because of its prescription usage in European and Latin American countries. Darvon, Talwin, Equanil, Valium, and Xanax are other examples of Schedule 4 drugs. For Schedule 4 drugs, the prescription order may be either written or oral (that is, telephoned to the pharmacy). In addition, the patient may (if authorized by the practitioner) have the prescription refilled up to five times and at any time within six months of the date of the initial dispensing. Import agents registered with the U.S. Drug Enforcement

Agency may import these substances into the United States unless they are narcotic-based.

Schedule 5 drugs Drugs that have a low, but very real, potential for abuse relative to substances in Schedule 4. The substances have a currently accepted use for treatment in the United States and a limited physical or psychological dependence potentiation when abused, relative to the substances listed in Schedule 4. Schedule 5 includes some prescription drugs and many over-the-counter narcotic preparations, including antitussives (cough medicines, particularly with codeine) and antidiarrheals. Even here, however, the law imposes restrictions beyond those normally required for over-the-counter sales; for example, the patient must be at least 18 years of age, must offer some form of identification, and must have his or her name entered into a special log maintained by the pharmacist as part of a record. Import agents registered with the U.S. Drug Enforcement Agency may import these substances into the United States unless they are narcotic-based.

Schistosoma A genus of parasites or flukes belonging to the family Schistosomatidae, class Trematoda, that thrives on blood; the blood fluke.

schizophrenia (schizophrenic disorders) A group of related disorders of unknown cause characterized by specific forms of disordered thinking, affect, and behavior. Clinically, patients exhibit disturbances of content of thought with delusions, such as the feeling that thoughts have been inserted into their head are now being broadcast out into the world. Speech may be coherent in actual words used but entirely unassociated with plausible thoughts or reality. Alternatively, the patient may be mute or completely incoherent. Perception is disordered by all forms of hallucinations. Affect may be flat or inappropriate to the situation. There is loss of a feeling of identity, and self-direction may be disturbed. All activity may be disturbed so that the ability to work or carry a task to completion is severely impaired. Interpersonal relations are abnormal and may take the form of social withdrawal and emotional detachment. The patient may be catatonic or otherwise unaware of his or her surroundings. In general, these disturbances are present for six months before the diagnosis of schizophrenia is accepted. Prognosis is usually poor, but over a 25- to 30-year period about one-third of patients show recovery or remission. Schizophrenia occurs equally in males and females and at any age, but the usual age of admission to a hospital is 28 to 34.

The relation of safe sex and first-episode schizophrenia (as compared with more chronic schizophrenia) has been the subject of recent research. It is noted that the first episode of schizophrenia can be a traumatic and frightening occurrence in a young person's life. The first episode comprises the prepsychotic period and the first five years after onset of psychosis; it is the period when the most severe deterioration in functioning takes place. It is also a time when young people with schizophrenia struggle with the developmental tasks of young adulthood, including those related to sexuality. Studies show that persons with schizophrenia are often involved in unprotected sex and become at risk for HIV infection. Research reports show a need for safe sex intervention. However, to date, there are only a few reports on programs for clients with schizophrenia, and they show limited success. Published data on work with first-episode schizophrenia and safe sex interventions are scarce.

Awareness of HIV and symptoms in schizophrenia, that is, AIDS content in psychosis and sexuality and first-episode clients, is important. Briefly, clinical experience indicates that clients with schizophrenia often experience AIDS-related content in their psychotic experiences. Clinicians report, however, that delusional and hallucinatory content related to AIDS may not be reality-based and may indicate that a patient is acutely psychotic. With regard to sexuality and first-episode clients, hypersexuality has been reported in first-episode patients. These symptoms have been shown to become more prominent with increased levels of psychosis and often lead to unsafe sex practices. Patients have also reported hallucinations and delusions with homosexual content. As the psychotic material remitted, these fears subsided, only to reappear at the start of a relapse. Fear of being homosexual has also been reported. It is not clear whether the studies reported no homosexual activity or whether there was only discomfort in discussing homosexual behavior.

Although coping with the diagnosis and symptoms of schizophrenia may overshadow sexual concerns for first-episode patients, learning about safe sex practices is both appropriate and necessary. Interventions designed to encourage safe sex practices for first-episode clients take place in both group therapy and individual treatment. Psychosocial interventions are generally varied, depending on where the patient is in the course of the illness. Safe sex interventions are called for when patients are in the "healing" phase, when psychotic symptoms are beginning to remit. This may occur when patients are receiving inpatient or outpatient treatment. Within the confines of a safe therapeutic environment, safe sex practices are discussed with all clients, regardless of whether they are currently sexually active. The rationale is that this is such a crucially important subject that it concerns everyone. For those patients who are sexually active, there may be additional work focusing on their unique situation.

An important process in treatment is helping patients reintegrate their identify. Reintegration of identity often becomes the content of phase-of-illness-related psychosocial interventions. It is during the healing phase that there is a need for returning to a normal lifestyle and redefining the sense of self. Along with returning to school, work, and households at whatever level possible, patients rekindle old relationships and form new ones. When sex is involved in relationships, education about HIV protection is crucial. An assertive role for the clinician is generally advised. If the patient is reluctant to introduce the subject of safe sex, therapeutic timing and close attention to individual needs have been shown to help ease the process. The mode of treatment, group or individual therapy, may call for somewhat different approaches. In groups, the power of the group is called on; in individual treatment, it is the one-to-one therapeutic alliance that becomes the foundation on which safe sex practices are established and monitored. Ultimately it is the responsibility of the clinician to see that the subject of safe sex becomes an integral component of the treatment plan for first-episode patients.

SCID   See SEVERE COMBINED IMMUNODEFICIENCY.

screening   The testing, usually by using one diagnostic procedure including laboratory studies, of large groups of people to determine the presence of a particular disease or of certain risk factors known to be associated with that disease. In an HIV/AIDS context, *screening* may entail mandatory HIV screening, screening of blood donors for HIV, screening of sperm for HIV, and/or screening through voluntary testing. Screening can also involve one person's being screened for virus. Some have advocated mandatory screening for HIV infection in large portions of the population (either of the population at large or of well-defined subgroups). In psychiatry screening is the initial examination to determine mental status and appropriate initial therapy. See MANDATORY TESTING; PRIVACY.

SDF-1   See STROMAL CELL–DERIVED FACTOR 1.

seborrhea   See SEBORRHEIC DERMATITIS.

seborrheic dermatitis   An acute or chronic inflammatory skin disease suspected to be due to a fungus, characterized by dry, moist, or greasy scaling and yellow or brown-gray crusted patches. It is called dandruff when it occurs on the scalp. It tends to involve the scalp but may include parts of the face, ears, genitalia, umbilicus, and even arms or legs. Generalized seborrheic dermatitis requires careful attention and skin hygiene. Oils and lotions can make the condition worse. The skin is kept as dry as possible. Topical cortisone or miconazole preparations may be required.

seborrheic eczema   See SEBORRHEIC DERMATITIS.

second generation   A drug that is in the same class (i.e., NONNUCLEOSIDE REVERSE TRANSCRIPTASE INHIBITOR; PROTEASE INHIBITOR) as already used drugs but has a promise of producing greater benefits or fewer side effects than previously approved drugs in that class.

secondary care setting   A place where patients are referred for special care beyond primary health care; a hospital.

secondary effect   A by-product or complication of drug use which does not occur as part of the drug's primary pharmacological activity. Secondary effects are unwanted consequences and may therefore be classified as adverse effects.

secondary immune response   The heightened response of the immune system to the second, or subsequent, occasion on which it encounters a specific antigen, toxin, bacterium, or other microorganism.

secondary infection   An infection contracted in addition to (and often due to the compromised immunity caused by) AIDS. Among the most common are MONONUCLEOSIS, TUBERCULOSIS, and PNEUMONIA.

secondary prophylaxis   A prophylactic medicine or measure (prophylactic treatment) to prevent an infection from recurring. Generally, the treatment must be taken for life. Also known as suppressive or maintenance therapy. See PRIMARY PROPHYLAXIS.

secondary response   The immune response that follows a second or later encounter with a particular ANTIGEN. MEMORY CELLS from the PRIMARY RESPONSE are the only part of the IMMUNE SYSTEM that take part in the body's response. As a result, the body can quickly defeat many pathogens that an individual is exposed to more than one time.

second-line therapy   A therapy used after an initial or first-line treatment has failed.

secretory leukocyte protease inhibitor (SLPI)   A protein in SALIVA that according to test tube studies inhibits HIV. The protein attaches to white blood cells and prevents HIV from infecting those cells. Current studies are focusing on whether SLPI has an application as an anti-HIV treatment or as a viricidal adjunct to safer sex.

Section 1619 of the Social Security Act   See SOCIAL SECURITY ACT, SECTION 1619.

sedative   Quieting, soothing, tranquilizing; an agent that has such an effect. Sedatives may be general, local, nervous, or vascular. Cardiac sedatives decrease the heart's force; nervous sedatives affect the nervous system.

segregation In an HIV/AIDS context, the separation of people with HIV/AIDS from the general population within a large custodial institution like a prison or military organization. Segregation addresses the AIDS epidemic by imposing restrictions on individuals as a means to prevent transmission of the virus. Segregation is similar to QUARANTINE.

Today, most knowledgeable people believe that the segregation of HIV-infected people or people with AIDS is ineffective, impractical, and unsound, medically and ethically. In addition, it could convey a false sense of security, causing those who believe that the risk is reduced to take fewer precautions to avoid infection. Confining individuals who engage in behaviors that transmit HIV cannot control such a widespread epidemic. Other factors to be considered are the logistics of testing, the possibility of inaccurate test results, and the sheer challenge of finding housing for all infected personnel.

seizure There are two types of brain activity that are commonly known as seizures. A convulsion, or episode of uncontrolled movements of the arms and legs accompanied by unconsciousness and loss of control over urine or stool is called a grand mal seizure. Petit mal seizures may also be called absence attacks, when individuals may suddenly simply stare off into space without realizing that they are doing so and having no recollection of doing so when it is called to their attention. Seizures in HIV-positive people are generally grand mal seizures. The usual cause of seizures in people with HIV is an OPPORTUNISTIC INFECTION such as TOXOPLASMIC ENCEPHALITIS, CRYPTOCOCCAL MENINGITIS, lymphoma, or an opportunistic tumor in the brain. Less commonly, seizures are caused by an imbalance of ELECTROLYTES or by medications. Recurrent seizures can usually be controlled with such drugs as Dilantin and phenobarbital. Anyone who has recurrent seizures should be careful about his or her physical circumstances: working on ladders, for instance, or driving. In many states, it is illegal for a person with seizures to drive until the seizures have been controlled for at least one year.

selective serotonin reuptake inhibitor (SSRI) A drug that blocks the neurons of the brain from reabsorbing serotonin, a neurotransmitter. This leads to the accumulation of serotonin in the brain and increased serotonin stimulation. These medications have replaced older ANTIDEPRESSANTS because they have far fewer side effects. Increasing serotonin activity when a patient is depressed appears to improve the patient's condition in many cases. Minor side effects include sleep disturbances and appetite suppression.

selenium A chemical element resembling sulfur. It is poisonous to certain animals that feed on plants grown in soil that contains an excess of it. Selenium is one of several antioxidants that people with HIV are often advised to take because of serious deficiencies and increased need for a number of nutrients.

self-disclosure The act of making something known about oneself. There are many factors that influence the decision to reveal whether one is HIV-positive or HIV-negative to one's partner; to a date, a boss, or one's parents, children, family, or friends. These factors include understanding why it is important to tell a particular person at this point in one's life. Individuals are generally advised to consider the emotional maturity of the person to whom they are disclosing information and to be prepared for questions. People often want to know all of the details of the process behind the disclosure. How did this happen? How long have you been this way? It is also important to think about whom the individual you are telling would then tell. Would keeping the status a secret be too large a burden for the person being told the status? What happens if one does not disclose?

For example is missing work for doctor's appointments going to cause problems in work attendance? Individuals are encouraged to check with their peers to receive encouragement on the topic and to ask how they have handled self-disclosure issues. Thinking about self-disclosure can be preparation for possible negative reactions that may (or may not) lie ahead. A second advantage of self-disclosure for HIV-positive persons is that it generally contributes to the development of a positive self-identity as an HIV-positive person. Through self-disclosure individuals commit to living in the world as HIV-positive individuals, being involved with others who are HIV-positive, and helping other HIV-positive individuals do the same in their life. It also helps to make an individual aware of the many times disclosure can protect him or her from passing the virus to another person. Self-disclosure applies not just to HIV but to many other areas of life that may be affected by acknowledging personal issues in public spaces.

self-insemination   A woman's introduction of donated sperm into her own body without the help of a doctor.

To inseminate herself, a woman should have no fertility problems and her menstrual cycle should be fairly regular. Charting one's basal temperature and mucus consistency for a few months is the first step. This will indicate when one is likely to ovulate. Finding a fertile man who is willing to donate sperm is the next step. When one knows from past cycles that one is about to ovulate, the sperm donor must masturbate into a clean (preferably boiled, but cooled) jar. Within an hour after ejaculation, the woman sucks the semen into a needleless hypodermic syringe (some women use an eye dropper or a turkey baster), gently inserts the syringe into her vagina while lying flat on her back with her rear up on a pillow. She then empties the syringe into the vagina to deposit the semen as close to the CERVIX as possible. The woman should continue lying down comfortably for about 10 minutes, so that as little sperm as possible leaks out of the vagina. It is generally recommended that this procedure be repeated with fresh sperm samples in two or three days, during and after the time the woman ovulates. Most woman become pregnant after trying self-insemination during three to five cycles.

semen   A thick, opalescent fluid, produced in the male reproductive organs, that is ejaculated through the PENIS during orgasm. Semen is the secretory product of various organs (the prostate, bulbourethral glands, seminal vesicles, and others) plus spermatozoa and ranges in color from milky white to yellow to grayish. Besides living sperm, semen contains water, three simple sugars (to provide nourishment for the sperm), alkalis (to buffer the acidity of the urethra and the vagina),

prostaglandins (substances that cause the contractions of the uterus and fallopian tubes and are thought to aid in the sperm's passage to the womb), vitamin C, zinc, cholesterol, and a few other elements. Healthy semen, in other words, does not contain anything that is harmful to health. In the age of AIDS, however, it is important to remember that, along with blood and vaginal secretions, semen is one of the primary carriers of HIV (it can also carry the organisms that cause GONORRHEA, HEPATITIS B, and CHLAMYDIA, among other illnesses). Use of CONDOMS and vaginal SPERMICIDAL CREAM or jelly can reduce women's chances of acquiring the virus during sexual intercourse; use of condoms can reduce men's chances also. Treating gonorrhea, chlamydial infections, trichomonas, and other sexually transmitted diseases in HIV-infected men significantly reduces the amount of HIV in semen. It does not, however, eliminate HIV completely, so BAREBACK activities should not be performed even when on HAART medications. Slang terms include cum, scum, spunk, load, spooge, and jism.

sensitivity   The degree of accuracy of a clinical test. Also, responsiveness to an ALLERGEN.

sensitization   The stimulation of allergic ANTIBODY production or DELAYED-TYPE HYPERSENSITIVITY by an initial encounter with a specific allergenic substance or hapten. Synonymous with PRIMARY RESPONSE.

sensuality   The quality of responsiveness to the senses; the capacity to experience sensual gratification. "Sensual" is sometimes used to refer to physical pleasure that is not overtly sexual, such as that derived from stroking.

sentinel animal   A susceptible animal used as an alarm for the presence of a HOT AGENT, since no instrument can detect a hot agent.

sepsis   Pathologic state, usually febrile, resulting from the presence of microorganisms or their poisonous products in the bloodstream. May be manifested as cellulitis (local dissemination of infection), lymphangitis or lymphadenitis (dispersion along lymphatic channels), or bacteremia (widespread dissemination by way of the bloodstream).

septicemia Presence of pathogenic bacteria in the blood. If allowed to progress, the organisms may multiply and cause an overwhelming infection and death. Symptoms usually include chills and fever, petechiae (small, purplish, hemorrhagic spots on the skin), purpuric pustules, and abscesses. Shock may be present.

Septra See TRIMETHOPRIM/SULFAMETHOXAZOLE.

sequencing This term is used in two instances. First, it refers to a type of therapy known as sequencing therapy: the act, by a physician or medical provider, of using various drugs in a specific sequence for specific reasons. In HIV treatment a patient's virus may become resistant to particular drugs. The virus may also become resistant to particular classes of drugs after use. Sequencing involves evaluating the patient's virus, identifying what it may already be resistant to, and determining the best treatment given the virus and patient allergies or reactions. The process attempts to reserve the maximal number of future drugs to use, while maximizing the reduction of the virus in the patient.

Second, *sequencing* refers to the process of determining the AMINO ACID sequence of a protein to identify the genetic code of a particular organism. It is done to ascertain the genetic code of viruses to determine how to treat infection. It is performed to discover the genetic code of humans to identify where certain inherited traits are established in the code. It may also be called reading the codons.

sero- A prefix referring to blood serum.

seroconcordance Having sex only with persons with the same HIV status.

seroconversion The process by which a person's ANTIBODY status converts from negative to positive, with the appearance of antibodies in the blood in response to infection or vaccination. The immune system usually takes several days or weeks to recognize a foreign substance like a virus and to produce antibodies to it. After transmission of the HIV virus, it may take several months or more for antibodies to develop.

serodiscordant relationships Couples in whom one partner has tested positive for HIV and the other partner has not tested positive. Being part of a serodiscordant couple can cause a great deal of stress for both people in the relationship. The HIV-positive person often fears infecting the other partner or the other partner's leaving out of fear of the virus. The HIV-negative partner often fears becoming infected or the infected partner's dying. Studies have shown that sex is often strained and sometimes nonexistent among serodiscordant partners, particularly heterosexual couples who have disclosed their serostatus. Consistent usage of CONDOMS has shown to reduce SEROCONVERSION in HIV-negative partners significantly. Despite this fact, studies have shown that nearly half of all serodiscordant couples, both heterosexual and homosexual, report that UNSAFE SEX occurs in their relationships on an irregular basis.

serologic Relating to serology, the branch of medicine concerned with blood SERUM, the clear fluid portion of blood.

serologic study A study that compares the characteristics of the blood SERUM of individuals, especially those markers that indicate exposure to a particular agent of disease.

serologic test Any test performed on blood SERUM, the clear, liquid portion of the blood. Often such tests are performed to determine the presence of antibodies, which would indicate the presence of an ANTIGEN such as a microbe. Such a test has been conducted on blood if a patient's lab report includes the phrase *positive* (or *negative*) *serology*.

serologic testing See SEROLOGIC TEST.

seronegative Testing negative for antibodies to a substance or organism in the blood, such as HIV; not having such antibodies present. Synonymous with ANTIBODY negativity. In the context of HIV, the term indicates "not infected," HIV-NEGATIVE.

seropositive Testing positive for antibodies to a substance or organism in the blood, such as HIV; having such antibodies present in the blood. In the context of HIV, the term indicates HIV infection (HIV-POSITIVE).

seroprevalence The number of people with evidence of antibodies against the causative agent of a disease in a given population over a specific period or at a particular time. For HIV, the rate at which a given population tests positive on the ELISA test for HIV antibodies. The seroprevalence rate is nearly the same as the rate of HIV infection in a given population, leaving out mainly those who were recently infected.

seroreverter A person whose ANTIBODY status has changed from positive to negative. The term is used to describe perinatally exposed infants who are not truly infected and become HIV antibody negative as they lose maternal HIV antibody.

serostatus The condition of having or not having detectable antibodies to a microbe in the blood as a result of infection. One may have either a SERONEGATIVE (uninfected) or SEROPOSITIVE (infected) serostatus.

Serostim Serostim is a trademarked name for a recombinant form of Human Growth Hormone that is used to treat HIV wasting syndrome. There was some concern and controversy in 1991 when counterfeit packages of Serostim, an injectable drug, turned up in the U.S. market. Somewhere between the manufacture and recipient, some person or group had replaced the Serostim with a fake powder later shown to be HCG, a hormone used by bodybuilders predominately. This incident has pointed out the lack of regulation in the drug distribution system by the FOOD AND DRUG ADMINISTRATION or other U.S. federal agencies. Although the manufacture of drugs is regulated, the distribution of the drugs is not. Any person or company can register as a distributor in many states. Counterfeiters have found plenty of opportunity to create falsely labeled drugs or drugs that have been watered down to create more of the substance, thereby increasing their profits. The federal government has not cracked down on the distribution system, leaving this to the individual states to license the distributors and regulate them, causing problems such as that with Serostim.

sertraline A widely used antidepressant, also used to treat obsessive-compulsive disorder. Sertraline belongs to a class known as serotonin reuptake inhibitors. It is chemically unrelated to tricyclic, tetracyclic, or other classes of antidepressants. It has become widely used because it is effective and tends to have fewer side effects than other older antidepressants. The side effects that occur most frequently are dry mouth, headache, dizziness, tremors, nausea, diarrhea, fatigue, insomnia, difficulty ejaculating, and sleepiness. (Brand name is Zoloft.)

serum The clear portion of any body fluid, separated from its solid elements; for instance blood serum. In medical usage the term usually refers to (human) blood serum. Also, blood serum from an animal that has been immunized against a pathogenic organism, used for passive immunization of humans. In ordinary usage "serum" is sometimes a synonym for "vaccine."

serum glutamic oxalacetic transaminase (SGOT) See ASPARTATE AMINOTRANSAMINASE.

serum glutamic pyruvic transaminase (SGPT) See ASPARTATE AMINOTRANSAMINASE.

serum protein Any protein in blood serum.

serum sickness An adverse immunologic response to a foreign ANTIGEN, usually a heterologous protein.

seven-year itch See SCABIES.

severe combined immunodeficiency (SCID) A combination of rare congenital disorders characterized by impairment of both HUMORAL and CELL-MEDIATED IMMUNITY, manifested as lack of ANTIBODY formation in response to the presence of ANTI-GENS, lack of delayed hypersensitivity, and inability to reject foreign tissue transplants. Without restoration of immune function or isolation in a gnotobiotic (germfree) environment, death usually occurs by the first birthday as a result of OPPORTUNISTIC INFECTION.

sex   The word often used to refer to either of the biological categories male and female, with the physical and behavioral traits that distinguish them. It is also the general term for erotic activity of any kind.

sex club   A private facility dedicated to the promotion and pursuit of sexual pleasure (e.g., bathhouses, orgy rooms).

sex industry   The area of commercial enterprise based on the exploitation of interest in sex—pornography, prostitution, sex clubs, sex toys, devices, and so forth. See SEX WORKERS.

sex negativism   The conviction that most sexual thoughts, beliefs, and behaviors are repugnant, immoral, and not to be trusted or tolerated. Such attitudes, grounded in religious belief, personal distaste, or psychological disturbance, have always existed, but they are particularly inappropriate and destructive as a response to the AIDS crisis, since they devalue and discourage any pragmatic approach to the problem.

sex toy   Any object used during sexual activity to enhance sensual experience. Sex toys include dildos, vibrators, specially made CONDOMS, provocative undergarments, and erotic pictures, as well as scented massage oils and feathers. Whether an object is a sex toy is largely the judgment of the user.

sex worker   A worker in the sex industry who provides sexual services for money or other considerations. Sex workers include prostitutes, exotic dancers, strippers, madams, nude models, escorts, porn actors, and workers in massage parlors. Sex work is a form of labor, and like most labor in capitalist economies, it is often alienated (that is, the

worker has little or no control over working conditions and the way the work is organized). A distinction is made between voluntary and forced sex work. Forced prostitution is a form of aggravated sexual assault.

In some countries, sex workers are screened for HIV, and those found to have the virus are detained in special facilities where they are supposed to be rehabilitated or retrained. The right to protection against HIV/AIDS, the consequences of unsafe sex, and the principles and practices of safe sex are examples of training content. In other places, people with HIV are prevented from working in the sex industry by imprisonment or detention in medical or quarantine facilities. Specific legal, or quasi-legal, actions are often taken to prevent HIV-infected workers from continuing to work. These include closing commercial sex venues, taking police action again sex workers suspected of carrying HIV, and screening photos of HIV-infected sex workers on television in the form of community service announcements. There are few protests in either industrialized or developing countries against the idea that the removal of people with HIV from the sex industry is sound policy.

The scapegoating of prostitutes for sexually transmitted diseases has a long history. Because the public has traditionally been poorly informed about the reality of sex work, it is hardly surprising that, as the AIDS epidemic grew, the scapegoating of prostitutes for AIDS became more and more commonplace. In the 1970s many organizations, were formed not only to work for women's rights but also to address the issues of sex work. Today such organizations as COYOTE (Call Off Your Old Tired Ethics) exist worldwide. Most of them are working to prevent the scapegoating of sex workers for AIDS and other sexually transmitted diseases, and to educate sex workers, their clients, and the general public about prevention of these diseases.

sexology   The scientific study of sex.

sexual abuse   The forced participation of an unwilling individual in sexual activity by use of direct or implied threats. Abuse may involve actual physical contact, acts of exhibitionism or indecent exposure, rape, sexual assault, or sexual molestation. The active person may be male, female, adult, or child, and the abused person may be of the same or opposite sex of the abuser.

sexual apartheid The practice of selecting sex partners based on their HIV status. Prevention activists disagree on whether it is morally acceptable to select on the basis of SEROSTATUS. Others go further, saying that HIV-mixed marriages should be discouraged.

sexual assault See RAPE.

sexual behavior Sexual activities, ranging from touching, caressing, and looking to teasing, kissing, massaging, licking, sucking, and penetrating. What an individual does during sex, what an individual feels about her or his sexuality, how s/he wants to explore it, who s/he is with, how much love and understanding s/he feels, how comfortable all parties involved are with their bodies, how each party feels that day are matters of personal preference and ingenuity. Sexual behavior is also a reflection of sexual drives and satisfactions, both of which generally evolve throughout an individual's lifetime.

sexual double standard The traditional view that sexual freedom is acceptable for men but not for women. In most Western countries it has become less prevalent than it was two or more decades ago.

sexual dysfunction Any condition that prevents normal sexual functioning, up to and including sexual intercourse. Dysfunction may be temporary or persistent; it may have physiological or psychological origins. The use of some prescription drugs may cause sexual dysfunction in some people (in some cases, similar drugs without this side effect may be substituted). To some extent, sexual dysfunction is culturally defined. Recognized forms of sexual dysfunction include, for women, anorgasmia, painful intercourse, and vaginismus; for men, impotence, premature ejaculation, and retarded ejaculation.

sexual ethics A moral code of sexual behavior; guidelines for treating partners with kindness and

decency, playfulness and pleasuring. A sexual ethics might include the following: remember the Golden Rule; take time to make yourself desirable; ask for what you want; make sure that was a yes; take no for an answer; take responsibility; respect your partner's nakedness; remember to say thank you; keep some things private. To some degree, AIDS has given rise to a new consciousness of sexual ethics and etiquette. One means of reducing the sexual transmission of HIV is to practice safe sex, and safe sex guidelines are, in many ways, a form of sexual etiquette.

sexual etiquette Guidelines for sexual conduct. See SEXUAL ETHICS.

sexual fulfillment A feeling of contentment after a pleasurable and satisfying sexual encounter. There is a feeling of intense fulfillment in the orgasmic and resolution phases of the sexual response cycle.

sexual health As contrasted with sexual dysfunction, a lack of problems in sexual desire and sexual response. The WORLD HEALTH ORGANIZATION has defined three elements of sexual health: a capacity to enjoy and control sexual behavior in accordance with a social and personal ethic; freedom from fear, shame, guilt, false beliefs, and other psychological factors inhibiting sexual relationships; and freedom from organic disorder, disease, and deficiencies that interfere with sexual and reproductive functions. Today, it is understood that sexual health is inextricably linked to total well-being—emotional and physical. The better informed we are sexually, the greater our potential health benefit. It is known that sexual problems can also be connected to depression, fatigue, headaches, diabetes, heart attacks, cholesterol, and arthritis, as well as HIV/AIDS.

A common response to the discovery of HIV infection is to shun sexual relations for some period of time. This is often a symptom of depression and may be accompanied by a poor appetite and sleep disturbances. Sexual dysfunction is also a normal, and usually temporary, initial response to learning of HIV infection. HIV+ people may need to go through the stages of grieving both in anticipation of their own death and for the loss of their identity as healthy and whole before they can actively continue healthy and safe relationships in which affection and sexuality are experienced.

sexual identity   One's sexual self-definition. An individual's sexual identity is influenced by biological and psychological components. In addition to biological gender, there are three psychological components of sexual identity: (1) gender identity (a secure sense of one's genital maleness or femaleness); (2) sexual preference; and (3) gender role identity and gender role behaviors, traits, and interests that are socially considered to be gender specific.

sexual intercourse   The physical act of sexual coupling. Sexual intercourse can be carried on by persons of the same sex or persons of the opposite sex. Genital contact between individuals is commonly involved. For heterosexuals, sexual intercourse is most commonly sexual contact that involves insertion of an erect penis into a vagina. In ANAL INTERCOURSE a man's penis is inserted in his partner's rectum. In oral intercourse the mouth of one partner is used to stimulate the genitals of the other partner.

sexual orientation   See SEXUAL PREFERENCE.

sexual pleasure   See SEXUAL FULFILLMENT.

sexual preference   The sexual orientation one prefers in choosing his or her sex partners.

sexual risk reduction   See RISK REDUCTION.

sexual transmission   See TRANSMISSION.

sexuality   The sexual aspect of being; the capacity to respond to erotic stimuli, experience sexual feeling, and act sexually. As an aspect of being human, sexuality does not entail any specific set of behaviors or sexual preference. There are biological, cultural, psychological, and social dimensions to human sexuality, all of which help to shape an individual's attitude toward the body and his or her sense of sexual self.

Sexuality, in our culture, has perhaps been the subject of more moralizing, and the source of more conflicted emotions and psychological distress than any other human activity. This has complicated thinking about sexually charged issues and sometimes, as in the AIDS epidemic, impeded the search for a rational approach to a serious problem.

sexually transmitted disease (STD)   Any of a group of diseases, affecting both men and women, that are spread from person to person during any kind of heterosexual or homosexual activity. Some STDs can spread through skin-to-skin contact with an infected person's genital area—not just through intercourse. Sexually transmitted diseases include AIDS, CHANCROID, chlamydiosis, infestation with PUBIC LICE, GENITAL WARTS (HPV), GONORRHEA, GRANULOMA INGUINALE, HEPATITIS B (HBV), HERPES SIMPLEX, LYMPHOGRANULOMA VENEREUM, NONGONO-COCCAL URETHRITIS, PELVIC INFLAMMATORY DISEASE, SYPHILIS, and VAGINITIS (YEAST INFECTIONS, TRICHOMONIASIS). Although each STD presents unique diagnostic, therapeutic, and prevention challenges, all STDs share a common mode of transmission. Populations at risk for one STD are at risk for others, and the presence of one infection may influence the acquisition and course of another.

All STDs are preventable. Reducing the risk of contracting one requires taking certain precautions (see SAFE SEX). Because routes of transmission are similar for HIV and other STDs, similar prevention methods work to prevent those who have HIV from acquiring another STD or transmitting HIV to their partners, and to prevent those who are HIV-negative from acquiring HIV/STDs. Decreasing the frequency of partner change, seeking STD treatment early (as soon as any symptom appears), and using condoms consistently are actions under an individual's control that can minimize STD/HIV transmission risk. However, because some women may have little control over whether a male partner uses a condom, there is clearly an urgent need for better female-controlled prevention methods. Vaginal MICROBICIDES that are safe and acceptable are undergoing testing, mainly in developing countries, as a way to limit the heterosexual spread of HIV. At the community level, STD/HIV prevention methods include adding HIV/STD education to the information taught in schools, improving the quality of STD/HIV counseling and treatment among primary care providers, and increasing access to reproductive health care among those who are uninsured. Expanded access to substance abuse treatment may have an indirect effect on STD prevention at the community level as expanded services decrease an important driving force for high-risk sexual behavior.

At the minimum, these diseases cause discomfort. Left untreated, some STDs can cause serious long-term health problems. For example, gonorrhea and chlamydial infections can cause pelvic inflammatory disease, infertility, and ECTOPIC PREGNANCY. Several common STDs adversely affect pregnancy, resulting in spontaneous abortion, stillbirth, and premature delivery. Genital infections due to HUMAN PAPILLOMAVIRUS are associated with CERVICAL CANCER, one of the most common cancers in women throughout the world today. Moreover a pregnant woman can pass an infection to her baby. Infections in newborns include syphilis, herpes, gonococcal conjunctivitis (an eye disease that can lead to blindness), and chlamydial pneumonia, an infection of the lungs that can develop into a chronic respiratory disease.

The possibility that STDs act as "cofactors" to facilitate HIV spread was an important public health question in the 1990s. HIV has spread at a startling rate through heterosexual contact in some parts of the developing world such as sub-Saharan Africa, where other STDs are very prevalent. Studies have now conclusively shown that untreated STDs in a community enhance the spread of HIV. Improved STD services at the community level have been shown to result in lower rates of new HIV cases than in areas where "usual care" for STDs is delivered. At the individual level, treatment of gonorrhea, chlamydia, and genital ulcers has been shown to result in lowering of the amount of HIV in vaginal secretions. Thus, it is clear that untreated STDs make those who are HIV-infected more likely to pass along HIV to their sex partners. It is also clear that untreated STDs make those who are HIV-negative more susceptible to acquiring HIV infection from an HIV-positive partner. This *epidemiologic synergy* between HIV and other STDs makes early STD diagnosis and treat-

ment high priorities wherever HIV poses a threat to public health. In the United States, meeting this priority will require better access to high-quality reproductive health care for both HIV-positive and HIV-negative women.

Researchers have been concerned about the possibility that STDs might accelerate the progression of HIV disease. This concern is based on observations that activation of the body's immune system, through either infections or administration of vaccines, may temporarily increase viral load. Although the clinical importance of such viral load increases is not definitively known, studies of HIV-positive persons with tuberculosis—an infection that may cause increases in HIV viral load—have demonstrated more rapid HIV disease progression. Researchers have questioned whether similar effects could be caused by STDs. An increase in the amount of genital secretions has been noted with several different STDs, but it is not clear whether this increase in HIV replication is confined to the genital compartment or is more widespread in the body. Because some STDs, such as syphilis, cause widespread immune stimulation, an increase in plasma viral load would be predicted.

Standard treatment regimens for most STDs are effective in those who also have HIV infection.

Initial reports focusing on the interaction of HIV and syphilis indicated that those with HIV and syphilis might suffer complications of syphilis more frequently than those without HIV who acquire syphilis. However, a recent study evaluating the response to treatment for early-stage syphilis among those who were HIV-positive and HIV-negative found that there was no major difference between groups. Most experts currently recommend a spinal tap to rule out evidence of central nervous system infection in HIV-positive individuals who have a positive blood test result for syphilis but who do not have clinical signs (either a genital ulcer or a characteristic syphilis rash) suggesting that their infection was recently acquired.

Effective treatments for most sexually transmitted diseases do exist and the diseases are not always fatal. AIDS is similar to these diseases in that it is passed from person to person sexually. It is different from other sexually transmitted diseases however because to date there is no effective treatment for AIDS and it is always fatal.

sexually transmitted infections (STIs) See SEXUALLY TRANSMITTED DISEASE.

sexually transmitted vaginitis See SEXUALLY TRANSMITTED DISEASE.

Sezary syndrome A form of cutaneous T-CELL LYMPHOMA characterized by exfoliative dermatitis (shedding), severe itching, peripheral lymphadenopathy, and abnormal hyperchromatic mononuclear cells in the lymph nodes, skin, and peripheral blood.

SGA See SUBSTANTIAL GAINFUL ACTIVITY.

shark cartilage Shark cartilage—which is exactly what it sounds like—is rich in an ANGIOGENESIS-inhibiting protein called cartilage-derived inhibitor. Angiogenesis is the process whereby new blood vessels are formed to feed cancers, particularly solid tumors, such as KAPOSI'S SARCOMA. To date, studies of shark cartilage as a MONOTHERAPY for Kaposi's sarcoma in PWAs have been disappointing.

sharps container A specialized container designed for the disposal of used needles, blades, and contaminated fluids. They are ubiquitous in doctors' offices and hospitals.

Shigella A genus of non-lactose-fermenting non-motile, gram-negative rods belonging to the family Enterobacteriaceae. It contains a number of species that cause digestive disturbance ranging from mild diarrhea to a severe and often fatal dysentery.

shigellosis The disease produced by organisms of the genus *Shigella*.

shingles Known medically as zoster or herpes zoster, it causes the eruption of acute, inflammatory blisters or vesicles along the area of an affected nerve. The blisters generally form pustules, then dry and scab, leaving scarring. Shingles scars always appear darker or lighter than the surrounding skin area and never fade. In most cases the rash stays in the area of the body where it first appeared. The shingles rash seldom lasts longer than three weeks. However, the pain can continue after the rash has healed, because of the irritation of the nerves involved. The pain can occur and cease for a long time.

The disease represents reactivation of VARICELLA-ZOSTER VIRUS, usually acquired in childhood (when it appears as chicken pox). Shingles can be spread by person-to-person contact if someone has not been exposed to the virus. It is possible for someone who has never had chicken pox to contract it through contact with someone who is currently having a shingles episode. People who are immunosuppressed can have recurrences of shingles, though this does not typically occur in healthy adults. It is a member of the HERPES family of viruses but is not sexually transmitted. Standard treatment is with FAMCICLOVIR or ACYCLOVIR.

shiitake mushrooms One of several immune system stimulants that serve to boost CD4+ counts. Shiitake mushrooms *(Lentinus edodes)* are a traditional Asian herbal remedy containing *Lentinan edodes* mycelia (LEM), which can be extracted as a powder. Test tube studies in Japan have shown that pretreatment of T CELL cultures with LEM protects them from both free-viral and cell-to-cell HIV infection; it has been suggested that E-P-LEM interferes in HIV interaction with the cellular CD receptor.

SHIV See SIMIAN/HUMAN IMMUNODEFICIENCY VIRUS.

shoot up In slang, to inject (illicit) drugs intravenously.

shooting gallery A location where drug addicts meet to SHOOT UP intravenous drugs, often sharing needles.

short-term memory (STM) A memory storage capacity, also called working memory, consisting of a central "executive," visuo-spatial "sketchpad," and articulatory loop used for storing small amounts of information for periods of time ranging from a few seconds to a few minutes. It is limited to about seven or eight items of information. Information in short-term memory is rapidly forgotten unless it is refreshed by rehearsal (a method of exercising memory), following which it may eventually be transferred to long-term memory. Various memory defects occur in HIV/AIDS and the OPPORTUNISTIC INFECTIONS that often accompany HIV/AIDS.

sho-saiko-to (SSKT) Sho-saiko-to (SSKT) is a central formula in traditional Chinese medicine and is readily available in many countries in Asia. While SSKT is a combination of seven ingredients in precise proportion, it is speculated that the most active component is scutellariae, from which baicalein is derived. Baicalein has been synthesized in a highly purified form and is being investigated at the National Cancer Institute. Studies of the effect of SSKT on lymphocytes from HIV-infected individuals have shown a greater inhibition of HIV REVERSE TRANSCRIPTASE and reductions in P24 ANTIGEN levels in HIV-SEROPOSITIVE asymptomatic people than in people with AIDS. To date, however, there exist insufficient data to support use of SSKT as an anti-HIV therapy.

SI See SELF-INSEMINATION.

SIDA The acronym for AIDS in French, Spanish, and other Romance languages.

side effect A normal, expected, and predictable response to a drug that accompanies the principal (intended) response sought in treatment. Side effects are part of a drug's pharmacological activity and are thus unavoidable. Most side effects are undesirable. The majority cause minor annoyance and inconvenience; some may cause serious problems in managing certain diseases; a few can be hazardous.

sigmoidoscope A flexible or rigid instrument used to examine the lower (sigmoid) COLON. See ENDOSCOPY.

sigmoidoscopy Inspection of the sigmoid colon (the S-shaped lower portion of the descending colon, located between the iliac crest and the rectum) using a SIGMOIDOSCOPE.

sign An indication of a disease or disorder. See SYMPTOM.

significance See STATISTICAL SIGNIFICANCE.

sildenafil citrate The first oral drug for male impotence, Viagra *(Sildenafil citrate)* works by dilating blood vessels in the penis, allowing the inflow of blood needed for an erection. PROTEASE INHIBITORS appear to increase blood levels of Viagra by inhibiting liver enzymes that would normally eliminate Viagra. Care needs to be taken when combining Viagra with protease inhibitors, consult your medical care provider.

Silence = Death An early symbol of AIDS, the powerful slogan Silence = Death emerged in 1987. It was used frequently by ACT-UP members in posters for demonstrations and in flyers and leaflets. The slogan was initially positioned below a point-up pink triangle, a symbol of gay liberation since the 1970s. The pink triangle was an effort to reclaim the symbol that homosexuals were forced to wear in Nazi concentration camps, much as Jews were forced to wear a yellow Star of David. The point-up triangle was used instead of the traditional point-down triangle to incite active fighting back against forces of silence in the epidemic. The declaration that silence about the AIDS epidemic would lead to death was used to demonstrate the U.S. government's lack of discussion or action against the growing epidemic, the press's refusal to print information about the disease, and the lack of organized medical treatment of the disease. The poster and slogan have never been attributed to any particular author. The slogan is still used today by the group ACT-UP as well as other organizations.

silent reservoirs Within the body, populations of infected cells in which a virus could survive for long periods despite the potent effects of antiretroviral drugs and restart the infection if HIGHLY ACTIVE ANTIRETROVIRAL THERAPY (HAART) were to be stopped. Reservoirs of virus carry serious implications for the idea of ridding the body of virus.

To reproduce, all viruses must insert their genes into active cells that contain the necessary parts for the production of new viral genes and that are capable of synthesizing large amounts of viral protein. In contrast, resting cells cannot support viral replication. They are not targeted by most viruses and less often infected by them. HIV is one of the rare viruses that both recognizes and infects resting cells, in this case, resting CD4+ T CELLS.

Although HIV can infect these cells, all of the steps necessary for replication cannot be completed. Viral RNA is copied into DNA by the reverse transcriptase enzymes carried into the cells within the viral particles, but the process appears to stop there. The newly synthesized viral DNA does not go into the nuclei of these cells but integrates into the cells' chromosomes. The unintegrated DNA remains outside the nucleus and rests. It may activate later, making it a latent infection.

Initially it was felt that this population of latently infected T cells was not very important: If the viral DNA remained unintegrated and inactive, the cells could not be involved in the production of a new virus. However, it was later found that these cells could become producers of new viruses. When these latent cells encounter antigens they recognize, they become activated and begin to mount a response to the antigen. As this activity begins, viral replication also begins. The latent, unintegrated viral DNA is carried into the cell nucleus and integrated. At this point the production of viral proteins and the assembly of new virus begins.

Researchers first thought this source of new virus was not a significant contribution to the overall infection and that the amount of new virus coming from these cells would be very small in comparison to the huge amounts being produced in chronically infected T cells and macrophages.

The initial thought that these cells did not survive long after becoming latently infected was changed with the advent of HAART. With the ability to suppress viral replication, complete removal of the virus from the human body became at least a theoretical possibility, and the issue of viral reservoirs became very important. With patients adhering rigidly to potent HAART regimes, some research groups estimated that in as few as three or four years, all chronically infected T cells and macrophages in the blood and lymphoid tissues would die out. And, if these were the only cells carrying the virus, eradication would have been

achieved. It soon seemed likely that the virus could also live in other cells and tissues where it could survive for this length of time despite HAART and serve as reservoirs from which infection could start again if HAART were to be stopped.

Reservoirs of HIV have been discovered in various places in the body, including brain tissue. Brain tissue is protected from direct exposure to many substances in the blood by a barrier most antiretroviral drugs cannot cross. This is referred to as the blood-brain barrier. Similar barriers are known to protect other tissues, including testes and retina, making these sites other potential reservoirs for HIV. HIV in these protected sites is extremely hard to detect. The size and amount of virus in these areas of the body remains unknown.

The importance of this and other reservoirs in rekindling infection after HAART is only beginning to be studied. Additional sources of virus are likely to be found. It has become clear that current treatment is not sufficient to cleanse the virus from the human body. More potent drugs and other treatments will need to be developed to remove the virus from these reservoirs. And if this proves to be impossible, then new antiretroviral drugs that are easier to take but equally as strong or stronger than existing drugs will be needed to control the virus for a lifetime.

Silybum marianum   See SILYMARIN.

silymarin   The seeds of milk thistle (*Silybum marianum*) have been cultivated for centuries as a medicinal remedy, and are considered by some to have liver-protecting properties. An extract is available under the name silymarin; proponents suggest that it is useful for liver-based problems, including cirrhosis, jaundice, chronic hepatitis, and damage due to drugs, alcohol, and poisoning from chemicals and diarrhea. Some reports have suggested that silymarin may stimulate certain immune functions and may protect the liver during hepatitis. To date, no studies of silymarin in PWAs have been conducted. No toxic effects of silymarin have been reported, although it is possible that because of its purported effect on the liver and kidneys, the compound may effect the absorption of other medications. Silymarin concentrations vary in milk thistle capsules, pills, and teas, and should be taken only upon the advice of an herbalist or physician.

simian acquired immunodeficiency disease See SIMIAN IMMUNODEFICIENCY VIRUS.

simian acquired immunodeficiency virus See SIMIAN IMMUNODEFICIENCY VIRUS.

simian/human immunodeficiency virus (SHIV) A genetically engineered virus used in research for new drugs and possible vaccine treatments. Potential new treatments are tested on macaques. SHIV is created from the ENVELOPE of HIV and the CORE of SIV. It is a variety of virus that mimics the subtype C of the virus found predominantly in Africa.

simian acquired immunodeficiency syndrome (SAIDS) An AIDS-like immunodeficiency syndrome found in some macaque monkeys infected with SIV, a RETROVIRUS related to HIV.

simian immunodeficiency virus (SIV) Any of a group of viruses found in monkeys structurally similar to the HUMAN IMMUNODEFICIENCY VIRUS (HIV). It has long been suspected that HIV evolved from SIV-1, a simian immunodeficiency virus, perhaps as a result of humans' becoming infected with monkey viruses that mutated inside their bodies. HIV-2 more closely resembles SIV than does HIV-1, the virus that infects most people in the United States. Both HIV viruses are thought to have been derived from SIV that infected either chimpanzees or macaques. It is known that a chimpanzee has had AIDS, confirming for the first time that HIV-1, the human virus responsible for most of the world's AIDS burden, can jump between species. Moreover, the human virus that infected the chimp has changed dramatically since it was experimentally injected into the animal in 1984. About 20 percent has mutated into a different form. This finding also suggests there may be a way to test future human treatments and vaccines on chimps.

simian retrovirus A form of AIDS found in monkeys and apes that does not affect humans.

simian T-cell lymphotrophic virus (STLV) See SIMIAN IMMUNODEFICIENCY VIRUS (SIV).

simvastatin A lipid level–lowering drug used to lower a person's CHOLESTEROL or TRIGLYCERIDE level when diet and exercise are not effective. (The trade name is Zocor.) See STATINS.

single-agent therapy Treatment with one drug at a time; also known as MONOTHERAPY.

sinusitis Infection of the sinuses, the air sacs next to the nasal passages, usually as a result of a cold or allergy. Sinusitis is common, especially in people with HIV infection, although the reason for this is obscure. Symptoms are pus drainage from the nose, headache, face pain, and fever. The usual treatment is with ANTIBIOTICS taken by mouth, such as TRIMETHOPRIM-SULFAMETHOXZOLE, AMOXICILLIN, ERYTHROMYCIN, cephalexin (Keflex), CIPROFLOXACIN (Cipro), or TETRACYCLINE. Some people do not respond to these drugs, and their sinuses need to be drained.

SIV See SIMIAN IMMUNODEFICIENCY VIRUS.

skilled nursing facility (SNF) A facility that provides skilled nursing (such as that given by RNs) and related services requiring the most intense and professional nursing home care. Also called an extended care facility. Costs of a stay in an SNF are covered by MEDICARE, MEDICAID, and some private health insurance.

skin The layer of tissue between the body and its environment is a major organ of the body. Skin functions include protection against injuries and parasitic invasion, regulation of body temperature, aid in elimination, and prevention of dehydration. The skin is a reservoir for food and water, a sense organ, and a source of antirachitic vitamin, which it produces when exposed to sunlight.

The term *skin* is also slang for condom.

skin disorder The skin and mucosa are the body's first line of defense against countless microbial threats such as bacteria, fungi, protozoa, and viruses. But this defense depends on a functional immune system. When the immune system is suppressed, disorders of the skin may appear. Organ transplantation and cancer patients who undergo immunosuppressive therapies may experience skin disorders such as KAPOSI'S SARCOMA or herpes outbreaks. In HIV, lesions, dry skin, and blisters are common early in the course of the infection and may recur or become chronic. Skin diseases in HIV infection include MOLLUSCUM CONTAGIOSUM, HERPES SIMPLEX VIRUS (HIV), HERPES ZOSTER (shingles), HAIRY LEUKOPLAKIA, and FOLLICULITIS. Viral skin disorders common in HIV-infected people are not ordinarily life-threatening, but they can cause significant pain, illness, and cosmetic frustration. In some cases, viral skin diseases can spread to infect other parts of the body, possibly resulting in life-threatening conditions such as HIV encephalitis. Early detection, prophylaxis, and treatment of skin diseases are recommended. See SALLOWNESS; SKIN RASH.

skin rash   Texture and temperature of skin are important signs of underlying conditions. Rashes and their causes, like scars, are diagnostic. Redness is usually seen in inflammation, skin disease, chronic alcoholism, vasomotor disturbances, and pyrexia, as well as sunburn. Local redness with pain indicates inflammation. Lesions, bumps, dry skin, or blisters are common in early HIV infection and may be caused by a number of conditions or infections, including HERPES ZOSTER, HERPES SIMPLEX, dermatitis, etc. See SALLOWNESS; SKIN DISORDER.

skin test   A test of the immune system by means of injections of certain proteins just below the surface of the skin. If the immune system is intact, a rash appears within 48 hours at the site of injection.

skip-generation parenting   A situation in which children are raised by grandparents instead of parents. Although data are scarce, it appears that when parents die of AIDS, children most often go to live, at least at first, with grandmothers or aunts. The problem of skip-generation parenting is not, however, solely attributable to HIV disease. Use of drugs, especially crack cocaine, has devastated many families. Grandparents—and especially grandmothers, since women have traditionally

taken on the role of family care giving—have taken over when their own children have been unable to take on parenting responsibilities or when they have chosen to move their children to a safer environment. This problem has particularly affected African-American communities.

Two general outcomes are predictable. First, some of these grandparents, no matter how willing and devoted they are, will be unable to continue to bear the burdens of child raising—and many of these children have severe behavior or academic problems—because of illness, age, emotional exhaustion, and poverty. Second, there will be no new generation of grandparents to take the place of this generation. The mothers and fathers lost to AIDS will become a lost generation of grandparents.

slim disease   See HIV WASTING DISEASE.

slow virus   A virus, such as HIV, that produces disease with a greatly delayed onset and protracted course. Diseases of a chronic degenerative nature that are now suspected to be due to slow viruses include subacute sclerosing panencephalitis and progressive multifocal leukoencephalopathy.

SMART (Strategies for Management of Antiretroviral Therapy)   A clinical trial sponsored by the Community Programs for Clinical Research on AIDS (CIPRA) of a size and duration designed to provide high-quality data about what happens to people who have been on antiretroviral therapy for more than a couple of years. Study plans include enrolling 6,000 people and following them for as long as nine years. The trial is the first randomized comparison of two viable but competing strategies for how to treat HIV. The study is open to both treatment-naïve and treatment-experienced HIV-positive people above the age of 13 who have CD4 counts above 350 cells/mm. The only other requirement is a willingness to have an open mind about the optimal way to use antiretroviral therapy for the best long-term outcome. Participants are randomly assigned to one of two camps—one group will follow the classic path of making every effort to keep their viral loads undetectable at all times (the viral suppression group), and the other will follow a strategy of avoiding treatment, despite detectable viral load numbers, as long as their CD4 counts stay above 250 cells/mm (drug conservation group). The trial has been characterized as a comparison of continuous versus episodic therapy or the "hit hard" versus the "go slow" school of thought. It has the historic potential to produce a body of information with broad and lasting significance, not only for the health of the participants, but for the millions of HIV-positive people in the world who will eventually face the need to begin treatment. For further information, visit the SMART Study website at www.smart-trial.org.

smoking   Tobacco smoking is harmful not only to smokers but also to those who live or work with them, regardless of HIV status. It has been associated with a higher risk of HIV infection. There are conflicting data on the effects of smoking on HIV disease progression, and the effects of preexisting smoker's leukocytosis (see below) do not seem to be protective.

Some studies point to increased risks for certain OPPORTUNISTIC INFECTIONS in HIV-infected smokers, especially PCP. However, the only infections in which this association has been proved are anogenital abnormalities and cancers. Other studies have shown that current smokers are more likely to develop oral CANDIDIASIS and oral HAIRY LEUKOPLAKIA, but less likely to develop cytomegalovirus disease. Heavy smokers (more than one pack a day) have been shown to be more likely to develop bacterial pneumonia compared with light smokers, nonsmokers, or ex-smokers. Finally, studies have shown that ex-smokers are more likely to develop PNEUMOCYSTIS CARINII PNEU-MONIA (PCP) than nonsmokers. Despite the long time it takes many smoking-related problems to develop, smoking is by no means without health risks for the immunocompromised person.

The association between smoking and HIV infection may have a biological basis. In many, smoking degrades the lining of the oral cavity or leads to minuscule ulcerations that could facilitate HIV transmission. Smoking has a number of known negative biological effects that may affect the progression of HIV disease. These include decreased lung function, chronic inflammatory disease of the lower airways, gum and oral diseases such as periodontis, various cancers, and a lowered ability to heal wounds. Along with the chronic inflammation of the lungs, which can lead to chronic bronchitis or emphysema, smoking causes an elevation of the body's white blood cell count, a condition known as smoker's leukocytosis.

sneeze   Sneezing has not been identified as a route of transmission for HIV/AIDS. To date, the virus has not been found in mucus from the nose.

sobriety   A state of complete abstinence from psychoactive substances by an addicted individual, in conjunction with a satisfactory quality of life.

social disease   A venereal or sexually transmitted disease.

social kiss   See DRY KISS.

Social Security   The United States' most extensive program to provide income for older and disabled Americans. It is paid for by a tax on workers and their employers. Qualified workers are eligible for old age and disability benefits. Benefits are also available for the spouse and dependents of a retired or disabled worker. When a worker dies, benefits can be collected by surviving family members who qualify. Over 95 percent of American workers, including household help, farm workers, self-employed persons, employees of state and local government, and (since 1984) federal workers, participate in the program. Railroad workers are covered by a separate federal program, railroad retirement, that is integrated with Social Security. The program is complicated, and the law and regulations change from time to time. Contact your local office of the Social Security Administration (SSA) for literature about Social Security benefits or to ask specific questions about your own case. They are listed in the United States Government section of your telephone directory. Or call 1-800-772-1213.

Social Security Act, Section 1619   This section allows for continued payment of SUPPLEMENTAL SECURITY INCOME (SSI) benefits to working disabled recipients, without regard to the SUBSTANTIAL

GAINFUL ACTIVITY (SGA), trial work period, and extended-period-of-eligibility limitations imposed by the companion SOCIAL SECURITY DISABILITY INSURANCE (SSDI) program. Section 1619 allows disabled workers whose earnings raise them over the SSI eligibility level to continue as SSI recipients for purposes of MEDICAID coverage if Medicaid-purchased care is what is enabling them to "work their way off welfare" and if they cannot otherwise secure such medical care.

Social Security Act, Title II The OLD AGE, SURVIVORS, AND DISABILITY INSURANCE SECTION of the Social Security Act.

Social Security Act, Title IV-A The AID TO FAMILIES WITH DEPENDENT CHILDREN (AFDC) section of the Social Security Act.

Social Security Act, Title XIV The AID TO THE PERMANENTLY AND TOTALLY DISABLED (APTD) section of the Social Security Act.

Social Security Act, Title XVI The SUPPLEMENTAL SECURITY INCOME (SSI) section of the Social Security Act.

Social Security Act, Title XVIII The MEDICARE section of the Social Security Act.

Social Security Act, Title XIX The MEDICAID section of the Social Security Act.

Social Security Act, Title XX Formerly, the section of the Social Security Act under which grants to states were provided for social services to the needy; since replaced by the Social Services Block Grant (SSBG) program, which is itself often referred to as "Title XX."

Social Security Administration (SSA) See SOCIAL SECURITY.

Social Security Disability Insurance (SSDI) A federal income insurance program operated by the Social Security Administration for workers whom it determines are disabled. There are several means by which people become eligible for SSDI. Most qualify by working and paying Social Security taxes, which earns "credits" toward eventual benefits. Disabled widows and widowers age 50 or older, may be eligible for a disability benefit earned on the Social Security record of a decreased spouse. Disabled children age 18 or older (whose disability must have originated before age 22) may be eligible for dependents' benefits on the Social Security record of a parent who is getting retirement or disability benefits or who has died. Children under the age of 18 qualify for dependents' benefits on the record of a parent who is getting retirement or disability benefits or on the record of a parent who has died.

social service Activity that serves the common good of society. The term covers private and public efforts, volunteer and professional services, small enterprises, and large organized programs but is most often used to refer to large-scale welfare programs carried on under professional auspices by trained personnel, either run by a government agency or paid for by public funds.

social status The position of an individual in relation to society. Calculations of social status, while inexact, encompass class, race, economic, and cultural factors and are largely expressions of society's biases, good and bad.

social withdrawal A state of living or being disposed to live in isolation, rather than in companionship with others or in a community.

sodomy Legally, a sexual act involving oral-genital, anal-oral, or anal-genital contact.

soluble CD4 A CD4 CELL that is capable of being dissolved or liquefied. CD4 has been subverted in man to serve as the receptor for HIV as it commandeers T-cells to serve as viral factories. As new viruses burst out, the T-cells rupture and die. The idea that CD4 could block the virus dates to the mid-to-late 1980s. CD4 quickly became one of the most intensively studied receptors of any enveloped virus, Research continues to date.

soluble factors   Certain proteins and other substances (e.g., IL-2, TUMOR NECROSIS FACTOR, ALPHA INTERFERON) found in the blood. They may have either helpful or harmful effects on disease progression.

solvent   A liquid that can dissolve other substances and hold them in solution. Ethyl alcohol and Campho-Phenique are solvents used to kill organisms on the skin. The latter is used primarily for cold sores. Camphor is the primary ingredient. It can be used as a counterirritant and as a moth repellent.

somatic   Related to the body, as opposed to the soul; physical instead of psychic.

somatic cell   Any cell of the body that is not a germ cell. A germ cell has only one set of CHROMOSOMES, whereas all somatic cells have two sets of chromosomes. Egg cells and sperm cells are considered germ cells.

somatic cell gene therapy   A genetic treatment that involves the insertion of GENES into SOMATIC CELLS for therapeutic purposes, for example, to induce the treated cells to produce a protein that the body is missing. It has been used in the treatment of autoimmune diseases and cancer. Inserting a particular gene into somatic cells affects only the patient being treated. It does not affect the genetic makeup of a patient's offspring and generally does not change all, or even most, cells in the patient. Therefore, it is considered an extension of normal medical care and does not generally fall under the moral and legal controls of other genetic engineering. It is being studied for potential use in the treatment of HIV.

somatic mutation   A process of change occurring in any nongerm cell. These changes may or may not be passed on to progeny during reproduction.

somatic therapy   Generally, any treatment focusing on the body. Examples of somatic therapy are MASSAGE THERAPY, ROLFING, and THERAPEUTIC TOUCH. It can also refer specifically to a treatment that is a holistically oriented therapy. In this sense

somatic therapy attempts to integrate the mental, physical, spiritual, and emotional aspects of the individual. It teaches the patient to focus awareness on the body to become aware of any ills or complaints that he or she may be unaccustomed to recognizing and to work on the causes of these ills.

somatostatin   A HORMONE that inhibits the release of SOMATOTROPIN. It is a hypothalamic peptide that also inhibits the secretion of insulin and gastrin. It is used in the treatment of certain tumors. It is an injection drug that has been used in HIV infection for its antidiarrheal properties.

somatrem   See HUMAN GROWTH HORMONE.

somatropin   See HUMAN GROWTH HORMONE.

somewhat risky sex   ORAL-GENITAL SEX without swallowing semen or INTERCOURSE without ejaculation. See RISK; SAFE SEX; UNSAFE SEX.

sonogram   See ULTRASOUND.

sonography   See ULTRASONOGRAPHY.

sore throat   Any inflammation of the tonsils, pharynx, or larynx.

soul kiss   See WET KISS.

South America   See CARIBBEAN; LATIN AMERICA.

Southern blot technique   A procedure, used to separate and identify DNA sequences, in which DNA fragments are separated by ELECTROPHORESIS onto an agarose gel, blotted onto a nylon or nitrocellulose membrane, and hybridized with labeled nucleic acid probes. It is used to test newborns for HIV antibodies.

SPD 756 (formerly known as BCH-13520)   A nucleoside analog being developed for HIV/AIDS by Shire Pharmaceuticals. It has been shown IN VITRO to retain efficacy against resistant clinical isolates including highly resistant strains of HIV.

SPD 756 entered phase I trials during the third quarter of 2001.

specificity The ability of a clinical test to correctly identify a subject who is not infected.

spending down Reducing income to the eligibility level for MEDICAID by deducting incurred medical bills.

sperm The male germ cells, or gametes. See SPERMATOZOON.

spermatozoa See SPERMATOZOON.

spermatozoon A mature male sperm cell that is formed within the seminiferous tubules of the TESTES. It consists of a head with a nucleus, a neck, a middle piece, and a tail and resembles a tadpole in shape. Spermatozoa make up the element of semen that pierces the envelope of the ovum to achieve fertilization.

spermicidal See SPERMICIDE.

spermicidal jelly, cream, or foam See SPERMICIDE.

spermicidal jelly See SPERMICIDE.

spermicide A chemical product that kills sperm or other organisms, such as viruses or bacteria, on contact. It is used to prevent pregnancy and some SEXUALLY TRANSMITTED DISEASES. CONTRACEPTIVE creams, jellies, foams, and lubricants contain spermicide, of which NONOXYNOL-9 is probably the best known. Spermicides can be used separately or, most effectively, with barrier contraceptives.

Many experts recommend the use of a spermicidal jelly or cream in conjunction with CONDOM use. In heterosexual sex, when used with a condom, the spermicide should be put directly inside the vagina. The amount of spermicide in a spermicide-lubricated condom is not sufficient to provide protection against many viruses. It is unknown whether any of the commercially used spermicides can be used to protect against HIV. In some research, spermicides have caused vaginal sores or irritation in some women and irritation of the penis in some men. These sores or irritations may make it easier for HIV or other viruses to enter the bloodstream. Research continues into whether a spermicide that will protect women against HIV infection can be developed. Research has concentrated in this area, as it is easier for women to control the use of the spermicide than to convince a man to wear a condom in many cultures.

spinal fluid See CEREBROSPINAL FLUID.

spinal tap A procedure, also called a lumbar puncture, for obtaining CEREBROSPINAL FLUID, the fluid that surrounds the brain and the spinal cord. The procedure involves inserting a needle into the middle of the back and into the MENINGES, the membrane that contains the cerebrospinal fluid. The needle is inserted between the L_3 and L_4 vertebrae. The fluid is then analyzed for evidence of infection of the brain or spinal cord. This is the only manner of detecting some infections. Repeat spinal taps then measure the effectiveness of treatment in these illnesses. In CRYPTOCOCCAL MENINGITIS, spinal taps are performed in order to drain some fluid to prevent the pressure on the brain from building up too much. Despite sounding unpleasant and risky, a spinal tap is a well-established medical procedure and is rarely associated with any important complications. The most common complaint is of headache after the procedure, which is less likely to occur if the person lies flat once the spinal tap is completed.

spiramycin An ANTIBIOTIC produced from a member of the *Streptomyces* bacteria. It is administered orally.

spirulina See BLUE-GREEN ALGAE.

spit See SALIVA.

spleen A glandlike lymphoid organ with immunologic and nonimmunologic functions, not all of which are understood. It removes worn-out cells from the circulatory system and is a graveyard for RED BLOOD CELLS, reintroducing iron from hemoglobin after red cell death. As do the LYMPH NODES, the spleen produces LYMPHOCYTES and is important early in life. Removal of the spleen has been shown to be associated with overwhelming bacterial infection in infants, children, and young adults. In HIV, spleen removal leads to an increase in level of circulating lymphocytes. Because CD4 counts can sometimes double, the measurement used to track HIV then becomes the percentage of CD4 cells in relation to all red blood cells.

splenic fever   See ANTHRAX.

splenomegaly   Enlargement of the SPLEEN. In HIV this can be caused by the HIV infection itself, IDIO-PATHIC THROMBOCYTOPENIC PURPURA (ITP), cirrhosis of the liver, or certain chronic infections. The spleen may or may not return to normal size when treatment of HIV is begun.

sponge   A CONTRACEPTIVE in the form of a polyurethane disc that contains SPERMICIDE and fits over the CERVIX.

sponsor   In the context of HIV and AIDS, an organization that develops a drug and usually pays the extensive bills to do so. Almost always the sponsor is a pharmaceutical company. Occasionally, a government agency or private nonprofit organization can be a sponsor. The term also refers to a person in a 12-step program who generally has at least one year of sobriety who offers support to another member.

sputum   The mucous matter that collects in the respiratory and upper digestive passages and is expelled by coughing and/or throat clearing. It is expectorated phlegm.

sputum analysis   A method of detecting certain infections (especially TUBERCULOSIS) by culturing of sputum and microscopic examination.

sputum examination   See SPUTUM ANALYSIS.

sputum test   See SPUTUM ANALYSIS.

SPV-30   An extract of the European boxwood tree. SPV-30 reputedly has anti-HIV properties and is sold in the United States by some AIDS buyers' clubs and a few pharmacies. For a limited time, it was available in America through a large informal trial protocol. The trial showed no positive results and no further research studies have been conducted with the food supplement.

squalamine   A compound from the immune defense system of the sand shark that, in laboratory experiments, has demonstrated activity against a broad range of bacteria and fungi. Sharks are unusual in that they appear to lack cellular immunity, do not reject grafts, and do not mount an antibody response when vaccinated; they maintain health even though they appear profoundly immunocompromised.

squamous cell   A flat, scalelike epithelial cell.

squamous intraepithelial lesion   Abnormalities in cells, revealed by PAP SMEAR, that may indicate cancer. Pap smears can be done on both the cervical and anal regions. See ANAL INTRAEPITHELIAL LESION; CERVICAL CANCER.

squamous-cell carcinoma   A cancer developing from squamous EPITHELIAL tissue.

SSA   See SOCIAL SECURITY.

SSDI   See SOCIAL SECURITY DISABILITY INSURANCE.

SSI   See SUPPLEMENTAL SECURITY INCOME.

SSI/SSP   The combined total SSI and SSP income eligibility level for poor, aged, and disabled people. The figure varies by state and with living arrangements.

SSP   See STATE SUPPLEMENTARY PAYMENT.

staging   Determining what stage in its progression a disease has reached, in order to tailor treatment accordingly.

standard of care   The level of care and treatment that all patients who have a particular condition should receive. Any care below that level is to be considered substandard. Various organizations, from the CENTERS FOR DISEASE CONTROL AND PREVENTION and the FOOD AND DRUG ADMINISTRATION to the American Medical Association to patients' rights groups adopt varying guidelines that they term standard of care.

standard therapy   A treatment that is FOOD AND DRUG ADMINISTRATION-approved for a particular condition and that is widely used as the first treatment for that particular condition.

Staphylococcus   A bacterium that consists of GRAM-POSITIVE spherical cells that divide in multiple planes to form irregular clusters resembling bunches of grapes. They are found on the skin, skin glands, and mucous and nasal membranes, as well as various food products.

Staphylococcus aureus   A species of *Staphylococcus* commonly found on the skin and mucous membranes, especially those of the mouth and nose. They cause serious suppurative (pus-forming) conditions and systemic diseases. *Staphylococcus aureus* is responsible for BOILS and FOLLICULITIS. In injection drug use, staphylococcal organisms can enter the bloodstream, causing a serious condition known as endocarditis, a swelling of the interior lining of the heart. Various strains of the species produce toxins that cause food poisoning and toxic shock syndrome.

state supplementary payment (SSP)   A state welfare payment added to the basic federal SSI allowance, raising the minimum income for poor, aged, blind, and disabled people.

statins   Also called statin drugs, the statins suppress cholesterol production by inhibiting the enzyme HMG CoA reductase. There are five generic statins—simvastatin (Zocor), pravastatin (Pravachol), fluvastatin (Lescol), atorvastatin (Lipitor), and lovastatin (Mevacor)—used currently for treating high cholesterol level. They lower LDL cholesterol level more than other types of drugs. They work by slowing the production of cholesterol and by increasing the liver's ability to remove the LDL cholesterol already in the blood. They also reduce TRIGLYCERIDE levels while raising HDL cholesterol ("good" cholesterol) level by a small amount. Some of the drugs have shown the ability to prevent heart attacks.

Many people who are HIV-positive and taking HAART may also need to take a statin drug to control the high cholesterol level that is common when taking HAART. Liver enzyme levels should be monitored when patients are on the statins. Statins are processed in the body by the same enzyme that processes some of the PROTEASE INHIBITORS and NUCLEOSIDE ANALOGS. As a result, fluctuations in the level of any of these drugs in the body may occur. Use of statins to control high cholesterol and triglyceride levels by HIV-positive people has been less of a concern in drug interactions than initially thought. Statins are usually given in a single dose at the evening meal or at bedtime. This dosage allows the drug to take advantage of the fact that the body makes more cholesterol at night than during the day.

statistical significance   In terms of comparative experimental research, such as drug testing, the result of an analytical evaluation of the results of a comparative trial or survey. Data yielding a difference in outcome depending on treatment or environmental factors are considered statistically significant if mathematical formulae indicate that there is less than a one-in-twenty (5 percent) chance that the same results would occur through random accident.

statute of limitations   A legal time limit during which, in criminal law, charges may be brought, and in tort law, claims or lawsuits may be brought. If a claim or lawsuit is not brought during the time allowed by law, the plaintiff or injured party loses the right to do so. In medical negligence claims, the statute of limitations usually starts from the time the wrong occurred or was or should have been discovered.

stavudine   A NUCLEOSIDE ANALOG similar in structure to ZIDOVUDINE, DIDANOSINE, and ZALCITABINE. U.S. Public Health Service guidelines indicate that the best way to use stavudine (as well as other HIV medications) is in combination with other drugs. It is often combined with zidovudine or LAMIVUDINE and a PROTEASE INHIBITOR. The two-drug combination of zidovudine and stavudine alone is not recommended, as they do not work well together. As the years have passed since the introduction of stavudine, several side effects have been connected to its use. PERIPHERAL NEUROPATHY is the most common. Doses of stavudine can be lowered somewhat if doing so decreases the symptoms; otherwise a change in drugs is recommended. Pancreatitis (inflammation of the pancreas) has occurred with stavudine as well as elevated liver enzyme levels. Both of these organ functions should be checked regularly when taking stavudine. Fatal lactic acidosis has occurred in pregnant women receiving the combination of didanosine and stavudine. Although it is not yet certain, some researchers have found that long-term use of stavudine may be a risk factor for some of the symptoms of LIPODYSTROPHY, such as loss of tissue from the face.

STD   See SEXUALLY TRANSMITTED DISEASE.

steatosis   The collection of excessive amounts of fats inside liver cells, which can also be referred to as fatty liver. By itself the condition is not threatening, though it usually indicates other problems. Causes of steatosis include HEPATITIS, alcoholism, malnutrition, pregnancy, and drug toxicities. Treatment involves eliminating the cause of the fat buildup, and prognosis is good if the condition is recognized and the problem has not continued over many years.

In HIV-positive people steatosis is one of the results attributed to MITOCHONDRIAL TOXICITY that has occurred after lengthy periods on NRTIs or reactions to NRTI drugs.

stem cell   The cells of which all immune cells are descendants; found in the BONE MARROW in small pools, stem cells multiply and mature, when needed, into functional CD4+, T and other white and red blood CELLS. Stem cells have often been thought to be the best reservoirs for harboring anti-HIV GENES. They have been notoriously difficult to identify and purify, but a newly developed simple method for isolating and maintaining them in culture dishes has enabled new research.

Researchers are currently trying to insert disease-resistant genes into the body's blood-forming cell "factories" to help cells counter HIV infection. The goal is to be able to reconstitute the immune system of HIV-infected patients with genetically modified HIV-resistant T cells. To deliver the therapeutic genes to the stem cells, the genes are enclosed in a harmless virus, an engineered adeno-associated virus (AAV). One of the genes being used makes T cells HIV-resistant through coding for the intracellular production of antibodies against HIV. In laboratory experiments, AAV has effectively transported such ANTIBODY-coding genes into test-tube grown cells, and the antibody produced inside these cells has successfully blocked HIV growth. Researchers intend to carry out these same experiments using stem cells isolated from fragments of HIV-positive patients' bone marrow. Eventually, the HIV-resistant stem cells will be returned to the patients, where they are expected to "home" back to the bone marrow and, as needed, multiply and develop into mature immune cells that are resistant to HIV.

Researchers are also trying to combine different methods of gene therapy against HIV. One strategy is to deliver different types of anti-HIV genes at the same time, all capable of inhibiting HIV growth by blocking either the function of one HIV gene or the function of one of the virus's protein components. Each kind of anti-HIV gene targets a single but critical step in the HIV's life cycle.

Because HIV inserts its genes into its host cell's own genetic material, which other viruses such as those that cause cold, flu, and herpes do not do, it functions, in a sense, as a contagious genetic disease. This is one of the reasons why strategies such as gene therapy, which are typically applied to inherited single-gene abnormalities, are so attractive as potential anti-HIV therapeutics.

sterility   Inability of the female to become pregnant or for the male to impregnate a female; also, condition of being free from living microorganisms.

sterilization   The destruction of all MICROORGANISMS in, on, or about an object by employing various means such as chemical agents (alcohol, ethylene oxide gas, phenol), high-velocity electron bombardment, steam, or ultraviolet light radiation. Also, the act or process by which an individual is made incapable of reproduction or fertilization (e.g., castration, tubectomy, vasectomy).

sterilizing immunity A term used to describe a treatment or vaccine that completely prevents the establishment of an infection.

steroid A member of a large family of structurally similar lipid substances. Steroid molecules have a basic skeleton consisting of four interconnected carbon rings. Different classes of steroids have different functions. All sex HORMONES are steroids. Anabolic steroids increase muscle mass. Antiinflammatory steroids, or CORTICOSTEROIDS, can reduce swelling, pain, and other manifestations of inflammation; when physicians use the term *steroid*, they are generally referring to this category. When lay people use the term, they are generally thinking of anabolic steroids. Side effects of steroids may include an increased appetite, mood changes, fluid retention, acne, increased blood pressure, elevated blood sugar level, intestinal ulcers, and lowered resistance to infection.

Stevens-Johnson syndrome A form of erythema multiforme (eruption of dark red papules or tubercles) that is sometimes fatal. It is characterized by systemic exfoliative mucocutaneous lesions, some of which may be severe, on or in the ears, nose, lips, eyes, anus, genitals, lungs, gastrointestinal tract, heart, and kidneys. In HIV it can be caused on rare occasions by reactions to certain drugs such as Bactrim or nevirapine. This condition must be treated and use of the drug discontinued immediately.

stigma More than a decade into the pandemic, HIV and AIDS still carry an enormous social stigma, harming persons who are infected, persons perceived to be infected, and uninfected family members and caregivers as well. Transmission of HIV in this country has been, and still is for some,

associated exclusively in the public mind with "immoral" or discreditable behavior like homosexuality and injection drug use. The linkage of AIDS with behaviors that society has marginalized and rejected has created a climate of fear and loathing in which it is permissible for those infected with HIV/AIDS to be despised, shunned, and even assaulted—verbally, physically, and economically. It is not surprising that some persons affected by HIV have taken the stigma and sense of shame that often accompany it as part of their own sense of identity.

To some extent, the law mitigates this situation by providing people affected with some recourse against discrimination and by giving them some control over access to medical information about themselves. Recent changes in federal laws have expanded markedly protection against HIV-related discrimination. See AMERICANS WITH DISABILITIES ACT; FAIR HOUSING AMENDMENTS ACT OF 1988; REHABILITATION ACT OF 1973.

stimulant Any agent temporarily increasing functional activity. Stimulants may be classified according to the organ upon which they act as follows: bronchial, gastric, cerebral, intestinal, nervous, motor, vasomotor, respiratory, and secretory.

STI See STRUCTURED TREATMENT INTERRUPTION.

stomach A dilated, saclike distensible portion of the alimentary canal between the esophagus and the intestines, located below the diaphragm, to the right of the spleen, and partly under the liver. The stomach's basic function is as an organ of digestion.

stomatitis Any of numerous inflammatory diseases of the mouth. Causes vary and include mechanical trauma, irritants, allergy, vitamin deficiency, and infection.

straight Slang for a person who prefers sex with a person of the opposite sex; nonhomosexual.

strain A subgroup or form of a species. HIV has several strains, or subtypes, called GROUP M, N, and O.

Strategies for Management of Antiretroviral Therapy   See SMART.

stratification   The classification or separation of people in a study into subgroups based on some characteristic such as income, drug use, or another unifying characteristic.

streetwalker   See PROSTITUTE.

Streptococcus pneumonia   See PNEUMOCOCCUS.

streptomycin   A bacterial ANTIBIOTIC derived from the soil microbe *Streptomyces griseus*. It belongs to the AMINOGLYCOSIDE class. It is used mainly in the treatment of TUBERCULOSIS. Streptomycin was the first drug with proven effectiveness against the MYCOBACTERIA that cause tuberculosis, but because of its toxicity and the development of alternatives, it is no longer first-line therapy for tuberculosis or other bacterial infections. Streptomycin is available as a solution for intramuscular injection. Nausea, vomiting, vertigo, flushing, skin rashes, and swelling are common side effects. Less frequently, deafness, severe peeling of the skin, anaphylactic shock, muscle weakness, vision impairment, and bone marrow toxicity occur. Rarely, kidney toxicity may occur.

stress   The result produced when a structure, system, or organism is acted upon by forces that disrupt equilibrium or produce strain. In health care, the term denotes the physical (gravity, mechanical force, pathogen, injury) and psychological (fear, anxiety, crisis, joy) forces that are experienced by individuals. It is generally believed that biological organisms require a certain amount of stress in order to maintain their well-being. When more stress occurs than the system can handle, it produces pathological changes. The amount of stress humans can withstand without having a pathological reaction to it varies from individual to individual and from situation to situation.

stressor   A factor that produces STRESS.

stroke   A suddenly occurring acute vascular lesion of the brain, such as a hemorrhage, embolism, or thrombosis, producing a condition characterized by paralysis and neurologic damage, often irreversible. Symptoms can include focal weakness, speech impediment, and impaired consciousness. Also called a CEREBROVASCULAR ACCIDENT.

stroke syndrome   The condition produced by a STROKE.

stromal cell–derived factor 1 (SDF-1)   A CHEMOKINE that binds to the CXCR-4 receptor site and interferes with HIV's fusion with uninfected cells. This blocking seems to occur strictly in T-TROPIC strains of HIV.

Strongyloides stercoralis   A nematode, or roundworm, occurring in tropical and subtropical countries and in the southern United States that infests dogs, primates, and humans. It causes the infection STRONGYLOIDIASIS.

strongyloidiasis   An infection caused by infestation with nematodes of the genus *Strongyloides*. Infestation may persist for years because of the nature of the life cycle. Infection can occur indirectly by larvae of a new generation developed in the soil. It may also occur directly by infected larvae developed without an intervening adult phase or by autoreinfection, in which the female inhabits the intestines of the host, and larvae develop within the feces of the host, penetrate the mucosa, and migrate through the venous system to the lungs, causing hemorrhage (pulmonary strongyloidiasis), then migrate back to the intestines through blood-lung interactions. Autoreinfection is the cause of the most serious human infections and the majority of fatalities. It was thought this illness would be a major problem in HIV-positive people early in the epidemic, because extended problems with this illness are typically seen in immunosuppressed people. It has not, however, proved to be any worse in HIV-infected individuals than in HIV-negative people. Their life cycle allows for massive infection sufficient to cause overwhelming systemic infection with fever, severe abdominal pain, shock, and possibly death. The condition is also called strongyloidosis; disseminated strongyloidosis is somewhat more common in HIV-positive people than in HIV-negative individuals. See STRONGYLOIDES STERCORALIS.

strongyloidosis   See STRONGYLOIDIASIS.

structured treatment interruption (STI)   Discontinuation of a treatment regimen, as contrasted to continued exposure to that regimen. The duration of a structured treatment interruption varies from case to case, as do the clinical risks, benefits, and implications. STIs are sometimes seen as a way to turn back the clock, undoing the damage wreaked by poor past treatments that allowed the evolution of drug resistance.

The original targets for STIs were patients who were experiencing multiple treatment failures who had no residual therapeutic options. The principle behind STI in this scenario is a possible reversion of the mutant virus to the wild type, leading to a potential restoration of drug susceptibility to allow the recycling of antiretroviral drugs. However, the reversion to the wild type is usually seen in plasma virus but not in cell-associated virus.

STI in fully suppressed patients supports a very different strategy. The idea is that STI may be able to augment the length and strength of host immune responses to HIV and increase immunologic control of the infection. Results in a few uncontrolled studies indicate that STI is safe; most patients experience a rapid rebound of plasma HIV RNA and a rapid decline in CD4 cells during therapeutic or drug holidays. After the reconstitution of treatment there are prompt reduction in viral load and an increase in CD4 cells. STI makes the most sense for acute HIV infection when antiretroviral therapy is initiated before deletion of host HIV cytotoxic T lymphocyte (CTL) responses. Promising data report attenuated rises of HIV RNA levels observed after repeated STIs in acute HIV infection. Note that even though the viral load set point can be lowered by STI during acute infection, uncontrolled studies suggest that such results may not apply to chronic infection. The first prospective, randomized controlled trial comparing continuous HAART to STI reports that regardless of the drug regimen, viral load rebounds to values similar to baseline values during each therapy interruption. The rate of viral load rebound did not change significantly during subsequent interruptions. Restarting therapy, however, suppressed viral load to values similar to the ones seen in the continuous HAART group.

Finally, STIs are also being evaluated as a means to reduce pill burden and drug toxicity. For instance, STI strategies have proved helpful in diminishing the lipid abnormalities of HIV patients on long-term HAART. In areas with limited resources, such strategies offer the possibility of increasing access to antiretroviral therapy. Many questions remain before the full adoption of STI in HIV patient management. What are the long-term effects on viral load and CD4 counts? What are the effects of therapeutic holidays in viral genotype and phenotype? What happens during STI in the different HIV compartments and reservoirs? The first STI studies appear to challenge the assumption that only harm would occur after interrupting HIV treatment and to support the evidence that STI strategies may assist patient management.

Theoretical objections to the treatment interruption approach to eliminating drug-resistant HIV have been raised. Exposing HIV to antiviral medications sets it down evolutionary pathways that become irreversible as mutations accumulate. It is not true that drug resistance mutations consistently yield an HIV that is less fit than the wild type. The later mutations that arise in response to AZT monotherapy are notorious for creating a faster-growing HIV, at least in the test tube. Other primary resistance mutations have their deleterious effects compensated for by secondary mutations. Note too that individual strains of HIV most likely do not "disappear" during either treatment or drug interruption. The genetic sequencing and viral culture assays used to determine HIV drug resistance have limits to their sensitivity. They are not able to detect HIV subpopulations existing below about 10 percent of the total viral population in someone's body. The overgrowth of wild-type HIV after therapy is stopped may merely conceal the survival of the more slowly replicating drug-resistant strains. If the eclipsed HIV subpopulations do not exist in actively replicating form, they may exist in a dormant form, hidden in quiescent white blood cells with latent HIV infection. These cells can survive for years, even decades, and the HIV within them can suddenly spring forth whenever the cells are activated to fight infection.

stud   Slang for a virile man, or one who has sex with many partners.

subacute encephalitis   See HIV ENCEPHALOPATHY.

subclinical infection   An infection, or phase of infection, without apparent symptoms or signs of disease.

subcutaneous   Under the skin, as a subcutaneous injection.

subepidemic   A secondary or subordinate epidemic; within the context of HIV, a secondary epidemic existing at the same time as HIV. For example, while HIV is the most serious danger facing gay men who have unprotected sex, it is far from being the only one. Prevention experts warn that those who slip from safe sex standards run the risk of starting—or spreading—a subepidemic of other sexually transmitted diseases such as HEPATITIS A, HEPATITIS B, HEPATITIS C, CHLAMYDIA, GONORRHEA, HERPES, and SYPHILIS.

subsidized employment   A job in which an employee does not fully "earn his own way," in which the paycheck is actually partial or full "disguised charity"; the term is applied by SOCIAL SECURITY to handicapped workshops and the like, where people are employed for charitable, morale, or therapeutic reasons. By extension, the term can be applied to situations in which a no-longer-productive deteriorating worker is continued on the payroll for altruistic purposes.

substance abuse   See ADDICTION; DRUG ABUSE.

substantial gainful activity (SGA)   A SOCIAL SECURITY term for work that brings an income of over $300 monthly, the limit of eligibility for disabled persons for SSDI.

subtype   A group of related STRAINS (or isolates) of HIV that can be classified by their degree of similarity. There are currently three strains of HIV: M, N, and O. Strain M consists of at least 10 subtypes, which are labeled A through J. Isolate O also consists of several subtypes. Subtype B of group M is the major subtype of the virus found in the United States. See CLADE; GROUP M, N, AND O.

subunit vaccine   A vaccine that contains only portions of a surface molecule of a disease-producing MICROORGANISM.

sucralfate   A medicine consisting of a complex formed from sucrose octasulfate and polyaluminum hydroxide. It is effective in treating peptic ulcers by forming a coating over them that stays in place for more than eight hours. (Trade name is Carafate.)

suffering   A state of severe pain and/or distress that leads to the deterioration of the patient's health.

suicide   The intentional and voluntary taking of one's own life. While many states continue to bar physicians from helping mentally competent, terminally ill adults to hasten their deaths, physician-assisted suicide still occurs in the United States. It is also a fact that while society may not approve of assisted suicide, books such as Derek Humphry's *Final Exit: The Practicalities of Self-Deliverance and Assisted Suicide for the Dying* and Sherwin B. Nuland's *How We Die: Reflections on Life's Final Chapter* continue to enjoy immense popularity. Additionally, suicide hot lines are supported in many states and counties nationwide. Psychologists and others continue to debate about whether or not assisted suicide is ever a rational choice. Some believe that suicide can be a rational act and that psychologists and other mental health professionals should be allowed to help such patients without fear of legal or professional repercussions. Others argue that suicide is a symptom of mental illness and that helping someone to commit it should continue to be banned. With regard to AIDS, many feel that suicide is a normal reaction to specific situations.

Attempts to define rational suicide outline three basic criteria. First, the patient should have a hopeless condition, which includes a low quality of life and psychological as well as physical pain. Second, the patient should be free of coercion, whether coercion consists of internal factors like ageist or able-ist beliefs or external factors like greedy relatives or cost-conscious medical professionals or institutions. Third, the patient should be engaged in sound decision making. Sound decision making, in turn, should include the following five sub-criteria: (1) the patient should be mentally competent, which eliminates patients with treatable depression and other judgment-clouding impairments; (2) the patient should nonimpulsively consider other options, such as psychotherapy, antidepressants, assisted living, or support groups; (3) the decision should be consistent with the patient's values; (4) the patient should consider the impact suicide will have on significant others; and (5) the patient should consult with others, such as religious leaders, disability advocates, physical therapists, or hospice personnel.

sulfa drug   A drug of the sulfonamide group possessing bacteriostatic properties. Sulfa drugs are among the most common ANTIBIOTICS used in the treatment of OPPORTUNISTIC INFECTIONS. Sulfa is a substance to which approximately 25 percent of HIV-positive people are allergic. Patients can experience some reaction to the drug on taking it. There are strategies that may lessen or manage this problem; desensitization or TREATING THROUGH, for example, is a relatively simple and safe way of overcoming sulfa allergies. See DAPSONE; SULFADIAZINE; TRIMETHOPRIM-SULFAMETHOXAZOLE.

sulfadiazine (SFDZ)   A derivative of sulfonamide that appears as a white or yellowish powder. Sulfadiazine is used to treat urinary tract infections, chancroid, and trachoma. With pyrimethamine, it is used to treat TOXOPLASMOSIS. It is also occasionally used to treat malaria resistant to chloroquine; with streptomycin, to treat meningitis; and with penicillin, ear infections. It is administered orally. The most common side effects are allergic reactions, including skin rashes, itching, anaphylactic shock, swelling, sensitivity to light, joint pain, fever, and chills. The most serious side effects are blood disorders, including reduced counts of red blood cells, white blood cells, and platelets. Other side effects include headache, peripheral neuropathy, mental depression, convulsion, weakness, hallucinations, ringing in the ears, vertigo, insomnia, and kidney

toxicity. Rarely, goiter production, changes in urination, and low-blood-sugar levels have occurred in people taking the drug.

Sulfadiazine is one of a number of sulfa drugs that work by interfering with FOLIC ACID (vitamin B) metabolism in susceptible organisms, preventing them from multiplying. Because parasites can rapidly develop resistance to sulfadiazine, the drug is usually used with pyrimethamine for toxoplasmosis. The activity of the combination, called sulfadoxine, against the parasite greatly exceeds that of either drug alone. Because both drugs cross the BLOOD-BRAIN BARRIER, the combination is effective against toxoplasmosis encephalitis, a serious and potentially fatal infection of the brain.

sunlight   Even before studies were published about the effect of sunlight on HIV, AIDS-knowledgeable physicians were cautious about the dangers of sunlight to persons with AIDS or ASYMPTOMATIC HIV INFECTION. It had long been known that ultraviolet light can damage or suppress the Langerhans cells of the skin. These cells are an important part of the immune system, and are cells which HIV is known to infect. Strong sunlight, probably the ultraviolet rays, can impair immune response. Laying out in the sun or playing volleyball in one's swimsuit for hours at a time are examples of activities about which to be worried. T-HELPER CELL counts drop almost invariably after someone spends a long weekend at the beach. While regular exposure during daily activities is not of concern, it is noted that a number of drugs used by persons with HIV/AIDS make the skin much more sensitive to the sun than usual. Additionally, in the late 1980s, researchers at the CENTERS FOR DISEASE CONTROL AND PREVENTION found that the onset of AIDS as well as almost all opportunistic infections, peak in the summer, when ultraviolet exposure from sunlight is highest. In addition to being harmful to persons with HIV/AIDS, sunlight can provoke HERPES outbreaks.

superantigen   A foreign material produced by infectious MICROORGANISMS. Superantigens have the ability to activate many different T CELLS, resulting in large amounts of CYTOKINE production and large-scale activation of the immune system.

This activation may result in shock. Many toxins that cause food poisoning in humans are super-antigens. Unlike normal ANTIGENS, they are not processed and associate with MHC Class II molecules outside the peptide binding groove; recognition also is not MHC-restricted.

superinfection　A new, second infection caused by an organism different from that which caused an initial infection. The microbe responsible is usually resistant to the treatment given for the initial infection.

superoxide dismutase　One of the major cellular antioxidant enzymes. It removes surplus peroxide, an oxidizing free radical. Superoxide dismutase comes in two forms, one containing copper and zinc and the other containing manganese.

Supplemental Security Income (SSI)　A federal welfare program, operated by the SOCIAL SECURITY Administration with general revenues, that makes monthly payments to people with low incomes and limited assets who are 65 or older, blind, or disabled. As its name implies, it supplements existing, but inadequate income. The level varies from state to state and can go up every year based on cost-of-living adjustments. In addition to low income, people on SSI must have limited assets.

support group　A group whose purpose is to give emotional and psychological encouragement and confidence to its members. Support groups are often associated with psychotherapy, but many have been formed by people in similar difficulties or with similar problems, for mutual benefit. See SUPPORT NETWORK.

support network　A therapeutic term for a group of interconnected or cooperative individuals who give each other mutual encouragement and support. A support network tends to be an informal group linked by ties of friendship or family, rather than a purposely created formal support group.

suppository　A cylinder or cone made of a semi-solid substance infused, generally, with medicine, such as soap, glycerinated gelatin, or cocoa butter, for introduction into the rectum, vagina, or urethra, where it dissolves. Suppositories are not recommended as barriers against the transmission of HIV or AIDS.

suppression　The elimination of detectable viral load or viral replication in a person's blood.

suppressor cell　See SUPPRESSOR T CELL.

suppressor T cell　Any of a subset of T LYMPHOCYTES that suppress antibody synthesis by B CELLS or inhibit other cellular immune reactions. In the process CD8+ cells not only kill HIV-infected cells but also secrete factors that suppress HIV replication in both blood and lymph cells. The process seems to occur because the factors that are secreted, called beta-CHEMOKINES, typically "call" inflammatory cells to the site of the infection. Some of these factors then apparently block HIV replication by occupying receptors necessary for the entry of particular strains of HIV into their target cells.

suppurate　To form or emit a flow of pus.

surgeon general　The title of the chief medical officer in the United States Army, Air Force, Navy, and PUBLIC HEALTH SERVICE.

surgical glove　A sterile, nonporous latex glove that covers the whole hand, worn by doctors and other medical personnel for surgery, examinations, and other medical procedures and in handling medical waste, blood products, and so forth. These gloves are often used for FIST- or FINGER-FUCKING and other HIGH-RISK SEX practices. Some users cut off the hand area and use the wrist/forearm area (flattened, slit lengthwise and opened) to create a DENTAL DAM/oral shield. Surgical gloves can be bought at most medical suppliers and chemists.

surrogacy　A legal arrangement under which a person or institution assumes responsibility for an adult individual judged incompetent to care for himself or to look after his affairs. There are different types of surrogacy, including attorney-in-fact, conservatorship, and guardianship. See SURROGATE.

surrogate A person or institution appointed by a court to look after the affairs of one judged incompetent because of illness, age, or some other condition. Forms of surrogacy include attorney-in-fact, conservatorship, and guardianship. The legal process to appoint surrogates, and the legal powers granted to them vary from state to state. In California, for example, individuals demonstrating continuing grave disability as a result of mental illness may be placed under a conservatorship, subject to yearly review and renewal by the court. Anyone may file a petition for conservatorship on behalf of a gravely disabled person, and the court will investigate the need and the qualifications of the proposed conservator. If there is "clear and convincing evidence" that a gravely disabled person is so incompetent as to be unable to care for him or herself, the court may appoint a temporary conservator who will serve until the investigation is complete. A surrogate may be charged with the obligation to make health care decisions for the person judged incompetent, and be empowered to give informed consent on his or her behalf.

surrogate marker A blood or other lab test measurement that indicates the presence and action of a virus, such as HIV, that is difficult to monitor directly. Ever since AIDS was recognized in 1981, the medical establishment has grappled with how exactly to describe the disease and monitor its progression. A major obstacle is that measuring the amount of HIV in the human body is extremely difficult. HIV is notoriously difficult to track, since it mutates rapidly, and it is difficult to grow in the test tube. No reliable, standardized lab test that measures HIV accurately is yet available, so many health care workers have been monitoring HIV disease progression by measuring quantities, other than virus levels, that reflect HIV activity, such as that of T4 CELLS. These are referred to as surrogate markers because they provide information on HIV through its secondary effects on the immune system. This information can guide treatment decisions and monitor the efficacy of treatments.

Researchers and activists are constantly engaged in debates about which markers are the most reliable, practical, and predictive of HIV progression. As with most aspects of AIDS, the dialogue about surrogate markers resonates with political implications. For instance, the use of surrogate markers to measure an experimental drug's efficacy may significantly shorten human trials and enable the drug to be made available more expediently. Additionally, the use of surrogate markers as a way of defining AIDS will directly determine who receives an AIDS- or HIV-positive diagnosis, who receives financial entitlements, who receives medical treatment, how research efforts are conducted, and how the scope of the epidemic is understood. Most surrogate markers are components of the immune system. These include different types of cells, such as T4 and T8 cells. In addition, proteins secreted by immune system cells, such as NEOPTERIN and BETA-2 (B2) MICROGLOBULIN, are used as surrogate markers. A fluctuation in a single marker may not be significant when a number of other markers remain steady. T cells are currently used as the surrogate marker that most closely measures HIV progression. See IMMUNOLOGIC MARKERS; VIROLOGIC MARKERS.

surveillance In public health terms, the process of monitoring conditions such as epidemics. According to the World Health Organization (WHO), "public health surveillance is the collection of information of sufficient accuracy and completeness regarding the distribution and spread of infection to be pertinent to the design, implementation, or monitoring of prevention and control programmes and activities." Public health surveillance involves an assessment of the existing distribution and scope of infection and its likely spread in the population and is an important first step in responding to a disease. As people infected with HIV can remain asymptomatic for a very long time and because infection can be detected only with a specific test, testing has became the central issue in monitoring HIV/AIDS.

Surveillance is a term often associated with intrusions into individual privacy. For the purpose of public health surveillance it is sufficient to know how many people are infected. It is not necessary to know the identities of the infected people. See PRIVACY.

surveillance case definition The AIDS case definition used for surveillance purposes. As

AIDS cases are diagnosed among various subpopulations, epidemiologists have come to recognize a wide spectrum of clinical signs and symptoms that may be associated with the disease. This diversity has resulted in changes in the case definition used for surveillance purposes, which in turn has led to changes in the prevalence of AIDS across risk categories.

The original surveillance definition for AIDS was developed primarily through studies of the natural history of the disease among homosexual and bisexual men and reflected the disease as it appeared in those individuals. It is now understood that there may be very different manifestations of the underlying immune defect across risk categories, including the "wasting syndrome" and HIV encephalopathy, which are now included in the surveillance definition of AIDS. The addition of IDUs, women, and children to the population to define the illness led to these changes.

The objectives of the most recent revisions were (1) to track more effectively the severe disabling morbidity associated with infection with HUMAN IMMUNODEFICIENCY VIRUS (HIV); (2) to simplify reporting of AIDS cases; (3) to increase the sensitivity and specificity of the definition through greater diagnostic application of laboratory evidence for HIV infection; and (4) to be consistent with the then-current diagnostic practices, which in some cases included presumptive (without confirmatory laboratory evidence) diagnosis of AIDS-indicative diseases (e.g., PNEUMOCYSTIS CARINII PNEUMONIA and KAPOSI'S SARCOMA).

Clinicians were cautioned not to rely on the revised definition alone to diagnose serious disease caused by HIV infection in individual patients because there may be additional information that would lead to a more accurate diagnosis. It was emphasized that the diagnostic criteria accepted by the AIDS surveillance case definition should not be interpreted as the standard of good medical practice. The Social Security Administration (SSA) disappointed many physicians by promptly accepting this definition and no others for its definition of AIDS for potential disability claims. Several other diseases may result from HIV infection; however, SSA does not view these as AIDS-defining illnesses. See AIDS CASE DEFINITION.

survey   A comprehensive appraisal of an area of research, particularly into a particular disease or health condition, especially its epidemiological aspects.

survival   Continued life, especially under conditions in which death would be expected to occur; a measure of drug efficacy consisting of the length of life of a person on a drug.

survival (or survivor) benefit   The amount payable to a beneficiary from an annuity or insurance policy when the policyholder dies.

survival rate   The percentage of a particular study group that survives over a given time.

susceptibility testing   See PHENOTYPIC ASSAY.

susceptible host   Any organism that is easily invaded by a parasitic organism.

Sutherlandia frutescens   A flowering plant native to South Africa that is currently undergoing testing in humans as a supplement to treat HIV. A plant that has been used for centuries by the San peoples of Southern Africa for medicinal purposes, it recently received broad attention because several medical doctors in South Africa are testing the supplement in humans. As with any supplement, there is likely to be no rush to prove its success as it cannot be patented by anyone, because it is a plant. According to the company Phyto Nova, which produces the supplements and is testing it, it contains several chemicals that are already used in the treatment of various illnesses. *Sutherlandia frutescens* was used by the Zulus in the early 20th century during influenza outbreaks.

sweats   See NIGHT SWEATS.

swing party   A party at which participants may engage in sexual acts.

swinger   Person who engages in sex at swing parties.

swollen glands A common way to refer to enlarged lymph nodes. Lymph nodes are the rounded bodies consisting of an accumulation of lymphatic tissue found at intervals in the course of the lymphatic vessels. In the context of HIV/AIDS, *swollen glands* generally refers to the condition of the lymph nodes in the region of the neck, the armpit, or the groin.

Soon after AIDS was identified as a new disease, physicians noticed that a large group of previously healthy homosexual men were seeking treatment for persistently swollen glands not explained by specific illnesses or drug use. The epidemiological characteristics of this population were identical with those of the population of AIDS patients. As the epidemic progressed, similar findings were reported among injection drug users, hemophiliacs, and the heterosexual partners of some AIDS patients. When the blood test for HIV-1 antibodies became available, researchers demonstrated that LYMPHADENOPATHY (chronically swollen lymph nodes) was a frequent consequence of infection with the virus.

Initially, it was believed that people who had persistent lymphadenopathy were more likely to have opportunistic infections than HIV-infected patients whose glands remained normal. Researchers in 1987 found that in the absence of other symptoms, persistently swollen glands are not indicative of a declining immune system. Swollen glands may also be enlarged salivary glands, which also occur more frequently in HIV infection.

symptom Any phenomenon or circumstance accompanying something and serving as evidence of it. In medicine, a phenomenon that arises from and accompanies a particular disease or disorder and serves as an indication of it. For example, genital ulcers are one symptom of HERPES SIMPLEX, and a slowly progressive neurologic dysfunction is one symptom of PROGRESSIVE MULTIFOCAL LEUKOEN-CEPHALOPATHY (PML), an opportunistic infection caused by the Creutzfeldt-Jakob virus.

symptomatic hyperlactatemia A less severe form of LACTIC ACIDOSIS, in which too much lactic acid has built up in a person's blood. This occurs in HIV-positive people who have taken NRTI drugs for several years or who have allergic-type reactions to NRTIs. It does not happen to everybody, and researchers are as yet unsure what triggers it in some people and not in others. Its symptoms are nausea, abdominal pain, vomiting, shortness of breath, sudden weight loss, burning or tingling sensation, and profound muscular weakness.

symptomology The complex of symptoms of a disease; also, the branch of medicine concerned with symptoms, their production, and the indications they furnish.

synapse The point of junction between two neurons in a neural pathway, where the termination of the axon of one neuron comes into close proximity to the cell body or dendrites of another. At this point, an electrical impulse traveling in the first neuron initiates an impulse in the second neuron. The impulses travel in one direction only. Synapses are susceptible to fatigue, offer resistance to the passage of impulses, and are markedly susceptible to the effects of oxygen deficiency, anesthetics, and other agents, including therapeutic drugs and toxic chemicals.

syncytium (pl. syncytia) A giant cell. Syncytia are multicellular clumps formed when cells fuse with each other. Cells infected with HIV often fuse with nearby uninfected cells, forming large giant cells called syncytia. Research has shown these giant cells cause cell death in uninfected cells that are attached to them.

At some point in the cycle of HIV illness, the HIV mutates and begins to attach to MACROPHAGES by using the CXCR-4 coreceptor. When this occurs, VIRAL LOAD increases greatly and patients begin to suffer more OPPORTUNISTIC INFECTIONS. This phase of the virus life causes syncytia. Syncytia have also been correlated to a rapid disease progression in HIV-infected people.

HIV strains can be classified as non-syncytia-inducing (NSI) and syncytia-inducing (SI). SI STRAINS invade T CELLS by binding to CXCR-4 and CD4 receptors. NSI strains infect MACROPHAGES and CD4 cells by binding to the CCR5 and CD4 receptors. See CCR5; NON-SYNCYTIUM-INDUCING VIRUS.

syndrome A group of symptoms and diseases that together are characteristic of a specific condition.

synergism   Cooperative interaction; interaction between two or more agents (e.g., drugs) that produces an effect greater than the sum of their individual effects. Also called SYNERGY.

synergy   See SYNERGISM.

synovir   See THALIDOMIDE.

synthetic baryta   See BARIUM SULFATE.

synthetic CD4   See CD4, SYNTHETIC.

syphilis   An infectious sexually transmitted disease caused by a spirochete (a type of bacterium), *Treponema pallidum*, that, if left untreated, can cause chronic infection of multiple organ sites, including the central nervous system. Syphilis is characterized by lesions that may involve any organ or body tissue. Syphilis usually appears initially as a single painless ulcer. This ulcer may not be noticed if it is inside the vagina, anus, urethra, or mouth. Syphilis may remain asymptomatic for years.

If untreated, syphilis progresses through three clinical stages: primary (initial painless ulcerative lesions at the site of inoculation); secondary (widespread mucocutaneous lesions and generalized regional lymphadenopathy generally visible, particularly on the palms of the hands, with frequent relapses); and tertiary (destructive lesions involving many organs and tissues, including the heart and central nervous system). When untreated in pregnant women, it can result in a life-threatening congenital infection in the newborn. Tertiary syphilis develops in 25 percent of patients if it is untreated.

Syphilis is usually transmitted through sexual contact (both heterosexual and homosexual) but may be acquired in utero or by direct contact with infected tissue or blood. Diagnosis usually is based on a serologic test, run along with a confirmatory test. Treatment failures do occur and may be more common in HIV illness. Penicillin is the preferred drug for treatment. It is the only therapy that has been widely used for patients with neurosyphilis, congenital syphilis, and syphilis during pregnancy. All sexually active patients with syphilis and their partners should be tested for HIV. Neurosyphilis

should be considered in the differential diagnosis of neurologic disease in HIV-positive persons.

Congenital syphilis is particularly virulent and can be deadly for the baby. It must be treated with intravenous penicillin. This type of syphilis is seen most often in the southern United States.

syphilitic chancre   The syphilis ulcer, the first symptom of syphilis.

syringe   Instrument for injecting fluids into cavities or vessels. A hypodermic is a syringe, fitted with a needle, used to administer drugs by injecting them into the SUBCUTANEOUS TISSUE. An oral syringe is made of plastic or glass, and is not fitted with a needle. It is graduated and is used to dispense liquid medication to children. The tip is constructed to prevent its breaking in the child's mouth.

syringe access   See NEEDLE ACCESS.

syringe exchange program   See NEEDLE EXCHANGE PROGRAM.

syringe sharing   See NEEDLE SHARING.

systemic   Relating to the entire organism, as distinguished from any of its individual parts. A systemic therapy is one that the entire body is exposed to, rather than just the tissues affected by a disease.

systemic chemotherapy   Treatment with antitumor or anticancer medication by introducing it into the veins for distribution to all tissues via general circulation.

systemic disease   Any pathologic condition involving the entire organism as distinct from an individual organ system or part.

systemic lupus erythematosus   An immune disease of unknown etiology characterized by fever, muscle pains, joint pains, skin rashes, anemia, and low white blood cell counts. It affects connective tissue as well as the kidneys, spleen, skin, heart, and the nervous system.

T

T cell   LYMPHOCYTE that travels from the BONE MARROW via the blood and enters the THYMUS, after which it enters into circulation again and settle in the spleen and LYMPH nodes. T cells are essential elements in cellular immunity against viruses, parasites, fungi, and malignant cells, and may be rendered ineffective by HIV. T cells also release factors that induce proliferation of T lymphocytes and B LYMPHOCYTES. T lymphocytes are found primarily in the blood, lymph, and lymphoid organs.

Immature T cells are called thymocytes. Mature T cells are "ANTIGEN-specific," meaning that each one responds only to one antigen. Unlike B cells, T cells do not recognize native antigen conformation directly, but only in association with self-antigens of the major histocompatibility complex. There are two major subsets of T cells: those expressing the accessory molecule CD4 and those expressing CD8. The former are mainly T helper cells; the latter are generally effector cells recognizing and destroying infected cells (i.e., cytotoxic cells). T helper cells recognize a specific MHC-antigen complex on the surface of a B cell and then induce its maturation and proliferation into specific antibody-screening (plasma) cells. While in the thymus, a T cell "learns" during T-cell maturation both to treat its body's Class I molecules as "self-antigens" and to recognize as foreign a specific epitope of a "non-self antigen." T cells do not produce antibody, but antibody production by B cells often requires T-cell help. T-cell receptors bind antigen on the surfaces of other cells only after it has been degraded or otherwise processed by that cell, and only after it has become physically associated with molecules of the MHC. MHC restriction refers to the process during T-cell maturation in the thymus when an individual's T cells come to recognize, and be activated by, antigen. Self-restriction occurs when T cells preferentially recognize foreign antigens encountered during their own development in the thymus. Cytotoxic T cells recognize tumor or virus-infected cells by their surface antigens in combination with their MHC markers, and will kill them. Other T cells (macrophage-activating cells) produce lymphokines, which promote macrophage activity. Suppressor T cells specifically suppress the immune response, probably through antigen-presenting cells and/or through more direct interactions with T-helper cells or B cells.

T cells are normally repopulated without regard to subset—that is, both CD4 and CD8 cells are produced to replace their loss. In people with HIV infection, CD4+ T cells are selectively infected by the virus, resulting in the preferential killing of these cells. The process of "blind T cell homeostasis" replaces lost CD4+ T cells with both CD4+ T cells and CD8+ T cells. The result is a gradual increase in the ratio of CD8+ T cells, even while the total T-cell count remains constant. Ultimately, for unknown reasons, blind T-cell homeostasis fails and CD8+ T cells, as well as CD4+ T cells, start to decrease in number.

T lymphocyte   See T CELL.

T lymphocyte proliferation assay   A test used to measure the response of T cells to antigens or microbes, such as HIV.

T1 cell   The cytotoxic T cells involved in cell-mediated immunity.

T4 cell   A LYMPHOCYTE and the most important cell in the specialized immune response, also known as a "helper" or CD4 cell. Helper T cells induce, help, and coordinate the specialized immune response, which cannot function without them. T4 cells also stimulate the production of B cells. They have an identifying surface structure called CD4 or T4.

T4 count   See T4-CELL COUNT.

T4 lymphocyte   See T4 CELL.

T4-cell count   A measure of the immune system; the number of T4 LYMPHOCYTES present in a microliter of blood. A normal range is anywhere from 500 to 1,500. T4 counts are the best known and most widely used SURROGATE MARKERS. Since HIV attacks T4 cells, comparing the number of existing T4 cells to the normal range (and to previous counts) is commonly used to predict progression of disease; T4 counts have been correlated with survival. T4 levels can be reported in the following ways: absolute number of T4 cells; percentage of T4 cells of all lymphocytes; and ratio of T4 to T8 cells.

To date, most research exploring T4 cells as surrogate markers for HIV disease has involved only gay and bisexual men. This information has been applied to women. Such extrapolation of research findings is common in HIV and many other areas. Research on surrogate markers in women is needed to confirm treatment recommendations such as PCP PROPHYLAXIS and anti-HIV therapies such as AZT and ddI.

T4-cell percentage   The percentage of the total number of LYMPHOCYTES that is T4 cells. The general average is between 35 percent and 65 percent. Note that the total number of lymphocytes varies widely from day to day. Note too that the count varies more than the percentage because of the way it is calculated. A change of three percentage points is considered significant, and a reduction of such size may indicate HIV progression even if absolute T4 counts remain steady. In general, the percentages are more stable than the absolute numbers.

T4-celi test   T4-cell tests are significantly limited. First, T4 counts may include nonfunctioning cells, since the mechanism that counts the cells does not distinguish between healthy T4 and HIV-impaired cells. Second, it is well known that T4 counts can fluctuate dramatically even in the course of a single day, and different labs may well report different counts for the same blood sample. For individuals being tested, it is important to have blood drawn at approximately the same time of day each time, if possible, and to have samples sent to the same lab. For diagnostic purposes, the trend in T4 counts over time is more meaningful than any single T4 value. See T4-CELL COUNT.

T4:T8 ratio   See T-CELL HOMEOSTASIS; T-CELL RATIO.

T8 cell   Also known as a CD8 or "suppressor/cytotoxic" cell, this LYMPHOCYTE suppresses or "turns off" the immune system when an infection has been suppressed. Without T8 cells, our immune systems would remain activated and might attack the healthy parts of our bodies. The suppressor T cell has the same identifying surface structure, called CD8 or T8, as the killer T cell. Standard lymphocyte typing does not therefore distinguish between suppressor T cells and killer T cells.

Much emphasis has been placed on the ratio of T8 cells to T4 cells. Normally, a person should have twice as many T4 CELLS as T8 cells, a ratio of 2:1. However, during HIV progression, the proportion of T4 cells decreases dramatically, and a person may have twice as many T8 cells as T4 cells. This inversion has also been interpreted as a bad sign, and some people advocate tracking the ratio of these cells. See also T-CELL HOMEOSTASIS.

Absolute T8 count, although not altogether well understood, has also been endorsed as a good surrogate marker by some AIDS clinicians.

T8 lymphocyte   See T8 CELL.

T20   See ENFUVIRTIDE.

T1249   Trimeris's second-generation experimental fusion inhibitor. As does the related T20, T1249 binds to gp41, part of the HIV envelope protein; gp41 holds the cell membrane and HIV together when the two are fusing. Once bound to T1249, gp41 cannot jackknife to draw cell and virus together. Administration is by subcutaneous injection. T1249 has a longer half-life than T20, which may allow T1249 to be injected less frequently. Information about toxicity and side effects is pending.

Tagamet   See CIMETIDINE.

tardive dyskinesia   Involuntary movements, generally of the muscles in the face or mouth. It is usually the consequence of long-term administration of certain psychoactive drugs.

tat   A gene of HIV that regulates viral activity.

tat antagonist   See TAT INHIBITOR.

tat gene   The HIV gene that enables HIV replication by encoding a transactivating genetic element of the virus that increases the production of cellular and viral proteins.

tat gene inhibitor   See TAT INHIBITOR.

tat inhibitor   One of a group of drug compounds that interfere with HIV replication by eliminating or disabling the TAT GENE. Also known as tat ANTAGONISTS or antitat compounds.

tattoo   An indelible body marking produced by injecting minute amounts of pigments into the skin. When tattooing is done commercially, sterile procedures should be used. Still, there is a risk that infectious hepatitis or HIV or both may be transmitted. Tattoos are usually done for decorative purposes, by those who find it attractive, but they may also be used cosmetically, to conceal a corneal leukoma, to mask pigmented areas of skin, or to color skin to look like the areola in mammoplasty.

Taxol   A chemotherapeutic drug used for the treatment of solid tumors. Taxol is an experimental treatment for KAPOSI'S SARCOMA. It works by interfering with internal cell structures, which are necessary for cell division. Consequently, it is highly toxic to rapidly dividing cells, such as those in tumors or in normal BONE MARROW. It has a long list of side effects, the most serious of which is severe and potentially fatal allergic reactions. Bone-marrow toxicity, resulting in a deficiency of white blood cells called NEUTROPENIA, is also common but is manageable and reversible. PERIPHERAL NEUROPATHY is the most common neurological side effect. Neuropathy is generally cumulative with repeated doses, and more likely to occur in people at risk for it, for instance those who have experienced neuropathy as a side effect of other therapy. Other side effects include irregular heart rhythm, hair loss, diarrhea, skin rashes, nausea, vomiting, stomach irritation, and seizures. Taxol is available as a solution for INTRAVENOUS injection. (Brand name is Paclitaxal.)

T-cell count   The number of T lymphocytes in a cubic millimeter of blood. See T CELLS.

T-cell homeostasis   Research indicates that the body's complex mechanisms that normally maintain levels of T cells, known as homeostasis, may contribute to the development of the abnormalities in T-cell numbers seen in HIV-infected people (i.e., falling CD4+ and rising CD8+ counts) and that the ultimate failure of T-cell homeostasis contributes to the onset of AIDS. Failure of T-cell homeostasis appears to represent a recognizable and clinically significant landmark in the natural history of HIV infection. Because of this, some researchers advocate measurements of all T-cell subsets, not just CD4+ cells. See T-CELL RATIO.

T-cell leukemia   See T-CELL LYMPHOMA.

T-cell lymphoma   An acute or subacute disease associated with a human T cell virus and characterized by LYMPHADENOPATHY, hypercalcemia, hepatosplenomegaly, skin lesions, and peripheral blood involvement. Also called T-CELL LEUKEMIA. Only some are associated with human T-cell leukemia virus types 1 and 2.

T-cell ratio   The relative proportions of T4 LYMPHOCYTES (helper cells) and T8 LYMPHOCYTES (suppressor cells) in the blood.

T-cell receptor   T CELLS need to recognize a wide variety of antigens, doing so through the cooperation of a membrane receptor (TCR) and accessory molecules. The genes encoding the receptor resemble those for antibodies and comprise variable and constant regions. As in that system, production of the TCR repertoire involves both germ-line diversity and gene rearrangements. ANTIGEN recognition by the T-cell receptors involves their binding that antigen (often a peptide fragment) when presented on another cell's surface stably bound to a protein encoded by the organism's major histocompatibility complex. Antigen-binding by the TCR activates a protein tyrosine kinase (enzymes providing a central switch mechanism in cellular signal transduction pathways, often involved in cell fate determination) and a generation of phosphatidyl-derived second messengers (a messenger produced by phospholipase, the activity as a breakdown of the major cell membrane phospholipid phosphatidy-linositol).

T-cell restriction   Alternative for MHC-RESTRICTION (major histocompatibility complex) of T CELL.

T-cell subset   Subpopulation of T lymphocytes, including T4 (CD4) or helper cells, which are the major regulatory cells, and T8 (CD8) or suppressor cells.

T-cell test   A test to determine T-cell count, used to monitor the immune status of someone who has HIV. See T4-CELL COUNT; T4-CELL TEST; T-CELL COUNT.

TCR   See T-CELL RECEPTOR.

T-dependent/independent   T-dependent ANTIGENS require immune recognition by both T and B CELLS to produce an immune response. T-independent antigens can directly stimulate B cells to produce specific ANTIBODY.

tears   Drops of the watery secretion of the lacrimal glands, tears are secreted continuously into the eyes. HIV has been recovered from tears but is unproved as a route of transmission of the virus. HIV is present in many body fluids, but the principal forms of transmission are limited to direct exposure to contaminated blood, sexual contact with exposure to secretions, and exchange of blood from mother to child during pregnancy or shortly thereafter.

Teldrin   See CHLORPHENIRAMINE.

telomere   A complex of repetitive DNA sequences that cap the ends of chromosomes. Telomeres play a role in cellular replication via the telomerase enzyme, which helps determine whether cells are able to replicate. Telomeres shorten each time a cell divides and signal cell senescence (loss of function) when they reach a critical length.

temazepam   A psychoactive-sedative compound, a member of a class of psychoactive drugs called BENZODIAZEPINES. All of these drugs reduce anxiety or cause drowsiness to some degree. Compared with other benzodiazepines, temazepam is relatively long-acting and is useful for people who wake up too early. Its primary disadvantage is that it can cause a hangover the day after its use. Temazepam is available as capsules for oral administration. The most common side effects are dizziness and daytime drowsiness. Other side effects include lethargy, hangover, anxiety, diarrhea, euphoria, weakness, confusion, and vertigo. (Trade name is Restoril.)

Temporary Assistance for Needy Families (TANF)   A plan that replaced the AID TO FAMILIES WITH DEPENDENT CHILDREN (AFDC) program. Whereas AFDC provided direct cash assistance to families, TANF consists of block grants to the states, which were required to have their own welfare reform plans in place by July 1, 1997. New features include a requirement that most adult recipients must be working within two years of beginning welfare assistance and a lifetime limit of five cumulative years of cash assistance for each family. States can exempt up to 20 percent of their caseload from this five-year limit, but alternatively they can impose a shorter time limit on welfare recipients. States have the option of further restrictions: They can deny benefits to children born to welfare recipients, can deny benefits to unwed parents under age 18, and can maintain recipients who move in from another state at the benefit level that applied in their former state for one year. However, states must still follow the former AFDC rules with regard to eligibility for Medicaid.

tenidap A drug extensively tested for treating arthritis, tenidap is a drug under development that works to inhibit TUMOR NECROSIS FACTOR.

tenofovir Tenofovir is a nucleotide analog reverse transcriptase inhibitor (NtRTI). It is slightly different in makeup than nucleoside reverse transcriptase inhibitors (NRTI). Tenofovir is the first NtRTI that has been approved for the treatment of HIV. It was approved in October 2001. One major difference is that tenofovir is metabolized by the kidney. So it does not affect the liver's ability to metabolize other drugs.

Studies have shown it to be a very potent drug against HIV. It is closely related to the drug adefovir, which was not approved for treatment of HIV but is now used to treat hepatitis B (HBV). Tenofovir is also being tested for use by HBV patients. It is thought that it may be able to treat NRTI-resistant viruses, but studies have not been completed in this area. It is currently being used as a second- or third-line treatment strategy because it has been shown to be so powerful.

Tenofovir has been well tolerated by patients in research studies. Some people show higher liver enzymes as well as increased bilirubin levels. There have been studies in animals that show tenofovir may cause decreases in bone density. This effect has not been seen yet in humans. Tenofovir may also in rare instances raise creatinine levels, but it has not been seen in any great degree. Tenofovir will raise the levels of ddI in the blood but has not reportedly effected other HIV medicines. It should be used with care when mixed with other drugs that metabolize in the kidneys, as that may cause a rise or lowering of the drug availability. It has not been studied in pregnant women or in children, so dosing is unknown for these groups. It is a once a day medicine that will benefit those that struggle to maintain medicine regimens.

It has been tested extensively in animals because it was shown to be effective against various viral infections. It has also been shown to prevent SIV infection in monkeys that took the drug after being injected with SIV. Researchers may soon look at the role of tenofovir as a treatment for post-HIV exposure to prevent the virus from establishing infection. (The trade name is Viread. It was also known as bis-POC PMPA during development.)

teratogenicity The ability to cause malformations in a fetus. It is distinct from mutagenicity, which causes genetic mutations in sperm, eggs, or other cells. Teratogenicity is a potential side effect of many drugs, such as THALIDOMIDE.

terbinafine A drug being studied for possible treatment of oral CANDIDIASIS resistant to fluconazole. It is already available as a pill or topical ointment for use in the treatment of athlete's foot and fungal nail infections. A rare side effect of terbinafine is a rash. If a rash develops, use of the drug should be discontinued.

terfenadine A relatively new, long-lasting ANTIHISTAMINE used to treat the symptoms of seasonal allergies. In people with HIV, the drug is also used to reduce certain drug-induced allergic side effects, including skin rashes, redness, swelling, hives, and breathing difficulties. The main difference between this drug and the older antihistamines is that it causes less drowsiness and is often suitable for people who need to stay alert. Terfenadine is available as regular and extended-release tablets for oral administration. Common side effects include nausea and loss of appetite. (Brand names are Contact Allergy Formula, Seldane, and Seldane-D.)

terminal Pertaining to the end phase; in medical terms, leading ultimately to death.

testes See TESTICLES.

testicles The male sex glands, or testes, which produce both sperm and testosterone. Located in the scrotum. Slang terms include *balls, family jewels, nuts,* and *orchids.*

testicular atrophy A wasting away, or decrease in size and function, of the TESTICLES.

testicular cancer Cancer of the TESTICLES.

testing See HIV TESTING; MANDATORY TESTING; PRIVACY.

testosterone A naturally occurring male hormone, found in both men and women. Testosterone is responsible for the masculinizing and tissue-building (anabolic) changes that occur in males during adolescence, including the growth of the reproductive tract and the development of secondary sexual characteristics. When administered as a drug it can cause gain in lean body mass, increased sex drive, and possibly aggressive behavior. Many men with HIV have low testosterone levels caused by HIV suppression of normal endocrine-gland function or by drugs (like KETON-CONAZOLE) used to treat opportunistic infections. These deficiencies are associated with the loss of both energy and lean tissue mass in HIV-related weight loss. Testosterone and other ANABOLIC STEROIDS are often prescribed as part of TESTOSTERONE REPLACEMENT THERAPY.

Oral and injectable testosterone have long been available to treat testosterone deficiencies. Synthetic forms are also available. The advantages of these include lower risk of liver toxicity and fewer of the masculinizing side effects common when injectable testosterone is used. Recently, a daily-wear, no-adhesive transdermal (through the skin) testosterone patch has become available. It is applied to the scrotum and provides serum testosterone levels that mimic the normal daily pattern in healthy adults. This form of delivery also avoids the peaks and troughs in blood levels that occur with testosterone injections. For treatment of HIV-related weight loss, one manufacturer recently started a CLINICAL TRIAL of a rub-on testosterone gel. Testosterone patches are already approved for use in hypogonadal wasting. The rub-on gel must

be applied to a shaved scrotum, while the patches can be placed anywhere on the body.

For treatment of HIV-related weight loss, testosterone is effective only for people with abnormally low testosterone levels. For maximum effect against wasting, both adequate nutrition and exercise should be combined with testosterone therapy. The hormone makes cells ready to build tissue but has little effect without the proper building blocks or exercise. Prolonged use of oral testosterone, however, as of other oral anabolic steroids, has been associated with severe liver toxicity and liver cancer.

Not much is known about how the use of testosterone and other anabolic steroids affects HIV replication, disease progression, or survival. Even less is known about the use of anabolic-steroid therapy in HIV-positive women.

testosterone replacement therapy The therapeutic use of testosterone to substitute for natural testosterone that is either absent or diminished. Also used as an approach to managing weight loss.

tetracycline Any of a group of broad-spectrum ANTIBIOTICS belonging to certain species of *Streptomyces.* They may also be produced semisynthetically. Tetracyclines are effective against a variety of organisms, including GRAM-NEGATIVE and GRAM-POSITIVE BACTERIA, CHLAMYDIAS, MYCOPLASMAS, RICKETTSIAS, and some viruses and protozoa.

Th0 response An immune response that involves aspects of both Th1 and Th2 branches of the immune system. TH0 cells produce cytokines that are characteristic of both TH1 and TH2 response.

Th1 cell A subdivision of the helper T cell involved in cell-mediated immunity and characterized by its production of IFN-γ and IL-2. The cytotoxic T cells involved in this response are known as T1.

Th1 response An acquired immune response whose most prominent feature is high cytotoxic T LYMPHOCYTE activity relative to the amount of antibody production. The Th1 response is promoted by T4 Th1 T-helper cells.

Th2 cell   A type of T-HELPER CELL that stimulates B CELLS to produce immunoglobin gamma E, immunoglobin gamma G, and proinflammatory effects in allergy and other ANTIBODY responses. They are characterized by their production of IL-4, IL-5, IL-6, and IL-10. The suppressor T cells involved in this response are known as T2 cells.

Th2 response   An acquired immune response whose most prominent feature is high ANTIBODY production relative to the amount of cytotoxic T-LYMPHOCYTE activity. The Th2 response is promoted by T2 Th2 T-HELPER CELLS.

thalidomide   A drug made infamous in the early 1960s when it caused severe birth defects in children born to women who took it during pregnancy, thalidomide has been found to effectively heal severe mouth and throat ulcers in people with HIV infection. For the many patients with HIV infection who suffer from these ulcers, eating can be excruciatingly painful, which exacerbates wasting and debilitation. Thalidomide is the first treatment shown in a scientific study to heal these ulcers. Because of its potential toxicity, treatment should be carefully monitored and limited in its duration. Possible serious side effects include irreversible, painful peripheral nerve damage, rash, birth defects and sleepiness.

Thalidomide is also currently being investigated for use against primary HIV infection and AIDS-related wasting syndrome. Since the sixties, thalidomide has been found to be relatively safe in nonpregnant populations and effective in treating a number of clinical conditions, many of which are similar to each other and to symptoms observed in HIV patients. A common link may be TUMOR NECROSIS FACTOR ALPHA, a CYTOKINE, or intracellular messenger, that is possibly a key element in both wasting syndrome and HIV activation. Thalidomide has been found to selectively inhibit TNF production and release. It is a possible alternative to the immensely expensive human growth hormone, another experimental antiwasting treatment. (Trade name is Synovir.)

THC   See DELTA-9 TETRAHYDROCANNABINOL; DRONABINOL; MARIJUANA.

T-helper cell   See T4 CELL.

T-helper cell count   See T4-CELL COUNT.

T-helper lymphocyte   See T4 CELL.

T-helper to T-suppressor ratio   See T-CELL HOMEOSTASIS; T-CELL RATIO.

therapeutic drug   A drug having medicinal or healing properties.

therapeutic drug monitoring   Measuring of the blood levels of the medication(s) an individual is taking for a given condition or conditions. At issue are the desired blood levels for maximal treatment effectiveness and the patient's blood levels. Also at issue are toxicity, side effects, and drug interactions.

therapeutic holiday   See STRUCTURED TREATMENT INTERRUPTIONS.

therapeutic index   The ratio obtained by dividing the lethal dose (LD-50) of a drug by its MINIMUM EFFECTIVE DOSE (MED-50). If the ratio is equal to 10 or more, it indicates that a lethal dose is at least 10 times the minimum effective dose.

therapeutic touch   Popularized by nursing professor Dolores Krieger, therapeutic touch is practiced by registered nurses and others to relieve pain and stress. The practitioner assesses where the person's energy field is weak or congested and then uses his or her hands to direct energy into the field to balance it.

therapeutic vaccine   A vaccine administered after infection with a disease-causing microorganism to modify the immune response to make it more effective. Therapeutic vaccination is a well-known medical technique first introduced a century ago for the treatment of chronic staphylococcal infections, syphilis, and tuberculosis. These early efforts with therapeutic vaccination were only marginally successful; they almost faded from use when antibiotics were introduced in the late 1940s. However, therapeutic vaccination today remains the standard of care for those believed to be infected with rabies and for babies born to mothers infected with hepatitis B virus. In diseases against which therapeutic vaccination does work, the vaccine retards early infection before the development of a natural immune response.

Within the context of HIV, an injected therapy consisting of synthetic HIV antigen (e.g., gp160) is administered to people who already have HIV. It is supposed to heighten and broaden the immune response to HIV, helping to halt disease progression. Since general immune stimulation via IL-2 or other agents has not offered much hope of directly restricting HIV, researchers all along have been considering ways to construct a strong specific anti-HIV immune defense. Therapeutic vaccines are the major strategy that has been proposed to preferentially increase surviving CD4 CELLS that could orchestrate a new defense against HIV.

After introduction of new foreign proteins (antigen) to the body, naive CD4 cells sensitive to portions of that protein eventually are activated and multiply to construct new immune defenses. The therapeutic vaccine concept is to improve on the immune defense against a particular already-existing infection by inoculating pieces of the infectious agent's protein presented in a way to trigger new naive cell activation. An immune-enhancing adjuvant is frequently used to help this process along. In 1996 investigators presented evidence that therapeutic vaccines can reduce the extent and duration of genital herpes outbreaks in people with frequent eruptions and in infected guinea pigs.

Most prominent researchers have always been skeptical of the validity of the therapeutic vaccine approach for HIV. One of the common arguments against this approach is that vaccines are not promising because the body already sees lots of HIV antigen—adding a little extra is not likely to make any difference. There is also a serious objection concerning viral diversity: Even if an induced immune response is effective, won't HIV merely mutate to rearrange the bit of viral protein that triggers the attack? Indeed, the field of therapeutic vaccines for HIV is littered with failures, despite clear demonstrations that the vaccines provoke new immune responses against HIV. To date, the most extensively tested product has been a gp160 (HIV envelope protein) inoculant made by bio-engineered insect cells, developed by Micro-GeneSys. Studies showed that the MicroGeneSys vaccine, though clearly "immunogenic," completely flopped in a placebo-controlled trial. After following 608 volunteers (with starting CD4 counts of a⁺ least 400) for three to five years, researchers concluded that the bimonthly injections of the vaccine were safe, but no difference existed between the placebo and vaccine groups in terms of occurrence of opportunistic infections, drop in CD4 count, rise in plasma HIV levels, or other measures of disease progression. A similar 278-person, 3-year Canadian trial had equally negative results. Findings of both trials were presented at the Eleventh International Conference on AIDS, July 7–12, 1996.

Three other, more naturally structured vaccine products (Immuno AG's gp160 produced by mammalian cell cultures, a hybrid canary pox virus with a gp160 envelope, and British Biotech's virus-like particles consisting of yeast protein particles coated with HIV p24 core protein) have also failed. Nonetheless those interested in this approach remain hopeful.

therapeutic window (therapeutic ratio) The range of dosages of a drug that achieve clinical efficacy but do not cause intolerable side effects; the difference between the minimal and maximal effective doses.

therapy The TREATMENT of a disease or pathological condition.

THF See THYMIC HUMORAL FACTOR.

thiazide diuretic One of a group of related chemicals that stimulate secretion of urine, resulting in loss of water from the body; a diuretic. Thiazides are used to treat swelling due to congestive heart failure or chronic liver or kidney disease. Brand names vary as per different types—bendromethiazide, hydrochlorothiazide, hydroflumethiazide, chlorothiazide, methyclothiazide, trichlormethiazide, chlorthalidone, and metalazone.

thiethylperazine A compound belonging to a class of psychoactive drugs called phenothiazines, used as an antinausea/antivomiting agent. Although the mechanism by which these drugs work is unknown, they have potent effects on the CENTRAL NERVOUS SYSTEM and other organs and can reduce blood pressure, stop seizures, and control nausea and vomiting. Occasional cases of drowsiness, dizziness, headache, fever, and restlessness have been reported in people using thiethylperazine. Serious side effects, such as convulsions and involuntary muscle movements, are uncommon, but they have occurred. Thiethylperazine is available in tablets for oral administration and as a solution for intramuscular injection (Trade name is Torcan.) Other phenothiazines include compazine, phenergan, reqian, tiqan, and zofran.

thioctic acid A natural thiol (sulfur-containing) antioxidant that has a potent neutralizing effect on many free radicals. Thioctic acid may have some activity against HIV.

third spacing Massive hemorrhagic bleeding under the skin.

third-line treatment The third preferred therapy for a particular condition; used when first- and second-line therapy fail or the patient cannot tolerate the side effects of first- and second-line treatments.

3′-deoxy-3′ fluorothimidine (FLT) A NUCLEOSIDE ANALOG (like AZT, ddI, and ddc) that has been under investigation for the treatment of HIV. It has been touted as the most potent nucleoside analog and is 2 to 10 times more potent than AZT. It has a long half-life and good brain penetration but causes significant toxicity to BONE MARROW, and therefore can cause severe ANEMIA (low red blood cell counts) and LEUKOPENIA (low white blood cell counts). It is hoped research will show

that toxicity may be prevented by using low doses, or managed with colony-stimulating factors.

3TC See LAMIVUDINE.

thrombocytopenia An abnormally low count (penia) of thrombocytes (or platelets), cells in the blood which facilitate clotting. The usual count of thrombocytes is 150,000 to 300,000 per milliliter of blood. Lower counts of 80,000 to 120,000 per milliliter are common in people with HIV infection. When the count is very low, from 5,000 to 25,000 per milliliter, bleeding problems may occur. People with HIV infection have thrombocytopenia because their bodies produce antibodies against their own platelets. Recent data suggest that in HIV there is diminished platelet production and decreased platelet survival, possibly resulting from direct infection of megakaryocytes (large BONE MARROW cells with large or multiple nuclei that give rise to blood platelets essential for the clotting mechanism of blood).

Presentation is generally made on laboratory testing. Bruising easily, epistaxis (hemorrhage from nose), gingival, or rectal bleeding may be present. Platelet counts as low as 10,000 are often without symptoms. Petechiae (small, purplish, hemorrhagic spots on the skin that appear in certain severe fevers and are indicative of great prostration) and ecchymoses (skin discoloration consisting of large, irregularly formed hemorrhagic areas) may be seen. Platelet counts of <100,000 define thrombocytopenia. Bone marrow biopsy often reveals decreased megakaryocytes. Some people have no symptoms but must still be careful to avoid cuts or anything that could cause bleeding.

Treatment of immune thrombocytopenia has been limited in the past by short duration of response, high cost, and sometimes serious side effects of the available therapies. There are several possible approaches to the management of thrombocytopenia in HIV: ZIDOVUDINE; PREDNISONE; intravenous GAMMA GLOBULIN; splenectomy (the surgical removal of the spleen); danazol; low-dose splenic irradiation; and no therapy. These approaches have met with some success. A conservative approach with careful observation and education for nonbleeding patients is recommended. Zidovudine, if tolerated, should be initiated because it has been found to increase platelet production in HIV-infected patients with and without thrombocytopenia. Patients with dangerously low platelet counts (<10,000) or significant bleeding should be hospitalized. In hospitalized patients, IV gamma globulin followed by platelet transfusion generally results in rapid correction. Prednisone is then begun, and the patient is discharged. Outpatient follow-up must be close, and the goal should be to taper the prednisone to the lowest possible dose that will keep the patient symptom-free and the platelet count >15,000.

thrombopenia See THROMBOCYTOPENIA.

thrush An infection of the mouth or pharynx caused by the fungus CANDIDA ALBICANS. See ORAL CANDIDIASIS; CANDIDIASIS.

thymic hormone Any of the hormones produced by the THYMUS. They are believed to play a role in the maturation of T LYMPHOCYTES and overall modulation of the immune system. Versions of several are under study as anti-HIV therapies—THYMOPENTIN and thymosis-α1 in particular.

thymic humoral factor (THF) A synthetic thymic peptide being examined as an anti-HIV treatment.

thymic humoral factor gamma 2 (THF g²) A thymic peptide that has been developed as an immune-modulating treatment for HIV. The hope is that it will stimulate an infected person's immune system to fight HIV and diseases associated with it.

thymic peptide Peptide produced in the THYMUS gland. Although the importance of thymic peptides remains in dispute, several investigators have reported that they can assist development of immature precursor cells into fully competent T CELLS. They also regulate the functioning of T-cells once they have matured.

Thymic peptide-based drugs have been developed as immune-modulating treatments, in the hope that they will stimulate HIV-infected persons' immune systems to fight the virus and diseases associated with it. These drugs include THYMIC HUMORAL FACTOR GAMMA 2, THYMOPENTIN, THYMOSIN ALPHA 1, THYMOMODULIN, and THYMOSTIMULIN.

thymidine One of the basic components of DEOXYRIBONUCLEIC ACID (DNA), thymidine is the nucleoside that the NUCLEOSIDE ANALOGS AZT and D4T mimic.

thymine A nucleic acid base in deoxyribonucleic acid (DNA) that pairs with ADENINE.

thymomodulin A THYMIC PEPTIDE, a natural extract of calf THYMUS. In Italy, where it has been approved (under the trade name Leucotrofina), it is used to treat bacterial and viral infections, food allergies in children, and immunodeficiencies in the elderly. Unlike most synthetic peptides, thymomodulin is an oral drug. It is made into syrup from the filtered freeze-dried calf thymus extract.

thymopentin A small, synthesized thymic peptide drug, also known as TP-5 or Timunox. Thymopentin has been studied more extensively than most other thymic peptide drugs, but the results have been ambiguous due to the studies' small size and flawed design.

thymopoietin A THYMIC PEPTIDE that stimulates differentiation of thymocytes.

thymo-ripoff See RIPOFF.

thymosin A THYMIC PEPTIDE that adjusts immune response when aberrations occur. Thymosin boosts the number of RECEPTORS on T CELLS, especially for ALPHA-INTERFERON and IL-2. It also increases the efficiency of T cells' response to signaling agents and causes cells to produce more of them. Intercellular signaling molecules (CYTOKINES) like alpha-interferon and IL-2 commonly have severe adverse effects. These agents are released during disease to help bolster the inflammatory response, which causes a variety of flulike symptoms. Thymosin, in contrast, circulates in the blood at comparatively constant levels. In clinical trials to date, no serious side effects have been noted. Since thymosin promotes the action of alpha-interferon and IL-2, it is speculated that combining it with these could allow lower dosages to be used, resulting in both greater safety and greater efficacy.

The pharmaceutical development path of alpha-thymosin has been characterized by disappointments, discouragements, and contradictory data. Despite the problematic aspects of past thymosin trials, however, some believe that the drug merits further study, since it is an open question whether thymosin works or not.

thymosin alpha 1   A small synthetic peptide, first produced in the 1970s. It has been licensed in Italy for the treatment of primary immunodeficiencies and as a booster for influenza vaccine in renal dialysis patients. The drug is being tested in ongoing CLINICAL TRIALS for activity against chronic HEPATITIS B and C, HIV infection and certain forms of cancer. It is by far the most thoroughly studied of all the THYMIC PEPTIDE drugs, but published reports from ongoing trials remain inconclusive.

thymostimulin   A THYMIC PEPTIDE also known as Tp-1, thymostimulin is, like THYMOMODULIN, a natural extract from calf THYMUS.

thymus   The thymus is an organ making up part of the lymph system. It is located in the center of the chest, just behind the sternum. It is where T CELLS grow and mature before traveling to other parts of the body. In children, the thymus weighs 5 to 10 grams. It will grow slightly through a person's adolescence, becoming approximately 50 grams, then decreasing in size, becoming a small, fatty tissue. By the time of a person's death it is usually so small as to be unseen on X rays. Stem lymphocyte cells travel from the bone marrow to the lymph system, going to the thymus. There they differentiate into T4 or T8 CELLS before using the lymph vessels to travel to the spleen, liver, and other locations. The thymus is also the location where T cells that might have negative reactions to the person's own body are removed from the lymph system.

Some treatments have been tried that would maintain or increase the size of the thymus, thereby hopefully increasing production of T cells. These have been unsuccessful so far. Some practitioners of natural medicine believe stimulating the thymus through massage of the area, or vibratory rapping on the chest, can stimulate activity and maintain the thymus's health. Patients with myasthenia gravis, an autoimmune disease of the muscles and nerves, often have the thymus removed as it becomes tumorous.

thymus-dependent antigen   ANTIGEN that depends on T-CELL interaction with B CELLS for antibody synthesis, (e.g., erythrocytes, SERUM proteins, and HAPTEN-carrier complexes).

thymus-independent antigen   ANTIGEN that can induce an immune response without the apparent participation of T LYMPHOCYTES.

thyroid stimulating hormone   Hormone secreted by the anterior lobe of the pituitary that stimulates the thyroid gland. Abbreviated TSH.

thyroxine (T_4)   A hormone secreted by the thyroid gland that increases energy production and protein synthesis.

TIA   See TRANSIENT ISCHEMIC ATTACK.

T.I.D. *(ter in die)*   Latin phrase that translates as "three times a day." The letters *T.I.D.* often appear in a pharmacist or doctor's prescription instructions.

Tinactin   See TOLNAFTATE.

tinea   Any fungal skin disease. Also called RINGWORM.

tinidazole   An antiprotozoal used as a first-line therapy for a variety of parasitic and amoebic infections. (Trade name is Fasigyn.)

tipranavir (PNU-140690 and TPV)   An experimental PROTEASE INHIBITOR (PI) from Boehringer-Inglheim. It is currently in phase II/III trials. It has shown fairly typical PI side effects of diarrhea, nausea, and headaches. This drug has been demonstrated to speed up the CYTOCHROME P450 process that other PIs slow so it may not be suitable unless proper dosing and drug compatibility can be worked out before the FOOD AND DRUG ADMINISTRATION approval process. It is different in design from current PIs in that it is a nonpeptidic PI. This means it bonds differently than current PIs and has a very different resistance profile. It has been shown to be effective in studies against virus that has become resistant to other PIs.

Title II   See SOCIAL SECURITY ACT, TITLE II.

Title IV-A   See SOCIAL SECURITY ACT, TITLE IV-A.

Title VI   See PUBLIC HEALTH SERVICE ACT, TITLE VI.

Title XIV   See SOCIAL SECURITY ACT, TITLE XIV.

Title XVI   See PUBLIC HEALTH SERVICE ACT, TITLE VI; SOCIAL SECURITY ACT, TITLE XVI.

Title XVI state   A state that gives MEDICAID to all SSI recipients under Title XVI of the federal SOCIAL SECURITY ACT. This benefit is not automatic—it requires aged, blind, and disabled recipients to apply separately for Medicaid at a state welfare office, bringing proof of SSI eligibility.

Title XVIII   See SOCIAL SECURITY ACT, TITLE XVIII.

Title XIX   See SOCIAL SECURITY ACT, TITLE XIX.

Title XX   See SOCIAL SECURITY ACT, TITLE XX.

TJ-9   A preparation of a traditional Asian medicine known as sho-saiko-to (SSKT), or xiao chai hu tang. SSKT is a blend of seven medicinal herbs including bupleurum, *Scutelaria radix,* pinellia, fresh ginger, ginseng, jujube, and glycyrrhizin. It has been used for thousands of years to treat what the Chinese call lesser yang disorders, which include fevers, influenza, bronchitis, respiratory ailments, malaria, jaundice, and hepatitis. SSKT appears to be fairly safe, although it has been reported to induce pneumonitis in a few elderly

patients. IN VITRO data suggest that the blend may have anti-HIV activity by directly inhibiting REVERSE TRANSCRIPTASE and by decreasing TNF-alpha and free-radical promotion of viral replication. The data also suggest that the herbal formula is strongly synergistic with AZT. It may also have some immune modulatory effects.

T-killer cell   A type of LYMPHOCYTE, or white blood cell, that kills foreign organisms after being activated by T-HELPER CELLS.

TLC G-65   Liposomal gentamicin. See GENTAMICIN.

TMC 125   An experimental NNRTI from a Belgian company, Tibotec-Virco, which was bought by Johnson & Johnson. It is in PHASE II trials and has shown some promising results against virus that has become resistant to other NNRTIs.

TMC 126, 114   Two new drugs from Tibotec-Virco. Both are protease inhibitors. They are both in PHASE II trials in Europe. Both have good resistance profiles that are different from those of currently available protease inhibitors. TMC 114 is thought to be a molecule that could adapt itself to fight the changing virus. TMC 125 is being tested for the same mutability.

TMP-SMX   See TRIMETHOPRIM-SULFAMETHOXAZOLE.

TNF   See TUMOR NECROSIS FACTOR.

TNF inhibitor   See TUMOR NECROSIS FACTOR (TNF) INHIBITOR.

tolerability   Ability to be tolerated. In HIV/AIDS, factors that influence tolerability include a regimen's pill burden, dosing frequency, taste, convenience, toxicity and side effects, and drug interaction profile.

tolerance   In cell biology, the condition in which responsive cell clones have been eliminated or inactivated by prior contact with ANTIGEN, with the result that no immune response occurs on administration of antigen. See IMMUNE TOLERANCE.

tolnaftate A synthetic antifungal agent appearing as a white-to-creamy-white powder. It is used topically in treating various forms of TINEA. (The trade name is Tinactin.)

tomography A method of producing images of the interior of the body using computer and X-ray technology. See COMPUTERIZED AXIAL TOMOGRAPHY.

toot See COCAINE.

top In sexual intercourse, a slang term for the partner who penetrates the body of the other.

In regard to sexually transmitted diseases, many sexually active men, both hetero- and homosexual, who prefer the top role mistakenly perceive themselves not to be at risk as tops. This is the "top mentality." It is also often assumed that it is the job of the top to be responsible for safety. See BOTTOM.

top mentality See TOP.

topical Pertaining to a specific surface area.

topical microbicide An antibacterial or antifungal compound that can be applied directly to the lining of the vagina before intercourse to thwart sexually transmitted microbes that cause diseases such as gonorrhea, syphilis, genital herpes, chlamydia, hepatitis B, and HIV infections. Today, the development of safe, effective, female-controlled topical microbicides that will block the transmission of HIV and other STD agents is a global priority and a central focus of the STD research program of the National Institute of Allergy and Infectious Diseases (NIAID). The goal is to develop safe antimicrobial products that effectively fight a combination of infectious agents, whether they are viral, bacterial, or protozoan.

The currently available mechanical and chemical products thought to prevent STD/HIV transmission have limitations. A major drawback of the male condom is that it cannot be used at the discretion of a woman without her partner's knowledge or consent, and personal, social, or cultural barriers often interfere with her ability to negotiate its use. Existing spermicides have not been clinically evaluated, and issues of safety and efficacy for STD/HIV prevention remain unresolved.

topoisomerase An enzyme that uncoils the tightly wound DNA in cells' nuclei so that cell division and replication can take place.

topotecan An experimental anticancer chemotherapy that inhibits TOPOISOMERASE I and blocks cell division. It is a possible therapy for HIV, having been found to inhibit HIV replication in the lab, and PROGRESSIVE MULTIFOCAL LEUKOENCEPHALOPATHY (PML), an opportunistic virus infection of the brain.

torulosis See CRYPTOCOCCOSIS.

total parenteral nutrition See PARENTERAL NUTRITION.

toxic Poisonous.

toxic reaction An unintended, sickening, sometimes severe and dangerous physiological reaction to a toxic substance in vitamin, drug, or other substance. See SIDE EFFECT.

toxic shock syndrome A rare disease—an extreme toxic reaction—caused by toxins that are produced by certain strains of *Staphylococcus aureus* bacteria. It is characterized by acute fever, diarrhea, vomiting, and myalgia (tenderness or pain in the muscles), followed by hypotension and possible death due to shock. Most cases have been attributed to toxins found in tampons, but cases also have been diagnosed in nonmenstruating women and in men.

toxic side effect See SIDE EFFECT.

toxicity Poisonousness, of a chemical, drug, or other substance.

toxin A chemical that is poisonous to cells.

toxoid A toxin with its toxicity destroyed but still capable of inducing the formation of antibodies on injection.

Toxoplasma gondii The organism that causes TOXOPLASMOSIS, one of the most common causes of inflammation of the brain in people with AIDS. *Toxoplasma gondii* is an intracellular, non-host-specific, widespread sporozoan species that is parasitic in a number of vertebrates, including humans. The sexual cycle of *Toxoplasma gondii,* leading to the production of oocysts, develops exclusively in cats and other felines. An oocyte is a cell undergoing meiosis during oogenesis (the production of ova, involving usually both meiosis and maturation). It enters the body through the mouth and digestive tract from contaminated meat or contact with cat feces. It then travels through the blood to the brain, where it invades and kills neuronal cells.

toxoplasmic encephalitis The most common form of TOXOPLASMOSIS in people with HIV infection.

toxoplasmosis Widespread infection of an organ, usually the brain, or the whole body with the parasite TOXOPLASMA GONDII. *Toxoplasma gondii* is found in many mammals and birds, but the definitive host is cat excrement, which, with raw meat, is the most common source of infection. About 30 percent of all adults in the United States have *Toxoplasma gondii* in their bodies, but the majority are unaware of it. The parasite remains dormant and rarely causes disease unless the immune system is weakened. When symptoms do appear, they may range from a mild, self-limited disease similar to mononucleosis to a more severe, disseminated disease causing extensive damage to the brain, central nervous system, liver, and lungs. Encephalitis, hepatitis, or pneumonia are examples of such disseminating diseases. In people with HIV infection, the most common form of toxoplasmosis is an infection of the brain called TOXOPLASMIC ENCEPHALITIS.

Common symptoms of toxoplasmic encephalitis include headache, confusion, and fever. Focal neurologic deficits occur in most patients. Since *T. gondii* is the most common opportunistic pathogen of the brain in people with AIDS, the practice of presumptive treatment of patients with a characteristic finding on COMPUTERIZED AXIAL TOMOGRAPHY (CT) SCAN, MAGNETIC RESONANCE IMAGING (MRI) (one or more contrast-enhancing focal lesions), and toxoplasma serological test results is widely accepted. The

absence of detectable antitoxoplasma immunoglobulin G (IgG) antibodies does not exclude the diagnosis. The limitations of the serodiagnosis method have been documented. Note that POLYMERASE CHAIN REACTION (PCR) is a noninvasive technique that confirms the presence or absence of *T. gondii* DNA. This sensitive DNA test may be more effective in diagnosing toxoplasmosis than older methods.

Studies have documented that people who experience immune recovery while on potent antiretroviral therapy may safely discontinue primary prophylaxis for toxoplasmosis. Additionally, data demonstrate that PCP prophylaxis with trimethoprim/sufamethoxazole (TMP/SMX) or cotrimoxazole confers cross-protection against toxoplasmosis. TMP/SMX is the recommended prophylactic agent for toxoplasmosis for all patients with CD4 counts below 100 cells/mm and a previous episode of toxoplasmic encephalitis. For people who cannot tolerate TMP/SMX, current guidelines from the U.S. Department of Health and Human Services recommend several alternative prophylactic regimens, which are based on data from clinical studies.

Empirically treated patients should show a clear clinical response within 14 days, and there should be a clear radiographic response of all lesions within three weeks. In patients who do not respond to therapy, brain biopsy should be considered relatively early in the course of treatment (seven to 10 days) with or without a change in treatment. The optimal treatment for toxoplasmic encephalitis is the combination of pyrimethamine plus sulfadiazine, or for patients intolerant to sulfonamides, pyrimethamine plus clindamycin.

Patients intolerant of or refractory to first-line therapies may benefit from other agents that have shown activity in several small or nonrandomized studies.

Current guidelines recommend discontinuing secondary prophylaxis (maintenance therapy) for toxoplasmosis in people with a sustained (e.g., six months) increase in CD4 cell counts to above 200 cells/mm in response to HAART—if they complete their initial therapy and have no symptoms or signs attributable to these pathogens.

tranquilizer A drug that acts to reduce mental tension and anxiety-without interfering with normal mental activity. The use of tranquilizers has facilitated the treatment of severely disturbed psychiatric patients. Drugs in use include chlordiazepoxide (Librium), chlorpromazine (Thorazine), diazepam (Valium), meprobamate (Miltown, Equanil), alprazolam (Xanax), and reserpine (Serpasil). Side effects, particularly from chlorpromazine and reserpine, have included jaundice, nausea, rashes, and in some instances severe mental depression.

transactivator (TAT-3) gene   See TAT GENE.

transamination   The transfer of an amino (NH_2) group from an amino acid to a carbon chain to form a non-essential amino acid; takes place in the liver.

transcription   The process by which a cell reproduces genetic material. Specifically, the synthesis of RNA molecules from a DNA template.

transfer factor   In immunology, a factor present in LYMPHOCYTES that have been sensitized to ANTIGENS, which can in humans be transferred to a nonsensitized recipient. Thus the recipient will react to the same antigen that was originally used to sensitize the lymphocytes of the donor. In humans, the factor can be transferred by injecting the recipient with either intact lymphocytes or extracts of disrupted cells.

transformation zone   The area of the cervix where squamous cells and columnar cells meet; a common site of dysplasia; the area where abnormalities detected by Pap smear arise.

transfusion, analogous   Blood TRANSFUSION in which the patient receives his or her own blood, donated several weeks before an elective surgical procedure. The blood may also be collected at the site of surgery during the procedure. Transfusion with autologous blood is the safest form of transfusion. Before 1985, autologous blood transfusions were rarely used, and many blood centers in the United States did not have procedures for handling predeposited blood. From the perspective of the HIV epidemic, the infrequent use of autologous transfusion is regrettable. Autologous blood trans-

fusion would have been especially beneficial between 1978 and 1985 when the prevalence of HIV in the blood supply was greatest but before a specific test was available to screen donor blood. Although current testing procedures have rendered the United States blood supply extremely safe, a patient may opt for this procedure because of fear of exposure to the human immunodeficiency virus and other bloodborne infections.

transfusion, blood   The replacement in the body of blood or one of its components. The modern era of blood transfusion started during World War II, when battlefield medicine became sophisticated in the use of blood and plasma. Today, blood transfusion is a highly complex field, combining the latest knowledge of immunology and physiology with practical management of a wide range of services. The key concept in modern transfusion medicine is the provision of integrated blood transfusion services. An integrated system, a reality in industrialized countries, seeks to ensure a timely supply of adequate amounts of safe blood and blood products, where needed and at an affordable cost. The integrated system must manage donor recruitment, collection, testing and storage of blood, preparation of appropriate blood products and their appropriate use, and complex record-keeping and logistical tasks. In many developing countries, even in the major hospitals, there are no such systems. Blood is obtained from a donor, subjected (or not) to simple tests of compatibility and safety and infused into the recipient. The people of the developing world therefore rarely receive the full benefits of blood transfusion, and often suffer risks that have for the most part been eliminated in more developed countries.

Effective and safe transfusion therapy requires a thorough understanding of the clinical condition being treated. In advanced countries today, there is very little chance of getting HIV from a blood transfusion. Clotting factors obtained from donated blood are equally safe. Nearly all the people infected with HIV through blood transfusions received those transfusions before 1985, the year it became possible to test donated blood for HIV. Since mid-1983, all blood donations in the United States have come from volunteers who are questioned about their risks for HIV infection. People at increased risk of infection are not allowed to donate blood. Since mid-1985, all donated blood has been tested for HIV and other viruses (seven different tests are now conducted on each blood sample). Blood that tests positive for HIV is destroyed. Donors are confidentially told that they are infected with HIV and are not allowed to donate blood again. There is no risk of getting infected by giving blood because a new, sterile needle is used for each blood donation.

transfusion-associated AIDS   Acquired immunodeficiency syndrome developed as a result of a transfusion with HIV-infected blood or blood components. Widespread, accurate blood-testing procedures have greatly reduced the risk of becoming infected with HIV through a BLOOD TRANSFUSION.

transgender   The term, broadly defined, refers to someone whose core gender identity does not coincide with the birth gender. Transgendered people include transsexuals, cross-dressers, intersexuals, and those people whose gender roles are ambiguous. The term transgendered is used to make it clear that gender, not sexual orientation, is the main issue that these individuals are facing.

HIV in the transgender population has not been studied extensively. Some reports indicate that transgendered people have a high risk for contracting HIV. Issues such as identity confusion or conflict, shame and isolation, secrecy, and fear of discovery and rejection all can lead people to make decisions that may not value their own life. In a study conducted in Minneapolis, transgendered people said it was easier to have unsafe sex or share in injection drug use (IDU) than to protect themselves because feelings of shame and confusion lead to low self-esteem.

Transgender people are represented in all demographic groups, Euro-American, Latino/a, African American, and all ages. A large percentage of transgendered people are involved in sex work, because of discrimination faced in other employment areas. Links between sex work as a career choice and drug and alcohol use are well established. Both drug and alcohol use and sex work can lead to impaired choices in using safe sex to protect oneself. As a result of fear, ignorance, or other factors, education aimed at the transgender community has been largely overlooked outside a few metropolitan areas.

transient HIV infection   HIV infection that becomes undetectable in infants. Clearance of HIV infection in an infant born in 1991 was reported by National Institutes of Health–supported investigators in 1995. The boy was born to an HIV-infected mother; no HIV could be found in his blood when he was born, but viral culture tests at day 19 and day 51 did reveal the virus. Later attempts to find HIV using HIV-culture techniques, polymerase chain reaction, and antigen searches did not reveal any virus. Today he is healthy and has no evidence of HIV infection. Researchers noted the similarity of the child's experience to the likely outcome of HIV exposure after immunization—transient infection with no later evidence of virus or disease. How HIV is cleared in such cases is not known. The data do not suggest that infection in infants will automatically disappear but do raise numerous questions about the frequency and mechanism of transient HIV infections, the implications for pregnant women and their children, the HIV disease process and the body's immune response.

Three possible explanations may suggest how the transient HIV infection may have occurred. One is that the boy's immune response to HIV either eliminated or is totally suppressing the virus. A second is that the immune response could come from maternal antibodies passed during pregnancy and/or from his immune system. A third theory is that he may have been infected with a defective form of HIV that could not adequately replicate. Each theory requires more evidence and testing.

transient ischemic attack (TIA)   Temporary interruption of blood supply to the brain. The symptoms and signs of neurologic deficit may last from a few minutes to hours but are not persistent. There is no evidence of residual brain damage or neurologic damage after an attack.

translation   In cell biology, the process of formation of a peptide chain from individual amino acids to form a protein molecule.

transmissible   Capable of passing from one person to another through means other than casual contact.

transmissibility   The property of a disease-causing organism that enables it to spread from person to person.

transmission   Throughout the world, people can contract HIV infection in three possible ways: through sexual contact, either homosexual or heterosexual; through contact with blood or other body fluids, blood products, or tissues of an infected person; or through transfer of the virus from an infected mother to her infant before or during birth or shortly after birth through breastfeeding. Note that the transfer of the virus from one person to another in a population is known as *horizontal transmission,* as distinguished from *vertical transmission,* the transfer of the virus from one generation to another. Sexual transmission and blood-to-blood transmission are both examples of horizontal transmission; perinatal transmission is an example of vertical transmission.

Discussion of these modes of transmission is followed by discussion of transmission from HIV-positive patients to health care workers and transmission from HIV-positive health-care workers to patients. Other secondary routes of transmission are also mentioned. The entry concludes with an overview of how HIV is not transmitted. Note that perinatal transmission is treated in greater depth elsewhere in this work, in the entries on PREGNANCY and WOMEN.

Transmission Through Sexual Activity

This can occur via intercourse and other direct contact with infectious areas (blisters, open sores, rashes, mucous patches), warts, or infected mucous membranes in the urethra, cervix, anus, throat, or eyes. Heterosexual contact is the leading means of HIV transmission worldwide and the fastest growing mode of HIV transmission in the United States.

Bidirectional transmission   *Bidirectional* is an adjective meaning capable of reacting or functioning in two, usually opposite, directions. In the context of HIV/AIDS, bidirectional transmission relates to the capacity of the virus to be passed or spread from one individual to another bidirectionally—between men and women, women and men, men and men, and women and women. HIV/AIDS is a disease that does not have sexual preferences. This is evident in the course of the disease in Africa, where the rate of the infection is equal for the two sexes. It is also evident in the course of the disease in the United States, where the profile of the disease has changed dramatically since the first decade of the epidemic. Additionally, it is evident in the continued evolution of the disease in the rest of the industrialized world, where the incidence of AIDS cases associated with heterosexual transmission has been on the rise since 1991. In the early years of the epidemic, it was assumed that the risk of transmission from an infected female to an uninfected male was less than the risk of transmission from an infected male to an uninfected female. It was also assumed that it was easier for men to give HIV/AIDS to women than for women to give HIV/AIDS to men, and easier for men to give HIV/AIDS to men than for women to give HIV/AIDS to women. Similarly it was also assumed that it was easier for women to give HIV/AIDS to their fetus than for them to pass it to their infants in childbirth. Today many of these assumptions have been called into question. Today we know that many factors may alter an individual's susceptibility and HIV's infectiousness, and we know that gender is but one of the many factors associated with sexual transmission. These factors include the following:

- The presence of either acute HIV infection or advanced HIV disease in the infected partner increases the risk of sexual transmission.

- The presence of genital tract infections in either partner increases the risk. The risk of transmission markedly increases if yeast infection or genital sores or ulcers are present. Such sores can be caused by ulcer-producing sexually transmitted diseases (STDs) such as syphilis, herpes, and chancroid. Sores or ulcers in the uninfected partner facilitate contact between that person's CD4 lymphocytes and macrophages and HIV from the infected partner; sores in the infected person provide additional avenues for release of HIV, exposing the uninfected partner to a greater dose of virus.

- STDs that do not produce ulcers, such as gonor-rhea, chlamydia, and trichomoniasis, also increase the risk of acquiring HIV. This is thought to occur because these diseases cause inflamma-tion of the mucous membranes of the genital tract. Inflammation is a normal immune response to infection or injury, but it activates and attracts a large number of white blood cells, including monocytes, macrophages, and T lym-phocytes, to the inflamed area. In the HIV-infected partner this increases the amount of free virus and the number of virus-infected cells in genital secretions. In the HIV-negative partner the risk of acquiring HIV infection is increased because the inflammation of the genital tract concentrates cells susceptible to HIV infection in the genital tissues.

- Anal intercourse and probably intercourse dur-ing menstruation also increase the risk of sexual transmission. The rectal lining is thin and con-tains many lymphocytes, macrophages, and other cells that HIV can infect. Anal intercourse also easily causes tears in the rectal lining that result in direct contact between infected semen and the blood of the receptive partner.

- Number of instances of intercourse is related to risk. The greater the number of exposures to infected semen or vaginal secretions, the higher the risk of HIV transmission.

- Genetic characteristics of the particular HIV strain to which a person is exposed, as well as genetic characteristics of the exposed person, affect the risk of HIV transmission.

- Some studies have shown that the use of oral contraceptives, diaphragms, cervical caps, or intrauterine devices increases the risk of HIV transmission.

- A risk of HIV transmission exists even during safe sex; minimizing the risk requires that con-doms be used consistently and correctly

Sexual transmission from men to women This process is fairly well understood. Semen from an infected man contains HIV that is mostly associated with infected LYMPHOCYTES also present. HIV intro-duced into the VAGINA must make its way into the bloodstream to initiate viral reproduction. Small breaks in the lining of the vagina are the presumed main route of entry into the bloodstream.

Studies indicate that sexual transmission from men to women may be substantially more effec-tive than transmission from women to men, par-ticularly in the strains of HIV that are widespread in the developed nations. It has been estimated that there is anywhere from a 3- to 19-fold excess risk for male-to-female over female-to-male sex-ual transmission among HIV-discordant couples. This difference has not been documented in Africa, where over 50 percent of those with both HIV and AIDS are women, where heterosexual intercourse is the most common means of trans-mission of HIV for both sexes and where homo-sexual sex is taboo. Other studies indicate that women may be more susceptible to infection than men after a single exposure, a difference that may be attributable to the greater number of potential entry sites in the vagina than on the surface of the penis and to the fact that the vagina is exposed to a greater volume of infectious material during intercourse than the penis is.

Sexual transmission from women to men Although this is known to occur, the means are less clear. Women can and do transmit other SEXU-ALLY TRANSMITTED DISEASES (STDS) to men as well as to other women, and there are documented cases of woman-to-man transmission of HIV. HIV, like CHLAMYDIA, GONORRHEA, HERPES, SYPHILIS, and other STDs, can thrive in the vaginal juices, mucous tissues in the vagina, blood (including menstrual blood), and breast milk. STDs are easily passed between partners of either sex through open sores. Studies have also demonstrated a clear relationship between HIV infection in men and the presence of genital ulcers. Researchers hypothesize that genital ulcers in men serve the same function as breaks in the lining of the vagina by providing the virus a portal into the bloodstream.

Other factors undoubtedly influence transmis-sion during heterosexual genital intercourse. The presence of menstrual fluids, simultaneous infec-tion with other organisms, cutaneous conditions, prior exposure to chemical irritants that disrupt the skin, and other conditions may all play a part.

Heterosexual transmission is the most common route of HIV infection for women worldwide and is rapidly becoming the most common in the United States as well. HIV transmission from men to women and from women to men has occurred mainly through vaginal intercourse.

Homosexual/bisexual transmission For the first decade of the epidemic, male homosexuals and bisexuals, as well as injection drug users, were considered at high risk for HIV infection. Indeed, the development of the epidemic was often linked to these so-called high-risk groups, including, in addition to homosexuals and bisexuals, blood donors, hemophiliacs, Haitian immigrants, low-income women, prostitutes, and partners of individuals in high-risk groups. In the United States, the incidence rates among gay and bisexual men have declined, indicating changes in the epidemiology of AIDS in the United States. In the second decade of the epidemic, the focus shifted from high-risk groups to high-risk behavior, and, while homosexuals and bisexuals pose continuing challenges, as do injection drug users, concerns about heterosexual transmission, perinatal transmission, AIDS and adolescents, and AIDS in children equaled if not outweighed concerns about homosexual and bisexual transmission.

Sexual transmission from women to women As noted above, women can and do transmit STDs to other women during sexual activity. Cases of woman-to-woman transmission of HIV have been reported, and it is now believed that the virus can indeed be transmitted in this way, although very little is known about the process. Researchers agree that while cervical secretions can carry HIV, menstrual blood does not carry it in the same potency as circulatory blood, which has a higher living cell density than other body fluids. The CDC has so far not identified any high-risk sexual behavior between women and finds no reason to believe that lesbians are a risk group.

Transmission via Contaminated Blood and Blood Products

HIV is present in blood of both asymptomatic and symptomatic people as free virus particles and in infected cells. The number of free virus particles in the blood can rise to extremely high levels during the period of acute infection. Then, within weeks, viral levels decrease and the virus nearly disappears from the blood. As the disease progresses, however, the number of CD4 cells in the blood drops and the number of free virus particles progressively rises again. In advanced HIV disease there may be as many as a million free virus particles per milliliter of blood, as a large proportion of CD4 cells are infected, each of which can produce thousands of virus particles daily.

Transmission by blood and body fluids can occur very efficiently through transfusion of HIV-contaminated blood or blood products or through the sharing of needles and other equipment used to inject drugs. Although safety has been a concern since the beginning of the era of transfusion medicine and although it is not unique to the AIDS epidemic, the advent of AIDS and HIV infection raised new concerns about the safety of the blood supply in the United States. Early in the epidemic, suspicions arose that AIDS could be transmitted by transfusion. In the spring of 1983, cases of AIDS diagnosed among hemophiliacs were thought to be related to clotting factor concentrates made from contaminated blood. Although the etiologic or causative agent of AIDS had not been identified in the early 1980s and no specific diagnostic tests were available, reports of cases among transfusion recipients and hemophiliacs prompted blood banks to institute a variety of procedures to reduce the risk of AIDS associated with blood transfusions. Such procedures included efforts to exclude donors who were members of groups at high risk for the disease, studies of the use of tests that measured factors considered to be surrogate markers of AIDS (e.g., antibody to HEPATITIS B core ANTIGEN, T lymphocyte ratios), the increased use of autologous donation (providing one's own blood for personal use), and the reduction of unnecessary transfusions of blood and blood components.

After the etiologic agent, HIV, was identified and blood tests for the antibody to the virus became available in March 1985, blood collection organizations added this serologic test to their screening procedures. Despite the high sensitivity of HIV antibody tests, they do not detect all infected donors. A variable length of time elapses between acquisition of the virus and development of a detectable antibody response. Generally, this period is no more than a few months. During this so-called window period, the blood collected from an infected donor may test negative and thus go undetected by the serologic screening mechanisms employed in most blood banks. As of this writing, the current incidence of HIV infection from antibody-negative blood in the United States is not known.

Although HIV antibody tests cannot eliminate the possibility of transfusion-associated HIV infection, they have vastly improved the safety of the blood supply. Additional methods to detect infected units are being explored to increase the sensitivity of serologic testing. These include those based on recombinant DNA technology, synthetic peptides, and gene-amplification techniques. Other safeguards include improved donor screening and recruitment.

Substance abusers compose a population severely affected by AIDS. The spread of AIDS in the substance-abusing population occurs via two primary vectors. Substance abusers transmit the HIV virus to other abusers through the use of unclean intravenous needles or other blood-contaminated drug apparatus. In addition, as with other populations at risk for AIDS, substance abusers spread HIV to other drug users and nonusers alike through unsafe sexual practices. The use of IV drugs without cleaning needles between uses and users is the prominent risk in the former category. Two drug injection practices in particular set the stage for HIV transmission during needle sharing: the initial drawing of blood into the barrel of the syringe to verify that the needle is inserted into a vein and the practice of refilling the syringe repeatedly with blood after drug injection to rinse out any remaining drug. Hygienic needle use is hard to achieve for a variety of reasons. It does not occur frequently enough to alter significantly the spread of HIV through blood and needles. The AIDS risk-reduction message has, to date, not reached drug users with the same impact as it has reached gay and bisexual men. Many counselors and epidemiologists consider substance users to be the "second wave" of the AIDS epidemic.

Transmission from Mother to Child During Pregnancy, Birth, and Postpartum Period

In the mid-1980s, the idea that AIDS would become an epidemic of women and children would have been met with considerable skepticism. But increasingly women and children are becoming infected. Women are more vulnerable to HIV infection than men, in part because the direction of sexual spread favors male-to-female transmission. Worldwide, it is the second most common mode of transmission after sexual transmission. About 25 percent to 35 percent of babies born to HIV-infected women have HIV infection. The time from birth to the development of AIDS varies from weeks to years.

The vast majority of AIDS cases in children are a result of transmission from mother to child during pregnancy or birth. Note that a woman can also transmit the virus to her infant during the postpartum period, the interval after birth, through breast-feeding. Clinical studies have found HIV in fetuses well before delivery, in umbilical cord blood obtained from the placenta, and in maternal blood lost during delivery. Exposure to any of these sources of virus is a potential means of infection.

Transmission from mother to child during pregnancy It is possible to transmit the virus to the fetus in the uterus, before birth, but at present it is unclear when the transmission of HIV actually occurs. The virus has been isolated from the placenta, the amniotic fluid, and the fetal tissue. Infection may occur prenatally, at delivery, or through breast-feeding. The risk in each pregnancy may depend on such factors as how advanced the disease is, the woman's immunological state, or the gestational age of the infant at birth. The rate of transmission ranges widely. Studies have shown that women with HIV base their reproductive choices on the same criteria used by noninfected women of similar socioeconomic and psychosocial status. When providers are able to identify which fetus is infected or will be infected, women can incorporate that knowledge into their decision making. Amniocentesis, cordocentesis, and chorionic virus sampling have all been explored as prenatal HIV diagnostic techniques, but because of the blood-borne nature of the virus they themselves involve risk of transmission.

The question of whether infected mothers will give birth to infected infants has attracted enormous emotional attention in the HIV/AIDS pandemic. As early as 1982, only a few months after AIDS had been described as a new disease in adults by the United States Centers for Disease Control, children with AIDS were reported in North America and Europe. Even though the virus responsible for the disease had not yet been identified, the pediatricians involved were certain that the children had been infected either by their mothers during pregnancy or through blood transfusions. Even though the description differed from that of genetic immune deficiencies, these reports were initially received with skepticism by the medical community, in part because these cases had been identified almost simultaneously in different geographical areas under widely differing circumstances. Today we know that factors associated with perinatal transmission include the characteristics of the mother's infection (her clinical status during pregnancy, and her immune response to the virus), the integrity of the placental barrier, the virus itself, and the child's clinical status during exposure to HIV.

We now know that fetuses can be infected with HIV as early as eight weeks after conception. By then, they already have the receptors that enable HIV to penetrate their T cells. However, HIV transmission also seems to occur at a later stage in pregnancy, as indicated by both the absence of clinical signs of infection in the newborn and the low number of viruses in the blood, which therefore creates difficulties in detection by polymerase chain reaction or viral culture. Some children not infected during pregnancy probably become infected during birth.

One of the central difficulties confronting researchers seeking to uncover how HIV passes from mother to child is the determination of whether or not HIV has passed or not. Babies do not come into this world complete with their own ready-made immune systems. They inherit some antibodies from their mothers. Others they develop themselves. It takes more than a year for a child's immune system to mature, and this process is by no means uniform. Some maternal antibodies disappear more quickly than others. Some of the child's own antibodies take longer to develop than others. Although a reliable indicator of HIV infection in an adult, the presence of HIV antibodies provides no reliable indication about an infant's HIV status. And because newborns lack fully developed immune systems, they naturally remain at high risk of contracting some of the opportunistic infections normally associated with HIV during the first 15 months of life.

Some of the other questions that remain follow. What precisely is the risk of perinatal HIV transmission? What are the exact factors influencing this transmission? Does pregnancy affect the course of HIV infection, and, conversely, does HIV influence the evolution and outcome of pregnancy? What strategies could prevent or control the perinatal transmission of HIV? Issues related to transmission of HIV infection from pregnant women to their infants continue to be studied to generate interest and discussion. The relationship between a pregnant woman's plasma HIV levels and transmission of the virus to her baby has aroused interest. Researchers have sought to discover whether higher HIV levels in blood plasma correlate with an increase of mother-to-child transmission. They have also sought to discover whether a threshold viral load exists below which HIV transmission does not occur. A related question has also been asked: does an AZT-reduced reduction in a woman's viral load lead to a reduced risk of her baby's contracting HIV before and during birth? Today, the predictive power of viral load has been established, but it is noted that although the predictive value is good, it is not absolute. Today it is thought that transmission at delivery is not necessarily tied to high maternal viral load during delivery and that events during delivery that expose the baby to maternal blood or cervicovaginal secretions might promote transmission.

Transmission from mother to child during birth
While we know that it is possible for HIV to pass from a pregnant woman to her fetus, we do not know for sure how HIV passes from a woman to her fetus during pregnancy and/or during delivery. We do know that a woman is most likely to transmit the HIV virus to the fetus either immediately after she is infected or during childbirth. A low CD4 cell count (below 300), anemia, inflammation of the placenta, the presence of other infections, and advanced AIDS in a woman may each increase the risk of transmission to the fetus and affect a woman's health and the progress of her pregnancy.

Every infant born to an HIV+ woman will have its mother's antibodies in its blood and may test positive for HIV for a period of time even if it is not infected. Because the current standard antibody test cannot distinguish between the mother's and the infant's antibodies, it has been necessary to wait a few months to determine whether the infant is infected. New tests have been developed that can determine HIV infection in infants as young as three to six months, and researchers are seeking tests that can reliably detect infection in a fetus. Testing, however, is a complex issue. Some policy makers advocate routine testing of all newborns for HIV as a means of assessing the percentage of reproductive-age women who are infected with HIV. Those concerned with women's rights strenuously oppose any testing that is done without the informed consent of the mother. They argue persuasively that the time and money involved in widespread testing could better be spent on prevention, education, and treatment of HIV disease.

A study reported in the *New England Journal of Medicine* reported that the amount of HIV in the blood of perinatally infected infants peaks at one to two months of age and then declines slowly to level off at 24 months at relatively high concentrations compared to those for an adult. Peak VIRAL LOADS at one month of age suggest that the majority of the infected infants were exposed around the time of delivery. The same study also reported that a small number of infected infants had high blood levels of HIV at birth, indicating that some may have become infected in utero. Researchers note that the dynamics of viral replication in HIV-infected infants are distinctly different from those observed in infected adults. Following a dramatic rise in viremia during their first month of life, the viral burden remains very high in infants in contrast to the sharp decline usually seen in adults. This persistently high viremia may partially explain the more rapid progression of AIDS observed in infants compared to adults and further underscore the need for early antiretroviral therapy.

A research report published in the July 26, 1997 issue of the *British Medical Journal* notes that cleansing the birth canal with an inexpensive antiseptic solution dramatically reduced post-birth infections, hospitalizations, and deaths. The investigators report that washing the birth canal with a very safe solution—0.25 percent chlorhexidine in sterile water—at each vaginal examination before delivery, and then wiping the babies with the solution after delivery, significantly reduced postpartum infectious problems in both mothers and babies. Perhaps most significant was their finding that infant deaths related to sepsis, or bacteria in the bloodstream, were reduced threefold among babies in the intervention phase of the trial. Chlorhexidine has a long track record of safety, and the investigators noted no adverse reactions to the solution among mothers or babies. The low cost, simplicity, and safety of this approach suggests that it may have a role in reducing illness and death associated with perinatal bacterial infections, which exact a considerable toll among women and neonates, especially in the developing world. Specifically, the cost of the antiseptic solution used in the study, and the cotton to apply it, was less than 10 cents per patient, making this a feasible approach for the most resource-poor settings.

Transmission from mother to child during breast-feeding In the developed world, breast-feeding has been advocated over formula for some time: It promotes mother-child bonding and may promote parenting skills. Today, there are a number of documented cases of HIV transmission through breast-feeding, but the mechanism for transmission is unclear. Although the virus has been isolated from breast milk, many women also have cracks and abrasions on the nipple and surrounding areas. For this reason, breast-feeding is not recommended for HIV-infected women in developed countries.

The World Health Organization (WHO), however, feels that the morbidity and mortality associated with the use of formula in developing countries outweighs the risk of transmission through breast-feeding. For two decades, doctors and public health agencies had offered uniform advice to new mothers in developing countries: Breast-feed your babies to protect their health. But now, the AIDS pandemic is upsetting that simple equation. Studies have shown that mothers infected with the AIDS virus can transmit it through breast milk at significant rates. Based on such findings, the United Nations recently estimated that one-third of all infants with HIV got the virus through their mother's milk. To a growing number of researchers and advocates of breast-feeding, the implications of such studies are as compelling as they were once unthinkable—infant formula, a product whose misuse in developing countries with poor sanitation was once blamed by opponents for killing 1 million babies a year—may now be a powerful weapon to reduce childhood deaths from AIDS. Doctors in industrialized nations have long recommended that HIV-infected mothers use formula. But as women in developing countries become aware of the risks of breast-feeding, they face excruciating choices and confront societal taboos. Physicians in the developing world are also torn. In many instances, advising new mothers to use formula would be impractical: Many lack the means to sterilize bottles or the money to afford formula. Additionally, the majority of pregnant women in developing countries are not tested for HIV and thus are unaware of the risks they and their newborns face.

Although the data are incomplete, some experts say, in the vast majority of the developing world, more infants will be imperiled by renewed promotion of bottle-feeding, with its accompanying risks of diarrhea and dehydration, than by the danger of HIV transmission through breast-feeding. These experts contend that in 90 percent of the developing world, the protection afforded by breast-feeding against the diseases of the developing world is higher than the rate of HIV transmission. Some advocates of breast-feeding are prepared to work with formula makers, their sworn enemies for decades, on combating the growing threat. Meanwhile, the United Nations has come under criticism from scientists who say that the group, in its zeal to promote breast-feeding, has not confronted the HIV issue. Others say that it is imperative to find alternatives to breast-feeding, including ways to make safe, affordable formula widely available.

Transmission from mother to child during the postpartum period A baby born to an HIV-infected woman will test positive for HIV at birth whether or not the infant is actually infected because the positive antibodies are transferred from the mother. Since it takes more than a year for a child's immune system to develop, these antibodies may last in the child's bloodstream well into the second year of life.

In poorer countries, most babies born to HIV-infected mothers will not be infected, but they will probably become orphans because their mothers, and often their fathers, are infected and will die before they are grown.

The relationship between a pregnant woman's plasma HIV levels and transmission of the virus to her baby has aroused interest. Researchers have sought to discover whether higher HIV levels in blood plasma correlate with an increase of mother-to-child transmission. They have also sought to discover whether a threshold viral load exists below which HIV transmission does not occur. A related question has also been asked: does an AZT-reduced reduction in a woman's viral load lead to a reduced risk of her baby's contracting HIV before and during birth? Today, the predictive power of viral load has been established, but it is noted that although the predictive value is good, it is not absolute.

Transmission from HIV-positive Patients to Health Care Workers

The transmission of HIV from an infected patient to an uninfected health care worker is possible if the health care worker accidentally cuts himself or herself during surgery or is stuck by a needle that contains infected blood from the patient. This kind of on-the-job exposure to HIV is known as occupational exposure. It can also occur if a health care worker has open wounds or skin abrasions that have contact with an infected patient's blood or other virus-laden body fluids. Exposure to any infectious agent that involves a cut, abrasion, or break in the skin—including a break caused by a needle stick—is referred to as percutaneous exposure.

Transmission from HIV-positive Health Care Workers to Patients

In the United States, the only verified case of transmission from a health care worker to patients involved a dentist who infected six of his patients. The mode of transmission in this case remains unknown. Testing of the dentist's 1100 patients revealed nine who were HIV-infected. Infections in three of them proved to be unrelated to the dentist: not only did all three have a history of recognized risk factors, but molecular analyses showed that the viral strains present in these three patients were only distantly genetically related to the viral strain present in the dentist. Viruses isolated from the remaining six patients, however, were closely related to the virus from the dentist.

Secondary Routes of Transmission

Aside from the three primary routes of transmission, HIV may be transmitted through nonsexual contact with body fluids and secretions other than blood, including cerebrospinal fluid, donated sperm, transplanted organs, and vaginal and cervical secretions. Other body fluids such as tears and urine are as yet unproven routes of transmission. Transmission via saliva may be possible through deep kissing—French or tongue kissing—which could lead to infection, especially if open sores were present on the lips, tongue, or mouth. Note that to date this route of transmission has not been confirmed.

How HIV Is Not Transmitted

The major myth is that HIV infection is easy to contract. Unlike in the plague or malaria, insects do not spread it. Unlike in the common cold, sneezing does not spread it. Unlike in cholera, it is not spread by water. If it were spread in any of these ways, the pattern of the epidemic would be far different from what it is: either entire households would be affected, or individuals would be affected randomly, or the epidemic's spread would be determined by climate, altitude, quality of the water supply, and other such environmental factors. That is not the case for the epidemic of HIV. HIV is spread in specific ways: sexual contact, blood-to-blood contact, and mother-to-infant transmission. These modes were established early in the epidemic, and continuing surveillance over a period of more than 20 years (ca. 1980 to date) has revealed no additional routes of transmission. There is no evidence that HIV is transmitted by casual contact, including talking or shaking hands, hugging or ordinary kissing; sharing kitchens, lunchrooms, dishes, or eating utensils; touching floors, walls, door knobs, or toilet seats; sharing offices, rest rooms, computers, telephones, or writing utensils; being bitten by mosquitoes, fleas, bed-bugs, and other insects. Note that if precautions are taken to prevent blood-to-blood contact, there is no evidence that HIV transmission occurs in a nonsexual, non-needle-sharing relationship with a person who is HIV-positive. See BLOOD; DRUG ABUSE; DRUG ADDICTION; INTERCOURSE; NEEDLE SHARING; PREGNANCY; RISK; SAFE SEX; SPERM; STIGMA; TRANSFUSION, AUTOLOGOUS; TRANSFUSION, BLOOD; TRANSIENT HIV INFECTION; TRANSPLANT; UNSAFE SEX; UNIVERSAL PRECAUTIONS; WOMEN.

transplantation   See ORGAN TRANSPLANTATION.

transplant-associated AIDS   AIDS acquired via an organ TRANSPLANT. See TRANSMISSION.

transsexual   An individual who is biologically of one sex but identifies with the other. (This identification may have more to do with socially constructed gender roles than biological sex differences). Male-to-female transsexuals may have had surgery for breast implants, removal of the testes and penis, and construction of a synthetic vagina. Even without surgical intervention, these individuals often take estrogen and/or progesterone to support desired secondary sexual characteristics, such as absence of facial hair, enlarged breasts, and change in voice quality. Female-to-male transsexuals support desired secondary sexual qualities by taking androgens.

Hormone use in male-to-female transsexuals, beside having its pros and cons in itself, may complicate the treatment of HIV and AIDS. Addressing the use of hormones enables the clinician to correctly calculate the dosing schedule of drugs, to monitor complications accurately, and to achieve desired therapeutic effects while reducing unwanted complications. The clinician must also be on the lookout for drug interactions and the risk of breast and possibly other cancers, all of which may be affected by hormones, and must monitor the unknown effect of estrogens and progestins themselves on immune response.

transvestite   A man who obtains erotic enjoyment from dressing in women's clothes.

trauma   Any damage or injury to the body caused by something outside the body; also, and by extension, any psychological injury caused by an extremely stressful or upsetting event or experience. See POST-TRAUMATIC STRESS SYNDROME; TRAUMATIC EVENT.

traumatic event   An event or experience that causes psychological TRAUMA.

Traumatic events or experiences have come to mean those that are outside the usual range of human experience, those that would be markedly distressing to almost anyone. These events or experiences are so overwhelming that emotional reactions and affects may be extraordinarily deep and long lasting, evoking stressful feelings and other responses, and perhaps affecting patterns of behavior, long after the traumatic event has occurred. See POST-TRAUMATIC-STRESS SYNDROME; TRAUMATIC EVENT.

traumatic lesion   A scratch, scrape, or chafing on the body. See LESION; TRAUMA.

travel restrictions   The exclusion from the United States of aliens infected with the human immunodeficiency virus (HIV). Few issues in immigration law have caused as much controversy in recent years as the issue of travel restrictions. Seemingly a straightforward question, the issue is actually quite complex and has a long and volatile history. Should persons with HIV/AIDS be allowed to travel without restriction to the United States to professional, business, or scientific conferences? Is this a question of the public interest? Or a question of the rights of persons with HIV/AIDS? Should nonimmigrants be allowed in the United States without restriction for the purpose of receiving medical treatment? What is the role or purpose of special visas, waivers, and quotas? Are these initiatives based on the best medical thinking, on sound public policy, or on prejudice? These are some of the questions that have been debated by the United States government, public health and medical authorities, the news media and AIDS activists, as well as persons with HIV/AIDS during the first and second decades of the epidemic.

The regulation of IMMIGRATION on the basis of contagious diseases dates to the adoption and ultimate codification in 1952, as part of the Immigration and Naturalization Act (INA), of specific exclusions for aliens suffering from such contagious diseases as leprosy and tuberculosis. The provision was revised in 1961 to reflect changes in medical language and to incorporate more precise language. The language of the provision is that "aliens who are afflicted with any dangerous contagious disease" shall be excluded from the United States. Determination and designation of which diseases are "dangerous contagious diseases" are left to the United States Public Health Service. In mid-1987, the Public Health Service added AIDS to

the list. Soon thereafter, despite considerable opposition from AIDS and immigration advocates, doctors and public interest organizations, the Public Health Service replaced AIDS on the list with Human Immunodeficiency Virus (HIV) infection, further expanding the definition of persons considered to be afflicted with a contagious disease. On July 8, 1987, the Immigration and Naturalization Service and the State Department began testing aliens seeking admission to the United States for HIV. This set the stage for what was to become a hotly contested congressional battle following the enactment of the 1990 Immigration Act to statutorily exclude HIV-infected aliens.

The Immigration Act of 1990 completely revised the grounds of exclusion and provided for the exclusion of aliens on health-related grounds who, according to Public Health Service regulations, have been determined to have a "communicable disease of public health significance." The act also permitted, for the first time, a waiver of health-related exclusion grounds for permanent resident and immigrant visa applicants. In January 1991, the Public Health Service announced its intention to remove HIV from its list of communicable diseases because it had determined that HIV is not spread by casual contact. After critical public response, the Public Health Service decided to postpone finalizing its rule.

In 1993, the Public Health Service drafted new regulations that would have removed HIV from the list of contagious diseases and, as a result, two congressional bills were introduced containing language that would deem HIV a communicable disease of public health significance for purposes of exclusion. The ensuing congressional debate led to the enactment of the National Institutes of Health Revitalization Act of 1993, which specifically codified HIV-infection as a ground of exclusion.

Current law now provides for the statutory exclusion of HIV-infected immigrants and nonimmigrants. Any person who is determined to have a communicable disease of public health significance that includes infection with the etiological agent (HIV) for acquired immune deficiency syndrome (AIDS) is excludable. Certain classes of aliens are eligible for waivers that permit nonimmigrants entry to the United States on a temporary basis and that permit immigrants the right to be admitted and remain permanently. In this context, nonimmigrants are those persons, non-citizens and non-residents seeking to enter the United States on a temporary basis for a variety of reasons, including business, pleasure, and schooling. Immigrants, on the other hand, are those persons wishing to enter the United States with the intent to remain permanently. "Excludability" and "inadmissibility" are terms used interchangeably. Although a medical examination is required for all applicants applying for immigrant visas, a medical examination is not mandatory for nonimmigrant visa applicants. However, if a consular officer suspects that an applicant is HIV-infected, a medical examination to determine whether or not the applicant is eligible for a visa may be requested. Although the grant of a waiver to nonimmigrants is discretionary in nature, there are standard factors considered by consular officers in reaching their determination. These factors include whether the person, (1) is currently afflicted with symptoms of the disease; (2) is coming to the United States for a short visit; (3) has insurance or assets that will enable the person to pay medical expenses should he or she become ill; and (4) whether there is a reason to believe that the person poses a danger to the public health in the United States. See IMMIGRATION.

treat through The action of continuing treatment for a particular illness despite the patient developing an reaction to a drug used in the treatment of the original illness. In HIGHLY ACTIVE ANTIRETROVIRAL THERAPY (HAART) a patient may develop a reaction to a particular drug used in the treatment regimen. One drug that causes this to occur with some frequency is abacavir. Bactrim is another such drug. Both these drugs may produce a rash and a fever when initially taken. However, in the majority of patients, these symptoms can be overcome, and the treatment continued if the patient continues to take the medication. In some people this is not possible, so it is always important to speak with your medical provider in these cases. This process of continuing treatment allows the body to adjust to the medication, and the reaction lessons as time goes on.

treatment Medical, surgical, dental, or psychiatric management of a patient. Today, "treatment"

is often broadly interpreted to encompass the nutritional, psychological, psychosocial, and spiritual management of a patient. Treatment also refers to any specific procedure or substance, or course of such procedures or substances, used for the cure or the amelioration of a disease or pathological condition. An overview of primary HIV/AIDS care follows, with a focus on the medical management of persons with HIV/AIDS.

Five key components of HIV care include: (1) the prevention of TRANSMISSION; (2) the preservation of the immune function; (3) PROPHYLAXIS against OPPORTUNISTIC INFECTION; (4) early diagnosis and treatment of opportunistic infection; and (5) optimizing the quality of life. Medical management of HIV infection consists of monitoring CD4 count; offering antiretroviral therapy when CD4 count falls below 500; initiating prophylaxis against PNEUMOCYSTIS CARINII PNEUMONIA (PCP) at a CD4 count of 200 or less; and initiating prophylaxis against MAC at a CD4 count of 50 or less. Additionally, the HIV-infected individual must be monitored closely for the development of opportunistic processes.

Treatment generally begins with an initial patient visit in which a general history of the patient is examined. Specific questions are indicated regarding mode of infection and possible dates of infection. Occurrence of any HIV-related problems or AIDS-defining illness must be documented. Current medication should be noted, including vitamins or other substances taken for nutritional or medicinal purposes. Special attention should be paid to sexually transmitted diseases and fungal, parasitic, and mycobacterial infections. Dates and treatment should be noted. A review of systems is conducted, and the patient is asked about his or her experience of fatigue; weight loss, anorexia; anxiety, depression; fever, chills, night sweats; adenopathy; skin rash; bruises or other skin lesions; headache, sinusitis; blurring of vision or other visual changes; oral sores; dysphagia or odynophagia; shortness of breath or dyspnea on exertion; cough; abdominal pain; nausea, vomiting, diarrhea, constipation; rectal sores, genital sores; arthritis, muscle weakness; forgetfulness; and lack of coordination. A psychosocial history is also taken, and patients should be asked about familiarity and experiences with others having HIV infection. A dialogue regarding individual expectations of immediate and long-term prospects should be initiated and continued throughout treatment. Patients may have strong feelings regarding the level of intervention they desire, particularly in regard to life-prolonging measures. A complete physical examination and laboratory tests are also commonly part of the initial patient visit.

Follow-up visits are generally scheduled as soon as possible after lab results have become available. Particular emphasis should be given to the psychosocial dimensions of the patient's response to HIV infection. A review of systems should be performed at each visit, and a physical examination is also indicated at each visit. Laboratory results are reviewed and interpreted at the follow-up examination.

Prevention is a key concept in the care of HIV-infected individuals—the prevention of viral transmission, prevention of illness by immunizing patients, and prevention of opportunistic infections. Prophylactic regimens vary from opportunistic infection to opportunistic infection. Common opportunistic infections include *Pneumocystis carinii* pneumonia, MYCOBACTERIUM AVIUM COMPLEX, and TOXOPLASMOSIS ENCEPHALITIS, fungal infections, and herpes simplex.

Antiretroviral therapy involves the use of one or more of the four antiretroviral medications currently available to physicians—zidovudine, didanosine, zalcitabine, and stavudine. All are REVERSE TRANSCRIPTASE inhibitors. There are three major considerations in the evaluation of antiretroviral therapy: the TOXICITY of the medications; the duration of effectiveness of the currently available drugs, especially in advanced disease; and the fact that reverse transcriptase inhibitors do not completely suppress viral replication. Questions about the optimal usage of antiretroviral agents remain.

Treatment for common HIV-associated infections and conditions is also a part of the management of HIV/AIDS. CANDIDIASIS, COCCIDIOIDOMYCOSIS, *CRYPTOCOCCUS NEOFORMANS, CRYPTOSPORIDIUM, ISOSPORA BELLI,* and *MICROSPORIDIA,* CYTOMEGALOVIRUS, herpes simplex, HISTOPLASMOSIS, KAPOSI'S SARCOMA, HIV-related lymphoma, *Mycobacterium avium* complex, *Mycobacterium tuberculosis, Pneumocystis carinii,* PROGRESSIVE MULTIFOCAL LEUKOENCEPHALOPATHY, THROMBOCYTOPENIA, *Toxoplasma gondii,* and VARICELLA ZOSTER are common HIV-associated infections. Common complaints of HIV-infected individuals include dermatologic complaints; diarrhea; fatigue; fever; hepatomegaly/elevated liver enzymes; headaches, seizures and focal neurologic findings; odynophagiz/dysphagia; peripheral neuropathy; and respiratory complaints. Issues specific to the treatment of women with HIV/AIDS include gynecologic concerns; gynecologic infections; menstrual disorders; cervical dysplasia and neoplasia; pregnancy; prenatal care; opportunistic infection prophylaxis in pregnancy; intrapartum considerations; and postpartum considerations.

Issues specific to the treatment of infants and children with HIV/AIDS include when to consider testing and the challenge of providing comprehensive and anticipatory health maintenance, including prophylaxis and treatment of common pediatric HIV-associated infections and conditions.

Increasingly, the medical management for persons with HIV/AIDS involves experimental and nontraditional treatments for HIV/AIDS. In the 1980s, science could offer nothing to people with the AIDS virus. Today, the problem is just the opposite. There are numerous approved drugs and treatments on the market and many possible regimens for using them. These drugs include nucleoside/nucleotide reverse transcriptase inhibitors, nonnucleoside reverse transcriptase inhibitors, and protease inhibitors. There are a broad array of experimental drugs under study—fusion inhibitors, nucleoside reverse transcriptase inhibitors, nonnucleoside reverse transcriptase inhibitors, protease inhibitors, budding and assembly inhibitors, cellular metabolism modulators, therapeutic vaccines, and cytokines. Clinical trials for adults and adolescents, for women and children provide unparalleled opportunities to learn about opportunistic infections, HIV-related disorders, and HIV infection. There is no question but that scientists have made significant progress in their quest to answer what are the central strategic questions: How should the treatments be used, in what order, and in what combinations, at what stages of the illness?

AIDS researchers are the first to admit that the latest treatments could ultimately prove disappointing. First, the virus can evolve rapidly in the body to become resistant to drugs, limiting how long even the best ones will work. Second, most AIDS treatments, including the new ones, seem to work best in people who are not too sick to begin with. For the many thousands who have already progressed to severe illness, science does not hold out as much hope. Finally, tapping into the latest developments is complicated and expensive. Those with access to experimental treatments and nutritional counseling have largely been middle-class white men, while the virus is afflicting more and more poor women and minorities. This "knowledge gap" is emerging as an enormous problem. Many people with the virus don't know they have it, much less what kinds of treatment are available.

treatment access   Despite the fact that there have been vast improvements in treatment access since the first decade of the epidemic, access to treatment remains one of the more controversial areas in HIV-related research today. In the early 1980s, the medical and scientific communities were not prepared to tackle the unexpected AIDS epidemic. The slow, methodical path that experimental therapies went through from initial conception to final approval was clearly inadequate. Efforts of community groups and AIDS service organizations, among others, led to significant changes in the way clinical research is performed. Still, as the second decade of the epidemic nears its end, many aspects of CLINICAL TRIALS, drug testing, and development remain a source of confusion, frustration, and at times, anger among people living with HIV.

Of particular concern is the exclusionary nature of many clinical trials. In the past, this has been a source of frustration for women who have been discriminated against in clinical research, mainly because of pregnancy-related concerns. This has been done to protect the fetus from potentially harmful new drugs. Also in the past, children were discriminated against in clinical research—the focus was always on men first. Because children are very different from adults, most children's therapies need to be tested separately. The exclusionary nature of many clinical trials has also been the source of tremendous frustration for many people who have been willing to enter trials, only to be rejected because their CD4+ count is too high or too low, or because they have taken AZT or some other drug in the past. Although trials will always involve specific exclusion and inclusion criteria, researchers and persons with HIV/AIDS hope that they will become more open in the near future,

thereby increasing access to treatment for men, women, and children.

The red-tape of the United States drug testing and development bureaucracy has historically thwarted access to promising new drugs for persons with HIV/AIDS. Today, the FOOD AND DRUG ADMINISTRATION has approved several mechanisms for distributing experimental drugs before those drugs are approved for general sale, including compassionate use, parallel track, and treatment IND. Also today, persons with HIV/AIDS can make use of the growing network of community-based research groups in the United States whose top priority is the prevention of OPPORTUNISTIC INFECTIONS. Supporters of the CRI movement insist that it is doing an end run around federal incompetence and indifference. They insist that through community-based research, persons with HIV/AIDS can save their own lives, and encourage persons who want to survive AIDS to make contact with the community-based research group in his or her area.

treatment guidelines   Guides for the medical, surgical, dental, or psychiatric management of a patient, generally including a series and sequence of treatment procedures for a future course of action based on an individualized evaluation of what is needed to restore the health and function of a patient.

treatment IND (Investigational New Drug)   See INVESTIGATIONAL NEW DRUG.

treatment IND status   See INVESTIGATIONAL NEW DRUG.

treatment plan   A projected series and sequence of treatment procedures for an individual patient, based on an evaluation of what is needed to restore or improve his or her health and functioning.

treatment use regulations   FOOD AND DRUG ADMINISTRATION rules under which drug manufacturers apply to distribute drugs for the treatment of the desperately ill when the drugs have been approved only for CLINICAL TRIALS. In some cases, these rules also cover drugs that have been approved for use but not for the disease for whose treatment it is being proposed. A change in the rules in June 1987 allowed for the early release of anti-AIDS drugs.

TREC (T-cell receptor-rearrangement excision cells) T cells begin production in the bone marrow, where they are called progenitor cells. When these cells are to become T cells, they leave the bone marrow and migrate to the THYMUS. In the thymus, T cells become either CD4 or CD8 cells, depending on the markers they acquire that allow various antigens to lock onto the cells. These T-cell receptors, where antigens lock on, are arranged randomly in the thymus. Many differently shaped T cells are made this way. Up to 95 percent of the T cells created by the thymus are later destroyed in the thymus because the randomization makes them contain receptors that would match up with those in their own body, causing many problems. This is the last job of the thymus, to destroy these self-reactive T cells. The remaining 5 percent of T cells leave the thymus to protect the body from various antigens.

These T cells are called NAÏVE T CELLS because they have not been exposed to an antigen that matches their receptor. Scientists in the late 1990s found a way to track these naïve T cells. They can be tracked because these naïve T cells leave behind some extra DNA that researchers can locate. These extra sections of DNA are called T-cell receptor-rearrangement excision cells (TREC). TREC is divided each time a T cell divides and new cells are created from the naïve cells. That way scientists can measure the "age" of the T cells and see new naïve T cells in older patients. Most of the body's T cells are produced in childhood. It was thought that the thymus stopped production of T cells at the time. However, researchers learned by tracking TREC that these cells are produced slowly and steadily throughout life. In HIV patients, TREC levels decrease as the disease progresses. This leads researchers to believe that HIV damages the thymus in some manner. However, with treatment of HAART, naive T-cell production has been shown, through TREC testing, to increase again to age-normal levels. Research studies have shown that rapid drops in TREC are correlated with viral progression in HIV-positive people.

Treponema pallidum The microorganism that causes SYPHILIS; sometimes referred to as a spirochete because of its shape.

tretinoin A derivative of VITAMIN A being tested as a topical and oral treatment for KAPOSI'S SARCOMA. Although the oral form appears to have an effect on the disease, it also has serious side effects, including severe nausea and vomiting, intolerable headaches, malaise, altered blood calcium levels, and inflammation of the pancreas.

triage The classifying of sick, injured, or wounded persons according to the severity (and survivability) of their conditions and the urgency of their medical needs; the assignment of priority for treatment. Triage promotes the most efficient use of health care resources when time, personnel, facilities, and equipment are limited.

trial The experimental testing of a drug under controlled conditions. See DRUG TRIAL; MANAGEMENT TRIALS.

trial accrual The number of persons enrolled in a CLINICAL TRIAL at a given time.

tribadism A sexual act between two women involving rubbing their bodies together.

Trichomonas A genus of parasitic protozoa, most commonly sexually transmitted, that cause an infection of the urogenital tract, mainly in women, in whom it causes a copious yellow or green vaginal discharge with a fishy odor and extreme itching. Occasionally it is present and asymptomatic. Diagnosis is by examination of vaginal secretions and findings of motile trichomonads. It may coexist with other vaginal PATHOGENS. It may be a marker for the presence of additional sexually transmitted infections, particularly GONORRHEA and CHLAMYDIA. Treatment is with metronidazole. For women who can not tolerate metronidazole, garlic suppositories are a home remedy that is reported to work well.

Trichomonas vaginalis A species of parasitic protozoan flagellates, belonging to the genus *Tri-*

chomonas, commonly found in the urethra and vagina of women and in the urethra and prostate gland of men. It is the causative agent of TRICHOMONIASIS VAGINITIS.

trichomoniasis A form of vaginitis caused by the protozoan TRICHOMONAS VAGINALIS.

trichomoniasis vaginitis Acute or subacute urethritis or vaginitis due to infection with *TRICHOMONAS VAGINALIS* that does not invade the tissue or mucosa but causes an inflammatory reaction. Infection is venereal or by other forms of contact. It is usually asymptomatic but may produce vaginitis, with vulvar and vaginal pruritus, vaginal discharge of white or yellowish viscid fluid containing mucus and pus, and rarely purulent urethritis in males.

trichosanthin (compound q, GLQ-223) The active ingredient derived from the root of the Chinese cucumber plant. Trichosanthin has been studied as an anti-HIV therapy and has been shown to kill HIV-infected macrophages. Trichosanthin has had harmful side effects in clinical trials, such as high fever and inflammation. Chinese and U.S. researchers continue to conduct experiments to study the drug.

trifluorothymidine See TRIFLURIDINE.

trifluridine An antiviral used for topical treatment of infections caused by HERPES SIMPLEX VIRUS. In people infected with HIV, it has been used topically to treat skin, genital, and perianal HSV infections resistant to acyclovir. Trifluridine works by interfering with DNA synthesis in infected cells. It has been shown to be effective for treatment, but not prevention, of herpes virus infections. It is not effective against bacterial, fungal, or chlamydial infections. Available as a sterile solution for administration into the eyes. The most common effect of the optical solution is mild, transient burning when dropping it into the eye. Also called TRIFLUOROTHYMIDINE. (Trade name is Viroptic.)

triglyceride A combination of glycerol with three of five different fatty acids. These substances,

triacylglycerols, are also called neutral fats. A large portion of the fatty substance in the blood is composed of triglycerides. Because these lipids are not soluble in water, they are transported in combination with proteins. About one or two grams of triglycerides per kilogram of body weight are ingested daily in the usual diet in the United States. In addition, they are produced in the liver from carbohydrates.

trimethoprim An antimicrobial agent that enhances the effect of sulfonamides and sulfones.

trimethoprim-sulfamethoxazole (TMP/SMX) A first-line combination drug for *PNEUMOCYSTIS CARINII PNEUMONIA* prophylaxis and treatment. Possible side effects include skin rash, pruritus, cytopenia, liver abnormalities, and gastrointestinal upset. This commonly used combination antibiotic has a variety of interactions and toxicities that need to be monitored. The most common side effect associated with the sulfa component is a skin rash, usually allergic in nature, which on rare occasions spreads to other body surfaces and becomes the life-threatening Stevens-Johnson syndrome. It is also known that the drug can increase the skin's sensitivity to ultraviolet light, so excessive exposure to the sun should be avoided while taking it. Common drugs that have been reported to interact with TMP/SMX's liver effects include Coumadin (an anticoagulant) and Dilantin (an anticonvulsant). Elevated potassium levels sometimes also occur when on TMP/SMX. High potassium may lead to abnormal heart rhythms and contractions. In the presence of kidney disease, TMP/SMX can accumulate and cause greater toxicity. Kidney-toxic drugs (e.g., amphotericin, foscarnet) and AMINOGLYCOSIDE ANTIBIOTICS (amikacin, gentamicin, paromomycin, streptomycin) pose a special problem for people taking TMP/SMX, as does potassium supplementation. Finally, TMP/SMX increases the effect of the anticonvulsant Dilantin by inhibiting the liver's ability to break down the drug. (Trade names are Bactrim, Septra, and Cotrimoxale.)

trimetrexate An antineoplastic agent and antiprotozoal "orphan" drug used in the treatment of moderate-to-severe PNEUMOCYSTIS CARINII PNEU-MONIA. Often used as "SALVAGE THERAPY" for people with PCP who do not respond to or who are intolerant of standard treatments. Trimetrexate causes severe bone marrow, liver, kidney, and gastrointestinal toxicities. It must be administered along with LEUCOVORIN (folinic acid) to ameliorate these adverse effects. (Trade name is Neutrexin.)

Trimox   See AMOXICILLIN.

trip   A vernacular term used to denote a drug-induced period of hallucination or euphoria.

triple helix   A genetically engineered modification to DNA, now in development. Naturally occurring DNA consists of two interlocking strands (the famous double-helix structure). Scientists have now developed the means to attach a third strand, effectively blocking transcription—in other words, preventing the organism from reproducing. They are now working to synthesize small strands of modified DNA targeting specific sequences of the HIV genome.

In the same way that RNA-targeted therapeutics are more efficient than drugs that bind with proteins, synthesized triple helix promises to be more efficient than the controversial antisense. The compound would bind to the DNA itself, rather than to the thousands of RNA transcripts. Thus less drug would be needed and greater efficacy achieved—transcription of the unwanted gene would cease completely. This technology is at an early stage of development and many biochemical obstacles remain.

triple therapy   A three-drug combination of antiviral medications, one of them usually from the potent PROTEASE INHIBITOR family of compounds, recommended for all people with AIDS. The rationale behind this approach is that triple therapy with three antiviral drugs greatly decreases a person's risk of getting sicker or dying of AIDS. See HAART.

Trizivir   An HIV medicine that is a combination of three antiviral medicines made by GlaxoSmithKline: ZIDOVUDINE (AZT), LAMIVUDINE (3TC), and ABACAVIR.

It has made pill loads manageable for many people who had difficulty taking the multiples of pills often required in HAART treatment. It cannot be used by people of low body weight, who require lowered doses of medication. It can cause all of the side effects that the individual drugs can cause. Therefore, someone who is allergic to abacavir should not take Trizivir. No difference in drug availability has been found in people taking Trizivir and people taking individual doses of the three separate medicines.

Important interim results from a Phase III randomized, double-blind comparison of three protease inhibitor–sparing regimens for the initial treatment of HIV infection were released by the Department of Health and Human Services in March 2003. It was reported that in antiretroviral treatment–naive patients, a combination of three nucleoside analogs, Trizivir, was inferior to two other efavirenz-containing treatment regimens being evaluated in the study. The data met pre-specified guidelines for stopping this one arm of the study based on virologic failure. There were no concerns about the toxicity of the study drugs. As of this writing, these findings have not been presented at a scientific meeting, peer reviewed, or published. See http://www.nlm.nih.gov/databases/alerts/clinical_alerts.html or http://www.niaid.nih.gov/daids/default.htm for further information.

trough level   The minimal concentration of a drug in blood plasma, which occurs before the next time that drug is administered. Sometimes abbreviated as CMIN. Achieving an adequate trough level that retains sufficient antimicrobial activity is important to preventing the rise of drug-resistant microbes.

TSS   See TOXIC SHOCK SYNDROME.

T-suppressor lymphocyte   See T8 CELL.

tubal pregnancy   Pregnancy in which the egg is fertilized and remains in the fallopian tube, which later ruptures. See ECTOPIC PREGNANCY.

tubal surgery   Surgery on the fallopian tubes, generally performed to reverse the effects of PELVIC INFLAMMATORY DISEASE (scarring and infertility).

tubercle A granulomatous lesion caused by infection with *Mycobacterium tuberculosis*. Tubercles vary in size and in histologic component proportions but tend to be circumscribed, firm, spheroidal lesions that generally consist of three zones: an inner focus of necrosis; a middle zone consisting of an accumulation of large mononuclear phagocytes, or macrophages; and an outer zone consisting of mostly LYMPHOCYTES with a few MONOCYTES and plasma cells. Where healing has begun, fibrous tissue forming at the periphery may form a fourth zone. "Tubercle" is also used nonspecifically to refer to any granuloma.

tuberculin unit The unit of measurement for doses of tuberculin purified protein derivative (PPD), used to test for TUBERCULOSIS.

tuberculosis (TB) A bacterial infection, usually in the lungs (where it is infectious), caused by *Mycobacterium*, most commonly *Mycobacterium tuberculosis*. It may also occur outside the lungs. Tuberculosis is far more frequent in people with HIV infection than in the general population. It is transmitted when a person with active TB coughs or sneezes, releasing microscopic particles in the air. These, also called droplet nuclei, contain live tubercle bacteria and may cause infection when inhaled by another person. Once infected by TB, most people remain healthy and develop only latent infection. In this state they are neither sick nor infectious, but they do have the potential to become sick and infectious with active TB. Many researchers compare HIV disease to tuberculosis as both HIV and the tuberculosis bacterium tend to become resistant to drugs.

The immunological factors that allow latent TB infection to develop into active disease are unknown. It is known that HIV-positive people have a higher risk of developing active TB disease. It is also believed that some people with active HIV will develop active disease from a newly acquired infection due to their inability to mount a sufficient immune response.

Although TB is spread through the air, infection usually occurs only after prolonged exposure to someone with active TB. Documented TB outbreaks have been primarily associated with hospitals, clinics, nursing homes, prisons, shelters for the homeless, and other places where persons who may have TB congregate.

The most common site of active TB is the lungs. This is called pulmonary TB. However, TB may affect any part of the body (extrapulmonary TB), including the skin, bone marrow, liver, spleen, kidney, bones, and even the breast and may occur simultaneously as pulmonary and extrapulmonary disease. General symptoms of disease include fever, NIGHT SWEATS, dramatic weight loss, and a feeling of malaise. Symptoms of TB in the lungs include these, an otherwise unexplained cough lasting longer than three weeks, and bloody sputum. Since the symptoms of TB can mirror the symptoms of a number of other infections, it is important that TB be considered along with *PNEUMOCYSTIS CARINII* PNEUMONIA and other mycobacterial infections such as *Mycobacterium avium intracellulare*.

Clinical manifestations of active TB in persons with HIV infection can vary considerably depending on the stage of disease. TB can occur early in HIV disease, when CD4 cell counts average 300 to 400. At this stage of HIV disease, TB is usually localized in the lungs and the sputum specimen is smear positive (infected matter is visible over solid culture media). As the CD4 count declines, the presentation of TB may change, with more extrapulmonary disease, miliary lung involvement, negative sputum smears, and atypical chest X-ray patterns.

In HIV-infected people who develop active TB, levels of HIV in the bloodstream increase five- to 160-fold, findings which help explain why HIV-infected people with active TB have a poorer prognosis than HIV-infected people without TB. Research has shown that high levels of HIV in the blood correlate with an increased risk that an HIV-infected person will develop AIDS or die. The fact that active TB disease boosts HIV levels in the blood underscores the importance of diagnosing and effectively treating tuberculosis in HIV-infected people. These facts also highlight the importance of preventive TB therapy in HIV-infected people. Such therapy may not only help to control the spread of TB, but also prevent the increased replication of HIV associated with active TB.

The PPD (purified protein derivative) skin test is the first step in diagnosing TB. PPD is injected under the skin of the forearm. After 48 to 72 hours, the injection site will be indurated (i.e., have developed a red hard bump) if there is TB infection. This induration is caused by an immune response; immunosuppressed persons may have little or no reaction to the test, even if they have been exposed to TB. According to the CENTERS FOR DISEASE CONTROL AND PREVENTION (CDC), an HIV-infected individual with an induration of greater than or equal to 5 mm is considered to be infected with TB. Some researchers believe that even the 5 mm cutoff may underestimate the rate of true TB infection and suggest that a 2 mm induration be considered a positive skin test in HIV-infected patients. A positive PPD skin test does not mean that the person has active TB, only that the individual has been infected with the bacteria that causes TB. Lack of response to PPD skin test is more frequent when CD4 cells drop below 200.

Along with a PPD test, an HIV-positive individual should receive an anergy test (skin reaction) to verify immune competence. An anergy test consists of two or three common ANTIGENS, usually candida, mumps, or tetanus toxoid, which are injected under the skin. If there is a reaction to the antigens, the person is considered nonanergic, and the TB skin test results are considered reliable. If there is no reaction to either the antigens or the PPD, the person is considered anergic. A negative PPD reaction should never be used to exclude the diagnosis of TB infection in persons who are anergic.

A person who has a positive skin test or who has symptoms of active TB should have a chest X ray and sputum sample analysis. The sputum will be examined microscopically for the presence of ACID FAST bacilli (AFB) and cultured for TB.

TB is treated with a combination of several ANTIBIOTICS. Combination antibiotic therapy given intermittently (less than daily) has recently been shown to be an effective initial treatment for persons with HIV-related TB. Prior to this finding, the standard of care was to prescribe multidrug therapy for several months before switching to intermittent therapy for the remainder of a typical nine-month course of treatment. When effective therapy is given, symptoms typically improve within four weeks and sputum cultures become negative within three months. The standard treatment of drug-sensitive TB in HIV-positive people generally includes isoniazid, rifampin, pyrazinamide, and ethambutol. TB treatment regimens that contain rifampin are far superior to those that do not contain rifampin. Rifampin-containing regimens are usually much shorter (six to nine versus 18 to 24 months) and have faster clearance of the tubercule bacterium from the sputum, higher cure rates, and fewer relapses.

Rifamycins, the class of drugs that includes rifampin and rifabutin pose a significant problem for TB patients who are also HIV-positive. Rifampin and rifabutin heighten the activity of the liver's drug-metabolizing CYTOCHROME P450 enzyme system, leading to subtherapeutic blood levels of the anti-HIV PROTEASE INHIBITORS (saquinavir, indinavir and ritonavir). At the same time, the protease inhibitors inhibit the P450 enzymes, causing higher levels of rifampin and rifabutin with an accompanying increased risk of serious side effects (including bone marrow suppression and inflammation of various tissues and organs). In late 1996, the CDC issued guidelines for HIV-positive patients with tuberculosis who also require treatment with protease inhibitors.

The CDC recommends completion of a six-month TB regimen containing rifampin for all HIV-positive patients with active TB regardless of CD4 cell count. For TB patients already on protease inhibitor therapy, the CDC believes one option is discontinuing therapy with protease inhibitors and completing a six-month course with a rifampin-containing TB regimen. A second option is to switch from rifampin to rifabutin (150 mg per day) and to indinavir from other protease inhibitors, and suggests treating patients with a four-drug rifabutin-containing TB regimen for nine months. The CDC also recommends measuring rifabutin plasma concentrations. A third option is a four-drug rifampin-containing regimen for two months or until the sputum culture has converted to negative, followed by 16 months of continued TB treatment with isoniazid at 15 mg/kg of body weight and ethambutol at 50 mg/kg, given twice weekly. Some experts also recommend adding a third drug such as streptomycin for the continuation phase. This regimen allows for reintroduction of protease inhibitor therapy after the second month of TB therapy. This third option is not recommended for patients with INH-resistant TB.

The agency's advice is based on the best guesses of experts in the fields of HIV, TB, and drug metabolism. The regimens have not been formally tested since most trials of protease inhibitors excluded patients requiring rifamputin or rifabutin. The recommendations serve as a good starting point that will encourage practitioners who care for people with TB not to withhold potent antiretroviral therapy from patients who also have HIV. As TB is known to accelerate the rate of HIV disease, intervention with protease inhibitor therapy in this patient population is considered crucial.

TB is considered multidrug resistant (MDR-TB) if it does not respond to two or more standard anti-TB drugs. MDR-TB usually occurs when treatment is interrupted thus allowing mutations to occur which confer drug resistance. Resistance may also be the consequence of inadequate care and follow-up that resulted in undermedication of TB. However, primary infection with MDR-TB can occur as well. MDR-TB strains are difficult to treat with the existing range of medicines. In most cases, MDR-TB has led to death in people with AIDS. MDR-TB has serious public health implications due to the rapid progression to life threatening disease, the efficient transmission to others, and delays in diagnosis.

PROPHYLAXIS with anti-TB drugs can prevent the development of active TB. Therefore, TB screening should be a routine part of HIV clinical management. Persons with HIV are more likely to suffer adverse reactions to anti-TB drugs and therefore require careful monitoring. The BACILLE CALMETTE-GUÉRIN (BCG) vaccine is the only TB vaccine currently available. BCG is widely used in parts of Africa and Asia where TB is endemic. BCG is not recommended for anyone who is immunocompromised, due to reported incidents of disseminated infection with the Calmette-Guérin bacillus. BCG vaccination should only be given to immune competent children who are at unavoidable risk of exposure to TB and for whom other methods of prevention and control have failed or are not feasible.

tubuloplasty A surgical operation to reconstruct the fallopian tubes and restore fertility.

tumescence A swollen and enlarged condition. The penis is tumescent when sexually aroused.

tumor Any abnormal growth, whether or not cancerous or a threat to health.

tumor necrosis factor (TNF) A CYTOKINE produced in response to infection by circulating white blood cells called MONOCYTES. TNF helps activate T CELLS; it may also stimulate HIV activity. TNF levels are very high in people with HIV and the molecule is suspected of playing a part in HIV-related WASTING, NEUROPATHY, and DEMENTIA.

TNF is one of a wide variety of cytokines produced by the immune system, each with differing effects on immune function. These cytokines also have effects on body metabolism that parallel their role in immune response. The observed metabolic effects of chronic exposure to TNF include fever, anorexia, hypermetabolism, and, finally, wasting. TNF can furthermore trigger the release of other factors implicated in wasting and other symptoms, among them such cytokines as INTERLEUKIN-1, endocrine hormones, PROSTAGLANDIN E2, and the LEUKOTRIENES. It has also been shown to activate latent HIV infection within cells.

The list of therapies promoted as TNF reducers or inhibitors is quite long; it includes thalidomide, pentoxifylline (Trental), ketotifen, tenidap (an antiarthritis medication), vesnarinone, OPC-8212 (an oral agent used in Japan as a treatment for congestive heart failure), cyclosporine, peptide T, sulfasalazine, thorazine, many antioxidants, corticosteroids, anti-TNF monoclonal antibodies, recombinant TNF soluble receptors, marijuana, glycyrrhizin, sho-saiko-to (SSKT, a Chinese herbal formulation), L-carnitine, and use of hyperthermia and hyperbaric oxygen therapy. Most of these therapies have been reported to reduce TNF in the test tube. Whether any achieves this in the body is hard to tell—there are conflicting reports about several of the therapies mentioned. Even when there is a broad consensus that a given disease elevates TNF, there is always a study or two that contradict that conclusion.

These discrepancies could be due to a number of factors. First, TNF has a very short half-life, and if blood samples are not tested right away, assays will probably not detect it. Second, TNF quickly binds to soluble and cellular receptors (which makes it undetectable in many tests), but this does not mean that it cannot cause damage. There are several laboratory tests that measure TNF, both free and bound, but researchers do not agree on which to use.

tumor necrosis factor (TNF) inhibitor   Drugs that work to inhibit TUMOR NECROSIS FACTOR.

turmeric   See CURCUMIN.

tumor-specific antigen   A cell surface ANTIGEN that is expressed on malignant but not normal cells.

turned on   A slang term for sexually excited.

12-step program   A self-help program to achieve a goal, usually sobriety, organized in a set number of stages (often but not always 12). These programs are carried out by members of such groups as Alcoholics Anonymous (AA; the original 12-step program), Narcotics Anonymous (NA), Overeaters Anonymous (OA), and so forth. In most, the focus is on a mind-body-spirit approach to a behavioral problem.

typhoid fever   An acute infectious disease acquired by ingesting food or water contaminated by human waste matter. It is characterized by sustained bacteremia and infestation of the PATHOGEN within the mononuclear phagocytic cells of the liver, LYMPH NODES, SPLEEN, and PEYER'S PATCHES of the ileum, accompanied by fever, rash, headache, malaise, and abdominal pain. Diagnosis is made by isolation of the bacteria from the blood.

typhus   Any of a group of infectious diseases caused by RICKETTSIA. Typhus is characterized by great prostration, severe headache, generalized maculopapular rash, sustained high fever, and usually progressive neurologic involvement, ending in a crisis in 10 to 14 days. Three diseases are included in this group: epidemic (louse-borne) typhus, caused by *Rickettsia prowazekii*; Brill-Zinsser disease (recrudescent typhus), caused by *Rickettsia prowazekii*; and murine (flea-borne) typhus, caused by *Rickettsia typhi*. Although clinically and pathologically similar, they differ in intensity of symptoms severity and mortality rate. Broad spectrum antibiotics, such as tetracyclines and chloramphenical, give excellent results. Prognosis is variable. Mortality may be quite high in epidemic typhus and almost nonexistent in murine typhus.

U

U89 See ABACAVIR.

U90 See DELAVIRDINE.

ubiquinone A lipid-soluble QUINONE (important small hydrophobic component of the electron transport chain) also known as COENZYME Q10, present in virtually all cells. It is a collector of reducing equivalents during intracellular respiration. It is converted to its reduced form, ubiquinol, while involved in this process.

UC781 An experimental NONNUCLEOSIDE REVERSE TRANSCRIPTASE INHIBITOR (NNRTI) from the Crompton Corporation. It was initially developed to fight fungi in food crops but has shown some promise in HIV control. It is being looked at specifically for development in a topical microbicide.

ulcer An open sore or lesion of the skin or mucous membrane, accompanied by the sloughing of inflammatory necrotic tissue. It may discharge pus if it becomes infected. Trauma, caustics, intense heat or cold, and arterial or venous stasis are some causes of simple ulcers (local ulcers with no severe inflammation or pain). Ulcers may also occur as a complication of varicose veins, in which stasis of blood leads to inflammation, necrosis, and sloughing of tissue, or they may be caused by a specific disease such as SYPHILIS or lupus. Ulcers of the stomach or duodenum are caused by the effect of gastric acid and pepsin. The secretion from these sores contains the causative agent *Treponema pallidum.*

ulceration The development or formation of an ulcer; an ulcer.

ultrasensitive Usually refers to viral load tests that can detect 50 or fewer copies of HIV RNA per cubic millimeter.

ultrasonic cardiography See ECHOCARDIOGRAPHY.

ultrasonography The use of ultrasonic waves to make an image of an organ or tissue by recording the echoes or pulses of the waves as they are reflected by the tissues.

ultraviolet Beyond the visible spectrum at its violet end; said of radiation whose wavelength is between that of violet light and roentgen rays (X RAYS).

ultraviolet light Some people in the HIV community believe that there is a danger in exposure to sunlight and artificial tanning lights and that their potential for immune suppression and viral activation may play a role in accelerating the virus's activity. It is a generally held belief that ultraviolet (UV) radiation harms the immune system. However, studies have not shown any clinical difference in those who have exposure to tanning beds and those HIV positive people who do not. A significant number of HIV-infected individuals have dermatological conditions that may be treated with PUVA (psoralen ultraviolet-A light) therapy. These include psoriasis and eosinophillic folliculitis. Some treatments of seasonal affective disorder (SAD) have been treated with UVB light. Tanning beds typically employ UV lights of both ranges, and both are received through sunlight also.

umbilicus The umbilical cord, the structure that connects the fetus to the placenta.

unblind   To reveal the treatment assignment of an individual patient or group of patients to an individual or group of individuals associated with the trial (e.g., patients, study physicians, or a treatment effects monitoring committee) who have heretofore been denied this information.

uncontrolled clinical trial   A clinical trial that does not involve a control treatment. Also, any research study in which there are no participants taking a placebo or an alternate therapy and followed over the same period as those in the treated group.

undetectable   See LIMIT OF DETECTION.

unemployed parent   In the AFDC (AID TO FAMILIES WITH DEPENDENT CHILDREN) program, the highest-earning parent unemployed over 30 days, whose unemployment qualifies even a two-parent family for AFDC and MEDICAID, if they are also poor.

uniform treatment allocation   A scheme in which the assignment probability of any one treatment group is the same as that of every other treatment group in a trial.

universal precautions   In 1985, the CENTERS FOR DISEASE CONTROL AND PREVENTION (CDC) developed the strategy of "universal blood and body fluid precautions" to address concerns regarding transmission of HIV in the HEALTH CARE setting. Now referred to simply as "universal precautions," the concept stresses that all patients should be assumed to be infectious for HIV, HBV, and other bloodborne PATHOGENS. In hospitals and other health care settings, universal precautions should be followed when workers are exposed to blood, certain other body fluids (amniotic fluid, pericardial fluid, peritoneal fluid, pleural fluid, synovial fluid, cerebrospinal fluid, semen, and vaginal secretions), or any body fluid visibly contaminated with blood. Since HIV and HBV transmission has not been documented from exposure to feces, nasal secretions, sputum, sweat, tears, urine, and vomitus, universal precautions do not apply to these fluids, or to saliva, except in the dental setting, where it is likely to be contaminated with blood. The precautions recommend that because the unpredictable nature of exposures encountered by emergency and public safety workers may make differentiation between hazardous and nonhazardous body fluids difficult or impossible, these workers should treat all body fluids as potentially hazardous when they encounter them. Part I of the CDC's published "Guidelines for Prevention of Transmission of Human Immunodeficiency Virus (HIV) and Hepatitis B Virus (HBV) to Health-Care and Public-Safety Workers" addresses disinfection (of equipment and surfaces), decontamination (of hands, soiled linen, protective clothing), and disposal (of needles and sharps, infective waste). Fire and emergency medical procedures and equipment are also addressed (gloves, masks, eyewear, gowns, resuscitation equipment), as are other considerations, such as handling bodies, autopsies, and forensic requirements. Part II, "Recommendations for Preventing Transmission of Human Immunodeficiency Virus (HIV) and Hepatitis B Virus (HBV) During Exposure-Prone Invasive Procedures," discusses infection control during surgery and other invasive procedures, including oral, cardiothoracic, colorectal, and obstetric/gynecologic procedures, as well as digital palpation of needle tips in body cavities or any procedure involving simultaneous presence of a health care worker's fingers and a needle or other sharp instrument in a poorly visualized or highly confined anatomic site.

The most commonly referenced principles of universal precautions include appropriate handwashing, protective barriers, and care in the use and disposal of needles and other sharp instruments. These should be maintained rigorously in all health care settings. Proper application of universal precautions is designed to minimize the risk of transmission from patient to health care worker, health care worker to patient, and patient to patient. "Recommendations for Preventing Transmission of Human Immunodeficiency Virus and Hepatitis B Virus to Patients During Exposure-Prone Invasive Procedures" were published in the *Morbidity and Mortality Weekly Report (MMWR)* 40 (no. RR-8), 1991.

The CDC's "Guidelines for Prevention of Transmission of Human Immunodefiency Virus and Hepatitis B Virus to Health-Care and Public-Safety

Workers" was published in *MMWR* 38 (No. S-6), 1989 (http://www.cdc.gov/epo/mmwr/preview/mmwrhtml/00001450.htm).

unlabeled uses Generally accepted uses of a drug that are not currently included in FOOD AND DRUG ADMINISTRATION approved labeling.

unprotected sex Sexual intercourse without the use of a condom or other prophylactic or contraceptive device.

unsafe sex Dangerous or risky sex. Unsafe sex is essentially UNPROTECTED SEX.

While the concept of "SAFE SEX" has been around since the early 1980s and the basic priorities of prevention have changed little since then, there is currently disagreement about how "safe" and "unsafe" should be defined. The biggest arguments involve oral sex, the condom-every-time message, and the pros and cons of negotiation between partners. Ultimately the arguments are over a question on which no one is an expert: how much risk is acceptable? For years the major prevention organizations and government agencies said none. By most accounts, a significant number of men, both gay and straight, have simply ignored the advice or have set a goal of safer rather than absolutely safe sex. It is difficult to draw conclusions, however, since for many reasons government agencies remain reluctant to fund research into infection trends, risk, and prevention, so most information remains anecdotal.

up-regulation An increase in the rate at which a process occurs, a substance is released, and so on.

uracil One of the pyrimidine nucleic acid bases that make up nucleotides, the building blocks of genetic material. Uracil takes the place of thymine (T) in RNA.

Ureaplasma A genus of GRAM-NEGATIVE bacteria found in the human genitourinary tract, throat, and/or rectum. *Ureaplasma* may be sexually transmitted and is a cause of nongonococcal urethritis. Left untreated, infection can lead to inflammation of the prostate in men and pelvic inflammatory disease in women.

uremia A toxic condition caused by chronic or acute renal failure, resulting in an excessive amount of nitrogenous substances in the blood that are normally excreted by the kidneys; the constellation of symptoms associated with this condition, including anorexia, nausea, and vomiting.

ureter The long tube that carries urine from the kidney to the bladder.

urethra The tube that carries urine from the bladder out of the body. In the female it ends at the urethral opening in the vestibule between the vagina and clitoris. In the male it goes through the penis, where it also serves as the passage for semen.

urethritis Infection of the urethra.

uridine A nucleoside of uracil.

urinalysis A laboratory test performed on urine to detect disease.

urinary tract The four-part system, including two kidneys, two ureters, the bladder, and the urethra, that creates, processes, and removes urine from the body.

urinary tract infection (UTI) Infections of the urinary tract are usually caused by bacteria, such as *Escherichia coli*, which travel from the colon to the urethra and bladder (and occasionally to the kidneys). Low resistance, poor diet, stress, and damage to the urethra from childbirth, surgery, catheterization, and so on can predispose individuals to infection. Often a sudden increase in sexual activity triggers symptoms. UTIs recur frequently in males and females. Pregnant women are especially susceptible (pressure of the growing fetus keeps some urine in the bladder and uterus, allowing bacteria to grow), as are postmenopausal women (because of hormonal changes). Older men are susceptible due to benign enlarged prostates. This can cause obstruction of the urethra and lead to infection. The incidence and severity of UTIs in HIV-positive people is somewhat greater than in the general population. HIV-positive women get more frequent infections at a younger age than their counterparts. UTIs may also be referred to as bladder infections.

urine A yellow fluid, produced in the kidneys and passed through the urinary tract, in which waste is excreted from the body. In healthy persons, urine is amber color with a slightly acid reaction. Urine is sterile and nontoxic, except in one who is suffering from an infection. Changes in the quantity, color, transparency, odor, proteinuria (the amount of protein found in urine), specific gravity, or acidity of urine are often significant as indicators of the presence of certain substances or of certain conditions or diseases.

urine culture A laboratory test that shows what bacteria are present in a sample of urine by creating ideal conditions for their growth.

urophilia The erotic attraction to urine; the desire to be urinated upon or to urinate upon a sex partner.

urticaria Itchy, raised swollen areas on the skin or mucous membranes, often a manifestation of an allergic reaction. Commonly referred to as *hives*.

us and them The "us"/"them" dichotomy is part of the familiar system of social classification—the way "difference" or "differentness" is conceived and made sense of—to which the discourse of AIDS, like other social discourse, is assimilated. Other such oppositions are "self and other," "heterosexual and homosexual," "homosexual and general population," "active and passive," and so forth. The effect of such reflexive opposition is to isolate the self ("general population") from the other ("AIDS victims"), justifying indifference to or unequal treatment of the other. See STIGMA.

uterus The major female reproductive organ that nurtures the fetus during pregnancy. The lining of the uterus is excreted during the menstrual period. This is a possible site of infection.

UTI See URINARY TRACT INFECTION.

uveitis Inflammation of the uvea, the vascular middle coat of the eye within the outer part (the sclera). Anterior uveitis is an inflammation of the frontal membranes (e.g., the iris and the choroid). Pain and redness characterize the condition.

VA   See DEPARTMENT OF VETERANS AFFAIRS.

vaccination   The act of receiving or administering a VACCINE, for the purpose of provoking active immunity against a specific infection or disease.

vaccine   A suspension of infectious agents, or some part of them, given for the purpose of establishing resistance to an infectious disease. Vaccines stimulate an immune response in the body by creating antibodies or activated T lymphocytes (see T CELL) capable of controlling the organism. The result is more or less permanent protection against a disease. There are four general classes of vaccines: those containing living attenuated infectious organisms; those containing infectious agents killed by physical or chemical means; those containing living fully virulent organisms; or those containing soluble parts of microorganisms. Vaccines are given by mouth or by injection. BCG (bacillus of Calmette and Guérin), cholera, DPT (diphtheria, pertussis, tetanus), hemophilus influenza B, hepatitis B, influenza, measles, mumps, plague, pneumococcal vaccine, polio, rabies, Rh immune globulin rubella (German measles), smallpox, typhoid, and yellow fever are examples of vaccines. The age administered and booster schedule vary for each vaccine.

Dr. Jonas Salk, the famous polio researcher, was the first to suggest vaccination of HIV-infected people with HIV vaccine products. Today most clinicians, researchers, and scientists would agree that a preventive HIV vaccine is the world's best hope of ending the AIDS pandemic. Many scientists currently believe that finding a safe and effective vaccine is possible. The need for an HIV vaccine is most acute in developing countries, where 90 percent of all new HIV infections are occurring. And the epidemic is expanding rapidly in many of those countries. For worldwide use, an anti-HIV vaccine should be inexpensive and easy to administer; should be easy to transport and store; should include long-lasting immunity with a single immunization and require few, if any, booster doses; should be compatible with other vaccines; and should provide protection against many strains of HIV.

In 1997 then-president Bill Clinton challenged scientists and researchers to develop an AIDS vaccine within 10 years. Researchers remain hopeful of achieving that goal, noting that progress toward the development of a vaccine to prevent HIV infection or of slowing the progression of disease if the vaccinated person does become infected is encouraging. Diverse approaches to vaccine design are being actively pursued, including advances and refinements of vaccines based on HIV surface proteins, DNA vaccines, vaccines using HIV functional proteins, combination vaccines, and novel vaccines that stimulate both components of the immune system (antibody and cell-mediated responses). The pipeline of innovative concepts continues to generate new possibilities for a preventive vaccine. Several experimental approaches have shown considerable promise in animal model tests; several of these candidates will soon move, or already have moved, into phase I safety trials in humans. In addition, expansion of trials of candidate vaccines that are already being tested in humans will be considered in the next few years.

HIV is very different from all other viruses against which vaccines have been developed, and HIV infection is different in important ways from other viral infections. These differences include the following:

• Since the immune system of an HIV-infected individual does not spontaneously clear the virus from his or her body, the question of what constitutes an effective immune response to HIV is unanswered. Cell-mediated immunity is thought to be more important than antibody-mediated immunity to controlling HIV infection. In contrast, existing vaccines primarily stimulate antibody-mediated immunity and only to a lesser degree cell-mediated immunity. Furthermore, there is no ideal animal model available that exactly mimics the human immune response.

- Compared to most other viral infections, HIV infection establishes itself quickly in the body. A successful HIV vaccine might have to prepare the immune system to respond exceptionally quickly to the virus.

- HIV mutates frequently. This means that although all HIV particles have the same basic structure, their various proteins can differ slightly from one virus particle to the next. Whereas the immune responses generated by a vaccine would recognize the proteins of the HIV strain(s) used to make the vaccine, they might not recognize genetic variants of HIV.

- There are multiple subtypes of HIV worldwide. It is unlikely that a single vaccine will protect against all of them. Thus, several vaccines will probably be needed, each protecting a few subtypes or perhaps even only one of them.

- Other than the rare, protected, impractical, and costly chimpanzee, no animal has yet been found to experience an AIDS-like immune deficiency when given HIV. The best animal model currently available is the macaque infected with the simian immunodeficiency virus (SIV), which results in an AIDS-like disease. SIV is closely related to HIV, but it is nevertheless a different virus. So although vaccine experiments with SIV are useful, they cannot indicate the safety or effectiveness of a vaccine designed for use against humans.

In addition to the difficulties noted, ethical, legal, and economic hurdles have dampened the pharmaceutical industry's interest in development of an HIV vaccine.

To date, some of the most central issues remain unsolved. Researchers have yet to agree on the so-called correlates of protection, what sort of measurable immune response—blood-borne versus mucosal, antibody versus cellular—a vaccine should trigger to confer protective immunity to HIV. Vaccines against other diseases have been developed without settling the "correlates" question, but human testing of HIV vaccines is bogged down by this controversy. Additionally, scientists have not created a generally accepted animal model for more direct testing of vaccine-generated protection.

There are several obstacles in developing a vaccine to prevent AIDS. One obstacle is that HIV is genetically diverse in populations and also mutates within infected individuals. This means that a vaccine will need to protect a person against many different strains of the virus. In addition, HIV infects helper T cells, the immune cells that orchestrate the immune response. It is very difficult to design a vaccine that, to be effective, must activate the very cells that are infected by the virus.

A second obstacle is that HIV is transmitted both as free virus as well as by infected cells. This suggests that both arms of the immune system—antibodies that clear free virus and cell-meditated responses that kill HIV-infected cells—may have to be stimulated to provide protection. More information on the immunological characteristics of HIV infection and ways to induce broadly reactive immune responses is needed.

A third problem is that the most common means of human infection is sex. During sex the virus directly infects cells in the mucous membranes of the sexual organs. It is likely that cytotoxic lymphocytes (CTLs) in the bloodstream are not enough to achieve full protection from sexual exposure of HIV. The activation of specific mucosal responses will be required too. Stopping this route of infection—ensuring mucosal protection whether through vaccines or topical anti-HIV microbicides—calls for cellular immunity, a quite distinct arm of the immune system that employs antibodies in the fluid surrounding mucous membranes as well as marauding white blood cells called killer T cells. (Virus that is transmitted directly into the bloodstream as a free-floating particle is easier to stop: An effective vaccine must produce the kind of antibodies that circulate in the blood, ready to neutralize the invader before it infects cells.)

Fourth, we do not know at this point whether a vaccine that works in the United States will also work in other countries. To develop a vaccine to prevent AIDS, studies need to include populations around the world, sometimes with the same candidate vaccines or strategies. In a similar vein, we do not know now whether a vaccine that works in one racial or ethnic population will work in other racial or ethnic populations. To develop a vaccine to prevent AIDS HIV clinical studies need to include participants from different races and ethnicities reflective of not only the U.S. population but global populations. Recruitment efforts for an efficacy trial must therefore include various racial and ethnic populations, including those people at an increased risk of becoming infected with HIV.

A final obstacle is a risk inherent to all killed-virus vaccines. Suppose by accident some virus escapes being killed? The 1950s witnessed such a catastrophe when a manufacturing error loosed into the population a number of doses of Salk vaccine that contained live virus; they caused a rash of vaccine-induced polio that almost derailed the fight against the disease. With AIDS, the consequences of such a mistake could even be more devastating. All viruses subvert cells by ordering them to make new viral offspring instead of new cells. But the AIDS virus takes subdivision one step further: It not only invades the cell, it splices the genes into those on the cell and then hides there indefinitely, invisible to the immune system. All it might take to cause disease, then, is a single escapee, just one live virus.

Participants in the AIDS vaccine wars have included researchers who focus on primates as well as those who focus on people already infected with the virus. In 1986, Daniel Zagury of Pierre and Marie Curie University in Paris and Robert Gallo of the National Cancer Institute, began a series of experiments to try to immunize humans against HIV. Their experiments involved injecting people who already had symptoms with a genetically engineered vaccine containing an HIV envelope protein. The vaccine incorporated the HIV protein into the harmless vaccinia virus, originally used in smallpox inoculations, which has become an all-purpose carrier for engineered vaccines. Soon afterward, Zagury expanded the study to include uninfected volunteers. One year later, albeit with the help of an impractical regimen of booster shots, it was clear that the vaccine could indeed beef up immune defenses against HIV. Zagury himself served as one of the volunteers in the experiment.

Jonas Salk, who died in 1995, took a rather similar tack, arguing that since AIDS symptoms typically do not develop until years after the initial infection, there may be a way to augment the body's immune defenses before it's too late. He called this approach immunotherapy, to distinguish it from what people conventionally think of as a vaccine. Salk began with the premise that once in the body, HIV's main mode of spread is not through the bloodstream but from cell to cell. Infected cells often fuse with healthy ones to form unwieldy clumps filled with virus. By destroying diseased cells much of the resident virus may also be destroyed. Salk's team, who continue his research, thus hopes to prevent disease in people already infected by shoring up their immune system's ability to destroy infected cells—so-called cellular immunity. The researchers are relying on the proven techniques that served Salk so well with his polio vaccine. In contrast to Zagury and others who are using genetically engineered vaccines containing pieces of HIV, Salk's preparation contains the actual killed virus. In a further departure from the approach favored by others, Salk's killed virus contains no envelope proteins. Salk's team is after the destruction of infected cells rather than free-floating virus, so the loss of the outer proteins may not be crucial.

To learn more about HIV vaccine clinical trials, go to http://www.nih.niaids.gov/vaccines, the National Institutes of Health website.

vaccine development When scientists first proved in 1984 that HIV causes AIDS, a vaccine race quickly spun into action with high hopes that the world would soon have a means to stop the epidemic. To date, an HIV/AIDS vaccine remains an elusive goal. An understanding of AIDS vaccine development begins with discussion of the process of vaccine development itself.

In the face of any infectious disease, vaccine development begins with the observation that some infected people recover from infection and are protected thereafter from development of the same infection. Microbiologists then isolate and identify the microbe responsible for the infection.

Next, they must determine which proteins belonging to the microbe are the most important for stimulating the protective immune response.

Other scientists, meanwhile, study the immune response itself to determine its nature. They want to know, for example, whether antibody-mediated immunity or cell-mediated immunity is more important in conferring protection against the microbe. This information is known as the correlates of immunity. Identifying the correlates of immunity may require several years of research.

Knowledge about the microbe's antigens and its correlates of immunity is then used to develop candidate vaccines. These in turn are tested in laboratory animals, a phase of vaccine development known as preclinical testing. Preclinical testing is essential for demonstrating the safety and degree of protection offered by a candidate vaccine before the vaccine is tested in humans.

Not just any species of laboratory animal can be used for preclinical vaccine testing. It must be an animal that when infected by the microbe contracts a disease that is similar to the disease in humans, and, in the case of HIV, it must do so within a practical period of time. Furthermore, the animal should have an immune response to the microbe that is similar to the immune response in humans: that is, the correlates of immunity should be the same in the animal and humans.

During preclinical testing, researchers give the candidate vaccine to animals and study the strength and durability of the resulting immune response. They wait weeks, months, or even years, and then expose vaccinated and unvaccinated animals to a live form of the microbe to measure the candidate vaccine's success in protecting the animal against the specific disease. Scientists refer to this step as challenging the animals.

If animal testing shows that a candidate vaccine is safe and effective, a vaccine developer (in the United States it is usually a pharmaceutical company) applies to the U.S. FOOD AND DRUG ADMINISTRATION for approval to begin testing in humans. The pharmaceutical company must also develop a safe, efficient, and cost-effective method for manufacturing the candidate vaccine in large quantity. No effective vaccine against HIV/AIDS has yet been developed. Developing one is a particularly difficult challenge because the virus is constantly mutating. To be effective, a vaccine would have to protect against a variety of types. One obstacle to developing a vaccine is the lack of a laboratory animal that develops AIDS after infection with HIV. Such an animal would make it much easier to test potential vaccines. Since that animal has not been found yet, scientists have to rely on human volunteers. Moreover, the biggest scientific obstacle faced in developing an HIV vaccine is that the correlates of immunity—the specific immune responses that might protect an individual from HIV—have thus far proven elusive. Tough questions such as What if a flawed vaccine caused a volunteer to develop AIDS? and How do you determine whether a vaccine works? raise serious barriers to research, and many fear that there may never be an effective vaccine against HIV. At the very least, it will take years to develop.

Developing a vaccine against the AIDS virus has been the chief goal of AIDS vaccine science. The traditional view of an HIV/AIDS vaccine required that it provided "sterilizing immunity," which means that it would prevent an individual from becoming infected with the virus. Vaccines for other viral diseases only prevent the development of acute illness, not infection itself, but this approach has been perceived as extremely risky in the case of HIV. One of the new goals of HIV/AIDS vaccine development is to prevent "disease," not infection. Another goal of vaccine research today is the development of vaccine-like agents designed to boost the defenses of people who are already infected.

Investigators have observed that a high HIV setpoint (the HIV level attained after primary infection) is associated with rapid disease progression, while a low setpoint is associated with slow progression. If a drug or vaccine is developed that can push down this initial steady state, disease progression might be slowed to a very low rate, even though an individual would remain chronically infected. Since viral load also is associated with infectiousness, a vaccine that merely limited the HIV setpoint would have substantial epidemiological impact by reducing the rate of HIV transmission. The most immediate implication for HIV vaccine research is the possibility of using plasma viral load as an endpoint measurement for vaccine evaluation studies in primates.

In another retreat from the absolutism of sterilizing immunity, the National Institute of Allergy and Infectious Diseases (NIAID) is now talking of "preventive trials" as opposed to "vaccine trials." Purportedly, this new emphasis is a recognition that behavioral modification and physical and chemical barriers are also keys to preventing HIV infection.

In an interview published in the September 1995 issue of *AIDS Agenda,* Dr. Jack Killen, director of NIAID's division of AIDS, reported that many remain optimistic that an effective vaccine against HIV can be developed. Killian outlined the criteria of an "ideal" HIV vaccine. An ideal HIV vaccine would be safe and produce few side effects; produce strong immune responses against all subtypes of HIV to which an individual is likely to be exposed; provide long-lasting protection against all potential routes of infection, especially infection at the vaginal and rectal mucosa; be inexpensive to manufacture; and be easily stored and administered anywhere in the world.

Dr. Killen felt that progress toward such a vaccine would be made in incremental steps, through fundamental research and clinical trials of multiple vaccine approaches. He claimed that the biggest scientific obstacle faced in developing an HIV vaccine was the fact that the correlates of immunity—the specific immune responses that might protect an individual from HIV—have thus far proved elusive. Continuing advances in our understanding of the basic biology of HIV disease would facilitate the design of a safe and effective vaccine.

Scientists have been searching for an HIV vaccine since 1987, when the first clinical trial opened at the National Institutes of Health. But so far, researchers have been stumped. Nine subtypes of the virus, which mutate once they are inside the body, make developing a working vaccine challenging.

There are four core goals of HIV vaccine clinical trials: safety, sterilizing immunity to HIV or reversal and clearance of HIV infection, long-term control of HIV infections, and new scientific knowledge about potential vaccine safety and efficacy. Additionally, HIV vaccine clinical trials have three goals related to global use: practicality for global use and impact, effectiveness in many countries and communities, and use of vaccines with broader prevention and treatment efforts.

Clinical trials test the safety and effectiveness of a drug, vaccine, or medical device. Doctors and other health professionals run clinical trials according to strict rules set by the U.S. Food and Drug Administration. FDA rules ensure that the people who agree to participate in the studies are treated as safely as possible.

There are two types of HIV vaccine clinical trials: therapeutic and preventive. Therapeutic vaccines are for people who are already infected with HIV. Therapeutic vaccines test to see whether a vaccine will prevent HIV from weakening the immune system of the person it resides in. A preventive vaccine would protect a person from becoming infected with the virus, even if the person were exposed to it. It should be noted that with many diseases, individuals can be exposed to the virus that causes the disease but not become infected.

There are three phases of clinical trials. Phase I trials of HIV vaccine candidates are conducted domestically and internationally with people who have a low risk of becoming infected with HIV. Phase I trials have a small number of participants, usually fewer than 50 people. These studies test vaccines for safety and ability to stimulate an immune response and provide data that will assist in determining which vaccine should be advanced into larger phase II trials. Phase I trials usually last 12 to 18 months.

Phase II trials usually have hundreds of participants (both low- and high-risk individuals) and are conducted at a larger number of U.S. and international sites. Phase II trials expand on testing in phase I trials to include people who engage in behavior that puts them at high risk for acquiring HIV; test subjects may include injection drug users and people who have unprotected sex and/or multiple sex partners. Phase II trials usually last about two years.

Phase III trials are conducted on a large scale with thousands of participants at many sites. Participants include people who engage in high-risk behavior. The purpose of phase III trials is to determine efficacy (how well or efficiently a vaccine works) and what type of immune response occurs. Phase III trials usually last three to four years.

Each trial has different guidelines about who can be enrolled. Most studies, however, require that participants be in good health and between the ages of 18 and 60 years. A history of serious allergic reactions or some medical conditions may exclude a participant as well as use of certain prescription medications.

Before joining a clinical trial, a potential participant must be informed of all the risks and of his or her responsibilities as a participant. Informed consent requires the participant's signed agreement to participate in the trial. Before signing any documents, participants are asked whether they understand and accept every component of the trial. A written description of the study, along with the opportunity to ask questions, are always provided to a potential volunteer before the trial begins. A volunteer may say no to participating at any time and may drop out of the trial at any time.

Institutional review boards (IRBs), data monitoring committees, Food and Drug Administration inspections, and community advisory boards (CABs) provide four means of protection for volunteers. Scientists, doctors, and others from the local community, including lay persons, serve on IRBs to review and monitor their hospital's or research institution's medical research involving people. They monitor studies to help make sure that there is the least possible risk to volunteers and that the risks are reasonable in relation to the expected benefits. IRBs make sure that volunteer selection is fair and that informed consent is obtained correctly.

Data monitoring committees are used mainly when one treatment is being compared with another treatment and in studies in which treatments are selected for patients at random. These committees are particularly important in double-blind studies of treatments for serious or life-threatening diseases. These experts review information from studies to make sure they are being done in a way that is safest for the volunteers. During a study, if the committee finds that the treatment is harmful or of no benefit, it stops the study. If there is evidence that one treatment gives a greater benefit than another, the committee stops the study, and all volunteers are offered the better treatment.

The Food and Drug Administration routinely inspects the records of various scientists, clinics, and other research sites involved in a study. It aims to make sure volunteers are being protected and stud-

ies are being done correctly. From time to time, such inspections are done in response to complaints.

Almost every trial has a community advisory board, which is a voluntary organization of individuals who are participating in a clinical trial or who are members of the local community who are interested in HIV clinical trials. CABs serve as the eyes and ears of the community, providing education and serving as the liaison between vaccine volunteers and the staff at the trial site.

Several approaches have been used in the preparation of the various candidate vaccines that have undergone either phase I or phase I and phase II testing in humans—subunit vaccines based on HIV envelope proteins, synthetic peptide vaccines, recombinant subunit vaccines, and live recombinant vector vaccines.

- Candidate vaccines based on the gp120 envelope protein have been among the most widely tested. Two of them have gone through phase I and phase II testing, but in June 1994 the National Institutes of Health decided not to proceed with phase III testing. The vaccines were faulted for their inability to produce neutralizing antibodies and to elicit cell-mediated immune responses.

- Synthetic peptide candidate vaccines consist of short chains of amino acids, peptides, which are assembled by machines. The structure of the synthetic peptides mimics that of small fragments of certain HIV proteins. These fragments are believed to be those to which neutralizing antibodies bind. The so-called V3 loop, for example, is a fragment of the HIV gp120 envelope protein that is important to that protein's function. At least two candidate synthetic peptide vaccines mimicking portions of the V3 loop that are common to several strains of HIV have undergone early testing in humans. However, this type of vaccine has elicited only weak antibody responses and has not stimulated cell-mediated immunity.

- Recombinant subunit vaccines use viral proteins produced by using recombinant DNA technology. Recombinant gp160 proteins and p24 proteins have been tested in early clinical trials. Their apparent drawback resides in a component of the recombinant product that is subtly different from that of the natural HIV proteins. As a result, the antibodies elicited by the recombinant proteins did not effectively neutralize strains of HIV that are commonly transmitted.

- Live recombinant vector vaccines use a non-disease-causing virus—an avirulent virus, other than HIV, in which certain genes from HIV have been inserted through recombinant DNA technology. The avirulent virus serves merely as a vehicle, or vector, that carries the HIV genes, along with its own, into body cells. There, the avirulent virus replicates harmlessly but produces both its own proteins and those encoded by the HIV genes. In theory, all the viral proteins should elicit an immune response, including a response against HIV proteins. Vaccinia and canarypox viruses are two live recombinant vector vaccines currently undergoing development and early testing.

Vaccine strategies undergoing laboratory study include attenuated live-HIV vaccines, DNA vaccines, and pseudovirions.

- Attenuated live-virus vaccines use a weakened form of the virus. The virus actually replicates within cells of the host, but without causing disease. In this way, attenuated live-virus vaccines imitate a natural infection and activate both cell-mediated and antibody-mediated arms of the immune system. As a result, these vaccines are very effective—attenuated live-virus vaccines are used to protect children against measles, mumps, rubella, and polio and were successful in eradicating smallpox. The feasibility of an attenuated live-HIV vaccine has been tested by using simian immunodeficiency virus (SIV) in macaques. Note that attenuated live-virus vaccines carry an important risk: they can sometimes mutate back to a virulent form.
- DNA vaccines are made up of rings of harmless bacterial DNA that also include one or two viral genes. The viral genes are spliced into the rings of bacterial DNA by recombinant techniques. When the vaccine is injected into muscle, the DNA rings are taken up by body cells. If all goes well, the cells begin producing the viral proteins,

which then elicit immune responses that will protect against the virus. Furthermore, because the cells that have taken up the DNA produce viral proteins, the proteins are displayed on the cell surface, which activates the cell-mediated immune response. Thus, they can elicit both cell-mediated and antibody-mediated immune responses. DNA vaccines have a number of advantages over other types of vaccines: they may be safer for individuals with a compromised immune system, they are easier to prepare, and they do not require refrigeration. For these reasons, DNA vaccines could potentially be produced in large quantities and distributed worldwide at reasonable cost.

- Research on attenuated live-virus HIV candidate vaccines has led to the finding that the gag gene of HIV may itself direct the assembly of viruslike particles. These particles—known as pseudovirions, or false viruses—have much of the outer structure of a normal HIV particle but do not contain genetic material. Pseudovirions, therefore, cannot replicate, but they do display many important HIV antigens.

Today there are numerous groups involved in vaccine advocacy. These include community groups, such as the AIDS Vaccine Advocacy Coalition (AVAC); government agencies, such as the Centers for Disease Control and Prevention, Food and Drug Administration, National Institutes of Health, and United States Agency for International Development; and international agencies, such as, Global Alliance for Vaccines and Immunizations, Global Fund for AIDS, Tuberculosis and Malaria, International AIDS Vaccine Initiative, and the United Nations Programme on HIV/AIDS. Other key players include various bodies of the National Institutes of Health (NIH), such as the AIDS Vaccine Research Committee (an advisory group); the Comprehensive International Program of Research on AIDS (a program); the HIV Vaccine Trials Network, an NIH-funded trial network; the National Cancer Institute, an NIH institute; and the Office of AIDS Research, an NIH office; as well as the Vaccine Research Center, an NIH center. Note too the involvement of the U.S. military at the Walter Reed Army Institute of Research.

vaccine memory The ability of the body to recall memory cells to fight antigen that the body has been vaccinated against.

vaccinia Vaccinia virus is the virus used in the smallpox VACCINE. Since smallpox has been eliminated in the world, except in laboratory samples, it is little used currently in general medicine. It is under development as a vector (a transporter that carries a virus to the body) in a number of vaccines for other diseases. The variety of vaccinia that is being tested in new vaccines is a much less virulent strain of the virus than was used in the smallpox vaccine.

vaccinology A science encompassing all aspects of vaccine from its conception in the laboratory to its production by companies and its application and distribution in the field.

vacular myelopathy See MYELOPATHY.

vacuole A clear place in the substance of a cell. Sometimes it is degenerative in character; sometimes it surrounds a foreign body and serves as a temporary stomach for digestion of that foreign matter. Also, minute space found in any tissue.

vagina The organ in women leading from the vulva to the uterus. The vagina serves as the passage for the intromission of the penis, for the reception of semen, and for the discharge of the menstrual flow, as well as the passageway through which the fetus is delivered. Slang terms include beaver, box, cunt, honey pot, manhole, pussy, quiff, quim, and Velcro triangle.

vaginal candidiasis See CANDIDIASIS.

vaginal discharge Abnormal vaginal secretions. Healthy vaginal secretions are made up of aging cell cast off from the vaginal walls, secretions from the cervix that help protect the uterus from infection and aid in fertility, and chemicals produced by vaginal bacteria and fungi. Normal vaginal secretion is clear and/or white. Different conditions can cause the discharge to become different colors. If a color change from what is normal for an individual occurs, a doctor should perform an examination to determine the cause. Any abnormal aromas of the vaginal area also need to be investigated by a doctor. Abnormal discharge can be due to infection and is frequently associated with pain, burning, itching, and painful urination. PELVIC INFLAMMATORY DISEASE (PID), HERPES GENITALIS, other STDs, infection of the inside of the uterus, and inflammation of the vagina due to lack of estrogen are other possible causes of vaginal discharge.

vaginal douche See DOUCHE.

vaginal fluid All women secrete moisture and mucus from membranes that line the vagina. Vaginal fluids provide lubrication, help keep the vagina clean, and maintain the acidity of the vagina to prevent infections. The walls of the vagina may be almost dry to very wet. The vagina tends to be dry before puberty, during lactation, and after menopause, as well as during the part of the menstrual cycle right after the flow. It tends to increase in moisture around ovulation time, during pregnancy, and when the person is sexually aroused. When a woman is under stress, secretion also increases. The discharge is clear or slightly milky and may be somewhat slippery or clumpy. When dry it may be yellowish. Vaginal fluids normally cause no irritation or inflammation of the vagina or vulva.

Many bacteria grow in the vagina of a normal, healthy woman. Some of them help to keep the vagina somewhat acidic in order to prevent yeast, fungi, and other harmful organisms from multiplying out of proportion. These harmful organisms may secrete wastes that, in large amounts, irritate the vaginal walls and cause infections. At such times, there may be an abnormal discharge, mild or severe itching and burning of the vulva, chafing of the thighs, and, occasionally, frequent irritation.

HIV was first detected in the cervical secretions of HIV-infected women in 1986. Scientists reported that the virus could be cultured from secretions throughout the menstrual cycle, an indication that the presence of the virus was not merely the result of contamination with menstrual blood. Since that time it has been learned that all body fluids of infected individuals contain some amount of HIV. This is because all fluids are derived from blood, which is created in the bone marrow, that is, lymph tissue, which has the greatest concentration of HIV in the body. In male-to-female transmission of HIV, contact with infected semen leads to entry to a small opening, possibly in the cervical wall, where the blood vessels are closer to the surface. Female-to-male transmission probably results when cervical and vaginal fluids that contain HIV enter through the urethra or possible tiny cuts on the surface of the penis. As concerns prevention, although condoms and female condoms reduce the risk of infection with HIV and other venereal diseases, they do not eliminate it. The only way to eliminate risk is to prevent all exposure to infectious semen, blood, and vaginal fluids.

vaginal intercourse In heterosexual sexual intercourse, the insertion of the penis into a woman's vagina.

vaginal opening The opening to the vagina, closely protected by the labia minora.

vaginal secretion See VAGINAL FLUID.

vaginal thrush See CANDIDIASIS.

vaginal-manual intercourse A sexual practice involving placing a portion of or the entire hand in a partner's vagina.

vaginal yeast infection See CANDIDIASIS.

vaginitis An inflammation or infection of the vagina. Vaginitis occurs when the normal environment of the vulva and vagina is disturbed, usually by common bacteria. Although the vagina resists disease as well as the rest of the body, vaginal imbalance and lowered resistance to infection can be caused by poor diet; lack of sleep, exercise or cleanliness; and stress. Causes of vaginitis include trichomona virus, candida, bacterial vaginosis, and several other possibilities. The presence of vaginal pathogens may predispose women to increased frequency of herpes outbreaks or recurrences of GENITAL WARTS.

vaginosis See BACTERIAL VAGINOSIS.

valaciclovir A medication used in the treatment of HERPES ZOSTER (shingles) and HERPES SIMPLEX (genital herpes). It inhibits the replication of viral DNA that is necessary for viruses to reproduce themselves. Valaciclovir is actually a prodrug, meaning that it is not active itself against the virus. Rather, in the body it is converted to ACYCLOVIR, which is active against the viruses. It has been shown to be more effective at lower doses than acyclovir. Valaciclovir, therefore, is active against the same viruses as acyclovir but has a longer duration of action. (Trade name is Valtrex.)

valganciclovir A PRODRUG form of ganciclovir, which is taken orally. Through absorption in the body, the drug converts rapidly into ganciclovir. It has been approved for the treatment of CYTOMEGALOVIRUS (CMV) in HIV patients. It does not cure people of CMV but does slow or stop the progression of the disease, which otherwise would lead to blindness in many people. If people are taking AZT and ddI, their dosages of those drugs must be changed, as valganciclovir alter their metabolism. Side effects are similar to those of ganciclovir, so people who have had allergies to one drug should not take the other. Common side effects include diarrhea, nausea, headache, and sometimes neutropenia. Currently the drug is taken twice a day, an improvement over the intravenous administration ganciclovir, formerly used to treat CMV. (Trade name is Valcyte.)

valley fever See COCCIDIOIDOMYCOSIS.

variable In research studies, an element or condition that changes or may change in a measurable way in relation to other elements, providing a means to value and compare results. An *independent variable* is controlled by the investigator directly to allow examination of its effects; *a dependent variable* is one which is influenced by the independent variable. See DRUG TRIAL.

varicella-zoster virus (VZV) Also known as human herpesvirus-3 (HHV-3). VZV is a virus related to the HERPES SIMPLEX viruses. It is responsible for two different illnesses in humans: chicken pox (varicella) and SHINGLES (HERPES ZOSTER). Upon initial infection the virus causes chicken pox, a rash of pustules that begins typically on the body, moving outward to the arms, legs, and face. These pustules then crust over and typically disappear. It is highly contagious at this point and can be spread through the air by sneezing and coughing. After the illness ends, the virus does not leave the body. It lies dormant in the ganglia, the "nerve roots," of the spinal cord. When the VZV is reactivated, it causes pain and a rash in the area supplied by the affected sensory nerves. This is commonly called SHINGLES. The virus typically reactivates in later years or when people have immune disorders. Shingles can be contagious to children or adults who have not had chicken pox if they have contact with the broken blisters caused in shingles. Someone who has had shingles is most unlikely to contract it again; it recurs in only 4 percent of adults. People with compromised immune systems may, however, have recurring cases, though in a different location from the first outbreak.

vas deferens   The tube that transfers sperm from the testicles to the seminal vesicles.

vasectomy   The surgical severing of the vas deferens, usually as a means to prevent conception. Vasectomy leaves the man's genital system basically unchanged. His sexual hormones remain operative, and there is no noticeable difference in his ejaculate because sperm makes up only a small part of the semen. A vasectomy does not offer protection from HIV transmission during a sexual encounter. The semen of an HIV-positive man can transmit HIV regardless of whether or not a man has had a vasectomy.

VD   See SEXUALLY TRANSMITTED DISEASE.

VDRL   See VENEREAL DISEASE RESEARCH LABORATORIES TEST.

vector   A carrier or means of transport. A disease vector is a carrier that moves a disease-causing agent from one organism to another. An example

of a disease vector is a mosquito. A viral vector is an engineered virus used to introduce genes into an organism; it can also be a live virus used in a vaccine to insert an antigen into an organism and generate an immune response.

vector vaccine   A vaccine using a non-disease-causing virus or bacterium to transport HIV or other foreign genes into the body. The GENOMES of these "vector" viruses, including HIV DNA, integrate into the host cell's genetic machinery.

Venereal Disease Research Laboratories (VDRL) test   A laboratory test, named after the Venereal Disease Research Laboratory of the U.S. PUBLIC HEALTH SERVICE, where it was developed, for the presence of antibodies in the blood to *Treponema pallidum*, the MICROORGANISM that causes SYPHILIS. It is the only test for syphilis that uses spinal fluid in deriving its results.

venereal wart   See GENITAL WART.

verification   The process by which a benefits program or agency checks an applicant's claim of eligibility (establishes citizenship, residency, age, disability, income, and so forth).

vertical transmission   The transmission of a pathogen, or disease-causing agent, from a mother to fetus or baby during pregnancy, birth, or breast-feeding. See TRANSMISSION.

Veterans Administration   See DEPARTMENT OF VETERANS AFFAIRS.

Viagra   See SILDENAFIL.

Viatical settlements   See LIFE INSURANCE.

victim   A person who suffers from a destructive or injurious action or agency. Since the beginning of the AIDS epidemic, much energy has been expended in preventing people from referring to people living with AIDS, or HIV as "victims" or "sufferers." The emphasis today is on the empowerment of persons who are HIV+ or have AIDS:

people with HIV/AIDS are able to speak for or about themselves, and are able to determine policy despite their biased status. The term has also been condemned by AIDS activists, medical workers, and service providers because it elicits an improper emotional attitude in both volunteers and the so-called experts.

A second concern about the term "victim" is its relationship to violence. In this society, violence against persons who are HIV+ or have AIDS has occurred throughout the epidemic in varying degrees. "Blaming the victim" is a means by which society tells persons with HIV/AIDS that they caused it or brought it on themselves in some way. It is a myth that supports violence against persons with HIV/AIDS, violence which has been perpetrated by individuals and institutions. AIDS activists have, in many ways, successfully challenged victim-blaming views. People with HIV/AIDS have emerged; hiding is no longer an acceptable means for people with HIV/AIDS to protect themselves and their fellow PWAs (Persons With AIDS) from violence. Awareness of the "blame the victim" mentality is the first step toward prevention of AIDS-related violence.

victimization   To apply "victim" status to another person or to a group of people; as regards the AIDS epidemic, the victimization of persons who are HIV+ or have AIDS. See VICTIM.

vidarabine   An antiviral agent that inhibits DNA synthesis and is effective in the treatment of HERPES SIMPLEX and HERPES VARICELLA ZOSTER VIRUS. It has also been shown to be effective against HERPES SIMPLEX ENCEPHALITIS. Also called ADENINE ARABINOSIDE and ARA-A. (Trade name is Vira-A.)

Videx   See DIDEOXYINOSINE.

vif gene   One of nine genes that make up the two identical strands of RNA that compose HIV. The vif gene encodes a protein that determines how infective the virus will be. Deletion of the vif gene from the virus produces a viral particle that is a thousandfold less infective than the normal virus.

villoma   See PAPILLOMA.

villous papilloma   See PAPILLOMA.

villous tumor   See PAPILLOMA.

vinblastine   An anticancer agent used for the treatment of Hodgkin's disease, lymphoma, testicular cancer, and breast cancer. In people with HIV, it is used for the treatment of KAPOSI'S SARCOMA. Vinblastine belongs to a class of cancer drugs called vinca alkyloids, which are naturally occurring chemicals isolated from the periwinkle plant. Vinca alkyloids stop the growth of tumors by preventing cells from dividing. Although vinblastine can be used by itself to treat cancers, it is used more frequently in combination with other chemotherapy drugs. Vinblastine is available as a solution for intravenous injection. The most common side effect is reduction in the number of white blood cells, which occurs, to some extent, in virtually everyone using the drug. Hair loss occurs commonly. Constipation, loss of appetite, nausea, vomiting, abdominal pain, sore mouth, jaw pain, diarrhea, stomach bleeding, and rectal bleeding may occur. In general, side effects occur most frequently when large doses of the drug are used.

vincristine   An anticancer agent used for the treatment of a wide variety of cancers including LEUKEMIA and HODGKIN'S DISEASE. In people who have HIV infection it is used primarily as part of combination therapy for NON-HODGKIN'S LYMPHOMA and KAPOSI'S SARCOMA. Vincristine belongs to a class of cancer drugs called vinca alkyloids, which are naturally occurring chemicals isolated from the periwinkle plant. Vinca alkyloids stop the growth of tumors by preventing cells from dividing. Vincristine has a relatively low toxicity to normal cells in the BONE MARROW when compared to VINBLASTINE and is often the drug of choice for people with impaired bone marrow function. The most serious side effects of vincristine are hair loss and neurological impairment, which is often progressive. PERIPHERAL NEUROPATHY, a condition characterized by tingling numbness or pain in the extremities, is the most common side effect. See VINBLASTINE.

vincristine sulfate   A drug that prevents the development, growth, or proliferation of malignant cells, obtained from the periwinkle plant *Vinca rosea*. It has similar activity to VINBLASTINE but is more useful in the treatment of acute leukemia and lymphocytic lymphosarcoma. See VINCRISTINE.

Vira-a   See VIDARABINE.

Viracept   See NELFINAVIR.

Viral care   See CAPSID.

viral DNA   See DEOXYRIBONUCLEIC ACID.

viral encephalitis   ENCEPHALITIS caused by a VIRUS.

viral envelope   The outer shell of HIV. It is composed of two layers of fatty molecules called LIPIDS. Embedded in the viral envelope are proteins from the host cell, as well as 72 copies (on average) of a complex HIV protein that protrudes from the envelope surface. This protein, known as ENV, consists of a cap made of three or four molecules called GLYCOPROTEIN 120 (GP120) and a stem consisting of three or four GP41 molecules that anchor the structure in the viral envelope. Much of the research to develop a vaccine against HIV has focused on these envelope proteins.

viral fitness   The inherent ability of a virus to replicate and cause disease. In HIV patients who have been taking HAART, the virus that is left in the body after use of HAART is less fit than WILD-TYPE VIRUS that has not been treated. Studies showing these results may influence some patients to remain on therapy even if the DRUG REGIMEN is beginning to fail because their treated virus is less likely to replicate than the wild-type virus, which would return if they stopped treatment.

viral hepatitis   HEPATITIS caused by one of several types of VIRUSes. Hepatitis A, B, C, D, E, and G are all blood-borne viruses that can be transmitted sexually.

viral infections   Microorganisms such as viruses, bacteria, parasites, and fungi all cause OPPORTUNISTIC INFECTIONS, or SECONDARY INFECTIOUS DISEASES, in persons with AIDS. Examples of infections caused by viruses include CYTOMEGALOVIRUS, HERPES SIMPLEX VIRUS, VARICELLA-ZOSTER, EPSTEIN-BARR VIRUS, and ADENOVIRUSES.

viral interference   The inhibition of the multiplication of one type of VIRUS by the presence of another virus in the same cell.

viral load   The quantity of free virus in plasma as measured by the concentrations of HIV RNA. Treatment-associated reductions in viral load have been shown to correlate with protection from AIDS and AIDS-related death. Today, HIV viral load is increasingly employed as a SURROGATE MARKER for disease progression. It is important as a direct measure of the number of cells that are being infected and killed by HIV each day. Imagine a train, heading toward a particular destination called AIDS. The CD4 count can be imagined as a measure of the current distance to the destination and viral load as a measure of the speed of the train in getting there.

Viral load is measured by POLYMERASE CHAIN REACTION, BRANCHED DNA, and NASBA ASSAY tests and is expressed in number of HIV copies or equivalents per milliliter of blood. Approximately 1 percent to 2 percent of HIV in the body is in the blood. The other 98 percent is in lymph tissue. The blood assays are thought to depict the activity in the lymph areas accurately. Diagnostic techniques that measure the amount of HIV in the blood provide a quick assessment of the effectiveness of antiviral therapies without the need to wait for clinical ENDPOINTS (the onset of OPPORTUNISTIC INFECTIONS or death). For individual patients and their physicians, these tests may ultimately provide a way to track disease progression more clearly. An increase in someone's HIV population might indicate that current treatment has lost its effectiveness and thus point to the need to alter antiviral therapy.

Viral load is commonly checked before initiation of therapy, four to eight weeks after initiating therapy, and then every three or four months. After a patient starts a new antiviral, a consistent decrease in viral load should be seen. If viral load creeps up or increases dramatically, and assuming the patient is taking the antiviral properly, the antiviral is seen to have failed. Physicians can then think about adding or switching therapies. Research has gone back and forth between viral load and CD4 counts as the best marker of progression in HIV disease. Studies have also found that prediction of disease progression can be optimized by measuring viral load and CD4+ T-cell count before, and viral load shortly after, treatment begins. Findings indicate that AIDS is more likely to develop in individuals who have high viral loads and low CD4+ T-cell counts than in those with high viral loads and relatively higher CD4+ T-cell counts. The extent to which viral load is a stable marker in the majority of patients continues to be studied. Research has shown that HIV can be suppressed but has not shown how long and for whom. It is clear that present antiviral therapy needs further refinement, and that better understanding of the variation in viral load and its causes is needed.

viral load assay   See VIRAL LOAD.

viral load blip   Temporary spike in viral load to above 50 copies/mL that returns to undetectable levels on the next viral load test. Viral load blips are detected in 30 percent–50 percent of patients whose viral load is otherwise stable and fully suppressed. Rises in viral load may be caused by variations in the tests themselves or anything that stimulates the patient's immune system such as a vaccination or infection. Additional causes of an increase in viral load are medication noncompliance and drug–drug interactions, which may lead to resistant virus. The frequency at which blips are detected depends on the frequency at which viral load testing is performed. Even though viral load blips are most frequent among patients with more drug experience, it seems that patients who have blips are at greater risk of virologic failure than patients who do not. How to respond to these blips is still unclear because most patients who have them do return to undetectable viral levels but some do not. The role of the blips in predicting treatment failure is also unclear. The current recommendations for any REBOUND in viral load are to confirm the rise with a second test performed two weeks later and in the meantime to attempt to identify potential causes of the blip. Clinicians also recommend delaying viral load testing for at least two weeks after vaccination or infection. Several investigators agree that a viral load result of 400 copies/mL is the most suitable definition of virologic failure at present.

viral load test   See VIRAL LOAD.

viral suppression   Viral suppression is a goal of highly active antiretroviral therapy (HAART), as well as other medical therapy in HIV. Suppression is measured differently for different people. VIRAL LOAD is usually given in VIRIONS per milliliter of blood. So a count of 100,000 means 100,000 virions/mL of blood.

Changes in viral load are stated in terms of logarithmic (log) changes. *Log* is a mathematical term that represents a large number measured by a factor of 10. So if you have a viral load of 100,000 and your viral load change is −1.0 log, then your new viral load would be 10,000. A 1 log increase or decrease equals a tenfold (multiplied 10 times) adjustment, which is another way this change is often expressed. In someone who has an extremely high viral load, above 1,000,000, anything less than 10,000 viral load would be a successful result of therapy.

Many doctors seek a viral load drop of 10 times, or 1.0 log, the first month of therapy. Then they seek to suppress the viral load to below the detectable level of viral load tests within three to six months. This gives CD4 cells time to regroup and produce at a rate that can boost the body's defenses. Some people who have HIV never achieve a viral load below the 400 count that is considered the measurable level. This may mean that they have some drug resistance or are not adhering to the drug schedule. In 90 percent of people who have a drop of viral load an increase in CD4 cells also occurs.

The ultrasensitive viral load assay is more expensive and is not performed unless specifically requested. It measures viral load to less than 50 copies/mL. The standard viral load measurement tests cannot detect viral activity accurately below 400 copies/mL. Therefore, patients are generally told they have less than 400 copies/mL, or below the level of quantification, as their viral load result. If someone says an individual has an undetectable viral load, this is not quite correct. The person still has a virus that can be passed to other people, even if the viral load is below the level the test can measure.

viral test Generally, a blood test for HIV activity, and for other markers of disease severity or progression. These tests are critically important for developing new drugs and for patient care. Reliable tests might shorten the time required to show which drugs are good candidates from years to months, allowing many more potential treatments to be tested. Better viral tests could also improve medical care with the drugs we already have by showing when a course of treatment is working for an individual and when it is not, so that the physician will have rational guidance on when to add or switch therapies. Examples of viral tests include PCR (POLYMERASE CHAIN REACTION), quantitative PCR, QC-PCR (quantitative competitive PCR), BRANCHED DNA ASSAY (bDNA), P24 ANTIGEN TEST, and VIRAL CULTURES. See VIRAL ASSAY.

Viramune See NEVIRAPINE

viremia The presence of a VIRUS in blood or blood plasma. Viremia may be a qualitative as well as a quantitative measure of virus.

virion A complete viral particle existing outside a cell.

virologic failure The failure to achieve the desired degree of viral suppression (less than 50 copies/mL on some tests, less than 400 copies/mL on the most common viral load assays) or a viral rebound in a patient whose viral load had previously not been quantifiable.

virology Study of VIRUSes and viral diseases.

virucide An agent that destroys or inactivates a VIRUS.

viruria Presence of a virus in the urine as measured by urinalysis done on a sample provided by a patient.

virus Any of a large group of submicroscopic agents, or MICROBES, capable of infecting plants, animals, and bacteria, characterized by a total dependence on living cells for reproduction and a lack of independent metabolism. Unlike bacteria, viruses can neither survive nor reproduce unless they live in a cell. Viruses consist of a core of genetic material, either RNA or DNA, surrounded by a protein coat. HIV is a virus that lives in CD4 LYMPHOCYTES in humans. Viruses may be named and classified according to the host they dominate, or according to their origin, mode of transmission, manifestations, and geographic location where they were first isolated.

virus-hunting Nearly discredited by the failed war on cancer, virus-hunting is the attempt to link viruses and illness. In large part due to AIDS, virus-hunting has enjoyed a spectacular revival in the 1980s and 1990s. Within the context of AIDS, virus-hunting has become a public scientific controversy. On one side stand microbiologist Peter Duesberg and a circle of defenders who believe that the HUMAN IMMUNODEFICIENCY VIRUS (HIV) has not been proved to cause AIDS. These "dissidents" argue that HIV is an innocent bystander in the AIDS epidemic, and assert that millions of dollars have been poured into research to find vaccines and therapies, and thousands of people are poisoning themselves with toxic medications, all in the goal of obstructing a virus that doesn't make anyone sick. On the other side are mainstream AIDS researchers who insist that HIV is the primary cause of AIDS.

visceral leishmaniasis Leishmaniasis caused by *Leishmania donovani.*

visna A viral disease that affects sheep. The primary target is the CENTRAL NERVOUS SYSTEM. It is characterized by asymptomatic onset and partial paralysis of the hindlimbs, progressing to total paralysis and death.

visualization The act of viewing or sensing a picture of an object.

One of many different methods used to reach a state of relaxation. With eyes closed, one becomes completely relaxed either by another method or, for example, by visualizing walking down a shaded stairway, becoming more and more relaxed as one descends into comforting darkness.

Once relaxed, an image is brought to mind that may represent the desired change in any number of ways. Some people see themselves as being completely healthy. Others imagine the healing white blood cells as white knights charging forth, conquering the invading infections and visualizing the "bad guys" in full retreat. For those who may have trouble focusing clearly on an image, the suggestion is made to draw the desired image on paper to give it more substance and reality. The practice of visualization or imagery is recognized as one of the most powerful healing techniques available today.

vitamin   Any of a group of organic substances other than proteins, carbohydrates, fats, minerals, and organic salts that are essential for normal metabolism, growth, and development of the body. Vitamins are not sources of energy; nor do they contribute significantly to the substance of the body, but they are indispensable for the maintenance of health. Effective in minute quantities, they act principally as regulators of metabolic processes and play a role in energy transformation, usually acting as coenzymes in enzymatic systems. Vitamins may be fat-soluble or water-soluble. Fat-soluble vitamins are processed by the liver. They are generally stored for long periods in the body for use when needed. Water-soluble vitamins are processed in the kidney. They are not stored to a great extent in the body, so frequent consumption is necessary. When present in excess of the body's needs, they are excreted in the urine. See MINERALS.

vitamin A   Vitamin A, also known as retinol, was first isolated in 1913. When its chemical structure was first defined, its discoverer won the Nobel Prize in chemistry because it was the first vitamin isolated and described chemically. Vitamin A is essential for vision, for adequate growth, and for the proper development of cells and body tissues. It is particularly important in the formation of epithelial cells, which are the linings of the body (skin, cornea, and mucous membranes, among others). Deficiencies in vitamin A can cause night blindness, tumors of the eyes, and reductions in levels of white cells and red blood cells. Resistance to infection is impaired. Thus vitamin A deficiency can result in more, and more severe, diseases of many types. Vitamin A deficiency has also been related to the development of a variety of cancers. Several illnesses can cause deficiencies, particularly stomach, intestinal, and liver diseases. This is because vitamin A is fat-soluble and must be absorbed and processed in the liver, where it is stored for future use. Level of vitamin A has been shown to be deficient in many HIV-positive people. Supplementation in HIV-positive people has shown no direct influence on CD4 counts or viral load numbers. However, many practitioners believe vitamin A can act as an ADJUVANT to a healthy immune system. Beta-carotene is a PROFORM of vitamin A. It is the supplement most often used when adding vitamin A to the diet. Because beta-carotene is also a coloring (yellow-orange), one sign of excess of vitamin A is orange coloring of the skin. An excess of vitamin A can lead to severe health problems; it can cause toxicity quite quickly over the course of a few days of oversupplementation. Beta-carotene has been studied extensively and is thought to help prevent some cancers. It is not automatically stored in the body since it is a PRODRUG and is excreted when it is not needed. However, it has been linked to lung cancer in people who use tobacco. Smokers should not supplement vitamin A with beta-carotene. Foods rich in beta-carotene include carrots, yellow and dark green leafy vegetables (e.g., spinach, broccoli), pumpkin, apricots, and melon. Retinol is found in liver, egg yolk, fish, whole milk, butter, and cheese.

vitamin B complex   A group of water-soluble vitamins isolated from liver, yeast, and other sources. Among the B vitamins are thiamine (vitamin B_1), riboflavin (vitamin B_2, niacin (vitamin B_3), pyridoxine (vitamin B_6), biotin, pantothenic acid (vitamin B_5), FOLIC ACID (or folate, vitamin B_9), and cyanocobalamin (vitamin B_{12}). The vitamin B complex affects growth, appetite, lactation, and the gastrointestinal, nervous, and endocrine systems; aids in marasmus; stimulates appetite; aids metabolism of carbohydrates; and stimulates biliary action. B vitamins are also used as adjuncts to some antituberculosis drugs.

Deficiency disorders include beriberi, pellagra, digestive disturbances, enlargement of the liver, disturbance of the thyroid, degeneration of sex glands, and neurological disturbances. Vitamin B deficiencies induce edema; affect the heart, liver, spleen, and kidneys; enlarge the adrenals; and cause dysfunction of the pituitary and salivary glands. Dietary sources of thiamine include red meat, whole grains, potatoes, peas, beans, nuts, and yeast. As this nutrient is water-soluble, it can be lost when food is cooked in liquids.

Natural sources of riboflavin (B_2) include dairy products, meat, fish, and green leafy vegetables. Whole grain cereals are also good sources, as are egg whites. Vitamin B_2 is broken down by heat, so exposure during cooking (by broiling, for instance) can deplete it. Vitamin B_2 is given to alcoholics to reduce delirium tremens (DTs).

Deficiencies in vitamin B_6 are common in HIV-positive people. Foods rich in B_6 include meat, fish, egg yolks, beans, fruits, and vegetables. Liver is a good source, as are whole grain cereals. Losses occur during cooking. However, an excess of vitamin B_6 can lead to neurologic damage. It is given to people who are taking ISONIAZID for tuberculosis.

Studies have shown 25 percent of HIV-positive people have deficiencies in vitamin B_{12}. It has an important function in nerve and spinal cord health. It is provided in the diet by meat, fish, and eggs, so vegetarians are particularly at risk of deficiency. AZT and d4T cause the creation of large red blood cells, as also occurs in deficiencies of B_{12}. This is called pernicious anemia and causes a lack of oxygen in the blood. However, it has not been shown that these two issues are the same problem.

Folate can be found in leafy vegetables, organ meats, and yeast, which are good dietary sources. Alcohol causes deficiencies of FOLIC ACID. It plays an important role in the metabolism of DNA and RNA, the carriers of genetic information in all living things. Women should take extra folic acid before and during pregnancy to ensure proper fetal development. The other B vitamin levels are rarely deficient. They are readily available in most B supplements and a variety of food sources.

vitamin C (ascorbic acid) A vitamin necessary for the formation of collagen, the intercellular substance of connective tissue, which is essential to maintenance of the integrity of intercellular cement in many tissues, especially capillary walls. Deficiency leads to scurvy, a disorder of skin and bone that causes capillary bleeding. Except guinea pigs, primates are the only mammals who cannot make it in their bodies. Few nutrients are as active in human metabolism as ascorbic acid. It is known to be the most important water-soluble antioxidant and cofactor in cellular metabolism. Researchers have clearly demonstrated that the immune system is sensitive to intake levels of vitamin C and that numerous immunological functions are dependent on it for their mediation. Vitamin C is possibly the most often used dietary supplement, particularly by immune-suppressed individuals and those suffering from other degenerative illnesses. Vitamin C can be purchased in tablet, capsule, or powdered form. If vitamin C powder is taken dissolved in water or juice, it should be drunk with a straw, as ascorbic acid can, over time, erode tooth enamel. The major side effects of an excess of vitamin C, and that in extremely high doses, are diarrhea and oxalate kidney stones.

vitamin D A generic name for a group of steroid-like substances with antirachitic (curing rickets) activity, vitamin D is essential in calcium and phosphorus metabolism and supports healthy bone growth. It also plays an important role in the proper functioning of muscles, nerves, blood clotting, cell growth, and energy utilization. Deficiency disorders include imperfect skeletal formation, bone diseases, rickets, and caries (erosion of teeth). Vitamin D is most readily received from milk products and sunlight. Excessive consumption of vitamin D can cause calcium levels in the blood that reach toxic, life-threatening levels.

vitamin E A fat-soluble vitamin, composed of a group of compounds called tocopherols. Seven forms of tocopherol exist in nature: alpha, beta, delta, epsilon, eta, gamma, and zeta. Of these, alpha-tocopherol is the most potent form and has the greatest nutritional and biological value. Tocopherols occur in highest concentrations in cold-pressed vegetable oils, seeds and nuts, and soybeans. Wheat germ oil is the source from which vitamin E was first obtained. The vitamin is necessary for all oxygen-consuming life forms. Vitamin E is an ANTIOXIDANT, which means it opposes oxidation of substances in the body. Oxidation involves a compound called an oxidizer that attacks another compound, removing an electron from it. Vitamin E protects other substances by being oxidized itself, taking the brunt of any attack on lipids or other components of the membranes. Vitamin E prevents saturated fatty acids and VITAMIN A from breaking down and combining with other substances that may become harmful to the body. Fat oxidation results in the formation of FREE RADICALS. Free radicals are highly destructive molecules that can alter DNA and cause extensive damage to the body, from blood clots to cancer. The VITAMIN B COMPLEX and ascorbic acid are also protected against oxidation when vitamin E is present in the digestive tract. Fats and oils containing vitamin E are less susceptible to rancidity than those devoid of vitamin E. Vitamin E is also of great importance in energy production. It plays an essential role in the cellular respiration of all muscles, especially cardiac and skeletal. The vitamin makes it possible for these muscles and their nerves to function with less oxygen, thereby increasing their endurance and stamina. It also causes dilatation of the blood vessels, permitting a fuller flow of blood to the heart. Vitamin E is a highly effective antithrombin in the bloodstream, inhibiting coagulation of blood by preventing formation of clots. It also aids in conducting nourishment to the cells, strengthening the capillary walls, and protecting the red blood cells from destruction by poisons in the blood. Vitamin E prevents both the pituitary and the adrenal hormones from being oxidized and promotes proper functioning of linoleic acid and unsaturated fatty acid. Since aging in the cells is due primarily to oxidation, vitamin E may be useful in retarding that process. Vitamin E is also necessary for the proper focusing of the eyes in middle-aged people. The vitamin stimulates urine excretion, which helps cardiac patients whose body tissues contain an excessive amount of tissue fluid. Finally, vitamin E may be involved in calcium metabolism, correcting deposition in the body of either too little or too much calcium. Vitamin E is an antioxidant that has been theorized to have a beneficial effect on the functioning of the immune system. Studies at Tulane University suggest that vitamin E increases AZT's ability to fight symptoms caused by HIV. Vit-amin E may also reduce the bone marrow toxicity caused by AZT. Studies have shown a deficiency in vitamin E in most HIV-positive people. Moderate amounts of supplementation have shown no side effects in HIV-positive individuals, so many physicians and alternative medical practitioners recommend supplements of this vitamin. Vitamin E has been shown to be an anticoagulant so hemophilia patients and people with low platelet counts should not use it. Because vitamin E is contained in the capsules of amprenavir, supplements are not needed.

vitamin K A fat-soluble vitamin produced by bacteria in the intestines. Vitamin K is needed primarily for the blood clotting mechanism that prevents bleeding to death as a result of cuts and wounds, as well as internal bleeding. The best dietary sources of vitamin K_1 are green leafy vegetables such as turnip greens, spinach, broccoli, cabbage, and lettuce. Other rich sources are soybeans, beef liver, and green tea. Deficiencies of vitamin K are rare and most frequently develop from malabsorption or prolonged antibiotic therapy coupled with compromised dietary intake. There are no known deficiencies due specifically to HIV.

Vitamin PQQ A recently discovered substance called pyrroloquinoline quinone (PQQ) has been confirmed as another vitamin, according to Japanese researchers. Below-normal amounts of this substance have been shown to cause reduced fertility and roughened fur in lab mice. Vitamins that have significant obvious effects in mice have been established to have similar effects on humans. If further studies reveal the same correlation between mice and humans in this case, it would confirm PQQ as the first vitamin to be discovered since 1948.

vitreous humor The gellike substance that fills the eyeball between the lens and the retina.

Vocational Rehabilitation Act of 1973 One of two federal statues that address the issue of employment of people with disabilities (the other is the AMERICANS WITH DISABILITIES ACT). Congress passed the Rehabilitation Act to promote the hiring of the disabled and to prohibit employers who receive funds under the act from discriminating against disabled workers who are otherwise able to perform their duties. Following a case brought by an employee with tuberculosis against a Florida school board [*Arline v. School Bd. of Nassau County,* 480 U.S. 273 (1987)], the act was amended to state that while a person with a contagious disease such as AIDS does qualify as disabled, the act does not apply to individuals who pose a health or safety threat to others or who are unable to perform their duties due to illness. Both statutes require "reasonable accommodation" of the employee's disability.

volunteer organizations   The "AIDS service industry," which emerged in the 1980s, spawned a vast array of volunteer organizations, which differ in mission, purpose, target audience, structure, staff, and funding. National, regional, and local in scope, volunteer organizations include the broad array of AIDS Service Organizations (ASOs), many of which are educational and support agencies for people with HIV/AIDS, as well as AIDS advocacy and/or activist groups (i.e., groups which promote the urgent need for biomedical research on AIDS and groups which provide updated information on experimental drug treatments for persons with HIV or AIDS), and specialized groups, such as organizations comprised of people who have been diagnosed as having AIDS, or HIV, or others which provide education and support to women with AIDS. See VOLUNTEERS.

volunteers   The backbone of AIDS SERVICE ORGANIZATIONS (ASOs), volunteers have been, and continue to be, the primary workforce in the AIDS service industry. This work has been characterized as a cultural response to both disease and shifting mores. Volunteers typically provide their services and/or time willingly and without pay. They care for people with HIV-related illnesses and provide a broad range of other client services, including meeting food and medical needs, daily living, prevention education, legal, and social needs of persons with HIV/AIDS. Other volunteers provide specialized services to people of color and drug users. Other volunteers may be involved with advocacy; fund-raising; counseling; community,

professional or general public education; policy-making; or public relations. Volunteers pursue their work in the AIDS service industry for a variety of reasons, ranging from the altruistic to the political to the self-interested. Feeling more personally engaged and less hopeless are just two possible positive outcomes of pursuing this kind of work.

vomiting   Ejection through the mouth of the gastric contents and, in cases of bowel obstruction, intestinal contents. It may result from any number of causes, from viruses to virus symptoms to nervousness; or allergies. It constitutes a serious problem in advanced HIV disease. Controlling the vomiting can improve absorption of food and medicine.

voyeur   One who obtains erotic enjoyment from watching others naked or engaging in sexual acts.

vpr gene   One of nine genes that make up the two identical strands of RNA that compose HIV. The vpr gene encodes a protein that appears to be involved in regulating viral replication early in the HIV life cycle.

vpu gene   One of nine genes that compose the two identical strands of RNA that make up HIV. The vpu gene encodes a protein that is thought to be involved in new VIRUS assembly and release. It is unique to HIV-1.

V3 loop   Also known as the third variable loop, it is a portion of the HIV ENVELOPE PROTEIN, gp20, which plays a central role in enabling HIV VIRIONS to bind to uninfected cells. The V3 loop is believed to trigger a strong antibody response, and several candidates for VACCINE DEVELOPMENT are focusing on this area. One drawback is that the amino acid sequence of the V3 loop can mutate considerably in HIV. Some scientists believe that the V3 loop is simply a decoy of the virus to ward off the antibodies that would interfere in the infection and REPLICATION of the virus.

vulva   The external female sex organs, including the outer and inner lips of the vagina and the clitoris.

vulvovaginal candidiasis See CANDIDIASIS.

vulvovaginal condition A condition that affects all of a woman's external and internal genital organs. The vulva is composed of the outer and inner lips of the external organs; the vagina is the internal organ. The term is typically used to describe a condition that affects the whole of a woman's genital area.

VX-497 An inosine monophosphate dehydrogenase (IMPDH) inhibitor from Vertex Pharmaceuticals. It is in PHASE II trials for treatment of HEPATITIS C. It has been shown also to have effects on the overproduction of lymphocytes and their migration. This effect is believed to lower the inflammatory response of the liver. It is also being considered for use in immunosuppressive operations such as transplantation.

VZV See VARICELLA-ZOSTER VIRUS.

waiver The procedure by which rules of regulatory and benefits programs can be set aside in extraordinary circumstances, usually for experimental, research, demonstration, or compassionate purposes.

Walter Reed Classification System A standard scale of measurement of the progression and severity of HIV disease. It distinguishes six stages following exposure. Stage 1: infection; flulike syndrome characterized by fever, myalgia, malaise, and lymphadenopathy; SEROCONVERSION. Stage 2: chronic LYMPHADENOPATHY. Stage 3: T4 count below 400. Stage 4: reduced delayed hypersensitivity response to common allergens. Stage 5: complete anergy and appearance of chronic viral or fungal infections of mucous membranes. Stage 6: AIDS as defined by CENTERS FOR DISEASE CONTROL AND PREVENTION standards; the presence of OPPORTUNISTIC INFECTIONS in sites other than the skin or mucous membranes. The length of time a patient stays in each stage is still relatively unclear. See AIDS CASE DEFINITION; AIDS-DEFINING ILLNESS.

wart A circumscribed elevation of the skin resulting from an increase in size or bulk of the epidermis and protuberances in the layer just under the epidermis. Warts are caused by a PAPILLOMAVIRUS. Genital, plantar, seborrheic, and venereal are four common types of warts.

waste See MEDICAL WASTE.

wasting An involuntary loss of 10 percent or more of usual body weight, including lean tissue. It can be caused by a variety of conditions associated with disease and drug therapy. Wasting and weight loss accompany most major infections. In HIV/AIDS, weight loss in the absence of an identifiable cause may result directly from HIV, which can infect intestinal cells, causing inflammation and diarrhea. Wasting was added to the CENTERS FOR DISEASE CONTROL AND PREVENTION definition of AIDS in 1987 after an evaluation of diseases found often in INJECTION DRUG USERS.

wasting syndrome HIV- or AIDS-associated WASTING, known as wasting syndrome, is a major cause of illness and death in patients with late-stage HIV infection. It is defined, for Social Security disability purposes, as the documented involuntary loss of more than 10 percent of body weight, plus more than 30 days (not necessarily continuous) of either diarrhea, weakness, or fever that is not derived from another cause. Wasting is linked to disease progression and death. Loss of just 5 percent of body weight can have the same negative effects.

Several factors may lead to wasting syndrome. Low food intake can have a great effect. HIV can decrease appetite, particularly when combined with any of the OPPORTUNISTIC INFECTIONS (OIs). HIV-positive people are like other people when they are ill and often do not feel like eating. Also some HIV medicines must be taken on an empty stomach. Scheduling medication periods along with a regular eating schedule has proved difficult for many people. Some of the OIs directly affect the mouth, esophagus, or stomach, making eating painful or difficult at best.

Another factor in wasting is poor nutrient absorption by HIV-positive people. People usually absorb nutrients from the small intestine. In HIV-positive people several illnesses can interfere with the intestine in absorbing nutrients. Parasites in particular can cause havoc. In addition, the diarrhea and cramps caused by some medications make absorption difficult because calories and nutrients are being voided from the body.

Because of the increased activity of the body in fighting the virus, HIV-positive individuals probably need to derive more nutrients and minerals from their food intake. This necessity may lead the body to reduce stores of fat and muscle mass in seeking the needed energy to fight the virus. When all these factors are added up, it is easy to see how wasting can play a large role in disease progression. For example, infections may increase the body's energy requirements. These same infections can interfere with nutrient absorption and cause tiredness. The fatigue can reduce appetite and make people less able to spend time grocery shopping or cooking. They eat less, thereby accelerating the whole disease process.

Hormone levels can affect metabolism. Some studies have related the wasting in men to decrease in the production of testosterone during HIV. When given testosterone, men regained lean body mass and had more energy. Women also are noted to have a lower level of testosterone in HIV infection. Whether this is a sign of the problem or part of the problem as a whole is still unclear.

Treatment for wasting can involve several options. In some people treatment with HIGHLY ACTIVE ANTIRETROVIRAL THERAPY (HAART) reduces the loss of nutrients and allows the body to slow down metabolism because chemicals other than the body's own defenses are fighting the virus. In other people supplements such as Ensure or Advera can keep nutrient levels high through an easy to ingest fluid. The FDA has licensed a recombinant form of HGH to use as a treatment for HIV wasting syndrome called SEROSTIM. It does in some cases encourage lean muscle mass gain, but not all people are helped in this manner.

Other medications include DRONABINOL, which is a synthetic marijuana pill that increases appetite. Megesterol acetate was the first treatment for wasting and is still used. It is a very strong appetite stimulant. It tends primarily to add fat in weight gain, so it may not be the most helpful means in the long run of building lean muscle mass. Various steroids have also been used to assist people to gain muscle mass, including oxandralone, testosterone, and nandralone. Thalidomide has also been used to increase hunger but is generally used very sparingly as it has several severe side effects.

water sports   A 20th-century slang term for sexual activities that involve URINE; also known as golden showers. The HIV viral load found in urine is extremely low. Activity of this nature, although not completely safe, is not known to have caused HIV transmission. See TRANSMISSION.

water-based lubricant   See LUBRICANT.

weakness   A subjective symptomatic condition; a feeling of lack of strength compared to normal. The cause may be organic or a combination of an organic and a mental state. If it is unremitting, it requires careful investigation with special attention given to potentially lethal causes that may be curable, such as anemia, cancer, neurologic conditions, or certain parasitic or infectious diseases.

weight loss   Weight loss (as distinct from WASTING SYNDROME) is common in people with HIV/AIDS. Weight loss can be intentional or unintentional. People with HIV infection lose weight for different reasons: difficulty eating (perhaps because an infection in the mouth, such as thrush, makes eating difficult), lack of appetite, apathy and depression, prolonged diarrhea, nausea and vomiting, HIV itself, OPPORTUNISTIC INFECTIONS that affect various organs of the body, and fever. Treatments vary, depending on the cause, and include diet adjustments, appetite stimulants, small but frequent meals, high-calorie and protein foods, nutritional supplements, or intravenous feeding (a procedure called parenteral hyperalimentation or total PARENTERAL NUTRITION). An adequate exercise program is also especially important for people with HIV infection and AIDS. Diarrhea, nausea, and vomiting, can be treated with drugs. If fever is a factor in weight loss, treatment will try to reduce fever with aspirin, acetaminophen, or ibuprofen and will try to eliminate the cause of the fever.

well-being   *Well-being* is a relative term. HIV affects not only the body but the emotions and has obvious consequences for personal relationships. In the context of HIV/AIDS well-being depends not only on fighting the disease, but on preserving mental health, keeping from giving in to hopelessness and depression. See WELLNESS.

wellness   A condition reflecting the overall quality of life, rather than merely the absence of a (medically treatable) disorder of an individual. Maintaining optimal physical health through adequate nutrition and exercise and good mental health all contribute to wellness. Today, HIV and AIDS have added yet another dimension to the concept of wellness. See WELL-BEING.

Western blot   See WESTERN BLOT TEST.

Western blot test   The second of two tests that are used to determine whether a person is HIV-positive. It is not a test specific to HIV but rather a method of testing blood for specific proteins to determine whether antibodies to the virus are in the blood. When used in conjunction with the ELISA test, it offers relative assurance of a person's HIV status (see BLOTTING METHODS). The ELISA is an easier, less expensive test to perform and so is usually done first. The ELISA can produce false-positive or false-negative readings, as can any test, so the Western blot is used as a confirmatory test. When the two tests are run together, they give a fairly secure idea of whether someone is HIV-positive or negative at that moment in time.

The Western blot test involves putting the blood sample on a strip of paper (made out of nitrocellulose), which is embedded with HIV antigens. The blood moves along the paper, and a visible band appears in places where HIV antibodies from the patient bind with the antigens. If no bands appear, then the person is HIV-negative. If three bands appear, then the person is considered HIV-positive. If one or two bands appear, then the result is considered indeterminate and the patient is advised to return in six months for a retest to determine HIV status.

Western Europe   In sheer numbers the HIV epidemic in Western Europe is minor in comparison to that in Southern Africa and the Caribbean. France, Italy, and Spain have the largest numbers of HIV-positive people; 130,000 in Spain, 100,000 in Italy and in France. Switzerland, Spain, and Portugal all have rates of infection of 0.5 percent. Those are the highest in the region. Spain and Italy have rates of 0.4 percent. All of those numbers are below the numbers discussed even in some parts of Eastern Europe. Overall the rate of infection in Western Europe is 0.3 percent. There are close to 600,000 people living with HIV in the region.

In Western Europe the HIV epidemic has followed the same pattern that it has in North America. It began early in the 1980s, seen almost completely in people reporting homosexual behavior. It raged out of control, spreading to the INJECTION DRUG USER (IDU) population, then with the advent of HIGHLY ACTIVE ANTIRETROVIRAL THERAPY (HAART) a large drop in the death rates was seen. After spending relatively large amounts of funds on education, these countries also saw declining HIV infection rates until 2000. At that point some of these countries saw a rise in the rate of new infections as a result of unsafe sexual practices among men having sex with men (MSM).

In these countries the change in the epidemic has reflected large decreases in the rate of infection among IDUs and MSM, but a rising number of cases spread through heterosexual activities. This is particularly true in the United Kingdom, where there was a 130 percent increase in such cases between 1997 and 2000. Belgium, Norway, and Ireland report similar changes in their statistics. Statistics from blood donation centers show a decrease in the number of donors who are HIV-positive, though the numbers have remained somewhat high in Greece and Portugal in comparison to those in the other countries. The exceptions are in the southern countries that have the higher rates of infection, where IDUs are still increasingly testing positive for HIV.

Many of the Western European nations provide extended medical care to all their citizens, and this system has allowed access to HAART medications that have not been available in many regions of the world. It has also meant a greater portion of their budget is expended on medical care than previously. Europe has also spent large sums of money on education and on prevention of HIV in other countries. This is true of Scandinavian countries that have so far have not had large numbers of HIV-positive people. The proportion of HIV-positive individuals in Sweden, Norway, and Finland has been 0.1 percent or less of the total population.

A problem of recent vintage has been the dual infections seen in southern Europe of HIV and LEISHMANIASES. Leishmaniasis is a protozoan illness that damages the immune system and causes boils, scarring, and other problems on the hands, face, and other extremities. Spain, Portugal, Italy, and Greece have seen an increasing rate of this sickness as the range of the sandfly that passes the protozoan between humans had increased.

wet kiss   A kiss in which each partner sticks his or her tongue in the other's mouth, making exchange of saliva likely. Also called a FRENCH KISS.

wet mount   The most important diagnostic procedure to detect the cause of VAGINITIS or VAGINAL DISCHARGE. Often called the saline wet mount test, because it uses a saline (salt) solution. A cotton-tipped stick is dipped in saline and then mixed with a bit of vaginal discharge. It is examined immediately under the microscope for one of three common causes of vaginitis: TRICHOMONIASIS; CANDIDIASIS; or hemophilus vaginals. In some cases a woman's sex partner's urine is also examined to make certain that she is not being constantly reinfected as a consequence of sexual activity.

wet sex   Any kind of sexual activity in which bodily fluids are exchanged.

whey   Recent experiments have suggested that whey, a protein that can be extracted cheaply from the waste product from cheese making, could provide a weapon in the battle against AIDS. Researchers have found that whey seems to block HIV from entering CD4 cells, the white blood cells that are the main target when the virus infects the body. Researchers think it might eventually be prepared as an ointment, for use along with condoms, to block transfer of the virus during sexual intercourse. Other virologists think that whey might also be used as a wash for newborns to prevent them from being infected with HIV after passing through the birth canal. They speculate that it might be able to prevent mother-to-baby transmission of the virus that way. The milk protein will have to be tested to see how it affects normal tissues and whether it is toxic. It is also not clear that blocking the receptors in CD4 cells will be sufficient to prevent infection completely because the virus can invade a few other kinds of cells. Research has shown that whey protein increases the GLUTATHIONE levels in the body; other research has shown that increased glutathione levels indicate long-term health in HIV-positive individuals.

Whipple's disease   A malabsorption syndrome characterized by abnormal skin pigmentation, diarrhea, weight loss, weakness, arthritis, lymphadenopathy, and lesions of the central nervous system.

white blood cell   A blood cell whose primary function is to fight infections. See LYMPHOCYTE.

white matter   Another term for white nerve fibers (as opposed to cell bodies, which appear as gray). The white appearance is due to myelin, a fatty substance that surrounds axons, acting as an insulator to enhance electrical conduction of action potentials. Gray matter in the brain is primarily found in the outer layers of the cerebrum and in some deeper areas; gray matter also makes up the inner core of the spinal cord. White matter disease is disease that affects those neurons that have myelinated axons. An example of white matter disease in HIV/AIDS is PROGRESSIVE MULTIFOCAL LEUKOENCEPHALOPATHY (PML), a neurological disease believed to be caused by reactivation of latent JC VIRUS infection, resulting in demyelination of neurons in the central nervous system. Initially brain lesions occur around blood vessels. Note that JC virus infects oligodendrocytes, the cells in the brain that produce myelin.

WHO   See WORLD HEALTH ORGANIZATION.

whole-killed virus vaccine   A vaccine composed of an intact, but killed, virus.

wild-type virus   HIV that is distinctive to an individual's body. Individuals have in their body a dominant variety of the virus. It is that quasi species of the virus that is found to be the most advantageous for reproduction in that body, before anything is done or any drug is taken to attack it.

It is also a term used to refer to a variety of the virus that is most represented in the population at large that is used in a laboratory to test antiretrovirals or other treatment. So all treatments are based on a similar virus that is often referred to as wild-type virus.

Because HIV mutates both independently and through drug interference, there is never just one single virus in the body; there are many different varieties. It is therefore a mixture of viruses called quasi species. Before antiretroviral therapy is started, a person's wild-type virus is the most abundant in the body and dominates all quasi species in the body. There are thought to be around 10–12 quasi species in a person's body at the time before drug therapy is started. Some of these variants do not reproduce as well, or cannot compete as well, as the wild-type virus. When wild-type virus is discussed, recognize that this is an "antibiotic virgin" virus that is being spoken about.

After drug intervention, the virus left active in the body is virus that can compete against the drugs used to fight the wild-type virus. This is known as resistance (see DRUG RESISTANCE). It is quite easy for the virus to become resistant to one drug (see MONOTHERAPY); for that reason HIV-positive people taking medication generally use three or more drugs. If someone has resistance to one or more of the antiretroviral drugs and has unprotected sex or shares needles with someone who is not infected with the virus, he or she may infect the partner with a drug-resistant variant—a strain of HIV containing mutations that cause resistance to one or more antiretrovirals. It also may be possible for someone already infected to become infected again, with a variant that is resistant to antiretrovirals.

Someone who has been taking medication acquires resistance to a particular drug (see GENOTYPIC TESTING) or drug regimen sometimes when he or she stops using his or her current medication, the wild-type virus returns as the dominant virus in the body. This does not happen every time but does occur. This process makes the use of the regimen or medication effective again. Other times a different or even a drug-resistant virus has become more adept or more capable of becoming the dominant virus; it would not be a wild-type virus.

will 1) A legally enforceable declaration of what people want done with their property and their instructions concerning other matters when they die. Wills can be changed or revoked before the author dies. 2) The mental capacity used in choosing or deciding upon an act or thought. 3) The power of controlling one's own actions or emotions.

Having a will is important for a variety of reasons. When a person dies without having formally signed or "executed" a will, state law determines how the property is distributed. In some cases, distribution is in accord with what the deceased person would have wanted; in other cases, not. State laws vary, but all of them mandate distributions to lawful relations by marriage or blood only, with nothing going to friends or lovers, no matter what their relationships with the deceased.

Other important reasons for having a will relate to the disposition of remains and conduct of memorial services. Local medical examiners' offices, hospitals, and funeral homes look almost exclusively to family members for direction on such issues as funeral plans, burial vs. cremation, post-funeral possession of the ashes of a cremated deceased, and all of the small decisions involved in each of these issues. Unless there is clear agreement between family members and surviving friends or lovers, the latter are likely to be excluded from decision making when the deceased might have preferred either that they share responsibility or that the decisions be left in their hands entirely. This is true even if the deceased has made his or her wishes known explicitly, but not in a will, which is legally enforceable.

It is important that a will and related documents (LIVING WILL, POWER OF ATTORNEY, etc.) be made at a time and under circumstances that do not invite an inference of undue influence by a potential beneficiary. It is on this issue that most AIDS-related challenges have arisen.

von Willebrand's disease   A congenital bleeding disorder, von Willebrand's disease usually affects people at an early age, and the symptoms decrease with age or during pregnancy. It is considered a milder form of blood clotting disorder than hemophilia. It is characterized by prolonged periods of bleeding and a deficiency of coagulation factor VIII in the blood. It is associated with increased bleeding during surgery or trauma and excessive loss of blood during menstruation.

window period The time in which a person is infected with HIV but has not produced enough antibodies to be found in tests of blood, body fluids, or tissues. The window period is usually from several weeks to six months.

woman-to-man transmission See TRANSMISSION.

woman-to-woman transmission See TRANSMISSION.

womb See UTERUS.

women HIV/AIDS in women has long been a neglected aspect of the HIV epidemic. Until recently, little scientific attention has been paid to many fundamental questions about HIV disease in women. Scientists still do not know exactly how HIV is transmitted from men to women, and many questions remain about the course of HIV disease in women. Women desperately need methods to prevent heterosexual HIV transmission that are under their own control. And although a number of MICROBICIDES are under development, at best it will be several years before any is licensed and widely available.

HIV infection among women often represents a threat to two or more people—a mother and her progeny. Indeed, the growing HIV case rate in women has implications for children, since the overwhelming majority of HIV-positive children have acquired the virus from the mother. The incidence of HIV infection continues to grow among women, and the rate at which it is growing is now higher than that among men. In 1995, heterosexual transmission overtook INJECTION DRUG USE (IDU) as the leading cause of HIV infection in women. Today, HIV infection has increased among women in the United States, and in some developing countries it is even more prevalent in women

than in men. In the United States, HIV infection is more likely to occur among women of color, particularly African-American and Hispanic women.

Discussion of women and HIV disease follows, and takes into account women's vulnerability to HIV infection; the prevention of HIV transmission in women; the course of HIV infection in women; differences in the "natural history" of HIV infection in women and people of color; biologically unique aspects of HIV disease in women; and the medical management of women with HIV disease. Discussion of women in clinical trials concludes the entry.

Both biological and psychosocial factors place women at higher risk than men of acquiring HIV infection. In biological terms, when an HIV-infected male ejaculates during intercourse, the several milliliters of semen he releases are rich in both free virus and virus-infected LYMPHOCYTES and MACROPHAGES. This semen is in contact with a broad surface of mucosal tissue in the vagina and the cervix. These tissues contain high numbers of CD4 lymphocytes, which can become infected by HIV from the semen; however, it is believed that most of the transmission is into dendritic cells and/or macrophages, not CD4s. When an HIV-infected woman has intercourse with an uninfected man, the primary sources of transmission from her to him are free virus and virus-infected cells present in the vaginal and cervical secretions. These secretions mainly have contact with the skin of the penis. If the skin is intact, the virus cannot penetrate it. HIV-infected vaginal secretions have little access to the mucosal tissue lining the male's urethral canal, making transmission of the virus a less likely event. Note too that sexual intercourse is rarely a single event for two members of a sexually active couple. Each instance of unprotected sexual intercourse with an infected female statistically increases the risk that an uninfected male will acquire HIV. Thus, in the long run the rate of female-to-male HIV transmission becomes similar to the rate of male-to-female transmission. This explains why the prevalence of HIV infection is similar in men and women in the developing world today.

A number of psychosocial factors also increase a woman's vulnerability to HIV infection. Some women have little or no control over the means to practice low-risk sexual behavior. There is nothing they can do to protect themselves without the knowledge and consent of their male sexual partner. Second, because of their inferior social standing in relation to men virtually worldwide, women are generally unable to negotiate the frequency and nature of sexual interactions. Sometimes they are not even able to choose who their partner will be. Third, other important sources of HIV infection for women living in developing countries include transfusions with untested or poorly tested blood, nonsterile medical equipment used during childbirth, and reused, unsterilized needles and syringes used to inject medications. Fourth, lesbian and bisexual women are also at risk for HIV/AIDS. Transmission of HIV during homosexual sex between women is uncommon (although it has been reported) and remains fairly unresearched. However, lesbians may engage in the same high-risk behavior as heterosexual women, and because they often socialize with bisexual men, as well as gay men, they may be at higher risk than heterosexual women when having unprotected sex with an infected man.

All sexually active women, including pregnant women, should consider themselves at risk for HIV infection. The level of risk for a woman who is not an injection drug user varies greatly, depending on her sexual practices and the risk factors of the men with whom she associates. For a woman who has no sexual relations, the risk is virtually nil. For a woman in a stable monogamous relationship, the risk is small, although it depends on her partner's faithfulness. For a woman who engages in casual sex with multiple partners, the risk can be very high. Here, the level of risk rises with the prevalence of HIV infection in her social circles and geographic area. The safest course for a woman who wants to be sexually active is to enter into a monogamous, committed, and mutually faithful relationship; before entering such a relationship, both she and her partner should undergo HIV testing twice, over the course of six weeks to three months (completely abstaining from risky sexual behavior and drug use in the interval), and receive negative results on both blood tests. Only after both partners have tested negative for HIV, and after sufficient trust in fidelity has been established between them can they forgo safe sex practices and engage in unprotected sex with each other and

only with each other. Under all other circumstances, sexually active women should always practice safe sex—use a male latex or polyurethane condom or a female condom during every act of vaginal or rectal intercourse. During oral–penile sex, use a male condom; during oral–vaginal sex, use a latex or polyurethane barrier such as a condom split lengthwise to form a sheet.

In general, with regard to the course of HIV disease in woman, studies have shown that women have poorer survival rates than men. Some investigators have speculated that this might be due to social factors such as limited access to health care and lower socioeconomic status, including homelessness, domestic violence, and lack of social support. The rates of disease progression do not appear to differ significantly in men and women. Psychological factors play a significant role in the course of HIV disease in women. For example, women who are not pregnant are usually diagnosed later in the disease than men, largely because HIV infection is still regarded by many as a disease of men and gay men. This delays the start of antiretroviral therapies and the use of prophylaxis for opportunistic infections in women. Older women are usually diagnosed and treated even later because they and their doctors have still lower expectations of HIV infection; their way of life is assumed to present none of the risk factors associated with HIV infection. As a second example, women have less access than men to routine and state-of-the-art HIV/AIDS care. They are often less mobile than men and more likely to face language and cultural barriers, all of which reduce access to health care and interfere with their ability to comply with demanding treatment regimens. Third, there are few support groups organized for women with HIV disease. Fourth, women often neglect their own health care to take care of others. And, last, fewer than 10 percent of all participants in HIV-related clinical trials are women. Given that such trials are often portals to expert care and promising new drugs, women are disadvantaged by their absence. Additionally, to this day, the number of women enrolled in clinical trials is too low to allow statistical calculations that might reveal whether the response of women to a treatment is different from the response of men.

In recent years, new information has become available suggesting that the "natural history" of

HIV infection, that is, the way in which HIV can make people sick, may be different in women and in people of color when compared to white men. However, the recommendations followed by doctors to determine treatment for individuals with HIV infection are based mostly on studies of viral load and treatment in HIV-infected white men. There are three areas in which there is evidence of differences between women and men: levels of VIRAL LOAD, T-cell counts in people with or without HIV infection, and level of T-cell counts at which AIDS develops. The differences found between whites and people of color include viral load differences and differences in rate of decline of T cells.

- Recent studies suggest that viral load tends to be lower in women than in men, in people of color than in whites, and in persons reporting a history of injection drug use.

- Some data have suggested that for women with HIV infection, remaining alive is predicted more by the T-cell count than by the viral load. Well-controlled studies also show that CD4 is a better predictor of survival for women than it is for men.

- Today we know that the "normal" T-cell levels in women and men are different. In people without HIV infection, the T-cell levels are about 100 cells/mm higher in women than in men. The differences in T-cell counts may matter if they mean that women can acquire AIDS- or HIV-related diseases at higher T-cell counts than men. Alternatively, women's higher T-cell counts may "protect" them by preventing the development of AIDS for a longer period after becoming infected with HIV. T-cell counts do not appear to differ by race, however, at least across the Caucasian, African-American, and Latino groups in the United States.

These findings have led some physicians and scientists to question whether it is appropriate to assume that the information gained from studies of white men should be used to develop the treatment recommendations for women and people of color. There are three major measures that physicians and other health care providers use to recommend treatment to HIV-infected individuals:

clinical disease, T-cell count, and viral load. It is clear that HIGHLY ACTIVE ANTIRETROVIRAL THERAPY (HAART) should be recommended and provided to any person with clinical disease. It is less clear at what T-cell or viral load level treatment should be first recommended. Because of recent information suggesting gender and racial differences in T cells and viral load, there has been concern that the current treatment recommendations may not be correct for women and people of color; the scientific community is currently trying to determine whether the current treatment recommendations are correct for them.

There are several biological unique aspects of HIV disease in women, many of which stem from the fact that the HIV-related conditions that occur uniquely in women involve infections or malignancy of the female reproductive tract. Most of these gynecological problems also occur in HIV-negative women. They include certain vaginal infections (genital ulcers of unknown origin, vaginal candidiasis, or yeast infection of the vagina, and bacterial vaginosis and trichomoniasis); PELVIC INFLAMMATORY DISEASE; precancerous cellular changes of the cervix (CERVICAL INTRAEPITHELIAL NEOPLASIA [CIN]; and menstrual disorders. CIN progresses more rapidly to invasive cervical cancer in women infected with HIV. Note that CIN occurs less frequently in women in developed countries, as a result of more widespread medical management, among other factors. Since few studies have compared the incidence of these conditions in women with and without HIV disease, a debate continues over whether they actually occur more frequently in women who are HIV-infected. It is well agreed, however, that these diseases are more aggressive in women infected with HIV.

Consideration of gynecological and family planning needs is often a component of the medical management of women with HIV disease. Women who are HIV-positive should receive a complete gynecological exam, including a PAP SMEAR test, during their initial medical visit. A second Pap test should be done six months later. If both tests reveal no sign of CIN, women with symptomatic HIV disease can later be given annual Pap tests. However, HIV-positive women should receive subsequent Pap tests every six months if they have symptomatic HIV disease or if they show evidence of HIV infection, as suggested by the presence of CIN through a positive Pap test result or the finding of genital warts. The initial medical evaluation of HIV-positive women should also include the following: a complete menstrual, sexual, obstetrical, and gynecological history; breast and pelvic exams; and screening for vaginitis, urinary tract infection, syphilis, gonorrhea, and chlamydia.

Nonpregnant HIV-positive women should receive prophylaxis for PNEUMOCYSTIS CARINII PNEUMONIA and for MYCOBACTERIUM AVIUM COMPLEX on the same basis as men. However, certain prophylactic drugs must be prescribed with caution during pregnancy because of risks to the fetus. Women should be offered antiretroviral therapy with the same standards of care that are used for men; they must also have the same opportunities as men to participate in clinical trials.

Weight loss and WASTING are common complications of HIV disease. Wasting is a life-threatening condition that results in the loss not only of fat tissue but also of muscle. Use of the male sex hormone testosterone is widely accepted for the treatment of HIV-associated wasting syndrome in men and women, but it is not yet approved by the U.S. FOOD AND DRUG ADMINISTRATION. Its possible role in the treatment of wasting is even less well established in women than in men. In addition, it has a number of side effects in women such as suppression of menstruation, hair loss, and growth of facial hair. Megestrol acetate (Megace) is an appetite stimulant also used in the treatment of HIV-associated wasting. Megestrol acetate is a progestin, a chemical related to progesterone, a hormone produced by the ovaries. When taken by women, megestrol acetate produces significant irregular vaginal bleeding. The use of megestrol acetate alone and in combination with testosterone for the treatment of wasting in HIV-positive men and women is being studied.

In recent years, consideration of menopausal issues has become more important as HIV-positive women live longer and as more women who are nearing menopause or are postmenopausal become infected. To date there has been no documented association between HIV disease and premature ovarian failure. *Menopause* is defined as the permanent cessation of menstruation caused by the loss of ovarian function. Women who are HIV-positive can receive hormone replacement therapy for managing the symptoms of natural or premature menopause. There are several alternatives to hormone replacement therapy that are also available to HIV-positive women, including progestin-only regimens; nonhormonal lubricants and or moisturizers or Estring for the management of urogenital atrophy; bisphosphonates for the prevention or treatment of osteoporosis; and selective estrogen receptor modulators that offer bone and cardiovascular benefit. Symptoms of menopause can be overlooked in HIV-positive women or can be attributed to the symptoms of HIV infection. Menopausal symptoms include hot flashes, sweating, cystitis, atrophic vaginitis, urethritis, vaginal dryness and itching, and discomfort during urination or intercourse.

Discussion of HIV/AIDS in women would be incomplete without mention of the importance of enrollment in both pharmaceutical and government-sponsored HIV clinical trials. To date, women remain underrepresented in CLINICAL TRIALS. It has been established that both structural and attitudinal barriers prevent women from enrolling in clinical trials. Recent studies have identified reasons for not participating, including lack of information about clinical trials, lack of interest in participating, and fear of side effects. Studies have also shown that lack of child care, lack of transportation, and amount of time required for participation were less frequently cited as reasons for not participating. Additionally, studies have shown that among the women enrolled in clinical trials, the greatest facilitator to participation in a trial was the support and/or recommendation of the primary care provider: Women enrolled in clinical trials have also identified the support of the research staff as a major facilitator to participation. Finally, studies have shown perceived barriers to participation from the provider's side—gender prejudice in the medical profession, lack of knowledge about available studies, and lack of coordinated care. Representation in clinical research ensures equal access to investigational medications; it also ensures the availability of accurate information regarding side effects and pharmacokinetics in women as the face of the epidemic changes. See LESBIANS; PREGNANCY; TRANSMISSION.

work incentives SOCIAL SECURITY has designed a number of special rules, called "work incentives," that provide cash benefits and continued MEDICARE or MEDICAID coverage while a recipient works. (The rules are different for Social Security and SUPPLEMENTARY SECURITY INCOME [SSI] beneficiaries.) Work incentives are particularly important to people with HIV disease who, because of the recurrent nature of HIV-related illnesses, may be able to return to work following periods of disability.

workers' compensation A no-fault system of injury compensation for the protection of employees while engaged in the employer's business. It requires only that an injured party show that the accident occurred in the workplace. Once the causation threshold is met, administrative compensation is available in an expedited fashion for economic costs. In the United States, insurance and, when necessary, tort litigation are two means by which the cost of accidents is shifted from injured individuals to a broader pool of others.

If one contracts HIV at the workplace, the injured health care provider may choose to bring a lawsuit against a hospital, or to sue manufacturers of needles or other equipment. Lawsuits against hospitals are not easy. First, it will be somewhat difficult to define the standard of care that was violated, and, if the duty of care is not easily defined, it will likely be difficult to prove negligence. Even more important, infected health care workers must prove that their infection occurred at the workplace. While most providers should recall and report needle-stick injuries that occur, these accidents rarely are witnessed. Since transmission of HIV occurs much more commonly through sexual or parenteral transmission outside the workplace, infected health care workers will face the prospect of proving that this more common form of transmission is not the cause of their HIV infection. Hospitals will resist establishment of a legal presumption that infected health care workers contracted the virus at work, and may, in fact, investigate the private lives of litigants. Thus, the causation question represents a significant threshold to successful suits.

In light of this, some health care workers may choose to sue manufactures of needles or other equipment. These suits would be based on a claim that the equipment was designed in a substandard fashion, increasing the risk of injury.

Presumably, however, tort litigation will not play an important role in compensation of injured health care workers. Indeed, many health care workers may be unable to sue employers because of the availability of workers' compensation benefits and the attendant exclusivity doctrine that prohibits suits against employers who provide such benefits. Many health care workers, and especially support staff, nurses, and physicians employed by hospitals are eligible for workers' compensation benefits. In the past, workers' compensation boards have provided benefits for workers' infected with HEPATITIS B, and indeed have developed presumptions regarding infectious causation. This relaxation of causation standards makes workers' compensation a much more attractive alternative for shifting the costs of accidents.

This is not to say that workers' compensation is a panacea for the costs associated with occupational infection with HIV. First, workers' compensation has generally performed poorly in compensating for occupational disease. Second, benefits will be small in general, especially for nurses and physicians in training who will have their compensation pegged to the salary they are earning at the hospital and not to the much larger salary they expect once their training is completed. Third, self-employed physicians and nurses will not be as eligible for benefits and will likely have to seek other alternatives.

The foregoing assumes that the health care worker has information regarding the HIV status of a patient. This is not the case in many needle-stick or other types of accidents that occur. In these situations, health care workers will want to know the HIV status of the patient. Such testing is generally prohibited without the patient's consent. A constitutional analysis also favors nontesting because it would be easier to perform serial antibody testing on the potentially infected health care worker. These arguments are complicated somewhat by the fact that some individuals do not immediately develop antibodies. Some state legislatures have balanced trade-offs and require testing of patients who may have exposed an emergency, or "first response," to health care workers. Moreover, some courts have characterized exposed parties' interests as superior to privacy rights in cases of rape and other exposures of body fluids. The law in this matter is unsettled.

works Slang term for apparatus (needle, syringe, spoon, bottle cap, cotton, for filtering the heated drug) used to prepare and inject INTRAVENOUS drugs. Sharing works exposes users to HIV. Needle sharing and having unprotected sex with someone who shares drug paraphernalia are the most common ways that HIV infection is spread among women. Needles and other works, to be cleaned, must be soaked in rubbing alcohol or household bleach for at least 10 minutes. The alcohol or bleach should not be injected. Works should then be washed thoroughly in running water. Bleach and water must not be reused. Cookers must be cleaned with bleach-soaked cotton, then rinsed with water. The cotton must be discarded after use.

World AIDS Day A day when the world is encouraged to focus its attention on the global plague of HIV/AIDS, the tragic human losses it has caused, and the memory of those who have died. Generally, it is held on December 1.

World Health Organization (WHO) The World Health Organization came into being on July 22, 1946, as one of the charter organizations of the United Nations. There are currently 193 members of WHO, four more than the number of member nations of the United Nations. The initial charter of WHO, which has not been amended since 1946, includes provisions declaring the rights of all people, including "enjoyment of the highest attainable standard of health," which is "fundamental to the attainment of peace and security and is dependent upon the fullest co-operation of individuals and States." These statements lead WHO to monitor and track all diseases and to try to implement programs and policies to affect and promote health for all peoples. In 1969 WHO implemented specific International Health Regulations; among these are guidelines for international aircraft, vaccinations, and statistical compilation. WHO has been at the forefront of working in HIV and AIDS across most of the globe and maintains statistics of AIDS cases worldwide. WHO, in conjunction with the joint UN agency UNAIDS, has been instrumental in providing HIV and AIDS education in many places that could not otherwise afford programs.

worried well Persons who are healthy but who live in fear of AIDS. Because of their anxiety or imagined illness, they may frequent medical care facilities seeking reassurance. Signs of this fear include a decision that the only way to be safe from AIDS is to abstain from sex completely; loss of interest in sex; diminution of sex drive; impotence or lack of orgasm; unsociability and loneliness; curtailment of friendship with gay or bisexual persons or activity in the gay or bisexual community; sadness, anxiety, or depression for no apparent reason; sleeplessness, nightmares, or loss of appetite without an apparent cause; constant anxiety about health despite physicians' assurances that medical conditions, if any, are not AIDS-related; refusal to believe negative results of HIV antibody tests; feelings of self-rejection because of homosexuality or bisexuality; self-blame for having had lovers who were gay or bisexual injection drug users; guilt about one's history of injection drug use; psychosomatic symptoms that are known to be signs of AIDS, such as night sweats or seemingly inexplicable weight loss; strong feelings of regret or guilt over past sexual behavior. See FEAR OF AIDS.

X See MDMA.

X ray A high-energy electromagnetic wave varying in length from 0.05 to 100 angstrom units. X rays are produced by bombarding a target in a vacuum tube with high-velocity electrons. Because of their ability to penetrate most solid matter to some extent and to act on photographic film, X rays are used to produce images of the interior of the body to enable medical diagnosis and therapy.

Xanax See ALPRAZOLAM.

xenogeneic Pertaining to the relationship that exists between members of genetically different species.

xerosis Dryness of the skin, mouth, or eyes; abnormal except in the aged, in whom it is the result of normal sclerosis of tissues.

yeast Any of several fungi of the genus *Saccharomyces*. Most familiar are the yeast that are used in the preparation of beer. Yeasts that can cause illness in HIV-positive individuals include CANDIDA ALBICANS and CRYPTOCOCCUS. Candida can cause mucosal infections in the throat, vagina, and anogenital areas. *Cryptococcus* can cause pneumonia and meningitis when it becomes disseminated in the body.

yeast infection A term typically used to refer to an infection of the vagina. Studies show that 85 percent of all women suffer from a vaginal yeast infection at least once. Symptoms of a yeast infection can include itching and burning in the vagina; itching and burning of the skin area around the vagina; swelling and redness of the skin area around the vagina; a thick, white vaginal discharge that looks like cottage cheese; and pain during sexual intercourse. Some causes of yeast infections include some medications, diabetes, and pregnancy. It is simply an imbalance of the commonly found natural fungi in the vagina. Women should consult a doctor if these infections occur regularly. Yeast infections in HIV-positive women occur much more frequently than in HIV-negative women.

Yersinia enterocolitica A type of intestinal bacterium that can cause diarrhea and occasionally systemic infections, particularly in immune impaired people. Outbreaks are related to poor refrigeration of cheese, and occur irregularly in the United States.

yogurt Milk that has been fermented by a mixture of bacteria and yeasts forms a custardlike product. The milk is defatted and soured with *Lactobacillus acidophilus* and other bacteria. These are not bacteria typically found in the intestine, but some people and marketers attempt to market yogurt as providing or replenishing bacteria needed for the health of the intestine.

Yogurt is thought to possibly aid digestion. It contains the B-complex vitamins and has a higher percentage of VITAMINS A and D than does the milk it was made from. It is also high in protein. Its calcium is thought to benefit women. Many people that support alternative and natural health regimens believe yogurt can help the body in numerous ways.

Z

Zalcitabine (ddC) A seldom used NUCLEOSIDE ANALOG that inhibits infection of new cells by HIV. It is most commonly known as ddC. It was the third drug approved in the United States for treatment of HIV. ddC was at one time an important part of combination anti-HIV treatment. Side effects of ddC include skin eruptions, canker sores, general inflammation of the mouth, nausea, pancreatitis, and fever. Long-term use of ddC increases risk of PANCREATITIS; however, the main side effect over time has been PERIPHERAL NEUROPATHY. As a result, this drug is not to be combined in treatment with d4T. Peripheral neuropathy usually ceases after treatment with ddC is stopped but may not completely disappear for several months. Combining ddC with ddI, d4T, or 3TC is not recommended, as these drugs do not work well together: ddC is also not recommended for cancer patients who receive radiation therapy as the drug breaks down under these conditions. ddC can be taken on a full or an empty stomach. It cannot be absorbed properly when any antacid is taken; individuals should inform the doctor if they are taking prescription or over-the-counter antacids. (The trade name is Hivid.)

zaleplon (Sonata) A hypnotic used to treat insomnia. (Trade name is Sonata.)

zap In the vocabulary of protest, agitation, and other forms of public activities, a small strike against a selected target. The major victories of AIDS activists in transforming clinical research policy were won by a combination of tactics that included zaps in the form of telephone campaigns, street protests, and so forth. See ACT-UP.

ZDV See ZIDOVUDINE.

Zerit See STAVUDINE.

Ziagen See ABACAVIR.

zidovudine (ZDV or AZT) A synthetic thymidine (one of the basic components of DNA) that inhibits the growth and development of HIV, the virus that causes AIDS. Originally named azidothymidine (AZT) or azido-deoxythymidine, it is properly called zidovudine, but is almost universally referred to as AZT (a practice followed in this encyclopedia). It was the first antiretroviral therapy and the first anti-AIDS drug approved by the FOOD AND DRUG ADMINISTRATION. It is marketed under the trade name Retrovir. For a complete discussion of zidovudine, see AZT.

zinc An essential trace mineral occurring in the body. Outside of iron, zinc is found in larger amounts than all other trace minerals. It is present in all tissues. Zinc stimulates the activity of approximately 100 different enzymes, which promote chemical reactions in the body. Zinc is believed to be an important component of healthy immune systems. Studies have shown that it helps support normal growth and development during pregnancy through adolescence. It is needed for healing of wounds to the body as well as in the maintenance of the smell and taste senses.

Zinc is found in a wide variety of foods. Oysters contain more zinc per serving than any other food, but red meat and poultry provide the majority of zinc in the American diet. Other good food sources include beans, nuts, certain seafood, whole grains, fortified breakfast cereals, and dairy products. Zinc absorption is greater from a diet high in animal protein than a diet rich in plant proteins. Phytates, which are found in whole grain breads, cereals, legumes, and other products, can decrease zinc absorption.

Zinc deficiency most often occurs when zinc intake is inadequate or poorly absorbed. Signs of zinc deficiency include growth retardation, hair loss, diarrhea, delayed sexual maturation and impotence, eye and skin lesions, and loss of appetite. Maternal zinc deficiency can slow fetal growth. Since many of these symptoms are general and are associated with other medical conditions, do not assume they are due to a zinc deficiency. It is important to consult with a medical doctor about medical symptoms so that appropriate care can be given.

Low zinc status has been observed in 30 percent to 50 percent of alcoholics. Alcohol decreases the absorption of zinc and increases loss of zinc in urine. In addition, many alcoholics do not eat an acceptable variety or amount of food, so their dietary intake of zinc may be inadequate. Diarrhea results in a loss of zinc. HIV positive individuals who experience chronic diarrhea as a result of medications, should make sure they include sources of zinc in their daily diet and may benefit from zinc supplementation. A medical doctor can evaluate the need for a zinc supplement if diet alone fails to maintain normal zinc levels in these circumstances.

Zinc is required for the development and activation of T-lymphocytes, a kind of white blood cell that helps fight infection. When zinc supplements are given to individuals with low zinc levels, the numbers of T-cell lymphocytes circulating in the blood increase and the ability of lymphocytes to fight infection improves. Zinc is found in great quantities in the thymus, where these T-cells are produced. Many of the hormones produced by the thymus also require zinc to travel in the body, therefore increasing it's importance in the immune system.

Although HIV positive people have been shown to have lowered levels of zinc, it is unclear whether this is through poor absorption of the mineral or a result of the illness itself. Many activists believe zinc supplementation can be beneficial, however, there can be too much zinc in the body also, which causes levels of copper to drop to low levels leading to other complications and illnesses. Consulting a doctor regarding supplementation of diet is important.

zinc finger Chains of AMINO ACIDS found in cellular proteins that bind to DNA or messenger RNA, and play important roles in a cell's life cycle. They also appear to play a role during the earlier stages of cell infection. They are called zinc fingers because they capture and help package HIV genetic material into newly budding virions. Zinc fingers can have a number of structures. In HIV's zinc finger, four amino acids are responsible for capturing the zinc ion. The sequence is unique, found elsewhere only in other lentiviruses, the family of retroviruses that includes HIV-1 and 2, cancer-causing HTLV, feline immunodeficiency virus, and murine leukemia virus, to name a few.

Data presented by researchers from the National Cancer Institute at the Thirty-fifth Annual Interscience Conference on Antimicrobial Agents and Chemotherapy held in September 1995 indicate that HIV's zinc fingers may be the next antiviral target. The two zinc fingers in HIV's nucleocapsid (NC), a core viral protein, are involved in binding and packaging viral RNA into new virions budding from an infected cell. To date, experiments in which the zinc fingers have been deleted have shown that new budding virions do not incorporate RNA, which instead spills out of the infected cell. The NC protein and zinc fingers also play some role in the process of reverse transcription, although its exact nature is unclear. Some speculate that it may anchor the RNA molecule while the REVERSE TRANSCRIPTASE enzyme builds HIV DNA from the RNA template. HIV that lacks zinc fingers is unable to infect new cells. The zinc fingers are therefore essential for two phases of the viral life cycle.

Research findings indicate that HIV may not be able to mutate and escape the effects of drugs targeting its zinc fingers. Moreover, since HIV's zinc fingers are identical, one antiviral compound could inhibit both. Research is under way to find such a compound.

zinc finger inhibitors A group of drugs with the potential to disrupt HIV's replicating abilities. The phrase *zinc finger* refers to the loops resembling fingers that form when amino acids are linked together by zinc atoms. Drugs are being formulated to interrupt the formation of the fingerlike nucleocapsid protein through which HIV conveys genetic material to new virus being created in infected cells. Results of testing patients with zinc finger inhibitors has not proven highly effective, but manufacturers have several compounds that are from this group of drugs that are being tested for anti-HIV activity.

Zintevir (AR-177) An experimental NUCLEOTIDE REVERSE TRANSCRIPTASE INHIBITOR no longer in trials because of poor results and sale of the original developing company, Aronex.

zip code genocide An expression sometimes used by dismayed AIDS activists in the first decade of the epidemic, to refer to proposed public health policies that would explicitly have confined money spent on fighting the disease to certain geographical areas in which it was, at that time, concentrated. It was feared that such policies would create virtual AIDS ghettos, with disastrous social and economic effects on those within, while trivializing the seriousness of the problem by implying that the danger was confined to a few marginal neighborhoods and groups of people, while the rest of the population shared little risk.

In the first decade of the AIDS epidemic it was often observed that AIDS was settling into certain narrow geographic and cultural parameters (minority populations in specific urban areas), and that many other areas and demographic groups were virtually untouched. Sequestering the disease epidemiologically and putting money where the problems were—in specific neighborhoods in Houston, New York, Miami, San Francisco, and other cities—was often proposed as a preventative measure. It was pointed out, however, that identifying certain groups, whether infected or not, through such demographic means as zip code distribution was likely to lead to serious consequences—decreased property values, rejection of insurance coverage, higher rates of unemployment, and other forms of social and economic ostracism. Indeed it was predicted that in cities less tolerant than San Francisco, targeted groups might find their neighborhoods increasingly "ghettoized" and isolated from the larger community. Today, such segregationism is generally viewed as a dangerous idea that has racist and homophobic undertones. Also, much progress has been made in AIDS

education, helping to lessen discrimination against groups severely affected by the epidemic. This was accomplished largely by shifting the focus from HIGH-RISK GROUPS to HIGH-RISK BEHAVIORS.

Zithromax See AZITHROMYCIN.

Zocor See SIMVASTATIN.

Zoloft See SERTRALINE.

zolpidem A sleeping pill that is often prescribed for HIV patients who have trouble sleeping because of pain. Ambien works well for most people and does not cause drowsiness the following day. It cannot be taken with some PROTEASE INHIBITORS because they cause increase of the drug in the body and may lead to overdose in some situations. (Trade name is Ambien.)

zoning districts See ZONING RESTRICTIONS.

zoning ordinances See ZONING RESTRICTIONS.

zoning restrictions Zoning or land use ordinances generally divide a community into districts and designate uses appropriate to each. There are always districts limited to residential uses, and frequently single-family and multifamily residences are assigned to separate districts. Ordinances may define the type of family permitted in residential districts and may limit the number of unrelated people who may live together. Thus they may effectively prohibit informal group living arrangements for people with HIV who wish to live together, as families in family residences, in hospices, or in group homes or similar facilities.

Zoning ordinances may provide specifically for group homes by allowing them as "special-use" or "special exception" dwellings in residential districts, if they are considered compatible with the neighborhood. A special-use designation is allowed in a zoning district only after it has been approved by the local zoning agency or municipal governing body. Although special-use provisions do not on the surface present a serious obstacle to group homes for people with HIV, opponents of such homes may use these provisions to block their establishment in locations where they are needed.

Some areas specifically allow group homes as permitted uses in residential districts but limit the number of such homes or the extent to which they can be concentrated. State legislation that prohibits the exclusion of group homes from residential districts may contain similar restrictions.

Zoning restrictions on group homes and unrelated families may not serve a constitutionally acceptable purpose. They may also deny equal protection of the laws guaranteed by the Fourteenth Amendment, although the courts have been divided on the Fourteenth Amendment's application to zoning. Given the uncertainty of constitutional protection, advocates are relying on the FAIR HOUSING ACT to oppose discriminatory zoning practices. Although the act does not expressly prohibit zoning discrimination, it does prohibit acts that "otherwise make unavailable or deny" housing because of a handicap, such as HIV or AIDS. The courts have held that this language applies to discrimination that occurs through zoning ordinances.

Zovirax   See ACYCLOVIR.

APPENDIXES

I. Frequently Used Abbreviations
II. Statistics

I. HIV/AIDS Surveillance in the United States. (Source: Centers for Disease Control and Prevention)
1. Persons reported to be living with HIV infection and with AIDS, by area and age group, reported through December 2001
2. AIDS cases and annual rates per 100,000 population, by area and age group, reported through December 2001, United States
3. HIV infection cases by area and age group, reported through December 2001, from areas with confidential HIV infection reporting
4. AIDS cases and annual rates per 100,000 population, by metropolitan area and age group, reported through December 2001, United States
5. AIDS cases by age group, exposure category, and sex, reported through June 2001, United States
6. HIV infection cases by age group, exposure category, and sex, reported through December 2001, from areas with confidential HIV infection reporting
7. AIDS cases by sex, age at diagnosis, and race/ethnicity, reported through December 2001, United States
8. HIV infection cases by sex, age at diagnosis, and race/ethnicity, reported through December 2001, from areas with confidential HIV infection reporting
9. Pediatric AIDS cases by exposure category and race/ethnicity, reported through December 2001, United States

III. Selected Resources for Practitioners, Researchers, and Persons with HIV/AIDS

APPENDIX I
FREQUENTLY USED ABBREVIATIONS

ACT-UP	AIDS Coalition to Unleash Power
ACTG	AIDS clinical trial group
ADAP	AIDS Drug Assistance Program
AHCPR	Agency for Health Care Policy and Research
AIDS	acquired immunodeficiency syndrome
AIN	anal intraepithelial neoplasia
AmFAR	American Foundation for AIDS Research
AMA	American Medical Association
ARC	AIDS-related complex
ART	antiretroviral therapy
ASO	AIDS service organization
AZT	zidovudine, Retrovir
BID	twice a day
BV	bacterial vaginosis
CAT	computerized axial tomography; computer-assisted tomography (see CT)
CBC	complete blood count
CDC	[U.S.] Centers for Disease Control and Prevention
CFS	chronic fatigue syndrome
CID	Center for Infectious Diseases (of CDC)
CIN	cervical intraepithelial neoplasia
cis	carcinoma in situ
CMV	cytomegalovirus
CNS	central nervous system
CPCRA	Community Programs for Clinical Research on AIDS
CSF	cerebral spinal fluid
CSW	commercial sex worker
CT	computerized tomography (formerly CAT [see CAT])

DAIDS	Division of AIDS (U.S. National Institute of Allergy and Infectious Diseases)
ddC	2′, 3′-dideoxycytidine (Zalcitabine)
ddI	2′, 3′-dideoxyinosine (Didanosine)
DFA-TP	direct fluorescent antibody staining for *Treponema pallidum*
d4T	stavudine, Zerit
DHHS	U.S. Department of Health and Human Services
DNA	deoxyribonucleic acid
DSMB	data and safety monitoring board
EBV	Epstein-Barr virus
ELISA	enzyme-linked immunosorbent assay
FDA	[U.S.] Food and Drug Administration
FTA-ABS	fluorescent treponemal antibody absorption
G6PD	glucose-6 phosphate dehydrogenase
GI	gastrointestinal
GMHC	Gay Men's Health Crisis
GRID	gay-related immunodeficiency disease
GUD	genital ulcer disease
HAART	highly active antiretroviral therapy
HBV	hepatitis-B virus
HCV	hepatitis-C virus
HHV	human herpes virus
HIV	human immunodeficiency virus
HIV+	HIV-positive
HIV−	HIV-negative
HPV	human papillomavirus
HRT	hormone replacement therapy
HSV	herpes simplex virus
IAVI	international AIDS vaccine initiative
IDU	injection drug user
IFA	immunofluorescence antibody
IgG	immunoglobulin G

IM	intramuscular	OI	opportunistic infection
IND	Investigational New Drug	PACTG	pediatric AIDS clinical trials group
INH	isoniazid	PAP	Papanicolaou (Pap test, Pap smear)
IRB	Investigational Review Board	PCP	*Pneumocystis carinii* pneumonia
IV	intravenous	PCR	polymerase chain reaction
IVDU	intravenous drug user	PEP	post-exposure prophylaxis
KS	Kaposi's sarcoma	PGL	persistent generalized
LIP	lymphocytic interstitial pneumonia		lymphadenopathy
LP	lumbar puncture	PHS	[U.S.] Public Health Service
MAC	*Mycobacterium avium* complex	PI	protease inhibitor
MAI	*Mycobacterium avium intracellulare*	PID	pelvic inflammatory disease
MACS	multicenter AIDS cohort study	PML	progressive multifocal leukoen-
MDR	multidrug-resistant		cephalopathy
MHA-TP	microhemagglutination assay for	PMS	premenstrual syndrome
	Treponema pallidum	PWA	Person with AIDS; person living with
MHC	major histocompatibility complex		AIDS
MMWR	*Morbidity and Mortality Weekly Report*	QD	once a day
MRI	magnetic resonance imaging	RNA	ribonucleic acid
MSM	men who have sex with men	SIV	simian immunodeficiency syndrome
NGO	nongovernmental organization	SSI	supplemental security income
NHL	non-Hodgkin's lymphoma	SSDI	supplemental security disability
NIAID	National Institute of Allergy and		income
	Infectious Diseases (of NIH)	STD	sexually transmitted disease
NICHD	National Institute of Child Health and	STI	sexually transmitted infection
	Human Development (of NIH)	STI	structured treatment interruption
NIH	[U.S.] National Institute of Health	TAT 3	transactivator gene
NLM	National Library of Medicine (of NIH)	TB	tuberculosis
NNRTI	nonnucleoside reverse transcriptase	TID	three times a day
	inhibitor	TMP/SMX	trimethoprim-sulfamethoxazole
NRTI	nucleoside reverse transcriptase	3TC	lamivudine, Epivir
	inhibitor	UNAIDS	Joint United Nations Programme on
NtRTI	nucleotide reverse transcriptase		HIV/AIDS
	inhibitor	VAIN	vaginal intraepithelial neoplasia
OB/GYN	obstetrics/gynecology; obstetrician/	VIN	vulvar intraepithelial neoplasia
	gynecologist	WHO	[U.N.] World Health Organization

APPENDIX II
STATISTICS
I. HIV/AIDS Surveillance in the United States.
(Source: Centers for Disease Control)

TABLE 1 PERSONS REPORTED TO BE LIVING WITH HIV INFECTION[1] AND WITH AIDS, BY AREA AND AGE GROUP[2], REPORTED THROUGH DECEMBER 2001[3]

Area of residence (Date HIV reporting initiated)	Living with HIV infection[4]			Living with AIDS[5]			Cumulative totals		
	Adults/ adolescents	Children <13 years old	Total	Adults/ adolescents	Children <13 years old	Total	Adults/ adolescents	Children <13 years old	Total
Alabama (Jan. 1988)	5,279	32	5,311	3,410	17	3,427	8,689	49	8,738
Alaska (Feb. 1999)	43	0	43	238	1	239	281	1	282
Arizona (Jan. 1987)	4,670	32	4,702	3,604	8	3,612	8,274	40	8,314
Arkansas (July 1989)	2,114	13	2,127	1,761	20	1,781	3,875	33	3,908
California	—	—	—	45,285	143	45,428	45,285	143	45,428
Colorado (Nov. 1985)	5,566	17	5,583	3,119	2	3,121	8,685	19	8,704
Connecticut (July 1992)[6]	26	74	100	6,071	52	6,123	6,097	126	6,223
Delaware	—	—	—	1,355	12	1,367	1,355	12	1,367
District of Columbia	—	—	—	7,130	75	7,205	7,130	75	7,205
Florida (July 1997)	22,844	201	23,045	38,306	436	38,742	61,150	637	61,787
Georgia	—	—	—	11,193	76	11,269	11,193	76	11,269
Hawaii	—	—	—	1,065	5	1,070	1,065	5	1,070
Idaho (June 1986)	336	2	338	233	0	233	569	2	571
Illinois	—	—	—	10,617	100	10,717	10,617	100	10,717
Indiana (July 1988)	3,476	25	3,501	2,928	16	2,944	6,404	41	6,445
Iowa (July 1998)	415	4	419	620	3	623	1,035	7	1,042
Kansas (July 1999)	985	9	994	1,036	2	1,038	2,021	11	2,032
Kentucky	—	—	—	1,859	14	1,873	1,859	14	1,873
Louisiana (Feb. 1993)	7,269	95	7,364	5,805	46	5,851	13,074	141	13,215
Maine	—	—	—	482	4	486	482	4	486
Maryland	—	—	—	11,172	116	11,288	11,172	116	11,288
Massachusetts	—	—	—	7,318	50	7,368	7,318	50	7,368
Michigan (April 1992)	5,106	74	5,180	4,861	23	4,884	9,967	97	10,064
Minnesota (Oct. 1985)	2,754	23	2,777	1,728	9	1,737	4,482	32	4,514
Mississippi (Aug. 1988)	4,228	37	4,465	2,320	21	2,341	6,548	58	6,606
Missouri (Oct. 1987)	4,395	37	4,432	4,531	17	4,548	8,926	54	8,980
Montana	—	—	—	172	0	172	172	—	172
Nebraska (Sept. 1995)	539	6	545	518	4	522	1,057	10	1,067
Nevada (Feb. 1992)	2,784	21	2,805	2,240	9	2,249	5,024	30	5,054
New Hampshire	—	—	—	505	2	507	505	2	507
New Jersey (Jan. 1992)	13,119	318	13,437	15,542	160	15,702	28,661	478	29,139

New Mexico (Jan. 1998)	672	0	672	1,035	5	1,040	1,707	5	1,712
New York (June 2000)	19,172	1,231	20,403	56,331	461	56,792	75,503	1,692	77,195
North Carolina (Feb. 1990)	9,819	91	9,910	5,371	31	5,402	15,190	122	15,312
North Dakota (Jan. 1988)	67	1	68	45	1	46	112	2	114
Ohio (June 1990)	5,976	61	6,037	4,868	37	4,905	10,844	98	10,942
Oklahoma (June 1988)	2,346	18	2,364	1,679	6	1,685	4,025	24	4,049
Oregon (Sept. 1988)[6]	4	13	17	2,213	5	2,218	2,217	18	2,235
Pennsylvania	—	—	—	12,533	147	12,680	12,533	147	12,680
Rhode Island	—	—	—	954	7	961	954	7	961
South Carolina (Feb. 1986)	6,677	67	6,744	5,143	29	5,172	11,820	96	11,916
South Dakota (Jan. 1988)	183	1	184	94	1	95	277	2	279
Tennessee (Jan. 1992)	6,036	59	6,095	5,005	16	5,021	11,041	75	11,116
Texas (Jan. 1999)[6]	10,390	256	10,646	24,819	117	24,936	35,209	373	35,582
Utah (April 1989)	697	8	705	1,086	3	1,089	1,783	11	1,794
Vermont	—	—	—	214	2	216	214	2	216
Virginia (July 1989)	7,990	53	8,043	6,373	70	6,443	14,363	123	14,486
Washington	—	—	—	4,417	9	4,426	4,417	9	4,426
West Virginia (Jan. 1989)	570	7	577	533	5	538	1,103	12	1,115
Wisconsin (Nov. 1985)	2,187	19	2,206	1,656	13	1,669	3,843	32	3,875
Wyoming (June 1989)	72	0	72	78	2	80	150	2	152
Subtotal	**158,806**	**2,905**	**161,711**	**331,471**	**2,410**	**333,881**	**490,277**	**5,315**	**495,592**
U.S. dependencies, possessions, and associated nations									
Guam (March 2000)	58	1	59	32	0	32	90	1	91
Pacific Islands, U.S.[7]	8	—	8	3	0	3	11	0	11
Puerto Rico	—	—	—	9,471	77	9,548	9,471	77	9,548
Virgin Islands, U.S. (Dec. 1998)	195	3	198	243	5	248	438	8	446
Total	**159,067**	**2,909**	**161,976**	**341,679**	**2,499**	**344,178**	**500,746**	**5,408**	**506,154**

[1] Includes only persons reported with HIV infection who have not developed AIDS.

[2] Age group based on person's age as of December 31, 2001.

[3] Persons reported with vital status "alive" as of the last update. Excludes persons whose vital status is unknown.

[4] Includes only persons reported from areas with confidential HIV reporting. Excludes 2,223 adults/adolescents and 54 children reported from areas with confidential HIV infection reporting whose area of residence is unknown or are residents of other areas.

[5] Includes 459 adults/adolescents and seven children whose area of residence is unknown.

[6] Connecticut has confidential HIV infection reporting for pediatric cases only; through September 2001, Oregon has confidential HIV infection reporting for children less than six years old. Texas reported only pediatric HIV infection cases from February 1994 until January 1999. Some persons who were children when HIV was initially diagnosed are now aged 13 years or older and are presented as adults/adolescents living with HIV.

[7] American Samoa began confidential HIV infection reporting in August 2001 and the Northern Mariana Islands began reporting in October 2001.

TABLE 2   AIDS CASES AND ANNUAL RATES PER 100,000 POPULATION, BY AREA AND AGE GROUP, REPORTED THROUGH DECEMBER 2001, UNITED STATES

Area of residence	2000		2001		Cumulative totals		
	No.	Rate	No.	Rate	Adults/adolescents	Children <13 years old	Total
Alabama	482	10.8	438	9.8	6,632	74	6,706
Alaska	23	3.7	18	2.8	490	5	495
Arizona	443	8.6	540	10.2	7,925	41	7,966
Arkansas	194	7.2	199	7.4	3,139	38	3,177
California	4,696	13.8	4,315	12.5	123,200	619	123,819
Colorado	339	7.8	288	6.5	7,351	30	7,381
Connecticut	614	18.0	584	17.1	11,972	176	12,148
Delaware	220	28.0	248	31.1	2,803	24	2,827
District of Columbia	873	152.9	870	152.1	13,796	173	13,969
Florida	4,905	30.6	5,138	31.3	83,888	1,436	85,324
Georgia	1,231	15.0	1,745	20.8	24,347	212	24,559
Hawaii	115	9.5	124	10.1	2,569	16	2,585
Idaho	22	1.7	19	1.4	514	3	517
Illinois	1,758	14.1	1,323	10.6	26,047	272	26,319
Indiana	382	6.3	378	6.2	6,466	49	6,515
Iowa	92	3.1	90	3.1	1,392	10	1,402
Kansas	127	4.7	98	3.6	2,453	12	2,465
Kentucky	210	5.2	333	8.2	3,648	27	3,675
Louisiana	661	14.8	861	19.3	13,350	125	13,475
Maine	40	3.1	48	3.7	995	9	1,004
Maryland	1,455	27.4	1,860	34.6	23,228	309	23,537
Massachusetts	1,185	18.6	765	12.0	16,797	211	17,008
Michigan	761	7.6	548	5.5	11,755	108	11,863
Minnesota	184	3.7	157	3.2	3,896	23	3,919
Mississippi	428	15.0	418	14.6	4,821	56	4,877
Missouri	452	8.1	445	7.9	9,594	60	9,654
Montana	16	1.8	15	1.7	338	3	341
Nebraska	77	4.5	74	4.3	1,157	10	1,167
Nevada	283	14.0	252	12.0	4,637	28	4,665
New Hampshire	30	2.4	40	3.2	910	9	919
New Jersey	1,875	22.2	1,756	20.7	43,068	756	43,824
New Mexico	144	7.9	143	7.8	2,179	8	2,187
New York	6,301	33.2	7,476	39.3	147,065	2,276	149,341
North Carolina	674	8.3	942	11.5	11,240	116	11,356
North Dakota	3	0.5	3	0.5	109	1	110
Ohio	588	5.2	581	5.1	11,834	124	11,958
Oklahoma	353	10.2	243	7.0	4,004	26	4,030
Oregon	208	6.1	259	7.5	5,039	17	5,056
Pennsylvania	1,658	13.5	1,840	15.0	26,033	336	26,369
Rhode Island	99	9.4	103	9.7	2,130	23	2,153
South Carolina	789	19.6	729	17.9	10,151	86	10,237
South Dakota	8	1.1	25	3.3	187	4	191
Tennessee	839	14.7	602	10.5	9,114	52	9,166
Texas	2,631	12.6	2,892	13.6	56,344	386	56,730
Utah	148	6.6	124	5.5	2,076	21	2,097
Vermont	38	6.2	25	4.1	422	6	428
Virginia	872	12.3	951	13.2	13,842	176	14,018
Washington	496	8.4	532	8.9	9,971	34	10,005
West Virginia	61	3.4	100	5.5	1,168	10	1,178
Wisconsin	213	4.0	193	3.6	3,737	31	3,768
Wyoming	11	2.2	5	1.0	189	3	192
Subtotal	**40,307**	**14.3**	**41,755**	**14.7**	**780,012**	**8,660**	**788,672**
U.S. dependencies, possessions, and associated nations							
Guam	13	8.4	12	7.6	58	0	58
Pacific Islands, U.S.	0	0.0	1	0.3	5	0	5
Puerto Rico	1,346	35.3	1,242	32.3	25,730	389	26,119
Virgin Islands, U.S.	34	28.1	35	28.6	501	17	518
Total[1]	**41,795**	**14.6**	**43,158**	**14.9**	**807,075**	**9,074**	**816,149**

[1] U.S. totals presented in this report include data from the United States (50 states and the District of Columbia), and from U.S. dependencies, possessions, and independent nations in free association with the United States. See Technical Notes. Totals include 777 persons whose area of residence is unknown.

TABLE 3 HIV INFECTION CASES[1] BY AREA AND AGE GROUP, REPORTED THROUGH DECEMBER 2001, FROM AREAS WITH CONFIDENTIAL HIV INFECTION REPORTING

Area of residence (Data HIV reporting initiated)	2001	Cumulative totals		
		Adults/ adolescents	Children <13 years old	Total
Alabama (Jan. 1988)	491	5,505	41	5,546
Alaska (Feb. 1999)	15	48	1	49
Arizona (Jan. 1987)	553	4,936	42	4,978
Arkansas (July 1989)	211	2,155	20	2,175
Colorado (Nov. 1985)	391	5,820	29	5,849
Connecticut (July 1992)[2]	4	0	108	108
Florida (July 1997)	5,744	23,325	232	23,557
Idaho (June 1986)	27	393	4	397
Indiana (July 1988)	394	3,688	39	3,727
Iowa (July 1998)	79	420	8	428
Kansas (July 1999)	103	1,015	14	1,029
Louisiana (Feb. 1993)	830	7,692	125	7,817
Michigan (April 1992)	674	5,858	118	5,976
Minnesota (Oct. 1985)	272	2,918	34	2,952
Mississippi (Aug. 1988)	408	4,447	49	4,496
Missouri (Oct. 1987)	481	4,571	47	4,618
Nebraska (Sept. 1995)	90	565	8	573
Nevada (Feb. 1992)	297	3,127	25	3,152
New Jersey (Jan. 1992)	1,571	14,770	403	15,173
New Mexico (Jan. 1998)	80	699	3	702
New York (June. 2000)	13,403	19,161	1,609	20,770
North Carolina (Feb. 1990)	1,046	10,730	123	10,853
North Dakota (Jan. 1988)	7	75	1	76
Ohio (June 1990)	831	6,344	80	6,424
Oklahoma (June 1988)	223	2,472	27	2,499
Oregon (Sept. 1988)[2]	1	0	17	17
South Carolina (Feb. 1986)	695	7,258	102	7,360
South Dakota (Jan. 1988)	14	200	5	205
Tennessee (Jan. 1992)	721	6,247	74	6,321
Texas (Jan. 1999)[2]	4,237	10,495	320	10,815
Utah (April 1989)	50	709	11	720
Virginia (July 1989)	879	8,609	75	8,684
West Virginia (Jan. 1989)	55	601	8	609
Wisconsin (Nov. 1985)	165	2,363	29	2,392
Wyoming (June 1989)	9	79	0	79
Subtotal	**35,051**	**167,295**	**3,831**	**171,126**
U.S. dependencies, possessions, and associated nations				
American Samoa (Aug. 2001)	1	1	0	1
Guam (March 2000)	19	63	1	64
Mariana Islands, U.S (Oct. 2001)	18	18	0	18
Virgin Islands, U.S (Dec. 1998)	24	206	4	210
Persons reported from states with confidential HIV reporting who were residents of other states[3]	462	2,520	87	2,607
Total	**35,575**	**170,103**	**3,923**	**174,026**

[1] Includes only persons reported with HIV infection who have not developed AIDS.

[2] Connecticut has confidential HIV infection reporting for pediatric cases only; through September 2001, Oregon has confidential HIV infection reporting for children less than six years old. Texas reported only pediatric HIV infection cases from February 1994 until January 1999.

[3] Includes 692 persons reported from areas with confidential HIV infection reporting, but whose area of residence is unknown. See Technical Notes.

[4] American Samoa began confidential HIV infection reporting in August 2001 and the Northern Mariana Islands began reporting in October 2001.

Metropolitan area of residence (with 500,000 or more population)	2000		2001		Cumulative totals		
	No.	Rate	No.	Rate	Adults/ adolescents	Children <13 years old	Total
Akron, Ohio	30	4.3	21	3.0	606	1	607
Albany-Schenectady, N.Y.	115	13.1	80	9.1	1,807	25	1,832
Albuquerque, N.Mex.	72	10.1	63	8.7	1,163	2	1,165
Allentown, Pa.	49	7.7	85	13.2	910	11	921
Ann Arbor, Mich.	35	6.0	14	2.4	412	9	421
Atlanta, Ga.	704	17.0	1,293	30.3	17,041	116	17,157
Austin, Tex.	179	14.2	208	15.8	4,046	27	4,073
Bakersfield, Calif.	82	12.4	106	15.7	1,124	8	1,132
Baltimore, Md.	967	37.8	1,287	50.0	15,580	212	15,792
Baton Rouge, La.	143	23.7	221	36.4	2,110	19	2,129
Bergen-Passaic, N.J.	210	15.3	187	13.6	5,608	83	5,691
Birmingham, Ala.	115	12.5	109	11.7	1,996	23	2,019
Boston, Mass.	1,013	16.7	659	10.8	14,758	187	14,945
Buffalo, N.Y.	81	6.9	136	11.7	1,945	19	1,964
Charleston, S.C.	116	21.1	55	9.9	1,608	12	1,620
Charlotte, N.C.	125	8.3	182	11.8	2,278	23	2,301
Chicago, Ill.	1,520	18.3	1,053	12.6	22,462	241	22,703
Cincinnati, Ohio	74	4.5	40	2.4	1,938	15	1,953
Cleveland, Ohio	163	7.2	212	9.4	3,533	43	3,576
Colorado Springs, Colo.	24	4.6	19	3.6	472	5	477
Columbia, S.C.	153	28.4	178	32.7	2,197	18	2,215
Columbus, Ohio	116	7.5	102	6.5	2,315	13	2,328
Dallas, Tex.	647	18.3	749	20.5	13,082	37	13,119
Dayton, Ohio	64	6.7	60	6.3	1,056	17	1,073
Daytona Beach, Fla.	80	16.1	107	21.0	1,237	14	1,251
Denver, Colo.	250	11.8	217	10.0	5,830	21	5,851
Detroit, Mich.	550	12.4	389	8.7	8,123	73	8,196
El Paso, Tex.	78	11.4	115	16.7	1,184	10	1,194
Fort Lauderdale, Fla.	855	52.4	689	41.3	13,345	249	13,594
Fort Wayne, Ind.	24	4.8	22	4.4	334	3	337
Fort Worth, Tex.	189	11.0	132	7.5	3,364	26	3,390
Fresno, Calif.	93	10.0	56	5.9	1,252	14	1,266
Gary, Ind.	59	9.3	54	8.5	783	6	789
Grand Rapids, Mich.	37	3.4	42	3.8	805	4	809
Greensboro, N.C.	96	7.6	124	9.8	1,784	21	1,805
Greenville, S.C.	119	12.3	107	10.9	1,607	7	1,614
Harrisburg, Pa.	69	11.0	123	19.5	1,134	8	1,142
Hartford, Conn.	235	20.4	195	16.8	4,158	46	4,204
Honolulu, Hawaii	84	9.6	52	5.9	1,838	13	1,851
Houston, Tex.	687	16.4	801	18.7	19,735	163	19,898
Indianapolis, Ind.	161	10.0	175	10.7	3,046	20	3,066
Jacksonville, Fla.	285	25.8	311	27.5	4,715	70	4,785
Jersey City, N.J.	220	36.1	256	42.1	6,735	120	6,855
Kansas City, Mo.	178	10.0	164	9.1	4,091	14	4,105
Knoxville, Tenn.	45	6.5	33	4.7	759	6	765
Las Vegas, Nev.	250	15.8	216	13.0	3,807	27	3,834
Little Rock, Ark.	54	9.2	81	13.7	1,125	14	1,139
Los Angeles, Calif.	1,644	17.2	1,391	14.4	43,252	236	43,488
Louisville, Ky.	91	8.9	149	14.5	1,779	17	1,796
McAllen, Tex.	40	7.0	51	8.6	420	10	430
Memphis, Tenn.	322	28.3	259	22.6	3,417	18	3,435
Miami, Fla.	1,303	57.5	1,232	53.8	24,868	489	25,357
Middlesex, N.J.	132	11.2	147	12.4	3,286	71	3,357
Milwaukee, Wis.	133	8.9	115	7.7	2,072	18	2,090
Minneapolis–Saint Paul, Minn.	169	5.7	135	4.5	3,465	17	3,482
Mobile, Ala.	99	18.3	86	15.8	1,275	16	1,291
Monmouth-Ocean, N.J.	129	11.4	126	11.0	2,942	62	3,004
Nashville, Tenn.	326	26.4	186	14.9	2,908	17	2,925
Nassau/Suffolk, N.Y.	246	8.9	350	12.6	6,889	113	7,002
New Haven, Conn.	312	18.3	348	20.3	6,789	124	6,913
New Orleans, La.	322	24.1	312	23.4	7,185	67	7,252

TABLE 4   AIDS CASES AND ANNUAL RATES PER 100,000 POPULATION, BY METROPOLITAN AREA AND AGE GROUP,
REPORTED THROUGH DECEMBER 2001, UNITED STATES *(Continued)*

Metropolitan area of residence (with 500,000 or more population)	2000		2001		Cumulative totals		
	No.	Rate	No.	Rate	Adults/ adolescents	Children <13 years old	Total
New York, N.Y.	5,412	58.1	6,152	65.9	124,201	2,036	126,237
Newark, N.J.	773	38.0	711	34.8	17,469	327	17,796
Norfolk, Va.	271	17.2	334	21.1	4,061	63	4,124
Oakland, Calif.	272	11.3	320	13.1	8,304	43	8,347
Oklahoma City, Okla.	204	18.8	120	11.0	1,894	7	1,901
Omaha, Nebr.	53	7.4	54	7.5	808	3	811
Orange County, Calif.	286	10.0	299	10.3	5,889	36	5,925
Orlando, Fla.	356	21.5	532	31.2	6,458	82	6,540
Philadelphia, Pa.	1,357	26.6	1,355	26.5	20,091	278	20,369
Phoenix, Ariz.	294	9.0	376	11.1	5,635	27	5,662
Pittsburgh, Pa.	106	4.5	146	6.2	2,496	18	2,514
Portland, Oreg.	174	9.0	220	11.2	4,089	8	4,097
Providence, R.I.	93	9.6	97	10.0	2,000	21	2,021
Raleigh-Durham, N.C.	145	12.1	159	12.9	2,151	22	2,173
Richmond, Va.	168	16.8	126	12.5	2,716	29	2,745
Riverside–San Bernardino, Calif.	399	12.2	392	11.5	7,260	59	7,319
Rochester, N.Y.	75	6.8	127	11.6	2,448	13	2,461
Sacramento, Calif.	171	10.4	130	7.6	3,331	24	3,355
Saint Louis, Mo.	246	9.4	282	10.8	4,966	41	5,007
Salt Lake City, Utah	131	9.8	111	8.2	1,805	14	1,819
San Antonio, Tex.	167	10.4	200	12.3	4,129	28	4,157
San Diego, Calif.	439	15.5	478	16.7	11,015	55	11,070
San Francisco, Calif.	762	44.0	596	34.6	28,391	47	28,438
San Jose, Calif.	110	6.5	120	7.2	3,241	14	3,255
San Juan, P.R.	872	44.3	701	35.3	16,130	242	16,372
Sarasota, Fla.	129	21.8	139	22.8	1,579	24	1,603
Scranton, Pa.	19	3.0	13	2.1	442	4	446
Seattle, Wash.	285	11.8	348	14.3	6,987	19	7,006
Springfield, Mass.	147	24.2	94	15.4	1,822	24	1,846
Stockton, Calif.	37	6.5	26	4.4	781	13	794
Syracuse, N.Y.	90	12.3	116	15.9	1,407	10	1,417
Tacoma, Wash.	58	8.2	67	9.3	897	9	906
Tampa–Saint Petersburg, Fla.	454	18.9	607	24.8	8,901	105	9,006
Toledo, Ohio	31	5.0	43	7.0	610	12	622
Tucson, Ariz.	74	8.7	122	14.1	1,633	10	1,643
Tulsa, Okla.	71	8.8	71	8.8	1,198	9	1,207
Vallejo, Calif.	64	12.3	90	16.9	1,465	11	1,476
Ventura, Calif.	42	5.5	33	4.3	846	3	849
Washington, D.C.	1,542	31.2	1,657	32.8	24,549	295	24,844
West Palm Beach, Fla.	538	47.4	459	39.4	7,912	206	8,118
Wichita, Kans.	45	8.2	17	3.1	746	2	748
Wilmington, Del.	173	29.4	197	33.1	2,235	17	2,252
Youngstown, Ohio	18	3.0	28	4.7	395	0	395
Metropolitan areas with 500,000 or more population	**33,916**	**18.7**	**34,732**	**19.0**	**676,768**	**7,700**	**684,468**
Central counties	*33,132*	*20.1*	*33,904*	*20.4*	*663,026*	*7,560*	*670,586*
Outlying counties	*784*	*4.7*	*828*	*4.9*	*13,742*	*140*	*13,882*
Metropolitan areas with 50,000 to 499,999 population	**4,493**	**9.2**	**4,690**	**9.5**	**77,206**	**834**	**78,040**
Central counties	*4,205*	*9.7*	*4,371*	*10.0*	*72,084*	*760*	*72,844*
Outlying counties	*288*	*5.2*	*319*	*5.7*	*5,122*	*74*	*5,196*
Nonmetropolitan areas	**3,083**	**5.4**	**3,278**	**5.8**	**48,865**	**510**	**49,375**
Total[1]	**41,795**	**14.6**	**43,158**	**14.9**	**807,075**	**9,074**	**816,149**

[1] Totals include 4,266 persons whose area of residence is unknown.

TABLE 5 AIDS CASES BY AGE GROUP, EXPOSURE CATEGORY, AND SEX, REPORTED THROUGH JUNE 2001, UNITED STATES

	Males				Females				Totals[1]			
	2001		Cumulative total		2001		Cumulative total		J2001		Cumulative total	
Adult/adolescent exposure category	No.	(%)	No.	(%)	No.	(%)	No.	(%)	No.	(%)	No.	(%)
Men who have sex with men	13,265	(42)	368,971	(55)	—	—	—	—	13,265	(31)	368,971	(46)
Injecting drug use	5,261	(16)	145,750	(22)	2,212	(20)	55,576	(39)	7,473	(17)	201,326	(25)
Men who have sex with men and inject drugs	1,502	(5)	51,293	(8)	—	—	—	—	1,502	(3)	51,293	(6)
Hemophilia/coagulation disorder	97	(0)	5,000	(1)	9	(0)	292	(0)	106	(0)	5,292	(1)
Heterosexual contact:	2,762	(9)	32,735	(5)	4,142	(37)	57,396	(41)	6,904	(16)	90,131	(11)
Sex with injecting drug user	549		9,821		937		21,736		1,486		31,557	
Sex with bisexual male	—		—		192		3,801		192		3,801	
Sex with person with hemophilia	5		69		8		425		13		494	
Sex with transfusion recipient with HIV infection	19		446		13		619		32		1,065	
Sex with HIV-infected person, risk not specified	2,189		22,399		2,992		30,815		5,181		53,214	
Receipt of blood transfusion, blood components, or tissue[3]	105	(0)	5,057	(1)	113	(1)	3,914	(3)	218	(1)	8,971	(1)
Other/risk not reported or identified[4]	8,909	(28)	57,220	(9)	4,606	(42)	23,870	(17)	13,515	(31)	81,091	(10)
Adult/adolescent subtotal	31,901	(100)	666,026	(100)	11,082	(100)	141,048	(100)	42,983	(100)	807,075	(100)
Pediatric (<13 years old) exposure category												
Hemophilia/coagulation disorder	0	(0)	229	(5)	0	(0)	7	(0)	0	(0)	236	(3)
Mother with/at risk for HIV infection:[4]	79	(85)	4,113	(88)	71	(87)	4,171	(95)	150	(86)	8,284	(91)
Injecting drug use	17		1,626		16		1,612		33		3,238	
Sex with injecting drug user	8		763		7		728		15		1,491	
Sex with bisexual male	2		91		3		95		5		186	
Sex with person with hemophilia	1		18		0		15		1		33	
Sex with transfusion recipient with HIV infection	0		11		0		14		0		25	
Sex with HIV-infected person, risk not specified	22		656		16		683		38		1,339	
Receipt of blood transfusion, blood components, or tissue	1		74		1		80		2		154	
Has HIV infection, risk not specified	28		874		28		944		56		1,818	
Receipt of blood transfusion, blood components, or tissue[3]	2	(2)	241	(5)	0	(0)	140	(3)	2	(1)	381	(4)
Other/risk not reported or identified[5]	12	(13)	78	(2)	11	(13)	95	(2)	23	(13)	173	(2)
Pediatric subtotal	93	(100)	4,661	(100)	82	(100)	4,413	(100)	175	(100)	9,074	(100)
Total	31,994		670,687		11,164		145,461		43,158		816,149	

[1] Includes one person whose sex is unknown.

[2] Includes persons known to be infected with human immunodeficiency virus type 2 (HIV-2). See MMWR 1995;44:603–06.

[3] Forty-one adults/adolescents and two children developed AIDS after receiving blood screened negative for HIV antibody. Thirteen additional adults developed AIDS after receiving tissue, organs, or artificial insemination from HIV-infected donors. Four of the 13 received tissue, organs, or artificial insemination from a donor who was negative for HIV antibody at the time of donation. See N Engl J Med 1992;326:726–32.

[4] Thirty-four adults/adolescents are included in the "other" exposure category who were exposed to HIV-infected blood, body fluids, or concentrated virus in health care, laboratory, or household settings, as supported by seroconversion, epidemiologic, and/or laboratory evidence. See MMWR 1993;42:329–31, MMWR 1993;42:948–51, and XI International Conference on AIDS; Vancouver, Canada: July 7–12, 1996;1:179 [abstract Mo.D.1728]. One person was infected following intentional inoculation with HIV-infected blood. Additionally, 221 persons acquired HIV infection perinatally and were diagnosed with AIDS after age 13. These 221 persons are tabulated under the adult/adolescent, not pediatric, exposure category. See Technical Notes.

[5] Includes five children who were exposed to HIV-infected blood as supported by seroconversion, epidemiologic, and/or laboratory evidence: 1 child was infected following intentional inoculation with HIV-infected blood and four children were exposed to HIV-infected blood in a household setting (see MMWR 1992; 41:228–31 and N Engl J Med 1993;329:1835–41). Twelve of the children had sexual contact with an adult with or at high risk for HIV infection (see Pediatrics 1998;102:e46).

TABLE 6 HIV INFECTION CASES[1] BY AGE GROUP, EXPOSURE CATEGORY, AND SEX, REPORTED THROUGH DECEMBER 2001, FROM AREAS WITH CONFIDENTIAL HIV INFECTION REPORTING[2]

	Males				Females				Totals[3]			
	2001		Cumulative total		2001		Cumulative total		2001		Cumulative total	
Adult/adolescent exposure category	No.	(%)	No.	(%)	No.	(%)	No.	(%)	No.	(%)	No.	(%)
Men who have sex with men	7,674	(32)	52,139	(43)	—	—	—	—	7,674	(22)	52,139	(31)
Injecting drug use	1,844	(8)	14,904	(12)	1,097	(10)	8,609	(17)	2,941	(8)	23,514	(14)
Men who have sex with men and inject drugs	614	(3)	6,651	(6)	—	—	—	—	614	(2)	6,651	(4)
Hemophilia/coagulation disorder	24	(0)	455	(0)	6	(0)	37	(0)	30	(0)	492	(0)
Heterosexual contact:	1,466	(6)	8,597	(7)	3,071	(28)	19,157	(39)	4,537	(13)	27,754	(16)
Sex with injecting drug user	208		1,694		544		4,594		752		6,288	
Sex with bisexual male	—		—		150		1,330		150		1,330	
Sex with person with hemophilia	4		17		13		147		17		164	
Sex with transfusion recipient with HIV infection	7		82		11		120		18		202	
Sex with HIV-infected person, risk not specified	1,247		6,804		2,353		12,966		3,600		19,770	
Receipt of blood transfusion, blood components, or tissue	47	(0)	447	(0)	52	(0)	467	(1)	99	(0)	914	(1)
Other/risk not reported or identified[4]	12,230	(51)	37,675	(31)	6,907	(62)	20,956	(43)	19,137	(55)	58,639	(34)
Adult/adolescent subtotal	23,899	(100)	120,868	(100)	11,133	(100)	49,226	(100)	35,032	(100)	170,103	(100)
Pediatric (<13 years old) exposure category												
Hemophilia/coagulation disorder	8	(3)	107	(6)	1	(0)	2	(0)	9	(2)	109	(3)
Mother with/at risk for HIV infection:	205	(73)	1,603	(83)	185	(71)	1,733	(87)	390	(72)	3,336	(35)
Injecting drug use	31		472		30		473		61		945	
Sex with injecting drug user	17		168		7		178		24		346	
Sex with bisexual male	2		19		0		15		2		34	
Sex with person with hemophilia	0		1		0		7		0		8	
Sex with transfusion recipient with HIV infection	0		8		0		5		0		13	
Sex with HIV-infected person, risk not specified	47		317		56		403		103		720	
Receipt of blood transfusion, blood components, or tissue	4		15		1		16		5		31	
Has HIV infection, risk not specified	104		603		91		636		195		1,239	
Receipt of blood transfusion, blood components, or tissue	2	(1)	21	(1)	2	(1)	26	(1)	4	(1)	47	(1)
Risk not reported or identified[4]	67	(24)	202	(10)	73	(28)	229	(12)	140	(26)	431	(11)
Pediatric subtotal	282	(100)	1,933	(100)	261	(100)	1,990	(100)	543	(100)	3,923	(100)
Total	24,181		122,801		11,394		51,216		35,575		174,026	

[1] Includes only persons reported with HIV infection who have not developed AIDS.

[2] See Table 3 for areas with confidential HIV infection reporting.

[3] Includes nine persons whose sex is unknown.

[4] For HIV infection cases, "risk not reported or identified" refers primarily to persons whose mode of exposure was not reported and who have not been followed up to determine their mode of exposure, and to a smaller number of persons who are not reported with one of the exposures listed above after follow-up. See Technical Notes.

TABLE 7 AIDS CASES BY SEX, AGE AT DIAGNOSIS, AND RACE/ETHNICITY, REPORTED THROUGH DECEMBER 2001, UNITED STATES

Male Age at diagnosis (years)	White, not Hispanic No.	(%)	Black, not Hispanic No.	(%)	Hispanic No.	(%)	Asian/Pacific Islander No.	(%)	American Indian/ Alaska Native No.	(%)	Total[1] No.	(%)
Under 5	535	(0)	2,165	(1)	783	(1)	17	(0)	12	(1)	3,515	(1)
5–12	346	(0)	498	(0)	284	(0)	10	(0)	6	(0)	1,146	(0)
13–19	916	(0)	1,020	(0)	570	(0)	26	(0)	23	(1)	2,555	(0)
20–24	7,938	(3)	7,590	(3)	4,520	(4)	181	(3)	84	(4)	20,337	(3)
25–29	38,967	(12)	26,595	(12)	17,138	(14)	675	(13)	351	(17)	83,794	(12)
30–34	71,345	(23)	46,088	(20)	28,377	(23)	1,161	(22)	536	(26)	147,600	(22)
35–39	71,995	(23)	51,302	(22)	27,047	(22)	1,169	(22)	473	(23)	152,124	(23)
40–44	52,653	(17)	41,395	(18)	19,215	(16)	927	(17)	303	(15)	114,585	(17)
45–49	32,116	(10)	24,839	(11)	10,937	(9)	558	(10)	134	(7)	68,635	(10)
50–54	17,498	(6)	12,959	(6)	5,861	(5)	301	(6)	63	(3)	36,718	(5)
55–59	9,337	(3)	6,987	(3)	3,242	(3)	177	(3)	37	(2)	19,801	(3)
60–64	5,139	(2)	3,819	(2)	1,769	(1)	76	(1)	18	(1)	10,829	(2)
65 or older	4,249	(1)	3,242	(1)	1,455	(1)	76	(1)	17	(1)	9,048	(1)
Male subtotal	**313,034**	**(100)**	**228,499**	**(100)**	**121,198**	**(100)**	**5,354**	**(100)**	**2,057**	**(100)**	**670,687**	**(100)**

Female Age at diagnosis (years)	No.	(%)	No.	(%)	No.	(%)	No.	(%)	No.	(%)	No.	(%)
Under 5	502	(2)	2,153	(3)	770	(3)	17	(2)	13	(3)	3,460	(2)
5–12	196	(1)	521	(1)	223	(1)	10	(1)	0	(0)	953	(1)
13–19	295	(1)	1,250	(1)	316	(1)	8	(1)	4	(1)	1,873	(1)
20–24	1,774	(6)	4,844	(6)	1,625	(6)	46	(6)	36	(8)	8,328	(6)
25–29	4,831	(16)	11,876	(14)	4,364	(15)	116	(14)	69	(14)	21,266	(15)
30–34	6,818	(22)	18,055	(21)	6,418	(22)	146	(18)	105	(22)	31,564	(22)
35–39	6,244	(20)	18,351	(22)	5,878	(21)	142	(18)	95	(20)	30,733	(21)
40–44	4,199	(14)	13,221	(16)	3,950	(14)	121	(15)	61	(13)	21,560	(15)
45–49	2,307	(7)	6,922	(8)	2,249	(8)	74	(9)	48	(10)	11,607	(8)
50–54	1,309	(4)	3,447	(4)	1,245	(4)	37	(5)	22	(5)	6,062	(4)
55–59	816	(3)	1,865	(2)	750	(3)	29	(4)	18	(4)	3,479	(2)
60–64	519	(2)	1,103	(1)	411	(1)	29	(4)	5	(1)	2,069	(1)
65 or older	1,044	(3)	1,073	(1)	355	(1)	28	(3)	4	(1)	2,507	(2)
Female subtotal	**30,854**	**(100)**	**84,681**	**(100)**	**28,554**	**(100)**	**803**	**(100)**	**480**	**(100)**	**145,461**	**(100)**
Total[2]	**343,889**		**313,180**		**149,752**		**6,157**		**2,537**		**816,149**	

[1] Includes 545 males and 89 females whose race/ethnicity is unknown.
[2] Includes one person whose sex is unknown.

TABLE 8 HIV INFECTION CASES[1] BY SEX, AGE AT DIAGNOSIS, AND RACE/ETHNICITY, REPORTED THROUGH DECEMBER 2001, FROM AREAS WITH CONFIDENTIAL HIV INFECTION REPORTING[2]

Male	White, not Hispanic		Black, not Hispanic		Hispanic		Asian/Pacific Islander		American Indian/ Alaska Native		Total[3]	
Age at diagnosis (years)	No.	(%)	No.	(%)	No.	(%)	No.	(%)	No.	(%)	No.	(%)
Under 5	214	(0)	906	(2)	299	(2)	5	(1)	2	(0)	1,429	(1)
5–12	123	(0)	244	(0)	127	(1)	5	(1)	1	(0)	504	(0)
13–19	872	(2)	1,654	(3)	249	(2)	8	(1)	20	(3)	2,825	(2)
20–24	5,725	(11)	6,271	(11)	1,403	(10)	74	(12)	119	(17)	13,720	(11)
25–29	10,326	(20)	8,729	(16)	2,507	(18)	141	(22)	165	(24)	22,147	(18)
30–34	11,490	(23)	10,637	(19)	2,999	(21)	160	(25)	155	(22)	25,752	(21)
35–39	9,582	(19)	10,249	(19)	2,775	(20)	99	(16)	118	(17)	23,121	(19)
40–44	5,907	(12)	7,485	(14)	1,790	(13)	65	(10)	61	(9)	15,526	(13)
45–49	3,258	(6)	4,479	(8)	1,039	(7)	41	(6)	34	(5)	8,968	(7)
50–54	1,693	(3)	2,288	(4)	488	(3)	20	(3)	13	(2)	4,573	(4)
55–59	757	(1)	1,104	(2)	241	(2)	8	(1)	8	(1)	2,150	(2)
60–64	382	(1)	543	(1)	133	(1)	4	(1)	3	(0)	1,081	(1)
65 or older	335	(1)	523	(1)	124	(1)	6	(1)	2	(0)	1,005	(1)
Male subtotal	**50,664**	**(100)**	**55,112**	**(100)**	**14,174**	**(100)**	**636**	**(100)**	**701**	**(100)**	**122,801**	**(100)**

Female	White, not Hispanic		Black, not Hispanic		Hispanic		Asian/Pacific Islander		American Indian/ Alaska Native		Total[3]	
Age at diagnosis (years)	No.	(%)	No.	(%)	No.	(%)	No.	(%)	No.	(%)	No.	(%)
Under 5	214	(2)	1,039	(3)	307	(6)	8	(4)	8	(3)	1,583	(3)
5–12	61	(1)	242	(1)	97	(2)	2	(1)	2	(1)	407	(1)
13–19	739	(7)	2,716	(8)	256	(5)	9	(4)	23	(9)	3,762	(7)
20–24	1,776	(16)	5,036	(15)	657	(12)	47	(22)	47	(18)	7,628	(15)
25–29	2,117	(19)	5,885	(17)	919	(17)	51	(24)	46	(18)	9,096	(18)
30–34	2,111	(19)	6,183	(18)	1,032	(19)	37	(17)	44	(17)	9,498	(19)
35–39	1,719	(16)	5,203	(15)	837	(15)	24	(11)	47	(18)	7,896	(15)
40–44	1,041	(9)	3,556	(10)	588	(11)	19	(9)	30	(11)	5,280	(10)
45–49	604	(6)	2,014	(6)	367	(7)	6	(3)	13	(5)	3,038	(6)
50–54	290	(3)	984	(3)	207	(4)	4	(2)	0	(0)	1,497	(3)
55–59	140	(1)	480	(1)	107	(2)	2	(1)	0	(0)	744	(1)
60–64	63	(1)	271	(1)	47	(1)	1	(0)	1	(0)	384	(1)
65 or older	101	(1)	258	(1)	34	(1)	6	(3)	0	(0)	403	(1)
Female subtotal	**10,976**	**(100)**	**33,867**	**(100)**	**5,455**	**(100)**	**216**	**(100)**	**261**	**(100)**	**51,216**	**(100)**
Total[4]	**61,641**		**88,981**		**19,629**		**852**		**962**		**174,026**	

[1] Includes only persons reported with HIV infection who have not developed AIDS.
[2] See table three for areas with confidential HIV infection reporting.
[3] Includes 1,514 males and 441 females, whose race/ethnicity is unknown.
[4] Includes nine persons whose sex is unknown.

TABLE 9 PEDIATRIC AIDS CASES BY EXPOSURE CATEGORY AND RACE/ETHNICITY, REPORTED THROUGH DECEMBER 2001, UNITED STATES

Exposure category	White, not Hispanic 2001 No.	(%)	White, not Hispanic Cumulative total No.	(%)	Black, not Hispanic 2001 No.	(%)	Black, not Hispanic Cumulative total No.	(%)	Hispanic 2001 No.	(%)	Hispanic Cumulative total No.	(%)
Hemophilia/coagulation disorder	0	(0)	159	(10)	0	(0)	34	(1)	0	(0)	37	(2)
Mother with/at risk for HIV infection:	25	(76)	1,197	(76)	100	(88)	5,110	(96)	22	(85)	1,900	(92)
Injecting drug use	5		493		24		1,966		4		755	
Sex with injecting drug user	9		242		4		741		2		495	
Sex with bisexual male	1		67		4		75		0		41	
Sex with person with hemophilia	1		19		0		6		0		8	
Sex with transfusion recipient with HIV infection	0		8		0		8		0		9	
Sex with HIV-infected person, risk not specified	4		155		27		895		7		274	
Receipt of blood transfusion, blood components, or tissue	0		43		2		75		0		34	
Has HIV infection, risk not specified	5		170		39		1,344		9		284	
Receipt of blood transfusion, blood components, or tissue	2	(6)	191	(12)	0	(0)	86	(2)	0	(0)	93	(5)
Risk not reported or identified[1]	6	(18)	32	(2)	13	(12)	107	(2)	4	(15)	30	(1)
Total	**33**	**(100)**	**1,579**	**(100)**	**113**	**(100)**	**5,337**	**(100)**	**26**	**(100)**	**2,060**	**(100)**

Exposure category	Asian/Pacific Islander 2001 No.	(%)	Asian/Pacific Islander Cumulative total No.	(%)	American Indian/Alaska Native 2001 No.	(%)	American Indian/Alaska Native Cumulative total No.	(%)	Cumulative totals[2] 2001 No.	(%)	Cumulative totals[2] Cumulative total No.	(%)
Hemophilia/coagulation disorder	0	(0)	3	(6)	0	(0)	2	(6)	0	(0)	236	(3)
Mother with/at risk for HIV infection:	3	(100)	36	(67)	0	(0)	29	(94)	150	(86)	8,284	(91)
Injecting drug use	0		6		0		14		33		3,238	
Sex with injecting drug user	0		6		0		6		15		1,491	
Sex with bisexual male	0		2		0		0		5		186	
Sex with person with hemophilia	0		0		0		0		1		33	
Sex with transfusion recipient with HIV infection	0		0		0		0		0		25	
Sex with HIV-infected person, risk not specified	0		9		0		4		38		1,339	
Receipt of blood transfusion, blood components, or tissue	0		1		0		1		2		154	
Has HIV infection, risk not specified	3		12		0		4		56		1,818	
Receipt of blood transfusion, blood components, or tissue	0	(0)	11	(20)	0	(0)	0	(0)	2	(1)	381	(4)
Risk not reported or identified	0	(0)	4	(7)	0	(0)	0	(0)	23	(13)	173	(2)
Total	**3**	**(100)**	**54**	**(100)**	**0**	**(0)**	**31**	**(100)**	**175**	**(100)**	**9,074**	**(100)**

[1] See Table 5, footnote 5 and Technical Notes.
[2] Includes 13 children whose race/ethnicity is unknown.

560

TABLE 10 PEDIATRIC HIV INFECTION CASES[1] BY EXPOSURE CATEGORY AND RACE/ETHNICITY, REPORTED THROUGH DECEMBER 2001, FROM AREAS WITH CONFIDENTIAL HIV INFECTION REPORTING[2]

Exposure category	White, not Hispanic 2001 No.	(%)	White, not Hispanic Cumulative total No.	(%)	Black, not Hispanic 2001 No.	(%)	Black, not Hispanic Cumulative total No.	(%)	Hispanic 2001 No.	(%)	Hispanic Cumulative total No.	(%)
Hemophilia/coagulation disorder	5	(6)	77	(13)	2	(1)	21	(1)	1	(1)	6	(1)
Mother with/at risk for HIV infection:	57	(71)	460	(75)	252	(74)	2,127	(87)	81	(68)	721	(87)
Injecting drug use	8		136		42		598		11		203	
Sex with injecting drug user	11		92		9		174		4		76	
Sex with bisexual male	0		8		1		17		1		5	
Sex with person with hemophilia	0		5		0		3		0		0	
Sex with transfusion recipient with HIV infection	0		3		0		4		0		5	
Sex with HIV-infected person, risk not specified	20		104		67		450		16		160	
Receipt of blood transfusion, blood components, or tissue	0		7		3		19		2		5	
Has HIV infection, risk not specified	18		105		130		862		47		267	
Receipt of blood transfusion, blood components, or tissue	2	(3)	22	(4)	1	(0)	13	(1)	1	(1)	11	(1)
Risk not reported or identified[3]	16	(20)	53	(9)	86	(25)	270	(11)	37	(31)	92	(1)
Total	80	(100)	612	(100)	341	(100)	2,431	(100)	120	(100)	830	(100)

Exposure category	Asian/Pacific Islander 2001 No.	(%)	Asian/Pacific Islander Cumulative total No.	(%)	American Indian/Alaska Native 2001 No.	(%)	American Indian/Alaska Native Cumulative total No.	(%)	Cumulative totals[2] 2001 No.	(%)	Cumulative totals[2] Cumulative total No.	(%)
Hemophilia/coagulation disorder	1	(50)	4	(20)	0	(0)	1	(8)	9	(2)	109	(3)
Mother with/at risk for HIV infection:	0	(0)	10	(50)	0	(0)	10	(77)	390	(72)	3,336	(85)
Injecting drug use	0		2		0		3		61		945	
Sex with injecting drug user	0		0		0		2		24		346	
Sex with bisexual male	0		2		0		1		2		34	
Sex with person with hemophilia	0		0		0		0		0		8	
Sex with transfusion recipient with HIV infection	0		0		0		1		0		13	
Sex with HIV-infected person, isk not specified	0		5		0		0		103		720	
Receipt of blood transfusion, blood components, or tissue	0		0		0		0		5		31	
Has HIV infection, risk not specified	0		1		0		3		195		1,239	
Receipt of blood transfusion, blood components, or tissue	0	(0)	1	(5)	0	(0)	0	(0)	4	(1)	47	(1)
Risk not reported or identified	1	(50)	5	(25)	0	(0)	2	(15)	140	(26)	431	(11)
Total	2	(100)	20	(100)	0	(0)	13	(100)	543	(100)	3,923	(100)

[1] Includes only persons reported with HIV infection who have not developed AIDS.
[2] See table 3 for areas with confidential HIV infection reporting.
[3] For HIV infection cases, "risk not reported or identified" refers primarily to persons whose mode of exposure was not reported and who have not been followed up to determine their mode of exposure, and to a smaller number of persons who are not reported with one of the exposures listed above after follow-up. See Technical Notes.
[4] Includes 17 children whose race/ethnicity is unknown.

**TABLE 11   ADULT/ADOLESCENT AIDS CASES BY SINGLE AND MULTIPLE EXPOSURE CATEGORIES,
REPORTED THROUGH DECEMBER 2001, UNITED STATES**

	AIDS cases	
Exposure category	No.	(%)
Single mode of exposure		
Men who have sex with men	351,612	(44)
Injecting drug use	156,869	(19)
Hemophilia/coagulation disorder	4,308	(1)
Heterosexual contact	88,163	(11)
Receipt of transfusion[1]	8,958	(1)
Receipt of transplant of tissues, organs, or artificial insemination[2]	13	(0)
Other[3]	256	(0)
Single mode of exposure subtotal	**610,179**	**(76)**
Multiple modes of exposure		
Men who have sex with men; injecting drug use	43,096	(5)
Men who have sex with men; hemophilia/coagulation disorder	208	(0)
Men who have sex with men; heterosexual contact	13,128	(2)
Men who have sex with men; receipt of transfusion/transplant	3,613	(0)
Injecting drug use; hemophilia/coagulation disorder	219	(0)
Injecting drug use; heterosexual contact	41,114	(5)
Injecting drug use; receipt of transfusion/transplant	1,766	(0)
Hemophilia/coagulation disorder; heterosexual contact	136	(0)
Hemophilia/coagulation disorder; receipt of transfusion/transplant	808	(0)
Heterosexual contact; receipt of transfusion/transplant	1,968	(0)
Men who have sex with men; injecting drug use; hemophilia/coagulation disorder	55	(0)
Men who have sex with men; injecting drug use; heterosexual contact	7,245	(1)
Men who have sex with men; injecting drug use; receipt of transfusion/transplant	656	(0)
Men who have sex with men; hemophilia/coagulation disorder; heterosexual contact	24	(0)
Men who have sex with men; hemophilia/coagulation disorder; receipt of transfusion/transplant	46	(0)
Men who have sex with men; heterosexual contact; receipt of transfusion/transplant	334	(0)
Injecting drug use; hemophilia/coagulation disorder; heterosexual contact	100	(0)
Injection drug use; hemophilia/coagulation disorder; receipt of transfusion/transplant	38	(0)
Injecting drug use; heterosexual contact; receipt of transfusion/transplant	1,193	(0)
Hemophilia/coagulation disorder; heterosexual contact; receipt of transfusion/transplant	40	(0)
Men who have sex with men; injecting drug use; hemophilia/coagulation disorder; heterosexual contact	20	(0)
Men who have sex with men; injecting drug use; hemophilia/coagulation disorder; receipt of transfusion/transplant	16	(0)
Men who have sex with men; injecting drug use; heterosexual contact; receipt of transfusion/transplant	200	(0)
Men who have sex with men; hemophilia/coagulation disorder; heterosexual contact; receipt of transfusion/transplant	6	(0)
Injecting drug use; hemophilia/coagulation disorder; heterosexual contact; receipt of transfusion/transplant	27	(0)
Men who have sex with men; injecting drug use; hemophilia/coagulation disorder; heterosexual contact; receipt of transfusion/transplant	5	(0)
Multiple modes of exposure subtotal	**116,061**	**(14)**
Risk not reported or identified[4]	80,835	(10)
Total	**807,075**	**(100)**

[1] Includes 41 adult/adolescents who developed AIDS after receiving blood screened negative for HIV antibody.
[2] Thirteen adults developed AIDS after receiving tissue, organs, or artificial insemination from HIV-infected donors. Four of the 13 received tissue or organs from a donor who was negative for HIV antibody at the time of donation. See *N Engl J Med* 1992;326:726–32.
[3] "Other" includes 221 persons who acquired HIV infection perinatally, but had AIDS diagnosed after age 13. See Technical Notes.
[4] See Technical Notes.

TABLE 12   DEATHS IN PERSONS WITH AIDS, BY RACE/ETHNICITY, AGE AT DEATH, AND SEX, OCCURRING IN 1999 AND 2000; AND CUMULATIVE TOTALS REPORTED THROUGH DECEMBER 2001, UNITED STATES[1]

Race/ethnicity and age at death[2]	Males			Females			Both sexes		
	1999	2000	Cumulative total	1999	2000	Cumulative total	1999	2000	Cumulative total
White, not Hispanic									
Under 15	8	3	575	4	8	427	12	11	1,002
15–24	22	18	2,567	14	10	501	36	28	3,068
25–34	666	431	55,693	151	117	4,857	817	548	60,550
35–44	1,907	1,568	83,459	329	263	5,576	2,236	1,831	89,035
45–54	1,310	1,147	38,845	160	146	2,247	1,470	1,293	41,092
55 or older	542	518	16,438	56	65	1,837	598	583	18,275
All ages	4,455	3,685	197,724	714	609	15,466	5,169	4,294	213,190
Black, not Hispanic									
Under 15	41	16	1,473	28	14	1,439	69	30	2,912
15–24	55	62	2,536	79	54	1,540	134	116	4,076
25–34	920	753	34,675	581	553	12,596	1,501	1,306	47,271
35–44	2,300	1,915	53,099	1,066	945	16,322	3,366	2,860	69,421
45–54	1,718	1,629	24,925	560	550	6,127	2,278	2,179	31,052
55 or older	749	687	10,634	232	223	2,701	981	910	13,335
All ages	5,783	5,062	127,450	2,546	2,339	40,752	8,329	7,401	168,202
Hispanic									
Under 15	11	5	637	14	7	587	25	12	1,224
15–24	21	22	1,373	17	10	501	38	32	1,874
25–34	461	353	21,010	163	119	4,762	624	472	25,772
35–44	1,007	847	27,892	303	250	5,359	1,310	1,097	33,251
45–54	562	576	11,729	176	154	2,058	738	730	13,787
55 or older	290	240	4,875	50	79	960	340	319	5,835
All ages	2,352	2,043	67,557	723	619	14,236	3,075	2,662	81,793
Asian/Pacific Islander									
Under 15	0	1	19	1	1	18	1	2	37
15–24	2	1	38	1	0	8	3	1	46
25–34	13	13	743	5	3	84	18	16	827
35–44	46	28	1,181	2	8	112	48	36	1,293
45–54	23	15	578	8	2	70	31	17	648
55 or older	8	10	267	2	5	57	10	15	324
All ages	92	68	2,828	19	19	351	111	87	3,179
American Indian/Alaska Native									
Under 15	0	0	13	0	0	8	0	0	21
15–24	0	1	26	0	0	3	0	1	29
25–34	13	5	398	4	3	79	17	8	477
35–44	24	19	430	8	3	81	32	22	511
45–54	12	10	151	1	5	31	13	15	182
55 or older	2	4	50	3	1	14	5	5	64
All ages	51	39	1,070	16	12	216	67	51	1,286
All racial/ethnic groups									
Under 15	60	25	2,717	47	30	2,480	107	55	5,197
15–24	100	104	6,545	111	74	2,554	211	178	9,099
25–34	2,074	1,555	112,577	904	795	22,380	2,978	2,350	134,957
35–44	5,287	4,378	166,172	1,710	1,469	27,459	6,997	5,847	193,631
45–54	3,629	3,379	76,275	905	857	10,535	4,534	4,236	86,810
55 or older	1,592	1,460	32,284	343	373	5,572	1,935	1,833	37,856
All ages	12,742	10,901	396,871	4,020	3,598	71,039	16,762	14,499	467,910

[1] Data tabulations for 1999 and 2000 are based on date of death occurrence. Data for deaths occurring in 2001 are incomplete and not tabulated separately, but are included in the cumulative totals. Tabulations for 1999 and 2000 may increase as additional deaths are reported to CDC.
[2] Data tabulated under "all ages" include 360 persons whose age at death is unknown. Data tabulated under "all racial/ethnic groups" include 260 persons whose race/ethnicity is unknown.

II. Life Expectancy and Causes of Death Worldwide.
(Source: World Health Organization)

TABLE 1   HEALTHY LIFE EXPECTANCY (HALE) IN ALL MEMBER STATES, ESTIMATES FOR 2000

			Healthy life expectancy[a] (years)								Expectation of lost healthy years at birth (years)		Percentage of total life expectancy lost	
		Total population At birth	Males				Females							
	Member State		At birth	Uncertainty interval	At age 60	Uncertainty interval	At birth	Uncertainty interval	At age 60	Uncertainty interval	Male	Females	Male	Females
1	Afghanistan	33.8	35.1	30.3–40.4	7.1	5.5–8.8	32.5	26.2–39.5	5.8	2.6–9.0	9.1	12.5	20.5	27.8
2	Albania	59.4	56.5	54.4–59.3	11.4	10.3–12.6	62.3	59.9–64.8	14.4	13.0–16.0	7.9	10.6	12.2	14.5
3	Algeria	58.4	58.4	55.8–61.9	11.1	9.4–13.1	58.3	54.5–62.2	11.0	8.9–12.9	9.7	12.9	14.3	18.1
4	Andorra	71.8	69.8	67.4–73.0	17.0	15.4–18.7	73.7	70.7–77.9	19.4	17.3–22.5	7.3	10.1	9.5	12.1
5	Angola	36.9	36.2	33.7–42.0	7.4	5.3–10.1	37.6	33.3–42.8	7.3	4.6–10.3	8.1	10.8	18.2	22.3
6	Antigua and Barbuda	61.9	61.7	58.4–64.8	14.8	13.5–16.3	62.1	59.0–65.2	15.4	14.1–16.9	10.1	14.5	14.1	18.9
7	Argentina	63.9	61.8	59.6–64.0	13.2	12.0–14.6	65.9	63.0–68.6	16.0	14.8–17.5	8.4	11.9	12.0	15.3
8	Armenia	59.0	56.9	55.0–58.6	9.7	8.8–10.6	61.1	58.1–64.1	12.0	10.9–13.1	7.5	10.1	11.7	14.2
9	Australia	71.5	69.6	67.8–71.5	17.0	16.1–18.1	73.3	69.8–75.4	19.5	18.7–20.6	6.9	8.8	9.1	10.7
10	Austria	70.3	68.1	66.9–69.4	15.2	14.5–16.0	72.5	70.3–74.3	18.4	17.8–19.2	6.8	8.9	9.0	10.9
11	Azerbaijan	55.4	53.3	50.6–56.3	12.2	10.8–14.0	57.5	54.3–60.8	14.6	12.9–16.5	8.4	11.4	13.6	16.5
12	Bahamas	58.1	57.2	54.0–60.5	12.4	10.2–14.7	59.1	54.2–64.0	12.0	10.1–15.2	10.8	15.7	15.9	21.0
13	Bahrain	62.7	63.0	61.0–65.2	11.3	9.8–12.8	62.3	59.1–65.1	11.4	10.2–12.6	9.7	12.4	13.3	16.6
14	Bangladesh	49.3	50.6	47.4–54.1	8.8	7.5–10.4	47.9	43.6–52.6	8.0	6.4–9.9	9.8	12.9	16.2	21.2
15	Barbados	63.3	62.3	59.7–65.0	13.4	12.1–14.9	64.3	60.9–67.7	16.1	14.1–18.4	9.3	13.4	13.0	17.2
16	Belarus	60.1	55.4	53.4–57.5	9.9	9.2–10.8	64.8	62.7–66.9	14.4	13.2–15.9	6.6	9.2	10.7	12.4
17	Belgium	69.4	67.7	66.2–69.2	15.3	14.5–16.2	71.0	69.0–73.0	18.0	17.2–18.7	6.9	9.9	9.2	12.2
18	Belize	59.2	58.0	55.2–61.0	12.7	11.2–14.1	60.4	55.6–64.9	13.6	11.0–16.4	11.1	14.3	16.1	19.2
19	Benin	42.5	43.1	39.8–46.5	8.4	6.7–10.1	41.9	37.5–46.5	7.4	3.9–10.5	8.5	11.9	16.5	22.0
20	Bhutan	49.2	50.1	44.8–55.1	9.3	7.5–11.1	48.2	43.5–53.7	8.8	6.1–11.7	10.3	14.3	17.0	22.9
21	Bolivia	51.4	51.4	47.4–55.5	9.8	8.3–11.5	51.4	47.1–55.9	10.0	8.0–11.8	9.5	12.1	15.6	19.1
22	Bosnia and Herzegovina	63.7	62.1	60.3–64.3	12.4	11.3–13.5	65.3	62.8–67.9	14.3	13.0–15.7	6.6	9.4	9.5	12.5
23	Botswana	37.3	38.1	34.3–42.0	8.3	6.4–10.1	36.5	33.2–40.0	8.9	6.3–11.5	6.5	7.9	14.6	17.7
24	Brazil[b]	57.1	54.9	51.4–58.1	10.7	9.2–12.0	59.2	54.8–64.1	12.6	9.8–15.2	9.5	12.7	14.8	17.6
25	Brunei Darussalam	64.9	63.8	61.5–66.0	13.3	12.0–14.6	65.9	62.4–69.6	15.1	13.8–16.5	9.6	12.7	13.1	16.2
26	Bulgaria	63.4	61.0	59.4–62.6	12.4	11.8–13.1	65.8	63.8–67.7	15.2	14.0–16.4	6.3	9.2	9.4	12.2
27	Burkina Faso	34.8	35.4	32.5–38.3	8.0	6.2–9.7	34.1	30.5–37.9	7.4	4.9–10.0	7.2	9.5	16.8	21.7
28	Burundi	33.4	33.9	30.4–37.5	7.6	6.0–9.1	32.9	29.3–36.9	7.7	5.4–10.3	6.7	8.5	16.5	20.5
29	Cambodia	47.1	45.6	43.1–48.0	9.0	7.8–10.3	48.7	45.4–52.4	10.1	8.0–12.2	7.8	9.8	14.7	16.8
30	Cameroon	40.4	40.9	37.6–44.0	8.4	6.2–10.6	39.9	36.7–43.2	8.0	5.7–10.5	8.1	10.5	16.5	20.8
31	Canada	70.0	68.3	66.9–69.7	15.4	14.6–16.3	71.7	70.0–73.5	17.8	17.0–18.6	7.7	9.8	10.2	12.0
32	Cape Verde	58.4	56.9	53.7–60.2	11.3	9.8–12.8	60.0	56.3–63.8	12.0	10.0–14.1	9.6	12.3	14.4	17.0
33	Central African Republic	34.1	34.7	31.6–38.2	8.2	6.6–9.8	33.6	30.3–37.3	7.9	5.9–9.8	6.9	8.9	16.7	20.9
34	Chad	39.3	38.6	35.3–43.7	7.4	5.5–9.4	39.9	36.1–44.5	7.5	4.6–10.5	8.7	11.2	18.4	22.0
35	Chile	65.5	63.5	61.5–66.0	13.1	11.8–14.5	67.4	64.5–70.3	15.7	14.4–17.1	9.0	12.1	12.4	15.2
36	China	62.1	60.9	59.5–62.5	11.8	10.8–12.8	63.3	59.1–65.8	14.3	13.6–15.1	8.0	9.7	11.6	13.2
37	Colombia	60.9	58.6	56.2–61.0	12.9	11.6–14.2	63.3	59.8–66.2	14.0	12.8–15.1	8.6	11.8	12.8	15.7
38	Comoros	46.0	46.2	42.8–49.6	8.0	6.6–9.5	45.8	41.4–50.3	7.7	5.4–9.9	9.1	12.3	16.4	21.1
39	Congo	42.6	42.5	39.3–47.0	8.7	7.0–11.0	42.8	39.1–47.2	8.9	6.1–11.7	7.7	10.1	15.3	19.1
40	Cook Islands	60.7	60.4	58.1–62.8	11.4	10.4–12.3	61.1	57.7–64.9	13.0	11.6–14.6	8.3	11.0	12.0	15.3
41	Costa Rica	65.3	64.2	61.9–66.9	14.0	12.4–15.6	66.4	63.1–69.2	15.6	14.2–17.1	9.2	12.4	12.6	15.7
42	Côte d'Ivoire	39.0	39.1	36.7–42.6	8.6	7.3–10.1	38.9	35.9–42.1	8.5	5.9–11.2	7.2	9.5	15.6	19.7
43	Croatia	64.0	60.8	59.5–62.0	11.4	10.8–12.1	67.1	64.7–69.2	15.2	14.6–15.8	9.0	10.6	12.9	13.6
44	Cuba	65.9	65.1	63.0–67.2	14.5	13.4–15.6	66.7	64.4–68.8	15.5	14.1–16.9	8.6	10.9	11.6	14.0
45	Cyprus	66.3	66.4	64.6–68.7	14.5	12.9–16.3	66.2	63.4–68.8	14.1	12.8–15.7	8.4	12.7	11.2	16.1
46	Czech Republic	65.6	62.9	61.3–64.4	13.0	12.2–13.8	68.3	65.7–70.5	15.8	15.2–16.4	8.6	9.9	12.0	12.6
47	Democratic People's Republic of Korea	55.4	54.9	51.5–58.4	11.1	10.0–12.4	56.0	52.2–59.8	12.1	10.6–13.8	9.6	11.2	14.8	16.7
48	Democratic Republic of the Congo	34.4	34.4	31.6–39.4	7.2	5.9–8.8	34.4	30.5–39.3	7.4	5.1–9.6	7.2	9.6	17.4	21.9
49	Denmark	69.5	68.9	67.5–70.3	15.7	14.9–16.6	70.1	68.2–72.0	16.5	15.8–17.3	5.3	8.4	7.2	10.7
50	Djibouti	35.1	35.6	31.3–40.4	7.4	5.5–9.5	34.6	30.1–39.6	7.0	4.6–9.6	7.8	10.1	18.0	22.5

[a] Healthy life expectancy estimates published here are not directly comparable to those published in the *World Health Report 2000,* due to improvements in survey methodology and the use of new epidemiological data for some diseases. See Statistical Annex notes (pp. 130–135). The figures reported in this table along with the data collection and estimation methods have been largely developed by WHO and do not necessarily reflect official statistics of Member States. Further development in collaboration with Member States is under way for improved data collection and estimation methods.

[b] Figures not yet endorsed by Member States as official statistics.

		Healthy life expectancy[a] (years)								Expectation of lost healthy years at birth (years)		Percentage of total life expectancy lost	
		Males				Females							
	Total population At birth	At birth	Uncertainty interval	At age 60	Uncertainty interval	At birth	Uncertainty interval	At age 60	Uncertainty interval	Male	Females	Male	Females
51 Dominica	64.6	63.2	59.7–66.1	14.4	13.1–15.9	66.1	63.3–69.3	16.4	14.8–18.1	9.4	12.2	13.0	15.6
52 Dominican Republic	56.2	54.7	50.9–58.2	12.3	11.0–13.5	57.7	53.4–61.9	13.0	11.0–15.0	10.8	14.0	16.4	19.5
53 Ecuador	60.3	58.4	55.4–61.3	12.7	11.3–14.0	62.2	58.6–66.0	14.4	12.4–16.5	9.9	12.0	14.5	16.2
54 Egypt	57.1	57.1	55.4–58.8	9.9	8.6–11.2	57.0	54.1–59.3	10.0	8.9–11.2	8.3	12.0	12.6	17.4
55 El Salvador	57.3	55.3	52.0–58.7	11.9	10.5–13.5	59.4	55.3–63.3	13.3	10.7–15.9	11.0	13.9	16.6	19.0
56 Equatorial Guinea	44.8	44.9	40.6–48.7	8.7	7.1–10.3	44.8	40.2–49.4	8.3	5.8–10.9	8.7	11.4	16.2	20.2
57 Eritrea	41.0	41.4	38.1–45.0	8.3	6.5–10.0	40.5	36.5–45.0	8.1	5.6–10.7	7.7	10.4	15.7	20.4
58 Estonia	60.8	56.2	54.7–57.6	10.0	9.1–10.9	65.4	62.5–67.7	14.8	14.0–15.8	9.3	11.0	14.2	14.4
59 Ethiopla	35.4	35.7	32.2–40.9	7.7	5.8–9.7	35.1	30.4–40.9	7.5	4.9–10.3	7.1	9.6	16.6	21.4
60 Fiji	59.6	58.7	55.9–61.3	11.2	9.6–12.7	60.5	56.9–64.3	12.7	10.8–14.4	8.3	10.7	12.3	15.1
61 Finland	68.8	66.1	64.9–67.2	14.8	14.0–15.4	71.5	69.9–73.0	17.9	17.4–18.5	7.6	9.5	10.3	11.7
62 France	70.7	68.5	67.4–69.5	16.6	15.9–17.2	72.9	71.4–74.5	19.4	18.9–20.0	6.7	10.2	8.9	12.2
63 Gabon	46.6	46.8	42.9–50.0	9.2	7.7–10.8	46.5	42.6–49.9	9.3	7.6–11.2	7.8	10.4	14.2	18.4
64 Gambia	46.9	47.3	44.1–50.6	8.5	6.8–10.3	46.6	42.4–50.8	8.1	6.0–10.5	8.6	12.1	15.4	20.6
65 Georgia	58.2	56.1	54.1–58.3	9.5	8.5–10.5	60.2	57.3–62.8	11.1	10.3–11.9	9.6	11.6	14.6	16.1
66 Germany	69.4	67.4	66.0–68.7	14.8	14.0–15.6	71.5	69.4–73.3	17.6	16.9–18.2	6.9	9.2	9.3	11.4
67 Ghana	46.7	46.5	43.4–49.7	8.9	6.9–10.8	46.9	43.5–51.1	9.0	6.5–11.3	8.5	11.0	15.5	18.9
68 Greece	71.0	69.7	68.5–70.8	16.0	15.2–16.6	72.3	69.9–74.0	17.6	17.1–18.3	5.7	8.5	7.6	10.5
69 Grenada	61.9	62.1	59.5–65.1	14.0	12.6–15.4	61.8	57.8–65.7	14.1	12.0–16.4	8.8	11.5	12.4	15.7
70 Guatemala	54.7	53.5	49.9–57.2	11.3	9.1–13.6	56.0	52.3–59.7	11.7	10.0–13.5	10.1	12.6	15.8	18.3
71 Guinea	40.3	40.4	36.7–44.0	7.3	5.6–9.1	40.1	35.9–45.5	7.0	3.9–10.3	8.6	11.9	17.5	22.8
72 Guinea-Bissau	36.6	36.7	33.6–39.8	7.2	5.1–9.1	36.4	33.0–40.3	7.1	4.1–10.1	7.7	10.5	17.4	22.3
73 Guyana	52.1	51.4	48.3–54.6	10.3	9.1–11.6	52.8	47.7–58.4	11.1	8.9–13.6	10.1	14.2	16.4	21.2
74 Haiti	43.1	41.3	37.0–46.2	7.8	6.1–9.5	44.9	38.8–51.1	8.5	5.7–11.4	8.4	11.2	16.9	20.0
75 Honduras	56.8	55.8	52.5–59.6	11.7	10.0–13.3	57.8	53.6–62.0	12.7	10.9–14.7	10.6	13.2	16.0	18.6
76 Hungary	59.9	55.3	53.7–56.9	9.4	8.3–10.3	64.5	61.8–66.7	13.8	13.0–14.6	11.0	10.7	16.5	14.2
77 Iceland	71.2	69.8	68.1–71.5	16.2	15.1–17.4	72.6	70.3–74.9	18.6	17.6–19.6	7.3	9.3	9.5	11.3
78 India	52.0	52.2	50.2–54.2	9.9	8.7–11.0	51.7	48.5–54.8	10.9	9.6–12.1	7.6	11.0	12.7	17.5
79 Indonesia	57.4	56.5	55.7–58.2	11.6	10.8–12.5	58.4	55.8–61.0	12.5	11.8–13.3	6.9	9.1	10.9	13.5
80 Iran, Islamic Republic of	58.8	59.0	56.4–61.6	11.3	9.7–12.9	58.6	55.3–61.9	11.4	10.0–12.7	9.1	11.4	13.3	16.2
81 Iraq	52.6	52.6	48.6–57.0	9.3	6.7–12.0	52.5	48.6–57.3	9.5	7.5–11.9	9.2	12.1	14.8	18.7
82 Ireland	69.3	67.8	66.3–69.1	14.3	13.5–15.1	70.9	68.6–72.7	16.9	16.2–17.6	6.3	8.8	8.5	11.0
83 Israel	69.9	69.3	67.7–71.0	16.2	15.2–17.3	70.6	68.3–72.9	17.1	15.8–18.4	7.3	10.0	9.6	12.4
84 Italy	71.2	69.5	68.4–70.8	16.3	15.6–17.2	72.8	70.5–74.5	18.8	18.1–19.4	6.4	9.6	8.5	11.6
85 Jamaica	64.0	62.9	59.8–65.8	14.6	13.5–15.9	65.0	62.1–68.1	15.7	13.7–17.7	10.0	11.5	13.7	15.1
86 Japan	73.8	71.2	69.9–72.5	17.6	16.8–18.4	76.3	74.6–77.8	21.4	20.3–22.5	6.3	8.4	8.1	9.9
87 Jordan	58.5	58.2	56.4–60.3	10.3	9.0–11.7	58.8	56.0–61.4	11.3	10.1–12.6	10.3	13.6	15.0	18.8
88 Kazakhstan	54.3	50.5	48.0–53.1	10.9	9.9–11.9	58.1	55.6–60.6	14.6	13.1–16.0	7.5	10.3	13.0	15.0
89 Kenya	40.7	41.2	38.7–44.4	9.3	8.0–10.7	40.1	36.7–43.8	9.1	7.0–11.0	7.0	9.4	14.5	19.1
90 Kiribati	53.6	52.8	49.6–56.1	10.7	9.2–12.2	54.4	50.7–57.9	11.4	9.3–13.3	7.6	10.1	12.6	15.7
91 Kuwait	64.7	64.6	62.1–66.8	12.4	10.8–13.8	64.8	61.4–68.0	13.0	10.7–15.0	9.6	12.0	13.0	15.6
92 Kyrgyzstan	52.6	49.6	46.5–53.1	8.5	6.2–10.9	55.6	51.2–60.1	11.8	9.7–13.9	10.4	13.2	17.4	19.2
93 Lao People's Democratic Republic	44.7	43.7	39.1–47.5	9.6	8.1–11.2	45.7	40.6–49.6	10.6	8.4–12.7	8.6	10.4	16.4	18.5
94 Latvia	57.7	51.4	49.0–53.5	9.1	7.9–10.0	63.9	60.9–66.5	14.4	13.5–15.4	12.8	11.6	19.9	15.3
95 Lebanon	60.7	60.3	57.6–63.1	11.3	9.6–12.8	61.1	57.4–65.1	12.2	10.3–14.3	8.9	12.2	12.8	16.7
96 Lesotho	35.3	36.1	33.1–39.7	8.7	6.8–10.6	34.5	31.2–38.7	8.8	6.4–11.3	5.9	7.7	14.1	18.2
97 Liberia	37.8	38.2	34.0–42.4	7.3	6.1–8.5	37.4	33.5–41.5	6.9	4.3–9.5	8.4	11.7	18.1	23.9
98 Libyan Arab Jamahiriya	58.5	58.4	55.7–61.4	10.6	9.0–12.4	58.6	55.2–62.5	11.3	9.2–13.4	9.2	12.4	13.6	17.4
99 Lithuania	58.4	53.6	51.6–55.5	10.1	9.0–11.0	63.2	60.2–65.9	14.2	13.2–15.2	13.3	14.0	19.8	18.2
100 Luxembourg	69.8	67.6	66.2–69.2	14.9	14.1–15.8	72.0	69.5–74.0	18.4	17.6–19.1	6.3	8.7	8.5	10.8

(continues)

TABLE 1   HEALTHY LIFE EXPECTANCY (HALE) IN ALL MEMBER STATES, ESTIMATES FOR 2000 *(Continued)*

	Member State	Total population At birth	Males At birth	Males Uncertainty interval	Males At age 60	Males Uncertainty interval	Females At birth	Females Uncertainty interval	Females At age 60	Females Uncertainty interval	Expectation of lost healthy years at birth (years) Male	Female	Percentage of total life expectancy lost Male	Female
101	Madagascar	42.9	43.2	40.6–46.1	8.0	6.4–9.5	42.6	38.0–47.3	7.5	4.6–10.9	8.5	12.0	16.5	22.1
102	Malawi	30.9	31.4	28.2–34.6	7.6	5.8–9.4	30.5	26.8–34.4	7.8	5.1–11.0	5.8	7.4	15.5	19.5
103	Malaysia	61.6	59.7	57.3–62.1	10.6	8.9–12.3	63.4	60.3–66.6	12.7	11.3–14.1	8.6	10.7	12.6	14.5
104	Maldives	52.4	54.2	50.3–58.2	10.1	8.4–11.9	50.6	46.4–55.9	8.6	6.1–10.8	10.4	13.8	16.1	21.5
105	Mali	34.5	34.8	31.5–39.3	7.1	5.9–8.9	34.1	29.5–38.9	7.2	4.3–10.1	7.9	10.5	18.5	23.5
106	Malta	70.4	68.7	67.3–70.2	15.6	14.7–16.5	72.1	69.7–74.1	17.7	16.9–18.5	6.7	8.6	8.9	10.7
107	Marshall Islands	56.1	54.8	51.9–57.9	10.4	8.8–12.2	57.4	54.3–60.3	12.3	10.6–14.2	7.9	10.4	12.7	15.3
108	Mauritania	41.5	42.1	37.7–46.3	7.8	5.7–10.0	40.8	35.5–46.0	7.1	3.7–10.3	9.6	12.7	18.5	23.8
109	Mauritius	60.5	58.6	55.6–61.3	10.1	8.6–11.5	62.5	58.4–66.3	12.3	10.1–14.6	9.1	12.2	13.4	16.3
110	Mexico	64.2	63.1	60.8–65.2	14.5	13.1–16.0	65.3	61.5–68.1	15.0	13.8–16.4	7.9	10.9	11.2	14.3
111	Micronesia, Federated States of	56.6	55.8	52.8–58.8	11.0	9.5–12.5	57.5	54.0–61.0	12.0	10.6–13.4	8.0	10.3	12.5	15.2
112	Monaco	71.7	69.4	67.5–72.1	17.2	16.0–18.8	73.9	71.1–76.7	20.2	18.4–22.4	7.4	10.5	9.6	12.4
113	Mongolia	52.4	50.3	46.3–54.3	10.8	9.0–12.6	54.5	50.8–58.2	12.7	10.4–15.1	10.9	12.4	17.8	18.5
114	Morocco	54.9	55.3	53.4–57.3	9.9	8.4–11.4	54.5	51.3–57.2	10.0	8.7–11.2	10.8	16.0	16.3	22.7
115	Mozambique	31.3	31.5	28.9–34.9	7.3	5.4–9.6	31.1	28.1–34.7	7.3	5.4–9.7	6.4	8.4	17.0	21.3
116	Myanmar	49.1	47.7	43.8–51.6	9.2	7.6–10.9	50.5	45.7–54.3	10.1	7.8–12.1	8.5	10.7	15.1	17.4
117	Namibia	35.6	36.5	32.5–41.2	9.2	7.4–11.0	34.7	31.4–38.8	9.1	6.6–11.7	6.3	7.9	14.8	16.6
118	Nauru	52.9	50.4	47.0–54.4	7.9	6.6–9.5	55.4	51.0–60.2	10.5	8.2–13.2	8.3	11.1	14.1	16.7
119	Nepal	45.8	47.5	44.4–51.1	10.2	8.3–12.0	44.2	39.1–49.8	9.6	6.3–12.7	11.0	13.8	18.8	23.9
120	Netherlands[b]	69.7	68.2	67.1–69.3	15.2	14.6–15.9	71.2	69.7–72.7	17.8	17.2–18.4	7.3	9.7	9.6	12.0
121	New Zealand	70.8	69.5	68.0–71.0	16.7	15.8–17.7	72.1	69.8–74.0	18.8	17.9–19.6	6.4	8.9	8.5	11.0
122	Nicaragua	56.9	55.8	51.8–60.3	11.3	9.6–13.4	58.0	54.3–62.4	12.5	10.6–14.7	10.6	13.0	16.0	18.3
123	Niger	33.1	33.9	30.9–37.7	6.6	3.8–9.3	32.4	27.1–37.6	5.8	3.2–8.4	8.8	11.5	20.7	26.2
124	Nigeria	41.6	42.1	39.2–45.0	8.4	6.8–10.0	41.1	37.7–45.0	8.2	6.4–10.1	7.7	10.3	15.5	20.1
125	Niue	61.1	60.8	57.1–64.2	13.0	11.4–14.7	61.4	58.6–65.2	13.8	11.9–16.2	8.7	11.4	12.6	15.6
126	Norway	70.5	68.8	67.0–70.5	15.8	14.8–16.8	72.3	70.2–74.6	18.2	16.9–19.5	6.9	9.1	9.2	11.2
127	Oman	59.7	59.2	57.2–61.4	10.3	8.8–11.9	60.3	56.6–63.1	12.0	10.5–13.5	10.3	13.2	14.8	17.9
128	Pakistan[b]	48.1	50.2	46.6–54.2	9.8	8.7–11.2	46.1	41.5–51.1	8.7	5.6–11.8	10.0	14.7	16.6	24.1
129	Palau	57.7	56.5	54.3–58.6	9.5	8.4–10.3	58.9	55.7–62.4	10.7	9.2–12.2	8.2	10.4	12.6	15.0
130	Panama	63.9	62.6	60.1–65.1	13.7	12.4–14.9	65.3	62.6–68.0	15.3	13.8–16.8	8.9	11.0	12.5	14.4
131	Papua New Guinea	46.8	46.6	42.8–50.5	9.2	7.7–10.6	47.1	43.6–50.9	10.5	8.7–12.1	8.5	10.4	15.4	18.1
132	Paraguay	60.9	59.9	56.7–63.4	12.3	10.4–14.3	61.9	58.8–65.5	14.0	12.4–15.6	10.3	12.3	14.7	16.6
133	Peru	58.8	57.8	55.2–60.6	12.0	10.5–13.6	59.8	56.2–63.6	13.6	11.6–15.8	8.9	11.8	13.4	16.4
134	Philippines	59.0	57.0	54.3–59.4	11.5	10.3–12.6	60.9	57.7–64.3	13.6	11.9–15.5	7.7	10.2	11.9	14.3
135	Poland	61.8	59.3	57.9–60.5	10.9	10.1–11.7	64.3	61.2–66.7	13.8	12.9–14.6	10.0	13.4	14.4	17.2
136	Portugal	66.3	63.9	62.5–65.4	13.6	12.7–14.4	68.6	66.2–70.5	16.0	15.3–16.7	7.8	10.7	10.9	13.5
137	Qatar	60.6	59.3	56.5–62.6	9.2	7.0–11.4	61.8	58.4–65.4	11.6	9.8–13.6	11.1	13.2	15.7	17.6
138	Republic of Korea	66.0	63.2	60.8–65.3	12.3	11.1–13.4	68.8	64.0–71.4	16.0	15.1–17.0	7.3	9.5	10.3	12.1
139	Republic of Moldova	58.4	55.4	52.4–57.9	10.2	8.8–11.4	61.5	59.1–64.3	12.5	11.1–13.9	7.7	8.9	12.3	12.7
140	Romania	61.7	59.5	57.4–61.4	12.1	11.0–12.9	64.0	61.6–66.8	14.4	13.1–15.7	6.8	9.5	10.2	12.9
141	Russian Federation	55.5	50.3	48.6–52.4	8.2	7.3–8.9	60.6	57.0–63.3	12.2	11.5–13.0	9.1	11.4	15.3	15.8
142	Rwanda	31.9	32.0	29.6–36.5	7.0	4.8–9.4	31.8	28.3–36.2	7.2	5.3–9.2	6.5	8.7	17.0	21.5
143	Saint Kitts and Nevis	59.6	57.6	54.7–60.7	10.3	9.4–11.3	61.5	57.8–65.6	12.6	10.8–14.5	8.4	10.5	12.8	14.5
144	Saint Lucia	62.0	60.7	58.1–63.0	12.5	11.3–13.8	63.3	60.0–66.5	13.9	12.1–15.6	8.5	10.9	12.2	14.7
145	Saint Vincent and the Grenadines	60.9	59.7	57.1–62.2	12.1	11.0–13.3	62.1	59.1–65.0	14.1	12.5–15.7	8.0	11.3	11.9	15.4
146	Samoa	59.9	58.2	55.6–60.6	12.3	10.9–13.7	61.6	59.0–64.4	14.3	12.7–16.0	8.5	11.3	12.7	15.6
147	San Marino	72.0	69.7	68.0–71.8	15.9	14.8–17.0	74.3	72.2–76.4	19.9	18.4–21.5	6.5	9.5	8.5	11.4
148	Sao Tome and Principe	50.0	50.3	46.8–53.6	9.6	8.0–11.0	49.7	44.8–54.7	9.2	7.5–10.6	10.0	12.2	16.6	19.8
149	Saudi Arabia	59.5	58.3	55.0–61.1	10.5	8.4–12.3	60.7	56.5–64.9	12.1	9.8–14.2	9.7	12.8	14.3	17.4
150	Senegal	44.9	45.2	42.1–48.0	8.4	6.8–9.8	44.5	40.9–48.4	8.0	5.0–11.1	8.8	11.6	16.3	20.7

[a] Healthy life expectancy estimates published here are not directly comparable to those published in the *World Health Report 2000*, due to improvements in survey methodology and the use of new epidemiological data for some diseases. See Statistical Annex notes (pp. 130–135). The figures reported in this Table along with the data collection and estimation methods have been largely developed by WHO and do not necessarily reflect official statistics of Member States. Further development in collaboration with Member States is underway for improved data collection and estimation methods.
[b] Figures not yet endorsed by Member States as official statistics.

	Member State	Total population At birth	Males				Females				Expectation of lost healthy years at birth (years)		Percentage of total life expectancy lost	
			At birth	Uncertainty interval	At age 60	Uncertainty interval	At birth	Uncertainty interval	At age 60	Uncertainty interval	Male	Female	Male	Female
151	Seychelles	58.7	57.0	54.1–59.7	9.4	7.2–11.5	60.4	57.1–64.0	10.7	8.8–13.1	9.5	13.8	14.3	18.6
152	Sierra Leone	29.5	29.7	26.4–36.0	6.5	4.7–8.8	29.3	25.2–35.1	6.0	2.9–9.5	7.3	9.6	19.6	24.6
153	Singapore	67.8	66.8	64.3–69.0	14.5	13.1–15.8	68.9	65.8–71.7	16.2	14.6–18.0	8.6	11.3	11.4	14.1
154	Slovakia	62.4	59.6	58.1–60.9	10.7	9.9–11.6	65.2	62.3–67.5	14.0	13.2–14.9	9.7	12.3	14.0	15.9
155	Slovenia	66.9	64.5	62.1–66.7	13.6	12.8–14.3	69.3	66.5–71.9	16.7	15.4–18.0	7.4	10.2	10.3	12.8
156	Solomon Islands	59.0	58.0	55.1–61.5	11.2	9.4–13.3	60.1	56.6–63.8	12.4	10.7–14.1	8.6	11.3	12.9	15.9
157	Somalia	35.1	35.5	32.5–38.9	7.3	5.2–9.5	34.7	30.6–38.8	6.4	2.6–9.7	8.3	11.2	18.9	24.4
158	South Africa	43.2	43.0	41.1–45.0	9.1	7.9–10.5	43.5	40.5–46.4	10.4	8.7–12.1	6.6	8.6	13.3	16.5
159	Spain	70.6	68.7	67.3–70.3	15.8	14.9–16.8	72.5	70.3–74.2	18.3	17.5–19.1	6.6	9.8	8.8	11.9
160	Sri Lanka	61.1	58.6	55.7–61.5	12.5	10.9–14.1	63.6	61.0–67.0	14.6	12.8–16.6	9.0	11.7	13.4	15.6
161	Sudan	45.1	45.7	42.2–49.3	8.3	6.5–10.1	44.4	39.2–50.2	7.8	5.8–9.6	9.8	13.4	17.6	23.1
162	Suriname	60.6	59.5	57.0–61.9	12.2	11.0–13.6	61.7	58.5–64.6	13.3	11.5–15.1	8.5	11.9	12.5	16.1
163	Swaziland	38.2	38.8	34.1–44.2	9.3	7.0–11.5	37.6	32.6–42.7	9.6	7.5–12.0	6.0	8.0	13.3	17.4
164	Sweden	71.4	70.1	68.7–71.6	16.8	15.9–17.7	72.7	70.6–74.6	18.7	18.0–19.4	7.2	9.2	9.3	11.3
165	Switzerland	72.1	70.4	68.7–72.1	17.0	16.1–17.9	73.7	71.3–75.7	19.7	19.0–20.4	6.2	8.8	8.1	10.7
166	Syrian Arab Republic	59.6	59.6	56.6–62.3	11.2	9.1–13.2	59.5	55.7–63.0	11.6	9.3–13.7	9.7	12.9	14.0	17.9
167	Tajikistan	50.8	49.6	46.2–53.2	9.0	7.1–11.0	52.0	47.8–56.1	10.3	7.7–12.8	10.8	12.7	17.9	19.7
168	Thailand	59.7	57.7	55.7–59.7	13.2	12.1–14.3	61.8	57.9–64.9	14.4	13.4–15.5	8.4	10.5	12.6	14.6
169	The former Yugoslav Republic of Macedonia	64.9	63.9	62.0–65.6	12.5	11.7–13.4	65.9	64.1–67.6	14.3	13.3–15.2	6.3	8.9	9.0	12.0
170	Togo	42.7	42.7	39.3–46.5	8.6	6.7–10.7	42.7	39.3–46.8	8.6	6.5–10.9	7.9	10.3	15.5	19.4
171	Tonga	60.7	59.3	57.0–61.9	11.6	10.3–13.0	62.0	58.4–65.2	13.6	12.3–15.0	8.1	10.8	12.0	14.9
172	Trinidad and Tobago	61.7	60.3	57.9–63.1	11.6	10.2–13.1	63.0	59.0–65.8	13.3	12.1–14.5	8.2	10.7	12.0	14.5
173	Tunisia	61.4	61.0	59.2–62.9	11.8	10.6–12.2	61.7	58.0–65.4	12.6	10.6–14.7	8.2	11.7	11.8	15.9
174	Turkey	58.7	56.8	55.4–58.2	11.2	10.3–12.1	60.5	57.4–63.2	13.4	12.7–14.2	10.0	12.0	14.9	16.5
175	Turkmenistan	52.1	51.2	48.3–54.3	8.8	7.5–10.3	53.0	50.1–56.7	9.5	7.9–11.1	8.8	11.9	14.7	18.3
176	Tuvalu	57.0	56.4	54.0–58.9	9.9	8.8–11.0	57.6	54.0–61.0	11.5	8.8–13.7	7.2	10.0	11.3	14.8
177	Uganda	35.7	36.2	33.4–39.8	7.7	6.2–9.3	35.2	31.1–39.6	7.4	4.9–10.0	7.2	9.4	16.7	21.1
178	Ukraine	56.8	52.3	51.0–53.7	8.1	7.3–8.9	61.3	58.0–63.5	11.8	11.3–12.5	10.3	12.0	16.4	16.4
179	United Arab Emirates	63.1	62.3	60.0–64.5	11.5	9.8–13.2	63.9	59.9–66.9	13.3	11.8–14.7	10.0	12.5	13.8	16.4
180	United Kingdom	69.9	68.3	66.8–69.7	15.3	14.4–16.1	71.4	69.2–73.1	17.4	16.7–18.1	6.5	8.5	8.7	10.6
181	United Republic of Tanzania	38.1	38.6	35.4–42.7	7.8	5.9–9.8	37.5	34.0–41.1	7.7	5.2–10.2	7.2	9.6	15.7	20.4
182	United States of America[b]	67.2	65.7	63.8–67.5	15.0	14.0–16.0	68.8	66.5–71.0	16.8	15.8–17.9	8.2	10.7	11.1	13.4
183	Uruguay	64.1	61.7	59.0–64.6	12.6	11.6–13.6	66.5	63.5–69.4	15.8	14.0–17.7	8.4	11.4	11.9	14.6
184	Uzbekistan	54.3	52.7	49.2–56.3	9.9	7.9–11.9	55.8	51.5–60.2	11.6	9.6–13.7	9.4	12.2	15.1	17.9
185	Vanuatu	56.7	56.0	52.6–59.7	10.9	9.4–12.6	57.4	53.6–61.8	11.7	9.9–13.8	8.2	10.8	12.8	15.8
186	Venezuela, Bolivarian Republic of	62.3	60.4	57.7–63.2	13.0	11.1–14.7	64.2	59.9–67.2	14.7	13.2–16.1	10.1	12.3	14.4	16.1
187	Viet Nam	58.9	58.2	55.6–60.7	11.4	10.3–12.6	59.7	56.5–62.8	12.3	10.3–14.2	8.5	11.3	12.7	15.9
188	Yemen	49.1	48.9	45.7–51.9	8.5	6.8–10.4	49.3	44.4–53.9	8.8	6.7–10.8	10.4	12.7	17.5	20.5
189	Yugoslavia	64.3	63.3	62.1–64.7	13.0	12.2–13.7	65.4	63.2–67.3	14.6	13.4–15.7	6.5	9.3	9.3	12.5
190	Zambia	33.0	33.7	30.6–37.0	8.2	6.8–9.6	32.3	28.9–36.1	8.5	5.5–11.5	5.5	7.2	14.1	18.3
191	Zimbabwe	38.8	39.6	37.4–41.9	9.3	7.7–10.8	38.1	34.7–41.3	9.7	8.0–11.4	5.8	7.9	12.8	17.1

TABLE 2　DEATHS BY CAUSE, SEX, AND MORTALITY STRATUM IN WHO REGIONS,[a] ESTIMATES FOR 2000

Cause[b]	Both sexes		Males		Females		AFRICA — High child, high adult	AFRICA — High child, very high adult	THE AMERICAS — Very low child, very low adult	THE AMERICAS — Low child, low adult	THE AMERICAS — High child, high adult
			Sex				Mortality stratum		Mortality stratum		
Population (000)	6,045,172		3,045,372		2,999,800		294,099	345,533	325,186	430,951	71,235
	(000)	% total	(000)	% total	(000)	% total	(000)	(000)	(000)	(000)	(000)
TOTAL DEATHS	55,694	100	29,696	100	25,998	100	4,245	6,327	2,778	2,587	510
I. Communicable diseases, maternal and perinatal conditions and nutritional deficiencies	17,777	31.9	9,282	31.3	8,495	32.7	2,893	4,597	203	475	185
Infectious and parasitic diseases	10,457	18.8	5,637	19.0	4,819	18.5	1969	3467	60	213	93
Tuberculosis	1,660	3.0	1048	3.5	613	2.4	146	235	2	33	22
STDs excluding HIV	217	0.4	119	0.4	97	0.4	43	58	0	1	0
Syphilis	197	0.4	118	0.4	79	0.3	42	56	0	0	0
Chlamydia	7	0.0	0	0.0	7	0.0	1	1	0	0	0
Gonorrhea	4	0.0	0	0.0	4	0.0	1	1	0	0	0
HIV/AIDS	2,943	5.3	1,500	5.0	1,443	5.6	517	1,875	15	34	23
Diarrheal diseases	2,124	3.8	1178	4.0	946	3.6	272	433	2	49	27
Childhood diseases	1,385	2.5	693	2.3	692	2.7	432	308	0	2	6
Pertussis	296	0.5	148	0.5	148	0.6	92	74	0	1	6
Poliomyelitis	1	0.0	0	0.0	0	0.0	0	0	0	0	0
Diphtheria	3	0.0	2	0.0	2	0.0	1	1	0	0	0
Measles	777	1.4	388	1.3	388	1.5	264	188	0	0	0
Tetanus	309	0.6	154	0.5	154	0.6	75	45	0	1	1
Meningitis	156	0.3	87	0.3	69	0.3	19	23	1	9	1
Hepatitis[c]	128	0.2	70	0.2	57	0.2	15	18	5	3	1
Malaria	1,080	1.9	522	1.8	558	2.1	489	477	0	1	1
Tropical diseases	124	0.2	76	0.3	48	0.2	33	30	0	20	3
Trypanosomiasis	50	0.1	32	0.1	18	0.1	25	24	0	0	0
Chagas disease	21	0.0	12	0.0	9	0.0	0	0	0	18	3
Schistosomiasis	11	0.0	8	0.0	3	0.0	3	2	0	1	0
Leishmaniasis	41	0.1	23	0.1	18	0.1	5	4	0	0	0
Lymphatic filariasis	0	0.0	0	0.0	0	0.0	0	0	0	0	0
Onchocerciasis	0	0.0	0	0.0	0	0.0	0	0	0	0	0
Leprosy	2	0.0	2	0.0	1	0.0	0	0	0	0	0
Dengue	12	0.0	8	0.0	4	0.0	0	0	0	0	0
Japanese encephalitis	4	0.0	1	0.0	2	0.0	0	0	0	0	0
Trachoma	0	0.0	0	0.0	0	0.0	0	0	0	0	0
Intestinal nematode infections	17	0.0	9	0.0	8	0.0	1	2	0	2	1
Ascariasis	6	0.0	3	0.0	3	0.0	0	1	0	1	0
Trichuriasis	2	0.0	1	0.0	1	0.0	0	0	0	0	0
Hookworm disease	6	0.0	4	0.0	2	0.0	1	1	0	0	0
Respiratory infections	3,941	7.1	2,121	7.1	1,821	7.0	460	622	115	104	43
Lower respiratory infections	3,,866	6.9	2,084	7.0	1,782	6.9	454	614	115	102	42
Upper respiratory infections	69	0.1	34	0.1	35	0.1	4	5	0	1	1
Otitis media	6	0.0	3	0.0	3	0.0	1	2	0	0	0
Maternal conditions	495	0.9	0	0.0	495	1.9	97	146	0	13	7
Perinatal conditions	2,439	4.4	1,307	4.4	1,133	4.4	296	281	17	106	28
Nutritional deficiencies	445	0.8	218	0.7	227	0.9	70	81	10	39	13
Protein-energy malnutrition	271	0.5	137	0.5	134	0.5	49	52	5	28	8
Iodine deficiency	9	0.0	5	0.0	5	0.0	1	2	0	0	0
Vitamin A deficiency	41	0.1	17	0.1	24	0.1	11	13	0	0	0
Iron-deficiency anemia	103	0.2	49	0.2	53	0.2	8	13	6	11	2

[a] See List of Member States by WHO Region and Mortality Stratum (pp. 168–169).

[b] Estimates for specific cause may not sum to broader cause groupings due to omission of residual categories.

[c] Does not include liver cancer and cirrhosis deaths resulting from chronic hepatitis virus infection.

Cause[b]	EASTERN MEDITERRANEAN		EUROPE			SOUTHEAST ASIA		WESTERN PACIFIC	
	Mortality stratum		Mortality stratum			Mortality stratum		Mortality stratum	
	Low child, Low adult	High child, high adult	Very low child, very low adult	Low child, low adult	Low child, high adult	Low child, low adult	High child, high adult	Very low child, very low adult	Low child, low adult
Population (000)	139,071	342,584	411,910	218,473	243,192	293,821	124,813	154,358	1,532,946
	(000)	(000)	(000)	(000)	(000)	(000)	(000)	(000)	(000)
TOTAL DEATHS	690	3,346	4,076	1,952	3,636	2,142	12,015	1,152	10,238
I. Communicable diseases, maternal and perinatal conditions and nutritional deficiencies	153	1,556	240	221	152	604	4913	131	1,454
Infectious and parasitic diseases	84	836	49	85	86	332	2,540	25	618
Tuberculosis	7	129	6	19	49	157	517	6	336
STDs excluding HIV	0	12	0	2	1	1	95	0	3
Syphilis	0	10	0	1	0	1	85	0	2
Chlamydia	0	0	0	0	0	0	4	0	0
Gonorrhea	0	0	0	0	0	0	2	0	0
HIV/AIDS	0	54	10	1	10	37	334	0	32
Diarrheal diseases	24	262	2	27	4	30	921	1	71
Childhood diseases	1	196	0	8	0	43	337	0	52
Pertussis	0	57	0	0	0	1	62	0	2
Poliomyelitis	0	0	0	0	0	0	0	0	0
Diphtheria	0	0	0	0	0	0	1	0	0
Measles	0	81	0	7	0	34	168	0	34
Tetanus	0	57	0	0	0	8	105	0	17
Meningitis	2	22	2	7	5	12	42	1	11
Hepatitis[c]	3	7	4	5	2	5	32	5	22
Malaria	0	47	0	0	0	8	43	0	13
Tropical diseases	1	5	0	0	0	0	30	0	2
Trypanosomiasis	0	1	0	0	0	0	0	0	0
Chagas disease	0	0	0	0	0	0	0	0	0
Schistosomiasis	1	2	0	0	0	0	0	0	2
Leishmaniasis	0	2	0	0	0	0	30	0	0
Lymphatic filariasis	0	0	0	0	0	0	0	0	0
Onchocerciasis	0	0	0	0	0	0	0	0	0
Leprosy	0	0	0	0	0	0	1	0	0
Dengue	0	1	0	0	0	1	10	0	1
Japanese encephalitis	0	0	0	0	0	0	0	0	3
Trachoma	0	0	0	0	0	0	0	0	0
Intestinal nematode infections	0	2	0	0	0	1	5	0	3
Ascariasis	0	1	0	0	0	0	1	0	1
Trichuriasis	0	0	0	0	0	0	0	0	1
Hookworm disease	0	0	0	0	0	0	3	0	0
Respiratory infections	40	330	168	86	44	142	1,221	102	463
Lower respiratory infections	39	327	165	85	42	141	1,199	101	439
Upper respiratory infections	1	3	3	1	1	1	22	1	24
Otitis media	0	0	0	0	0	0	1	0	0
Maternal conditions	3	62	0	2	1	21	122	0	19
Perinatal conditions	20	284	11	42	19	90	919	2	321
Nutritional deficiencies	5	43	11	6	2	19	110	1	32
Protein-energy malnutrition	2	23	3	2	1	8	66	1	22
Iodine deficiency	0	2	0	0	0	0	3	0	0
Vitamin A deficiency	0	6	0	0	0	0	10	0	0
Iron-deficiency anemia	1	8	8	3	2	6	27	0	7

(continues)

TABLE 2   DEATHS BY CAUSE, SEX AND MORTALITY STRATUM IN WHO REGIONS,[a] ESTIMATES FOR 2000 *(Continued)*

							AFRICA		THE AMERICAS		
	Sex						Mortality stratum		Mortality stratum		
Cause[b]	Both sexes		Males		Females		High child, high adult	High child, very high adult	Very low child, very low adult	Low child, low adult	High child, high adult
Population (000)	6045172		3045372		2999800		294099	345533	325186	430951	71235
	(000)	% total	(000)	% total	(000)	% total	(000)	(000)	(000)	(000)	(000)
II. Noncommunication conditions	**32855**	**59.0**	**16998**	**57.2**	**15856**	**61.0**	**1043**	**1286**	**2397**	**1779**	**276**
Malignant neoplasms	6930	12.4	3918	13.2	3011	11.6	228	305	652	371	50
Mouth and oropharynx cancers	340	0.6	242	0.8	98	0.4	11	22	11	10	2
Esophagus cancer	413	0.7	274	0.9	139	0.5	5	21	16	14	1
Stomach cancer	744	1.3	464	1.6	280	1.1	18	18	19	42	10
Colon/rectum cancer	579	1.0	303	1.0	276	1.1	11	15	77	26	3
Liver cancer	626	1.1	433	1.5	193	0.7	28	35	15	14	3
Pancreas cancer	214	0.4	114	0.4	100	0.4	3	5	34	13	1
Trachea/bronchus/lung cancers	1213	2.2	895	3.0	318	1.2	9	14	182	47	3
Melanoma and other skin cancers	65	0.1	35	0.1	30	0.1	4	5	13	5	0
Breast cancer	459	0.8	0	0.0	458	1.8	14	24	56	28	3
Cervix uteri cancer	288	0.5	0	0.0	288	1.1	21	38	6	17	6
Corpus uteri cancer	76	0.1	0	0.0	76	0.3	1	2	9	10	1
Ovary cancer	128	0.2	0	0.0	128	0.5	3	7	16	6	1
Prostate cancer	258	0.5	258	0.9	0	0.0	24	19	45	26	3
Bladder cancer	157	0.3	117	0.4	40	0.2	8	6	16	6	1
Lymphomas, multiple myeloma	291	0.5	173	0.6	118	0.5	18	19	47	16	3
Leukemia	265	0.5	145	0.5	119	0.5	8	12	27	18	3
Other neoplasms	115	0.2	59	0.2	56	0.2	1	2	10	9	2
Diabetes mellitus	810	1.5	345	1.2	465	1.8	19	35	76	120	23
Nutritional/endocrine disorders	224	0.4	103	0.3	121	0.5	17	20	29	24	6
Neuropsychiatric disorders	948	1.7	477	1.6	472	1.8	31	44	135	51	13
Unipolar depressive disorders	0	0.0	0	0.0	0	0.0	0	0	0	0	0
Bipolar affective disorder	4	0.0	1	0.0	3	0.0	0	0	0	0	0
Schizophrenia	17	0.0	8	0.0	9	0.0	0	0	1	0	0
Epilepsy	98	0.2	59	0.2	38	0.1	9	15	2	6	2
Alcohol use disorders	84	0.2	73	0.2	12	0.0	2	5	8	13	4
Alzheimer's and other dementias	276	0.5	93	0.3	183	0.7	2	3	61	7	1
Parkinson disease	90	0.2	44	0.1	45	0.2	2	2	16	2	0
Multiple sclerosis	17	0.0	6	0.0	10	0.0	0	0	3	1	0
Drug use disorders	15	0.0	14	0.0	2	0.0	0	0	2	1	0
Post-traumatic stress disorder	0	0.0	0	0.0	0	0.0	0	0	0	0	0
Obsessive-compulsive disorder	0	0.0	0	0.0	0	0.0	0	0	0	0	0
Panic disorder	0	0.0	0	0.0	0	0.0	0	0	0	0	0
Insomnia (primary)	0	0.0	0	0.0	0	0.0	0	0	0	0	0
Migraine	0	0.0	0	0.0	0	0.0	0	0	0	0	0
Sense organ disorders	7	0.0	3	0.0	4	0.0	0	0	0	0	0
Glaucoma	1	0.0	0	0.0	0	0.0	0	0	0	0	0
Cataracts	1	0.0	0	0.0	1	0.0	0	0	0	0	0
Hearing loss, adult onset	0	0.0	0	0.0	0	0.0	0	0	0	0	0
Cardiovascular diseases	16701	30.0	8195	27.6	8506	32.7	460	514	1138	786	98
Rheumatic heart disease	332	0.6	137	0.5	195	0.7	13	16	6	6	3
Ischemic heart disease	6894	12.4	3625	12.2	3269	12.6	162	167	581	306	29
Cerebrovascular disease	5101	9.2	2406	8.1	2695	10.4	137	166	197	229	24
Inflammatory heart disease	395	0.7	216	0.7	180	0.7	15	19	34	27	3

[a] See List of Member States by WHO Region and Mortality Stratum (pp. 168–169).
[b] Estimates for specific cause may not sum to broader cause groupings due to omission of residual categories.
[c] Does not include liver cancer and cirrhosis deaths resulting from chronic hepatitis virus infection.

Cause[b]	EASTERN MEDITERRANEAN		EUROPE			SOUTHEAST ASIA		WESTERN PACIFIC	
	Mortality stratum		Mortality stratum			Mortality stratum		Mortality stratum	
	Low child, Low adult	High child, high adult	Very low child, very low adult	Low child, low adult	Low child, high adult	Low child, low adult	High child, high adult	Very low child, very low adult	Low child, low adult
Population (000)	139,071	342,584	411,910	218,473	243,192	293,821	124,813	154,358	1,532,946
	(000)	(000)	(000)	(000)	(000)	(000)	(000)	(000)	(000)
II. Noncommunicable conditions	459	1,530	3,637	1,586	3,009	1,307	5,961	942	7,640
Malignant neoplasms	78	164	1,056	290	536	226	877	341	1,756
Mouth and oropharynx cancers	2	20	25	9	1?	18	152	6	34
Esophagus cancer	4	10	28	11	15	3	68	12	205
Stomach cancer	10	7	70	33	83	9	55	56	313
Colon/rectum cancer	5	7	141	29	67	23	32	44	100
Liver cancer	4	7	38	9	20	26	26	35	365
Pancreas cancer	2	1	52	12	30	4	11	20	26
Trachea/bronchus/lung cancers	11	20	206	59	109	35	118	62	339
Melanoma and other skin cancers	1	1	15	4	9	1	2	3	2
Breast cancer	5	12	91	21	43	26	78	12	46
Cervix uteri cancer	5	14	8	8	13	15	102	3	33
Corpus uteri cancer	1	1	16	6	13	2	2	3	9
Ovary cancer	1	3	26	5	17	7	17	5	15
Prostate cancer	3	4	71	9	14	6	15	11	9
Bladder cancer	3	9	37	9	18	5	15	6	18
Lymphomas, multiple myeloma	5	12	54	9	14	14	40	14	27
Leukemia	7	9	37	9	15	12	38	9	62
Other neoplasms	1	4	27	3	5	26	5	10	10
Diabetes mellitus	11	52	86	26	25	50	146	17	123
Nutritional/endocrine disorders	3	25	24	2	2	15	16	8	33
Neuropsychiatric disorders	11	73	158	27	33	51	169	20	131
Unipolar depressive disorders	0	0	0	0	0	0	0	0	0
Bipolar affective disorder	0	0	0	0	0	0	3	0	0
Schizophrenia	1	1	1	0	0	2	6	0	5
Epilepsy	2	5	6	5	4	5	19	1	18
Alcohol use disorders	0	2	13	5	9	5	7	1	11
Alzheimer's and other dementias	1	5	76	4	7	20	37	7	48
Parkinson disease	1	4	21	1	1	2	10	4	24
Multiple sclerosis	0	0	4	1	2	0	3	0	1
Drug use disorders	0	0	4	0	0	1	3	1	3
Post-traumatic stress disorder	0	0	0	0	0	0	0	0	0
Obsessive-compulsive disorder	0	0	0	0	0	0	0	0	0
Panic disorder	0	0	0	0	0	0	0	0	0
Insomnia (primary)	0	0	0	0	0	0	0	0	0
Migraine	0	0	0	0	0	0	0	0	0
Sense organ disorders	0	0	0	0	0	0	1	0	3
Glaucoma	0	0	0	0	0	0	0	0	0
Cataracts	0	0	0	0	0	0	0	0	1
Hearing loss, adult onset	0	0	0	0	0	0	0	0	0
Cardiovascular diseases	276	811	1,797	1,051	2,125	598	3,493	406	3,147
Rheumatic heart disease	4	17	12	10	16	11	106	3	110
Ischemic heart disease	136	288	762	472	1,115	237	1,706	140	792
Cerebrovascular disease	58	158	470	276	741	181	625	173	1,667
Inflammatory heart disease	4	12	28	23	26	13	111	8	74

(continues)

TABLE 2   DEATHS BY CAUSE, SEX AND MORTALITY STRATUM IN WHO REGIONS,[a] ESTIMATES FOR 2000 *(Continued)*

							AFRICA		THE AMERICAS		
							Mortality stratum		Mortality stratum		
		Sex					High child, high adult	High child, very high adult	Very low child, very low adult	Low child, low adult	High child, high adult
Cause[b]	Both sexes		Males		Females						
Population (000)	6,045,172		3,045,372		2,999,800		294,099	345,533	325,186	430,951	71,235
	(000)	% total	(000)	% total	(000)	% total	(000)	(000)	(000)	(000)	(000)
Respiratory diseases	3,542	6.4	1,891	6.4	1,651	6.3	101	131	172	170	16
Chronic obstructive pulmonary disease	2,523	4.5	1,367	4.6	1,156	4.4	51	63	124	76	6
Asthma	218	0.4	107	0.4	111	0.4	8	16	7	11	3
Digestive diseases	1,923	3.5	1,151	3.9	772	3.0	87	112	97	144	32
Peptic ulcer disease	237	0.4	140	0.5	96	0.4	6	10	6	11	4
Cirrhosis of the liver	797	1.4	531	1.8	266	1.0	31	38	30	58	17
Appendicitis	33	0.1	19	0.1	13	0.1	1	1	1	2	1
Diseases of the genitourinary system	825	1.5	447	1.5	378	1.5	54	67	57	49	14
Nephritis/nephrosis	620	1.1	327	1.1	293	1.1	35	44	31	38	12
Benign prostatic hypertrophy	35	0.1	35	0.1	0	0.0	3	4	1	2	1
Skin diseases	68	0.1	30	0.1	38	0.1	10	12	4	5	2
Musculoskeletal diseases	104	0.2	36	0.1	68	0.3	6	7	12	9	3
Rheumatoid arthritis	20	0.0	6	0.0	14	0.1	1	1	2	2	1
Osteoarthritis	4	0.0	1	0.0	3	0.0	0	0	1	1	0
Congenital abnormalities	657	1.2	341	1.1	315	1.2	30	36	15	40	16
Oral diseases	2	0.0	1	0.0	1	0.0	0	0	0	0	0
Dental caries	0	0.0	0	0.0	0	0.0	0	0	0	0	0
Periodontal disease	0	0.0	0	0.0	0	0.0	0	0	0	0	0
Edentulism	0	0.0	0	0.0	0	0.0	0	0	0	0	0
III. Injuries	**5,062**	**9.1**	**3,475**	**11.5**	**1,647**	**6.3**	**308**	**445**	**178**	**33.3**	**50**
Unintentional	3,403	6.1	2,262	7.6	1,141	4.4	196	245	119	185	29
Road traffic accidents	1,260	2.3	931	3.1	329	1.3	69	99	49	82	10
Poisoning	315	0.6	204	0.7	112	0.4	15	20	12	3	2
Falls	283	0.5	170	0.6	113	0.4	8	10	23	15	2
Fires	238	0.4	104	0.3	135	0.5	18	17	4	5	1
Drowning	450	0.8	301	1.0	148	0.6	44	40	5	20	2
Other unintentional injuries	857	1.5	553	1.9	304	12	42	60	26	60	12
Intentional	1,659	3.0	1,153	3.9	506	1.9	112	199	59	148	21
Self-inflicted	815	1.5	509	1.7	305	1.2	10	17	39	23	4
Violence	520	0.9	401	1.4	119	0.5	40	76	20	123	17
War	310	0.6	233	0.8	77	0.3	62	106	0	2	0

[a] See List of Member States by WHO Region and Mortality Stratum (pp. 168–169).
[b] Estimates for specific cause may not sum to broader cause groupings due to omission of residual categories.
[c] Does not include liver cancer and cirrhosis deaths resulting from chronic hepatitis virus infection.

Cause[b]	EASTERN MEDITERRANEAN Mortality stratum		EUROPE Mortality stratum			SOUTHEAST ASIA Mortality stratum		WESTERN PACIFIC Mortality stratum	
	Low child, Low adult	High child, high adult	Very low child, very low adult	Low child, low adult	Low child, high adult	Low child, low adult	High child, high adult	Very low child, very low adult	Low child, low adult
Population (000)	139,071	342,584	411,910	218,473	243,192	293,821	124,813	154,358	1,532,946
	(000)	(000)	(000)	(000)	(000)	(000)	(000)	(000)	(000)
Respiratory diseases	26	126	205	65	127	135	482	57	1,728
Chronic obstructive pulmonary disease	13	43	136	42	93	52	255	23	1,545
Asthma	5	17	14	9	11	22	35	7	55
Digestive diseases	23	123	185	81	112	115	367	46	399
Peptic ulcer disease	3	6	18	7	14	21	53	5	74
Cirrhosis of the liver	7	28	68	47	55	42	181	15	180
Appendicitis	0	1	1	1	1	1	18	0	6
Diseases of the genitourinary system	17	69	60	26	28	56	140	27	162
Nephritis/nephrosis	11	58	40	18	11	45	122	24	131
Benign prostatic hypertrophy	1	1	1	2	3	1	8	0	8
Skin diseases	0	5	8	1	2	5	6	1	8
Musculoskeletal diseases	1	3	18	2	4	10	3	5	20
Rheumatoid arthritis	0	0	4	1	1	2	1	2	2
Osteoarthritis	0	0	1	0	0	0	0	0	0
Congenital abnormalities	12	76	13	12	10	20	254	4	119
Oral diseases	0	0	0	0	0	0	1	0	0
Dental caries	0	0	0	0	0	0	0	0	0
Periodontal disease	0	0	0	0	0	0	0	0	0
Edentulism	0	0	0	0	0	0	0	0	0
III. Injuries	**79**	**259**	**199**	**143**	**475**	**231**	**1,141**	**78**	**1,144**
Unintentional	61	181	140	88	285	155	900	49	769
Road traffic accidents	40	51	46	20	55	115	320	16	288
Poisoning	2	16	6	14	89	4	78	1	53
Falls	4	17	48	11	17	8	31	8	81
Fires	4	20	3	4	15	7	121	2	19
Drowning	3	16	4	10	33	12	85	6	169
Other unintentional injuries	8	61	34	29	76	8	266	16	158
Intentional	17	78	59	55	190	76	241	30	376
Self-inflicted	7	16	54	25	107	19	150	28	315
Violence	7	24	4	11	62	11	66	1	58
War	3	36	0	17	20	45	18	0	2

III. HIV/AIDS Statistics Worldwide by Country.

(Source: Joint United Nations Programme on HIV/AIDS)

HIV/AIDS STATISTICS WORLDWIDE BY COUNTRY

Country	1. Estimated number of people living with HIV/AIDS, end 2001				2. Children orphaned by AIDS 2001		3. AIDS deaths 2001	4. Population 2001 (thousands)	
	Adults and children	Adults (15–49)	Adults (15–49) rate (%)	Women (15–49)	Children (0–14)	Orphans (0–14) currently living	Deaths Adults and children	Total	Adults (15–49)
Global total	**40,000,000**	**37,100,000**	**1.2**	**18,500,000**	**3,000,000**	**14,000,000**	**3,000,000**	**6,119,328**	**3,198,252**
Sub-Saharan Africa	**28,500,000**	**26,000,000**	**9.0**	**15,000,000**	**2,600,000**	**11,000,000**	**2,200,000**	**633,816**	**291,310**
Angola	350,000	320,000	5.5	190,000	37,000	100,000	24,000	13,527	5,767
Benin	120,000	110,000	3.6	67,000	12,000	34,000	8,100	6,446	2,929
Botswana	330,000	300,000	38.8	170,000	28,000	69,000	26,000	1,554	762
Burkina Faso	440,000	380,000	6.5	220,000	61,000	270,000	44,000	11,856	5,046
Burundi	390,000	330,000	8.3	190,000	55,000	240,000	40,000	6,502	2,887
Cameroon	920,000	860,000	11.8	500,000	69,000	210,000	53,000	15,203	7,065
Central African Republic	250,000	220,000	12.9	130,000	25,000	110,000	22,000	3,782	1,722
Chad	150,000	130,000	3.6	76,000	18,000	72,000	14,000	8,135	3,570
Comoros	...	...	...	...	...	...	...	727	351
Congo	110,000	99,000	7.2	59,000	15,000	78,000	11,000	3,110	1,364
Côte d'Ivoire	770,000	690,000	9.7	400,000	84,000	420,000	75,000	16,349	7,854
Dem. Republic of Congo	1,300,000	1,100,000	4.9	670,000	170,000	930,000	120,000	52,522	22,073
Djibouti	...	...	...	...	...	...	...	644	284
Equatorial Guinea	5,900	5,500	3.4	3,000	420	...	370	470	211
Eritrea	55,000	49,000	2.8	30,000	4,000	24,000	350	3,816	1,760
Ethiopia	2,100,000	1,900,000	6.4	1,100,000	230,000	990,000	160,000	64,459	28,952
Gabon	...	...	...	...	...	...	...	1,262	552
Gambia	8,400	7,900	1.6	4,400	460	5,300	400	1,337	647
Ghana	360,000	330,000	3.0	170,000	34,000	200,000	28,000	19,734	9,700
Guinea	...	...	...	...	...	...	...	8,274	3,868
Guinea-Bissau	17,000	16,000	2.8	9,300	1,500	4,300	1,200	1,227	557
Kenya	2,500,000	2,300,000	15.0	1,400,000	220,000	890,000	190,000	31,293	15,333
Lesotho	360,000	330,000	31.0	180,000	27,000	73,000	25,000	2,057	984
Liberia	...	...	...	...	...	...	...	3,108	1,518
Madagascar	22,000	21,000	0.3	12,000	1,000	6,300	...	16,437	7,538
Malawi	850,000	780,000	15.0	440,000	65,000	470,000	80,000	11,572	5,118
Mali	110,000	100,000	1.7	54,000	13,000	70,000	11,000	11,677	5,096
Mauritania	...	...	...	...	...	...	...	2,747	1,268
Mauritius	700	700	0.1	350	<100	...	<100	1,171	667
Mozambique	1,100,000	1,000,000	13.0	630,000	80,000	420,000	60,000	18,644	8,511
Namibia	230,000	200,000	22.5	110,000	30,000	47,000	13,000	1,788	820
Niger	...	...	...	...	...	...	...	11,227	4,831
Nigeria	3,500,000	3,200,000	5.8	1,700,000	270,000	1,000,000	170,000	116,929	53,346
Rwanda	500,000	430,000	8.9	250,000	65,000	260,000	49,000	7,949	3,756
Senegal	27,000	24,000	0.5	14,000	2,900	15,000	2,500	9,662	4,521
Sierra Leone	170,000	150,000	7.0	90,000	16,000	42,000	11,000	4,587	2,093
Somalia	43,000	43,000	1.0	...	...	...	...	9,157	4,015
South Africa	5,000,000	4,700,000	20.1	2,700,000	250,000	660,000	360,000	43,792	23,666
Swaziland	170,000	150,000	33.4	89,000	14,000	35,000	12,000	938	450
Togo	150,000	130,000	6.0	76,000	15,000	63,000	12,000	4,657	2,152
Uganda	600,000	510,000	5.0	280,000	110,000	880,000	84,000	24,023	10,290
United Rep. of Tanzania	1,500,000	1,300,000	7.8	750,000	170,000	810,000	140,000	35,965	16,701
Zambia	1,200,000	1,000,000	21.5	590,000	150,000	570,000	120,000	10,649	4,740
Zimbabwe	2,300,000	2,000,000	33.7	1,200,000	240,000	780,000	200,000	12,852	5,972
East Asia & Pacific	**1,000,000**	**970,000**	**0.1**	**230,000**	**3,000**	**85,000**	**35,000**	**1,497,066**	**833,058**
China	850,000	850,000	0.1	220,000	2,000	76,000	30,000	1,284,972	726,031
Dem. People's Rep. of Korea	...	...	...	...	...	...	...	22,428	11,876
Fiji	300	300	0.1	<100	...	–0	...	823	443
Hong Kong	2,600	2,600	0.1	660	<100	–0	<100	6,961	4,134
Japan	12,000	12,000	<0.1	6,600	110	2,000	430	127,335	59,109
Mongolia	<100	<100	<0.1	...	...	–0	...	2,559	1,416
Papua New Guinea	17,000	16,000	0.7	4,100	500	4,200	880	4,920	2,491
Republic of Korea	4,000	4,000	<0.1	960	<100	1,000	220	47,069	27,558
Australia & New Zealand	**15,000**	**14,000**	**0.1**	**1,000**	**<200**	**<1000**	**<100**	**23,146**	**11,845**
Australia	12,000	12,000	0.1	800	140	...	<100	19,338	9,933
New Zealand	1,200	1,200	0.1	180	<100	...	<100	3,808	1,911

HIV/AIDS STATISTICS WORLDWIDE BY COUNTRY *(continued)*

| Country | 5. Ranges of uncertainty around estimates | | | | | | 6. HIV prevalence rate (%) in young people (15–24) | | | |
| | Adults and children living with HIV/AIDS, end 2001 | | Deaths in adults (15–49) 2001 | | Deaths in children (0–14) 2001 | | Female | | Male | |
	Low estimate	High estimate	Low estimate	High estimate	Low estimate	High estimate	Low estimate	High estimate	Low estimate	High estimate
Global total	30,000,000	50,000,000	1,800,000	3,000,000	440,000	720,000	1.00	1.78	0.59	1.05
Sub-Saharan Africa	22,000,000	35,000,000	1,300,000	2,300,000	380,000	650,000	6.41	11.39	3.13	5.56
Angola	250,000	450,000	12,000	20,000	5,400	9,600	4.14	7.33	1.61	2.85
Benin	100,000	150,000	4,700	7,000	1,800	2,700	2.97	4.46	0.94	1.41
Botswana	260,000	390,000	17,000	26,000	3,900	5,900	29.99	44.98	12.86	19.29
Burkina Faso	350,000	660,000	26,000	39,000	9,400	14,000	7.78	11.67	3.18	4.77
Burundi	280,000	500,000	21,000	37,000	8,100	14,000	7.98	14.11	3.58	6.33
Cameroon	740,000	1,100,000	31,000	47,000	11,000	17,000	10.09	15.25	4.33	6.55
Central African Republic	200,000	300,000	14,000	21,000	3,900	5,900	10.83	16.25	4.66	6.99
Chad	96,000	200,000	6,600	14,000	2,200	4,600	2.79	5.77	1.55	3.20
Comoros	. . .	. . .	. . .	. . .	. . .	. . .	. . .	. . .	. . .	. . .
Congo	74,000	150,000	5,500	11,000	1,900	4,000	5.08	10.52	2.13	4.42
Côte d'Ivoire	620,000	930,000	47,000	71,000	13,000	19,000	6.67	9.95	2.34	3.49
Dem. Republic of Congo	960,000	1,700,000	63,000	110,000	25,000	45,000	4.27	7.55	2.11	3.74
Djibouti	. . .	. . .	. . .	. . .	. . .	. . .	. . .	. . .	. . .	. . .
Equatorial Guinea	3,800	8,000	170	360	<100	140	1.80	3.74	0.91	1.88
Eritrea	40,000	70,000	220	420	<100	<100	3.10	5.49	2.01	3.55
Ethiopia	1,500,000	2,700,000	84,000	150,000	33,000	58,000	5.65	9.99	3.17	5.62
Gabon	. . .	. . .	. . .	. . .	. . .	. . .	. . .	. . .	. . .	. . .
Gambia	5,400	11,000	180	380	<100	150	0.88	1.82	0.34	0.71
Ghana	260,000	390,000	16,000	30,000	3,800	5,700	2.08	3.86	0.95	1.76
Guinea	. . .	. . .	. . .	. . .	. . .	. . .	. . .	. . .	. . .	. . .
Guinea-Bissau	11,000	23,000	560	1,200	200	420	1.94	4.02	0.69	1.43
Kenya	2,000,000	3,000,000	120,000	180,000	33,000	50,000	12.45	18.67	4.80	7.21
Lesotho	230,000	480,000	13,000	28,000	3,100	6,500	24.75	51.40	11.31	23.49
Liberia	. . .	. . .	. . .	. . .	. . .	. . .	. . .	. . .	. . .	. . .
Madagascar	18,000	26,000	. . .	. . .	. . .	. . .	0.19	0.28	0.05	0.08
Malawi	720,000	1,100,000	48,000	72,000	16,000	24,000	11.91	17.87	5.08	7.62
Mali	73,000	150,000	5,200	11,000	1,800	3,800	1.35	2.81	0.89	1.84
Mauritania	. . .	. . .	. . .	. . .	. . .	. . .	. . .	. . .	. . .	. . .
Mauritius	460	940	<100	<100	. . .	. . .	. . .	. . .	. . .	. . .
Mozambique	860,000	1,500,000	50,000	80,000	10,000	25,000	10.56	18.78	4.41	7.84
Namibia	150,000	230,000	7,900	12,000	2,600	3,900	19.43	29.15	8.88	13.32
Niger	. . .	. . .	. . .	. . .	. . .	. . .	. . .	. . .	. . .	. . .
Nigeria	2,800,000	4,200,000	110,000	170,000	41,000	61,000	4.66	6.99	2.39	3.59
Rwanda	400,000	600,000	29,000	44,000	10,000	15,000	8.96	13.44	3.93	5.90
Senegal	21,000	32,000	1,500	2,300	430	650	0.43	0.65	0.15	0.22
Sierra Leone	110,000	230,000	5,200	11,000	2,100	4,400	4.88	10.19	1.61	3.36
Somalia	28,000	58,000	. . .	. . .	. . .	. . .	. . .	. . .	. . .	. . .
South Africa	4,000,000	6,000,000	280,000	420,000	26,000	48,000	20.51	30.76	8.53	12.79
Swaziland	130,000	200,000	7,600	11,000	2,000	3,000	31.59	47.38	12.18	18.27
Togo	120,000	180,000	7,400	11,000	2,300	3,400	4.75	7.12	1.64	2.46
Uganda	480,000	720,000	48,000	72,000	19,000	29,000	3.70	5.56	1.59	2.38
United Rep. of Tanzania	1,200,000	1,700,000	86,000	130,000	25,000	37,000	6.44	9.67	2.84	4.25
Zambia	930,000	1,400,000	70,000	110,000	22,000	34,000	16.78	25.18	6.45	9.68
Zimbabwe	1,800,000	2,700,000	120,000	190,000	35,000	52,000	26.40	39.61	9.90	14.85
East Asia & Pacific	700,000	1,300,000	24,000	44,000	1,200	2,200	0.06	0.10	0.12	0.22
China	800,000	1,500,000	23,000	42,000	720	1,300	0.06	0.11	0.11	0.20
Dem. People's Rep. of Korea	. . .	. . .	. . .	. . .	. . .	. . .	. . .	. . .	. . .	. . .
Fiji	200	400	. . .	. . .	. . .	. . .	. . .	. . .	. . .	. . .
Hong Kong	2,100	3,200	<100	<100	<100	<100	0.00	0.00	0.00	0.00
Japan	9,300	14,000	320	480	<100	<100	0.03	0.04	0.01	0.02
Mongolia	. . .	. . .	. . .	. . .	. . .	. . .	. . .	. . .	. . .	. . .
Papua New Guinea	11,000	22,000	500	1,100	<100	140	0.25	0.53	0.21	0.45
Republic of Korea	3,200	4,800	170	260	<100	<100	0.01	0.01	0.02	0.03
Australia & New Zealand	10,000	18,000	<100	140	<100	<100	0.00	0.01	0.01	0.02
Australia	9,600	14,000	<100	<100	<100	<100	0.01	0.02	0.09	0.14
New Zealand	960	1,400	<100	<100	<100	<100	0.01	0.02	0.04	0.06

(continues)

HIV/AIDS STATISTICS WORLDWIDE BY COUNTRY *(continued)*

7. HIV prevalence (%), selected populations

Country	Women in antenatal care clinics: urban areas				Women in antenatal care clinics: outside major urban areas				Male STI patients: major urban areas				Female sex workers: major urban areas			
	Year	Median	Min.	Max.	Year	Median	Min.	Max.	Year	Median	Min.	Max.	Year	Median	Min.	Max.
Global total																
Sub-Saharan Africa																
Angola	1999	3.4	3.4	3.5	1999	8.0	8.0	8.0	1992	2.5	2.5	2.5	1999	19.4	19.4	19.4
Benin	1999	2.3	2.3	2.3	1999	4.3	1.4	7.3	1999	3.9	3.9	3.9	1999	40.8	40.6	41.0
Botswana	2001	44.9	39.1	55.8	2001	34.8	25.8	50.9	2000	53.2	46.0	60.4	. . .	. . .	. . .	. . .
Burkina Faso	2000	6.3	4.8	7.2	2000	5.5	2.9	13.4	1991	17.5	17.5	17.5	1994	58.2	57.2	59.2
Burundi	1998	18.6	18.6	18.6	1998	19.7	19.7	19.7	. . .	. . .	. . .	. . .	1993	42.2	42.2	42.2
Cameroon	2000	9.0	4.0	13.6	2000	10.7	3.4	18.0	2000	22.0	22.0	22.0	1995	16.4	15.0	17.7
Central African Republic	1997	12.8	10.8	15.2	1997	12.2	5.3	22.0	1996	19.0	14.0	24.0	1989	18.9	18.9	18.9
Chad	2000	4.0	3.0	8.2	2000	6.4	2.3	11.1	. . .	. . .	. . .	. . .	1995	13.4	13.4	13.4
Comoros	1996	0.0	0.0	0.0	. . .	. . .	. . .	. . .	1996	0.0	0.0	0.0	1994	56.8	56.8	56.8
Congo	2000	10.0	5.4	14.6	1993	4.0	2.0	13.6	1990	16.4	16.4	16.4	1987	49.2	34.3	64.1
Côte d'Ivoire	2000	9.0	9.0	9.0	2000	8.8	7.1	10.3	2000	25.0	25.0	25.0	1999	36.0	36.0	36.0
Dem. Republic of Congo	1999	4.1	2.7	5.4	1999	8.5	8.5	8.5	1997	12.2	12.2	12.2	1997	29.0	29.0	29.0
Djibouti	1996	2.9	2.9	2.9	. . .	. . .	. . .	. . .	1996	22.2	22.2	22.2	1998	27.5	27.5	27.5
Equatorial Guinea	1999	3.3	. . .	. . .	1999	3.3	. . .	. . .	1996	3.0	2.8	3.2	. . .	. . .	. . .	. . .
Eritrea	2000	2.8	. . .	. . .	2000	2.8	. . .	. . .	1999	15.0	15.0	15.0	1999	5.8	5.8	5.8
Ethiopia	2000	14.9	10.1	17.4	2000	3.1	0.7	14.3	1992	37.5	32.0	43.0	1998	73.7	73.7	73.7
Gabon	1995	4.0	2.1	5.4	1993	1.2	1.2	1.2	1988	3.6	3.6	3.6	. . .	. . .	. . .	. . .
Gambia	2001	0.9	. . .	. . .	2001	1.3	0.5	2.8	1991	4.7	4.7	4.7	1993	13.6	13.6	13.6
Ghana	2000	3.8	1.3	4.0	2000	2.2	1.0	7.8	1999	39.0	39.0	39.0	1998	50.0	50.0	50.0
Guinea	1996	2.1	2.1	2.1	1996	1.9	0.7	2.3	1996	4.0	4.0	4.0	1994	36.6	36.6	36.6
Guinea-Bissau	1997	2.5	2.5	2.5	. . .	. . .	. . .	. . .	. . .	. . .	. . .	. . .	. . .	. . .	. . .	. . .
Kenya	2000	15.3	12.2	18.4	2000	14.0	3.3	31.0	1996	14.0	14.0	14.0	2000	27.0	24.1	51.8
Lesotho	2000	42.2	42.2	42.2	2000	19.0	12.3	26.0	2000	65.2	65.2	65.2	. . .	. . .	. . .	. . .
Liberia	1993	4.0	4.0	4.0	1998	10.1	10.1	10.1	1993	8.0	8.0	8.0	. . .	. . .	. . .	. . .
Madagascar	1996	0.0	0.0	0.0	1996	0.0	0.0	1.0	1998	0.0	0.0	0.0	1995	0.3	0.3	0.3
Malawi	2001	20.1	18.6	28.5	2001	16.1	4.5	35.8	1996	54.8	54.8	54.8	1994	70.0	70.0	70.0
Mali	2001	1.7	. . .	. . .	2001	1.7	. . .	. . .	. . .	. . .	. . .	. . .	2000	21.0	21.0	21.0
Mauritania	1994	0.5	0.5	0.5	. . .	. . .	. . .	. . .	1996	1.7	1.7	1.7	. . .	. . .	. . .	. . .
Mauritius	1999	0.0	0.0	0.0	. . .	. . .	. . .	. . .	1999	0.4	0.4	0.4	1998	7.5	7.5	7.5
Mozambique	2000	14.4	13.0	15.7	2000	10.6	4.0	31.2	1999	15.1	15.1	15.1	. . .	. . .	. . .	. . .
Namibia	2000	29.6	28.2	31.0	2000	17.3	6.6	32.5	1998	42.2	39.9	44.6	. . .	. . .	. . .	. . .
Niger	1993	1.3	1.3	1.3	1994	1.2	1.2	1.2	1992	4.1	4.1	4.1	1997	23.6	23.6	23.6
Nigeria	2001	4.2	1.3	14.3	2001	5.3	1.0	15.0	1995	3.0	3.0	3.0	1996	30.5	30.5	30.5
Rwanda	2000	23.0	23.0	23.0	1999	7.0	2.3	13.2	1996	41.8	29.1	54.5	. . .	. . .	. . .	. . .
Senegal	1998	0.5	0.5	0.5	1998	0.5	0.2	0.7	1998	3.0	0.0	4.1	1998	7.0	6.1	13.3
Sierra Leone	1997	7.0	. . .	. . .	1997	7.0	. . .	. . .	1992	3.3	3.3	3.3	1995	26.7	26.7	26.7
Somalia	1998	0.0	0.0	0.0	1999	0.7	0.4	1.7	1990	0.0	0.0	0.0	1990	2.4	2.4	2.4
South Africa	2000	24.3	8.7	36.2	2000	22.9	11.2	29.7	2000	64.3	64.3	64.3	2000	50.3	50.3	50.3
Swaziland	2000	32.3	32.3	32.3	2000	34.5	27.0	41.0	2000	48.9	48.9	48.9	. . .	. . .	. . .	. . .
Togo	1997	6.8	6.8	6.8	1997	4.6	3.0	8.2	1992	45.2	45.2	45.2	1992	78.9	78.9	78.9
Uganda	2000	11.3	10.7	11.8	2000	5.0	1.9	13.1	1999	23.0	23.0	23.0	. . .	. . .	. . .	. . .
United Rep. of Tanzania	2000	17.0	10.1	23.3	2000	14.0	2.7	32.1	1997	5.1	5.1	5.1	2000	3.5	1.0	6.0
Zambia	2001	30.7	30.7	30.7	1998	13.0	5.2	31.0	1991	59.7	59.7	59.7	1998	68.7	68.7	68.7
Zimbabwe	2000	31.1	30.0	33.5	2000	33.2	13.0	70.7	1995	71.1	71.0	71.2	1995	86.0	86.0	86.0
East Asia & Pacific																
China	2000	0.0	0.0	0.0	2000	0.5	0.5	0.5	2000	0.0	0.0	1.3	2000	0.0	0.0	10.3
Dem. People's Rep. of Korea	. . .	. . .	. . .	. . .	. . .	. . .	. . .	. . .	. . .	. . .	. . .	. . .	. . .	. . .	. . .	. . .
Fiji	. . .	. . .	. . .	. . .	. . .	. . .	. . .	. . .	. . .	. . .	. . .	. . .	. . .	. . .	. . .	. . .
Hong Kong	. . .	. . .	. . .	. . .	. . .	. . .	. . .	. . .	1994	0.1	0.1	0.1	1988	0.0	0.0	0.0
Japan	1999	0.0	0.0	0.0	1999	0.0	0.0	0.0	1989	0.0	0.0	0.0	1992	0.0	0.0	0.0
Mongolia	. . .	. . .	. . .	. . .	. . .	. . .	. . .	. . .	1989	0.0	0.0	0.0	1989	0.0	0.0	0.0
Papua New Guinea	1995	0.2	0.2	0.2	1992	0.0	0.0	0.0	1998	7.0	7.0	7.0	2000	16.0	16.0	16.0
Republic of Korea	. . .	. . .	. . .	. . .	. . .	. . .	. . .	. . .	. . .	. . .	. . .	. . .	. . .	. . .	. . .	. . .
Australia & New Zealand																
Australia	. . .	. . .	. . .	. . .	. . .	. . .	. . .	. . .	1996	0.6	0.5	0.7	. . .	. . .	. . .	. . .
New Zealand	. . .	. . .	. . .	. . .	. . .	. . .	. . .	. . .	1997	0.2	0.2	0.2	. . .	. . .	. . .	. . .

Note: For key to letters used after figures, see page 587.

HIV/AIDS STATISTICS WORLDWIDE BY COUNTRY *(continued)*

	7. HIV prevalence (%) *(con't.)*						8. Knowledge and behavior indicators								
	Injecting drug users: major urban areas				Don't know that a healthy-looking person can be infected with HIV/AIDS (%)(15–24)		Median age at first sex (20–24)			Reported higher-risk sex for adults (15–49) in the last year (%)			Reported condom use for adults (15–24) at last higher-risk sex (%)		
Country	Year	Median	Min.	Max.	Female	Year	Male	Female	Year	Male	Female	Year	Male	Female	Year
Global total															
Sub-Saharan Africa															
Angola	. . .	. . .	. . .	. . .	57.2	2000	. . .	. . .	. . .	. . .	. . .	. . .	. . .	. . .	. . .
Benin	. . .	. . .	. . .	. . .	59.1	1996	17.6	17.2	1996	38.2 *k*	9.3	1996	31.0	16.1	2001
Botswana	. . .	. . .	. . .	. . .	21.6	2000	. . .	17.4	1988	. . .	. . .	. . .	85.0 *a*	. . .	1996
Burkina Faso	. . .	. . .	. . .	. . .	58.0	1999	20.0	17.3	1999	28.2 *rw*	7.7 *r*	1999	58.7 *hr*	42.4 *hr*	1999
Burundi	. . .	. . .	. . .	. . .	33.4	2000	. . .	20.4	1987	8.9	3.1	1990	. . .	. . .	. . .
Cameroon	. . .	. . .	. . .	. . .	46.3	2000	17.0	16.3	1998	54.6	27.6	1998	5.2 *h*	2.7 *hr*	1998
Central African Republic	. . .	. . .	. . .	. . .	54.0	2000	. . .	16.0	1995	22.7	10.7	1995	. . .	12.8 *h*	1995
Chad	. . .	. . .	. . .	. . .	72.3	2000	18.4	16.0	1997	27.3 *w*	6.2	1997	5.4 *hr*	1.6 *hr*	1997
Comoros	. . .	. . .	. . .	. . .	45.2	2000	18.1	20.9	1996	. . .	. . .	. . .	45.0 *h*	21.7 *h*	1996
Congo	. . .	. . .	. . .	. . .	. . .	. . .	. . .	. . .	. . .	. . .	. . .	. . .	. . .	12.0	1999
Côte d'Ivoire	1995	75.0	75.0	75.0	49.0	2000	. . .	16.2	1999	87.4	29.9	1998	11.6 *hr*	1.0 *hr*	1998
Dem. Republic of Congo	. . .	. . .	. . .	. . .	. . .	. . .	. . .	. . .	. . .	. . .	. . .	. . .	. . .	. . .	. . .
Djibouti	. . .	. . .	. . .	. . .	. . .	. . .	. . .	. . .	. . .	15.0	3.0	1995	71.7	67.4	1995
Equatorial Guinea	. . .	. . .	. . .	. . .	53.7	2000	. . .	. . .	. . .	. . .	. . .	. . .	. . .	. . .	. . .
Eritrea	. . .	. . .	. . .	. . .	46.5	1995	. . .	17.9	1995	11.5 *w*		1995	. . .	. . .	. . .
Ethiopia	. . .	. . .	. . .	. . .	61.2	2000	. . .	18.1	2000	21.1 *xw*	8.2 *x*	2000	30.3	13.4	2000
Gabon	. . .	. . .	. . .	. . .	28.3	2000	15.7	16.2	2000	76.5	51.8	2000	48.4 *h*	31.7 *h*	2000
Gambia	. . .	. . .	. . .	. . .	47.4	2000	. . .	. . .	. . .	. . .	. . .	. . .	. . .	. . .	. . .
Ghana	. . .	. . .	. . .	. . .	26.1	1998	19.5	17.5	1998	. . .	. . .	. . .	29.9 *r*	14.3 *r*	1998
Guinea	. . .	. . .	. . .	. . .	41.6	1999	17.5	16.0	1999	47.4	12.4	1999	32.9 *r*	17.6 *r*	1999
Guinea-Bissau	. . .	. . .	. . .	. . .	69.3	2000	. . .	. . .	. . .	50.3	29.5	1990	. . .	. . .	. . .
Kenya	. . .	. . .	. . .	. . .	25.4	2000	16.2	17.3	1998	44.7	20.3	1998	42.4	16.0	1998
Lesotho	. . .	. . .	. . .	. . .	53.9	2000	. . .	. . .	. . .	52.6	28.4	1989	. . .	. . .	. . .
Liberia	. . .	. . .	. . .	. . .	69.2 *b*	2000	17.8	15.5	2000	. . .	. . .	. . .	. . .	. . .	. . .
Madagascar	. . .	. . .	. . .	. . .	72.5	2000	. . .	17.0	1997	24.5 *x*	7.1 *x*	2000	2.6 *x*	0.3 *x*	2000
Malawi	. . .	. . .	. . .	. . .	16.7	2000	17.7	17.1	2000	36.9 *x*	9.4 *x*	2000	38.9	28.7	2000
Mali	. . .	. . .	. . .	. . .	62.6	1996	18.7	15.9	1996	22.9		1996	33.9 *h*	11.7 *h*	1996
Mauritania	. . .	. . .	. . .	. . .	70.0	2000	. . .	. . .	. . .	7.1 *x*		2000	. . .	. . .	. . .
Mauritius	. . .	. . .	. . .	. . .	. . .	. . .	. . .	. . .	. . .	1.5 *a*	. . .	1996	26.3 *a*	. . .	1996
Mozambique	. . .	. . .	. . .	. . .	62.1	1997	. . .	16.0	1997	59.4	. . .	1997	. . .	. . .	. . .
Namibia	. . .	. . .	. . .	. . .	. . .	. . .	. . .	18.6	1992	. . .	. . .	. . .	. . .	. . .	. . .
Niger	. . .	. . .	. . .	. . .	77.9	2000	. . .	15.7	1998	16.3 *w*	2.3	1998	2.6 *h*	1.5 *h*	1998
Nigeria	. . .	. . .	. . .	. . .	55.0	1999	. . .	18.1	1999						
Rwanda	. . .	. . .	. . .	. . .	76.5	2000	20.6 *w*	20.3 *z*	2000	12.4	7.0	2000	50.3 *h*	14.7 *h*	2000
Senegal	. . .	. . .	. . .	. . .	55.1	1997	. . .	19.3	1997	33.0 *u*	10.0 *u*	1997	67.0 *h*	45.0 *h*	1997
Sierra Leone	. . .	. . .	. . .	. . .	64.7	2000	. . .	. . .	. . .	. . .	. . .	. . .	. . .	. . .	. . .
Somalia	. . .	. . .	. . .	. . .	89.3	2000	. . .	. . .	. . .	. . .	. . .	. . .	. . .	. . .	. . .
South Africa	. . .	. . .	. . .	. . .	>50.0 *c*	1998	. . .	. . .	. . .	. . .	. . .	. . .	. . .	. . .	. . .
Swaziland	. . .	. . .	. . .	. . .	81.5	2000	. . .	. . .	. . .	19.2	6.1	1991	. . .	. . .	. . .
Togo	. . .	. . .	. . .	. . .	32.6	1998	18.0	16.5	1998	35.3 *w*	16.4	1998	36.8 *h*	17.3 *h*	1998
Uganda	. . .	. . .	. . .	. . .	24.5	2001	19.4 *z*	16.7	2000	28.4 *x*	14.1 *x*	2000	58.9 *h*	37.8 *h*	2000
United Rep. of Tanzania	. . .	. . .	. . .	. . .	33.0	1999	17.5	17.4	1999	52.3 *w*	29.1	1999	34.0 *r*	22.8 *r*	1999
Zambia	. . .	. . .	. . .	. . .	25.3	2000	16.0	16.6	1996	43.2 *x*	29.3 *x*	1998	30.1	17.6	1998
Zimbabwe	. . .	. . .	. . .	. . .	26.0	1999	19.5	18.9	1999	42.5 *w*	16.0	1999	70.2	42.0	1999
East Asia & Pacific															
China	2000	0.2	0.0	20.5	. . .	. . .	. . .	. . .	. . .	. . .	. . .	. . .	. . .	. . .	. . .
Dem. People's Rep. of Korea	. . .	. . .	. . .	. . .	. . .	. . .	. . .	. . .	. . .	. . .	. . .	. . .	. . .	. . .	. . .
Fiji	. . .	. . .	. . .	. . .	. . .	. . .	. . .	. . .	. . .	. . .	. . .	. . .	. . .	. . .	. . .
Hong Kong	1997	0.0	0.0	0.0	. . .	. . .	. . .	. . .	. . .	. . .	. . .	. . .	. . .	. . .	. . .
Japan	1999	0.0	0.0	0.0	. . .	. . .	. . .	. . .	. . .	23.7	16.3	1996	. . .	. . .	. . .
Mongolia	. . .	. . .	. . .	. . .	43.3	2000	. . .	. . .	. . .	. . .	. . .	. . .	. . .	. . .	. . .
Papua New Guinea	. . .	. . .	. . .	. . .	54.0	1996	. . .	. . .	. . .	15.0	12.0	1994	38.0	12.0	1994
Republic of Korea	. . .	. . .	. . .	. . .	. . .	. . .	. . .	. . .	. . .	. . .	. . .	. . .	. . .	. . .	. . .
Australia & New Zealand															
Australia	1996	1.7	1.7	1.7	. . .	. . .	. . .	. . .	. . .	. . .	. . .	. . .	. . .	. . .	. . .
New Zealand	1997	0.4	0.3	0.5	. . .	. . .	. . .	17.2	1995	. . .	. . .	. . .	. . .	. . .	. . .

(continues)

HIV/AIDS STATISTICS WORLDWIDE BY COUNTRY *(continued)*

Country	1. Estimated number of people living with HIV/AIDS, end 2001					2. Children orphaned by AIDS 2001	3. AIDS deaths 2001	4. Population 2001 (thousands)	
	Adults and children	Adults (15–49)	Adults (15–49) rate (%)	Women (15–49)	Children (0–14)	Orphans (0–14) currently living	Deaths Adults and children	Total	Adults (15–49)
South & Southeast Asia	**5,600,000**	**5,400,000**	**0.6**	**2,000,000**	**220,000**	**1,800,000**	**400,000**	**1,978,430**	**1,031,463**
Afghanistan	. . .	. . .	. . .	. . .	. . .	. . .	. . .	22,474	10,435
Bangladesh	13,000	13,000	<0.1	3,100	310	2,100	650	140,369	72,340
Bhutan	<100	<100	<0.1	. . .	. . .	. . .	. . .	2,141	972
Brunei Darussalam	. . .	. . .	. . .	. . .	. . .	. . .	. . .	335	187
Cambodia	170,000	160,000	2.7	74,000	12,000	55,000	12,000	13,441	6,314
India	3,970,000	3,800,000	0.8	1,500,000	170,000	. . .	. . .	1,025,096	533,580
Indonesia	120,000	120,000	0.1	27,000	1,300	18,000	4,600	214,840	118,163
Iran (Islamic Republic of)	20,000	20,000	<0.1	5,000	<200	. . .	290	71,369	37,396
Lao People's Dem. Rep.	1,400	1,300	<0.1	350	<100	. . .	<150	5,403	2,542
Malaysia	42,000	41,000	0.4	11,000	770	14,000	2,500	22,633	11,868
Maldives	<100	<100	0.1	. . .	. . .	. . .	. . .	300	141
Myanmar	. . .	. . .	. . .	. . .	. . .	. . .	. . .	48,364	25,855
Nepal	58,000	56,000	0.5	14,000	1,500	13,000	2,400	23,593	11,106
Pakistan	78,000	76,000	0.1	16,000	2,200	25,000	4,500	144,971	67,964
Philippines	9,400	9,400	<0.1	2,500	<10	4,100	720	77,131	39,600
Singapore	3,400	3,400	0.2	860	<100	. . .	140	4,108	2,324
Sri Lanka	4,800	4,700	<0.1	1,400	<100	2,000	250	19,104	10,695
Thailand	670,000	650,000	1.8	220,000	21,000	290,000	55,000	63,584	36,636
Vietnam	130,000	130,000	0.3	35,000	2,500	22,000	6,600	79,175	43,343
Eastern Europe & Central Asia	**1,000,000**	**1,000,000**	**0.5**	**260,000**	**15,000**	**<5000**	**23,000**	**393,245**	**209,038**
Armenia	2,400	2,400	0.2	480	<100	. . .	<100	3,788	2,152
Azerbaijan	1,400	1,400	<0.1	280	. . .	. . .	<100	8,096	4,529
Belarus	15,000	15,000	0.3	3,700	. . .	. . .	1,000	10,147	5,397
Bosnia and Herzegovina	. . .	900*	<0.1*	. . .	. . .	. . .	. . .	4,067	2,292
Bulgaria	. . .	400*	<0.1*	. . .	. . .	. . .	. . .	7,867	3,915
Croatia	200	200	<0.1	<100	<10	. . .	<10	4,655	2,331
Czech Republic	500	500	<0.1	<100	<10	. . .	<10	10,260	5,233
Estonia	7,700	7,700	1.0	1,500	. . .	. . .	<100	1,377	702
Georgia	900	900	<0.1	180	. . .	. . .	<100	5,239	2,726
Hungary	2,800	2,800	0.1	300	<100	. . .	<100	9,917	5,001
Kazakhstan	6,000	6,000	0.1	1,200	<100	. . .	300	16,095	8,866
Kyrgyzstan	500	500	<0.1	<100	. . .	. . .	<100	4,986	2,627
Latvia	5,000	5,000	0.4	1,000	<100	. . .	<100	2,406	1,215
Lithuania	1,300	1,300	0.1	260	<100	. . .	<100	3,689	1,901
Poland	. . .	14,000*	0.1*	. . .	. . .	. . .	. . .	38,577	20,685
Republic of Moldova	5,500	5,500	0.2	1,200	–0	. . .	300	4,285	2,339
Romania	6,500	2,500	<0.1	. . .	4,000	. . .	350	22,388	11,761
Russian Federation	700,000	700,000	0.9	180,000	. . .	. . .	9,000	144,664	78,166
Slovakia	<100	<100	<0.1	<100	. . .	. . .	<100	5,403	2,934
Tajikistan	200	200	<0.1	<100	. . .	. . .	<100	6,135	3,111
Turkmenistan	<100	<100	<0.1	<100	. . .	. . .	<100	4,835	2,508
Ukraine	250,000	250,000	1.0	76,000	. . .	. . .	11,000	49,112	25,251
Uzbekistan	740	740	<0.1	150	<100	. . .	<100	25,257	13,395
Western Europe	**550,000**	**540,000**	**0.3**	**140,000**	**5,000**	**150,000**	**8,000**	**407,021**	**200,286**
Albania	. . .	. . .	. . .	. . .	. . .	. . .	. . .	3,145	1,692
Austria	9,900	9,900	0.2	2,200	<100	. . .	<100	8,075	4,058
Belgium	8,500	8,100	0.2	2,900	330	. . .	<100	10,264	4,987
Denmark	3,800	3,800	0.2	770	<100	. . .	<100	5,333	2,519
Finland	1,200	1,200	<0.1	330	<100	. . .	<100	5,178	2,462
France	100,000	100,000	0.3	27,000	1,000	. . .	800	59,453	29,001
Germany	41,000	41,000	0.1	8,100	550	. . .	660	82,007	40,191
Greece	8,800	8,800	0.2	1,800	<100	. . .	<100	10,623	5,269
Iceland	220	220	0.2	<100	<100	. . .	<100	281	144
Ireland	2,400	2,200	0.1	660	190	. . .	<100	3,841	2,022
Italy	100,000	100,000	0.4	33,000	770	. . .	1,100	57,503	28,018
Luxembourg	. . .	360	0.2	. . .	. . .	. . .	<100	442	221
Malta	. . .	240	0.1	. . .	. . .	. . .	<100	392	193
Netherlands	17,000	17,000	0.2	3,300	160	. . .	110	15,930	7,997
Norway	1,800	1,800	0.1	400	<100	. . .	<100	4,488	2,155
Portugal	27,000	26,000	0.5	5,100	350	. . .	1,000	10,033	5,089

HIV/AIDS STATISTICS WORLDWIDE BY COUNTRY *(continued)*

Country	5. Ranges of uncertainty around estimates						6. HIV prevalence rate (%) in young people (15–24)			
	Adults and children living with HIV/AIDS, end 2001		Deaths in adults (15–49) 2001		Deaths in children (0–14) 2001		Female		Male	
	Low estimate	*High estimate*	*Low estimate*	*High estimate*	*Low estimate*	*High estimate*	*Low estimate*	*High estimate*	*Low estimate*	*High estimate*
South & Southeast Asia	**4,100,000**	**7,800,000**	**250,000**	**450,000**	**29,000**	**56,000**	**0.36**	**0.64**	**0.22**	**0.38**
Afghanistan	. . .	. . .	. . .	. . .	. . .	. . .	. . .	. . .	. . .	. . .
Bangladesh	9,400	17,000	420	750	<100	<100	0.01	0.01	0.01	0.01
Bhutan	. . .	. . .	. . .	. . .	. . .	. . .	. . .	. . .	. . .	. . .
Brunei Darussalam	. . .	. . .	. . .	. . .	. . .	. . .	. . .	. . .	. . .	. . .
Cambodia	140,000	210,000	8,100	12,000	1,800	2,700	1.99	2.98	0.77	1.16
India	2,600,000	5,400,000	. . .	. . .	. . .	. . .	0.46	0.96	0.22	0.46
Indonesia	94,000	140,000	3,400	5,100	240	360	0.05	0.07	0.05	0.08
Iran (Islamic Republic of)	13,000	27,000	150	300	<100	<100	0.01	0.01	0.03	0.06
Lao People's Dem. Rep.	1,000	1,800	<100	<100	<100	<100	0.02	0.03	0.03	0.06
Malaysia	34,000	51,000	1,900	2,800	. . .	. . .	0.09	0.14	0.56	0.84
Maldives	. . .	. . .	. . .	. . .	. . .	. . .	. . .	. . .	. . .	. . .
Myanmar	180,000	420,000	8,400	13,000	1,200	1,700	. . .	. . .	. . .	. . .
Nepal	37,000	78,000	1,400	2,800	220	450	0.18	0.38	0.17	0.36
Pakistan	51,000	110,000	2,600	5,500	290	600	0.03	0.07	0.04	0.08
Philippines	7,500	11,000	570	860	. . .	. . .	0.01	0.02	0.01	0.02
Singapore	2,700	4,100	<100	160	<100	<100	0.12	0.19	0.12	0.17
Sri Lanka	3,800	5,800	200	300	<100	<100	0.03	0.04	0.02	0.03
Thailand	530,000	800,000	50,000	76,000	2,200	3,300	1.32	2.00	0.88	1.33
Vietnam	110,000	160,000	4,900	7,400	390	590	0.13	0.20	0.25	0.38
Eastern Europe & Central Asia	**720,000**	**1,300,000**	**15,000**	**30,000**	**<100**	**<100**	**0.19**	**0.34**	**0.75**	**1.33**
Armenia	1,900	2,900	<100	<100	<100	<100	0.05	0.07	0.18	0.27
Azerbaijan	1,000	1,800	<100	<100	<100	<100	0.01	0.02	0.04	0.08
Belarus	9,600	20,000	650	1,400	<100	<100	0.13	0.26	0.38	0.79
Bosnia and Herzegovina	. . .	. . .	. . .	. . .	. . .	. . .	. . .	. . .	. . .	. . .
Bulgaria	. . .	. . .	. . .	. . .	. . .	. . .	. . .	. . .	. . .	. . .
Croatia	140	280	<100	<100	. . .	. . .	0.00	0.00	0.00	0.00
Czech Republic	400	600	<100	<100	. . .	. . .	0.00	0.00	0.00	0.00
Estonia	5,600	9,800	<100	<100	<100	<100	0.45	0.79	1.80	3.17
Georgia	590	1,200	<100	<100	<100	<100	0.01	0.03	0.05	0.10
Hungary	2,000	3,500	<100	<100	. . .	. . .	0.01	0.03	0.07	0.12
Kazakhstan	4,200	8,800	210	380	<100	<100	0.02	0.04	0.09	0.17
Kyrgyzstan	330	680	<100	<100	<100	<100	0.00	0.00	0.00	0.00
Latvia	4,000	6,000	<100	<100	<100	<100	0.19	0.29	0.75	1.13
Lithuania	850	1,800	<100	<100	<100	<100	0.03	0.06	0.10	0.22
Poland	. . .	. . .	. . .	. . .	. . .	. . .	0.03	0.06	0.06	0.12
Republic of Moldova	3,600	7,400	200	410	<100	<100	0.09	0.18	0.30	0.62
Romania	4,200	8,800	230	470	. . .	. . .	. . .	. . .	. . .	. . .
Russian Federation	500,000	840,000	7,200	11,000	<100	<100	0.53	0.80	1.50	2.24
Slovakia	<100	<100	<100	<100	. . .	. . .	0.00	0.00	0.00	0.00
Tajikistan	130	270	<100	<100	<100	<100	0.00	0.00	0.00	0.00
Turkmenistan	<100	<100	<100	<100	<100	<100	0.00	0.00	0.00	0.00
Ukraine	180,000	320,000	7,900	14,000	<100	<100	0.63	1.12	1.41	2.50
Uzbekistan	480	1,000	<100	<100	. . .	. . .	0.00	0.00	0.01	0.01
Western Europe	**440,000**	**670,000**	**6,200**	**9,800**	**<100**	**<100**	**0.10**	**0.17**	**0.15**	**0.27**
Albania	. . .	. . .	. . .	. . .	. . .	. . .	. . .	. . .	. . .	. . .
Austria	7,900	12,000	<100	<100	. . .	. . .	0.10	0.14	0.18	0.27
Belgium	6,800	10,000	<100	<100	. . .	. . .	0.10	0.14	0.09	0.14
Denmark	3,600	5,500	<100	<100	. . .	. . .	0.05	0.08	0.11	0.16
Finland	970	1,500	<100	<100	. . .	. . .	0.02	0.03	0.03	0.04
France	81,000	120,000	640	960	<100	<100	0.14	0.21	0.21	0.31
Germany	33,000	49,000	530	790	. . .	. . .	0.04	0.05	0.08	0.12
Greece	7,000	11,000	Low	<100	. . .	. . .	0.05	0.08	0.11	0.16
Iceland	180	260	<100	<100	. . .	. . .	. . .	. . .	. . .	. . .
Ireland	1,900	2,900	<100	<100	. . .	. . .	0.04	0.06	0.05	0.07
Italy	84,000	130,000	880	1,300	. . .	. . .	0.21	0.31	0.23	0.34
Luxembourg	<100	<100	<100	<100	. . .	. . .	. . .	. . .	. . .	. . .
Malta	<100	<100	<100	<100	. . .	. . .	. . .	. . .	. . .	. . .
Netherlands	13,000	20,000	<100	130	. . .	. . .	0.07	0.11	0.16	0.24
Norway	1,400	2,100	<100	<100	. . .	. . .	0.03	0.05	0.06	0.09
Portugal	23,000	40,000	500	1,200	<100	<100	0.15	0.22	0.33	0.49

(continues)

HIV/AIDS STATISTICS WORLDWIDE BY COUNTRY *(continued)*

7. HIV prevalence (%), selected populations

Country	Women in antenatal care clinics: urban areas				Women in antenatal care clinics: outside major urban areas				Male STI patients: major urban areas				Female sex workers: major urban areas			
	Year	Median	Min.	Max.	Year	Median	Min.	Max.	Year	Median	Min.	Max.	Year	Median	Min.	Max.
South & Southeast Asia																
Afghanistan	...	...	...	...	...	...	...	...	...	...	...	...	...	...	...	...
Bangladesh	...	...	...	...	1989	0.00	0.0	0.0	1998	0.30	0.3	0.3	2000	20.0	20.0	20.0
Bhutan	...	...	...	...	1993	0.00	0.0	0.0	...	...	...	...	...	...	...	...
Brunei Darussalam	...	...	...	...	...	...	...	...	...	...	...	...	...	...	...	...
Cambodia	2000	2.7	2.7	2.7	2000	1.70	0.6	5.7	1994	8.50	8.5	8.5	2000	26.3	26.3	26.3
India	1999	2.0	0.0	3.3	2000	2.00	1.0	3.9	1999	3.60	0.8	64.4	1998	5.3	5.3	5.3
Indonesia	1999	0.0	0.0	0.0	1996	0.00	0.0	0.0	...	...	...	...	1998	0.2	0.2	0.2
Iran (Islamic Republic of)	1993	0.0	0.0	0.0	1994	0.00	0.0	0.0	...	...	...	...	1994	0.0	0.0	0.0
Lao People's Dem. Rep.	1998	0.0	...	...	...	...	...	...	...	...	...	...	2000	1.0	...	...
Malaysia	...	...	...	...	1996	0.10	0.0	0.7	1996	4.20	4.2	4.2	1996	6.3	6.3	6.3
Maldives	...	...	...	...	...	...	...	...	...	...	...	...	...	...	...	...
Myanmar	2000	2.8	2.0	3.5	2000	1.80	0.0	5.3	2000	12.60	12.1	13.0	2000	38.0	26.0	50.0
Nepal	1992	0.0	0.0	0.0	1992	0.00	0.0	0.0	2000	0.00	0.0	0.0	1999	36.2	36.2	36.2
Pakistan	1995	0.0	0.0	0.6	1999	0.00	0.0	0.0	1995	0.30	0.2	3.7	1995	0.0	0.0	0.0
Philippines	...	...	...	...	...	...	...	...	1994	0.00	0.0	0.0	1994	0.3	0.3	0.3
Singapore	1998	0.0	0.0	0.0	...	...	...	...	1998	0.70	0.7	0.7	1998	0.5	0.5	0.5
Sri Lanka	1996	0.0	0.0	0.0	1996	0.00	0.0	0.0	1998	0.10	0.1	0.1	1998	0.0	0.0	0.0
Thailand	2000	1.6	1.6	1.6	2000	1.50	0.4	5.3	2000	2.50	2.5	2.5	2000	6.7	6.7	6.7
Vietnam	1999	0.2	0.1	0.2	1999	0.00	0.0	0.3	1999	2.00	1.0	5.5	2000	11.0	11.0	11.0
Eastern Europe & Central Asia																
Armenia	1998	0.1	0.1	0.2	1998	0.00	0.0	0.0	1998	0.00	0.0	0.0	...	...	...	...
Azerbaijan	...	...	...	...	...	...	...	...	1995	0.00 *n*	...	...	...	...	...	...
Belarus	...	...	...	...	1996	0.04 *n*	...	...	1996	0.04 *n*	...	...	...	...	...	...
Bosnia and Herzegovina	...	...	...	...	...	...	...	...	...	...	...	...	...	...	...	...
Bulgaria	...	...	...	...	1997	0.01 *n*	...	...	1997	0.09 *n*	...	...	...	...	...	...
Croatia	...	...	...	...	...	...	...	...	...	...	...	...	...	...	...	...
Czech Republic	...	...	...	...	1996	0.005 *n*	...	...	1996	0.00 *n*	...	...	...	...	...	...
Estonia	...	...	...	...	...	...	...	...	1996	0.03 *n*	...	...	...	...	...	...
Georgia	1997	0.0	0.0	0.0	...	...	...	...	...	...	...	...	...	...	...	...
Hungary	...	...	...	...	1996	0.00 *n*	...	...	...	...	...	...	...	...	...	...
Kazakhstan	...	...	...	...	...	...	...	...	...	...	...	...	...	...	...	...
Kyrgyzstan	...	...	...	...	...	...	...	...	...	...	...	...	...	...	...	...
Latvia	...	...	...	...	1996	0.06 *n*	...	...	1996	0.05 *n*	...	...	1998	11.0	...	...
Lithuania	1996	0.0	0.0	0.0	1993	0.00 *n*	...	...	1996	0.00	...	...	...	...	...	...
Poland	...	...	...	...	...	...	...	...	...	...	...	...	...	...	...	...
Republic of Moldova	...	...	...	...	1995	0.00 *n*	...	...	1996	0.04 *n*	...	...	...	...	...	...
Romania	...	...	...	...	...	...	...	...	1996	0.50	...	...	...	...	...	...
Russian Federation	...	...	...	...	1998	0.005 *n*	...	...	1998	0.02 *n*	...	...	...	...	...	...
Slovakia	...	...	...	...	1995	0.00 *n*	...	...	1996	0.00 *n*	...	...	...	...	...	...
Tajikistan	...	...	...	...	...	...	...	...	...	...	...	...	...	...	...	...
Turkmenistan	...	...	...	...	...	...	...	...	...	...	...	...	...	...	...	...
Ukraine	1996	0.2	0.0	0.2	1996	0.05 *n*	...	...	1996	13.30	0.5	22.7	1995	0.0 *n*	...	...
Uzbekistan	...	...	...	...	...	...	...	...	...	...	...	...	...	...	...	...
Western Europe																
Albania	...	...	...	...	...	...	...	...	...	...	...	...	...	...	...	...
Austria	...	...	...	...	...	...	...	...	...	...	...	...	...	...	...	...
Belgium	...	...	...	...	...	...	...	...	...	...	...	...	...	...	...	...
Denmark	...	...	...	...	...	...	...	...	...	...	...	...	...	...	...	...
Finland	1994	0.0	0.0	0.0	1996	0.01 *n*	...	...	1996	0.10	...	...	...	...	...	...
France	1994	0.4	0.0	0.5	...	...	...	...	1993	4.20	3.7	8.0	1991	2.3	...	...
Germany	1997	0.1	...	...	1997	0.00	...	...	...	...	...	...	...	...	...	...
Greece	...	...	...	...	...	...	...	...	...	...	...	...	1991	0.0	...	...
Iceland	...	...	...	...	...	...	...	...	...	...	...	...	...	...	...	...
Ireland	...	...	...	...	...	...	...	...	...	...	...	...	...	...	...	...
Italy	1992	0.2	...	...	1993	0.10 *n*	...	...	1992	11.00 *n*	...	...	...	...	...	...
Luxembourg	...	...	...	...	...	...	...	...	...	...	...	...	...	...	...	...
Malta	...	...	...	...	...	...	...	...	...	...	...	...	...	...	...	...
Netherlands	1996	0.3	0.0	0.6	...	...	...	...	1996	3.30	...	...	1991	1.5	1.5	2.3
Norway	...	...	...	...	1996	0.01 *n*	...	...	1992	0.10	...	...	...	...	...	...
Portugal	1995	0.2	...	...	...	...	...	...	1992	5.80	...	...	1991	3.9	...	...

HIV/AIDS STATISTICS WORLDWIDE BY COUNTRY *(continued)*

Country	7. HIV prevalence (%) *(cont.)* Injecting drug users: major urban areas				8. Knowledge and behavior indicators Don't know that a healthy-looking person can be injected with HIV/AIDS (%) (15–24)		Median age at first sex (20–24)			Reported higher-risk sex for adults (15–49) in the last year (%)			Reported condom use for adults (15–24) at last higher-risk sex (%)		
	Year	Median	Min.	Max.	Female	Year	Male	Female	Year	Male	Female	Year	Male	Female	Year
South & Southeast Asia															
Afghanistan	...	...	...	...	...	...	...	...	...	...	...	...	...	...	...
Bangladesh	1998	2.5	2.5	2.5	76.6	2000	...	...	...	...	...	...	...	...	...
Bhutan	...	...	...	...	...	...	...	...	...	...	...	...	...	...	...
Brunei Darussalam	...	...	...	...	...	...	...	...	...	...	...	...	...	...	...
Cambodia	...	...	...	...	37.6	2000	...	21.9	2000	...	0.1 *x*	2000	...	0.5 *x*	2000
India	1996	3.5	3.5	3.5	~26.0	2000	21.0 *b*	18.0 *b*	2001	11.8	2.0	2001	51.2	39.8	2001
Indonesia	...	...	...	...	67.8	2000	...	20.4	1997	...	...	...	...	...	...
Iran (Islamic Republic of)	...	...	...	...	...	...	...	...	...	...	...	...	...	...	...
Lao People's Dem. Rep.	...	...	...	...	...	...	...	...	...	...	...	...	...	...	...
Malaysia	1996	16.8	16.8	16.8	...	...	...	...	...	...	...	...	...	...	...
Maldives	...	...	...	...	...	...	...	...	...	...	...	...	...	...	...
Myanmar	2000	47.6	37.1	58.1	...	...	...	...	...	...	...	...	...	...	...
Nepal	2000	50.0	50.0	50.0	71.0	2000	...	19.6	1996	...	...	...	...	...	...
Pakistan	2000	0.0	0.0	0.0	...	...	...	...	...	...	...	...	...	...	...
Philippines	1994	0.0	0.0	0.0	33.1	1999	...	...	1998	16.1	1.3	1990	...	...	...
Singapore	1994	0.2	0.2	0.2	...	...	...	...	...	16.2	1.0	1991	...	...	...
Sri Lanka	...	...	...	...	...	...	...	...	...	4.5	0.6	1997	44.4	...	1997
Thailand	2000	39.6	39.6	39.6	...	...	...	...	...	7.4	3.1	1990	...	...	...
Vietnam	2000	41.5	33.0	50.0	36.5	2000	...	...	...	12.0 *a*	...	1995	30.0 *a*	...	1995
Eastern Europe & Central Asia															
Armenia	1998	6.3	6.3	6.3	53.0	2000	...	19.7 *z*	2000	18.9	0.6	2000	43.3		2000
Azerbaijan	1995	0.0 *n*	...	...	64.4	2000	...	...	...	...	...	...	...	...	...
Belarus	1996	6.7 *n*	...	...	...	...	...	...	...	...	...	...	...	...	...
Bosnia and Herzegovina	...	...	...	...	26.4	2000	...	...	...	...	...	...	...	...	...
Bulgaria	...	...	...	...	...	...	...	18.7	1997	...	...	...	...	...	...
Croatia	1996	0.0 *n*	...	...	...	...	...	...	...	...	...	...	...	...	...
Czech Republic	1996	0.0 *n*	...	...	...	...	...	...	...	30.5	21.7	1994	41.3	35.0	1994
Estonia	...	...	...	...	...	...	...	18.4	1994	...	...	...	...	...	...
Georgia	...	...	...	...	53.7	2000	...	...	...	51.6 *u*	0.8 *u*	1997	79.1 *u*	...	1997
Hungary	...	...	...	...	...	...	18.0	18.5	1993	...	...	...	...	...	...
Kazakhstan	...	...	...	...	37.0	1999	18.6	20.0	1999	29.7	15.5	1999	58.3	18.7	1999
Kyrgyzstan	...	...	...	...	...	...	...	19.5	1997	...	...	...	...	...	...
Latvia	1997	0.0 *n*	...	...	...	...	18.2	18.5	1995	20.0	10.0	1997	69.0	66.3	1997
Lithuania	...	...	...	...	...	...	18.6	19.5	1995	...	...	...	...	...	...
Poland	1996	5.0 *n*	...	...	...	...	19.7	19.6	1991	...	...	...	...	...	...
Republic of Moldova	1996	1.1 *n*	...	...	21.2	2000	...	...	...	...	...	...	...	...	...
Romania	...	...	...	...	30.6	1999	17.3	19.5	1999	...	...	...	...	...	...
Russian Federation	1998	0.4 *n*	...	...	...	...	...	...	...	...	...	...	...	...	...
Slovakia	1996	0.0 *n*	...	...	...	...	...	...	...	...	...	...	...	...	...
Tajikistan	...	...	...	...	92.1	2000	...	...	...	...	...	...	...	...	...
Turkmenistan	...	...	...	...	58.0	2000	...	21.6 *b*	2000	...	4.5 *x*	2000	...	...	...
Ukraine	1998	8.6 *n*	...	...	34.0	2000	...	...	...	...	19.7	1999	...	...	...
Uzbekistan	...	...	...	...	59.0	2000	...	19.7	1996	...	...	...	...	...	...
Western Europe															
Albania	...	...	...	...	59.8	2000	...	...	...	...	...	...	...	...	...
Austria	1990	27.0	13.5	44.0	...	...	...	...	...	...	...	...	38.0 *a*	...	1992
Belgium	1989	4.0	4.0	4.0	...	...	18.1	18.7	1992	...	...	...	...	...	...
Denmark	...	...	...	...	...	...	17.5	17.0	1989	...	...	...	...	...	...
Finland	1995	0.1 *n*	...	...	...	...	18.0	18.0	1992	...	...	...	...	...	...
France	1990	3.0	...	...	...	...	17.9	18.4	1998	13.3	5.6	1990	64.7	50.2	1993
Germany	...	...	...	...	...	...	...	...	...	12.0	5.0	1990	...	...	...
Greece	1995	0.4	...	...	...	...	17.5	19.0	1990	22.1	5.8	1990	...	...	...
Iceland	...	...	...	...	...	...	16.8	16.9	1992	...	...	...	...	...	...
Ireland	...	...	...	...	...	...	...	...	...	...	...	...	...	...	...
Italy	1993	33.6	7.0	36.8	...	...	18.7	21.7	1996	...	...	...	...	...	...
Luxembourg	...	...	...	...	...	...	...	...	...	...	...	...	...	...	...
Malta	...	...	...	...	...	...	...	...	...	...	...	...	...	...	...
Netherlands	1996	5.1	...	...	...	...	18.3	18.3	1989	18.0	7.0	1989	...	...	...
Norway	...	...	...	...	...	...	18.3	17.6	1992	14.5	8.8	1992	8.4	5.3	1992
Portugal	1996	15.2	...	...	...	...	17.4	19.8	1997	...	...	...	...	...	...

(continues)

HIV/AIDS STATISTICS WORLDWIDE BY COUNTRY (continued)

Country	1. Estimated number of people living with HIV/AIDS, end 2001					2. AIDS orphans 2001	3. AIDS deaths 2001	4. Population 2001 (thousands)	
	Adults and children	Adults (15–49)	Adults (15–49) rate (%)	Women (15–49)	Children (0–14)	Orphans (0–14) currently living	Deaths Adults and children	Total	Adults (15–49)
Western Europe *(cont.)*									
Slovenia	280	280	<0.1	<100	<100	. . .	<100	1,985	1,047
Spain	130,000	130,000	0.5	26,000	1,300	. . .	2,300	39,921	20,794
Sweden	3,300	3,300	0.1	880	<100	. . .	<100	8,833	4,012
Switzerland	19,000	19,000	0.5	6,000	300	. . .	<100	7,170	3,437
TFYR Macedonia	<100	<100	<0.1	<100	<100	. . .	<100	2,044	1,079
United Kingdom	34,000	34,000	0.1	7,400	550	. . .	460	59,542	28,559
Yugoslavia	10,000	10,000	0.2	. . .	. . .	. . .	<100	10,538	5,341
North Africa & Middle East	**500,000**	**460,000**	**0.3**	**250,000**	**35,000**	**65,000**	**30,000**	**349,142**	**180,506**
Algeria	. . .	13,000*	0.1*	. . .	. . .	. . .	. . .	30,841	16,779
Bahrain	<1000	<1000	0.3	150	. . .	. . .	. . .	652	390
Cyprus	<1000	<1000	0.3	150	. . .	. . .	. . .	790	396
Egypt	8,000	8,000	<0.1	780	. . .	. . .	. . .	69,080	36,301
Iraq	<1000	<1000	<0.1	150	. . .	. . .	. . .	23,584	11,527
Israel	. . .	2,700	0.1	. . .	. . .	. . .	. . .	6,172	3,067
Jordan	<1000	<1000	<0.1	150	. . .	. . .	. . .	5,051	2,561
Kuwait	. . .	. . .	. . .	. . .	. . .	. . .	. . .	1,971	1,123
Lebanon	. . .	. . .	. . .	. . .	. . .	. . .	. . .	3,556	1,949
Libyan Arab Jamahiriya	7,000	7,000	0.20	1,100	. . .	. . .	. . .	5,408	2,952
Morocco	13,000	13,000	0.10	2,000	. . .	. . .	. . .	30,430	16,373
Oman	1,300	1,300	0.10	200	. . .	. . .	. . .	2,622	1,211
Qatar	. . .	. . .	. . .	. . .	. . .	. . .	. . .	575	350
Saudi Arabia	. . .	. . .	. . .	. . .	. . .	. . .	. . .	21,028	9,667
Sudan	450,000	410,000	2.60	230,000	30,000	62,000	23,000	31,809	15,496
Syrian Arab Republic	. . .	. . .	. . .	. . .	. . .	. . .	. . .	16,610	8,481
Tunisia	. . .	. . .	. . .	. . .	. . .	. . .	. . .	9,562	5,392
Turkey	. . .	3,700*	<0.1*	. . .	. . .	. . .	. . .	67,632	36,857
United Arab Emirates	. . .	. . .	. . .	. . .	. . .	. . .	. . .	2,654	1,533
Yemen	9,900	9,900	0.1	1,500	. . .	. . .	. . .	19,114	8,098
North America	**950,000**	**940,000**	**0.6**	**190,000**	**10,000**	**320,000**	**15,000**	**316,941**	**161,413**
Canada	55,000	55,000	0.3	14,000	<500	–0	<500	31,015	16,164
United States of America	900,000	890,000	0.6	180,000	10,000	–0	15,000	285,926	145,249
Caribbean	**420,000**	**400,000**	**2.3**	**210,000**	**20,000**	**250,000**	**40,000**	**32,489**	**17,183**
Bahamas	6,200	6,100	3.5	2,700	<100	2,900	610	308	170
Barbados	. . .	2,000*	1.2*	. . .	. . .	. . .	. . .	268	154
Cuba	3,200	3,200	<0.1	830	<100	1,000	120	11,237	6,121
Dominican Republic	130,000	120,000	2.5	61,000	4,700	33,000	7,800	8,507	4,561
Haiti	250,000	240,000	6.1	120,000	12,000	200,000	30,000	8,270	4,053
Jamaica	20,000	18,000	1.2	7,200	800	5,100	980	2,598	1,376
Trinidad and Tobago	17,000	17,000	2.5	5,600	300	3,600	1,200	1,300	748
Latin America	**1,500,000**	**1,400,000**	**0.5**	**430,000**	**40,000**	**330,000**	**60,000**	**488,031**	**262,151**
Argentina	130,000	130,000	0.7	30,000	3,000	25,000	1,800	37,488	18,741
Belize	2,500	2,200	2.0	1,000	180	950	300	231	119
Bolivia	4,600	4,500	0.1	1,200	160	1,000	290	8,516	4,131
Brazil	610,000	600,000	0.7	220,000	13,000	130,000	8,400	172,559	96,894
Chile	20,000	20,000	0.3	4,300	<500	4,100	220	15,402	8,121
Colombia	140,000	140,000	0.4	20,000	4,000	21,000	5,600	42,803	23,003
Costa Rica	11,000	11,000	0.6	2,800	320	3,000	890	4,112	2,204
Ecuador	20,000	19,000	0.3	5,100	660	7,200	1,700	12,880	6,874
El Salvador	24,000	23,000	0.6	6,300	830	13,000	2,100	6,400	3,289
Guatemala	67,000	63,000	1.0	27,000	4,800	32,000	5,200	11,687	5,459
Guyana	18,000	17,000	2.7	8,500	800	4,200	1,300	763	432
Honduras	57,000	54,000	1.6	27,000	3,000	14,000	3,300	6,575	3,214
Mexico	150,000	150,000	0.3	32,000	3,600	27,000	4,200	100,368	54,019
Nicaragua	5,800	5,600	0.2	1,500	210	2,000	400	5,208	2,539
Panama	25,000	25,000	1.5	8,700	800	8,100	1,900	2,899	1,549
Paraguay	. . .	. . .	. . .	. . .	. . .	. . .	. . .	5,636	2,836
Peru	53,000	51,000	0.4	13,000	1,500	17,000	3,900	26,093	13,878
Suriname	3,700	3,600	1.2	1,800	190	1,700	330	419	238
Uruguay	6,300	6,200	0.3	1,400	100	3,100	<500	3,361	1,625
Venezuela	. . .	62,000*	0.5*	. . .	. . .	. . .	. . .	24,632	12,985

HIV/AIDS STATISTICS WORLDWIDE BY COUNTRY *(continued)*

Country	5. Ranges of uncertainty around estimates						6. HIV prevalence rate (%) in young people (15–24)			
	Adults and children living with HIV/AIDS, end 2001		Deaths in adults (15–49) 2001		Deaths in children (0–14) 2001		Female		Male	
	Low estimate	High estimate	Low estimate	High estimate	Low estimate	High estimate	Low estimate	High estimate	Low estimate	High estimate
Western Europe *(cont.)*										
Slovenia	170	390	<100	<100	<100	<100	0.00	0.00	0.00	0.00
Spain	100,000	150,000	1,800	2,600	...	...	0.19	0.29	0.41	0.62
Sweden	2,600	4,000	<100	<100	...	...	0.04	0.05	0.05	0.08
Switzerland	15,000	23,000	<100	<100	<100	<100	0.32	0.47	0.37	0.55
TFYR Macedonia	<100	<100	<100	<100	...	...	0.00	0.00	0.00	0.00
United Kingdom	27,000	41,000	360	540	<100	<100	0.04	0.06	0.08	0.12
Yugoslavia	...	...	...	...			...	...	...	...
North Africa & Middle East	**320,000**	**680,000**	**16,000**	**32,000**	**3,900**	**8,100**	**0.23**	**0.41**	**0.08**	**0.15**
Algeria	8,600	18,000	...	...	...	...	...	...	...	...
Bahrain	...	...	...	...	...	...	...	...	...	...
Cyprus	...	...	...	...	...	...	...	...	...	...
Egypt	3,000	8,200	...	...	...	...	...	...	...	...
Iraq	650	1,400	...	...	...	...	...	...	...	...
Israel	...	...	...	...	...	...	...	...	...	...
Jordan	...	...	...	...	...	...	...	...	...	...
Kuwait	...	...	...	...	...	...	...	...	...	...
Lebanon	...	...	...	...	...	...	...	...	...	...
Libyan Arab Jamahiriya	4,600	9,500	...	...	...	...	...	...	...	...
Morocco	8,600	18,000	...	...	...	...	...	...	...	...
Oman	850	1,800	...	...	...	...	...	...	...	...
Qatar	...	...	...	...	...	...	...	...	...	...
Saudi Arabia	...	...	...	...	...	...	...	...	...	...
Sudan	280,000	580,000	11,000	23,000	3,900	8,100	2.04	4.23	0.70	1.46
Syrian Arab Republic	...	...	...	...	...	...	...	...	...	...
Tunisia	...	...	...	...	...	...	...	...	...	...
Turkey	...	...	...	...	...	...	...	...	...	...
United Arab Emirates	...	...	...	...	...	...	...	...	...	...
Yemen	6,400	13,000	...	...	...	...	...	...	...	...
North America	**760,000**	**1,100,000**	**12,000**	**18,000**	**<100**	**<100**	**0.16**	**0.29**	**0.33**	**0.58**
Canada	44,000	66,000	<500	<500	<100	<100	0.14	0.21	0.22	0.33
United States of America	720,000	1,100,000	12,000	18,000	<100	<100	0.18	0.27	0.38	0.57
Caribbean	**290,000**	**520,000**	**23,000**	**44,000**	**4,600**	**9,000**	**1.78**	**3.17**	**1.42**	**2.43**
Bahamas	4,600	9,500	360	740	<100	<100	1.97	4.09	1.72	3.56
Barbados	...	...	...	...	...	...	...	...	...	...
Cuba	2,100	4,400	120	180	<100	<100	0.03	0.06	0.06	0.12
Dominican Republic	100,000	150,000	5,600	8,300	720	1,100	2.22	3.30	1.69	2.51
Haiti	190,000	390,000	16,000	32,000	3,700	7,700	3.22	6.69	2.64	5.48
Jamaica	13,000	22,000	690	1,000	<100	130	0.69	1.03	0.66	0.98
Trinidad and Tobago	15,000	30,000	690	1,400	<100	140	2.09	4.37	1.56	3.27
Latin America	**1,200,000**	**1,800,000**	**42,000**	**80,000**	**3,500**	**6,600**	**0.26**	**0.46**	**0.39**	**0.69**
Argentina	110,000	170,000	1,500	4,500	<100	200	0.27	0.40	0.69	1.03
Belize	2,300	3,400	220	330	<100	<100	1.59	2.39	0.88	1.32
Bolivia	3,000	6,200	170	350	<100	<100	0.04	0.07	0.07	0.15
Brazil	490,000	730,000	7,000	20,000	330	1,500	0.38	0.58	0.51	0.77
Chile	11,000	23,000	160	1,000	<100	<100	0.08	0.17	0.23	0.48
Colombia	94,000	190,000	3,400	7,000	250	520	0.12	0.25	0.55	1.15
Costa Rica	7,200	15,000	540	1,100	<100	<100	0.18	0.36	0.38	0.79
Ecuador	13,000	27,000	1,000	2,100	<100	170	0.10	0.20	0.20	0.41
El Salvador	16,000	32,000	1,200	2,600	<100	210	0.23	0.48	0.50	1.04
Guatemala	44,000	91,000	2,800	5,800	590	1,200	0.55	1.14	0.59	1.22
Guyana	11,000	24,000	750	1,600	<100	200	2.60	5.41	2.13	4.43
Honduras	46,000	68,000	2,100	3,200	540	810	1.20	1.80	0.96	1.44
Mexico	97,000	170,000	3,600	8,000	<100	600	0.07	0.12	0.26	0.47
Nicaragua	3,800	7,800	230	480	<100	<100	0.05	0.10	0.15	0.31
Panama	18,000	33,000	1,200	2,200	<100	<100	0.90	1.60	1.35	2.40
Paraguay	...	...	...	...	...	...	...	...	...	0.16
Peru	38,000	68,000	2,600	4,600	210	370	0.13	0.23	0.30	0.53
Suriname	2,400	5,100	190	400	<100	<100	0.99	2.05	0.79	1.64
Uruguay	5,000	7,500	<500	<500	<100	<100	0.16	0.24	0.42	0.63
Venezuela	...	...	...	...	...	...	...	...	...	0.74

(continues)

HIV/AIDS STATISTICS WORLDWIDE BY COUNTRY (continued)

7. HIV prevalence (%), selected populations

Country	Women in antenatal care clinics: urban areas				Women in antenatal care clinics: outside major urban areas				Male STI patients: major urban areas				Female sex workers: major urban areas			
	Year	Median	Min.	Max.	Year	Median	Min.	Max.	Year	Median	Min.	Max.	Year	Median	Min.	Max.
Western Europe *(cont.)*																
Slovenia	...	...	...	...	1995	0.00 *n*	...	...	1996	0.00 *n*	...	...	...	...	...	...
Spain	1997	0.1	0.1	0.2	1996	0.15 *n*	...	...	1995	5.80 *n*	0.70	7.80	1995	2.0 *n*	...	...
Sweden	...	...	...	...	1995	0.01 *n*	...	...	1991	0.17 *n*	...	...	...	...	...	...
Switzerland	...	...	...	...	...	...	...	...	1997	1.80	0.00	10.3	...	...	...	...
TFYR Macedonia	...	...	...	...	...	...	...	...	...	...	...	...	...	...	...	...
United Kingdom	1997	0.2	0.0	0.5	1997	0.0	0.0	0.1	1997	0.70	...	...	1991	0.0	...	...
Yugoslavia	...	...	...	...	...	...	...	...	...	...	...	...	...	...	...	...
North Africa & Middle East																
Algeria	...	...	...	...	...	...	...	...	...	...	...	...	1988	1.2	0.4	1.9
Bahrain	1998	0.2	0.2	0.2	...	...	...	...	1998	0.00	0.00	0.00	...	...	...	...
Cyprus	...	...	...	...	1999	0.0	0.0	0.0	...	...	...	...	...	...	...	...
Egypt	1996	0.0	0.0	0.0	1993	0.0	0.0	0.0	1999	0.00	0.00	0.00	1999	0.0	0.0	0.0
Iraq	...	...	...	...	1999	0.0	0.0	0.0	...	...	...	...	...	...	...	...
Israel	...	...	...	...	...	...	...	...	...	...	...	...	...	...	...	...
Jordan	...	...	...	...	1999	0.0	0.0	0.0	...	...	...	...	...	...	...	...
Kuwait	1998	0.0	0.0	0.0	1999	0.0	0.0	0.0	1997	0.00	0.00	0.00	...	...	...	...
Lebanon	...	...	...	...	1995	0.0	0.0	0.0	...	...	...	...	...	...	...	...
Libyan Arab Jamahiriya	...	...	...	...	1998	0.0	0.0	0.0	...	...	...	...	...	...	...	...
Morocco	1999	0.1	0.0	0.7	1999	0.0	0.0	0.0	1999	0.40	0.10	1.30	...	...	...	...
Oman	...	...	...	...	...	...	...	...	...	...	...	...	...	...	...	...
Qatar	...	...	...	...	...	...	...	...	...	...	...	...	...	...	...	...
Saudi Arabia	...	...	...	...	...	...	...	...	...	...	...	...	...	...	...	...
Sudan	1998	0.5	0.5	0.5	1998	3.8	3.5	4.0	...	...	...	...	...	...	...	...
Syrian Arab Republic	1993	0.0	0.0	0.0	...	...	...	...	1999	0.00	0.00	0.00	1999	0.0	0.0	0.0
Tunisia	2000	0.2	0.2	0.2	1999	0.0	0.0	0.0	...	...	...	...	1999	0.0	0.0	0.0
Turkey	...	...	...	...	...	...	...	...	1992	0.10	...	...	1995	0.0 *n*	...	...
United Arab Emirates	...	...	...	...	...	...	...	...	...	...	...	...	...	...	...	...
Yemen	...	...	...	...	...	...	...	...	...	...	...	...	...	...	...	...
North America																
Canada	...	...	...	...	...	...	...	...	...	...	...	...	...	...	...	...
United States of America	...	...	...	...	...	...	...	...	...	...	...	...	...	...	...	...
Caribbean																
Bahamas	1995	3.6	3.6	3.6	1993	3.6	3.6	3.6	1990	8.40	8.40	8.40	1990	44.4	44.4	44.4
Barbados	1996	1.1	1.1	1.1	...	...	...	...	1988	4.70	4.70	4.70	...	...	...	...
Cuba	1996	0.0	0.0	0.0	...	...	...	...	1991	0.00	0.00	0.00	...	...	...	...
Dominican Republic	1999	1.2	1.2	1.2	1999	2.1	1.1	4.5	1999	4.40	4.40	4.40	1999	3.5	2.4	6.6
Haiti	2000	3.8	3.8	3.8	2001	3.4	0.0	6.1	2000	15.0	15.0	15.0	1992	65.0	65.0	65.0
Jamaica	1997	1.0	1.0	1.0	...	...	...	...	2000	3.00	3.00	3.00	1997	5.0	5.0	5.0
Trinidad and Tobago	1999	3.4	3.0	3.8	...	...	...	...	1996	5.80	5.80	5.80	1988	13.0	13.0	13.0
Latin America																
Argentina	1998	0.9	0.3	1.2	1998	0.2	0.0	0.5	1998	10.8	10.8	10.80	1993	2.6	2.6	2.6
Belize	1995	2.3	2.3	2.3	2000	1.4	1.4	1.4	...	...	...	...	...	...	...	...
Bolivia	1997	0.5	0.5	0.5	1988	0.0	0.0	0.0	1997	2.00	2.00	2.00	1997	0.0	0.0	0.0
Brazil	2000	1.6	0.1	4.0	2000	0.4	0.4	0.4	1996	1.50	1.00	1.90	1998	17.8	17.8	17.8
Chile	1999	0.1	0.1	0.1	1999	0.0	0.0	0.0	1999	3.50	3.50	3.50	...	...	...	...
Colombia	2000	0.1	0.1	0.1	2000	0.1	0.1	0.2	2000	0.10	0.10	0.10	1994	0.9	0.6	1.1
Costa Rica	1997	0.3	0.3	0.3	1997	0.1	0.1	0.1	1994	3.10	3.10	3.10	1995	0.9	0.9	0.9
Ecuador	2001	0.7	0.0	1.3	...	...	...	...	1993	3.60	3.60	3.60	2001	1.1	1.0	1.7
El Salvador	1997	0.2	0.2	0.3	...	...	...	...	1996	5.70	5.30	6.00	1993	1.1	1.1	1.1
Guatemala	1998	0.9	0.4	1.4	1999	0.0	0.0	1.0	1991	0.70	0.70	0.70	1998	4.7	4.7	4.7
Guyana	1997	3.8	3.8	3.8	...	...	...	...	1997	25.0	25.0	25.0	2000	45.0	45.0	45.0
Honduras	1998	2.9	0.7	5.0	1998	3.0	3.0	3.0	1991	11.2	11.2	11.2	1999	7.7	7.7	7.7
Mexico	1994	0.6	0.6	0.6	...	...	...	...	2000	17.4	17.4	17.4	1999	0.3	0.3	0.3
Nicaragua	...	...	...	...	...	...	...	...	...	...	...	...	1990	1.6	1.6	1.6
Panama	1994	0.3	0.3	0.3	1997	0.9	0.9	0.9	...	...	...	...	...	...	...	...
Paraguay	1992	0.0	0.0	0.0	...	...	...	...	...	...	...	...	1987	0.1	0.1	0.1
Peru	1999	0.3	0.3	0.3	1999	0.0	0.0	0.0	1990	18.7	18.7	18.7	1998	1.6	1.6	1.6
Suriname	1998	1.4	1.4	1.4	...	...	...	...	1990	1.10	1.10	1.10	1990	2.6	2.6	2.6
Uruguay	1991	0.0	0.0	0.0	1991	0.0	0.0	0.0	1991	1.30	1.30	1.30	1997	0.5	0.5	0.5
Venezuela	1996	0.0	0.0	0.0	1996	0.0	0.0	0.0	...	...	...	...	1996	1.1	1.1	1.1

HIV/AIDS STATISTICS WORLDWIDE BY COUNTRY (continued)

| | 7. HIV prevalence (%) (cont.) | | | | 8. Knowledge and behavior indicators | | | | | | | | | |
| | Injecting drug users: major urban areas | | | | Don't know that a healthy-looking person can be infected with HIV/AIDS (%) (15–24) | | Median age at first sex (20–24) | | | Reported higher-risk sex for adults (15–49) in the last year (%) | | | Reported condom use for adults (15–24) at last higher-risk sex (%) | | |
Country	Year	Median	Min.	Max.	Female	Year	Male	Female	Year	Male	Female	Year	Male	Female	Year
Western Europe (cont.)															
Slovenia	1996	0.6	...	...	...	...	17.0	18.0	1994	12.4	6.2	1996	16.9	17.9	1996
Spain	1996	31.0	...	...	...	...	18.7	20.1	1995	18.0	4.8	1995	49.4 e	32.5	1996
Sweden	1995	5.3	...	...	...	...	...	17.1	mid-1990s	13.0	7.0	1989	...	...	...
Switzerland	1997	1.4	0.0	16.7	...	...	18.3	18.6	1994	15.9	8.1	1994	56.7	36.9	1994
TFYR Macedonia	...	...	...	...	...	...	...	...	...	...	...	...	...	...	...
United Kingdom	1997	3.4	...	...	...	...	17.1	17.4	1991	26.9	6.8	1991	23.2	17.5	1991
Yugoslavia	...	...	...	...	34.8	2000	...	...	...	36.3	16.7	1997	35.7	44.0	1997
North Africa & Middle East															
Algeria	...	...	...	...	...	...	...	...	...	...	...	...	...	...	...
Bahrain	1999	0.0	0.0	0.0	...	...	...	...	...	...	...	...	...	...	...
Cyprus	...	...	...	...	...	...	...	...	...	...	...	...	...	...	...
Egypt	1999	0.0	0.0	0.0	...	...	...	...	...	...	...	...	...	...	...
Iraq	...	...	...	...	...	...	...	...	...	...	...	...	...	...	...
Israel	...	...	...	...	...	...	...	...	...	...	...	...	...	...	...
Jordan	...	...	...	...	43.0	1997	...	...	...	...	...	...	...	...	...
Kuwait	...	...	...	...	...	...	...	...	...	...	...	...	...	...	...
Lebanon	...	...	...	...	...	...	...	...	...	22.4a	...	1996	69.3a	...	1996
Libyan Arab Jamahiriya	...	...	...	...	...	...	...	...	...	...	...	...	...	...	...
Morocco	...	...	...	...	...	...	...	...	...	...	...	...	...	...	...
Oman	...	...	...	...	...	...	...	...	...	...	...	...	...	...	...
Qatar	...	...	...	...	...	...	...	...	...	...	...	...	...	...	...
Saudi Arabia	...	...	...	...	...	...	...	...	...	...	...	...	...	...	...
Sudan	...	...	...	...	...	...	...	...	...	3.0	1.0	1995	20.0	16.7	1995
Syrian Arab Republic	1999	0.0	0.0	0.0	...	...	...	...	...	...	...	...	...	...	...
Tunisia	1997	0.3	0.3	0.3	...	...	...	...	...	...	...	...	...	...	...
Turkey	1992	0.0	0.0	0.0	37.8	1998	...	...	...	...	...	...	...	...	...
United Arab Emirates	...	...	...	...	...	...	...	...	...	...	...	...	...	...	...
Yemen	...	...	...	...	...	...	...	...	...	...	...	...	...	...	...
North America															
Canada	...	...	...	...	...	...	...	17.8	mid-1990s	8.4	6.0	1997	72.3	71.9	1997
United States of America	...	...	...	...	...	...	...	17.2	mid-1990s	11.0 amx	...	1997	65.0 amx	...	1997
Caribbean															
Bahamas	...	...	...	...	...	...	...	...	...	...	...	...	...	...	...
Barbados	...	...	...	...	...	...	...	...	...	...	...	...	...	...	...
Cuba	...	...	...	...	9.6	2000	...	...	...	48.6	14.4	1996	...	...	...
Dominican Republic	...	...	...	...	11.2	2000	...	18.7	1996	14.8 k	9.8	1995	44.5	12.4	1996
Haiti	...	...	...	...	32.0	2000	...	18.2	2000	55.4	31.9	2000	25.5 h	14.4 h	2000
Jamaica	...	...	...	...	...	...	...	17.1	1997	...	...	...	...	38.3	1997
Trinidad and Tobago	...	...	...	...	5.1	2000	...	19.4	1987	...	...	...	...	...	...
Latin America															
Argentina	1995	92.0	92.0	92.0	...	...	...	...	...	...	...	...	<55.0 a	...	1995
Belize	...	...	...	...	...	...	...	...	...	...	...	...	...	...	...
Bolivia	...	...	...	...	45.6	2000	...	19.6	1998	28.3 k	...	1999	36.4 h	12.8 h	1998
Brazil	1999	42.0	42.0	42.0	21.0	1996	...	18.7	1996	37.9 w	14.1	1996	56.0	30.3	1996
Chile	...	...	...	...	...	...	...	...	...	28.0	6.0	1997	33.0	18.0	1997
Colombia	...	...	...	...	15.8	2000	...	18.4	2000	...	29.1 x	2000	...	23.0 h	2000
Costa Rica	...	...	...	...	...	...	...	...	...	21.4	12.5	1995	55.3	42.0	1995
Ecuador	...	...	...	...	41.0	1999	...	19.3	1999	...	...	...	...	...	...
El Salvador	...	...	...	...	32.0	1998	...	18.7	1998	...	...	...	...	...	...
Guatemala	...	...	...	...	56.0	1995	...	19.0	1999	...	...	...	...	4.36	1999
Guyana	...	...	...	...	15.8	2000	...	...	...	...	...	...	...	...	...
Honduras	...	...	...	...	22.2	1996	15.7	18.4	1996	...	...	...	...	...	...
Mexico	...	...	...	...	...	...	...	20.7	1987	15.4	...	1997	62.8 a	...	1997
Nicaragua	...	...	...	...	25.4	1998	15.8	18.1	1998	...	...	...	...	6.4 h	1998
Panama	...	...	...	...	...	...	...	17.9	...	...	...	...	...	...	...
Paraguay	...	...	...	...	26.7 d	1998	...	17.9	1996	...	...	...	...	79.1	1996
Peru	1990	28.1	28.1	28.1	28.2	2000	...	19.6	2000	13.6	1.5	1996	41.6 e	17.9	2000
Suriname	...	...	...	...	29.8	2000	...	...	...	...	...	...	...	...	...
Uruguay	1997	24.4	24.4	24.4	...	...	...	...	...	...	...	...	...	...	...
Venezuela	...	...	...	...	...	...	...	...	...	...	...	...	...	...	...

(continues)

KEY TO TABLE OF COUNTRY-SPECIFIC HIV/AIDS ESTIMATES AND DATA, END 2001

a   the proportion of both sexes combined
m   the median of a number of subnational surveys
u   urban samples
x   underestimation of true value due to survey methodology
w   15–59-year-olds
*   No country-specific models provided

HIV prevalence rate (%), data from selected populations

r   data from rural studies
n   a nationwide number without rural-urban breakdown

Don't know a healthy-looking person can be infected with HIV/AIDS (15–24) (%)

b   15–49-year-olds
c   15–19-year-olds
d   15–35-year-olds

Median age when first sexually active (20–24)

b   15–49-year-old females; 15–54-year-old males
z   25–29-year-olds

Reported higher-risk sex for adults (15–49) in the last year (%)

r   non-cohabiting regular partners who are assumed to be "high-risk"
k   15–64-year-olds

Reported condom use for adults (15–49) during last higher-risk sexual act (%)

e   an older survey (based on the 1–4 years preceding the stated survey)
h   only those people who have heard of AIDS
r   non-cohabiting regular partners who are assumed to be "high-risk"

APPENDIX III
SELECTED RESOURCES FOR PRACTITIONERS, RESEARCHERS, AND PERSONS WITH HIV/AIDS

These listings represent a selection of the resources available and are by no means complete. Inclusion in these listings does not imply endorsement by the authors or publisher.

1. TELEPHONE LISTINGS

Associations and Organizations

ACT-UP-New York
212/966-4873

AIDS Resource Foundation for Children (ARFC)
201/483-4250

American Cancer Society
800/227-2345

American Civil Liberties Union (ACLU)
212/549-2500

American College of Obstetricians and Gynecologists (ACOG)
202/638-5577

American Foundation for AIDS Research (AmFar)
800/39-AMFAR

American Holistic Medical Association (AHMA)
703/556-9728

American Holistic Nurses Association
800/278-2462

American Hospital Association (AHA)
312/422-3000

American Institute for Teen AIDS Prevention
440/774-5411

American Medical Association (AMA)
800/AMA-3211

American Public Health Association (APHA)
202/777-2500

American Red Cross
800/797-8022

American Society of Alternative Therapists
978/281-4400

Center for Infectious Diseases (CID)
See CENTERS FOR DISEASE CONTROL AND PREVENTION (CDC)

Center for Substance Abuse Prevention
See NATIONAL INSTITUTES OF HEALTH (NIH)

Centers for Disease Control and Prevention (CDC)

24-hour hot line	800/342-2437
Public inquiries	800/311-3435
In Spanish	800/344-7432 (Mon-Fri 8-2 Eastern)
For the hearing-impaired	800/243-7889 (Mon-Fri 10-10 Eastern)
Center for Infectious Diseases (CID)	800/311-3435
National AIDS Information Clearinghouse	800/458-5231
National Center for Health Statistics (NCHS)	301/436-8500

Children's AIDS Fund
703/471-7350

Department of Agriculture (DA)
703/305-2039
Food Nutrition Information Center   301/504-5719

Department of Health and Human Services (HHS)
877/696-6775

Department of Housing and Urban Development (HUD)
800/569-4287

Department of Veterans Affairs (VA)
800/827-1000

Elizabeth Glaser Pediatric AIDS Foundation
888/499-HOPE

Food and Drug Administration (FDA)
888/INFO-FDA

Gay and Lesbian Medical Association
415/255-4547

Gay Men's Health Crisis (GMHC)
800/243-7692

Lambda Legal Defense and Education Fund
212/809-8585

Mobilization Against AIDS
415/863-4676

Names Project Foundation (NPF)
404/688-5500

National AIDS Information Clearinghouse
See CENTERS FOR DISEASE CONTROL
AND PREVENTION (CDC)

National Association of People With AIDS (NAPWA)
202/898-0414

National Association of Public Hospitals and Health Systems
202/585-0100

National Cancer Institute (NCI)
See NATIONAL INSTITUTES OF HEALTH (NIH)

National Center for Health Statistics (NCHS)
See CENTERS FOR DISEASE CONTROL
AND PREVENTION (CDC)

National Center for Lesbian Rights (NCLR)
415/392-6257

National Gay and Lesbian Task Force (NGLTF)
202/332-6483

National Hemophilia Foundation
800/424-2634

National Hospice and Palliative Care Organization
800/658-8898

National Institutes of Health (NIH)
301/496-4000
Center for Substance Abuse Prevention,
workplace hotline
800/729-6686

National Cancer Institute (NCI)
800/4-CANCER

National Institute of Child Health and Human Development (NICHD)
800/370-2943

National Institute of Mental Health (NIMH)
301/443-1124

National Institute of Drug Abuse (NIDA)
800/843-4971

National Library of Medicine (NLM)
888/346-3656

National Pediatric and Family HIV Resource Center
800/362-0071

National Resource Center on Women and AIDS
202/872-1770

National Minority AIDS Council (NMAC)
202/483-6622

National Native American AIDS Prevention Center
510/444-2051

National Women's Health Network
202/628-7814

Physicians for Human Rights (PHR)
617/695-0041

Project Inform
415/558-8669

Red Cross
See AMERICAN RED CROSS

Social Security Administration (SSA)
800/772-1213

Teen AIDS Hotline
800/234-TEEN

Women Organized to Respond to Life-Threatening Diseases (WORLD)
510/986-0340

Education for Physicians/Practitioners

HIV Telephone Consultation Service for Health Care Providers
800/933-3413 (Mon.-Fri., 7:30-5 Pacific)

National Clinicians' Post-Exposure Prophylaxis Hotline
888/448-4911

AIDS Education and Training Centers

Alabama, Georgia, North Carolina, South Carolina
404/727-2929

Arkansas, Louisiana, Mississippi
504/568-3855

Connecticut, Maine, Massachusetts, New Hampshire, Rhode Island, Vermont
617/566-2994

Florida
813/974-4430

Illinois, Iowa, Minnesota, Missouri, Wisconsin
312/996-1364

Nevada, Arizona, Hawaii, California
415/502-8196

New Jersey
201/972-3690

New York, Virgin Islands
212/305-0030

North Dakota, South Dakota, Utah, Colorado, New Mexico, Nebraska, Kansas, Wyoming
303/315-2515

Ohio, Michigan, Kentucky, Tennessee
313/962-2000

Pennsylvania, Delaware, Maryland, Virginia, West Virginia, Washington, D.C.
412/624-1895

Puerto Rico
787/759-6528

Texas, Oklahoma
214/590-5529

Washington, Alaska, Montana, Idaho, Oregon
206/720-4250

Clinical Trials

AIDS Clinical Trials Information Service
800/TRIALS-A (Mon.-Fri. 9-7 Eastern)

Community Programs for Clinical Research on AIDS
301/628-3361

Community Research Initiative on AIDS
212/924-3934

National Institutes of Health (NIH) AIDS Trials
800/243-7644

Pharmaceutical Information

Carl Vogel Foundation
202/289-4898

DAAIR, Direct Access Alternative Information Resources
212/725-6994

Healing Alternatives Foundation
415/626-2316

PWA Health Group
212/255-0520

Stadtlanders Pharmacy
800/238-7828 TDD 800/336-8675

Payment Assistance Programs and Expanded Access Programs (by manufacturer)

Abbott (clarithromycin)
800/711-7193

Amgen (filgrastim)
800/272-9376

Astra (foscarnet)
800/488-3247

Bristol-Myers Squibb (didanosine, stavudine, nystatin)
800-272-4878

GlaxoSmithKline (acyclovir, atovaquone, primethamine, zidovudine, TMP/SMX)
888/825-5249

Fujisawa (pentamidine)
800/477-6472

Gilead Sciences, Inc. (cidofovir)
800/226-2056

Janssen (itraconazole)
800/544-2987

Bayer (ciprofloxacin)
800/468-0894

Merck (indinavir)
800/850-3430

Ortho Biotech (erythropoetin)
800/553-3851

Pfizer/Agouron (nelfinavir, fluconazole, streptomycin)
800/254-4445

Pharmacia (rifabutin)
800/242-7014

Hoffman-LaRoche (flucytosine, saquinavir, larium, gancyclovir, zalcitabine)
800/285-4484

Boehringer Ingelheim/Roxane (dronabinol, nevirapine)
800/274-8651

Schering-Plough (alfa-Interferon-2b)
800/521-7157

Medlmmune (trimetrexate)
877/633-4411

Journals and Newsletters

ACRIA Update
212/924-3934

AIDS Treatment News
800/TREAT-1-2

Bulletin of Experimental Treatments for AIDS (BETA)
415/487-8060

GMHC Treatment Issues
212/367-1456

HIV Impact
800/444-6472

MMWR Reports on HIV/AIDS: Morbidity and Mortality Weekly Report
404/639-4198

NUMEDX.com
212/845-7147

Poz Magazine
800/9-READ-POZ

Treatment Action Group TAGline
212/253-7922

State HIV/AIDS Hot lines

Centers for Disease Control and Prevention (CDC)
800/342-2437
   For a printed list: 800/458-5231

Local numbers
   Local phone directory (see Health Care [under State Government in Blue Pages])

2. WEBSITES

General Guides

AIDS.org
http://www.aids.org

AIDS Education Global Information System
http://www.aegis.com/
http://www.aegis.com/topics/sida/

AIDS Resource Sampler
http://nnlm.gov/pnr/samplers/aidspath.html

AIDS Treatment Information Service
http://www.hivatis.org/

The Body: A Multimedia AIDS and HIV Resource
http://www.thebody.com/index.shtml

CDC National Prevention Information Network
http://www.cdcnpin.org/rellinks.htm

Grupo de Trabajo sobre Tratamientos del VIH
http://www.gtt-vih.org/welcome2.html

HIV i-base
http://www.i-base.org.uk/

HIV InSite
http://hivinsite.ucsf.edu/InSite

HIV and Hepatitis.com
http://www.hivandhepatitis.com/

Journal of the American Medical Association (JAMA), HIV/AIDS site
http://www.ama-assn.org/special/hiv/

Lycos Health with WebMD: AIDS/HIV
http://webmd.lycos.com/condition_center?doi=hiv

National AIDS Resource Center
http://www.aids-ed.org/

NLM's ATIS-supported HIV/AIDS articles
http://tcxt.nlm.nih.gov/atis/list.html

Yahoo! Health: Diseases and Conditions: AIDS/HIV
http://dir.yahoo.com/Health/Diseases_and_Conditions/AIDS_HIV/

Medical Associations and General Information

American Cancer Society
http://www.cancer.org

American College of Obstetricians and Gynecologists (ACOG)
http://www.acog.org

American Holistic Nurses Association
http://www.ahna.org

American Medical Association (AMA)
http://www.ama-assn.org

American Public Health Association (APHA)
http://www.apha.org

American Red Cross
http://www.redcross.org

American Society of Alternative Therapies
http://www.asat.org

Centers for Disease Control
http://www.cdc.gov

WONDER on the Web (CDC publications)
http://wonder.cdc.gov/

Department of Agriculture (DA) Food Nutrition Information Center
http://www.nal.usda.gov/fnic/etext/000062.html

Department of Health and Human Services (HHS)
http://www.os.dhhs.gov

HIV/AIDS Bureau
http://hab.hrsa.gov/

Department of Housing and Urban Development (HUD)
http://www.hud.gov

Department of Veterans Affairs (VA)
http://www.va.gov

Food and Drug Administration (FDA)
http://www.fda.gov

Food Nutrition Information Center
See DEPARTMENT OF AGRICULTURE

Gay and Lesbian Medical Association
http://www.glma.org/

National Association of Public Hospitals and Health Systems
http://www.naph.org

National Cancer Institute (NCI)
http://www.nci.nih.gov

National Center for Health Statistics
http://www.cdc.gov/nchs/

National Center for HIV, STD and TB Prevention
http://www.cdc.gov/nchstp/od/nchstp.html

National Gay and Lesbian Task Force (NGLTF)
http://www.ngltf.org

National Hemophilia Foundation
http://www.hemophilia.org/home.htm

National Hospice and Palliative Care Organization
http://www.nhpco.org

National Institute of Justice (NIJ)
http://www.ncjrs.org/nijhome.htm

National Institutes of Health (NIH)
http://www.nih.gov

National Institute of Child Health and Human Development (NICHD)
http://www.nih.gov/nichd

National Institute on Drug Abuse (NIDA)
http://www.nida.nih.gov

National Institute of Mental Health (NIMH)
http://www.nimh.nih.gov

National Library of Medicine (NLM)
http://www.nlm.nih.gov

Physicians for Human Rights
http://www.phrusa.org/

Public Health Service
http://www.hhs.gov/phs/

Social Security Administration (SSA)
http://www.ssa.gov

United States Public Health Service
See PUBLIC HEALTH SERVICE

World Federation of Hemophilia
http://www.wfli.org/

World Health Organization (WHO)
http://www.who.int/en/

HIV/AIDS Agencies and Organizations

AIDS Alliance for Children, Youth & Families
http://www.aids-alliance.org/

AIDS Resource Foundation for Children
http://www.aidsresource.org/

American Academy of HIV Medicine
http://www.aahivm.org/new/index.html

American Foundation for AIDS Research (AmFar)
http://www.amfar.org

Association of Nurses in AIDS Care
http://www.anacnet.org/

Centers for Disease Control and Prevention (CDC)
http://www.cdc.gov
http://www.cdc.gov/spanish/

Global AIDS Program (GAP)
www.cdc.gov/nchstp/od/gap

Center for Infectious Diseases (CID)
http://www.cdc.gov/ncidod/ncid.htm

Division of HIV/AIDS Prevention (DHAP)
http://www.cdc.gov/nchstp/hiv-AIDS/dhap.htm

Elizabeth Glaser Pediatric AIDS Foundation
http://www.pedAIDS.org

Fight AIDS at Home
http://www.fightaidsathome.org/

Harvard AIDS Institute
http://www.hsph.harvard.edu/hai/

HIV Continuing Medical Education (CME)
http://www.hivcme.com/

International AIDS Vaccine Initiative
http://www.iavi.org/

Jewish AIDS Network
http://www.jewishaidsnetwork.org/welcome.html

Joint United Nations Programme on HIV/AIDS (UNAIDS)
http://www.unaids.org/

International AIDS Economics Network
http://www.iaen.org/index.htm

International Association of Physicians in AIDS Care
http://www.iapac.org/

National AIDS Treatment Advocacy Project (NATAP)
http://www.natap.org/

National Institute of Allergy and Infectious Diseases (NIAID)
http://www.niaid.nih.gov

Division of AIDS (DAIDS)
http://www.niaid.nih.gov/daids/

Project Inform
http://www.projectinform.org

UNAIDS
See JOINT UNITED NATIONS PROGRAMME ON HIV/AIDS

Publications

ACRIA Update
http://www.acria.org/treatment/treatment_edu_ACRIA_update.html

AIDS Book Review journal
http://www.uic.edu/depts/lib/aidsbkrv/

AIDS Daily Summary
http://www.cdcnpin.org/news/start.htm

AIDS Treatment News
http://www.aids.org/immunet/atn.nsf/page

AVERT.org World AIDS Statistics
http://www.avert.org/statindx.htm

Body Positive
http://www.thebody.com/bp/bpix.html

Bulletin of Experimental Treatments for AIDS (BETA)
http://www.sfaf.org/beta/

GMHC Treatment Issues
http://www.gmhc.org/living/treatmnt.html

HIV Impact
http://www.omhrc.gov/OMH/sidebar/omh-publications.htm

MMWR Reports on HIV/AIDS: Morbidity and Mortality Weekly Report (CDC, Division of HIV/AIDS [DHAP])
http://www.cdc.gov/epo/mmwr/mmwr.html

NUMEDX.com
http://www.numedx.com/

Poz Magazine
http://www.poz.com

SIDAahora
http://www.thebody.com/bp/bpix.html#sidaahora

Treatment Action Group TAGline
http://aidsinfonyc.org/tag/taglines/taglines.html

Conference Coverage and Publications

AIDS 2002 Barcelona 14th International AIDS Conference
http://www.aids2002.org/Home.asp

AIDS 2000 13th International AIDS Conference in Durban
http://www.thebody.com/confs/durban/aids2000.html

CDC Conference Calendar
http://www.cdcnpin.org/db/public/ccmain.htm

International AIDS Society Conference Calendar
http://www.ias.se/event/calendar.asp?pageid=420&category_id=3

AIDS Consumer and Patient Organizations

Actúa
http://interactua.net/

AIDS Action Council
http://www.aidsaction.org

Asian & Pacific Islander Wellness Center
http://www.apiwellness.org/

Asian & Pacific Islander Coalition on HIV/AIDS
http://www.apicha.org/apicha/main.html

Being Alive
http://www.beingalivela.org/index.html

Children with AIDS Project
http://www.aidskids.org/

Critical Path AIDS Project in Philadelphia
http://www.critpath.org/

Drug Infonet
http://www.druginfonet.com/

Drug Interactions
http://www.tthivclinic.com/interact_tables.html

Filipino Task Force on AIDS
http://www.ftfa.org/

Hispanic AIDS Forum
http://www.hispanicfederation.org/agencies/haf.htm

HIV Medication Guide
http://www.jag.on.ca/hiv/
http://www.jag.on.ca/vih/index.htm (French)
http://www.thebody.com/estrategias.html (Spanish)

Minority AIDS Project
http://www.map.org

National Association of People with AIDS (NAPWA)
http://www.napwa.org

National Minority AIDS Council
http://www.nmac.org/

National Native American AIDS Prevention Center
http://www.nnaapc.org/

National Pediatric AIDS Network
http://www.npan.org

Project Inform
http://www.projinf.org/
http://www.projinf.org/spanish/

Clinical Trials

Adult AIDS Clinical Trials Group
http://aactg.s-3.com/

AIDS Clinical Trials Information Service
http://www.actis.org/

AIDS Treatment Data Network
http://www.AIDSnyc.org/network

Canadian HIV Trials Network
http://www.hivnet.ubc.ca/ctn.html

Clinical Trials
http://www.clinicaltrials.gov

Community Programs for Clinical Research on AIDS (CPCRA)
http://www.cpcra.org

HIV/AIDS Treatment Information Service (ATIS)
http://www.hivatis.org

National AIDS Treatment Advocacy Project (NATAP)
http://www.natap.org/

Databases

AIDSLINE
http://www.ncbi.nim.nih.gov/entrez/query.fcgi

AIDS Drugs Structures
http://chem.sis.nim.nih.gov/aidsdrg4.html

HIV/AIDS Therapeutics
http://www.fda.gov/oashi/aids/status.html

HIV Molecular Immunology Database
http://hiv-web.lanl.gov/immuno

HIV Sequence Database
http://hiv-web.lanl.gov/content/index

Newsgroups

AIDS Newsgroups
http://www.compassnet.com/~shall/Newsgroupmailletters.html

AIDS Discussion Groups
http://www.critpath.org/aric/pwarg/links05.htm

Newsgroup:alt.sex.safe
news:alt.sex.safe

Newsgroup:misc.health.AIDS
news:misc.health.AIDS

Newsgroup:sci.med.AIDS
news:sci.med.AIDS

Terminology

AEGIS AIDS Glossary
http://www.aegis.com/ni/topics/glossary/

AIDS 101 Glossary
http://www.critpath.org/research/gloss-vh.htm

AIDS Treatment Data Network Glossary: Conditions & Symptoms
http://www.AIDSnyc.org/network/oisgloss.html

CPCRA Glossary of Medical, Statistical, and Clinical Trials Terms
http://www.cpcra.org/gloss.html

Glossary of HIV/AIDS-Related Terms
http://glossary.hivatis.org/index.asp

Glossary of AIDS-related terminology
http://www.unaids.org/publications/glossary.asp
(English, French, Russian, Spanish)

HIV Vaccine Glossary
http://www.niaid.nih.gov/factsheets/GLOSSARY.htm

National Human Genome Reseach Institute Glossary
http://www.genome.gov/glossary.cfm

Safer Sex & Harm Reduction

10%
http://www.10percent.org/safe-sex.html

Center for AIDS Prevention Studies
http://www.caps.ucsf.edu/capsweb/

Coalition for Positive Sexuality
http://www.positive.org

Lesbian Safer Sex Page
http://safersex.org/women/lesbianss.html

North American Syringe Exchange Network
http://www.nasen.org

Safer Sex Page
http://www.safersex.org/

Community and Regional Aids Organizations and Services

ACT-UP
http://www.actupny.org

AIDS Project Los Angeles
http://www.apla.org/apla/

Community Health Project
http://www.chp-health.org

Consumer News
http://www.AIDSnyc.org/cnews

Direct Access Alternative Information Resources (DAAIR)
http://www.daair.org

Gay Men's Health Crisis (GMHC)
http://www.gmhc.org/GMHC

OneWorld
http://www.oneworld.net/partners

People With AIDS Coalition of Philadelphia
http://www.critpath.org/wtp/

People with AIDS Coalition Utah
http://www.pwacu.org/

People with AIDS Coalition of Vermont
http://www.vtpwac.org/

STOP AIDS Project, San Francisco
http://www.stopAIDS.org/

Treatment Action Group
http://www.thebody.com/tag/tagpage.html

Law and Legislation

American Civil Liberties Union (ACLU)
http://www.aclu.org

Americans with Disabilities Act (ADA)
http://www.usdoj.gov/crt/ada/adahoml.htm

Lambda Legal Defense and Education Fund
http://www.lambdalegal.org

Webber' Website: An AIDS/HIV law and policy resource
http://www.critpath.org/aidslaw

Alternative Medicine

Alternative Medicine Homepage
http://www.pitt.edu/~cbw/altm.html

Bastyr University AIDS Research Center
http://www.bastyr.edu/research/buarc

Institute for Traditional Medicine
http://www.itonline.org/

National Center for Complementary and Alternative Medicine
http://www.nccam.nih.gov/

Miscellaneous

AIDS Clock
http://www.unfpa.org/modules/aidsclock/index.html

AIDS History Center
http://www.aidshistory.org/aidshist.htm

Names Project Foundation (NPF)
http://www.aidsquilt.org

Pasteur Institure, Paris
http://www.pasteur.fr/

World AIDS Day
http://www.worldaidsday.org
http://www.avert.org/worldaid.htm

Around the World

AfriAfya
http://www.afriafya.org/

AIDSlink South Africa
http://www.aidslink.org.za/

Asian AIDS/HIV Information (AIDS information in Southeast Asian languages)
http://www.utopia-asia.com/aids.htm

Asian AIDS Resources
http://www.growthhouse.org/asianhiv.html

Doctors without Borders/Médecins Sans Frontières
http://www.doctorswithoutborders.org/

International Council of AIDS Service Organizations
http://www.icaso.org/

Secretariat of the Pacific, HIV/AIDS and STD Project
http://www.spc.org.nc/aids/

Southern Africa AIDS Information Dissemination Service
http://www.safaids.org.zw/safaidsweb/

Treatment Action Campaign
http://www.tac.org.za/

BIBLIOGRAPHY

The Act-Up/New York Women & AIDS Book Group. *Women, AIDS & Activism*. Boston: South End, 1990.

AIDS Community Research Initiative of America. "ACRIA Update" formerly *CRIA Update*.) ACRIA, Fall 1997–Summer 2002. Available on-line. URL: http://www.criany.org/treatment/treatment_edu_ACRIA_update.html. Downloaded on July 9, 2002.

AIDS Education Global Information System (AEGIS). "AEGIS AIDS Glossary," AIDS Education Global Information System. 1998. Available on-line. URL: http://www.aegis.org/ni/topics/glossary/. Downloaded July 9, 2002.

AIDS "Treatment Data Network" Descriptions of Opportunistic Infections and Conditions." AIDS Treatment Data Network, Sept. 9, 1999. Available on-line. URL: http://www.atdn.org/oisgloss.html. Downloaded on July 9, 2002.

———. "Descriptions of Drugs and Treatments." AIDS Treatment Data Network, April 25, 2002. Available on-line. URL: http://www.atdn.org/drugloss.html. Downloaded on July 9, 2002.

AIDS Virus Education and Research Trust. "AIDS in India." Available on-line. URL: http://www.avert.org/aidsindia.htm. Downloaded on July 30, 2002.

Allen, Karen. "Eastern Europe Hit Hard by HIV Rise." BBC News, July 4, 2002. Available on-line. URL: news.bbc.co.uk/2/low/health/2095501.stm. Downloaded on July 30, 2002.

Altman, Dennis. *AIDS in the Mind of America: The Social, Political, and Psychological Impact of a New Epidemic*. Garden City, N.Y.: Anchor/Doubleday, 1986.

Altman, Roberta, and Michael J. Sarg. *The Cancer Dictionary*. New York: Facts On File, 1992.

Alyson, Sasha, ed. *You Can Do Something About AIDS*. Boston: The Stop AIDS Project, Inc., 1988.

Ammer, Christine. *The New A-to-Z of Women's Health: A Concise Encyclopedia*. Rev. and expanded ed. New York: Facts On File, 1989.

Anastos, Kathryn. "Re-examining Treatment Recommendations for Women." *ACRIA Update* 9(1). Available on-line. URL: http://www.criany.org/treatment/treatment_edu_winterupdate99_00_re.htm. Downloaded on July 22, 2002.

Armstrong, Gregory, Laura A. Conn, and Robert W. Pinner. *"Trends in Infectious Disease Mortality in the United States During the 20th Century."* JAMA, The Journal of the American Medical Association 281 (Jan. 6, 1999): 61.

Arno, Peter S., and Karyn L. Feiden. *Against the Odds: The Story of AIDS Drug Development, Politics and Profits*. New York: HarperCollins, 1992.

Art & Understanding, Inc. *A & U: Art and Understanding, America's AIDS Magazine*. Albany, N.Y.: Art & Understanding, 2001–2002.

Aspaas, Helen Ruth. "AIDS and Orphans in Uganda: Geographical and Gender Interpretations of Household Resources." *The Social Science Journal* 36, no. 2: 201–226.

Baker, Ronald D., ed. *HIV and Hepatitis.com*. HIV and Hepatitis Treatment Advocates, Inc. 1999–2002. URL: http:www.hivandhepatitis.com. Downloaded on May 17, 2002.

Bartlett, John G., and Ann K. Finkbeiner. *The Guide to Living with HIV Infection*. Baltimore: Johns Hopkins University Press, 1991.

Bartlett, John G., and Joel E. Gallant. *Medical Management of HIV Infection, 2001–2002*. Baltimore: Johns Hopkins University Press, 2001.

BBC News Online "AIDS Races Through Eastern Europe." BBC News, Nov. 28, 2001. Available on-line. URL: http://news.bbc.co.uk/2/low/world/Europe/1680624.stm. Downloaded on July 30, 2002.

————. "Brazil to Break AIDS Patent." BBC News Online: Business, Aug. 23, 2001. Available on-line. URL: http://news.bbc.co.uk/2/low/business/1505163.stm. Downloaded on July 30, 2002.

————. "Russia's AIDS Catastrophe Growing." BBC News. Available on-line. URL: http://news.bbc.co.uk/2/low/health/1043675.stm. Downloaded on July 30, 2002.

————. "US Drops Brazil AIDS Drug Case." BBC News Online: Business, June 25, 2001. Available on-line. URL: http://news.bbc.co.uk/2/low/business/1407472.stm. Downloaded on July 30, 2002.

Bechtel, Stefan, and the Editors of *Prevention and Men's Health* magazines. *The Sex Encyclopedia: An A-to-Z Guide to the Latest Information on Sexual Health, Safety, and Technique from the Nation's Top Sex Experts.* New York: Simon & Schuster, 1993.

BETA: Bulletin of Experimental Treatments for AIDS. San Francisco: San Francisco AIDS Foundation 12(2) (April 1999)–115(2) (Spring 2002).

Blakslee, Dennis. "Adherence to Therapy: A Background Briefing." *JAMA: HIV/AIDS Resource Center.* Chicago: American Medical Association, May 19, 1998. Available on-line. URL: http://www.ama-assn.org/special/hiv/newsline/briefing/adhere.htm. Downloaded on Aug 2, 2002.

————. "AIDS Dementia Complex: A Background Briefing." *JAMA: HIV/AIDS Resource, Center.* American Medical Association, December 2, 1997. Available on-line. URL: http://www.ama-adssn.org/special/hiv/newsline/briefing/adc.htm. Downloaded on August 2, 2002.

————. "The Cytochrome P450 Enzymes: A Background Briefing." *JAMA: HIV/AIDS Resource Center.* American Medical Association, June 10, 1997. Available on-line. URL: http://www.ama-assn.org/special/hiv/newsline/briefing/cytochro.htm. Downloaded on August 2, 2002.

————. "Cytokines, Chemokines, and Host Defense: A Background Briefing." *JAMA: HIV/AIDS Resource Center.* American Medical Association, Oct. 7, 1996. Available on-line. URL: http://www.ama-assn.org/special/hiv/newsline/briefing/cyto.htm. Downloaded on August 2, 2002.

————. "The Elusive Functions of nef: A Background Briefing." *JAMA: HIV/AIDS Resource Center.* American Medical Association, July 25, 2000. Available on-line. URL: http://www.ama-assn.org/special/hiv/newsline/briefing/nefback.htm. Downloaded on August 2, 2002.

————. "Fusion and Fusion Inhibitors: A Background Briefing." *JAMA: HIV/AIDS Resource Center.* American Medical Association, Jan. 19, 1999. Available on-line. URL: http://www.ama-assn.org/special/hiv/newsline/briefing/fusion.htm. Downloaded on August 2, 2002.

————. "HIV Integrase: Activity and Inhibitors: A Background Briefing." *JAMA: HIV/AIDS Resource Center.* American Medical Association, April 6, 1998. Available on-line. URL: http://www.ama-assn.org/special/hiv/newsline/briefing/integrase.htm. Downloaded on Aug. 2, 2002.

————. "HIV's Silent Reservoirs: A Background Briefing." *JAMA: HIV/AIDS Resource Center.* American Medical Association, March 8, 2000. Available on-line. URL: http://www.ama-assn.org/special/hiv/newsline/briefing/reserv.htm. Downloaded on Aug. 2, 2002.

————. "Long-term Nonprogressors." *JAMA: HIV/AIDS Resource Center.* American Medical Association, September 18, 2000. Available on-line. URL: http://www.ama-assn.org/special/hiv/newsline/briefing/ltnps.htm. Downloaded on August 2, 2002.

————. "Macrophages: A Background Briefing." *JAMA: HIV/AIDS Resource Center.* American Medical Association, January 11, 2001. Available on-line. URL: http://www.ama-assn.org/special/hiv/newsline/briefing/mphages.htm. Downloaded on August 2, 2002.

————. "Mother-to-Child Transmission of HIV: A Background Briefing." *JAMA: HIV/AIDS Resource Center.* Chicago: American Medical Association, May 22, 2001. Available on-line. URL: http://www.ama-assn.org/special/hiv/newsline/briefing/mother.htm. Downloaded on August 2, 2002.

————. "The Thymus and Immunologic Reconstitution: A Background Briefing." *JAMA: HIV/AIDS Resource Center.* Chicago: American Medical Association, February 8, 1999. Available on-line. URL: http://www.ama-adssn.org/special/hiv/newsline/briefing/thymus.htm. Downloaded on August 2, 2002.

Bollag, Burton. "African Universities Begin to Face the Enormity of Their Losses to AIDS." *The Chronicle of Higher Education.* March 2, 2001. A45. Available on-line. URL: http://www.chronicle.com/weekly/v47/i25/25a04501.htm. Downloaded on July 30, 2002.

The Boston Women's Health Book Collective. *The New Our Bodies, Ourselves: Updated and Expanded for the '90s.* New York: Simon & Schuster, 1992.

Breitman, Patti, Kim Knutson, and Paul Reed. *How to Persuade Your Lover to Use a Condom … and Why You Should.* Rocklin, Calif.: Prima, 1987.

Brown, David. "AIDS Is Up Sharply in Eastern Europe." *The Washington Post,* November 29, 2001, p. A29.

————. "AIDS Shortening Life in 51 Nations." *The Washington Post,* July 8, 2002, p. A2.

Buckley, Stephen. "Brazil Becomes Model in Fight Against AIDS." Washingtonpost.com, Sept. 17, 2000. Washington Post, Inc. Available on-line. URL: http://www.washingtonpost.com/ac2/wp-dyn?pagename=article&node=&contentld=A20559-2000Sep16. Downloaded on July 30, 2002.

Burris, Scott, Harlon L. Dalton, Judith Leonie Millera, and the Yale AIDS Law Project, eds. *AIDS Law Today: A New Guide for the Public.* New Haven, Conn.: Yale University Press, 1993.

Butler, Sandra, and Barbara Rosenblum. *Cancer in Two Voices.* San Francisco: Spinsters, 1991.

Cadman, Jill, ed. *Positive Words.com* Dallabrida and Associates, 2002. Available on-line. URL: www.positivewords.com. Downloaded on May 17, 2002.

Califia-Rice, Patrick. *The Advocate Adviser.* Boston: Alyson, 1991.

Califia-Rice, Patrick, ed. *The Lesbian S/M Safety Manual: Basic Health and Safety for Woman-to-Woman S/M.* Denver: Lace, 1988.

Callen, Michael. *Surviving AIDS.* New York: Harper-Collins, 1990.

Campaign for Access to Essential Medicines. "New Drug for Visceral Leishmaniases Is First Step in Neglected Diseases but Much More Must Be Done." Médecins Sans Frontières. June 21, 2002. Available on-line. URL: http://www.accessmed-msf.org/prod/publications.asp?scntid=21620021450442&contenttype=PARA&. Downloaded on August 4, 2002.

Carmichael, Cynthia G., J. Kevin Carmichael, and Margaret A. Fischl. *HIV/AIDS Primary Care Handbook.* Norwalk, Conn.: Appleton & Lange, 1995.

Carr, Andrew. "HIV-Associated Lipodystrophy, Metabolic Complications and Antiretroviral Toxicities." Hivand-Hepatitis.com, Inc., 2001. Available on-line. URL: http://www.hivandhepatitis.com/hiv_and_aids/lipo/lipo7a.html. Downloaded on July 19, 2002.

Carrera, Michael A. *The Language of Sex: An A to Z Guide.* New York: Facts On File, 1992.

Caulfield, Charles R., with Billi Goldberg. *The Anarchist AIDS Medical Formulary: A Guide to Guerrilla Immunology.* Berkeley, Calif.: North Atlantic, 1993.

Centers for Disease Control and Prevention. "The Case Definition of AIDS Used by CDC for National Reporting (CDC reportable AIDS)," Document no. 03125, August 1, 1985.

———. "The Case Definitions for Infectious Conditions Under Public Health Surveillance". *Morbidity and Mortality Weekly Report* 46(RR-10) (May 2, 1997).

———. "CDC Guidelines for National Human Immunodeficiency Virus Case Surveillance, Including Monitoring for Human Immunodeficiency Virus Infection and Acquired Immunodeficiency Syndrome." *Morbidity and Mortality Weekly Report* 48(RR-13) (December 10, 1999).

———. "CDC Surveillance Summaries" *Morbidity and Mortality Weekly Report* 6(SS-3) (August 13, 1993).

———. "First Report of AIDS" *Morbidity and Mortality Weekly Report* 50(21) (June 1, 2001).

———. *HIV/AIDS Surveillance Report* 11(2) (1999):1–46.

———. *HIV/AIDS Surveillance Report* 12(2) (2000):1–47.

———. *HIV/AIDS Surveillance Supplemental Report* 7(1) (2001):1–16.

———. *Sexually Transmitted Disease Surveillance.* Atlanta: Department of Health and Human Services, Centers for Disease Control, 1999.

———. "Update on Acquired Immune Deficiency Syndrome (AIDS)—United States" *Morbidity and Mortality Weekly Report* 31 (1982): 507–514.

Cohn, D. J., E. J. Fisher, et al. "A Prospective Randomized Trial of Four Three-Drug Regimens in the Treatment of Disseminated *Mycobacterium avium* Complex Disease in AIDS Patients: Excess Mortality Associated with High-Dose Clarithromycin." *Clinical Infectious Diseases* 29(1): 125–133.

Collie, Tim. "AIDS in the Caribbean." June 8, 2001. *South Florida Sun-Sentinel on the Web.* Sun-Sentinel Co. Available on-line. URL: http://www.sun-sentinel.com/news/southflorida/sfl-aidsintheislands.story. Downloaded on July 30, 2002.

Condon, Lee. "Cruising for Safe Sex." *The Advocate,* March 13, 2001, pp. 37–38.

Corea, Gena. *The Invisible Epidemic: The Story of Women* and AIDS. New York: HarperPerennial, 1992.

Crimp, Douglas. *AIDS Demo Graphics.* Seattle: Bay Press, 1990.

Crimp, Douglas, ed. *AIDS: Cultural Analysis Cultural Activism.* Cambridge, Mass.: MIT Press, 1988.

DeCotiis, Sue. *A Woman's Guide to Sexual Health.* New York: Pocket Books, 1989.

Delacoste, Frederique, and Priscilla Alexander, eds. *Sex Work: Writings by Women in the Sex Industry.* San Francisco: Cleis, 1987.

Dempster, Carolyn. "Medicinal Plant 'Fights' AIDS." BBC News Online, Nov. 30, 2001. Available on-line. URL: http://news.bbc.co.uk/2/low/world/africa/1683259.stm. Downloaded on July 30, 2002.

Denenberg, Risa. *Gynecological Care Manual for HIV Positive Women.* Durant, Okla.: Essential Medical Information Systems, 1993.

Dietz, Steven D., and M. Jane Parker Hicks. *Take Those Broken Wings and Learn to Fly: The AIDS Support Book for Patients, Family and Friends.* Tucson: Harbinger House, 1989.

Douglas, Paul Harding, and Laura Pinsky. *The Essential AIDS Fact Book.* New York: Pocket Books, 1989.

Dunne, Bruce. "Power and Sexuality in the Middle East." The Middle East Research and Information Project. Available on-line. URL: http://www.merip.org/mer/mer206/bruce.htm. Downloaded July 31, 2002.

Eckert, Eric. "Diseased Societies." *World and I* 13, no. 10: 166–174.

Edison, Ted, ed. *The AIDS Caregivers Handbook.* New York: St. Martin's, 1988.

European Centre for the Epidemiological Monitoring of AIDS. *HIV/AIDS Surveillance in Europe: End-Year Report 2001.* Saint-Maurice: Institut de Veille Sanitaire, 2002.

Ewald, Paul W., and Gregory Cochran. "Catching On to What's Catching." *Natural History* 108: 34.

Faiola, Anthony. "Brazil to Ignore Patent on AIDS Drug." *The Washington Post* August 23, 2001, p. A20.

Fettner, Ann Giudici. *The Science of Viruses: What They Are, Why They Make Us Sick, How They Will Change the Future.* New York: William Morrow, 1990.

Flanders, Stephen, A., and Carl N. Flanders. *AIDS.* New York: Facts On File, 1991.

Ford, Earl S., Wayne H. Giles, and William H. Dietz. "Prevalence of the Metabolic Syndrome Among US Adults." *Journal of the American Medical Association* 287, no. 3 (January 16, 2002): 356–359.

Ford, Michael Thomas. *100 Questions & Answers About AIDS: What You Need to Know Now.* New York: Beech Tree, 1992.

Formichella, Annamaria, Susan McIntyre, and Marjorie Brant Osterhout. *Tell It Like It Is: Straight Talk About Sex.* New York: Avon, 1991.

"The XIV International AIDS Conference," AIDS 2002 Available on-line. URL: http://www.aids2002.com. Downloaded July 13, 2002.

Fraser, Tony. "Caribbean Officials Say New Deal for Cheaper HIV/AIDS Drugs Will Help Region-Wide Effort." Body Health Resources Corporation: CDC News Updates, July 22, 2002. Available on-line. URL: http://www.thebody.com/cdc/news_updates_archive/july22_02/caribbean_aids_drugs.html. Downloaded on July 30, 2002.

Froman, Paul Kent. *Pathways to Wellness: Strategies for Self-Empowerment in the Age of AIDS.* New York: Penguin, 1990.

Frumkin, Lyn, and John Leonard. *Questions & Answers on AIDS.* 2d ed. Los Angeles: PMIC, 1994.

Garbus, Lisa. "Eastern Europe and Central Asia." University of California–San Francisco: HIVInSite, December 2001. Available on-line. URL: hivinsite.ucsf.edu/InSite.jsp?page=cr-02-06. Downloaded on July 31, 2002.

Gay Men's Health Crisis. *GMHC Treatment Issues: The Gay Men's Health Crisis Newsletter of Experimental AIDS Therapies.* New York: GMHC, Treatment Education, 1(1) (November 1987)–to date.

Gaytoday. "HIV+ Positive Patients and Organ Transplants." 6(125). Kaiser Family Foundation. Available on-line. URL: http://www.gaytoday.com/health/072902he.asp. Downloaded on August 1, 2002.

Geballe, Shelley, Janice Gruendel, and Warren Andiman. *Forgotten Children of the AIDS Epidemic.* New Haven, Conn.: Yale University Press, 1995.

Glesby, Marshall J. "Lipid Abnormalities in HIV-Positive Patients." *Cardiology Review* 19(3) (suppl.).

Goldschmidt, Ronald H., and Betty J. Dong. "Treatment of AIDS and HIV-Related Conditions: 2001." *Journal of the American Board of Family Practitioners* 14(4): 283–309.

Greub, Gilbert, Jacques Fellay, and Amalio Telenti. "HIV Lipoatrophy and Mosquito Bites." *Clinical Infectious Diseases* 34, no. 2: 288–289.

Gupta, Rajan. "Risk Factors and Societal Response to HIV/AIDS in India." Available on-line. URL: http://t8web.lanl.gov/people/rajan/AIDS-india/MYWORK/hivindia2001.html. Downloaded on July 31, 2002.

Gutierrez, Estrella. "AIDS Increasing Among Poor in Latin America." AIDS Education Global Information Service (AEGIS). June 14, 1998. Available on-line. URL: www.aegis.com/news/ips/1998/IP980603.html. Downloaded on July 30, 2002.

Hatem al-Qadhi, Mohammed. "A Silent Threat in Yemen." United Nations Development Programme: *Choices Magazine.* December 2001. Available on-line. URL: http://www.undp.org/dpa/choices/2001/december/Choic1201p12E.pdf. Downloaded on July 31, 2002.

Hay, Louise L. *The AIDS Book: Creating a Positive Approach.* Santa Monica, Calif.: Hay House, 1988.

Heimel, Cynthia. *Sex Tips for Girls.* New York: Simon & Schuster, 1993.

HIV/AIDS Treatment Information Service. *Glossary of HIV/AIDS-Related Terms.* 4th ed. National Library of Medicine, 2002. Available on-line. URL: http://glossary.hivatis.org/index.asp. Downloaded on July 9, 2002.

HIV Positive. Alpharetta, Ga.: Positive Health Publications, 2001–2002 issues.

HIV Positive. "Pain & HIV/AIDS: Glossary." TRX Interactive Communications, Inc., 1997–2002. Available on-line. URL: http://www.hivpositive.com/f-painHIV/PAIN/glossary. Downloaded on February 2, 2001.

Hogan, Carlton, and Trustees of the University of Minnesota. *CPCRA Glossary of Medical, Statistical, and Clinical*

Research Terminology. Community Programs for Clinical Research on AIDS (CPCRA), Oct. 12, 2001. Available on-line. URL: http://sdmc.cpcra.org/gloss.html. Downloaded on July 9, 2002.

Htun, Thaung. "Burma/Myanmar and AIDS: The Silent Crisis." National Coalition Government of the Union of Burma. June 25, 2001. Available on-line. URL: http://www.ncgub.net/Views/Burma_Myanmar%20a nd%20Aids,%20The%20Silent%20Crisis%20by%20 DTH%2025%20june%202001.htm. Downloaded on July 30, 2002.

Huber, Jeffrey T., ed. *How to Find Information about AIDS.* 2d ed. New York: Harrington Park, 1992.

Humphry, Derek. *Final Exit: The Practicalities of Self-Deliverance and Assisted Suicide for the Dying.* New York: Dell, 1991.

Hwang, T. L., et al. "High dose Ara-C related leukoencephalopathy." *Journal of Neuro-Oncology* 3, no. 4 (April 1986): 335–339. Darien, Conn.: Cliggott Publishing, 15(1)–19(4). Available on-line. URL: http://www.medscape.com/viewpublication/91_index. Downloaded on July 9, 2002.

India Ministry of Health and Welfare. "HIV Estimates for year 2001." (undated). National AIDS Control Organisation. Available on-line. URL: http://naco.nic.in/ vsnaco/indianscene/esthiv.htm. Downloaded on July 30, 2002.

Institute for the Advanced Study of Human Sexuality. *The Complete Guide to Safe Sex.* Published for the PreVenT Group of Beverly Hills, Calif., by Specific Press, 1987.

———. *Safe Sex in the Age of AIDS.* Secaucus, N.J.: Citadel, 1986.

International Crisis Group. "Myanmar: The HIV/AIDS Crisis." Crisisweb.org, Apr. 6, 2002. Available on-line. URL: http://www.crisisweb.org/projects/asia/burma_ myanmar/reports/A400601_02042002.pdf. Downloaded on July 30, 2002.

International Gay and Lesbian Human Rights Commission. "AIDS Treatment Interrupted in Argentina . . . Again." IGLHRC World Watch, September 2000. Available on-line. URL: http://www.iglhrc.org/world/ southamerica/Argentina2000Sept.html. Downloaded on July 30, 2002.

The Jamaica Observer. "Caribbean AIDS Cases Now 420,000." December 1, 2001. *The Jamaica Observer* on the Web. Available on-line. URL: http://www. jamaicaobserver.com/news/html/20011130t190000-0500_17730_obs_caribbean_aids_cases_now_____.asp. Downloaded on July 30, 2002.

James, John S., ed. *AIDS Treatment News.* Vol. 1. Berkeley, Calif.: Celestial Arts, 1989.

———. *AIDS Treatment News.* Vol. 2. Berkeley, Calif.: Celestial Arts, 1991.

———. *AIDS Treatment News.* Vol. 3. Boston: Alyson, 1994.

———. "AIDS Treatment News Archive." *AIDS Treatment News,* May 15, 1998–present. Available on-line. URL: http://www.aids.org/immunet/atn.nsf/page. Downloaded on July 9, 2002.

Johnson, Elizabeth A. *As Someone Dies: A Handbook for the Living.* Santa Monica, Calif.: Hay House, 1987.

Johnston, William I. *HIV Negative: How the Uninfected Are Affected by AIDS.* New York: Plenum, 1995.

Joint United Nations Programme on HIV/AIDS. "The Status and Trends of "HIV/AIDS/STI Epidemics in Asia and the Pacific." Monitoring the AIDS Pandemic Network. October 4, 2001. October 4, 2001. Available on-line. URL: http://www.unaids.org/hivaidsinfo/statistics/MAP/ MAP2001FINAL.doc. Downloaded on July 30, 2002.

Kahn, Ada P., and Linda Hughey Holt. *The A-Z of Women's Sexuality.* New York: Facts On File, 1990.

Kain, Craig, ed. *No Longer Immune: A Counselor's Guide to AIDS.* Alexandria, Va.: American Association for Counseling and Development, 1989.

Kaplan, Helen Singer. *The Real Truth About Women and AIDS: How to Eliminate the Risks Without Giving Up Love and Sex.* New York: Simon & Schuster, 1987.

Kaposi's Sarcoma. *Clinical Oncology.* 2d ed. Ed. Martin D. Abeloff, et al. Churchill Livingstone: Philadelphia, 2000. *MDConsult.* November 28, 2001. Available on-line. URL: http://www.mdconsult.com/das/book/ view/14873785/897/1320.html. Downloaded on July 30, 2002.

Kazan, Amy. "AIDS Catches Burma's Junta Off Guard." *Financial Times (London).* May 16, 2002. Available on-line. URL: http://www.burmaproject.org/051602aids_ catches_junta_offguard.html. Downloaded on July 30, 2002.

Keith-Reid, Robert. "AIDS Crisis Looms: AIDS Could Devastate Most Pacific Island Nations." *Pacific Magazine. Sept. 2001.* Available on-line. URL: http:// www.pacificislands.cc/pm92001/pmdefault.cfm? articleid=6. Downloaded on July 30, 2002.

Keswania, Sanjay C. et. al., "HIV-associated Sensory Neuropathies." *AIDS.* 16, no. 16: 2,105–2,117.

Kinsella, James. *Covering the Plague: AIDS and the American Media.* New Brunswick, N.J.: Rutgers University Press, 1989.

Kirp, David L. *Learning by Heart: AIDS and Schoolchildren in America's Communities.* New Brunswick, N.J.: Rutgers University Press, 1989.

Kirschmann, Gayla J., and John D. Kirschmann. *Nutrition Almanac.* 4th ed. New York: McGraw-Hill, 1966.

Kramer, Larry. *Reports from the Holocaust: The Making of an AIDS Activist.* New York: St. Martin's, 1989.

Kübler-Ross, Elisabeth. *AIDS: The Ultimate Challenge.* New York: Macmillan, 1987.

———. *Death: The Final Stage of Growth.* New York: Simon & Schuster, 1975.

———. *On Death and Dying.* New York: Macmillan, 1969.

———. *On Life After Death.* Berkeley: Celestial Arts, 1991.

———. *Questions and Answers on Death and Dying.* New York: Macmillan, 1974.

———. *To Live Until We Say Goodbye.* Englewood Cliffs, N.J.: Prentice-Hall, 1976.

Kurth, Ann, ed. *Until the Cure: Caring for Women with HIV.* New Haven, Conn.: Yale University Press, 1993.

Kyle, Garland Richard. *Whatever Happened to Passion: Writings from the Epidemic Years.* San Francisco: Modern Words, 1992.

Lester, Bonnie. *Women and AIDS: A Practical Guide for Those Who Help Others.* New York: Continuum, 1989.

Levin, Bruce R., J. J. Bull, and Frank M. Stewart. "Epidemiology, Evolution, and Future of the HIV/AIDS Pandemic." *Emerging Infectious Diseases* 7, no. 3 (suppl. 3) (June 2001): 505–511.

Levine, Alexandra M. "HPV Infection and Cervical/Anal PrecursorLesions in the HAART Era." Medscape from WebMD. 2002. Available on-line. URL: http://www.medscape.com/viewarticle/440151/. Downloaded on December 12, 2002.

Lingle, Virginia A., and M. Sandra Wood. *How to Find Information About AIDS.* New York: Harrington Park, 1988.

Lu, Henry C. *Chinese System of Food Cures: Prevention & Remedies.* New York: Sterling, 1986.

Lucas, Gregory M. "Management of HIV Infection in Injection-Drug Users." Medscape by WebMD, October 28, 2001. Available on-line. URL: http://www.medscape.com/viewarticle/418652. Downloaded on July 30, 2002.

Macklin, Eleanor D. *AIDS and Families: Report of the AIDS Task Force Groves Conference on Marriage and the Family.* Binghamton, N.Y.: Harrington Park, 1989.

Maddow, Rachel. "In The Big House." *HIV PLUS.* January 2000, Issue 6. Available on-line. URL: http://www.aidsinfonyc.org/hivplus/issue6/report/picture.html. Downloaded on January 12, 2003.

Malinowsky H. Robert, and Gerald J. Perry *AIDS Information Sourcebook.* Phoenix: Oryx, 1988.

———. *AIDS Information Sourcebook.* 2nd ed. Phoenix: Oryx, 1989.

Mann, Jonathan, Daniel J. M. Tarantola, and Thomas W Netter, eds. *AIDS in the World.* Cambridge, Mass.: Harvard University Press, 1992.

Marquez, Patricio. "Fighting HIV/AIDS in the Caribbean." *en breve.* June 2002 no.4. The World Bank Group, June 2002, no. 4. Available on-line URL: http://Inweb18.worldbank.org/External/lac/lac.nsf/en+breve/5BB91428184D 782285256BD 1005F685E?OpenDocument. Downloaded on July 31, 2002.

Martelli, Leonard J., with Fran D. Peltz and William Messina. *When Someone You Know Has AIDS: A Practical Guide.* New York: Crown, 1987.

Marti, James E., *The Alternative Health Medicine Encyclopedia: The Authoritative Guide to Holistic & Nontraditional Health Practices.* Washington, D.C.: Visible Ink, 1995.

Mason, Susan E. and Rachel Miller. "Safe Sex and First-Episode Schizophrenia." *Bulletin of the Menninger Clinic* 65, no. 2 (Spring 2001): 179–193.

Maugh, Thomas H. "AIDS to Cut Africa Life Expectancy to Under 30." *Los Angeles Times,* July 7, 2000, p. A-1.

McCormack, Thomas P. *The AIDS Benefits Handbook.* New Haven, Conn.: Yale University Press, 1990.

———. "Returning to Work and Keeping Medicare and Medicaid." Louisiana State University: Medical and Public Health Law Site July 16, 2001. Available on-line. URL: http://biotech.law.Isu.edu/cphl/HIV/returning_to_work.htm. Downloaded on July 11, 2002.

McGregor, Liz. "Botswana Battles Against Extinction." *The Guardian (London),* July 8, 2002. Available on-line. URL: www.guardian.co.uk/international/story/0,3604,751071,00.html. Downloaded on July 13, 2002.

Medscape. "AIDS Reader." 8(1)–12(4). Available on-line. URL: http://www.medscape.com/viewpublication/93_index. Downloaded on July 9, 2002.

MedScape from WebMD. Available on-line. URL: http://www.medscape.com. Accessed on July 9, 2002.

Memorial Sloan-Kettering Cancer Center, Department of Public Affairs. "AIDS-Associated Kaposi's Sarcoma." Memorial Sloan-Kettering Cancer Center, August 1, 2001. Available on-line. URL: www.mskcc.org/mskcc/html/5422.cfm. Downloaded on November 11, 2001.

Mikluscak-Cooper, Cindy, and Emmett E. Miller. *Living in Hope: A 12-Step Approach for Persons at Risk or Infected with HIV.* Berkeley, Calif.: Celestial Arts, 1991.

Miller, Heather G., Charles E Turner, and Lincoln E. Moses, eds. *AIDS: The Second Decade.* Washington, D.C.: National Academy Press, 1990.

Miller, Norman, and Richard C. Rockwell, eds. *AIDS in Africa: The Social and Policy Impact.* Lewiston, N.Y.: Edwin Mellen Press, 1988.

Mitsuyasu, Ronald T. "Immune Reconstitution with Antiretrovirals, Immunotherapy, and After Structured Treatment Interruption." Medscape by WebMD, 2000.

Available on-line. URL: http://www.medscape.com/viewarticle/420611. Downloaded on March 6, 2001.

Moffatt, Betty Clare. *When Someone You Love Has AIDS: A Book of Hope for Family and Friends.* New York: NAL Penguin, 1986.

Moyle, Graeme. "Metabolic Disturbances, Mitochondrial Toxicity and Lipodystrophy." Hivandhepatitis.com, Mar. 6, 2002. Available on-line. URL: http://hivandhepatitis.com/2002conf/9thcroi/20.html. Downloaded on August 1, 2002.

Muir, Jim. "Tackling AIDS in Iran." BBC News Online, March 20, 2002. Available on-line. URL: http://news.bbc.co.uk/2/low/world.middle-east/1881115.stm. Downloaded on July 31, 2002.

National Institutes of Health, National Cancer Institute. *Advanced Cancer: Living Each Day.* National Institutes of Health, Public Health Service, U.S. Department of Health and Human Services, Revised February 1994. NIH Publication No. 94-856.

———. *Taking Time: Support for People with Cancer and the People Who Care About Them.* National Institutes of Health, Public Health Service, U.S. Department of Health and Human Services, 1990. NIH Publication No. 94-2059.

National Institutes of Health, National Institute of Allergy and Infectious Diseases, Office of Communications and Public Liaison. "Fact Sheet: HIV Vaccine Glossary." National Institutes of Health, May 2000. Available on-line. URL: http://www.niaid.nih.gov/factsheets/glossary.htm. Downloaded on July 9, 2002.

National Institutes of Health, National Institute of Allergy and Infectious Diseases, Division of AIDS. *Glossary of Terms Used in the Division of AIDS Informed Consents.* Bethesda, Md.: National Institutes of Health, n.d.

National Institutes of Health, Office of Dietary Supplements, Warren Grant Magnuson Clinical Center. "Facts About Dietary Supplements." National Institutes of Health. December 09, 2002. Available on-line. URL: http://www.cc.nih.gov/ccc/supplements. Downloaded on December 12, 2002.

National Public Radio. "NPR Special Report: AIDS 2002, XIV International AIDS Conference." National Public Radio, 2002. Available on-line. URL: http://www.npr.org/special/aids2002/index.html. Downloaded on July 11, 2002.

Nevid, Jeffrey S. *201 Things You Should Know about AIDS and other Sexually Transmitted Diseases.* Boston: Allyn & Bacon, 1993.

New Mexico AIDS Info Network. "KS (Kaposi's Sarcoma) Fact Sheet Number 508." Body Health Resources Corporation. August 22, 2001. Available on-line. URL: http:www.thebody.com/nmai/ks.html. Downloaded on November 28, 2001.

———. "Mitochondrial Toxicity. Fact Sheet Number 556." Body Health Resources Corporation. March 15, 2002. Available on-line. URL: http://www.thebody.com/nmai/mitochondria.html. Downloaded on July 19, 2002.

———. "New Drugs Against HIV: Reverse Transcriptase Inhibitors, Fact Sheet Number 402." AIDS Education and Training Center, January 18, 2002. Available on-line. URL: http://www.aidsinfonet.org/402-new-drugs.html. Downloaded on July 10, 2002.

Nichols, Eve K. *Mobilizing Against AIDS.* Cambridge, Mass.: Harvard University Press, 1989.

Norwood, Chris. *Advice for Life: A Woman's Guide to AIDS Risks and Prevention.* New York: Pantheon, 1987.

Nuland, Sherwin B. *How We Die: Reflections on Life's Final Chapter.* New York: Alfred A. Knopf, 1993.

Nungesser, Lon G. *Epidemic of Courage: Facing AIDS in America.* New York: St. Martin's, 1986.

O'Sullivan, Sue and Pratibha Parmar. *Lesbians Talks (Safer Sex).* London: Scarlet Press, 1992.

Pan American Health Organization. "Case Definition: Acquired Immunodeficiency Syndrome (AIDS)." *Epidemiological Bulletin.* 22(2) (June 2001). Available on-line. URL: http:www.paho.org/English/SHA/be_v22n2-SIDA. htm. Downloaded on December 13, 2001.

Patton, Cindy. *Fatal Advice: How Safe-Sex Education Went Wrong.* Durham, N.C.: Duke University Press, 1996.

———. *Inventing AIDS.* New York: Routledge, 1990.

———. *Sex and Germs: The Politics of AIDS.* Boston: South End Press, 1985.

Patton, Cindy, and Janis Kelly. *Making It: A Woman's Guide to Sex in the Age of AIDS.* Ithaca, N.Y.: Firebrand, 1987.

The PDR Family Guide to Women's Health and Prescription Drugs. Montvale, N.J.: Medical Economics, 1994.

Peak, Maitland J. "Summary of Fact Finding Mission to Tajikistan." Open Society Institute: Eurasianet.org, March 1, 2001. Available on-line. URL: http://www.eurasianet.org/policy_forum/tajikist030101_print.shtml. Downloaded on August 1, 2002.

Pelham, Nicholas. "Morocco Begins to Confront AIDS Issues." *The Christian Science Monitor.* Mar. 9, 2001. Available on-line. URL: http://www.emro.who.int/AIEC/NewsRoom-ChristianTimes.htm. Downloaded on July 31, 2002.

Perrow, Charles, and Mauro E Guillen. *The AIDS Disaster: The Failure of Organizations in New York and the Nation.* New Haven, Conn.: Yale University Press, 1990.

Phair, John P., and Edward King, eds. "HIV/AIDS Annual Update 2001." Medscape by WebMD. October 28,

2001. Available on-line. URL: http://www.medscape.com/viewpublication/534_about. Downloaded on July 31, 2002.

Pinckney, Cathey, and Edward R. Pinckney. *Do-It-Yourself Medical Testing.* 3rd ed. New York: Facts On File, 1989.

———. *The Parent's Guide to Medical Tests.* 3d ed. New York: Facts On File, 1986.

Pisani, Elizabeth, et. al. *HIV and AIDS in the Americas: An Epidemic with Many Faces.* United States Bureau of the Census. December 2001. Available on-line. URL: http://www.census.gov/ipc/www/hivaidinamerica.pdf. Downloaded on July 31, 2002.

Pomfret, John. "China Blocks Trip to U.S. by AIDS Award Honoree." *The Washington Post,* May 30, 2001, p. A14.

———. "The High Cost of Selling Blood: As Crisis Looms in China, Official Response is Lax." *The Washington Post,* Jan. 11, 2001, p. A1.

Porter, Charlene. "AIDS Will Cause Negative Population Growth, New Data Show." Washington, D.C.: United States Department of State, 2000? Available on-line. URL: http://usinfo.state.gov/regional/af/usafr/t0071002.html. Downloaded July 13, 2002.

Positives for Positives. Cheyenne, Wyoming: Positives for Positives, 2001–2002 issues.

Preston, Richard. *The Hot Zone.* New York: Random House, 1994.

Princeton, Douglas C. *Current Clinical Strategies: Manual of HIV/AIDS Therapy 2003 Edition.* Laguna Hills, Calif.: Current Clinical Strategies Publishing, 2002.

Project Inform. *The HIV Drug Book.* Rev. and updated ed. New York: Pocket Books, 1998.

———. *PI Perspective.* Project Inform, no. 11–34, 1991–2002. Available on-line. URL: http://www.projinf.org/pub/pip_index.html. Downloaded on July 11, 2002.

Projectinform.com. "Mitochondrial Toxicity and Lactic Acidosis." April 2001. Project Inform. Available on-line. URL: http://www.projectinform.org/pdf/mito.pdf. Downloaded on August 4, 2002.

Rebêlo, Paul. "Brazil Targets Another AIDS Drug." WiredNews, Aug. 29, 2001. Available on-line. URL: http://www.wired.com/news/print/0,1294,46353,00.html. Downloaded on July 30, 2002.

Reinisch, June M. *The Kinsey Institute New Report on Sex: What You Must Know to Be Sexually Literate.* New York: St. Martin's, 1991.

Rhea, Joseph C., J. Steven Ott, and Jay M. Shafritz. *The Facts On File Dictionary of Health Care Management.* New York: Facts On File, 1988.

Richardson, Diane. *Women & AIDS.* New York: Methuen, 1988.

Richter, Alan. *Dictionary of Sexual Slang: Words, Phrases & Idioms from ACIDC to Zig-zig.* New York: Wiley, 1993.

Rieder, Ines and Patricia Ruppelt. *AIDS: The Women.* San Francisco: Cleis, 1988.

Rodriguez, Ana. "Mitochondrial Toxicity." *Women Alive.* Body Health Resources Corporation, 2001. Available on-line. URL: http://www.thebody.com/wa/spring01/toxicity.html. Downloaded on Aug. 1, 2002.

Rolan, Michelle. "Safety and Efficacy of Solid Organ Transplantation in HIV-Positive Patients." *The PRN Notebook* 6, no. 1: 19–23.

Rudd, Andrea, and Darien Taylor, eds. *Positive Women: Voices of Women Living with AIDS.* Toronto: Second Story Press, 1992.

Rybacki, James J., and James W Long. *The Essential Guide to Prescription Drugs 1997.* New York: HarperCollins, 1996.

SAfAIDS News. Harare, Zimbabwe: Southern Africa AIDS Information Dissemination Service, 7(1)–9(4), 1999–2001. Available on-line. URL: http://www.safaids.org.zw/safaidsweb/publications/. Downloaded on July 11, 2002.

Scanlon, Valerie C., and Tina Sanders. *Essentials of Anatomy and Physiology.* 2d ed. Philadelphia: F. A. Davis, 1995.

Schütz, Malte. "Quick Reference Guide to Antiretrovirals." Medscape by WebMD June 1, 2002. Available on-line. URL: www.medscape.com/viewarticle/424023. Downloaded on July 9, 2002.

Schwartländer, B., et al. "Resource Needs for HIV/AIDS." *Science* June 29, 2001, p. 2,434–2,436.

"Secretariat of the Pacific Community." *Pacific AIDS Alert Bulletin* no. 18–23, AIDS/HIV and STD Project, 2001. Available on-line. URL: http://www.spc.int/aids/General_Info/english_pub.htm. Downloaded on July 30, 2002.

Senterfitt, Walt. *Co-Receptors and Chemokines: What Do They Have to Do with My Life Anyway? Being Alive Newsletter.* December 1997/January 1998. Available on-line. URL: http://www.beingalivela.org/news1297/1297_index.html. Downloaded on July 10, 2002.

Sharp, P. M., et al. "Origins and evolution of AIDS virus." *Biological Bulletin* 196 (1999): 338–342.

Shernoff, Michael, ed. *Counseling Chemically Dependent People with HIV Illness.* Binghamton, N.Y.: Harrington Park, 1991.

Shilts, Randy. *And the Band Played On: Politics, People, and the AIDS Epidemic.* New York: St. Martin's, 1987.

Siegel, Bernie S. Love, *Medicine and Miracles: Lessons Learned About Self-Healing from a Surgeon's Experience with Exceptional Patients.* New York: Harper & Row, 1986.

Singer, P. W. "AIDS and International Security." *Survival* 44, no. 1: 145–158.

Skelton, Chad. "New HIV "Superbug" Emerges in Vancouver." *Vancouver Sun,* August 9, 2001, p. A1.

Smith, Kathleen, et al. "Exaggerated Insect Bite Reactions in Patients Positive for HIV." *Journal of the American Academy of Dermatology* 29, no. 2 (pt. 1): 269–272.

Smith, Michael. Africans "Faced With Extinction." *The National Post,* July 8, 2002, p. A01.

Smith, Raymond A., ed. *Encyclopedia of AIDS: A Social, Political, Cultural, and Scientific Record of the HIV Epidemic.* Chicago: Fitzroy Dearborn, 1998.

Social Link: A Web Resource for Students of Social Work. *HIV/AIDS Dictionary.* Smith College, 1998. Available online. URL: http://sophia.smith.edu/~rflor/Dictionary. htm. Downloaded on July 9, 2002.

Soglin, Becky. "Ul Studies GBV-C Virus Effect on Survival of HIV Positive People." Press Release, University of Iowa Health Care Sept. 6, 2001. Available on-line. URL: http://www.uiowa.edu/~ournews/2001/september/0906gbv-c-virus.html. Downloaded on December 25, 2002.

Sontag, Susan. *AIDS and Its Metaphors.* New York: Farrar, Straus & Giroux, 1989.

———. *Illness as Metaphor.* New York: Farrar, Straus & Giroux, 1978.

Standish, Leanna J., Carlo Calabrese, and Mary Lou Galantino. *AIDS and Complementary & Alternative Medicine: Current Science and Practice.* Philadelphia: Churchill Livingstone, 2002.

Stephenson, Joan. "Apocalypse Now: HIV/AIDS in Africa Exceeds the Experts' Worst Predictions." *Journal of the American Medical Association* 284(5) August 2, 2000 Available on-line. URL: http://jama. ama-assn.org/issues/v284n5/ffull/jmn0802-5.html. Downloaded on July 13, 2002.

———. "HIV/AIDS Surging in Eastern Europe." *Journal of the American Medical Association* 284(24), Dec. 27, 2000. Available on-line. URL: http://jama.ama-assn.org/ issues/v284n24/ffull/jmn1227-1.html. Downloaded on July 13, 2002.

———. "Researchers Wrestle with Spread and Control of Emerging Infections." *Journal of the American Medical Association* 287(16), April 24, 2002. Available on-line. URL: http://jama.ama-assn.org/issues/v287n16/ffull/ jmn0424-1.html#a0. Downloaded on August 4, 2002.

Sternberg, Robert J., ed. *Encyclopedia of Human Intelligence.* New York: Macmillan, 1994.

Stine, Gerald J. *AIDS Update 2001: An Annual Overview of Acquired Immune Deficiency Syndrome.* Upper Saddle River, N.J.: Prentice Hall, 2001.

———. *AIDS Update 2002: An Annual Overview of Acquired Immune Deficiency Syndrome.* Upper Saddle River, N.J.: Prentice Hall, 2002.

Straus, Stephen E. "Human Herpesvirus Type 8." *Mandrell, Douglas and Bennett's Principles and Practice of Infectious Diseases.* 5th ed. Ed. Gerald L. Mandrell, John E. Bennett, and Raphael Dolin. Philadelphia: Churchill Livingstone, 2000. Available on-line. URL: http:www. mdconsult.com/das/book/view/14873785/883/1090. html. Downloaded on November 11, 2001.

Susman, Ed. "AIDS Patients Do Okay with Transplants." *United Press International.* Oct. 15, 2001. Available online. URL: http://www.thebody.com/cdc/news_ updates_archive/oct17_01/transplants.html. Downloaded on August 1, 2002.

Tauber, Jeffrey T. *Dictionary of AIDS Related Terminology.* New York: Neal-Schuman, 1993.

Tauber's Cyclopedic Medical Dictionary. 17th ed. Philadelphia: E. A. Davis, 1993.

Terl, Allan H. *AIDS and the Law: A Basic Guide for the Nonlawyer.* Taylor & Francis, 1992.

Thain, Michael, and Michael Hickman. *The Penguin Dictionary of Biology.* 9th rev. ed. New York: Penguin, 1995.

Tilleraas, Perry. *Living with HIV A Spiritual Response to HIV: The Twelve Steps.* Center City, Minn.: Hazelden Educational Materials, 1990.

The Times of India. "East Timor Sliding Towards AIDS Disaster: Minister". July 5, 2002. The Times of India on the Web. Available on-line. URL: http://timesofindia.indiatimes.com/articleshow.asp?art_id=1509 5756. Downloaded on July 30, 2002.

Trivieri, Larry, Jr., and John W. Anderson, eds. *Alternative Medicine: The Definitive Guide.* 2d ed. Berkeley, Calif.: Celestial Arts, 2002.

University of Alabama School of Medicine, Division of Continuing Medical Education. *HIV Information Network, Fax Newsletter.* Birmingham: University of Alabama, Birmingham, February 8, 2001–present.

University of California, San Diego, Antiviral Research Center. "UCSD Treatment Center News." UCSD Antiviral Research Center, 1999–present Available online. URL: http://www.avrctrials.org/Newsletter/ Newsletter.html. Downloaded on July 10, 2002.

University of Michigan Health System. "Barriers to Organ Transplantation for HIV-Infected Patients Unethical." UMHS News, July 25, 2002. Available on-line. URL: http://www.med.umich.edu/opm/ newspage/2002/transplanthiv.htm. Downloaded on August 3, 2002.

United Nations Programme on HIV/AIDS and World Health Organization. "AIDS Epidemic Update: December 2000." UNAIDS, 2001. Available on-line. URL:

www.unaids.org/2000/files/WAD_epidemic_report. pdf. Downloaded on March 6, 2001.

———."AIDS Epidemic Update: December 2001." UNAIDS, 2002. Available on-line. URL: http://www. unaids.org/epidemic_update/report_dec01/index.html. Downloaded on March 16, 2002.

———. "Keeping the Promise: Summary of the Declaration of Commitment on HIV/AIDS." Joint United Nations Programme on HIV/AIDS. June 2001. Available on-line. URL: http://www.unaids.org/barcelona/ presskit/keepingthepromise/JC668-keepingPromise-E.pdf. Downloaded on July 13, 2002.

———. "National Responses: Turning Commitment into Action." Joint United Nations Programme on HIV/AIDS. July, 2002. Available on-line. URL: http://www.unaids.org/barcelona/presskit/report.htm l. Downloaded on July 13, 2002.

U.S. Census Bureau, Population Division, International Programs Center, Health Studies Branch. "Country Profiles." U.S. Census Bureau, May 3, 2001. Available on-line. URL: http://www.census.gov/ipc/www/ hivctry.html. Downloaded on July 31, 2002.

U.S. Department of Health and Human Services. *Healthy People: The Surgeon General's Report on Health Promotion and Disease Prevention.* Washington, DC: U.S. Department of Health and Human Services, 1979.

———. *Healthy People 2000.* Washington, D.C.: U.S. Department of Health and Human Services, 1990.

———. *Healthy People 2010: With Understanding and Improving Health and Objectives for Improving Health.* 2d ed. Washington, D.C.: U.S. Government Printing Office, 2000.

U.S. Department of Health and Human Services, Centers for Disease Control and Prevention. National Center for HIV, STD, and TB Prevention. Division of HIV/AIDS Prevention. *HIV/AIDS Surveillance Report* 12 no. 1(2000).

U.S. Department of Health and Human Services, Office of Minority Health. *HIV Impact.* Washington, D.C.: U.S.

Department of Health and Human Services. Spring 2000–Spring 2002.

U.S. Department of Health and Human Services, Public Health Service, Agency for Health Care Policy and Research. *Evaluation and Management of Early HIV Infection.* AHCPR Publication No. 94-0572. Rockville, Md.: U.S. Department of Health and Human Services, 1994.

U.S. Department of Justice. "HIV in Prisons, 2000." *Bureau of Justice Statistics, Bulletin.* October 2002. Available on-line. URL: http://www.ojp.usdoj.gov/bjs/pub/pdf/hivp00.pdf. Downloaded on December 12, 2002.

Voelker, Rebecca. "HIV/AIDS in the Caribbean: Big Problems Among Small Islands." *JAMA, Journal of the American Medical Association* 285, no. 23: 2,961–2,965. Available on-line. URL: http://jama.ama-assn.org/ issues/v285n23/ffull/jmn0620-1.html. Downloaded on July 31, 2002.

Ward, Darrell E. *The AmFAR AIDS Handbook: The Complete Guide to Understanding HIV and AIDS.* New York: W.W. Norton, 1999.

Watstein, Sarah Barbara, and Robert Anthony Laurich. *AIDS and Women: A Sourcebook.* Phoenix: Oryx, 1991.

Whipple, Beverly, and Gina Ogden. *Safe Encounters: How Women Can Say Yes to Pleasure and No to Unsafe Sex.* New York: Pocket Books, 1989.

White, Evelyn C., ed. *The Black Women's Health Book.* Seattle: Seal Press, 1990.

Wilson, Josleen. *Woman: Your Body, Your Health: The Essential Guide for Well-Being.* New York: Harcourt Brace Jovanovich, 1990.

Wood, Gary James, and Robert Marks, with James W Dilley. *AIDS Law for Mental Health Professionals: A Handbook for Judicious Practice.* San Francisco: The AIDS Health Project, University of California-San Francisco, 1992.

Worthington, Rogers. "Proliferation of AIDS Casts a Cloud Over Haiti's Future." *Chicago Tribune.* November 20, 1994. Chicagoland North Section, p. 6.

INDEX

allogeneic transplantation 71
allopathy **22**
aloe vera 3, **23,** 200
Alonso, Kenneth 240
alopecia **23**
alpha interferon (IFN-α) **23,**
  260–261, 270
    drug interactions of 7, 479
    low-dose oral **290**
    for progressive multifocal
      leukoencephalopathy 400
alpha-tocopherol 524
alprazolam **23,** 60, 484
ALRT-1057. *See* alitretinoin
ALT. *See* alanine
  aminotransaminase
alternative delivery **23–24**
alternative delivery system (ADS)
  24
alternative health care. *See*
  alternative treatment
alternative insemination. *See*
  artificial insemination
alternative medicine **24,** 230–231,
  301, **329**
alternative therapy **316–317**
alternative treatment **24–26**
ALVAC-HIV **26**
alveolar proteinosis. *See* pulmonary
  alveolar proteinosis
alveolus (alveoli) **26**
Alzheimer's disease **26,** 226
AMA. *See* American Medical
  Association
Ambien. *See* zolpidem
AmBisome. *See* amphotericin B
ambulatory care **26**
Amcill. *See* ampicillin
AMD-3100 **26**
Amdoxovir. *See* DAPD
ameba. *See* amoeba
amebiasis **26**
amebic dysentery **26**
amebic hepatitis **26**
amenorrhea **26,** 310
America Responds to AIDS **26,**
  256, 263
American Association of Blood
  Banks **26–27**
American Bar Association (ABA)
  3, 179, 397
American Cancer Society 294
American College of Obstetricians
  and Gynecologists (ACOG) 421
American Dental Association
  (ADA) 428

American Foundation for AIDS
  Research (AMFAR) 330
American ginseng 201
American hemorrhagic fever virus
  43
American Hospital Association
  House of Delegates 368
American Medical Association
  (AMA) 294, 428
American Samoa 349
Americans with Disabilities Act
  (ADA) **27–28,** 145–146, 168
amikacin **28,** 499
Amikin. *See* amikacin
amino acid **28,** 542
amino acid sequence 442
amino acid therapy **28**
aminoglycosides **28,** 499
aminosalicylic acid **28**
Aminosidine. *See* paromomycin
  sulfate
amitriptyline **28,** 37, 38, 335
amniotic fluid **28**
amobarbital 56
amoeba (amoebae) **28–29**
amoebiasis. *See* amebiasis
amoebic dysentery. *See* amebic
  dysentery
amoebic hepatitis. *See* amebic
  hepatitis
amoxicillin **29,** 49
Amoxil. *See* amoxicillin
ampalaya 64
amphetamine **29**
Amphogel 103
amphotericin B **29–30**
    for cryptococcal infection 125,
      126
    and drug fever 155
    drug interactions of 1, 28, 185,
      499
    liposomal 30, **285**
ampicillin 29, **30**
ampicillin sodium **30**
amplification **30**
ampligen **30**
amprenavir **30,** 403, 525
AMS. *See* paromomycin sulfate
amyl nitrite **31**
amyl nitrite inhalant. *See* isobutyl
  nitrite inhaler
amylase **31**
Amytal. *See* amobarbital
anabolic **31**
anabolic steroids **31,** 358, 460, 475
anacidity, gastric. *See* achlorhydria

Anadrol. *See* oxymetholone
anal cytology test 32
anal eroticism **31**
anal intercourse **31–32,** 56–57,
  385, **417,** 446, 487
anal intraepithelial neoplasia (AIN)
  32, 235–236
anal neoplasia 198
anal-oral sex. *See* anilingus
anal sex. *See* anal eroticism; anal
  intercourse
analgesics **32**
    adjuvant **9,** 38
    equianalgesic **174**
    self-administration of 368
analogous transfusion **484**
analogue/analog **32**
anamnestic response. *See* secondary
  immune response
anaphylactic shock. *See* anaphylaxis
anaphylaxis **33**
Anaprox. *See* naproxen
Ancobon. *See* flucytosine
And the Band Played On (Shilts) 58
androgen **33**
anecdotal evidence **33**
anemia **33**
    AZT and 51–52
    Cooley's **122**
    macrocytic **294–295**
    megaloblastic **308**
    microcytic **314**
    pernicious 524
    treatment-associated 181
anergic. *See* anergy
anergy, clonal **108**
anergy test 502
angiogenesis **33,** 448
angiomatosis, bacillary **54–55**
Angola 12, 13
angular cheilitis. *See* perleche
angular cheliosis. *See* perleche
angular stomatis. *See* perleche
anilinctus. *See* anilingus
anilingus **33**
animal models **33,** 510, 512
animals
    and bestiality 60
    sentinel **441**
anion **33**
anion gap **34**
anogenital wart **34**
anomanual intercourse **34**
anonymous testing **34**
anorectal disease **34**
anorexia **34**